AIDS

Etiology, Diagnosis, Treatment and Prevention

AIDS

Etiology, Diagnosis, Treatment and Prevention

Fourth Edition

Edited by

Vincent T. DeVita, Jr., M.D.
Director
Yale Cancer Center
Professor of Medicine and Professor
  of Epidemiology and Public Health
Yale University School of Medicine
New Haven, Connecticut

Samuel Hellman, M.D.
A.N. Pritzker Distinguished Service Professor
Department of Radiation and Cellular Oncology
The University of Chicago
Chicago, Illinois

Steven A. Rosenberg, M.D., Ph.D.
Chief of Surgery
National Cancer Institute
Professor of Surgery
Uniformed Services University of the Health
  Sciences School of Medicine
Bethesda, Maryland

Associate Editors

James Curran, M.D.
Dean, Rollins School of Public Health
Emory University
Atlanta, Georgia

Max Essex, D.V.M., Ph.D.
Chairman, Harvard AIDS Institute
Chairman, Department of Cancer Biology
Harvard School of Public Health
Mary Woodard Lasker Professor of Health Sciences
Harvard University
Boston, Massachusettes

Anthony S. Fauci, M.D.
Director, National Institute of Allergy
  and Infectious Diseases
Chief, Laboratory of Immunoregulation
National Institute of Allergy and Infectious Diseases
National Institutes of Health
Bethesda, Maryland

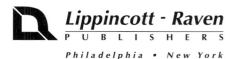

Lippincott - Raven
PUBLISHERS
Philadelphia • New York

With 86 contributors

161177

Developmental Editor: Eileen Jackson
Project Editor: Bridget H. Meyer
Production Manager: Caren Erlichman
Production Coordinator: David Yurkovich
Design Coordinator: Kathy Kelley-Luedtke
Indexer: Sandra King
Printer: Maple Press

Edition 4

Library of Congress Cataloging-in-Publication Data

AIDS: etiology, diagnosis, treatment, and prevention/edited by Vincent T. Devita, Jr.,
    Samuel Hellman; Steven A. Rosenberg: associate editors, James Curran, M. Essex,
    Anthony S. Fauci; with 86 contributors. -- 4th ed.
        p.   cm.
    Includes bibliographical references and index.
    ISBN 0-397-51538-3 (alk. paper)
    1. AIDS (Disease)   I. DeVita, Vincent T.   II. Hellman, Samuel.
III. Rosenberg. Steven A.
    [DNLM: 1. Acquired Immunodeficiency Syndrome.   WC 503 A2877 1997]
RC607.A26A346   1997
616.97'92--dc20
DNLM/DLC
for Library of Congress   96-17611
                                                                          CIP

9 8 7 6 5 4 3 2

Contributors

David M. Aboulafia, MD
Associate Clinical Professor
University of Washington
Attending Hematologist-Oncologist
Virginia Mason Clinic
Seattle, Washington

Donald I. Abrams, MD
Assistant Director, AIDS Program
San Francisco General Hospital
Professor of Clinical Medicine
University of California, San Francisco
San Francisco, California

Jonathan S. Allan, DVM
Scientist
Department of Virology and Immunology
Southwest Foundation for Biomedical Research
San Antonio, Texas

James E. Balow, MD
Clinical Director, NIDDK
National Institutes of Health
Bethesda, Maryland

David M. Bell, MD
Chief, HIV Infectious Branch
Hospital Infections Program
National Center for Infectious Diseases
Centers for Disease Control and Prevention
Atlanta, Georgia

Daniel R. Benson, MD
Professor, Department of Orthopaedics
Chief, Spine Trauma and Deformity
Sacramento, California

Elizabeth A. Bolyard, RN, MPH
Epidemiologist, HIV Infections Branch
Hospital Infections Program
National Center for Infectious Diseases
Centers for Disease Control and Prevention
Atlanta, Georgia

Bruce J. Brew, MBBS, MD, FRACP
Associate Professor of Medicine (Neurology)
Department of Neurology and Immunology
University of New South Wales
St. Vincent's Medical Center, Darlinghurst
Sydney, Australia
St. Paul's Hospital
University of British Columbia
Vancouver, British Columbia

Col. Donald Burke, MD
Walter Reed Army Institute of Research
Rockville, Maryland

Denise M. Cardo, MD
Medical Epidemiologist, HIV Infections Branch
Hospital Infections Program
National Center for Infectious Diseases
Centers for Disease Control and Prevention
Atlanta, Georgia

Susan Y. Chu, PhD
Associate Director, Center for Health Studies
Group Health Cooperative of Puget Sound
Seattle, Washington

Marinee K. L. Chuah, PhD
Center for Transgene Technology and Gene Therapy
Flemish Interuniversity Institute for Biotechnology
Campus Gasthuisberg University of Leuven
O&N Dienst Prof. Collen
Leuven, Belgium

Mary Lou Clements, MD, MPH
Professor of International Health
Head, Division of Vaccine Sciences
Director, Center for Immunization Research
Department of International Health
Johns Hopkins University
School of Public Health
Baltimore, Maryland

Jennifer L. Cleveland, DDS, MPH
Oral Health Program
Centers for Disease Control and Prevention
Chamblee, Georgia

Oren Cohen, MD
National Institute of Allergy and Infectious Diseases
National Institutes of Health
Bethesda, Maryland

Lawrence Corey, MD
University of Washington
Pacific Medical Center
Virology Division
Seattle, Washington

James W. Curran, MD
Dean, Rollins School of Public Health
Emory University
Atlanta, Georgia

Richard T. D'Aquila, MD
Infectious Disease Unit
Massachusetts General Hospital
Assistant Professor of Medicine
Harvard Medical School
Boston, Massachusetts

Richard T. Davey, Jr., MD
Laboratory of Immunoregulation
National Institutes of Health
Bethesda, Maryland

Catherine F. Decker, MD
Division of Infectious Diseases/
Department of Internal Medicine
National Naval Medical Center
Bethesda, Maryland

James F. Demarest, MD
National Institute of Allergy and Infectious Diseases
National Institutes of Health
Bethesda, Maryland

Don C. Des Jarlais, PhD
Director of Research
Beth Israel Medical Center
Chemical Dependency Institute
New York, NY

Beth A. Dillon, MSW
National Center for HIV, STD, and TB Prevention
Centers for Disease Control and Prevention
U.S. Public Health Service
Department of Health and Human Services
Atlanta, Georgia

Lynda S. Doll, PhD
Chief, Behavioral Intervention Research Branch
Division of HIV/AIDS
National Center for Infectious Diseases
Centers for Disease Control and Prevention
Atlanta, Georgia

John P. Doweiko, MD
Division of Hematology and Oncology
Division of Infectious Disease
Harvard Medical School
Boston, Massachusetts

Myron E. Essex, DVM, PhD
Department of Cancer Biology
Mary Woodward Lasker
Professor of Health Sciences
Chair, Harvard AIDS Institute
Harvard School of Public Health
Boston, Massachusetts

Anthony S. Fauci, MD
National Institute of Allergy and
Infectious Diseases
National Institutes of Health
Bethesda, Maryland

Martin S. Favero, PhD
Acting Director for Laboratory Science
Hospital Infections Program
National Center for Infectious Diseases
Centers for Disease Control and Prevention
Atlanta, Georgia

Harvey V. Fineberg, MD
Dean
Harvard School of Public Health
Boston, Massachusetts

Charles Flexner, MD
Division of Clinical Pharmacology
Johns Hopkins Hospital
Baltimore, Maryland

Thomas M. Folks, PhD
Chief, Retrovirus Diseases Branch
Division of AIDS, STD, TB, Laboratory Research
Center for Disease Control and Prevention
Lithonia, Georgia

Gerald Friedland, MD
Professor of Medicine and Epidemiology
and Public Health
Director, AIDS Program
Yale University School of Medicine
Yale-New Haven Hospital
New Haven, Connecticut

Christine Grady, RN, PhD
National Institute of Nursing Research
National Institutes of Health
Bethesda, Maryland

Cecilia Graziosi, PhD
National Institute of Allergy and Infectious Diseases
National Institutes of Health
Bethesda, Maryland

Deborah Greenspan, BDS, DSc, ScD(hc)
Department of Stomatology
University of California, San Francisco
San Francisco, California

John S. Greenspan, BSc, BDS, PhD, FRC(Path)
Professor and Chair
Department of Stomatology
School of Dentistry
University of California, San Francisco
San Francisco, California

Jerome E. Groopman, MD
Professor of Medicine
Chief, Division of Hematology and Oncology
New England Deaconess Hospital
Boston, Massachusetts

Clyde E. Hart
Retrovirus Diseases Branch
Division of AIDS, STD, and TB Laboratory Research
Centers for Disease Control and Prevention
Atlanta, Georgia

Barton F. Haynes, MD
Frederic M. Hanes Professor and Chairman
Department of Medicine
Duke University
Durham, North Carolina

Craig W. Hendrix, MD
Senior Scientist
Military Medical Consortium for
Applied Retroviral Research
Associate Professor Medicine
Division of Clinical Pharmacology
The Johns Hopkins University School of Medicine
Baltimore, Maryland

Martin S. Hirsch, MD
Infectious Disease Unit
Massachusetts General Hospital
Professor of Medicine
Harvard Medical School
Boston, Massachusetts

Derek Hodel
Director of Public Policy
Gay Men's Health Crisis
New York, New York

Scott D. Holmberg, MD, MPH
Chief, Special Studies Section
Division of HIV/AIDS
National Center for HIV, STD, and
*   TB Prevention (NCHSTP)*
Centers for Disease Control and Prevention
Atlanta, Georgia

David R. Holtgrave, PhD
Center for AIDS Intervention Research
Department of Psychiatry and Behavioral Medicine
Medical College of Wisconsin
Milwaukee, Wisconsin

Phyllis J. Kanki, DVM, SD
Associate Professor of Pathobiology
Harvard AIDS Institute
Harvard School of Public Health
Boston, Massachusetts

Joan C. Kaplan, PhD
Associate Professor of Microbiology
Infectious Disease Unit
Massachusetts General Hospital
Harvard Medical School
Charleston, Massachusetts

Gabor D. Kelen, MD, FRCP(C), FACEP
Professor and Chair
Department of Emergency Medicine
Johns Hopkins University School of Medicine
Baltimore, Maryland

Nancy B. Kiviat
HPV Research Group
Seattle, Washington

Jeffrey B. Kopp, MD
Senior Clinical Investigator
Kidney Disease Section/MDB/NIDDK
National Institutes of Health
Bethesda, Maryland

Donald P. Kotler, MD
Associate Professor of Medicine
Columbia University College of
*   Physicians and Surgeons*
St. Luke's-Roosevelt Hospital Center
New York, New York

Joseph A. Kovacs, MD
Critical Care Medicine Department
National Institutes of Health
Bethesda, Maryland

H. Clifford Lane, MD
National Institute of Allergy and
*   Infectious Diseases*
National Institutes of Health
Bethesda, Maryland

Tun-Hou Lee, DSc
Department of Cancer Biology
Harvard School of Public Health
Boston, Massachusetts

Stewart J. Levine
Critical Care Medicine Department
National Institutes of Health
Clinical Center
Bethesda, Maryland

Katherine Luzuriaga, MD
Department of Pediatrics
University of Massachusetts Medical School
Worcester, Massachusetts

Ruthanne Marcus
Yale University School of Medicine
Division of Epidemiology and Public Health
New Haven, Connecticut

Jonathan Mann, MD
Francois-Xavier Bagnoud Professor
*   of Health and Human Rights*
Francois-Xavier Bagnoud Center
*   of Health and Human Rights*
Cambridge, Massachusetts

Donald D. Marianos, DDS, MPH
Director, Division of Oral Health
National Center for Prevention Services
Centers of Disease Control and Prevention
Atlanta, Georgia

Henry Masur, MD
Critical Care Medicine
National Institutes of Health
Bethesda, Maryland

Francine E. McCutchan
Henry M. Jackson Foundation for
*   the Advancement of Military Medicine*
Rockville, Maryland

Thierry Mertens, MD, PhD
Head Evaluation
Development of Policy, Programme, and
*   Evaluation*
World Health Organization
Geneva, Switzerland

Julia A. Metcalf, MT
Laboratory of Immunoregulation
National Institutes of Health
Bethesda, Maryland

Ronald T. Mitsuyasu, MD
Director, UCLA CARE Center
Associate Professor of Medicine
Department of Medicine
UCLA School of Medicine
Los Angeles, California

Richard A. Morgan, PhD
Chief, Gene Transfer Technology
*   Section, CGTB, NCHGR*
Clinical Gene Therapy Branch
National Center for Human Genome Research
Bethesda, Maryland

Jeffrey Moulton Benevedes, PhD
Private Practice, San Francisco
San Francisco, California

Brigitta U. Mueller, MD
Visiting Scientist
National Cancer Institute
Bethesda, Maryland

David G. Ostrow, MD, PhD
Associate Professor of Psychiatry and
  Behavioral Medicine
Center for AIDS Intervention Research
Milwaukee, Wisconsin

Giuseppe Pantaleo, MD
Visiting Scientist
Laboratory of Immunoregulation
National Institute of Allergy and Infectious Diseases
National Institutes of Health
Bethesda, Maryland

Stephania Paolucci, MD
Laboratory of Immunoregulation
National Institute of Allergy and Infectious Diseases
National Institutes of Health
Bethesda, Maryland

George N. Pavlakis, MD, PhD
ABL-Basic Research Program
NCI-FCDRC
Frederick, Maryland

Carla B. Pettinelli, MD, PhD
Therapeutics Research Program
Division of AIDS
National Institute of Allergy and Infectious Diseases
Rockville, Maryland

Peter Piot, MD, PhD
Executive Director, Joint United Nations
  Programme on HIV
Geneva, Switzerland

Philip A. Pizzo, MD
Physician-in-Chief and Chair
Department of Medicine
Childrens Hospital
Boston, Massachusetts

Michael A. Polis, MD, MPH
Senior Investigator
National Institute of Allergy and
  Infectious Diseases, NIH
Laboratory of Immunoregulation
Bethesda, Maryland

Richard W. Price, MD
Professor of Neurology
University of California San Francisco
Chief of Neurology Service
San Francisco General Hospital
San Francisco, California

Michael O. Rigsby, MD
Assistant Professor of Medicine
Yale University School of Medicine
Director, HIV Program
West Haven VA Medical Center
West Haven, Connecticut

Michael S. Saag, MD
Associate Professor of Medicine
The University of Alabama at Birmingham
Department of Medicine
Birmingham, Alabama

Bijan Safai, MD, DSc
Professor and Chairman
Department of Dermatology
New York Medical College
Valhalla, New York

Timothy Schacker, MD
Acting Assistant Professor
Virology Research Clinic
University of Washington
Seattle, Washington

Steven Schnittman, MD
Therapeutics Research Program
Division of AIDS
National Institute of Allergy and.
  Infectious Diseases
Rockville, Maryland

James Shelhamer, MD
Deputy Chief, Critical Care Medicine
National Institutes of Health
Bethesda, Maryland

Louise Short, MD, MSc
Medical Epidemiologist
Hospital Infectious Program
National Center for Infectious Diseases
Centers for Disease Control and Prevention
Atlanta, Georgia

Michael C. Sneller, MD
Chief, Immunologic Diseases Section
Laboratory of Immunoregulation
National Institute of Allergy and
  Infectious Diseases
National Institutes of Health
Bethesda, Maryland

Cladd Stevens, MD
Head, Laboratory of Epidemiology
New York Blood Center
New York, New York

John Sullivan, MD
Professor of Pediatrics
Program in Molecular Medicine
University of Massachusetts
  Medical Center
Worcester, Massachusetts

Mauro Vaccarezza, MD
National Institute of Allergy and
  Infectious Diseases
National Institutes of Health
Bethesda, Maryland

Thierry VandenDriessche, PhD
Center for Transgene Technology and
  Gene Therapy
Flemish Interuniversity Institute for Biotechnology
Campus Gasthuisberg University of Leuven
O&N Dienst Prof. Collen
Leuven, Belgium

Sten H. Vermund, MD, PhD
Professor and Chair, Department of Epidemiology
Director, Division of Geographic Medicine
Department of Medicine
University of Alabama at Birmingham
Birmingham, Alabama

John J. Zurlo, MD
Penn State College of Medicine
University Hospital
Children's Hospital
The Milton S. Hershey Medical Center
Hershey, Pennsylvania

Preface

When the first edition of this textbook was published in 1985, approximately 7000 cases of AIDS had been reported in the United States. At that time, little was known concerning the details of the viral pathogenesis of the disease and no treatments existed that could impact on its relentless progression.

While much has been learned about AIDS in the intervening 11 years, the dramatic increase in recent HIV infection and AIDS cases worldwide has exceeded even the most dire of early predictions. Though the spread of the disease continues and is increasingly extending into the heterosexual population, significant insights are being developed concerning epidemiologic approaches to halt the spread of the disease and define new agents to use in its treatment.

For the preparation of this fourth edition, the editors relied upon the expertise of three worldwide experts to serve as Associate Editors, Dr. Anthony Fauci, Dr. Max Essex and Dr. James Curran. The current edition represents an attempt to present a concise but comprehensive summary of current scientific and clinical information related to HIV and AIDS. Our goal is to present existing knowledge concerning the understanding of the pathogenesis of the disease and current methods for the management of patients who contract AIDS. In each section of the text we have attempted to point to areas of current progress and opportunities for progress in the future as well.

The book is divided into five sections. The first section deals with our current understanding of the etiology and pathogenesis of the disease. This section is followed by a detailed consideration of the epidemiology of AIDS in the United States and throughout the world. Special attention has been paid to the heterosexual spread of AIDS and its transmission in adolescents, and maternal-fetal spread. Progress in the development of sensitive means for the diagnosis of HIV is dealt with in Section III of the textbook. The major portion of the book deals with the clinical manifestations and treatment of HIV infections, as presented in Sections IV and V. Each of the individual infectious and malignant complications of HIV infections is considered, as well as a detailed system-by-system analysis of its impact. The development of new agents for the treatment of HIV infection, as well as new approaches including gene therapy, are also dealt with in the final section of this text.

We present this book with the hope that it can be useful to clinicians and scientists as a comprehensive reference to help in the understanding of HIV infection and in the management of patients who develop the complex clinical problems associated with HIV infection.

Table of Contents

Color Figures

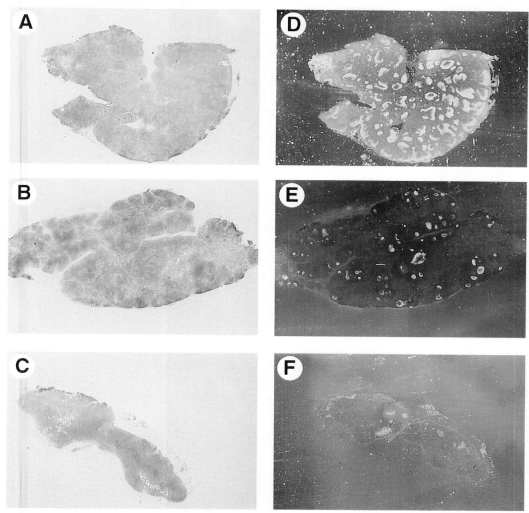

COLOR FIGURE 4-3. Excisional lymph node biopsies from HIV-infected individuals at various stages of disease. (**A**) Lymph node from a subject in early-stage disease with numerous large germinal centers invading the medulla, having irregular shapes, and a tendency to fuse. (**B**) Lymph node from a subject in intermediate-stage disease with large areas of tissue involution and focal fibrosis. (**C**) Lymph node from a subject in advanced stage disease. Most of the lymphoid tissue has been replaced by fibrotic tissue and fatty infiltration. (**D–F**) Dark-field images of in situ hybridization of the same lymph nodes shown in **A** through **C**. The location of HIV RNA is indicated by the silver grains, which appears as white dots. (**D**) The hybridization signal is mostly localized in the germinal centers, and HIV RNA corresponds to extracellular virions trapped in the FDC network; virus trapping is very efficient in this hyperplastic lymph node. (**E**) Reduction of trapping of virus is associated with follicular involution. (**F**) The trapping ability of the lymph node tissue virtually is lost completely in this lymph node that manifests lymphocyte depletion and follicular involution.

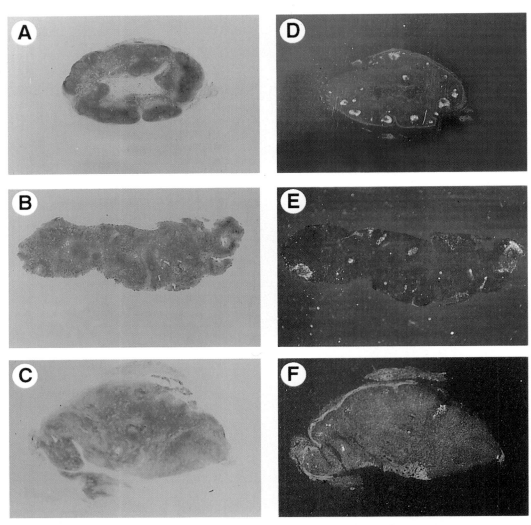

COLOR FIGURE 4-4. Lymph nodes from HIV-infected individuals who are long term non-progressors (LTNP). (**A**) Lymph node from a LTNP with numerous small germinal centers having regular shape. (**B**) Lymph node from a LTNP in which germinal centers are seen in half of the tissue section, whereas the other half contains non-organized lymphoid tissue. (**C**) Lymph node from a LTNP in which most of the tissue section is occupied by non-organized lymphoid tissue, whereas germinal center formation is minimal or absent. (**D–F**) in situ hybridization of the same lymph nodes shown in **A–C**. The location of HIV RNA is indicated by silver grains that appear as white dots. There are variable degrees of virus trapping, which in general is minimal and far lower than the degree of trapping noted in typical progressors early in the course of their disease. (Adapted from Schrager, LK, Young JM, Fowler MG, Mathieson BJ, Vermund SH. Long-term survivors of HIV-1 infections: definition and research challenges. AIDS 1994; 8:S95).

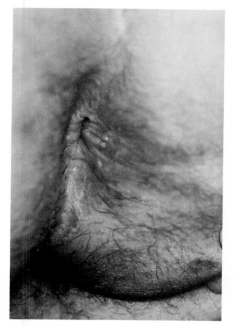

COLOR FIGURE 14.5-1. Zosteriform peri-rectal HSV infection in an HIV infected male.

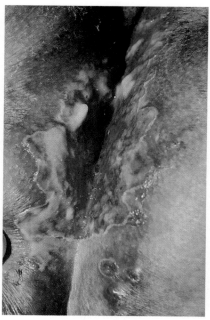

COLOR FIGURE 14.5-2. Acyclovir-resistant peri-rectal HSV2 infection in an HIV infected male.

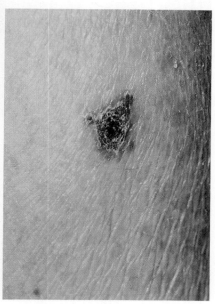

COLOR FIGURE 14.5-4. Ecthymatous zoster lesion in an HIV infected person (photo courtesy of Dr. David Spach).

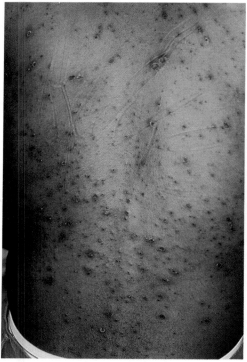

COLOR FIGURE 14.5-5. Disseminated hyperkeratotic zoser in an HIV infection person (photo courtesy of Dr. David Spach).

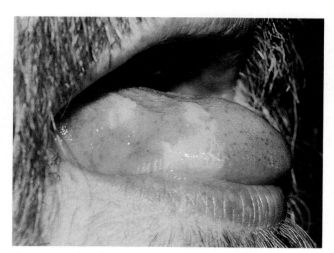

COLOR FIGURE 14.5-6. Oral hairy leukoplakia on the sides of the tongue in an HIV infected person (photo courtesy of Dr. David Spach).

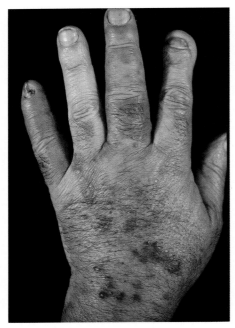

COLOR FIGURE 15.1-1. Classic Kaposi's sarcoma plaque and nodular lesion.

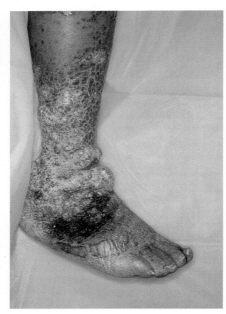

COLOR FIGURE 15.1-2. Classic Kaposi's sarcoma, showing extensive infiltration, tumor, and secondary lymphedema.

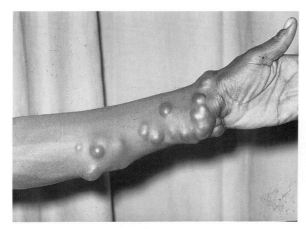

COLOR FIGURE 15.1-3. Endemic Kaposi's sarcoma, nodular form.

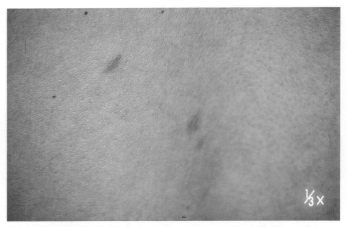

COLOR FIGURE 15.1-4. Early patch lesion of Kaposi's sarcoma in an AIDS patient.

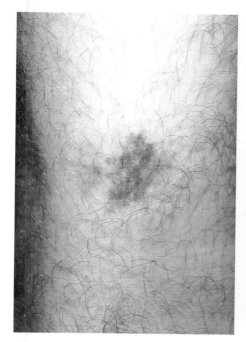

COLOR FIGURE 15.1-5. More advanced patch lesion of Kaposi's sarcoma in an AIDS patient.

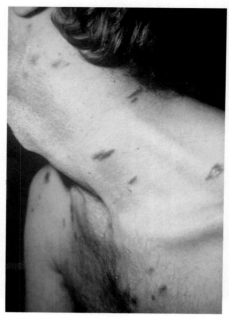

COLOR FIGURE 15.1-6. Patch lesions of Kaposi's sarcoma distributed symmetrically along Langer's (skin cleavage) lines.

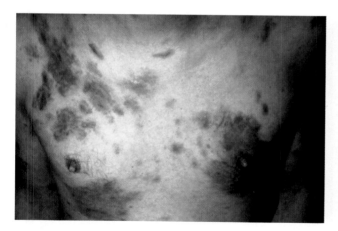

COLOR FIGURE 15.1-7. Hemorrhagic presentation of Kaposi's sarcoma in an AIDS patient.

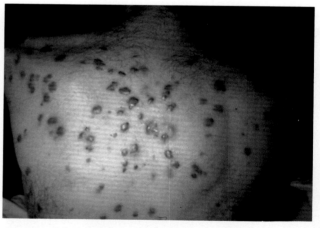

COLOR FIGURE 15.1-8. Extensive symmetric distribution of plaque and tumor lesions of Kaposi's sarcoma in an AIDS patient.

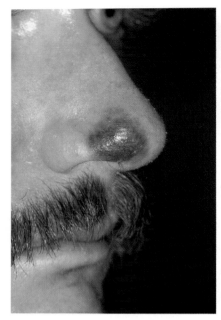

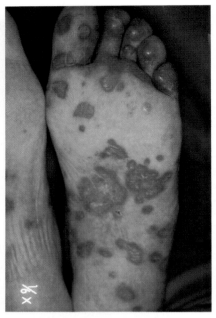

COLOR FIGURE 15.1-9. Large patch lesion of the nose, a common site for AIDS-related Kaposi's sarcoma.

COLOR FIGURE 15.1-10. Kaposi's sarcoma patches, plaques, and nodules on the sole of an AIDS patient.

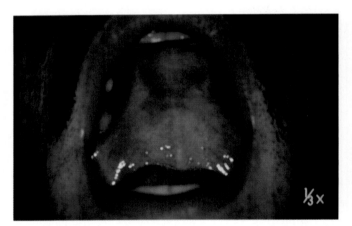

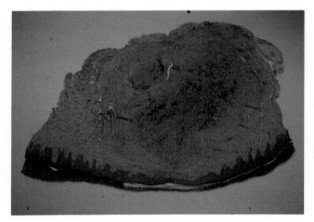

COLOR FIGURE 15.1-11. Involvement of the hard and soft palate by Kaposi's sarcoma.

COLOR FIGURE 15.1-13. Gross microscopic view shows the hemorrhagic and cellular nature of Kaposi's sarcoma.

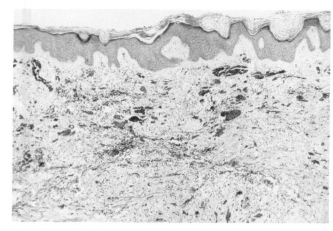

COLOR FIGURE 15.1-14. Low-power view of a patch lesion of Kaposi's sarcoma shows slit-like vascular spaces and inflammatory cell infiltrate of the dermis.

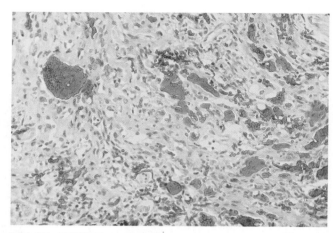

COLOR FIGURE 15.1-15. High-power view shows irregularly shaped vascular channels, extravasated erythyrocytes, and spindle cells of AIDS-associated Kaposi's sarcoma.

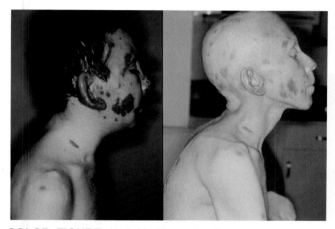

COLOR FIGURE 15.1-16. Extensive facial tumors of Kaposi's sarcoma before and after radiation therapy.

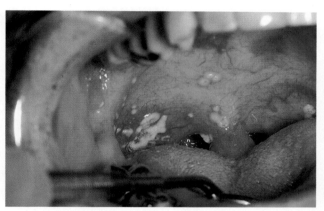

COLOR FIGURE 17-2. Pseudomembranous candidiasis, palate.

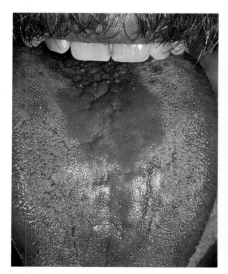

COLOR FIGURE 17-3. Erythematous candidiasis of the dorsal tongue.

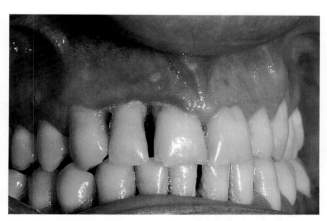

COLOR FIGURE 17-4. Necrotizing ulcerative periodontitis of the maxilla.

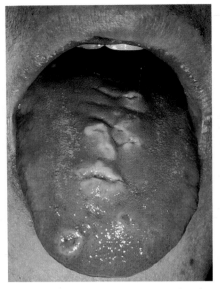

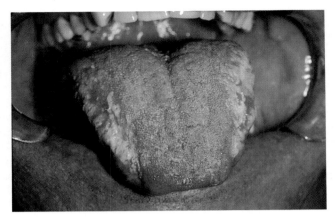

COLOR FIGURE 17-5. Herpes simplex on the dorsal tongue.

COLOR FIGURE 17-6. Hairy leukoplakia appears as bilateral thickening of the tongue.

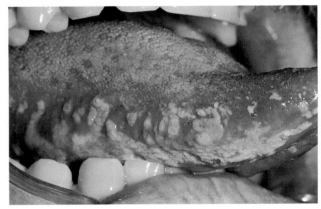

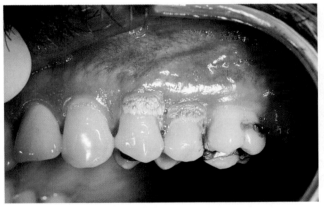

COLOR FIGURE 17-7. Hairy leukoplakia of the tongue.

COLOR FIGURE 17-8. Wart on the maxillary gingival margin.

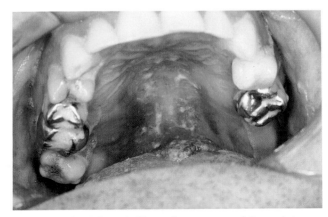

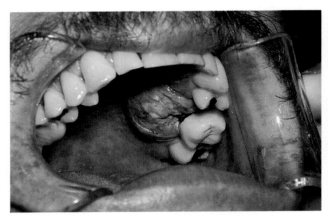

COLOR FIGURE 17-9. Kaposi's sarcoma of the palate.

COLOR FIGURE 17-10. Lymphoma of the palate.

PART I

Etiology and Pathogenesis

AIDS: Biology, Diagnosis, Treatment and Prevention, fourth edition, edited by Vincent T. DeVita, Jr., Samuel Hellman, and Steven A. Rosenberg. Lippincott–Raven Publishers, © 1997

CHAPTER 1.1

Origin of Acquired Immunodeficiency Syndrome

Myron E. Essex

If a "new" disease appears, the cause must also be new. If the new disease is infectious, as is acquired immunodeficiency syndrome (AIDS), the causative agent must have existed previously under one of several possible circumstances. First, the etiologic agent may represent a more virulent mutant variant or recombinant of an organism that was either previously infecting the same population without causing disease or had a distinctly different profile of disease pathology. Second, the organism may have been introduced from a relatively isolated population of people who had developed a resistance to the lethality of the agent. Third, the organism may have been introduced to humans from another species. This third explanation seems apparent for the human immunodeficiency virus type 2 (HIV-2) and is increasingly likely for HIV-1. Attempts to understand how HIVs and the related simian immunodeficiency viruses (SIVs) evolved are occasionally viewed as insensitive or irrelevant. Yet, understanding how human or nonhuman hosts evolved to resist the lethal effects of HIV or related viruses may provide valuable clues for the development of effective vaccines and drugs.

AIDS was first recognized as a new and distinct clinical entity in 1981.[1–3] The first cases were recognized because of an unusual clustering of diseases such as Kaposi's sarcoma and *Pneumocystis carinii* pneumonia in young homosexual men. Although such syndromes had occasionally been observed in distinct subgroups of the population (eg, older men of Mediterranean origin in the case of Kaposi's sarcoma, severely impaired cancer patients in the case of *P*

carinii pneumonia), the occurrence of these diseases in previously healthy young people was unprecedented. Because most of the first cases of this newly defined clinical syndrome to be described involved homosexual men, it seemed logical at first that the cause of this syndrome could be related to a lifestyle habit unique to that population. In the 1960s and 1970s, the revolution in sexual permissiveness brought with it an enhanced societal acceptance of homosexuality. The development of commercial bathhouses and other outlets for homosexual contact increased the incidence of promiscuity in self-selected segments of the male homosexual population. Such factors as frequent exposure to sperm, rectal exposure to sperm, and amyl or butyl nitrate "poppers," which were used to enhance sexual performance, were considered potential causes of AIDS. Yet, although it was apparent that AIDS was a new disease, most homosexual lifestyle habits had changed only in a relative sense.

AIDS cases were soon reported in other populations, including intravenous drug users[4] and hemophiliacs.[5–7] Although these groups were not necessarily exposed to amyl or butyl nitrate or to frequent contact with sperm, it was argued that they, like male homosexuals, may have been exposed to frequent immunostimulatory doses of foreign proteins and tissue antigens. Hemophiliacs used clotting factor preparations, which were prepared from the pooled blood of huge numbers of donors, and intravenous drug users often used needles contaminated with small amounts of blood from previous users, thereby increasing their exposure to foreign tissue antigens. Even independent of clinical AIDS, asymptomatic hemophiliacs and intravenous drug users were often found to have inverted ratios of helper to suppressor T lymphocytes, as did AIDS patients and a proportion of asymptomatic homosexual men. However, for patients not exhibiting the new syndrome, the distorted T-cell ratios were more often a result of an increase in the number of T-suppressor cells, as opposed to the absolute

Myron E. Essex: Mary Woodard Lasker Professor of Health Sciences, Chairman, Department of Cancer Biology, Harvard School of Public Health, Chairman, Harvard AIDS Institute, 665 Huntington Avenue, Boston, MA 02115.

decrease in T-helper cells seen in AIDS patients with progressing disease. The increase in T-suppressor cells is presumably a result of frequent antigenic stimulation.

Three new categories of AIDS patients were soon observed: blood transfusion recipients,[8,9] adults from Central Africa,[10–12] and infants born to mothers who themselves had AIDS or were intravenous drug users.[13–15] The patients with transfusion-associated cases were found to have received donations from an AIDS patient at least 3 years before symptoms developed.[8,9]

AN INFECTIOUS ETIOLOGY FOR AIDS

The developments just described, among others, made it clear that an infectious etiology for AIDS should be considered.[16] Several studies were initiated to determine seroprevalence rates for exposure to numerous microorganisms, especially viruses, and to compare exposure to given agents in AIDS patients and control subjects.[17] High on the list of candidate viruses was cytomegalovirus, because it was already associated with a less severe immunosuppression in kidney transplant patients; Epstein-Barr virus, presumably because it was a lymphotropic virus; and hepatitis B, because infection with this virus was known to occur at elevated rates in both homosexual men and recipients of blood or blood products. If one of these candidate viruses were to be etiologically involved, it would presumably have to be a newly mutated or recombinant genetic variant.

At the same time, my group,[18,19] Gallo and his colleagues,[20,21] and Montagnier and his colleagues[22] postulated that a variant T-lymphotropic retrovirus (HTLV) could be the etiologic agent of AIDS. Among the most compelling reasons for this hypothesis was that HTLV, discovered by Gallo and colleagues[23] in 1980, was the only human virus known to infect T-helper lymphocytes. It was already clear that T-helper lymphocytes became impaired or were eliminated in clinical AIDS.[13,24–26] HTLV was also known to be transmitted through the same routes as the etiologic agent of AIDS: by sexual contact, with transmission apparently more efficient from males; by blood; and by transmission from mothers to newborns.[27] Among animal retroviruses, the lymphotropic feline leukemia virus was known to be a major cause of lethal immunosuppression in cats.[28] Even HTLV-I, which causes leukemia or neurologic disease in only a fraction of infected individuals, was known to cause a nonlethal immunosuppression.[29]

Attempts to detect a virus related to HTLV-I or HTLV-II[30] met with partial success. Although antibodies cross-reactive with HTLV-I and HTLV-related genomic sequences were found in a minority of AIDS patients,[18,20–22] the reactivity was weak, suggesting either the coinfection of AIDS patients with an HTLV or the etiologic role of a distant, weakly reactive virus. Soon after, proof that the disease was linked to T-lymphotropic retroviruses was obtained by Gallo and his colleagues.[31–34] Further characterization of the agent, now termed human immunodeficiency virus type 1 (HIV-1),

revealed that it was only distantly related to HTLV yet was the same as the isolate detected earlier by Montagnier and his colleagues.[22]

ORIGINS OF HUMAN RETROVIRUSES

HTLV-I, the first human retrovirus identified, was known to be present at elevated rates in regions such as southwestern Japan, the Caribbean basin, northern South America, and Africa and at lower rates in most of North America and Europe. The theory that this virus originated in Africa was initially suggested by Gallo, who cited early reports of Africans in southwestern Japan.[35] Miyoshi and his colleagues then identified a virus related to HTLV-I in Asian monkeys.[36] This virus, designated simian T-cell leukemia virus (STLV), was later found in African monkeys and apes[37,38] and was associated with lymphoproliferative diseases in captive macaques.[39]

Seroepidemiologic studies in Old World primates from both Asia and Africa revealed that more than 30 species of monkeys and apes had widespread infection with an STLV[40] (Table 1.1-1). However, on further molecular characterization, it was recognized that the STLV viruses from Japanese macaques and related Asian species of monkeys were not as closely related to HTLV-I as were STLVs isolated from African primates such as chimpanzees and African green monkeys.[41] All isolates of HTLV-I, whether from Japanese, Caribbean, or African people, were highly related to African strains of STLV but not as highly related to Asian strains of STLV. This suggested that HTLV-I evolved from a subgroup of STLVs present in Africa but not in Asia. It also suggested that the STLV/HTLV-I family of retroviruses was present in numerous species of Old World monkeys for some time before it was introduced to humans from an African species of monkey or ape.

As a group, the STLV/HTLV-I viruses vary little from one isolate to another, but the HIV-1 viruses and the SIV/HIV-2 group of viruses vary highly from one isolate to another.[42,43] Although the HIV-1 viruses appear to cause AIDS or a related disease in a very high proportion of infected people, the STLV/HTLV-I viruses rarely cause lethal disease in people or monkeys.[44] SIVs appear to be nonvirulent in their natural African monkey hosts.[44,45] HIV-2 appears to be less virulent than HIV-1 but is associated with some cases of AIDS.[46–48] The high prevalence of infection with STLV in so many species of Old World monkeys also indicates that STLV only rarely causes lymphoma or other diseases under natural circumstances. Although it is unclear why STLV and HTLV-I are so limited in their pathogenicity, evolutionary pressure within the monkey species may have selected for a virus that was not highly virulent. An STLV of low virulence may then have been transmitted to humans, in whom it remained a virus of limited virulence.

HTLV-II, the second human retrovirus detected,[30] was only about 40% to 50% related to HTLV-I at the genomic level.[49] HTLV-II was also found at high prevalence in

TABLE 1.1-1. *Retroviruses related to HTLV and HIV in subhuman primates*

Region	Species	HTLV-1	HTLV-2	HIV-1	HIV-2
Africa	Chimpanzee	+	–	+	–
Baboon		+	–	–	–
Green monkey		+	–	–	+
Mangabey		?	?	–	+
Asia	Macaque	+	–	–	–*
South America	Spider monkey	–	+	–	–
	Marmoset	–	–	–	–

+, contains simian retrovirus related to virus shown; –, no known simian virus related to virus shown; ?, not known.

*Although wild macaques examined have all been seronegative, monkeys in captivity have been infected with a virus that is essentially the same as the mangabey SIV and HIV-2.

selected human populations of New World origin.[50–52] The closest HTLV-II–related virus of subhuman primates was in a New World species, the South American spider monkey.[53]

Whereas substantial genetic variation is seen among different isolates of HIV-1, particularly in the envelope gene, the same degree of variation is not seen for HTLV-I. Presumably, the rate of genetic drift seen in retroviruses is related to their rate of replication. HIVs, as lenti-type retroviruses, have a greater ability to circumvent the usual rigid requirements for cell division of the retroviruses. The presence of regulatory genes that allow a rapid increase in replication rate are properties not associated with simpler retroviruses. This replication potential, along with a reverse transcriptase that is substantially more error-prone,[54] helps explain why genomic variation among HIVs is substantially greater than for other retroviruses. Although HIV-1 can replicate to high titers and be detected as free virus in serum or plasma, HTLV-I cannot. Because HTLV-I is apparently transmitted only in a cell-associated manner (both between individuals and within the body), the rate of evolutionary diversion of this virus should be considerably less. Very different and more rapid evolutionary development would occur in the case of HIV-1.

DIVERSION AMONG HUMAN LENTIVIRUSES

Based on relatedness of nucleotide sequences and the diversion seen among HIV isolates, it is possible that HIV-1 and HIV-2 originated quite recently.[55] The first documented infection with HIV-1, based on antibody detection, occurred in 1959.[56]

Nucleotide sequence drift is most rapid in the *env* gene, in which variation occurs at a rate about three times that seen in the *pol* gene; *gag* has an intermediate rate. The average differences between HIV-1 *env* sequences deviate up to about 1% per year.[43] The higher degree of conservation observed among samples from clustered patients, compared with random donors in the same geographic area, was used as evidence for a rare case of dental exposure.[57] *Env* gene variations of 5% or more can be seen in viruses isolated from the same individual.

Cultivation in vitro appears to select initially for more highly related strains and to diminish subsequent rates of diversion.[58–60] This may be similar to an in vivo selection pressure exerted as a result of a host immune response.

ORIGIN OF HIV-1

After HIV-1 was recognized as the probable cause of AIDS, it soon became apparent that this virus was new to populations in the Western hemisphere. This raised the question of whether HIV-1 was also new in Old World human populations or whether it had recently been introduced from another species. If HIV-1 had been present in some human populations in Africa to the point of evolutionary equilibration (as had HTLV-I), it probably would have been limited to isolated tribes of people, and selection for host immunity as well as selection of an avirulent virus would have occurred. Such isolation seemed essential for evolutionary equilibration to have occurred, because, in both the United States and Haiti, blacks were just as likely as whites to develop clinical AIDS after exposure to HIV-1.

The possibility that HIV-1 or a related virus was present in human populations in central Africa at the same time or even before AIDS was diagnosed in the United States seemed even more probable after what was apparently the same syndrome was reported in Africans who sought treatment in Europe. Subsequently, it was recognized that HIV-1 infection and clinical AIDS were rapidly spreading in Central Africa (Table 1.1-2).

Serum samples collected from Africans at earlier periods were also examined for the presence of antibodies reactive with HIV-1. In some cases, the examination of stored samples suggested elevated rates of infection in Africa during the period 1965 to 1975. Subsequently, it was revealed that most of those surveys were conducted with first-stage tests that were imperfect, and the reactors were mostly false-positive cases, caused either by contamination of the HIV antigen or by "sticky sera" containing antibodies that reacted nonspecifically because of repeated freezing and thawing and maintenance under poor conditions.

TABLE 1.1-2. *Estimates of representative seroprevalence in Africa and Asia*

Region	Country	Seropositivity Rate (%) HIV-1 1985–1988	HIV-1 1990–1993	HIV-2 1985–1988	HIV-2 1990–1993
Central Africa	Burundi	5–10	10–20	<1	<1
	Congo	1–5	5–10	<1	<1
	Kenya	1–5	10–20	<1	<1
	Malawi	5–10	>20	<1	<1
	Mozambique	1–5	10–20	1–5	1–5
	Uganda	10–20	>20	<1	<1
	Zaire	5–10	5–10	<1	<1
	Zambia	10–20	10–20	<1	<1
West Africa	Burkina Faso	<1	5–10	1–5	1–5
	Gvinea Bissau	<1	<1	10–20	10–20
	Ivory Coast	1–5	>20	1–5	1–5
	Senegal	<1	1–5	1–5	1–5
Asia	Northern Thailand	<1	5–10	<1	<1
	Western India	<1	5–10	<1	1–5

While examining sera taken from African patients in the period 1955 to 1965, we found one antibody-positive sample that was clearly specific.[56] When tested by radioimmunoprecipitation, this sample was found to contain high titers of antibodies that were reactive with virtually all the major antigens of HIV-1 detectable by this technique: gp160, gp120, p55, gp41, p27, p24, and p17. However, this sample represented only a rare positive reactor in a high-risk group of individuals exposed to venereal infections and AIDS-like illnesses in a region that subsequently had high rates of infection with HIV-1. Positive results were obtained from fewer than 1% of sick individuals tested from Kinshasa, Zaire, which is now classified as a region of moderate to high prevalence. This suggests that the virus was only rarely present at that time in places that would now be considered within the AIDS belt of Africa (see Table 1.1-2). We speculated that HIV-1 or a virus very similar to it had moved to the cities of this region of Africa before the mid-1950s, either by introduction from subhuman primates or by migration of a few resistant carriers from a previously isolated tribe or tribes. Population redistribution was occurring at that time, with movement of previously isolated people into the newly expanding cities. Still, it seems unlikely that HIV-1 would have been present, as such, for many generations in isolated tribal regions. If this were so, we would expect to find Africans who show greater resistance to infection and disease development, owing to genetic evolution of the human species. However, in prospective studies conducted to date, exposed Africans appear to develop clinical AIDS and other signs and symptoms of HIV disease as rapidly as individuals in the United States or Europe.[61] Furthermore, as has been mentioned, the degree of genomic variation seen in African isolates of HIV-1 is greater than that seen in isolates from Europe or the United States.

A virus that could be a progenitor of HIV-1 has been isolated from a chimpanzee in central Africa[62] (Fig. 1.1-1A). This find-

ing, combined with the knowledge that all HIV-1 viruses tested appear to be avirulent when inoculated into chimpanzees, is also compatible with a subhuman primate origin for HIV-1. Some African isolates of HIV-1 appear to be as close to the chimpanzee isolate as to other prototype strains of HIV-1.[63,64]

DISTRIBUTION AND TRANSMISSION OF HIV-1 SUBTYPES

It is now apparent that the HIV-1s isolated from infected people in the United States and Europe are closer to each other than to typical HIV-1s from people in Africa or Asia. This has led to the classification of HIV-1s into subtypes or clades.[65] Such subtypes, designated A through K, have envelope gene sequences that vary by 20% or more between subtypes (Fig. 1.1-2A). All the HIV-1s isolated from the United States and western Europe through 1994 have been of a single subtype, HIV-1 B (Table 1.1-3). It is probable that new subtypes of HIV-1s will appear in the West in the future.

Most of the HIV-1 subtypes have been found in sub-Saharan Africa. On the African continent in general, subtypes A, C, and D have been found more frequently than others, although most of the others have also been described as occasional isolates. The highest rate of spread of HIV-1 for Africa appeared during the 1980s, at about the same time the epidemic was spreading in the United States and Europe.

In Asia, the introduction and spread of HIV-1 appeared about a decade later than in the West. In Thailand, HIV-1 subtype B was detected in intravenous drug users during the mid-1980s. During the late 1980s, subtype E was first detected. By the early to middle 1990s, HIV-1 subtype E had spread very rapidly among heterosexuals in Thailand, with the highest rates occurring in the northern regions of the country (Fig. 1.1-3).[66] Although it apparently was present earlier in the region, HIV-1 subtype B never spread to cause a major heterosexual epidemic as did subtype E.

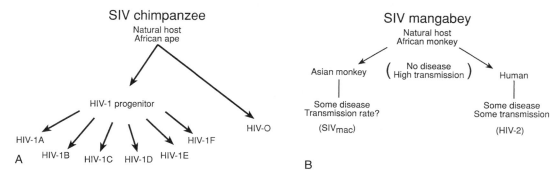

FIG. 1.1-1. Probable entry of HIV-1, HIV-2, and HIV-O from subhuman primate hosts. **(A)** HIV-1 and HIV-O originating from chimpanzees. **(B)** HIV-2 originating from mangabey and subsequently infecting Asian macaques as well as humans.

A similar situation occurred in India, with HIV-1 subtypes B and C. Although B apparently was introduced earlier and expanded among intravenous drug users, this subtype did not appear to spread as rapidly among heterosexuals as did HIV-1 C. Previously associated with a massive heterosexual epidemic in southeastern Africa, subtype C also caused a rapidly-spreading heterosexual epidemic in western India, evidently originating from the Bombay region.[66,67] The results in Africa and Asia suggest that HIV-1 subtypes A, C, D, and E are well adapted for heterosexual transmission but subtype B is less efficiently transmitted by this route (see Table 1.1-3). Whenever HIV-1 moves very rapidly through a new population, as has happened in Asia for subtypes E and C, the viruses isolated show relatively less diversity.[66]

An even more distant subtype, designated HIV-O, has been detected in Cameroon.[64] The viruses isolated from this subtype are less related to HIV-1 subtypes A through H than the other subtypes are related to each other, yet HIV-O is more related to HIV-1 than to HIV-2 (see Figure 1.1-2B).[68]

To emphasize this distance, HIV-1 subtypes A through H are designated the major group, and HIV-O is designated the outgroup.[69] Although HIV-1 subtypes A through H probably had a common human progenitor ancestor, HIV-O probably entered independently from a chimpanzee host, and HIV-2s almost certainly entered independently from mangabey monkey species native to West Africa.[70] Although some HIVs apparently entered human populations independently from subhuman primate hosts, others presumably emerged as recombinants from within a single human host.[71] HIV-1 subtype E, for example, is a recombinant with a *gag* and *pol* gene region from HIV-1 subtype A but a distinctly different envelope, presumably from a different human progenitor virus that has not yet been identified. Although rare, dual infections have been described with different clades of HIV-1 in the same human host.[72] Instances of dual infection with HIV-1 and HIV-2 have also been described,[73] although infection with one type appears to offer some protection against subsequent infection with another.[74]

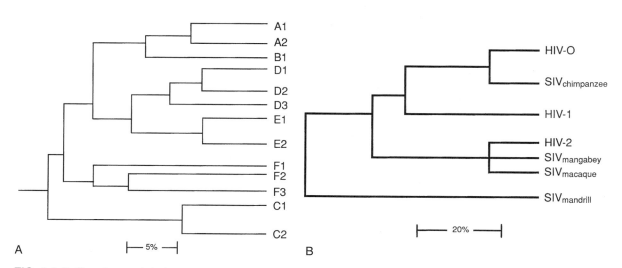

FIG. 1.1-2. Genotype relatedness among primate retroviruses. **(A)** Relatedness among envelope genes of representative HIV-1 viruses from different clades. **(B)** Relatedness among genomes of HIV-1, HIV-2, HIV-O, and different SIV viruses.

TABLE 1.1-3. *Geographic localization of HIV-1 according to transmission mode and genetic subtype*

Major Epidemic Pattern	Geographic Region	HIV-1 Subtype				
		A	B	C	D	E
Heterosexual hosts	Sub-Saharan Africa	+	—	+	+	+
	Southeast Asia	—	—	—	—	+
	India	—	—	+	—	—
Intravenous drug user and/or homosexual hosts	North America	—	+	—	—	—
	Western Europe	—	+	—	—	—
	Southeast Asia	—	+	—	—	—
	India	—	+	—	—	—

The movement and distribution of HIV-1 subtypes throughout the world is often perplexing, particularly because subtypes such as E through H are isolated more frequently in Asia, South America, and eastern Europe than in Africa, where they presumably originated.[75,76] However, the viruses that have been isolated and characterized were acquired for analysis after extensive regional selection bias and inadvertent clustering.

EMERGENCE OF HIV-1 DISEASE PHENOTYPES

In concert with the rapid diversion observed in virus isolates from different geographic regions, major differences can also be observed between genomes of viruses infecting the same individual. With the high replication potential observed for HIV-1s, an individual infected 5 to 10 years previously can harbor more than a million distinct genotypes.

One of the most perplexing aspects of AIDS as an infectious disease is the fact that clinical signs and symptoms rarely appear until several years after the initial infection. During this period, the host immune system presumably responds to the high rates of virus replication with continuous, vigorous immunoselection cycles, which allow the survival and expansion of immunoresistant variants. However, phenotypic variants with different cell tropisms and cytopathic properties have also been well characterized.

After infection by sexual contact, the HIV-1 viruses that can be isolated during the first few months or years, before clinical disease appears, have been designated "slow-low,"

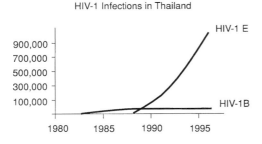

FIG. 1.1-3. Estimated prevalence of HIV-1 B and HIV-1 E in Thailand over the last decade.

because they grow poorly in cell culture.[77] Conversely, HIV-1 viruses isolated from patients with clinical disease have been designated "rapid-high" because they grow much more efficiently.[77] The slow-low HIV-1s also grow better in monocytes than in established T4-lymphoid cell lines, whereas the rapid-high viruses grow well in human T4 cell lines but poorly or not at all in fresh monocytes.[78] With the assumption that the HIV-1 viruses causing the initial infection were of a single genotype or of limited diversity, the infecting monocyte-tropic phenotype HIV-1s eventually give rise to dominant lymphotropic phenotype HIV-1s in about half of infected patients.[79]

Apparently by a form of convergent evolution for lymphotropism and disease induction, the differences in cell tropism can also be mapped to a relatively few point mutations in the *env* gene.[80] Some, but not all, of the same lymphocyte cell tropism properties are also linked to the ability of the virus to cause syncytia in vitro, giving rise to the designations syncytium-inducing and non–syncytium-inducing HIV-1.

Differences between HIV-1s can also be observed in the ability of the virus to kill fresh T4 lymphocytes.[81] The ability to grow in and kill fresh lymphocytes is not limited to those viruses that cause syncytia or those that grow in established T-cell lines. Both lymphotropic and monocyte-tropic viruses can infect and kill fresh uncultured human lymphocytes, but some HIV-1s also replicate efficiently in such cells without exhibiting a cytotoxic effect.[81] Whether the cytotoxic properties of HIV-1s also more commonly emerge as the disease progresses (as do the syncytium-inducing properties) remains to be determined. Recent in vivo studies revealed that efficient killing of T cells may be an important property of HIV-1 for disease development.[82,83] However, at least some of the amino acid residues that can control HIV-1 cytotoxicity are independent of those that cause lymphotropism or syncytium induction.[84]

Host selection of HIV-1s may partially explain the high rates of heterosexual transmission seen with subtypes C and E.[85] HIV-1 subtype B, the only dominant subtype in the West to date, appears to have undergone counterselection to lose the phenotypic property of efficient heterosexual transmission. If efficient heterosexual transmission requires a particular genotype for vaginal infection, such sequences may have been partially lost by these HIV-1 B strains that have been repeatedly passaged by blood exposure or rectal intercourse. Many strains of HIV-1 within non-B subtypes, on the other hand, could theoretically maintain vaginal phenotypic properties through regular heterosexual transmission in Africa and Asia.[86]

HIV-RELATED RETROVIRUSES OF MONKEYS

Soon after the recognition of clinical AIDS in humans, several clinical reports described outbreaks of severe infections, wasting disease, and death in colonies of Asian macaques housed at primate centers in the United States.[87,88] Such diseases were subsequently designated simian AIDS, or SAIDS. As with human AIDS, numerous possible causes were considered. After the recognition that SAIDS appeared to be of infectious origin, cytomegalovirus of monkeys was considered as a possible etiologic agent.

We investigated the possibility that rhesus and related species with SAIDS housed at the New England Regional Primate Research Center were infected with T-lymphotropic retroviruses related to HIV, because several other exogenous retroviruses had been found in subhuman primates, including the Mason-Pfizer type D virus of rhesus,[89] the gibbon ape leukemia virus[90] and a related simian sarcoma virus found in a woolly monkey,[91] and a recently described STLV in numerous Old World species.[36,39] Seroepidemiologic screening revealed that a proportion of the SAIDS monkeys had antibodies that cross-reacted with HIV[92] and that healthy rhesus monkeys had no such antibodies. Although the antibodies cross-reacted with core antigens of HIV-1, they showed only very weak cross-reactivity with the envelope antigens. However, the same antibody-positive rhesus sera reacted well with putative virus envelope antigens in reverse transcriptase-containing cultures of indicator human T4 cells cocultivated with buffy coat lymphocytes from antibody-positive monkeys.[92] Further characterization of the cultures revealed the presence of type C virus-like particles and antigens detectable with antibodies from either SAIDS monkeys or humans with AIDS. The sizes of the protein antigens detected by radioimmunoprecipitation were similar to those of HIV-1. This primate virus was named STLV-III, because of its relation to HIV-1 (which was then called HTLV-III or LAV); it was later designated simian immunodeficiency virus, SIV (ie, SIV-2).[93] Virtually all sera from people with AIDS and from healthy carriers of HIV have antibodies to the core antigens of SIV.

At the same time, studies were conducted using colonized rhesus monkeys with SAIDS, wild-caught and colony-maintained African green monkeys (*Cercopithicus aethiops*), and other African monkey species (see Table 1.1-1). These studies were undertaken because human AIDS, although clearly present in Africa, had not yet been found in people in Asia. In a serologic survey, 20% to 70% of different groups of wild-caught African green monkeys were found to be seropositive.[45,94] These included monkeys from the eastern region of sub-Saharan Africa, extending from Ethiopia to South Africa, and from Senegal, in the western region of sub-Saharan Africa. Wild-caught African green monkeys were seropositive even more often than colony-maintained animals of the same species.

Unlike captive rhesus monkeys, whose SIV infection was associated with SAIDS, African monkeys infected with SIV appeared to remain healthy. Captive African green or mangabey monkeys infected with SIV revealed no disease symptoms. In addition, at least half of the healthy wild-caught African green monkeys showed evidence of exposure to SIV on the basis of antibodies. Although the possibility that SIV caused an unusual case of disease in this species obviously could not be ruled out, especially if the disease occurred after reproductive life, it seemed clear that SIV was not closely linked to an immunosuppressive syndrome in African monkeys as it was in macaques. The African green monkey species, for example, was thriving despite the massive losses imposed by humans using it as a source of food.

As with STLV and HTLV-I, the possibility that SIV may cause disease rarely in African monkeys in advanced age could not be ruled out. Yet it was clear that this species had evolved a resistance and that the virus did not regularly cause severe disease as it did in rhesus monkeys, and as HIV-1 did in people. In the case of HTLV-I and STLV in monkeys, it appeared that evolutionary adaptation had selected for a virus of low virulence. It is difficult to postulate why SIV in African monkeys apparently does not cause disease, whereas a closely related virus does cause disease in macaques. Because wild macaques do not appear to be infected with SIV, and because the virus is limited to a small set of African primates, it appears probable that the virus accidentally infected captive rhesus monkeys quite recently. One possible explanation is that African species evolved to manifest immune resistance, whereas the virus itself has retained its virulence and causes symptoms only if it infects a species with no previous experience with the virus, such as the macaque. This explanation is also compatible with the widespread distribution of the virus in a high proportion of African monkeys. However, it is unclear why a virus that has coexisted for this long with the African green monkey species is not widely distributed in more species of Old World primates. And in one species in which an SIV-related virus is present, humans in West Africa (see discussion in a later section), this virus is not as frequently associated with highly lethal disease as is HIV-1.[95]

More recent studies have revealed that the SIV present in macaques and mangabeys is closest to the best-characterized strains of HIV-2 from West African people.[96] Whereas the macaque virus may have come from human materials experimentally inoculated into laboratory animals, the mangabey virus is more likely to be a potential source of infection in humans, because its range includes West Africa.[70] To date, however, most mangabey studies have been done with captive animals, sometimes also including animals that were inoculated with materials from macaques or humans.

A wide range of African monkey species are infected with different SIVs. These include several species commonly described as African greens (eg, vervet, grivet, sabaeus, tantalus), as well as mona, diana, Syke's, mandrill, and sooty mangabey species.[97–101] Thus far, SIVs have not been described in Asian species or in baboons, although these species can be infected in captivity with some primate lentiviruses. As a group, the SIVs are more closely related to HIV-2s than to HIV-1s, although some, such as the mandrill SIV, are evolutionarily distant[98] (see Fig. 1.1-2B). The sooty mangabey monkey virus and the Senegalese human HIV-2, on the other hand, are essentially the same at the genetic level.[96,101] It is this virus that also apparently accidentally infected the Asian macaques in captivity[44] (see Fig. 1.1-2B).

Why the SIV infections cause no disease in African monkeys remains unexplained. The observations that African monkey viruses may be virulent in macaques suggest that evolutionary development of host resistance rather than true virus attenuation may have occurred, but few studies have directly addressed this quandary. Although limited studies to detect active immune responses in African monkeys have been disappointing, soluble SIV-inhibitory factors have been found.[102]

HIV-2

Because a relative of HIV-1 (SIV) had been found in wild African monkeys but was only about 50% related to HIV-1 at the genomic level, it seemed logical that viruses more highly related to SIV may also be present in human populations. Serum samples from West African prostitutes were examined to determine whether they had antibodies that were more highly cross-reactive with SIV than with HIV-1.[46] West Africa was chosen because, at that time, it was largely free of HIV-1 and clinical AIDS, and female prostitutes were selected because they represent a group at high risk for amplification of prevalence rates for infection with sexually transmitted viruses.

Through Western blot techniques, it became clear that a significant proportion of Senegalese prostitutes had antibodies that were highly reactive with all the major antigens of SIV detected by this technique.[46,103] These included the *gag*-encoded p24, the *pol*-encoded p64/53 and p34, and the *env*-encoded transmembrane protein p34. Yet, when the same SIV antigens were reacted by Western blotting with sera from HIV-1–infected individuals of either European or central African origin with classic disease manifestations, little or no reaction was seen with the envelope antigens. Because the transmembrane protein of SIV is usually smaller than the comparable protein of HIV-1, this is manifested as the loss of reactivity where it might be expected at gp41 and the acquisition of reactivity with gp32, the carboxyl-terminus peptide of the *env* gene of SIV.[46] The class of reactivity seen with serum samples from West African prostitutes was vir-

tually indistinguishable from that seen with serum samples from African monkeys or captive rhesus. Similar results were also obtained by radioimmunoprecipitation, except that this procedure readily detects the gp120 amino-terminus *env* glycoprotein that is often missed by Western blotting. In this case, serum samples from the West African prostitutes reacted very well with the gp120 and gp160 of SIV but reacted only infrequently and weakly with the gp120 and gp160 of HIV-1.[103]

With evidence that a virus more closely related to SIV than to HIV-1 was present in Senegalese prostitutes, more extensive studies were undertaken to determine whether the SIV-related virus was more widely distributed in Africa in general, particularly in West Africa. The screening of more than 2000 high-risk individuals from central Africa, including many persons with AIDS and other sexually transmitted diseases, revealed no evidence that the virus, termed HIV-2, was present in the same regions in which HIV-1 was rampant[104] (see Table 1.1-2). However, pockets of infection with HIV-2 were detected in Mozambique and in Angola; although distant from West Africa, these regions are often on the same trade routes as Guinea Bissau and Cape Verde, West African countries whose rates of infection are among the highest.[105] Within Senegal, prevalence rates for HIV-2 were substantially higher in the southern region of Casamance, which borders Guinea Bissau, than in the northern region.[106]

Infection with HIV-2 was also substantially higher in female commercial sex workers than in other population groups,[105] indicating that this virus is also sexually transmitted. However, HIV-2 is transmitted less efficiently than HIV-1, both perinatally and sexually.[107,108] Analysis of circulating lymphocytes by polymerase chain reaction techniques reveals that most HIV-2–infected carriers have lower proportions of infected cells than HIV-1–infected carriers or fewer copies of proviral genomes per infected cell, or both.[109,110] As with the infrequently pathogenic HTLV-I, but not with the highly virulent HIV-1,[106] the age-specific prevalence for HIV-2 increases with increasing age. This presumably happens because relatively few HIV-2–infected people are lost from the population because of death.

The observations that HIV-2–infected carriers have lower loads of virus and slower rates of sexual transmission between people are compatible with the observations that HIV-2s appear to evolve and deviate less rapidly than HIV-1s.[111] This does not appear to be caused by any reduction in the error rate of the HIV-2 reverse transcriptase.[112] The slower rates of HIV-2 replication and spread also help explain why the HIV-2 epidemic is largely restricted to West Africa. Further, even within West Africa some HIV-2s are essentially indistinguishable from the SIVs that occur naturally in a particular monkey species living in the same area.[113,114]

The lower rates of replication for HIV-2 may also help explain why this virus appears less virulent than HIV-1 within individual hosts. Case reports and cross-sectional studies reveal that some HIV-2–infected people develop clinical AIDS.[115,116] However, even early studies in HIV-2 endemic areas suggested that disease rates were much lower than expected, based on HIV-1–associated disease with proportional prevalence rates.[117] One possible explanation for this dichotomy was that HIV-2 entered the human population more recently than HIV-1. This possibility was largely dismissed after it was recognized that HIV-2 rates had stabilized in West Africa. It seems clear that HIV-2 had stabilized in some regions of West Africa before HIV-1 had even moved in.[107] Also, analyses of West African sera stored from earlier time periods have shown that HIV-1 has been present in the region for an extended period.[118]

Recently, a natural history study was completed that followed disease development for seroconverting commercial sex workers infected with either HIV-2 or HIV-1 in the same cohort.[95] HIV-2–infected individuals resisted clinical AIDS development much better than did HIV-1–infected women. HIV-2–infected individuals also had stable T4 helper cell numbers for prolonged periods and did not experience the high rates of skin test anergy seen with HIV-1–infected patients.[95,119] It is too soon to say whether the slower pace of disease development with HIV-2 is associated with complete long-standing resistance to AIDS or whether most HIV-2–infected people eventually succumb to disease. A small fraction of HIV-1–infected persons, perhaps 2% to 5%, remain healthy with stable T4 cell numbers for 10 to 15 years.[120] This small fraction appear to have a natural history that is similar to that of most HIV-2–infected individuals. However, for both HIV-2 and HIV-1 it is also too soon to conclude that all strains and clades in different geographic regions show the same patterns of virulence characterized by HIV-1 in the West and HIV-2 in Senegal.

AIDS DENIAL

The recognition that HIV-1 is the cause of AIDS was not easy for some to accept. A small group of scientists have persisted in denying this etiology despite the overwhelming evidence for causation. Various conspiracy theories have emerged suggesting that HIV-1 may have been deliberately created by germ warfare scientists. Although such proclamations seem silly or irrational to informed medical scientists, they can interfere with constructive attempts to educate appropriate population groups.

One reason why some have been reluctant to accept that AIDS is an infectious disease caused by HIV-1 is the very prolonged induction period combined with a very high mortality rate. Most infectious diseases occur after a short induction period. Even for the small number of viral infectious diseases that have a very long induction period, such as tropical spastic paraparesis, adult T-cell leukemia, or shingles, only a small fraction of infected people experience that clinical outcome. The definition of AIDS as an amalgamation of clinical outcomes ranging from tuberculosis and

chronic diarrhea to lymphoma and Kaposi's sarcoma also causes confusion for those considering HIV-1 as the single etiologic cause. The clinical definition becomes logical only if it is recognized that AIDS is fundamentally an irreversible destruction of the immune system. All of the other outcomes are secondary to the immune destruction.

Another problem in understanding the cause of AIDS may be a lack of appreciation of the discipline of epidemiology or dissension about the proper definition of cause. For epidemiologists, a very high-risk association, such as for tobacco and lung cancer, is sufficient to ascribe cause. By this logic, the causal association between HIV-1 infection and subsequent destruction of the immune system is overwhelming. In prospective cohort studies, almost all HIV-1–infected people eventually develop immune depletion. This association is much higher than for such viral infections as polio or influenza. Concerning time and spatial geographic associations, clinical AIDS rates have exactly paralleled HIV infection rates, whether in Bombay, San Francisco, or Nairobi, allowing for the 5- to 15-year induction period.

Until recently, a lack of understanding about how HIV-1 caused immune depletion also helped those who reject epidemiology to deny causation. This situation has changed dramatically with the recognition that HIV-1s can be highly lytic for T4 lymphocytes[81] and that very large numbers of T4 cells are killed by the virus in vivo.[82,83] Further, although the very low rates of infected circulating lymphocytes were interpreted by some as incompatible with destruction of large numbers of cells, recent studies reveal that most HIV-1 is in lymph nodes rather than blood and that 25% to 50% of lymph node T cells may be infected.[120,121]

HIV-1 is also highly unusual as a virus that targets T4 lymphocytes and macrophages, both essential components of the immune system. No other infectious organism has the same tropism for these particular cell compartments. HIV-1 is also transmitted in exactly the same way as clinical AIDS—by blood, by sexual contact, and from mother to infant. Taken together, these various correlations provide inescapable evidence that HIV-1 must be the cause of AIDS.

CONCLUSIONS

A large family of HIV-related retroviruses is present in humans and monkeys in sub-Saharan Africa. All members of this family have the same complex genomic structure, share at least 40% to 50% homology, and infect T lymphocytes through the CD4 receptor.

Although both HIV-1 and HIV-2 appear to have entered the human population several decades ago, HIV-1 is more virulent than HIV-2. Numerous SIV-type viruses are present at high rates in African monkeys, in whom they appear to cause little or no disease. Although SIV in African monkeys is more closely related to HIV-2 than to HIV-1, the viruses in mangabeys and macaques are essentially the same virus as HIV-2. The macaque virus also appears to have originated from either a human or an African monkey source, because Asian primates show no evidence of natural infection. A chimpanzee virus, which is a logical progenitor of HIV-1, has also been identified in Africa. It seems probable that additional HIV progenitor viruses will be identified in African primates. Understanding of how subhuman primates naturally resist disease from HIV-related viruses should facilitate the development of new ways to treat and prevent HIV disease in humans.

REFERENCES

1. Gottlieb MS, Schroff R, Schanker HM, et al. *Pneumocystis carinii* pneumonia and mucosal candidiasis in previously healthy homosexual men: evidence of a new acquired cellular immunodeficiency. N Engl J Med 1981;305:1425.
2. Masur H, Michelis MA, Greene JB, et al. An outbreak of community-acquired *Pneumocystis carinii* pneumonia: initial manifestation of cellular immune dysfunction. N Engl J Med 1981;305:1431.
3. Seigal FP, Lopez C, Hammer GS, et al. Severe acquired immunodeficiency in male homosexuals, manifested by chronic perianal ulcerative herpes simplex lesions. N Engl J Med 1981;305:1439.
4. Centers for Disease Control. Centers for Disease Control Task Force on Kaposi's sarcoma and opportunistic infections. N Engl J Med 1982;306:248.
5. Davis KC, Horsburgh CR, Jr, Hasiba U, et al. Acquired immunodeficiency syndrome in a patient with hemophilia. Ann Intern Med 1983;98:284.
6. Poon MC, Landay A, Prasthofer EF, et al. Acquired immunodeficiency syndrome with *Pneumocystis carinii* pneumonia and *Mycobacterium avium-intracellulare* infection in a previously healthy patient with classic hemophilia: clinical, immunologic, and virologic findings. Ann Intern Med 1983;98:287.
7. Elliot JL, Hoppes WL, Platt MS, et al. The acquired immunodeficiency syndrome and *Mycobacterium avium intracellulare* bacteremia in a patient with hemophilia. Ann Intern Med 1983;98:290.
8. Curran JW, Lawrence DN, Jaffe H, et al. Acquired immunodeficiency syndrome (AIDS) associated with transfusions. N Engl J Med 1984;310:69.
9. Jaffe HW, Francis DP, McLane MF, et al. Transfusion-associated AIDS: serologic evidence of human T-cell leukemia virus infection of donors. Science 1984;223:1309.
10. Piot P, Quinn TC, Taelman H, et al. Acquired immunodeficiency syndrome in a heterosexual population in Zaire. Lancet 1984;2:65.
11. Van de Perre P, Rouvroy D, Lepage P, et al. Acquired immunodeficiency syndrome in Rwanda. Lancet 1984;2:62.
12. Clumeck N, Mascart Lemone F, de Maubeuge J, et al. Acquired immune deficiency syndrome in Black Africans. Lancet 1983;1:642.
13. Rubinstein A, Sicklick M, Gupta A, et al. Acquired immunodeficiency with reversed T4/T8 ratios in infants born to promiscuous and drug-addicted mothers. JAMA 1983;249:2350.
14. Oleske J, Minnefor A, Cooper R Jr, et al. Immune deficiency syndrome in children. JAMA 1983;249:2345.
15. Scott GB, Buck BE, Leterman JG, et al. Acquired immunodeficiency syndrome in infants. New Engl J Med 1984;310:76.
16. Francis DP, Curran JW, Essex M. Epidemic acquired immune deficiency syndrome (AIDS): epidemiologic evidence for a transmitted agent. J Natl Cancer Inst 1983;71:1.
17. Rogers MF, Morens DM, Stewart JA, et al. National case-control study of Kaposi's sarcoma and *Pneumocystis carinii* pneumonia in homosexual men: part 2, laboratory results. Ann Intern Med 1983;99:151.
18. Essex M, McLane MF, Lee TH, et al. Antibodies to cell membrane antigens associated with human T-cell leukemia virus in patients with AIDS. Science 1983;220:859.
19. Essex M, McLane MF, Lee TH, et al. Antibodies to human T-cell leukemia virus membrane antigens (HTLV-MA) in hemophiliacs. Science 1983;221:1061.
20. Gelmann EP, Popovic M, Blayney D, et al. Proviral DNA of a retrovirus, human T-cell leukemia virus, in two patients with AIDS. Science 1983;220:862.
21. Gallo RC, Sarin PS, Gelmann EP, et al. Isolation of human T-cell leukemia virus in acquired immune deficiency syndrome (AIDS). Science 1983;220:865.
22. Barre-Sinoussi F, Chermann J-C, Rey F, et al. Isolation of T-lymphotropic retrovirus from a patient at risk for acquired immune deficiency syndrome (AIDS). Science 1983;220:868.
23. Poiesz BJ, Ruscetti FW, Gazdar AF, et al. Detection and isolation of type C retrovirus particles from fresh and cultured lymphocytes of a patient with cutaneous T-cell lymphoma. Proc Natl Acad Sci USA 1980;77:7415.
24. Ammann AJ, Abrams D, Conant M, et al. Acquired immune dysfunction in homosexual men: immunologic profiles. Clin Immunol Immunopathol 1983;27:315.
25. Fahey JL, Prince H, Weaver M, et al. Quantitative changes in T helper or T suppressor/cytotoxic lymphocyte subsets that distinguish acquired immune deficiency syndrome from other immune subset disorders. Am J Med 1984;76:95.
26. Lane HC, Masur H, Gelmann EP, et al. Correlation between immunologic function and clinical subpopulations of patients with the acquired immune deficiency syndrome. Am J Med 1985;78:417.
27. Essex M. Adult T-cell leukemia/lymphoma: role of a human retrovirus. J Natl Cancer Inst 1982;69:981.
28. Essex M. Horizontally and vertically transmitted oncornavirus of cats. Adv Cancer Res 1975;21:175.
29. Essex M, McLane MF, Tachibana N, et al. Seroepidemiology of HTLV in relation to immunosuppression and the acquired immunodeficiency syndrome. In: Gallo RC, Essex M, Gross L, eds. Human T-cell leukemia viruses. Cold Spring Harbor, NY: Cold Spring Harbor Press, 1984:355.
30. Kalyanaraman VS, Sarngadharan MG, Robert-Guroff M, et al. A new subtype of human T-cell leukemia virus (HTLV-II) associated with a T-cell variant of hairy cell leukemia. Science 1982;218:571.
31. Popovic M, Sarngadharan MG, Read E, et al. Detection, isolation, and continuous production of cytopathic retroviruses (HTLV-III) from patients with AIDS and pre-AIDS. Science 1984;224:497.
32. Gallo RC, Salahuddin SZ, Popovic M, et al. Frequent detection and isolation of cytopathic retroviruses (HTLV-III) from patients with AIDS and at risk for AIDS. Science 1984;224:500.
33. Schupbach J, Popovic M, Gilden RV, et al. Serological analysis of a subgroup of human T-lymphotropic retroviruses (HTLV-III) associated with AIDS. Science 1984;224:503.
34. Sarngadharan MG, Popovic M, Bruch L, et al. Antibodies reactive with human T-lymphotropic retroviruses (HTLV-III) in the serum of patients with AIDS. Science 1984;224:506.
35. Gallo RC, Sliski AH, de Noronha CM, et al. Origins of human T-lymphotropic viruses. Nature 1986;320:219.
36. Miyoshi I, Yoshimoto S, Fujishita M, et al. Natural adult T-cell leukemia virus infection in Japanese monkeys. Lancet 1982;2:658.
37. Saxinger CW, Lange-Wantzin G, Thomsen K, et al. Human T-cell leukemia virus: a diverse family of related exogenous retroviruses of humans and old world primates. In: Gallo RC, Essex ME, Gross L, eds. Human T-cell leukemia/lymphoma virus. Cold Spring Harbor, NY: Cold Spring Harbor Press, 1984:323.
38. Guo HG, Wong-Staal F, Gallo RC. Novel viral sequences related to human T-cell leukemia virus in T cells of a seropositive baboon. Science 1984;223:1195.
39. Homma T, Kanki PJ, King NW Jr, et al. Lymphoma in macaques: association with exposure to virus of human T lymphotropic family. Science 1984;225:716.
40. Hayami M, Komuro A, Nozawa K, et al. Prevalence of antibody to adult T-cell leukemia virus-associated antigens (ATLA) in Japanese monkeys and other non-human primates. Int J Cancer 1984;33:179.
41. Watanabe T, Seiki M, Hirayama Y, et al. Human T-cell leukemia virus type I is a member of the African subtype of simian viruses (STLV). Virology 1986;148:385.
42. Alizon M, Wain-Hobson S, Montagnier L, et al. Genetic variability of the AIDS virus: nucleotide sequence analysis of two isolates from African patients. Cell 1986;46:63.
43. Myers G, Pavlakis GN. Evolutionary potential of complex retroviruses. In: Levy J, ed. The Retroviridae (vol. 1). New York: Plenum Press, 1992: 51.

44. Essex M, Kanki P. Origins of the AIDS virus. Sci Am 1988;259:64.
45. Kanki PJ, Kurth R, Becker W, et al. Antibodies to simian T-lymphotropic virus type III in African green monkeys and recognition of STLV-III viral proteins by AIDS and related sera. Lancet 1985;1:1330.
46. Barin F, Mboup S, Denis F, et al. Serological evidence for a virus related to simian T-lymphotropic retrovirus III in residents of West Africa. Lancet 1985;2:1387.
47. Clavel F, Mansinho K, Chamaret S, et al. Human immunodeficiency virus type 2 infection associated with AIDS in West Africa. N Engl J Med 1987;316:1180.
48. Marlink RG, Ricard D, Mboup S, et al. Clinical, hematologic, and immunologic cross-sectional evaluation of individuals exposed to human immunodeficiency virus type 2 (HIV-2). AIDS Res Hum Retroviruses 1988;4:137.
49. Chen ISY, McLaughlin J, Gasson JC, et al. Molecular characterization of genome of a novel human T-cell leukaemia virus. Nature 1983;305:502.
50. Heneine W, Kaplan JE, Gracia F, et al. HTLV-II endemicity among Guaymi Indians in Panama. N Engl J Med 1991;324:565.
51. Hjelle B, Scalf R, Swenson S. High frequency of human T-cell leukemia-lymphoma virus type II infection in New Mexico blood donors: determination by sequence-specific oligonucleotide hybridization. Blood 1990;76:450.
52. Maloney EM, Biggar RJ, Neel JV, et al. Endemic human T cell lymphotropic virus type II infection among isolated Brazilian Amerindians. J Infect Dis 1992;166:100.
53. Chen YMA, Jang YJ, Kanki PJ, et al. Isolation and characterization of simian T-cell leukemia virus type II from New World monkeys. J Virol 1994;68:1149.
54. Bebenek K, Abbotts J, Roberts JD, et al. Specificity and mechanism of error-prone replication by human immunodeficiency virus-1 reverse transcriptase. J Biol Chem 1989;264:16948.
55. Smith TF, Srinivasan A, Schochetman G, et al. The phylogenetic history of immunodeficiency viruses. Nature 1988;333:573.
56. Nahmias AJ, Weiss J, Yao X, et al. Evidence for human infection with an HTLV-III/LAV-like virus in Central Africa, 1959. Lancet 1986;1:1279.
57. CDC Update: transmission of HIV infection during an invasive dental procedure—Florida. MMWR 1991;40:21.
58. Goodenow M, Huet T, Saurin W, et al. HIV-1 isolates are rapidly evolving quadrispecies: evidence for viral mixtures and preferred nucleotide substitutions. J Acquir Immune Defic Syndr 1989;2:344.
59. Balfe P, Simmonds P, Ludlam CA, et al. Concurrent evolution of human immunodeficiency virus type 1 in patients infected from the same source: rate of sequence change and low frequency of inactivating mutations. J Virol 1990;64:6221.
60. Delassus S, Cheynier R, Wain-Hobson S. Evolution of the HIV-1 nef and LTR sequences over a four year period in vivo and in vitro. J Virol 1991;65:225.
61. Mann JM, Bila K, Colebunders RL, et al. Natural history of human immunodeficiency virus infection in Zaire. Lancet 1986;2:707.
62. Huet T, Cheynier R, Meyerhaus A, et al. Genetic organization of a chimpanzee lentivirus related to HIV-1. Nature 1990;345:356.
63. de Leys R, Vanderborght B, Haesevelde MV, et al. Isolation and partial characterization of an unusual human immunodeficiency retrovirus from two persons of West-Central African origin. J Virol 1990;64:1207.
64. Nkengasong, JN, Janssens W, Heyndrickx L, et al. Genotypic subtypes of HIV-1 in Cameroon. AIDS 1994;8:1405.
65. Louwagie J, McCutchan F, Mascola J, et al. Genetic subtypes of HIV-1. AIDS Res Hum Retroviruses 1993;9:147.
66. Weniger BG, Takebe Y, Ou CY, et al. The molecular epidemiology of HIV in Asia. AIDS 1994;8:513.
67. Jain MK, John TJ, Keusch GT. Epidemiology of HIV and AIDS in India. AIDS 1994;8:561.
68. Gurtler LG, Hauser PG, Eberle J,, et al. A new subtype of human immunodeficiency virus type 1 (MVP-5180) from Cameroon. J Virol 1994;68:1581.
69. Charneau P, Borman AM, Quillent C, et al. Isolation and envelope sequence of a highly divergent HIV-1 isolate: definition of a new HIV-1 group. Virology 1994;205:247.
70. Hirsch VM, Olmsted RA, Murphey-Corb M, et al. An African primate lentivirus (SIV) closely related to HIV-2. Nature 1989;339:389.
71. Sharp P, Roberston D, McCutchan F, et al. Recombination in HIV-1. Nature 1995;374:124.
72. Artenstein AW, VanCott TC, Mascola JR, et al. Dual infection with HIV-1 of distinct envelope (env) subtypes in humans. J Infect Dis 1995;171:805.
73. Evans LA, Moreau J, Odehouri K, et al. Simultaneous isolation of HIV-1 and HIV-2 from an AIDS patient. Lancet 1988;2:1389.
74. Travers K, Mboup S, Marlink R, et al. Natural protection against HIV-1 infection provided by HIV-2. Science 1995; 268:1612.
75. Louwagie J, Delwart EL, Mullins JI, et al. Genetic analysis of HIV-1 isolates from Brazil reveals the presence of two distinct genetic subtypes. AIDS Res Hum Retroviruses 1994;10:561.
76. Bobkov A, Cheingsong-Popov R, Garaev M, et al. Identification of an HIV-1 env G subtype and heterogeneity of HIV-1 in the Russian Federation and Belarus. AIDS 1994;8:1649.
77. Asjo B, Albert J, Karlsson A, et al. Replication capacity of human immunodeficiency virus from patients with varying severity of HIV infection. Lancet 1986;2:660.
78. Cheng-Mayer C, Seto D, Tateno M, et al. Biologic features of HIV-1 that correlate with virulence in the host. Science 1988;240:80.
79. Tersmette M, Lange J, DeGoede R, et al. Association between biological properties of human immunodeficiency virus variants and risk for AIDS and AIDS mortality. Lancet 1989;1:983.
80. Shioda T, Levy J, Cheng-Mayer C. Small amino acid changes in the V3 hypervariable region of gp120 can affect T-cell line and macrophage tropism of human immunodeficiency virus type 1. Proc Natl Acad Sci USA 1992;89:9434.
81. Yu X, McLane MF, Ratner L, et al. Killing of primary CD4 T cells by non–syncytium-inducing macrophage-tropic human immunodeficiency virus type 1. Proc Natl Acad Sci U S A 1994;91:10237.
82. Wei X, Ghosh SK, Taylor ME, et al. Viral dynamics in human immunodeficiency virus type 1 infection. Nature 1995;373:117.
83. Ho DD, Neumann AV, Perelson AS, et al. Rapid turnover of plasma virions and CD4 lymphocytes in HIV-1 infection. Nature 1995; 373:123.
84. Yu XF, McLane MF, Essex M, et al. Amino acid variations in the V3 loop of human immunodeficiency virus type 1 gp 120 change virus replication and cytopathicity in primary CD4 and T lymphocytes. Submitted for publication.
85. Essex M. The AIDS vaccine challenge. Technol Rev 1994;97:23.
86. Kunanusont C, Foy HM, Kreiss JK, et al. HIV-1 subtypes and male-to-female transmission in Thailand. Lancet 1995;345:1078.
87. Letvin NL, Eaton KA, Aldrich WR, et al. Acquired immunodeficiency syndrome in a colony of Macaque monkeys. Proc Natl Acad Sci USA 1983;80:2718.
88. Henrickson RV, Maul DH, Osborn KG, et al. Epidemic of acquired immunodeficiency in rhesus monkeys. Lancet 1983;1:338.
89. Chopra HC, Mason MM. A new virus in a spontaneous mammary tumor of a rhesus monkey. Cancer Res 1970;30:2081.
90. Kawakami TG, Huff SD, Buckley PM, et al. C-type virus associated with gibbon lymphosarcoma. Nature New Biol 1972;235:170.
91. Theilen GH, Gould D, Fowler M, et al. C-type virus in tumor tissue of a woolly monkey (Lagothrix spp.) with fibrosarcoma. J Natl Cancer Inst 1971;47:881.
92. Kanki PJ, McLane MF, King NW Jr, et al. Serologic identification and characterization of a macaque T-lymphotropic retrovirus closely related to human T-lymphotropic retroviruses (HTLV) type III. Science 1985;228:1199.
93. Biberfeld G, Brown F, Esparza J, et al. WHO working group on characterization of HIV-related retroviruses: criteria for characterization and proposal for a nomenclature system. AIDS 1987;1:189.
94. Kanki PJ, Alroy J, Essex M. Isolation of T-lymphotropic retrovirus related to HTLV-III/LAV from wild-caught African green monkeys. Science 1985;230:951.
95. Marlink R, Kanki P, Thior I, et al. Reduced rate of disease development after HIV-2 infection as compared to HIV-1. Science 1994;265:1587.
96. Essex M. Simian immunodeficiency virus in people. New Engl J Med 1994;330:209.
97. Johnson PR, Fornsgaard A, Allan J, et al. Simian immunodeficiency viruses from African green monkeys display unusual genetic diversity. J Virol 1990;64:1086.
98. Tsujimoto H, Hasegawa A, Maki N, et al. Sequence of a novel simian immunodeficiency virus from a wild-caught African mandrill. Nature 1989;341:539.

99. Allan JS, Short M, Taylor ME, et al. Species-specific diversity among simian immunodeficiency viruses from African green monkeys. J Virol 1991;65:2816.

100. Muller MC, Saksena NK, Nerrienet E, et al. Simian immunodeficiency viruses from central and western Africa: evidence for a new species-specific lentivirus in tantalus monkeys. J Virol 1993;67:1227.

101. Peeters M, Janssens W, Fransen K, et al. Isolation of simian immunodeficiency viruses from two sooty mangabeys in Cote d'Ivoire: virological and genetic characterization and relationship to other HIV type 2 and SIV$_{SM/MAC}$ strains. AIDS Res Hum Retroviruses 1994;10:1289.

102. Ennen J, Finderklee H, Dittmar MT, et al. CD8+ lymphocytes of African green monkeys secrete an immunodeficiency virus-suppressing lymphokine. Proc Natl Acad Sci USA 1994;91:7207.

103. Kanki PJ, Barin F, Mboup S, et al. New human T-lymphotropic retrovirus related to simian T-lymphotropic virus type III$_{AGM}$ (STLV-II-I$_{AGM}$). Science 1986;232:238.

104. Kanki PJ, Allan J, Barin F, et al. Absence of antibodies to HIV-2/HTLV-4 in six Central African nations. AIDS Res Hum Retroviruses 1987;3:317.

105. Kanki PJ, Mboup S, Ricard D, et al. Human T-lymphotropic virus type 4 and the human immunodeficiency virus in West Africa. Science 1987;236:827.

106. Kanki PJ, Marlink R, Siby T, et al. Biology of HIV-2 infection in West Africa. In: Papas T, ed. Gene regulation and AIDS. Woodlands, TX: Portfolio Publishing Company of Texas, 1990:255.

109. Korber B, Kanki P, Barin F, et al. Genetic and antigenic variability in different HIV-2 isolates. In: Chermann J-C, Barre-Sinoussi F, eds. Fourth International Conference on AIDS and Associated Cancers in Africa. Paris, France: FRAMACOM, 1989:170.

110. Simon F, Matheron S, Tamalet C, et al. Cellular and plasma viral load in patients infected with HIV-2. AIDS 1993;7:1411.

111. Sankalé J-L, Sallier de la Tour R, Renjifo B, et al. Intrapatient variability of the human immunodeficiency virus type 2 envelope V3 loop. AIDS Res Hum Retroviruses 1995;11:617.

112. Bakhanashvili M, Hizi A. Fidelity of the RNA-dependent DNA synthesis exhibited by the reverse transcriptase of human immunodeficiency viruses types 1 and 2 and of murine leukemia virus: mispair extension frequencies. Biochemistry 1992;31:9393.

113. Marx PA, Li Y, Lerche NW, et al. Isolation of a simian immunodeficiency virus related to human immunodeficiency virus type 2 from a West African pet sooty mangabey. J Virol 1991;65:4480.

114. Gao F, Yue L, White AT, et al. Human infection by genetically diverse SIV$_{sm}$-related HIV-2 in West Africa. Nature 1992;358:495.

115. Poulsen AG, Aaby P, Fredericksen K, et al. Prevalence of and mortality from human immunodeficiency virus type-2 in Bissau, West Africa. Lancet 1989;1:827.

116. Le Guenno BM, Barabe P, Griffet PA, et al. HIV-2 and HIV-1 AIDS cases in Senegal: clinical patterns and immunological perturbations. J Acquir Immune Defic Syndr 1991;4:421.

117. Romieu I, Marlink R, Kanki P, et al. HIV-2 Link to AIDS in West Africa. J Acquir Immune Defic Syndr 1990;3:220.

118. Kawamura M, Yamazaki S, Ishikawa K, et al. HIV-2 in West Africa in 1966. Lancet 1989;1:385.

119. Marlink R. The biology and epidemiology of HIV-2. In: Essex M, Mboup S, Kanki PJ, et al, eds. AIDS in Africa. New York: Raven Press, 1994:47.

120. Pantaleo G, Graziosi C, Demarest JF, et al. HIV infection is active and progressive in lymphoid tissue during the clinically latent stage of disease. Nature 1993;362:355.

121. Embretson J, Zupancic M, Ribas JL, et al. Massive covert infection of helper T lymphocytes and macrophages by HIV during the incubation period of AIDS. Nature 1993;362:359.

AIDS: Biology, Diagnosis, Treatment and Prevention, fourth edition, edited by Vincent T. DeVita, Jr., Samuel Hellman, and Steven A. Rosenberg. Lippincott–Raven Publishers, © 1997

CHAPTER 1.2

Human Immunodeficiency Virus–Related Infections in Animal Model Systems

Jonathan S. Allan

A good estimate for the number of genetically distinct simian immunodeficiency viruses (SIVs) harbored by African monkeys approaches 30.[1] Why only two of these SIVs have found their way into human populations remains a mystery; in fact, more detailed studies may yield additional human equivalents. An important animal model, the SIV-macaque, appeared on the scene at about the same time as the human acquired immunodeficiency syndrome (AIDS) epidemic arrived.[2,3] Asian monkeys housed in primate colonies began dying of a slowly progressive immunodeficiency syndrome that turned out to be a monkey equivalent of AIDS. Since that time, these animal model systems have been rigorously exploited to address important issues of pathogenesis, vaccine development, antiviral drug development, immunotherapy, and gene therapy.

There are several useful lentiviral animal models that represent major opportunities for study of the temporal relation and roles of viral replication, immune depletion, and host immune responses in limiting or exacerbating infection (Table 1.2-1). The importance of animal models was brought to light in the debate over the future of human vaccine clinical trials; the decision not to proceed to phase III trials for human immunodeficiency virus (HIV-1) vaccine prospects was arrived at in part because of a lack of fundamental knowledge of the correlates of immunity associated with any perceived successes in animal models.[4] Nevertheless, a substantial database is accumulating in the animal model systems that can provide clues to our fundamental understanding of disease progression and eventually demonstrate the feasibility of safe and effective vaccines directed toward HIV-1.

With each new discovery emanating from animal studies have come setbacks. For example, reports of successful vac-

cine trials in monkeys were closely followed by studies reporting that the source of protection was immune responses to cellular proteins rather than to viral antigens.[5–8] The monkey viruses were grown in human cell lines, and anticellular responses proved most beneficial in preventing virus challenge in vaccinated monkeys. Administration of these vaccine formulations resulted in the induction of potent anticellular responses which proved to be protective against challenge with SIV_{mac} virus.

In this chapter, nonhuman lentiviruses, of which the simian lentiviruses form the largest group, are discussed in the context of their natural host, their ability to cause disease when introduced into a species other than the natural host, and what we may learn from animal model systems that may aid development of vaccines, drug treatments, models for transmission, and a fundamental understanding of host and viral determinants of disease. The reader is also referred to several excellent review articles that have been published.[9–14]

HIV-1 INFECTION

Chimpanzees

Soon after HIV-1 was identified as the etiologic agent responsible for AIDS, it was recognized that our closest relative, the chimpanzee, would be useful as an animal model for HIV-1. In 1984, transfusion of blood from AIDS patients into chimpanzees clearly demonstrated that HIV-1 was infectious in chimpanzees.[15] The chimpanzees mounted an antiviral antibody response, and virus could frequently be isolated from their lymphocytes. These early efforts have led to studies in more than 100 chimpanzees, most in vaccine-related investigations. Although chimpanzees remain persistently infected and virus can be recovered from the blood for more than 1 year after infection, no HIV-related disease has been observed in any of these animals. Several

Jonathan S. Allan: Department of Virology and Immunology, Southwest Foundation for Biomedical Research, 7620 Northwest Loop 410 at Military Drive, San Antonio, TX 78228.

TABLE 1.2-1. *HIV-related infections in animal models*

Virus	Host	Disease	Comments/Major Uses
HIV-1	*Chimpanzees*	None	Vaccines, drugs
	Gibbons	None	Endangered, not used in research
	Pigtailed macaques	None	Further development needed
	SCID-hu mice	Pathology in xenotissues	Some vaccine, drug studies
	Transgenic mice	Associated with transgene	Viral gene function
	Rabbits	None	Further development needed
HIV-2	*Sooty mangabeys*	Not done	Unnecessary
	Macaques	AIDS	Vaccines
	Baboons	AIDS*	Further development needed
SIV$_{mac/smn}$	*Sooty mangabeys*	None	Natural resistance and pathogenesis
	Macaques	AIDS	Vaccines, drugs and pathogenesis
	Baboons	None	Not in development, see HIV-2
	Humans	None	Laboratory accidental transmission
SIV$_{agm}$	*African green monkeys*	None	Natural resistance and pathogenesis
	Pigtailed macaques	AIDS†	Further development needed
SHIV recombinants	Macaques	None	Vaccines, further development
	Baboons	None	Vaccines, further development
Feline immunodeficiency virus	*Cats*	AIDS‡	Drugs

The natural host is italicized.
*Current studies indicate limited pathogenesis; further studies are warranted.
†Other macaques species do not develop immunodeficiency diseases when infected with SIV$_{agm.}$
‡Some AIDS-like pathology is evident althouh the extent and long clinical latency are problematic.

HIV-infected chimpanzees have remained asymptomatic for more than 10 years. Therefore, the chimpanzee's main role as a model has been for investigation of vaccine efficacy.

In 1990, a chimpanzee lentivirus was isolated from two chimpanzees, one living in Gabon and a second in a Belgian zoo.[16–18] The virus SIV$_{cpz}$ is the closest nonhuman primate lentivirus to HIV-1, and most investigators agree that HIV-1 probably arose by cross-species transmission of SIV$_{cpz}$ to humans. The natural host species for the primate lentiviruses are usually resistant to disease. Although the reasons for the lack of disease in naturally infected monkeys is an area for debate, the fact that chimpanzees are resistant to HIV-1–related disease is in agreement with this species as the natural host for the original virus.

Several important findings have resulted from vaccine trials in chimpanzees. In one study, immunization with subunit vaccine preparations consisting of HIV-1 gp120 elicited neutralizing antibodies in vaccinated chimpanzees and further protected these chimpanzees from challenge with a laboratory strain of HIV-1.[19] Protection correlated with the presence of neutralizing antibodies to the principal neutralizing domain of HIV-1, also known as V3. More recently, protection was achieved in chimpanzees immunized with HIV-1 gp120 from the MN strain and later challenged with a heterologous HIV-1 strain, indicating that it may be possible to induce broad protection against widely disparate virus types using subunit vaccine approaches.[20] Passive immunization with either a polyclonal pooled HIV-1–positive human immunoglobulin (HIVIG) or a monoclonal antibody to the V3 region of the HIV-1 envelope gp120 was successful in protecting chimpanzees from challenge.[21,22] These studies emphasize the possibility of using antibodies as pre-exposure and postexposure therapeutic modalities.

There are some major limitations to the HIV-chimpanzee model. The first is that these animals are endangered in the wild and are not sacrificed because of ethical considerations. The cost of maintaining these animals for their lifespan, which can approach 50 years, is enormous. Second, the small number of chimpanzees in captivity severely limits the possibility of statistically meaningful studies. Many of the vaccine trials conducted in chimpanzees have included only a single animal control; this limits interpretation of results and, from a statistical perspective, makes some of these studies suspect. In addition, because these primates are not euthanized, complete specimens cannot be retrieved to study tropism and virus load in experimentally infected animals. Studies with SIV$_{cpz}$ in chimpanzees have only recently been initiated on a limited basis, and it is too soon to determine whether SIV$_{cpz}$ is a better virus with which to study natural host resistance. Because HIV-1, the human version of SIV$_{cpz}$, has had ample time to adapt to humans and therefore may have become less able to infect and sustain itself in chimpanzees, use of SIV$_{cpz}$ may be employed to gain insights into natural resistance to HIV-1 in a natural host. However, it must first be conclusively demonstrated that chimpanzees truly are the natural host for HIV-1.

There are several theories proposed to explain the relative lack of HIV-1–related disease in experimentally infected chimpanzees, the most prevalent of which suggests that the virus is simply noncytopathic in chimpanzee cell cultures. The lack of cell killing seen in HIV-1–infected chimpanzee cells is consistent with fact that the CD4+ T cell populations are not depleted. However, two recent studies have demonstrated that some HIV-1 strains are cytopathic for chimpanzee lymphocytes, although it is too soon to determine whether they may induce immunodeficiency in chimpanzees.[23,24] Second, the virus may be much more restricted in cell tropism. The ability of HIV-1 strains to infect chimpanzee macrophage-monocyte populations is controversial, although several groups have shown some replication in chimpanzee macrophages.[25,26] Theoretically, it has been proposed that the macrophage represents a major reservoir for HIV-1 during periods of latency because these cells can harbor HIV without being killed, whereas CD4+ T cells in humans tend to be acutely susceptible to cytopathic effects of HIV. While their numbers last, the chimpanzee remains an important model for testing of vaccines and for immunotherapeutics.

Pigtailed Macaques

Because chimpanzees are somewhat limited in their usefulness for addressing issues of pathogenesis, the development of other nonhuman primate models for this and for vaccine testing has important implications. In 1992, investigators at the University of Washington Primate Center reported that the pigtailed macaque (*Macaca nemestrina*), a close cousin of the rhesus macaque (*Macaca mulatta*), could be persistently infected with a laboratory strain of HIV-1.[27] There was initially a high degree of enthusiasm for this model because (1) the animals could be sacrificed at the end of the study for more detailed analysis, (2) more animals could be incorporated into vaccine testing to ensure statistically relevant results, and (3) drugs specific for HIV-1 gene products such as the reverse transcriptase or viral protease could be tested directly in a more plentiful model.[28] Although some success with this model has been reported, further progress has been slow, and other groups have failed to reproducibly infect pigtailed macaques.[29,30] Limitations to this model include the lack of demonstrable disease and the fact that large concentrations of cell-associated virus are usually necessary to establish infection in these monkeys, which may hamper challenge studies for vaccine efficacy. Furthermore, HIV-1 replicates only poorly in macaque lymphocytes, which means that this model is not well suited for drug or immunotherapy studies in which the virus load in the peripheral blood may be a major indicator for efficacy. Whether this model achieves widespread use depends on the outcome from attempts to better adapt the HIV-1 virus to pigtailed macaques.

Other HIV-1 Primate Models

Another primate that supports HIV-1 infection and replication is also a member of the ape family, the gibbon (*Hylobates lar*). Gibbons were experimentally infected with a laboratory strain of HIV-1 (IIIB) and were shown to develop both humoral and cellular responses to HIV antigens while not developing disease.[31] Virus could be isolated for more than 1 year from four experimentally infected gibbons, indicating viral persistence. In this study, an HIV-1 vaccine (ISCOM) did not protect three gibbons from HIV-1 challenge. These apes are also endangered, and their numbers in captivity are even more limited than those of chimpanzees. These facts have precluded further use of these animals for laboratory research involving HIV.

Several other nonhuman primates have been evaluated for susceptibility to HIV-1 infection without success. In my laboratory, we inoculated three groups of two baboons (*Papio* spp.) with three different laboratory strains of HIV-1 (IIIB, SF2, and RF) and observed them for 37 weeks after inoculation.[32] None of the six animals developed significant antibody responses to HIV-1 antigens, and all attempts to isolate virus failed. However, when the lymph nodes of five inoculated baboons were examined by nested polymerase chain reaction at necropsy, HIV-1 viral DNA could be detected in all five animals, indicating that HIV-1 must have entered and replicated to a limited extent in these animals. Studies by other investigators were also unsuccessful in infecting baboons, even when the animals were immunosuppressed with corticosteroids.[33]

The nature of host range restriction when it comes to virus replication is currently unknown, yet several studies have pointed to the *gag-pol* gene region of the HIV genome as being essential as a determinant for virus infectivity related to host range.[34] This is also consistent with results suggesting that the virus may enter cells and undergo at least a single round of reverse transcription to a viral DNA form. The envelope from immunodeficiency viruses is obviously a major determinant of cell tropism, because binding to CD4 initiates the entry of the virus into these cells. The major use of baboons for HIV-1 studies comes from vaccine experiments. Various vaccine preparations, consisting mainly of HIV-1 envelope proteins, have been evaluated for immunogenicity in baboons.[35] For example, recombinant gp120 expressed in mammalian cells was found to be a potent immunogen for eliciting neutralizing antibodies in baboons. These studies have been instrumental in the design and formulation of vaccines being tested in humans.

Other studies have shown that HIV-1 is noninfectious in rhesus macaques,[33] and in our hands African green monkeys, a natural host for SIV_{agm}, are also resistant to infection with HIV-1.[36] These studies demonstrate that HIV-1 is severely restricted in its tropism to only a few nonhuman primates. Although this fact has significantly inhibited research in this area, we may yet learn what factors are responsible for this host-specific block to infection and how to adapt these factors to retard the progression of HIV-1 disease in humans.

SCID-hu Mice

A severe combined immunodeficiency (SCID) mice model has been developed as an adjunct to HIV-1 testing in primates. SCID mice are ideally suited for immune reconstitution studies because they lack qualitatively demonstrable humoral and cellular immune responses. Implantation of mice with peripheral blood mononuclear cells or tissue explants such as fetal liver, lymph node, or thymus from humans results in a chimeric, quasi-reconstituted human immune system in mice that has been shown to persist for as long as 5 to 11 months.[37,38] If implanted mice are infected with various strains of HIV-1, a discernible pathologic effect can be seen in lymphoid compartments of at least 25% of the infected animals.[39,40] This model has also been useful for drug testing because large numbers of animals can be incorporated. In one report, SCID-hu mice implanted with fetal liver and thymus maintained infection with HIV-1 for more than 6 months. The circulating human T-cell defects were similar to those found in AIDS patients, with an inversion of the ratio of helper to suppressor T cells.[40] Furthermore, the pathology seen in the thymus correlated with the HIV-1 strain used to infect the mice. Although minimal effects on thymus maturation were observed with a primary isolate, progressive deterioration in the CD4+ T-cell population in the peripheral blood was evident, similar to what is seen in HIV-1–infected humans.

SCID mice have been used to assess protective immunity elicited by vaccine candidates tested in humans.[41] Peripheral blood cells or serum from healthy human volunteers previously immunized with recombinant gp160 have been infused into mice that were then challenged with HIV-1. This system allows for a means of evaluating the protective human immune responses to certain vaccine candidates, although the system is an artificial one and reduction in cell killing or infectivity could similarly be tested in a cell culture system.

The SCID-hu model has also recently been developed to test gene therapeutic approaches for HIV-1. In one study, transduced human hematopoietic stem cells were used to reconstitute the T-lymphoid compartment in SCID mice.[42] In this case, the SCID-hu mouse acted as a recipient for human CD34+ hematopoietic progenitor cells, which were transduced in vitro with a retroviral vector carrying the gene of interest plus a neomycin resistance gene (neo^R). It is expected that relevant therapies that introduce genes into hematopoietic stem cells to provide either resistance to HIV-1 infection or resistance to HIV-1–related disease can be tested in this model before proceeding to humans. There are several limitations with this model, however. Implanted mice are relatively expensive, and sampling of blood and other tissues is limited by the animal's size. Second, disease manifestations of HIV-1 infection in reconstituted SCID-hu mice are poorly defined, although lymph node or thymus implants in SCID-hu mice do show pathology reminiscent of that seen in naturally infected humans. With the exception of some modified versions of SCID-hu mice, there has been only a limited immune response by these reconstituted human immune cells to infection. Even for drug studies, interpretation of trials may be limited by significant differences in metabolism and clearance of drugs in mice and in

humans. This model remains an artificial system, but it does have a role in HIV-1 investigations. Its limitations have thus far precluded its widespread use despite recent advances.

Transgenic Mice

Transgenic technology has allowed for the introduction of viral genes directly into mouse embryos; these genes are then carried in the germline for future generations. Transgenic mouse models have generated a wealth of knowledge concerning HIV-1 pathogenesis; accordingly, they have been the focus of recent reviews, and several important findings have emanated from this model.[13,14] In one study, after the complete DNA provirus of HIV-1 was introduced into mice, heterologous offspring from these transgenic parents developed disease signs that were similar to those seen in humans, including cachexia, skin manifestations, splenomegaly, lymphadenopathy, thymic atrophy, and pulmonary compromise.[43] In addition, HIV-1 could be recovered from the offspring by co-cultivation methods using human cell lines. Unfortunately, these animals were lost because of unrelated problems associated with their care, and further studies to address the effect of complete virus expression in mice have not been forthcoming. One major drawback to the use of mice to study pathogenesis is that the mouse cells are nonpermissive for HIV-1 infection. Even after human CD4 was transfected and expressed on mouse cells, HIV-1 was shown to bind but not to enter these cells.[44] It is still uncertain what factor is lacking in mouse cells that may be necessary to facilitate HIV-1 entry into cells.

This model has been useful for understanding how specific HIV-1 genes participate in the disease process. In one study, tat-expressing mice developed Kaposi's sarcoma–like lesions, and other constructs have led to various skin lesions.[45] Transgenic mice have also been developed to express the nef gene under the control of a murine enhancer-promoter for CD3 in order to target nef expression to T cells.[46] Expression of HIV-1 nef was mainly confined to the thymus and led to a substantial decline in CD4+ T-cell numbers in comparison with the CD8+ T cell population. In a similar nef study, T cells from transgenic mice failed to respond to mitogens, a defect that is commonly found in AIDS patients and may indicate dysregulation of the immune system coinciding with other manifestations of AIDS.[47] Other findings in transgenic mice have shed light on the expression of specific genes in the pathogenesis of HIV-1, including encephalitis, renal disease, and eye disorders.[48–50]

This model can teach us a great deal about how certain viral genes can disrupt normal tissue functions when they are expressed either early during development or later during maturation of tissue types. An obvious advantage of the transgenic mouse in comparison with the SCID mouse model is that not only can a particular gene be inserted into a mouse, but these mice can reproduce and the resulting mouse line can be maintained indefinitely. It is also important to understand the current limitations of this model.

Transgenic mice cannot be used for vaccine studies because HIV-1 does not infect and replicate in mouse cells, evenin the presence of human CD4. These mice are also relatively expensive to maintain, and the facilities and technology for their maintenance are still not in widespread use.

Rabbits

Rabbits have been investigated as an AIDS model for more than 7 years. Initial studies reported that rabbits could be productively infected with HIV-1 by intraperitoneal inoculation of HTLV-infected rabbit cells that had been superinfected with HIV-1.[51] Induction of chemical peritonitis appeared to be a prerequisite for HIV-1 infection.[52] Antibodies to HIV-1 were detected for more than 1 year in the serum of infected rabbits, as was HIV-1 p24 antigen. In addition, virus could be recovered by co-cultivation of rabbit and human CD4 T cells. More recently, infection of rabbits with cell-free HIV-1 resulted in seroconversion, some evidence of cytopathology in lymph nodes, demonstration of virus by reverse transcription, and amplification of viral DNA from rabbit cells recovered in bone marrow, brain, liver, spleen, lymph nodes, and from similar tissues after co-cultivation with human cell lines. Because seroconversion and virus recovery were seen only after a second inoculation of concentrated cell-free virus, the effect of multiple inoculations and of high levels of foreign antigens may have directly influenced immune responsiveness and pathology.[53] Another research team reported successful infection with HIV-1 only after superinfection with *Treponema pallidum*, *Mycobacterium avium* complex, *Candida albicans*, vaccinia virus, herpes simplex virus, Shope virus, or malignant catarrhal fever virus.[54] In this case, evidence of HIV-1 infection could be demonstrated only by polymerase chain reaction amplification of viral DNA from the rabbit's peripheral blood lymphocytes and by seroconversion with Western blotting, and all attempts to isolate virus failed.

In summary, attempts to productively infect rabbit cells have been mostly unsatisfactory. Although HIV-1 DNA can be detected in rabbit cells, cell-free virus has not routinely been recovered.[55,56] Recently, it has been reported that primary lymphocyte cultures from the peripheral blood of rabbits are readily infectable in vitro, but no free virus was observed, which strongly suggests that HIV-1 infection is mainly abortive, as in mice.[55]

Although studies are continuing to focus on further development of the rabbit model, this model has not lived up to initial expectations; in some laboratories, the necessity of superinfecting rabbits with other pathogens lessens the enthusiasm for such a model and raises further ethical concerns. Efforts to adapt HIV-1 strains for growth in rabbit cells are needed, and a greater understanding of the nature of the lack of productive HIV-1 infection in itself would be an important area of contribution by a rabbit model to the AIDS field.

HIV-2

Some of the animal model systems described for studying HIV-1 can also be adapted for use with HIV-2, including both mouse and rabbit models. HIV-2 is a second human lentivirus that is primarily restricted to people living in West African countries. The worldwide significance of this infection in humans is substantially less than that of HIV-1. Most studies indicate that HIV-2 is much less pathogenic than HIV-1 and also less transmissible.[57] The major difference between these viruses is their relation to the monkey viruses. HIV-1 is highly related to SIV_{cpz}, which is found in chimpanzees, whereas HIV-2 has a close cousin, SIV_{smm}, that is found in sooty mangabeys. Because the range of the sooty mangabey is restricted to the same geographic location as that of humans infected with HIV-2, most investigators agree that HIV-2 arose by cross-species transmission from these monkeys.[58,59] Although most strains of HIV-2 are only approximately 40% related to HIV-1 in the envelope gene, a much higher degree of relatedness of HIV-2 with SIV_{smm} and SIV_{mac} can be seen, which also supports the hypothesis that HIV-2 has its origins in these monkeys. It is obvious that animals suitable for HIV-2 studies are likely to be the same as those most suitable for use with SIV_{smm}-like viruses.

Macaques

Rhesus, cynomolgus, and pigtailed macaques have all been used as models for the study of HIV-2 pathogenesis and vaccine testing.[60–62] Although the development of a pathogenic model in monkeys has lagged behind the $SIV_{mac/smm}$ models in macaques, recent evidence indicates that the macaque has the potential to become a relevant and reproducible AIDS model for HIV-2. It is not surprising that HIV-2 can be adapted for use in monkeys because of its close relation to the monkey viruses. HIV-2 has been traced to humans as early as the 1970s, and it has probably undergone some adaptation in humans since its introduction from monkeys. Therefore, it is not unreasonable to assume that in order to develop this model in monkeys, HIV-2 would have to become more SIV_{smm}-like, although it is presently unknown what genetic factors would be important in this adaptive process.[1]

Several strains of HIV-2 have been used to infect macaques, including HIV-2 (EHO), and HIV-2 (ROD), HIV-2 (ben), HIV-2 (SBL-6669), HIV-2 (sbl/isy), and HIV-2 (NIH-Z).[29,62–64] In most instances, animals remained persistently infected without demonstrable disease. However, HIV-2 (EHO) is more cytopathic and replicates more efficiently in human and macaque lymphocytes than does the prototype virus HIV-2 (ROD). This has been shown by scientists at the University of Washington Primate Center, who have recently been successful in inducing HIV-2–related AIDS in six of six animals inoculated with HIV-2 that had been passaged in pigtailed macaques to enhance its pathogenicity.[62] A precipitous decline in CD4 T-cell numbers was also seen. Thus far, AIDS-like disease has been consistently observed only in pigtailed macaques, but cynomolgus monkeys have been shown to support replication of HIV-2. Other studies have also demonstrated reproducibility of the macaque model for infectivity, and in some cases a demonstrable decline in CD4 cell numbers has been seen without subsequent disease.[29]

Much of the HIV-2–related research in monkeys has focused on development of vaccines against HIV-2. For example, passive immunization of monkeys with pooled anti–HIV-2 serum, taken from monkeys experimentally infected with HIV-2, led to the protection in five of seven cynomolgus monkeys (*Macaca fascicularis*), whereas all six control animals became infected with HIV-2 challenge virus.[65] Similarly, vaccination with various immunogens (eg, ISCOMs, subunit envelope proteins) along with different adjuvants have been tested in monkeys.[64,66] In most cases, protection could be achieved on HIV-2 challenge. Further efforts to develop this model are necessary; the successes currently reported indicate the likelihood of a reproducible pathogenic model for HIV-2–related AIDS, especially for testing of vaccine candidates.

Baboons

Baboons have also been investigated as a possible model for HIV-2, but early attempts at establishing this model resulted in equivocal findings.[67,68] In one study, inoculation of HIV-2 (ROD) into two baboons led to a persistent but low-level infection without demonstrable disease. Levy's group has also pursued this model and initially reported the persistent infection of baboons with HIV-2 (UCI) isolates.[69] However, no disease was present after more than 2 years of observation. More recently, evidence of AIDS-like disease, including a loss in CD4 T-cell numbers, was reported in two of six baboons.[70] The pathogenicity of HIV-2 may be species-related, because only one species of baboons tested (*Papio hamadryas*) was noted to have clinical disease. Skin lesions that share similarities with lesions of Kaposi's sarcoma in AIDS patients were also observed in one of the infected animals. Perhaps the baboon model may be developed to address issues regarding the underlying mechanism of Kaposi's lesions in HIV-1–infected humans.

The long clinical latency period (>2 years), coupled with the fact that most baboons do not develop disease, indicates that further studies are needed to determine whether the HIV-2 baboon system can serve as an important model for pathogenicity or vaccine development. Among other considerations, the ability to demonstrate that a molecular cloned version of HIV-2 is infectious and pathogenic in baboons is necessary in order to study pathogenesis.

SIV$_{MAC/SMM}$

Several lentiviruses have been recovered from macaques that died of immunodeficiency-like diseases. Although they have been given various names (eg, SIV$_{mac}$ in rhesus monkeys, SIV$_{mne}$ in pigtailed macaques), they all essentially have their origins in African sooty mangabeys and, as such, represent almost identical versions of the SIV$_{smm}$ virus, as evidenced by their close genetic relations.[2,71,72] SIV$_{mac}$ was discovered at the New England Primate Center in 1984 and was quickly developed into the most comprehensive model for studying almost every aspect of pathogenesis and vaccine and drug development.[73] Like the presumed pattern with HIV-12, SIV$_{mac}$ infection in Asian macaques probably resulted after infection by SIV$_{smm}$ from sooty mangabeys. Evidence of an AIDS-like syndrome in macaques at the Tulane Primate Center was traced to iatrogenic dissemination. Homogenates of cutaneous leprosy material taken from mangabeys were inoculated into four macaques in an attempt to study the pathogenesis of leprosy; however, these tissues also harbored SIV$_{smm}$.[74] Other studies have demonstrated a naturally occurring virus in as many as 60% of captive sooty mangabeys housed at the Yerkes Primate Center.[75,76] Epidemiologic studies to determine the prevalence of SIV$_{smm}$ in the wild have been more difficult, but in one study as many as 10% of wild-caught mangabeys in Liberia had antibodies to SIV$_{smm}$.[77]

The SIV$_{mac/smm}$ virus group mirrors the biology of HIV-1 in almost every way. SIV$_{mac}$ infects CD4+ T cells, macrophages, and most of the other CD4+ cell populations shown to be infected with HIV-1.[78] Like HIV-1, SIV$_{mac}$ is highly cytopathic in both human and monkey lymphocytes and readily induces syncytia. From a pathologic perspective, the disease and tissues affected are somewhat specific to the virus strain but nonetheless provide a model for studying the various sequelae. For example, infection with SIV$_{mac/smm}$ results in central nervous system disease unassociated with opportunistic infections in more than 50% of infected monkeys.[79] The pathology associated with encephalopathy includes the appearance of large, multinucleated giants cells associated with perivascular macrophages, and infiltration with lymphocytes and macrophages is a common feature. Another pathologic finding in rhesus monkeys is the development of a granulomatous interstitial and alveolar pneumonia with evidence of SIV-infected macrophages and lymphocytes in the tissues. Enteropathy is also a common early manifestation of SIV infection and in some cases leads to chronic diarrheal disease.[80,81] Another rather common feature of SIV$_{mac/smm}$ infection is the appearance of B-cell lymphomas as a late manifestation of the immunodeficiency syndrome. In one study, 30% of infected monkeys developed B-cell lymphoma associated with Epstein-Barr virus infection; this is the most common lymphoma seen in humans and has been theorized to arise from an overall dysregulation of immune surveillance.[82]

One of the greatest contributions to our knowledge of AIDS is the finding that a molecularly cloned SIV$_{mac}$ 239 strain with a defined nucleic acid sequence is not only infectious when inoculated into macaques but has properties similar to those of the wild-type virus for inducing disease in monkeys.[83] The existence of an infectious and pathogenic molecular clone means that researchers can begin to dissect out the functional relation of the individual SIV$_{mac}$ genes in the pathogenic process. Although much has been learned about the expression and role of viral genes in the virus life cycle in vitro, it has been more difficult to establish a direct role for some these viral genes in the pathogenesis of AIDS. Part of the problem lies with the fact that several genes are likely to contribute in some way to the disease process, and deletion of any one gene may have only minor effects. Because disease is a complex process with many factors contributing to the ultimate fate of the animal, it becomes a difficult proposition to dissect out the genetic factors associated with AIDS. A major finding along these lines was the observation that a deletion in the *nef* gene of SIV$_{mac}$ resulted in an absolute loss of in vivo pathogenicity, which was not expected because studies at that time indicated that *nef* could actually be a negative regulator of virus expression.[84] It has been theorized that the *nef* gene plays a prominent role in vivo and that its absence leads to much lower virus loads. Studies in humans have been equivocal although one long-term nonprogressor had a deleted *nef* gene, which suggests a prominent role for *nef* in disease outcome.[85]

Another example of the use of SIV$_{mac}$ models in defining the roles of viral genes in infection and disease is the studies with the *vpr* gene. Early work indicated that *vpr* may be important for infection of macrophages.[86] More recently, it was suggested that *vpr* may be important in cellular differentiation,[87] but another study suggests that *vpr* may actually suppress cellular proliferation.[88] Inoculation of *vpr* mutants into rhesus macaques produced no observable effect on virus load, decline in CD4, or disease, but a double mutant containing deletions in both *vpr* and *vpx* genes severely attenuated SIV$_{mac}$ after it was inoculated into adult animals.[89] Nevertheless, triple mutants in the auxiliary genes *vpr, vpx,* and *nef* induced the immunodeficiency syndrome in newborn macaques in the same manner as the wild-type virus.[90] These studies point out that even with a well defined animal model it is still difficult to address gene expression and its function on the disease process.

Infection of mangabeys, on the other hand, leads to life-long infection in the absence of clinical disease—a common feature among African primates.[74,75] AIDS-like diseases have not been observed in these primates at either the Yerkes or Tulane primate centers. The reasons for host resistance have not been elucidated but theoretically are similar to those described for chimpanzees. A potent humoral immune response has been noted, although cytotoxic T-cell responses have not been thoroughly analyzed.

Attempts to infect African green monkeys with SIV$_{mac}$ strains have failed. In our laboratory, we have used both cell-free virus and virus-infected cells to infect young African greens, yet these animals never seroconverted and virus could not be recovered for several years after inoculation. On the other hand, baboons have been persistently infected with SIV$_{mac}$, with detectable antibody responses

and virus isolation at several time points, although disease still could not be demonstrated.

SIV$_{SMM}$ VARIANTS

Although SIV$_{mac}$ and SIV$_{smm}$ strains have been used extensively for almost all aspects of HIV-1–related research, a variant of SIV$_{smm}$, known as SIV$_{smm}$ PBj14, which was developed by serial passage of SIV$_{smm}$ 9 in pigtailed macaques at the Yerkes Regional Primate Research Center, is unique because of its tremendous virulence.[91] Intravenous inoculation of pigtailed macaques with the PBj14 strain typically results in severe disease within the first 7 to 14 days. In contrast to the development of opportunistic infections after a long incubation period in humans and in other species of monkeys, the disease seen in these monkeys is manifested as an acute gastroenteritis with severe wasting and electrolyte disturbances leading to death. The virus replicates to extremely high titers and is accompanied by the production of high concentrations of tumor necrosis factor-α and interleukin-6 in the plasma; this is consistent with notion that high levels of cytokines may be responsible for the acute inflammation even in the absence of diarrhea.[92,93] A striking pathologic feature of SIV$_{smm}$ PBj14 infection is the extensive lymphoid hyperplasia found in gut-associated lymphoid tissue. Another curious finding associated with this virus is its ability to induce activation and proliferation in resting T cells. SIV$_{smm}$ PBj14 is also cytopathic in pigtailed macaques for CD4+ T lymphocytes, as is its parental virus strain.[94]

In contrast, inoculation of SIV$_{smm}$ PBj14 into rhesus monkeys caused only 30% to 50% of the animals become ill and die, once again suggesting that even small differences in the host species are reflected in large variations in disease outcome. When sooty mangabeys, the natural host for SIV$_{smm}$, were inoculated with this variant, three of four animals developed clinical disease and died.[91] This finding indicates that, under the right experimental conditions, natural resistance to infection can be overcome, apparently as a function of the relative virulence of the virus.

In order to determine what subtle genetic differences between PBj14 and its parental strain SIV$_{smm}$ 9 account for this large difference in pathogenicity, molecular clones of the original viruses have been generated and analyzed.[95,96] There initially was a great deal of skepticism in the scientific community about whether SIV$_{smm}$ or any lentivirus could be directly responsible for such a rapid rate of AIDS induction and death in the natural host, especially because lentiviruses are generally considered to be slow viruses. However, molecularly cloned virus has also been shown to induce rapidly fatal disease in pigtailed macaques. The nucleotide sequence of one molecular clone showed two pronounced differences between PBj14 and its parental strain: a duplication in the NF-kB enhancer element in the long terminal repeat and an insertion in the V1 region of the envelope.[95] Although speculation initially centered on the duplication in this cellular transcriptional site as the cause of the accelerated pathogenesis, removal of one of the two sites had little or no effect on disease progression.[97]

Recently, a series of chimeric clones were generated between SIV_{smm} PBj14 and SIV_{smm} 9 in order to locate the region or regions of the virus that impart the pathogenic phenotype seen with PBj14.[98] Thus far, the *gag* gene as well as a portion of the envelope's transmembrane region and possibly a region of *nef*, *tat*, and *rev* appear to be required for development of the acute disease. These studies further suggest that dissecting out a particular biologic property may be a difficult endeavor. The fact that SIV_{smm} PBj14 appears to target the gut implies that the virus either selects for predetermined cells already destined for this tissue or somehow initiates the homing process through regulation of cellular functions.

SIV_{agm}

Simian immunodeficiency viruses from African green monkeys constitute the largest reservoir of naturally occurring primate lentiviruses. Regardless of the geographic region in sub-Saharan Africa, SIV_{agm} is found in almost 50% of free-ranging green monkeys.[1] The phylogenetic relations of SIV_{agm} to other primate lentiviruses indicate that the African green monkey virus may be a direct descendant from the earliest ancestral viral strains. Based on several lines of evidence, including our own, we have theorized that SIV_{agm} has been in the green monkey population for at least 1000 years. In part, we have based this conclusion on the fact that viruses isolated from all four subspecies of these monkeys vary according to their host.[99] In other words, a strong case can be made that virus and host co-evolved and co-diverged in the ancient past. Consistent with this theory is the finding that SIV_{agm} induces no overt clinical disease in African green monkeys.

Although we have come to expect that African nonhuman primates may share some characteristics that impart disease resistance, for the SIV_{agm} group it is still necessary to demonstrate that these viruses have one or several features that may be responsible for inducing disease species other than the natural host. The obvious choice for such a primate model is the macaque, because it has been shown to be susceptible to SIV_{smm}-related disease. However, induction of disease in macaques has not been an easy task. Attempts in our laboratory and several others have failed to demonstrate disease using a number of different SIV_{agm} isolates in either rhesus or cynomolgus macaques.[36,100,101] Serial passage of virus among experimentally infected rhesus monkeys to adapt SIV_{agm} to macaques also has failed to induce disease. Recently, however, a more classic AIDS-like disease was observed in pigtailed macaques inoculated with SIV_{agm} 90, whereas none of the infected African green monkeys was symptomatic.[102] As a final assessment, molecularly cloned virus was also shown to induce disease when inoculated intravenously into pigtailed macaques. Of eight monkeys inoculated with SIV_{agm}, five showed evidence of disease that included a significant decline

in CD4+ T cells, lymphopenia, thrombocytopenia, weight loss, and chronic diarrhea. On necropsy of three of these affected animals, tuberculosis, pneumocystis pneumonia, and lymphoma were diagnosed. Consistent with the results reported for SIV_{smm} studies, pigtailed macaques again appear to be genetically more susceptible to these primate viruses and therefore probably represent a more reproducible disease model.

Like the sooty mangabey model, the African green monkey–SIV_{agm} model can be exploited to understand the nature of host resistance to disease. There are several important components that contribute to pathogenesis, among them virus replication rate, cytopathicity, immune response, and cell tropism. These are not isolated topics but represent the outcome of host and virus interactions. Although it has been stated by several investigators that SIV_{agm} is noncytopathic in African green monkey lymphocytes,[103] our own recent research suggests that green monkey CD4 T cells do not grow in tissue culture and are lost soon after seeding. This loss of the target population in culture precludes the examination of SIV_{agm} for its ability to kill African green monkey CD4+ T cells. It would also explain the absence of syncytia formation in these primary cultures. We do know that these viruses are CD4+ T-cell tropic, and other studies indicate that SIV_{agm} replicates in both human and green monkey macrophages.[104] Genetically, the SIV_{agm} group of viruses varies in genetic makeup from SIV_{mac} in that they lack a classic *vpr* gene, and it has been suggested that this simple difference may in part explain lack of host disease.[105]

The replication rate and virus load in naturally infected monkeys have been more difficult to study, but data suggest that the virus replicates poorly in these animals compared with pigtailed macaques. Only low levels of virus could be detected in various tissues of infected green monkeys, and the lowest levels were found in the peripheral blood lymphocytes.[102] By conventional methods, virus could be isolated from the plasma of naturally infected green monkeys, although only 5 to 50 viral DNA copies were found per 10^5 cells, which is consistent with studies in asymptomatic HIV-1–infected people. However, very high levels of virus load (10^6 viral RNA copies per milliliter) have been found in plasma (M. Feinberg, personal communication, Office of AIDS Research, NIH, 1995). It is too soon to know what to make of these findings, although the high levels of free virus coupled with only low levels in the tissues suggests that the kinetics of virus clearance could differ in these animals from that in animals that develop disease. It may mean that the virus levels slowly rise in the plasma without a consequent removal by the reticular endothelial system in the liver and other organ systems. Consistent with this hypothesis is the relative lack of neutralizing antibodies in naturally or experimentally infected monkeys and the inherent cytopathic nature of infection, which together may lead to a lack of any inflammatory responses associated with SIV_{agm} infection. Further studies are needed, including study of cytotoxic T-cell responses, which are theorized to be both beneficial and paradoxically harmful in HIV-infected people. In addition, one research team has found a soluble factor produced by green monkey CD8+ T cells that appears to act in suppressing virus expression in infected cells.[106]

RECOMBINANT AND CHIMERIC VIRUSES

A major breakthrough in AIDS vaccine research came in 1992.[106,107] The construction of chimeric viruses (SHIV) consisting of the *env, tat, rev,* and *vpu* genes of HIV-1 inserted into the SIV_{mac} 239 provirus has led to the development of newer models for vaccine testing. In addition, other chimeras are being constructed to examine traits such as pathogenicity and host restriction in tropism. Previous studies in vitro have demonstrated that nonenvelope determinants are responsible for the restriction of HIV-1 infection to humans and apes and that these determinants map to the *gag-pol* gene region.[34] Genetically engineered SHIV strains have been shown to persistently infect both cynomolgus and rhesus macaques.[108] Virus could regularly be recovered from the animals' lymphocytes, and all animals seroconverted to both the HIV-1 envelope and SIV_{mac} *gag* proteins. Recently, we have demonstrated that these chimeras can also be used to infect baboons.[32] Two distinct SHIV strains, one containing the HIV-1 *env* from the IIIB strain and a second SHIV with an envelope from the HIV-1/SF2 strain, both reproducibly infected baboons. As with macaques, no disease was evident in the baboons for more than 1 year. Igarashi and coworkers recently demonstrated other SHIV constructs, which contain HIV-1 *nef* and *vpr* in addition to *env, vpu, rev* and *tat*, are similarly infectious for macaques; however, as with other SHIV strains, no disease has been observed.[109] As previously stated, the *nef* and *vpr* genes have been implicated as factors in determining disease progression. Because AIDS is the culmination of many factors, determination of which genes act in concert with others as part of the disease process awaits further testing. In another study, rhesus macaques were infected with two distinct strains of SHIV, one with a more classic T-cell–tropic HIV-1 envelope (SF33) and a second with an HIV-1 envelope (SF162) that defines a more macrophage-tropic phenotype. The syncytium-inducing T-cell–tropic SHIV recombinant replicated to higher levels, and virus was more easily recovered at most time points from infected monkeys.[110]

Chimeric viruses are beginning to be used to test vaccine candidates. A virus can be molecularly generated that has the HIV-1 envelope for which the vaccine is derived but is inserted into the SIV backbone in order to overcome host range restrictions and allow for replication in monkeys. One disadvantage to this model is that there is currently no disease association. Therefore, the end point for success or failure of a particular vaccine is limited to whether protection from infection can be achieved. It has been argued that the induction of sterilizing immunity necessary for this type of protection with vaccine candidates may be an unrealistic goal and that protection from disease induction may be more

reasonable. At present, the SHIV viruses can tell us only whether the animal is protected from infection as determined by virus isolation, antibody responses, and detection of viral DNA in tissues by polymerase chain reaction. Because the SIV_{smm}/SIV_{mac} model is well adapted and well characterized in monkeys, recombinants between HIV-1 and $SIV_{smm/mac}$ are reasonable choices in the design of such experiments. In a recent study, SHIV-infected macaques were challenged with SIV_{mac} 251 and were not protected, which would dictate that protection with attenuated viruses should include the envelope homologous to that used in challenge studies.[110] In this case, the challenge consisted of an SIV_{mac} envelope, and the great degree of variation between HIV-1 and SIV_{mac} envelopes would preclude any protection derived from the envelope genes.

OTHER NON-SIV MODELS

Several important nonprimate animal models are being investigated and are briefly mentioned here. A number of these models were being studied long before the discovery of AIDS in humans. Lentiviruses of ungulates (hoofed animals), for example, include the equine AIDS virus or equine infectious anemia virus, which causes blood disorders in horses and is transmitted by insect vector and dirty needles. The virus has a predilection for macrophages, as does HIV-1.[112] Similarly, sheep carry a lentivirus called visna virus that has several well defined clinical manifestations, including pulmonary involvement and, in some cases, neurologic disease. Another close cousin is the caprine arthritis encephalitis virus, which afflicts goats and induces the diseases from which its name is derived.[113]

Bovine immunodeficiency virus of cattle represents still another resource that can be used for AIDS research.[114,115] A direct correlation with any disease has been difficult to assess because animal herds usually have a high turnover rate, and most animals have dual infections with another retrovirus, bovine leukemia virus. Although significant progress has been made in regard to the molecular biology of bovine immunodeficiency virus, it role in pathogenesis is still obscure; some evidence suggests that the virus induces lymphadenopathy and central nervous system disease.

Obvious advantages to these ungulate models are that the animals are domesticated for ease of handling and the viruses they carry are not known to be harmful to humans; therefore, housing of these animals does not require special biosafety conditions to limit infection of humans. This is also a limitation, however, because the viruses are only distantly related to the simian and human viruses and there are significant differences in genomic organization. Vaccine or therapeutic agents found to be effective for the ungulate viruses may not be as useful for HIV-infected humans. Nonetheless, work in progress has helped increase our understanding of the pathogenesis of HIV and, in particular, studies have elucidated the nature of macrophage infection and its role in clinical outcome.

FELINE IMMUNODEFICIENCY VIRUSES

Although feline immunodeficiency viruses (FIVs) were not discovered until 1987, much effort has gone into development of this AIDS model and initially it provided hope that a small animal model would greatly facilitate the pace of AIDS research.[12] There are several obvious reasons why the cat model may be a useful one. First, cats have previously been bred under specific pathogen–free (SPF) conditions to study the biology of the feline leukemia virus, another feline retrovirus. The breeding colonies are already in place. Second, the relative cost of care and maintenance of cat colonies is substantially cheaper than for nonhuman primates.

Since its discovery, much has been learned about FIV. FIV shares genomic structural similarities with HIV having *gag, pol, env, rev,* and *vif* genes, yet there is essentially no similarity in genetic sequence between HIV and FIV.[116,117] This fact alone limits the direct application of vaccine trials in cats for use in humans. Although FIV has been shown to infect CD4+ T cells, macrophages, and astrocytes, the primary receptor for virus entry appears to be a non-CD4 protein that may be analogous to human CD9, suggesting that the FIV envelope may functionally act differently from gp120 of HIV-1 and therefore that the nature of neutralizing epitopes may be quite different.[118] Infection with FIV in some cases leads to a decline in CD4+ T-cell populations, although the pathogenesis of infection is less clear.

Some reports suggest that infection may lead to an AIDS-like disease in cats, but the time course may be much delayed compared with SIV infection.[119–121] Usually, a well defined, reproducible disease caused by infection of SPF cats with FIV has been obscured by the relatively long clinical latency period, which may vary from 3 to 5 years. The interpretation of most reports on the pathologic changes induced by FIV have been complicated by the presence of other ongoing infections such as feline leukemia virus. The pathologic changes that have been identified in FIV-infected cats have come from retrospective studies of naturally infected animals or from studies with non-SPF cats. In one study, comparison of colony-bred animals with random-source animals indicated a greater likelihood among the former group for pathology associated with infection; however, consistent immunodeficiency-like diseases have not been observed, and this fact has hampered efforts in this area.[119] Like HIV, FIV appears to be neurovirulent in regard to clinical alterations in function, including delayed visual and auditory potentials, behavioral changes, and changes in sleep patterns; this pattern may make the cat model useful for the study HIV-related central nervous system disease.[122]

The FIV model has been adapted for the study of maternal-infant transmission, with a reported transmission rate of 70%.[123,124] Furthermore, vaccine studies have shown that cats can be protected from FIV challenge by passive transfer of antibodies from FIV-infected cats.[125] The FIV model is most suited for study of the effects of certain drugs on FIV replication; for example, reverse-transcriptase–targeted nucleoside analogs can be tested in addition to nonnucleoside inhibitors.[126] Although this model has much to offer, the fact that there is no genetic similarity with HIV-1, coupled with a relative weak pathogenic potential, has limited its value for AIDS research.

SUMMARY

The large variety of potential animal model systems, each with unique features, allows for the expansion of our database and our overall knowledge concerning the pathogenesis of HIV and in its prevention and treatment. Each model has an abundance of limitations, and none can directly reproduce all of the manifestations of HIV-1–related disease. The SIV$_{mac/smm}$ model comes the closest in its application to vaccine strategies and to our basic understanding of immunopathogenesis. It is unlikely that further refinements in other animal systems can outstrip the wealth of information that has accumulated through SIV$_{mac}$ studies, although data derived from nonprimate models may well be useful for further study in the monkey systems. Refinements in the SHIV primate animal model may also lead to a better understanding of the genetic basis for disease and the host genetic factors that influence lentiviral pathogenesis.

REFERENCES

1. Allan JS. Viral evolution and AIDS. J NIH Res 1992;4:51.
2. Daniel MD, Letvin NL, King NW, et al. Isolation of a T-cell tropic HTLV-III–like retrovirus from macaques. Science 1985;228:1201.
3. Kanki PJ, McLane MF, King NW, et al. Serologic identification and characterization of a macaque T-lymphotropic retrovirus closely related to HTLV-III. Science 1985;228:1199.
4. Thompson C. Go-ahead for HIV vaccine trial in developing world. (News) Lancet 1994;344:1218.
5. Murphey-Corb M, Martin L, Davison-Fairburn B, et al. A formalin-inactivated whole SIV vaccine confers protection in macaques. Science 1989;246:1293.
6. Desrosiers RC, Wyand M, Kodama T, et al. Vaccine protection against simian immunodeficiency virus infection. Proc Natl Acad Sci USA 1989;86:6353.
7. Stott EJ. Anti-cell antibody in macaques. Nature 1991;353:393.
8. Langlois AJ, Weinhold KJ, Matthews TJ, Greenberg ML, Bolognesi DP. The ability of certain SIV vaccines to provoke reactions against normal cells. Science 1992;255:292.
9. Gardner MB. Simian and feline immunodeficiency viruses: animal lentivirus models for evaluation of AIDS vaccines and antiviral agents. Antiviral Res 1991;15:267.
10. Lackner A. Pathology of simian immunodeficiency virus induced disease. Cur Top Microbiol Immunol 1994;188:35.
11. Mc Cune JM. The SCID-hu mouse as a model for human immunodeficiency virus (HIV) infection. In: Gallo RC, Jay G, eds. The human retroviruses. San Diego: Academic Press, 1991.
12. Bendinelli M, Pistello M, Lombardi S, et al. Feline immunodeficiency virus: an interesting model for AIDS studies and an important cat pathogen. Clin Microbiol Rev 1995;8:87.
13. Klotman PE, Rappaport J, Ray P, et al. Transgenic models of HIV-1. AIDS 1995;9:313.
14. Brady HJM, Pennington DJ, Dzierzak EA. Transgenic mice as models of human immunodeficiency virus expression and related cellular effects. J Gen Virol 1994;75:2549.
15. Alter HJ, Eichberg JW, Masur H, et al. Transmission of HTLV-III infection from human plasma to chimpanzees: an animal model for AIDS. Science 1984;239:617.

16. Peeters M, Fransen K, Delaporte E, et al. Isolation and characterization of a new chimpanzee lentivirus (simian immunodeficiency virus isolate cpz-ant) from a wild-captured chimpanzee. AIDS 1992;6:447.
17. Peeters M, Honore C, Huet T, et al. Isolation and partial characterization of an HIV-related virus occurring naturally in chimpanzees in Gabon. AIDS 1989;3:625.
18. Huet T, Cheynier R, Meyerhans A, Roelants G, Wain-Hobson S. Genetic organization of a chimpanzee lentivirus related to HIV-1. (See comments) Nature 1990;345:356.
19. Berman PW, Gregory TJ, Riddle L, et al. Protection of chimpanzees from infection by HIV-1 after vaccination with recombinant glycoprotein gp120 but not gp160. Nature 1990;345:622.
20. Berman PW, Eastman DJ, Nakamura GR, et al. Apparent protection of MN-rgp120–immunized chimpanzees from infection with a primary isolate of HIV-1. In: Chanock RM, Brown F, Ginsberg HS, Norrby E, eds. Vaccines 95. Cold Spring Harbor, NY: Cold Spring Harbor Press, 1995:143.
21. Emini EA, Schleif WA, Nunberg JH, et al. Prevention of HIV-1 infection in chimpanzees by gp120 V3 domain-specific monoclonal antibody. Nature 1992;355:728.
22. Prince AM, Reesink H, Pascual D, et al. Prevention of HIV infection by passive immunization with HIV immunoglobulin. AIDS Res Hum Retroviruses 1991;7:971.
23. Watanabe M, Ringler DJ, Fultz PN, et al. A chimpanzee-passaged human immunodeficiency virus isolate is cytopathic for chimpanzee cells but does not induce disease. J Virol 1991;65:3344.
24. Shibata R, Hoggan MD, Broscius C, et al. Isolation and characterization of a syncytium-inducing macrophage/T-cell line––tropic human immunodeficiency virus type 1 isolate that readily infects chimpanzee cells in vitro and in vivo. J Virol 1995;69:4453.
25. Gendelman HE, Ehrlich GD, Baca LM, et al. The inability of human immunodeficiency virus to infect chimpanzee monocytes can be overcome by serial viral passage in vivo. J Virol 1991;65:3853.
26. Eibl MM, Kupcu Z, Mannhalter JW, Eder G, Schaff Z. Dual tropism of HIV-1 IIIB for chimpanzee lymphocytes and monocytes. AIDS Res Hum Retroviruses 1992;8:69.
27. Agy M, Frumkin L, Corey L, et al. Infection of Macaca nemestrina by human immunodeficiency virus type 1. Science 1992;257:103.
28. Frumkin LR, Agy MB, Coombs RW, et al. Acute infection of Macaca nemestrina by human immunodeficiency virus type 1. Virology 1993;195:422.
29. Otten RA, Brown BG, Simon M, et al. Differential replication and pathogenic effects of HIV-1 and HIV-2 in Macaca nemestrina. AIDS 1994;8:297.
30. Gartner S, Liu Y, Polonis V, et al. Adaptation of HIV-1 to pigtailed macaques. J Med Primatol 1994;23:155.
31. Lusso P, Markham PD, Ranki A, et al. Cell-mediated immune response toward viral envelope and core antigens in gibbon apes (Hylobates lar) chronically infected with human immunodeficiency virus. J Immunol 1988;141:2467.
32. Allan JS, Ray P, Broussard S, et al. Infection of baboons with simian/human immunodeficiency viruses. J AIDS Hum Retrovirol 1995;9:429.
33. Morrow JW, Homsy J, Eichberg JW, et al. Long-term observation of baboons, rhesus monkeys, and chimpanzees inoculated with HIV and given periodic immunosuppressive treatment. AIDS Res Hum Retroviruses 1989;5:233.
34. Shibata R, Kawamura M, Sakai H, Hayami M, Ishimoto A, Adachi A. Generation of a chimeric human and simian immunodeficiency virus infectious to monkey peripheral blood mononuclear cells. J Virol 1991;65:3514.
35. Haigwood NL, Nara PL, Brooks E, et al. Native but not denatured recombinant human immunodeficiency virus type 1 gp120 generates broad-spectrum neutralizing antibodies in baboons. J Virol 1992;66:172.
36. Allan JS. Pathogenic properties of simian immunodeficiency viruses in nonhuman primates. AIDS Res Rev 1991;1:191.
37. Mosier DE, Gulizia RJ, Baird SM, Wilson DB. Transfer of a functional human immune system to mice with severe combined immunodeficiency. Nature 1988;335:256.
38. Namikawa R, Kaneshima H, Lieberman M, Weissman IL, McCune JM. Infection of the SCID-hu mouse by HIV-1. Science 1988;242:1684.
39. Kaneshima H, Su L, Bonyhadi ML, Connor RI, Ho DD, McCune JM. Rapid-high, syncytium-inducing isolates of human immunodeficiency virus type 1 induce cytopathicity in the human thymus of the SCID-hu mouse. J Virol 1994;68:8188.
40. Kollman TR, Kim A, Pettoello-Mantovani M, et al. Divergent effects of chronic HIV-1 infection on human thymocyte maturation in SCID-hu mice. J Immunol 1995;154:907.
41. Mosier DE, Gulizia RJ, MacIsaac PD, Corey L, Greenberg PD. Resistance to human immunodeficiency virus 1 infection of SCID mice reconstituted with peripheral blood leukocytes from donors vaccinated with vaccinia gp160 and recombinant gp160. Proc Natl Acad Sci USA 1993;90:2443.
42. Akkina RK, Rosenblatt JD, Campbell AG, Chen IS, Zack JA. Modeling human lymphoid precursor cell gene therapy in the SCID-hu mouse. Blood 1994;84:1393.
43. Abramczuk JW, Pezen DS, Leonard JM, et al. Transgenic mice carrying intact HIV provirus: biological effects and organization of a transgene. J Acquir Immune Defic Syndr 1992;5:196.
44. Maddon PJ, Dalgleish AG, McDougal JS, Clapham PR, Weiss RA, Axel R. The T4 gene encodes the AIDS virus receptor and is expressed in the immune system and brain. Cell 1986;47:333.
45. Vogel J, Hinrichs SH, Reynolds RK, Luciw PA, Jay G. The HIV tat gene induces dermal lesions resembling Kaposi's sarcoma in transgenic mice. Nature 1988;335:606.
46. Skowronski J, Parks D, Mariani R. Altered T cell activation and development in transgenic mice expressing the HIV-1 nef gene. EMBO J 1993;12:703.
47. Lindemann D, Wilhelm R, Renard P, Althage A, Zinkernagel R, Mous J. Severe immunodeficiency associated with a human immunodeficiency virus 1 NEF/3'-long terminal repeat transgene. J Exp Med 1994;179:797.
48. Corboy JR, Buzy JM, Zink MC, Clements JE. Expression directed from HIV long terminal repeats in the central nervous system of transgenic mice. Science 1992;258:1804.
49. Kopp JB, Weeks BS, Marinos NJ, et al. HIV associated nephropathy in transgenic mice. Abstract. International Conference on AIDS 1991;7:64.
50. Iwakura Y, Shioda T, Tosu M, et al. The induction of cataracts by HIV-1 in transgenic mice. AIDS 1992;6:1069.
51. Kulaga H, Folks T, Rutledge R, Truckenmiller ME, Gugel E, Kindt TJ. Infection of rabbits with human immunodeficiency virus 1. J Exp Med 1989;169:321.
52. Filice G, Cereda PM, Varnier OE. Infection of rabbits with human immunodeficiency virus. Nature 1988;335:366.
53. Reina S, Markham P, Gard E, et al. Serological, biological, and molecular characterization of New Zealand white rabbits infected by intraperitoneal inoculation with cell-free human immunodeficiency virus. J Virol 1993;67:5367.
54. Tseng CK, Hughes MA, Hsu PL, Mahoney S, Duvic M, Sell S. Syphilis superinfection activates expression of human immunodeficiency virus-1 in latently infected rabbits. Am J Pathol 1991;138:1149.
55. Tseng CK, Leibowitz J, Sell S. Defective infection of rabbit peripheral blood monocyte cultures with human immunodeficiency virus type 1. AIDS Res Human Retroviruses 1994;10:285.
56. Hague BF, Sawasdikosol S, Brown TJ, Lee K, Recker DP, Kindt TJ. CD4 and its role in infection of rabbit cell lines by human immunodeficiency virus type 1. Proc Natl Acad Sci USA 1992;89:7963.
57. Marlink R, Kanki P, Thior I, et al. Reduced rate of disease development after HIV-2 infection as compared to HIV-1. Science 1994;265:1587.
58. Hirsch VM, Olmsted RA, Murphey-Corb M, Purcell RH, Johnson PR. An African primate lentivirus (SIVsm) closely related to HIV-2. Nature 1989;339:389.
59. Gao F, Yue L, White AT, et al. Human infection by genetically diverse SIVsm-related HIV-2 in west Africa. Nature 1992;358:495.
60. Biberfeld G, Emini EA. Progress with HIV vaccines. AIDS 1991;5(Suppl 2):S129.
61. Franchini G, Markham P, Gard E, et al. Persistent infection of rhesus macaques with a molecular clone of human immunodeficiency virus type 2: evidence of minimal genetic drift and low pathogenetic effects. J Virol 1990;64:4462.
62. McClure J, Steele J, Dorofeeva N, et al. In vivo passage of HIV-2EHO in Macaca nemestrina results in increased virulence. Abstract. Symposium on Nonhuman Primate Models of AIDS 1993;11:.
63. Putkonen P, Bottiger B, Warstedt K, Thorstensson R, Albert J, Biberfeld G. Experimental infection of cynomolgus monkeys (Macaca fascicularis) with HIV-2. J Acquir Immune Defic Syndr 1989;2:366.

64. Luke W, Voss G, Stahl-Hennig C, et al. Protection of cynomolgus macaques (*Macaca fascicularis*) against infection with the human immunodeficiency virus type 2 strain ben (HIV-2ben) by immunization with the virion-derived envelope glycoprotein gp130. AIDS Res Hum Retroviruses 1993;9:387.

65. Putkonen P, Thorstensson R, Ghavamzadeh L, et al. Prevention of HIV-2 and SIVsm infection by passive immunization in cynomolgus monkeys. (See comments) Nature 1991;352:436.

66. Putkonen P, Bjorling E, Akerblom L, et al. Long-standing protection of macaques against cell-free HIV-2 with a HIV-2 ISCOM vaccine. J Acquir Immune Defic Syndr 1994;7:551.

67. Nicol I, Flamminio-Zola G, Dubouch P, et al. Persistent HIV-2 infection of rhesus macaque, baboon, and mangabeys. Intervirology 1989;30:258.

68. Letvin NL, Daniel MD, Sehgal PK, et al. Infection of baboons with human immunodeficiency virus-2 (HIV-2). J Infect Dis 1989;156:406.

69. Castro BA, Nepomuceno M, Lerche NW, Eichberg JE, Levy JA. Persistent infection of baboons and rhesus monkeys with different strains of HIV-2. Virology 1991;184:219.

70. Barnett SW, Murthy KK, Herndier BG, Levy JA. An AIDS-like condition induced in baboons by HIV-2. Science 1994;266:642.

71. Benveniste RE, Arthur LO, Tsai C-C, et al. Isolation of a lentivirus from a macaque with lymphoma: comparison with HTLV-III/LAV and lentiviruses. J Virol 1986;60:483.

72. Lowenstine LJ, Lerche NW, Yee JL, et al. Evidence for a lentiviral etiology in an epizootic of immune deficiency and lymphoma in stumptailed macaques (*Macaca arctoides*). J Med Primatol 1992;21:1.

73. Simon MA, Brodie SJ, Sasseville VG, Chalifoux LV, Desrosiers RC, Ringler DJ. Immunopathogenesis of SIVmac. Virus Res 1994;32:227.

74. Murphey-Corb M, Martin LN, Rangan SR, et al. Isolation of an HTLV-III–related retrovirus from macaques with simian AIDS and its possible origin in asymptomatic mangabeys. Nature 1986;321:435.

75. Fultz PN, McClure HM, Anderson DC, Swenson RB, Anand R, Srinivasan A. Isolation of a T-lymphotropic retrovirus from naturally infected sooty mangabey monkeys (*Cercocebus atys*). Proc Natl Acad Sci USA 1986;83:5286.

76. Fultz PN, Gordon TP, Anderson DC, McClure HM. Prevalence of natural infection with simian immunodeficiency virus and simian T-cell leukemia virus type I in a breeding colony of sooty mangabey monkeys. AIDS 1990;4:619.

77. Marx PA, Li Y, Lerche NW, et al. Isolation of a simian immunodeficiency virus related to human immunodeficiency virus type 2 from a West African pet sooty mangabey. J Virol 1991;65:4480.

78. Kannagi M, Yetz JM, Letvin NL. In vitro growth characteristics of simian T-lymphotropic virus type III. Proc Natl Acad Sci USA 1985;82:7053.

79. Baskin GB, Murphey-Corb M, Roberts ED, Didier PJ, Martin LN. Correlates of SIV encephalitis in rhesus monkeys. J Med Primatol 1992;21:59.

80. Baskin GB, Murphey-Corb M, Watson EA, Martin L. Necropsy findings in rhesus monkeys experimentally infected with cultured simian immunodeficiency virus (SIV)/Delta. Vet Pathol 1988;25:456.

81. Heise C, P. V, Miller CJ, Halsted CH, Dandekar S. Simian immunodeficiency virus infection of the gastrointestinal tract of rhesus macaques. Am J Pathol 1993;142:1759.

82. Rezikyan S, Kaaya EE, Ekman M, et al. B-cell lymphomagenesis in SIV-immunosuppressed cynomolgus monkeys. Int J Cancer 1995;61:574.

83. Kestler H, Kodama T, Ringler D, et al. Induction of AIDS in rhesus monkeys by molecularly cloned simian immunodeficiency virus. Science 1990;248:1109.

84. Kestler HW, Ringler DJ, Sehgal PK, Daniel MD, Desrosiers RC. Importance of the *nef* gene for the maintenance of high virus loads and for development of AIDS. Cell 1991;65:651.

85. Kirchhoff F, Greenough TC, Brettler DB, Sullivan JL, Desrosiers RC. Brief report: absence of intact *nef* sequences in a long-term survivor with nonprogressive HIV-1 infection. (See comments) N Engl J Med 1995;332:228.

86. Westervelt P, Henkel T, Trowbridge DB, et al. Dual regulation of silent and productive infection in monocytes by distinct human immunodeficiency virus type 1 determinants. J Virol 1992;66:3925.

87. Levy DN, Fernandes LS, Williams WV, Weiner DB. Induction of cell differentiation by human immunodeficiency virus 1 vpr. Cell 1993;72:541.

88. Rogel ME, Wu LI, Emerman M. The human immunodeficiency virus type 1 vpr gene prevents cell proliferation during chronic infection. J Virol 1995;69:882.

89. Gibbs JS, Lackner AA, Lang SM, et al. Progression to AIDS in the absence of a gene for vpr or vpx. J Virol 1995;69:2378.

90. Baba TW, Jeong YS, Pennick D, Bronson R, Greene MF, Ruprecht RM. Pathogenicity of live, attenuated SIV after mucosal infection of neonatal macaques. Science 1995;267:1820.

91. Fultz PN, McClure HM, Anderson DC, Switzer WM. Identification and biologic characterization of an acutely lethal variant of simian immunodeficiency virus from sooty mangabeys (SIV/SMM). AIDS Res Hum Retroviruses 1989;5:397.

92. Fultz PN, Zack PM. Unique lentivirus-host interactions: SIVsmmPBj14 infection of macaques. Virus Res 1994;32:205.

93. Birx DL, Lewis MG, Vahey M, et al. Association of interleukin-6 in the pathogenesis of acutely fatal SIVsmm/PBj-14 in pigtailed macaques. AIDS Res Hum Retroviruses 1993;9:1123.

94. Fultz PN. Replication of an acutely lethal simian immunodeficiency virus activates and induces proliferation of lymphocytes. J Virol 1991;65:4902.

95. Dewhurst S, Embretson JE, Anderson DC, Mullins JI, Fultz PN. Sequence analysis and acute pathogenicity of molecularly cloned SIVSMM-PBj14. (See comments) Nature 1990;345:636.

96. Novembre FJ, Hirsch VM, McClure HM, Johnson PR. Molecular diversity of SIVsmm/PBj and a cognate variant, SIVsmm/PGg. J Med Primatol 1991;20:188.

97. Novembre FJ, Johnson PR, Lewis MG, et al. Multiple viral determinants contribute to pathogenicity of the acutely lethal simian immunodeficiency virus SIVsmmPBj variant. J Virol 1993;67:2466.

98. Novembre FJ, Saucier MM, Hirsch VM, Johnson PR, McClure HM. Viral genetic determinants in SIVsmmPBj pathogenesis. J Med Primatol 1994;23:136.

99. Allan JS, Short MS, Taylor ME, et al. Species-specific diversity among simian immunodeficiency viruses from African green monkeys. J Virol 1991;65:2816.

100. Johnson PR, Goldstein S, London WT, Fomsgaard A, Hirsch VM. Molecular clones of SIVsm and SIVagm: experimental infection of macaques and African green monkeys. J Med Primatol 1990;19:279.

101. Honjo S, Narita T, Kobayashi R, et al. Experimental infection of African green monkeys and cynomolgus monkeys with a SIVAGM strain isolated from a healthy African green monkey. J Med Primatol 1990;19:9.

102. Hirsch VM, Dapolito G, Johnson PR, et al. Induction of AIDS by simian immunodeficiency virus from an African green monkey: species-specific variation in pathogenicity correlates with the extent of in vivo replication. J Virol 1995;69:955.

103. Norley SG, Kraus G, Ennen J, Bonilla J, Konig H, Kurth R. Immunological studies of the basis for the apathogenicity of simian immunodeficiency virus from African green monkeys. Proc Natl Acad Sci USA 1990;87:9067.

104. Hartung S, Boller K, Cichutek K, Norley SG, Kurth R. Quantitation of a lentivirus in its natural host: simian immunodeficiency virus in African green monkeys. J Virol 1992;66:2143.

105. Fukasawa M, Miura T, Hasegawa A, et al. Sequence of simian immunodeficiency virus from African green monkey, a new member of the HIV/SIV group. Nature 1988;333:457.

106. Ennen J, Findeklee H, Dittmar MT, Norley S, Ernst M, Kurth R. CD8+T lymphocytes of African green monkeys secrete an immunodeficiency virus-suppressing lymphokine. Proc Natl Acad Sci USA 1994;91:7207.

107. Li J, Lord CI, Haseltine W, Letvin NL, Sodroski J. Infection of cynomolgus monkeys with a chimeric HIV-1/SIVmac virus that expresses the HIV-1 envelope glycoproteins. J Acquir Immune Defic Syndr 1992;5:639.

108. Sakuragi S, Shibata R, Mukai R, et al. Infection of macaque monkeys with a chimeric human and simian immunodeficiency virus. J Gen Virol 1992;73:2983.

109. Igarashi T, Shibata R, Hasebe F, et al. Persistent infection with SIVmac chimeric virus having *tat, rev, vpu, env* and *nef* of HIV type 1 in macaque monkeys. AIDS Res Hum Retroviruses 1994;10:1021.

110. Luciw PA, Pratt-Lowe E, Shaw KES, Levy JA, Cheng-Mayer C. Persistent infection of rhesus macaques with T-cell-line-tropic and macrophage-tropic clones of simian/human immunodeficiency viruses (SHIV). 1995;92–7490.

111. Letvin N, Li J, Halloran M, Cranage MP, Rud EW, Sodroski J. Prior infection with a nonpathogenic chimeric simian-human immunodeficiency virus does not efficiently protect macaques against challenge with simian immunodeficiency virus. J Virol 1995;69:4569.

112. Sellon DC, Fuller FJ, McGuire TC. The immunopathogenesis of equine infectious anemia virus. Virus Res 1994;32:111.

113. Zink MC, Johnson LK. Pathobiology of lentivirus infections in sheep and goats. Virus Res 1994;32:139.

114. Gonda MA, Oberste MS, Garvey KJ, et al. Development of the bovine immunodeficiency-like virus as a model of lentivirus disease. Dev Biol Stand 1990;72:97.

115. Gonda MA, Luther DG, Fong SE, Tobin GJ. Bovine immunodeficiency virus: molecular biology and virus-host interactions. Virus Res 1994;32:155.

116. Olmsted RA, Hirsch VM, Purcell RH, Johnson PR. Nucleotide sequence analysis of feline immunodeficiency virus: genome organization and relationship to other lentiviruses. Proc Natl Acad Sci USA 1989;86:8088.

117. Elder JH, Phillips TR. Molecular properties of feline immunodeficiency virus (FIV). Inf Agents Dis 1994;2:361.

118. Willett BJ, Neil JC. cDNA cloning and eukaryotic expression of feline CD9. Mol Immunol 1995;32:417.

119. English RV, Nelson P, Johnson CM, Nasisse M, Tompkins WA, Tompkins MB. Development of clinical disease in cats experimentally infected with feline immunodeficiency virus. J Infect Dis 1994;170:543.

120. Femenia F, Crespeau F, Fontaine JJ, Boucheix C, Parodi AL. Early haematological and pathological abnormalities of pathogen-free cats experimentally infected with feline immunodeficiency virus (FIV). Vet Res 1994;25:544.

121. Parodi AL, Femenia F, Moraillon A, Crespeau F, Fontaine JJ. Histopathological changes in lymph nodes of cats experimentally infected with the feline immunodeficiency virus (FIV). J Comp Pathol 1994;111:165.

122. Phillips TR, Prospero-Garcia O, Puaoi DL, et al. Neurological abnormalities associated with feline immunodeficiency virus infection. J Gen Virol 1994;75:979.

123. O'Neil LL, Burkhard MJ, Diehl LJ, Hoover EA. Vertical transmission of feline immunodeficiency virus. AIDS Res Hum Retroviruses 1995;11:171.

124. Sellon RK, Jordan HL, Kennedy-Stoskopf S, Tompkins MB, Tompkins WA. Feline immunodeficiency virus can be experimentally transmitted via milk during acute maternal infection. J Virol 1994; 68:3380.

125. Pu R, Okada S, Little ER, Xu B, Stoffs WV, Yamamoto JK. Protection of neonatal kittens against feline immunodeficiency virus infection with passive maternal antiviral antibodies. AIDS 1995; 9:235.

126. Hartmann K, Donath A, Beer B, et al. Use of two virustatica (AZT, PMEA) in the treatment of FIV and of FeLV seropositive cats with clinical symptoms. Vet Immunol Immunopathol 1992;35:167.

AIDS: Biology, Diagnosis, Treatment and Prevention, fourth edition, edited by Vincent T. DeVita, Jr., Samuel Hellman, and Steven A. Rosenberg. Lippincott–Raven Publishers, © 1997

CHAPTER 2

The Life Cycle of Human Immunodeficiency Virus Type 1

Thomas M. Folks and Clyde E. Hart

The human immunodeficiency virus (HIV) shares features common to all retroviruses. First, retroviruses are so named because of their ability to route genetic information from RNA to DNA. This is accomplished by a unique enzyme, reverse transcriptase (RT), which is encoded by a gene within the retroviral genome (Fig. 2-1).This gene (*pol*) and two others, *gag* and *env,* are the major coding regions for the structural proteins needed for retroviruses to maintain and complete a life cycle. Although the seven major genera of retroviridae are usually differentiated by the pathogenic processes they initiate in their hosts, all use the products of their *gag, pol,* and *env* genes to proceed through a single cycle of replication (Table 2-1). Although it is not the purpose of this review to discuss the Retroviridae in general, much of what we know regarding HIV is predicated on knowledge gained in other retroviral systems.

The binding of an extracellular infectious virion to a susceptible cell (Fig. 2-2) begins the afferent portion of the HIV retroviral life cycle. Binding occurs between the surface gp120 Env protein of the virus and the cellular CD4 molecule. This reaction permits the transmembrane gp41 Env molecule to fuse the viral lipid envelope with the cell membrane. Cytoplasmic penetration by the virus core results, liberating the viral genomic RNA as a nucleoprotein complex. The RNA is then rapidly converted by RT into a copy of double-stranded DNA and transported to the nucleus. Here, in association with viral integrase, the viral DNA is integrated by cleavage steps into the host chromosomal DNA. This begins the efferent portion of the life cycle. The provi-ral DNA now functions as a mammalian gene and can repli-cate synchronously with host chromosomal genes. Expression of the viral genes begins when the proviral DNA serves as a template for DNA-dependent RNA polymerase activity. Such activity results in production of viral messenger RNA (mRNA), a procedure that can be divided into early and late steps. Early steps involve production of viral regulatory factors that enhance and stabilize the later-stage mRNAs responsible for structural function. These structural proteins assemble around viral genomic RNA at the plasma membrane. The final step consists of proteolytic cleavage of Gag precursor molecules, which occurs as the particle buds free from the cell, incorporating the Env protein and a portion of the plasma membrane into its outer envelope coat.

The discussion that follows details these major steps in the HIV life cycle and includes additional information on viral functions that may contribute to apoptosis, exogenous factors influencing viral replication, and targets within the viral life cycle that are potentially vulnerable to therapeutic intervention.

BINDING AND ENTRY

One of the most fortuitous findings in AIDS research was that the molecule used to identify the cell type (CD4), which had been observed to be depleted during disease progression, was also the major receptor for HIV-1.[1–4] This not only revealed the tropism and cellular host range of HIV-1 but also led to an understanding of the role played by the HIV-1 envelope glycoprotein and its receptor. To date, seven cell-surface structures have been identified as retroviral receptors. Primate lentiviruses (HIV-1, HIV-2, and simian immunodeficiency virus [SIV]) share the CD4 molecule as their major receptor. CD4 is part of the immunoglobulin G superfamily; it is expressed on the surface of helper T lymphocytes and participates in normal class II major histo-

Thomas M. Folks and Clyde E. Hart: Retrovirus Diseases Branch, Division of AIDS, STD, and TB Laboratory Research, Centers for Disease Control and Prevention, Atlanta, GA 30333.

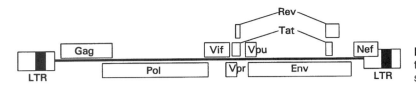

FIG. 2-1. Genomic organization of HIV-1. The relative sizes shown for the genes are not necessarily in scale to their actual sizes.

compatibility complex (MHC) recognition in association with T-cell responsiveness to foreign antigens. A number of other cell-surface molecules have been implicated as having accessory HIV-1 binding function, including MHC class I,[5] MHC class II,[6] leukocyte function–associated antigen 1 (LFA-1),[7] and, most recently, the cell surface peptidase, CD26.[8] However, no consistent experimental evidence supports any single accessory molecule for CD4.

The mature virion of HIV-1 makes primary contact with CD4 through a constellation of surface gp120 envelope glycoprotein spikes consisting of variable (V1 through V5) and conserved (C1 through C5) domains.[9,10] These glycoproteins are noncovalently linked to a transmembrane gp41 glycoprotein.[11] Critical binding may occur between the C3 and C4 domains of gp120[12,13] and the N-terminal extracellular domain of the CD4 molecule during primary attachment.[14] Although the V3 loop of gp120 does not bind to CD4, its role in overall virus binding and entry may be important. Certainly, syncytium induction,[15,16] neutralization,[17] and T-cell versus macrophage tropism[18,19] are dependent on the integrity of this region of gp120. Other cell-surface molecules, such as MHC class II HLA-DR, β_2-microglobulin, and CD44, which are "trapped" in the virion coat during budding (see later discussion), have also been considered as possible accessory ligands in virus binding.[20]

TABLE 2-1. *HIV-1 Structural and regulatory proteins*

Gene	Protein (kd) and Structure or Function
gag	Group-specific antigen. Encodes structural core matrix (17-kd), capsid (24-kd), and nucleocapsid (7-kd) proteins.
pol	Polymerase enzyme activity. Encodes the protease (10-kd), reverse transcriptase/RNase H (66-kd/51-kd) dimer, and integrase (32-kd) enzymes.
env	Envelope glycoproteins. Encodes transmembrane (41-kd) and external (120-kd) glycoproteins.
tat	Transactivator of transcription. Encodes a one-exon (14-kd) or two-exon (16-kd) protein that increases the overall level of steady-state HIV-1 RNA.
rev	Transactivator of structural gene expression. Encodes a 19-kd protein required for expression of HIV-1 unspliced and single-spliced mRNAs in the cytoplasm.

After gp120-CD4 binding, a number of events take place that position the virion for entry. Conformational changes may occur after binding that uncover domains of the gp41 transmembrane molecule.[21] It is theorized that exposure of the N-terminus of gp41, which contains a stretch of hydrophobic amino acids, allows the host cellular membrane to fuse with the lipid-envelope coat of the virion.[22] Cleavage of the gp120 V3 region by proteases (possibly as a second receptor) has been postulated[23] and may facilitate exposure of the fusogenic gp41 domain (Fig. 2-3).

Currently, no fusion receptor has been identified that could accommodate the gp41 hydrophobic domain, and the actual mechanism of virus-cell membrane fusion has not been described. In general, enveloped viruses enter a cell by either receptor-mediated, pH-dependent endocytosis or pH-independent membrane fusion. Most data support a membrane fusion mechanism for HIV-1,[24,25] and this process has been observed directly by electron microscopy. After insertion of the hydrophobic gp41 N-terminal domain into the lipid bilayer of the cell membrane, the viral membrane fuses with the cellular membrane. At this point, accessory cellular factors (receptors) may facilitate entry.

After fusion of viral and cellular membranes, the internal virion core is released into the cytoplasm as a ribonucleoprotein complex, allowing for reverse transcription of the genomic RNA. Not only are the Gag proteins important for assembly and release of HIV (see later discussion), but their association with the two-plus strands of the HIV genome are critical for reverse transcription and nuclear import of the preintegration complexes.[26] The p17 matrix protein has been shown to contain nuclear localization signals that are responsible for transport of the nucleoprotein complex to the nucleus.[27] The Vpr and Nef accessory proteins may facilitate this process.[28,29] In addition, the matrix protein may be responsible for transport of the preintegration complex in the absence of cell proliferation.[28]

REVERSE TRANSCRIPTION, NUCLEAR IMPORT, AND INTEGRATION OF VIRAL DNA

Subsequent to internalization and uncoating of the viral core, the HIV-1 nucleoprotein complex in the infected cell cytoplasm consists of Gag and Pol proteins and genomic viral RNA. The Pol protein containing the RT and ribonuclease H enzymatic activities (RT/RNase H), is a 66- and 51-kd heterodimer that uses the single-stranded genomic viral RNA to synthesize a double-stranded linear proviral

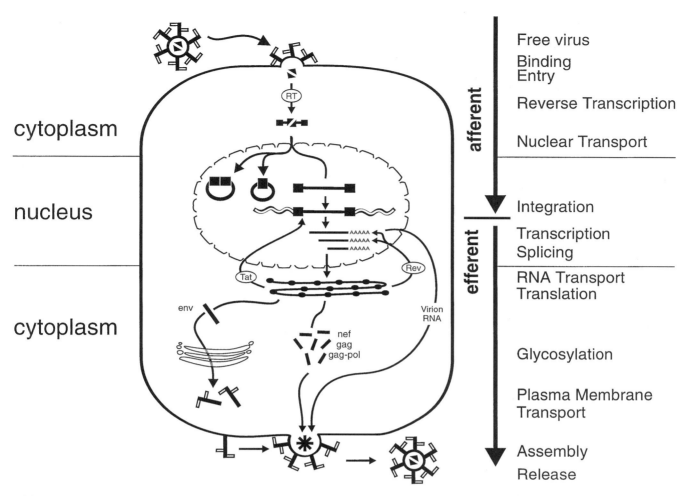

cytoplasm

nucleus

cytoplasm

Free virus

Binding
Entry

Reverse Transcription

Nuclear Transport

afferent

Integration

Transcription
Splicing

RNA Transport
Translation

Glycosylation

Plasma Membrane
Transport

Assembly
Release

efferent

env

Tat

Rev

Virion
RNA

nef
gag
gag-pol

FIG. 2-2. Life cycle of the human immunodeficiency virus. RT, reverse transcriptase; Tat and Rev, RNA-binding proteins; *env, nef, gag,* and *pol,* retroviral genes.

DNA. The reverse transcription process also generates the long terminal repeat (LTR) regions on both the 5′ and 3′ ends of the proviral DNA that are characteristic of retroviruses and necessary for integration of the proviral DNA into the cellular chromosomal DNA.

Reverse Transcription

The infecting HIV-1 virion carries the RT/RNase H enzyme and a cellular tRNA bound to the genomic RNA at the primer binding site for negative-strand DNA synthesis, the PBS(−). HIV-1 and other lentiviruses use tRNA^{lys} as a primer for the initiation of RNA-based DNA synthesis. The 18 nucleotides of the 3′ end of tRNA^{lys} bind to a perfect complementary region of the PBS(−) that is located immediately 3′ to the U5 region in the genomic viral RNA (Fig. 2-4). The RT enzyme initiates synthesis of the negative-strand proviral DNA at the PBS(−) by copying the R-U5 region at the 5′ end of the genomic RNA. The RNase H

activity degrades the R region RNA in the newly synthesized RNA-DNA hybrid. The RNase H degradation of the 5′ R region induces the newly synthesized negative-strand DNA (R-U5)+tRNA^{lys} to rehybridize to the intact 3′ R region of the same genomic RNA (intramolecular jump) or to the other copy of genomic RNA (intermolecular jump). Negative-strand DNA synthesis is then continued through the *env, pol,* and *gag* regions, including the PBS(−). RNase H degrades the RNA in the DNA-RNA hybrid except for a 16-base polypurine tract immediately 5′ to the U3 region. This polypurine tract, termed PBS(+), is used as the primer for initiation of positive-strand DNA synthesis. Positive-strand DNA synthesis begins by replication of the 3′ LTR and stops in the adjacent tRNA^{lys} primer. After RNase H removes the RNA primers in the PBS(+) and PBS(−), a final intramolecular jump occurs wherein the PBS(−) region in the newly synthesized positive-strand DNA hybridizes with the complementary PBS(−) in the negative-strand DNA. The RT enzyme completes the synthesis of both strands of DNA;

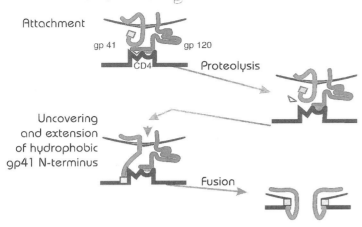

FIG. 2-3. HIV binding and fusion. Attachment of HIV to its receptor (CD4) begins with either free virus or cell-associated gp120 Env protein. Uncovering and extension of gp41 transmembrane protein allows hydrophobic N-terminus to penetrate cellular membrane. After a series of these interactions, viral lipid membrane fuses with cellular membrane, creating a "melting" or fusion event.

the negative strand is completed with synthesis of 5' LTR, and the positive strand is completed with the synthesis of all the protein coding regions and the 3' LTR.

The reverse transcription process is the point in the replication cycle that generates the rapid genomic variability characteristic of HIV-1. Some of the genetic heterogeneity may result from possible intermolecular strand switching of the RT/RNase H enzyme during synthesis of the negative-strand proviral DNA. Moreover, the RT enzyme is highly error-prone, in part because of the absence of 3'–5' exonuclease activity, which is required for the replacement of misincorporated bases. In vitro assays have reported an error rate of 1 per 6000

nucleotides[30] and an in vivo mutation rate of 1 base per HIV-1 genome.[31] This high error rate in replication has afforded the virus an intrinsic capacity to avoid immune surveillance, to quickly develop resistance to antiviral therapy, and to generate the diverse strains of HIV-1 worldwide that have impeded vaccine development.

Nuclear Transport of the Preintegration Complex

The product of reverse transcription, the double-stranded linear viral DNA, remains associated with the nucleoprotein complex, aptly termed the preintegration complex at this point in the virus life cycle. In addition to the double-stranded viral DNA, the preintegration complex contains the viral Gag matrix, Pol integrase, and Pol RT proteins that were present in the infecting virion.[26,32] The Gag matrix protein contains at least two nuclear localization signals that may be pivotal in targeting the nucleoprotein complex to the nucleus.[32] Recent data has indicated that the HIV accessory protein, Vpr, may be important for nuclear import of the preintegration complex. Nuclear localization signals in Vpr are similar to those in the Gag matrix protein,[33] and Vpr can substitute for the loss of nuclear import function of a mutated nuclear localization signal in the Gag matrix protein.[34]

Because HIV-1 can infect nondividing monocytes and macrophages in addition to activated CD4+ lymphocytes, the preintegration complex has to traverse an intact nuclear envelope for access to the host chromosomal DNA. Nuclear import of the preintegration complex is a two-phase process consisting of the initial prenuclear pore transport, which is independent of high-energy cofactors, and transport across the nuclear pore, which is dependent on high-energy cofactors.[32] Quiescent lymphocytes are believed to lack the undefined, high-energy cofactor because of their relatively low metabolic state, and they

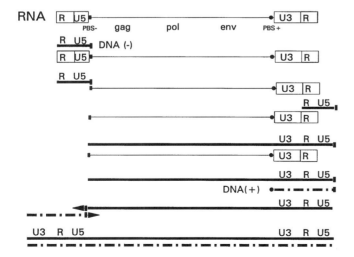

FIG. 2-4. Reverse transcription of HIV-1 genomic RNA. PBS(-) is the primer-binding site for negative-strand DNA synthesis; PBS(+) is the primer-binding site for positive-strand DNA synthesis.

are presumably unable to transport the preintegration complex across the nuclear pore.

Proviral DNA Integration

Once inside the nucleus, the linear double-stranded viral DNA associated with the preintegration complex is capable of integrating into the chromosomal DNA. Chromosomal integration of the viral DNA requires the *pol* gene–encoded 32-kd integrase enzyme contained in the preintegration complex. HIV-1 integrase removes the two nucleotides from the 3′ end of both viral DNA strands, producing recessed 3′ termini.[35] Integrase also generates the integration site by cutting the chromosomal DNA in a way that produces a 5′ five-nucleotide overhang on each of the newly formed chromosomal ends. Cellular DNA repair enzymes complete the integration process by ligating the recessed 3′ ends of viral DNA with the protruding 5′ ends of genomic DNA and filling the resulting five-nucleotide gap in the genomic DNA. The completed integration process results in a provirus minus two base pairs at the ends of both LTRs and an identical five-base pair sequence immediately upstream and downstream of the provirus. There is conflicting evidence on the necessity of an integrated provirus for viral replication. Experiments that detect high levels of unintegrated HIV-1 DNA in virus-producing cells have been interpreted to indicate that viral transcription and translation may occur with the use of an unintegrated viral DNA template. Infectious HIV-1 proviral DNA clones with integrase mutations support viral gene expression in transient DNA transfection assays, but these same integrase-defective DNA clones do not allow the spread of an HIV-1 infection throughout a cell culture.[36–38]

Until recently, the integration of HIV DNA was believed to occur randomly in the chromosomal DNA. However, a nonrandom integration of HIV-1 in the *fur* gene, located directly upstream from the *fos-fps* protooncogene, has been reported for non–B-cell lymphomas in four persons infected with HIV-1.[39] Previously, the tumor-inducing potential of HIV-1 was considered indirect, as in B-cell lymphomas and Kaposi's sarcomas, which do not contain integrated HIV DNA. The results by Shiramizu and colleagues suggest that HIV integration can directly induce lymphomagenesis through a nonrandom process.

REGULATION OF VIRAL TRANSCRIPTION

HIV-1 RNA transcription initiates in the 5′ LTR at the beginning of the R region and terminates in the 3′ LTR at the end of the R region. The combined effects of extracellular signals and cellular and viral factors control the amount and type of viral RNA transcripts produced in infected cells. As demonstrated in cell culture and in vivo, the cellular HIV-1 steady-state RNA levels range widely, from essentially a latent state (undetectable viral transcription) to a highly activated state of transcription that produces enormous levels of HIV RNA.

Basal Promoter Support of Transcription

There are multiple *cis*-acting regulatory sequences in the LTR that do not encode proteins but instead regulate viral RNA transcription. Many of the HIV-1 LTR regulatory elements are typical components of an RNA polymerase II enhancer-promoter, but other regions of the LTR proposed as putative regulatory elements have not been definitively characterized (Fig. 2-5). The TATA box and three SP1 binding sites are two important *cis*-acting regulatory elements in the U3 region of the HIV-1 LTR that control basal HIV-1 transcription.

The TATA box sequence (−24 to −27) facilitates assembly of transcription initiation complexes by binding the TATA-binding protein[40,41] of the transcription factor IID (TFIID) complex[42] during transcript initiation. Mutations in the HIV-1 TATA box result in a substantial decrease in basal transcription[43,44] and loss of viral infectivity.[45] However, even with a wild-type TATA sequence, investigations of the considerable low basal HIV-1 promoter activity in vivo have found that an intact TATA box is also required for efficient Tat transactivation.[44,46,47]

There are three SP1-binding sites (−46 to −78) in the HIV-1 LTR[48] that are also part of the basal HIV-1 transcription mechanism.[49] The three SP1 sites differ in their ability to support HIV-1 transcription and viral replication; site I (the most 3′ site) is dispensable in the presence of sites II and III, and site I alone does not support transcription or viral replication.[50–52] As with the TATA box, SP1 activity is reported to be essential for Tat transactivation[52,53] (see later discussion).

Besides the TATA box and SP1 sites, additional LTR sequences in the transcription initiation region may function in basal HIV-1 transcription. The −16 to +27 and the −38 to −16 LTR sequences are the targets of leader binding protein 1 (LBP-1)[54] or upstream binding protein (UBP-1).[55,56] The role of LPB-1 is unclear; when bound to sequences surrounding the transcription initiation site (−16 to +27), LPB-1 is important for support of basal transcription.[52,57] LBP-1 also has a weaker binding site around the TATA region (−38 to −16) that blocks the interaction of TFIID with the TATA box and inhibits transcription in vitro.[58] LBP-1 is not required for Tat transactivation and may, therefore, be involved in early HIV-1 transcription events. Many other LTR regions have been reported as putative transcription regulatory elements, but their precise roles in HIV transcription are yet to be determined.[59,60]

The NF-kB Enhancer and Activation of Transcription

The core enhancer region is the most defined element in the HIV LTR that responds to cellular activation signals by increasing viral transcription (see Fig. 2-5). The HIV-1 enhancer is composed of two 10-base pair elements in tan-

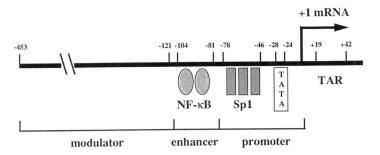

FIG. 2-5. Structural organization of the major *cis*-acting transcriptional regulatory elements of the HIV-1 long terminal repeat. NK-kB nuclear factor kB; TAR, *trans*-acting-response element.

dem (−105 to −96 and −91 to −82) that are binding sites for nuclear factor-kB (NF-kB).[61] NF-kB, originally identified as a cell-specific activation protein in B lymphocytes,[62] is a heterodimer composed of a 50-kd nucleic acid–binding protein and a 65-kd transactivation protein. Both subunits of NF-kB are now recognized as members of the *rel-dorsal* oncogene family.[63,64] Both the 50- and 65-kd subunits are capable of forming homodimers or heterodimers with other Rel proteins[64-66]; these protein complexes have differing capacities to bind and transactivate the HIV LTR through the NF-kB enhancer element.[64,67] NF-kB activity is strongly induced during T-lymphocyte activation by phorbol esters and cytokines and by HIV-1 infection.[68] Before activation, the NF-kB heterodimer is complexed to an inhibitor protein (IkB)[69-71] in the cytoplasm that blocks the nuclear localization signal and DNA-binding capacity of NF-kB.[65,69,72] In vitro studies have shown that phosphorylation of IkB results in the dissociation of the NF-kB : IkB complex.[73,74] The unbound NF-kB is then capable of transport to the nucleus, where it binds the NF-kB enhancer element and activates HIV transcription. There is no consensus on where in the virus life cycle the NF-kB enhancer element becomes an essential component of HIV transcription. In transient DNA transfection experiments using HIV-1 LTR recorder gene assays, the mutation of both NF-kB elements abolishes the response of the HIV-1 LTR to T-lymphocyte activators.[61,75,76] However, infection of activated T lymphocytes with HIV-containing mutated NF-kB elements results in very marginal, if any, decrease in virus production.[50] These results may indicate that the NF-kB elements are vital for activation of viral transcription in a cell with a latent HIV infection and that other transcription regulatory mechanisms may supersede the NF-kB element after the initial cell activation event.

Tat Transactivation

In addition to the upstream *cis*-acting elements just described, a major control element of HIV transcription is the *trans*-acting response element (TAR), which is located downstream of the transcription initiation site (see Fig. 2-5). The TAR region (+1 to +80) is the target for the viral transactivation of transcription protein, Tat. Tat transactivation

induces a dramatic overall increase in steady-state HIV RNA and is required for the high levels of virus production observed in human T-cell lines and activated human peripheral blood lymphocytes in culture. Although interest has been generated as the unique features of the HIV-1 Tat-TAR activation mechanism are discovered, three other lentiviruses, HIV-2, SIV, and equine infectious anemia virus, also encode a Tat protein–TAR mechanism that is very similar to the HIV-1 transactivation system.[77]

The full-length HIV-1 Tat protein (16 kd) is translated from two adjacent coding exons in a multispliced mRNA. The first exon, of 72 amino acids, contains functional domains for transactivation, TAR RNA binding (see later discussion), and nuclear localization. No definite function has been demonstrated for the second exon of HIV-1 *tat*. Transfection experiments using DNA plasmids that encode only the first exon of *tat* have shown that transactivation levels are not altered in the absence of the second exon. However, the second exon of HIV-2 and SIV *tat* is reported to be necessary for optimal transactivation.[78,79] Another report suggests that an Arg-Gly-Asp (RGD) sequence in the second exon of HIV-1 *tat* functions as a cell adhesion site for binding to cell-associated integrin molecules[80]; this sequence is absent in HIV-2 and SIV *tat*.[81]

Although a comprehensive effort has been made to define the molecular interactions involved in Tat transactivation of transcription, many aspects of this complex mechanism are not understood. However, one significant finding is that Tat, unlike other eukaryotic transcription factors, binds directly to the nascent leader RNA (TAR) to effect transactivation.[82-87] The HIV-1 TAR RNA region is predicted to form a stem-loop secondary structure (Fig. 2-6*A*) containing a three-nucleotide bulge region in the stem that binds Tat protein in vitro and is necessary for transactivation in vivo.[84-87] In addition to the viral Tat protein, the TAR RNA stem-loop binds nuclear proteins in vitro.[88-92] Mutational analyses of TAR RNA indicate that specific cellular protein–TAR RNA interactions at the TAR loop are especially critical for support of transactivation.[93-97] How these TAR RNA binding proteins work in concert with the viral Tat to increase steady state HIV-1 RNA is unknown. Results from a number of studies indicate Tat involvement in both transcript initiation and elongation.[59,60,98] It is not entirely

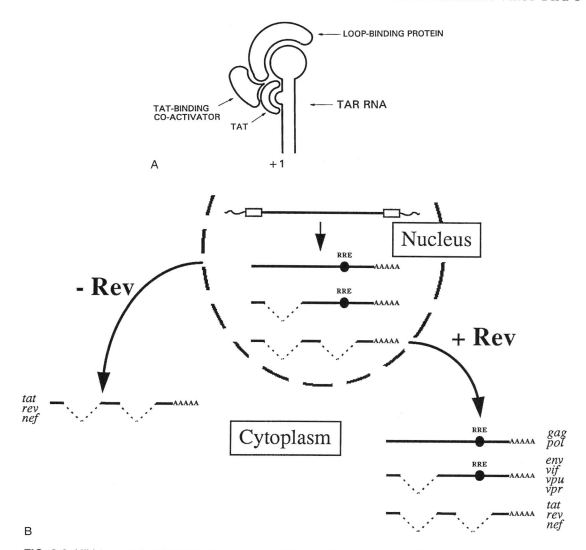

FIG. 2-6. HIV-1–encoded RNA binding proteins, Tat and Rev, are *trans*-acting regulatory factors that control steady state levels of transcription and mRNA splicing, respectively. (**A**) Tat transactivation of transcription requires the binding of Tat protein to a *trans*-acting–response element (TAR) RNA bulge region in concert with the binding of one or more cellular proteins to the loop region of TAR RNA. Cellular proteins that bind in the stem region of TAR RNA (not shown) and Tat-binding cellular proteins, co-activators, are also reported to be important for efficient Tat-directed transactivation. (**B**) Rev protein transactivation of expression of unspliced and single-spliced HIV-1 mRNAs containing the Rev-responsive element (RRE). In the presence of Rev, unspliced and single-spliced HIV-1 mRNAs in the nucleus are transported to the cytoplasm, allowing the translation of structural proteins encoded in the *gag, pol,* and *env* genes.

unlikely that Tat function in vivo may incorporate both of these mechanisms or exploit whichever one is more advantageous for a particular cell-type or cellular environment.

POSTTRANSCRIPTIONAL CONTROL OF HIV RNA EXPRESSION

The Tat-induced increase in HIV transcription results in an abundant pool of nascent viral RNA in the nucleus that must be processed and transported to the cytoplasm for viral protein synthesis to occur. In the eukaryotic nucleus, the RNA splicing

mechanism for splice-competent cellular transcripts is usually rapid and complete.[99–101] In an HIV-infected cell, both unspliced and spliced viral mRNAs must be coordinately produced from the same HIV proviral DNA. The discovery of the HIV-1 *rev* protein-coding sequence[102,103] has led to the identification of a second HIV-1–encoded transactivation mechanism that is required for the cytoplasmic expression of intron-containing, unspliced and single-spliced viral mRNAs (see Fig. 2-6B). Rev activity has also been confirmed in at least eight other retroviruses, including HIV-2, SIV, HTLV-I, and HTLV-II, and has been proposed in three more.[104]

The HIV-1 Rev protein is a 19-kd phosphoprotein encoded by two exons. In contrast to the situation with *tat*, both *rev* exons are required for function; one of two oligomerization domains spans the exon 1 and exon 2 splice junction, and the nuclear localization and activation domains are located in exon 2.[105] The oligomerization domains induce Rev protein multimers that are proposed to be the active form of the protein.[106,107] The nuclear localization domain of Rev includes an arginine-rich RNA binding domain, similar to Tat,[108] that binds to a *cis*-acting Rev response element (RRE) in viral RNA. The RRE RNA is a 234-nucleotide region located in the *env* gene that is predicted to form a stem-loop secondary structure.[106] The RRE is contained in all viral mRNAs that encode the unspliced *gag-pol* and single-spliced *vif, vpr,* and *vpu-env* genes (see Fig. 2-6*B*). Transcripts that encode *tat, rev,* and *nef* are multispliced mRNAs that do not contain the RRE RNA. The activation domain is a leucine-rich region that appears to mediate protein-protein interactions and is not involved with RRE binding. Rev protein that contains mutations in the activation domain binds RRE RNA but is functionally inactive.[106,109,110]

The purported mechanism of Rev activity is based on experiments that report a direct inhibition of splicing of RRE-containing mRNAs[111] or a selective transport of RRE-containing mRNAs from the nucleus that circumvents the splicing pathway.[112,113] Although the exact mechanism of Rev function is not determined, the final result of Rev activity is the cytoplasmic transport of viral mRNAs containing the structural *gag-pol* and *env* genes, which are absolutely essential for the production of infectious virions. Moreover, the absence of Rev activity has been proposed to play a role in HIV latency.[114,115] However, conflicting results are reported on Rev activity and the selective expression of multispliced HIV RNAs during the maintenance of clinical latency.[116–118]

TRANSLATIONAL CONTROL OF HIV PROTEIN SYNTHESIS

Most cellular mRNAs are monocistronic; they encode only one protein that can be translated in a relatively uninterrupted process. Many of the HIV mRNAs are multicistronic, with open reading frames that either partially overlap or are arranged in tandem. Ribosomal frame shifting and initiation site scan-through are two control mechanisms during viral protein synthesis that allow the translation of more than one protein species from a multicistronic mRNA. In addition to production of different viral proteins from one species of mRNA, appropriate stoichiometric amounts of these proteins must be maintained to ensure efficient virion assembly.[119]

Expression of Gag and Pol proteins from the same unspliced mRNA occurs by ribosomal frameshifting. *Gag* and *pol* genes are located in different reading frames, which overlap in their 3′ and 5′ regions, respectively (see Fig. 2-1).

In most translations of the Gag-Pol mRNA, the Gag protein is synthesized to completion and released from the ribosome. However, as the ribosome traverses the 3′ end of the *gag* open reading frame, a −1 frame shift can occur that puts the ribosome in the *pol* open reading frame. This results in a Gag-Pol fusion protein that is subsequently cleaved, by the viral-encoded protease, into the mature Gag and Pol proteins. Pol translation is totally dependent on the −1 frame shift because the *pol* gene does not have a functional AUG start site. The −1 frame shift is dependent on a specific heptamer sequence at the actual frame shift site and a predicted RNA stem-loop structure directly downstream of the heptamer.[120,121] The presence of the RNA stem-loop is predicted to cause a pause of the ribosome at the heptamer sequence and thereby allow the −1 frame shift in a limited number of translations.

Many of the spliced mRNAs of HIV-1 are multicistronic and are therefore capable of translating more than one protein.[122] The flanking sequences surrounding AUG start codons determine how efficient a particular start site is in initiating translation. If the most 5′ start site in a multicistronic mRNA is suboptimal, the ribosome may continue past this site and begin translation at a more efficient start site further downstream.[123] This suboptimal initiation site scan-through mechanism occurs readily in the translation of HIV-1 Env protein. All of the Env-encoding mRNAs contain the *vpu* start site upstream of the *env* start site.[124] The suboptimal status of the *vpu* start site, however, allows a majority of the ribosomes to scan through and find the strong *env* start site.[122,125] Because all HIV-1 regulatory genes (see Table 2-1) and accessory genes (Table 2-2) are encoded in multicistronic HIV-1 mRNAs,[122,125] the relative differences in the strengths of their respective translation start sites[122,124,125] suggest that translational control of these proteins is important in the virus life cycle.

Virion Assembly

Before the virion can be released from the cell, the structural viral proteins must coordinately assemble. HIV has been observed by electron microscopy to assemble both at the plasma membrane and within intracytoplasmic vacuoles. The actual mechanism responsible for this bidirectional trafficking is unknown. Nonetheless, as the major structural precursor proteins (55-kd Gag, 180-kd Gag-Pol, and gp160 Env) begin to accumulate, a number of steps are required for completion of the life cycle. First, the Gag (p55) polyprotein oligomerizes,[126] at which point the matrix (MA) domain of p55 (p17 processed matrix protein) is responsible for transport of the entire Gag protein to the plasma membrane.[127,128] As the polyprotein Gag complex approaches the cellular membrane and begins forming the inner framework of the virion, the nucleocapsid (NC) domain of p55 permits two copies of HIV genomic RNA to assemble around the "cys-His" box, which is an array of cysteines similar to a zinc finger motif.[129] Discrimination among multiple viral and

TABLE 2-2. *HIV-1 accessory genes*

Gene	Size	Contained in Virion	Function
vif (viral infectivity factor)	23 kd	No	Enhances efficiency of viral infection; enhances viral assembly through packaging of nucleoprotein core[177]
vpr (viral protein R)	14 kd	Yes	Localizes to nucleus; modifies cell cycle; reactivates virus from latency[29,162]; Imparts rapid growth advantage
vpu (viral protein U)	16 kd	No	Directs compartmental assembly; required for efficient maturation and release[178]; degrades CD4 in endoplasmic reticulum[179]; may have ion channel functionality[180]
nef (negative factor)	27 kd	?	Downregulates CD4 by endocytosis and lysosomal degradation[181,182]; shown to have kinase activity[183]; have cellular activating to induce viral replication from quiescent lymphocytes[163,164,184]

nonviral mRNAs and the full-length genomic RNA for Gag encapsidation lies in a *cis*-directed sequence designated psi. This site is located at the 5′ region of the HIV genome and is not present in spliced viral mRNA transcripts. To complete the encapsidation process, it is thought that the specific tRNA[lys] primer (necessary for priming negative-strand synthesis by RT) associates with the Pol domain in the larger Gag-Pol 180-kd polyprotein and is included in the infectious virion.[130,131] The capsid protein (CA) domain of Gag is essential for the morphogenesis of the mature, cone-shaped core.[132]

Virus Budding and Release

As a final step in the HIV life cycle, the infectious virus matures after it has been released from the plasma membrane. This occurs as a coordinated process by which the viral protease (located between the Gag and Pol domains) cleaves the Gag-Pol protein in an ordered fashion.[133] The conserved p2 domain of Gag is required to regulate this sequential proteolytic processing.[134] The protease begins its processing by cleaving the p55 Gag protein at the N-terminus of the p15 NC protein and then at the p24 CA.[135] P7 and p6 are the last proteins processed. The Pol polyprotein (RT and IN) remains inactive.

As the Gag and Gag-Pol proteins begin to encapsidate the HIV genomic RNA, the plasma membrane also begins to form a lipid bilayer around the viral core. Precursor gp160 Env undergoes glycosylation and oligomerization in the endoplasmic reticulum.[136,137] From this point, it is transported to the Golgi complex, where cellular enzymes process the glycoprotein to surface gp120 (SU) and transmembrane gp41 (TM).[138] Here, they associate noncovalently and are transported to the cell surface.[139] Critical to the final budding step is myristolation of the N-terminal glycine of the p17 MA protein.[127,140] This event culminates as the final process in condensing the inner core shell and linking it with the glycoprotein-incorporated lipid membrane.

Cell Activation

Because this chapter deals mainly with the HIV life cycle in T lymphocytes, it is important to understand the role of cellular activation on viral replication. The early events (afferent portion) of the viral life cycle (ie, binding, entry, and partial reverse transcription) are known to occur in the absence of activation. However, for efferent functions (integration, transcription, and translation) to efficiently take place, exogenous T-cell stimulation is required.[141–143] Several activation mechanisms are possible and may influence the viral life cycle. Probably the one that has the greatest positive effect on viral expression is activation through the T3-Ti specific antigen receptor on CD4+ lymphocytes.[144] Similar activation can be achieved through mitogens (eg, phytohemagglutinin, concanavalin A) and superantigens. Other exogenous factors (eg, cytokines, physiologic stimuli) also have been shown to have dramatic effects on HIV expression processes.[145] Some investigators have predicted that rapid progression in HIV disease, especially in Africa, may be linked to the activation status of the patients.[146]

T-cell lines have been developed to better understand these activation processes and have been extremely useful in synchronizing stages of the viral life cycle so that coordinate expression of the life cycle can be analyzed.[147–150] Second messenger signalling by Ca^{2+} and protein kinases is required for linking the exogenous stimulation to the viral life cycle–dependent events. Viral transcription is one of the best studied mechanisms that is dependent on cellular activation.[151] Intracellular second messenger pathways leading to NF-kB activation and other factors interacting with the viral LTR appear to be only a small segment of the control over the life cycle that T-cell activation can impart. Many believe that control of the viral life cycle through its dependence on cellular functions offers some of the greatest hope for therapeutic intervention.[141,152]

Role of Latency in the Life Cycle

Much attention has been focused on the afferent and efferent portions of the life cycle, primarily because of findings that throughout the course of HIV infection there is no microbiologic latent period associated with the clinical latent period.[153] However, there are microbiologically latent infected cells.[154] The greater issue is the role of these cells in pathogenesis and, more importantly, what we can understand about their origin. Clearly, HIV is replicating with virion turnover from the time of infection until the time of death of the patient.[153,155,156] Nevertheless, high ratios of viral DNA to viral RNA [154] and latent expressing cell lines [157] teach us that not every infected cell is programmed to immediately produce virus. It is probably premature to discard latency as not contributing to the pathogenic process, as some have indicated.[158] Instead, we should attempt to understand the factors or conditions that create the latent state. It may be that therapeutic intervention has great promise here.[159]

Several reports have described HIV-positive, functionally latent, CD4+ cells from AIDS patients.[160,161] The mechanisms controlling this postintegration, pretranscriptional "latent" event, however, are not understood.[157]

In vitro studies have recently implicated Vpr[29,162] and possibly Nef[163,164] in the control of transcriptional expression of HIV through cellular activation pathways. Many factors could be responsible for controlling expression[141] and inhibiting the efferent phase of virus replication. Understanding this portion of the life cycle may provide one of our clearest views yet into extending the clinically latent disease period.

Cell Death

Because HIV buds from the plasma membrane, there appears to be no selective advantage for the death of the virus-producing cell. However, direct cytotoxicity by replicating virus has been demonstrated.[165] Most of the direct killing effects have been attributed to the *env* gene products (gp120, gp160) and their affinity for CD4-positive cells.[166,167] Recently, the C-terminus of gp41 has been demonstrated to have a potent toxic effect on cells independent of CD4.[168,169]

Syncytium or multinucleated giant cell formation, resulting from fusion of HIV-infected and uninfected cells, has been shown to contribute to cell loss in culture. However, this process is not usually found in tissue of infected patients and may only be an artifact of in vitro virus propagation. Apoptosis or programmed cell death has been suggested to explain the loss of CD4+ cells seen in HIV infection.[170,171] Apoptosis differs from necrosis because the latter takes place faster, causing loss of plasma membrane integrity but no chromatin condensation. However, indirect effects of HIV infection resulting in the apoptotic process are thought to account for the majority of CD4 loss in vivo.[170,172] Such indirect effects include gp120-CD4 crosslinking followed by cell activation, autoantibodies, and cellular immune destruction. Recently, the HIV regulatory protein, Tat, has been implicated with the APO-1/Fas receptor (CD95) as a strong inducer of apoptosis.[173] This area of investigation continues to be intensely pursued to better understand CD4 depletion in AIDS and the role that products from the viral life cycle play in host pathogenesis.

Therapeutic Intervention of the Life Cycle

The most important reason for studying the HIV viral life cycle is to identify vulnerable steps that potential therapeutic intervention may successfully interrupt. To date, little success has been achieved toward this goal. The best known antiviral drugs are the nucleoside inhibitors (zidovudine, didanosine, and zalcitabine), which block reverse transcription by chain termination. However, resistance to these drugs develops rapidly.[174] Use of drugs that affect unique viral enzymes not present in mammalian cells is strongly desirable. For example, another unique viral enzyme (protease) is needed for nucleocapsid assembly and positioning during the final steps in budding and maturation and may provide a suitable therapeutic target.[175]

Many other new possibilities for intervention are emerging. A number of viral and nonviral intervention sites exist in the HIV life cycle (Fig. 2-7). Using the dependency of HIV on cellular activation, the viral life cycle can be divided into four areas: the viral afferent, cellular afferent, viral efferent, and cellular efferent portions. All of these areas can be strategically targeted to intervene in viral replication. A fifth area being tested is the extracellular component. An example of such therapeutic intervention is a design to inhibit the exogenous cellular activator, tumor necrosis factor-α.

Because excision of the viral genome from the host chromosome is not possible, some of the best opportunities in AIDS treatment lie in establishing a state of transcriptional latency.[176] Increased understanding of the role of HIV-dependent cellular activation pathways on viral transcriptional processes promises to yield important new therapeutic targets.

Cellular Targets

Viral Targets

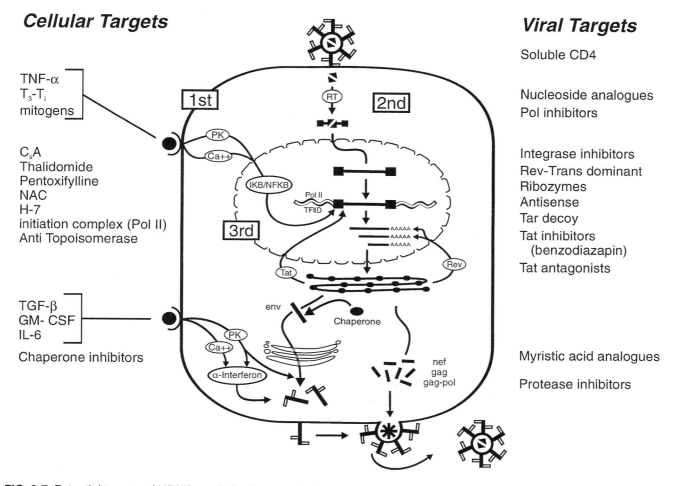

TNF-α
T_3-T_i
mitogens

C_sA
Thalidomide
Pentoxifylline
NAC
H-7
initiation complex (Pol II)
Anti Topoisomerase

TGF-β
GM- CSF
IL-6

Chaperone inhibitors

Soluble CD4

Nucleoside analogues
Pol inhibitors

Integrase inhibitors
Rev-Trans dominant
Ribozymes
Antisense
Tar decoy
Tat inhibitors
   (benzodiazapin)
Tat antagonists

Myristic acid analogues

Protease inhibitors

FIG. 2-7. Potential targets of HIV life cycle for therapeutic intervention. Boxes indicate cellular signalling pathways used by HIV for replication. The first defines cellular surface receptors; primary activation may take place by means of antigens, mitogens, or cytokines. The second refers to intracellular signals that transmit the first signal by means of kinases and ion flux. The third pathway is assembled in response to second messenger signalling and includes protein-DNA and protein-RNA interactions. Cellular and viral structures may serve as useful targets for intervention strategies in HIV life cycle disruption.

REFERENCES

1. McDougal JS, Kennedy MS, Sligh JM, et al. Binding of HTLV-III/LAV to T4+ T cells by a complex of the 110K viral protein and the T4 molecule. Science 1986;231:382.
2. Dalgleish AG, Beverly PC, Clapham PR, et al. The CD4 (T4) antigen is an essential component of the receptor for the AIDS retrovirus. Nature 1984;312:763.
3. Klatzmann D, Barre-Sinoussi F, Nugeyre MT, et al. Selective tropism of lymphadenopathy-associated virus (LAV) for helper-inducer T-lymphocytes. Science 1984;225:59.
4. Klatzmann D, Champagne E, Chamaret S, et al. T-lymphocyte T4 molecule behaves as receptor for human retrovirus LAV. Nature 1984;312:767.
5. Grassi F, Meneveri R, Gullberg G, et al. Human immunodeficiency virus type 1 gp120 mimics a hidden monomorphic epitope borne by class-I major histocompatibility complex heavy chains. J Exp Med 1991;174:53.
6. Mann DL, Read-Connole E, Arthur LO, et al. HLA-DR is involved in the HIV-1 binding site on cells expressing MHC class-II antigens. J Immunol 1988;141:1131.

7. Hildreth JEK, Orentas RJ. Involvement of a leukocyte adhesion receptor (LFA-1) in HIV-induced syncytium formation. Science 1989;244:1075.
8. Callebaut C, Krust B, Jacotot E, Hovanessian AG. T cell activation antigen CD26 as a cofactor for entry of HIV in CD4+ cells. Science 1993;262:2045.
9. Modrow S, Hahn BH, Shaw GM, et al. Computer-assisted analysis of envelope protein sequences of seven human immunodeficiency virus isolates: prediction of antigenic epitopes in conserved and variable regions. J Virol 1987;61:570.
10. Willey RL, Rutledge RA, Dias S, et al. Identification of conserved and divergent domains within the envelope gene of the acquired immunodeficiency syndrome retrovirus. Proc Natl Acad Sci USA 1986;83:5038.
11. Freed EO, Myers DJ, Risser R. Characterization of the fusion domain of the human immunodeficiency virus type 1 envelope glycoprotein. Proc Natl Acad Sci USA 1990;87:4650.
12. Felser JM, Klimkait R, Sliver J. A syncytia assay for human immunodeficiency virus type 1 (HIV-1) envelope protein and its use in studying HIV-1 mutation. Virology 1989;170:566.
13. Lasky LA, Nakamura G, Smith DH, et al. Delineation of a region of the human immunodeficiency virus type 1 gp120 glycoprotein critical for interaction with the CD4 receptor. Cell 1987;50:975.

14. Arthos J, Deen KC, Chaikin MA, et al. Identification of the residues in human CD4 critical for the binding of HIV. Cell 1989;57:469.
15. de Jong J-J, Goudsmit J, Keulen W, et al. Human immunodeficiency virus type 1 clones chimeric for the envelope V3 domain differ in syncytium formation and replication capacity. J Virol 1992;66:757.
16. Fouchier RAM, Groenink M, Kootstra NA, et al. Phenotype-associated sequence variation in the third variable domain of the human immunodeficiency virus type 1 gp120 molecule. J Virol 1992;66:3183.
17. Warren RQ, Anderson SA, Nkya WMMM, et al. Examination of sera for human immunodeficiency virus type 1 (HIV-1)–infected individuals for antibodies reactive with peptide corresponding to the principal neutralizing determinant of HIV-1 gp120 and for in vitro neutralizing activity. J Virol 1992;66:5210.
18. Chesebro B, Nishio J, Perryman S, et al. Identification of human immunodeficiency virus envelope gene sequence influencing viral entry into CD4-positive HeLa cells, T-leukemia cells, and macrophages. J Virol 1991;65:5782.
19. Moore JP, Nara PL. The role of the V3 loop of gp120 in HIV infection. AIDS 1991;5(Suppl 2):S21.
20. Orentas RJ, Hildreth JEK. Association of host cell surface adhesion receptors and other membrane proteins with HIV and SIV. AIDS Res Hum Retroviruses 1993;9:1157.
21. Sattentau QJ, Moore JP. Conformational changes induced in the human immunodeficiency virus envelope glycoprotein by soluble CD4 binding. J Exp Med 1991;174:407.
22. Gallaher WR. Detection of a fusion peptide sequence in the transmembrane protein of human immunodeficiency virus. Cell 1987;50:327.
23. Hattori T, Koito A, Takatsuki K, et al. Involvement of tryptase-related cellular protease(s) in human immunodeficiency virus type 1 infection. FEBS Lett 1989;248:48.
24. Maddon PJ, McDougal JS, Clapham PR, et al. HIV infection does not require endocytosis of its receptor, CD4. Cell 1988;54:865.
25. Hunter E, Swanstrom R. Retrovirus envelope glycoproteins. In: Swanstrom R, Vogt PK, eds. Retroviruses: strategies of replication. Berlin: Springer-Verlag, 1990:187.
26. Bukrinsky MI, Sharova N, Dempsey MP, et al. Active nuclear import of human immunodeficiency virus type 1 preintegration complexes. Proc Natl Acad Sci USA 1992;89:6580.
27. Bukrinsky MI, Haggerty S, Dempsey MP, et al. A nuclear localization signal within HIV-1 matrix protein that governs infection of non-dividing cells. Nature 1993;365:666.
28. Spina CA, Guatelli JC, Richman DD. Establishment of a stable, inducible form of human immunodeficiency virus type 1 DNA in quiescent CD4 lymphocytes in vitro. J Virol 1995;69:2977.
29. Levy DN, Refaeli Y, Weiner DB. Extracellular Vpr protein increases cellular permissiveness to human immunodeficiency virus replication and reactivates virus from latency. J Virol 1995;69:1243.
30. Ji J, Loeb LA. Fidelity of HIV-1 reverse transcriptase copying RNA in vitro. Biochemistry 1992;31:954.
31. Goodenow M, Huet T, Saurin W, Kwok S, Sninsky J, Wain-Hobson S. HIV-1 isolates are rapidly evolving quasispecies: evidence for viral mixtures and preferred nucleotide substitutions. J Acquir Immune Defic Syndr 1989;2:344.
32. Stevenson M. Identification of factors that govern HIV-1 replication in nondividing host cells. AIDS Res Human Retroviruses 1994;10:S11.
33. Myers G, Korber B, Wain-Hobson S, Jeang K-T, Henderson LE, Pavlakis GN, eds. Human retroviruses and AIDS. Los Alamos: Theoretical Biology and Biophysics, 1994.
34. Heinzinger NK, Bukrinsky MI, Haggerty SA, et al. The Vpr protein of human immunodeficiency virus type 1 influences nuclear localization of viral nucleic acids in nondividing host cells. Proc Natl Acad Sci USA 1994;91:7311.
35. Pauza CD. Two bases are deleted from the termini of HIV-1 linear DNA during integrative recombination. Virology 1990;179:886.
36. Engelman A, Englund G, Orenstein JM, Martin MA, Craigie R. Multiple effects of mutations in human immunodeficiency virus type 1 integrase on viral replication. J Virol 1995;69:2729.
37. Englund G, Theodore TS, Freed EO, Engleman A, Martin MA. Integration is required for productive infection of monocyte-derived macrophages by human immunodeficiency virus type 1. J Virol 1995;69:3216.
38. Wiskerchen M, Muesing MA. Human immunodeficiency virus type 1 integrase: effects of mutations on viral ability to integrate, direct viral gene expression from unintegrated viral DNA templates, and sustain viral propagation in primary cells. J Virol 1995;69:379.
39. Shiramizu B, Herndier BG, McGrath MS. Identification of a common clonal human immunodeficiency virus integration site in human immunodeficiency virus—associated lymphomas. Cancer Res 1994;54:2069.
40. Maldonado E, Ha I, Cortes P, Weis L, Reinberg D. Factors involved in specific transcription by mammalian RNA polymerase II: role of transcription factors IIA, IID, IIB during formation of a transcription-competent complex. Mol Cell Biol 1990;10:6335.
41. Peterson MG, Tanese N, Pugh BF, Tijan R. Functional domains and upstream activation properties of cloned human TATA binding protein. (Published erratum appears in Science 1990 Aug 24;249:844)
42. Reinberg D, Roeder RG. Factors involved in specific transcription by mammalian RNA polymerase II: purification and functional analysis of initiation factors IIB and IIE. J Biol Chem 1987;262:3310.
43. Bielinska A, Krasnow S, Nabel GJ. NF-kB-—mediated activation of the human immunodeficiency virus enhancer: site of transcriptional initiation is independent of the TATA box. J Virol 1989;63:4097.
44. Berkhout B, Jeang K-T. Functional roles for the TATA promoter and enhancers in basal and tat-induced expression of the human immunodeficiency virus type 1 long terminal repeat. J Virol 1992;66:139.
45. Lu Y, Stenzel M, Sodroski JG, Haseltine WA. Effects of long terminal repeat mutations on human immunodeficiency virus type 1 replication. J Virol 1989;63:4115.
46. Lu X, Welsh TM, Peterlin BM. The human immunodeficiency virus type 1 long terminal repeat specifies two different transcription complexes, only one of which is regulated by tat. J Virol 1993;61:1752.
47. Olsen HS, Rowen CA. Contribution of the TATA motif to tat-mediated transcriptional activation of human immunodeficiency virus gene expression. J Virol 1992;66:5594.
48. Jones KA, Kadonaga JT, Luciw PA, Tjian R. Activation of the AIDS retrovirus promoter by the cellular transcription factor, Sp1. Science 1986;232:755.
49. Harrich D, Garcia J, Wu F, Mitsuyasu R, Gonzalez J, Gaynor R. Role of Sp1-binding domains in vivo transcriptional regulation of the human immunodeficiency virus type 1 long terminal repeat. J Virol 1989;63:2585.
50. Leonard J, Parrot C, Buckler-White AJ, et al. The NF-kB binding sites in the human immunodeficiency virus type 1 long terminal repeat are not required for virus infectivity. J Virol 1989;63:4919.
51. Parrot C, Seidner T, Duh E, et al. Variable role of the long terminal repeat Sp1-binding sites in human immunodeficiency virus replication in T lymphocytes. J Virol 1991;65:1414.
52. Ross EK, Buckler-White AJ, Rabson AB, Englund G, Martin MA. Contribution of NF-kB and Sp1 binding motifs to the replicative capacity of human immunodeficiency virus type 1: distinct patterns of viral growth are determined by T-cell types. J Virol 1991;65:4350.
53. Berkhout B, Gatignol A, Rabson AB, Jeang K-T. TAR-independent activation of the HIV-1 LTR: evidence that tat requires specific regions of the promoter. Cell 1990;62:757.
54. Jones KA, Luciw PA, Duchange N. Structural arrangements of transcription control domains within the 5′-untranslated leader regions of the HIV-1 and HIV-2 promoters. Genes Dev 1988;2:1101.
55. Garcia JA, Wu FK, Mitsuyasu R, Gaynor RB. Interactions of cellular proteins involved in the transcriptional regulation of the human immunodeficiency virus. EMBO J 1987;6:3761.
56. Wu FK, Garcia JA, Harrich D, Gaynor RB. Purification of the human immunodeficiency virus type 1 enhancer and TAR binding proteins EBP-1 and UBP-1. EMBO J 1988;7:2117.
57. Boris-Lawrie KA, Brady JN, Kumar A. Sequences within the R region of the long terminal repeat activate basal transcription from the HIV-1 promoter. Gene Expr 1992;2:215.
58. Dayton AI, Sodroski JG, Rosen CA, Goh WC, Haseltine WA. The trans-activator gene of the human T cell lymphotropic virus type III is required for replication. Cell 1986;44:941.
59. Antoni BA, Stein SB, Rabson AB. Regulation of human immunodeficiency virus infection: implications for pathogenesis. Adv Virus Res 1994;43:53.
60. Jones KA, Peterlin BM. Control of RNA initiation and elongation at the HIV-1 promoter. Annu Rev Biochem 1994;63:717.
61. Nabel G, Baltimore D. An inducible transcription factor activates expression of human immunodeficiency virus in T cells. Nature 1987;326:711.
62. Sen R, Baltimore D. Multiple nuclear factors interact with the immunoglobulin enhancer sequences. Cell 1986;46:705.

63. Bou V, Villalobos J, Burd PR, Kelly K, Siebenlist U. Cloning of mitogen-inducible gene encoding a kB DNA-binding protein with homology to the rel oncogene and to cell-cycle motifs. Nature 1990;348:76.
64. Kieran M, Blank V, Logeat F, et al. The DNA binding subunit of NFkB is identical to factor KBF1 and homologous to the rel oncogene product. Cell 1990;62:1007.
65. Baeuerle PA, Baltimore D. A 65kD subunit of active NF-kB is required for inhibition of NF-kB by I-kB. Genes Dev 1989;3:1689.
66. Fujita T, Nolan GP, Ghosh S, Baltimore D. Independent modes of transcriptional activation by the p50 and p65 subunits of NF-kb. Genes Dev 1992;6:775.
67. Rattner A, Lorner M, Rosen PA, et al. Nuclear factor kB activates proencephalin transcription in T lymphocytes. Mol Cell Biol 1992;11:1017.
68. Bachelerie F, Alcami J, Arenzana-Seisdedos F, Virelizier J-L. HIV enhancer activity perpetuated by NF-kappa B induction on infection of monocytes. (See comments) Nature 1991;350:709.
69. Bauerle PA, Baltimore D. Activation of DNA-binding activity in an apparently cytoplasmic precursor of the NF-kB transcription factor. Cell 1988;53:211.
70. Inoue J, Kerr LD, Kakizuka A, Verma IM. IkB a 70 kd protein identical to the C-terminal half of p110 NF-kb: a new member of the IkBB family. Cell 1992;68:1109.
71. Kerr LD, Inoue J, Davis N, et al. The rel-associated pp40 protein prevents DNA binding of rel and NF-kB: relationship with IkBB and regulation by phosphorylation. Genes Dev 1991;5:1464.
72. Baeuerle PA, Baltimore D. I kappa B: a specific inhibitor of the NF-kappa B transcription factor. Science 1988;242:540.
73. Shirakawa F, Chedid M, Suttles J, Pollok BA, Mizel SB. Interleukin 1 and cyclic AMP induces kappa immunoglobulin light-chain expression via activation of an NF-kappa B-—like DNA-binding protein. Mol Cell Biol 1989;9:959.
74. Shirakawa F, Mizel SB. In vitro activation and nuclear translocation of NF-kappa B catalyzed by cyclic AMP-dependent protein kinase and protein kinase C. Mol Cell Biol 1989;9:2424.
75. Kawakami K, Scheidereit C, Roeder RG. Identification and purification of a human immunoglobulin-enhancer-—binding protein (NF-kB) that activates transcription from a human immunodeficiency virus type I promotor in vivo. Proc Natl Acad Sci U S A 1988;85:4700.
76. Franza BR, Josephs SF, Gilman MZ, Ryan W, Clarkson B. Characterization of cellular proteins recognizing the HIV enhancer using a microscale DNA-affinity precipitation assay. Nature 1987;330:391.
77. Peterlin BM, Adams M, Alonso A, et al. Tat trans-activator. In: Cullen BR, ed. Human retroviruses. Oxford: Oxford University Press, 1993:75.
78. Viglianta G, Mullins JI. Functional comparison of transactivation by simian immunodeficiency virus from rhesus macaques and human immunodeficiency virus type 1. J Virol 1988;62:4532.
79. Tong-Starksen S, Baur A, Lu XB, Peck E, Peterlin BM. Second exon of tat of HIV-2 is required for optimal transactivation of HIV-1 and HIV-2 LTRs. Virology 1993;195:826.
80. Brake DA, Debouk C, Biesecker G. Identification of an Arg-Gly-Asp (RGD) cell adhesion site in human immunodeficiency virus type 1 transactivation protein tat. J Cell Biol 111:1275.
81. Jeang K-T. HIV-1 tat: structure and function. In: Myers G, Korber B, Wain-Hobson S, Jeang K-T, Henderson LE, Pavlakis GN, eds. Human retroviruses and AIDS. Los Alamos: Theoretical Biology and Biophysics, 1994:III-11.
82. Berkhout B, Jeang K-T. Trans-activation of human immunodeficiency virus type 1 is sequence specific for both single-stranded bulge and loop of the trans-acting-—responsive hairpin: a quantitative analysis. J Virol 1989;63:5501.
83. Berkhout B, Silverman RH, Jeang K-T. Tat trans-activates the human immunodeficiency virus through a nascent RNA target. Cell 1989;59:273.
84. Dingwall C, Ernberg I, Gait MJ, et al. Human immunodeficiency virus 1 tat protein binds trans-activation-—response region (TAR) RNA in vitro. Proc Natl Acad Sci USA 1989;86:6925.
85. Feng S, Holland EC. HIV-1 tat trans-activation requires the loop sequence within TAR. Nature 1988;334:165.
86. Roy S, Delling U, Chen C-H, Rosen CA, Soneberg N. A bulge structure in HIV-1 TAR RNA is required for tat binding and tat-mediated trans-activation. Genes Dev 1990;4:1365.
87. Weeks KM, Ampe C, Schultz SC, Steitz TA, Crothers DM. Fragments of the HIV-1 Tat protein specifically bind TAR RNA. Science 249:1281.
88. Gatignol A, Buckler C, Jeang K-T. Relatedness of an RNA-binding motif in human immunodeficiency virus type 1 TAR RNA-binding protein TRBP to human P1/dsI kinase and Drosophila staufen. Mol Cell Biol 1993;13:2193.
89. Gatignol A, Buckler-White A, Berkhout B, Jeang K-T. Characterization of a human TAR RNA-binding protein that activates the HIV-1 LTR. Science 1991;251:1597.
90. Gatignol A, Kumar A, Rabson A, Jeang K-T. Identification of cellular proteins that bind to the human immunodeficiency virus type 1 trans-activation--response TAR element RNA. Proc Natl Acad Sci USA 1989;86:7828.
91. Gaynor R, Soultanakis E, Kuwabara M, Garcia J, Sigman D. Specific binding of HeLa cell nuclear protein to RNA sequences in the human immunodeficiency virus transactivating region. Proc Natl Acad Sci USA 1989;86:4858.
92. Han X-M, Laras A, Rounseville MP, Kumar A, Shank PR. Human immunodeficiency virus type I tat-mediated trans-activation correlates with the phosphorylation state of a cellular TAR RNA stem-binding factor. J Virol 1992;66:4065.
93. Marciniak RA, Calnan BJ, Frankel AD, Sharp PA. HIV-1 tat protein trans-activates transcription in vitro. Cell 1990;63:791.
94. Marciniak RA, Garcia-Blanco MA, Sharp PA. Identification and characterization of a HeLa nuclear protein that specifically binds to the trans-activation-—response (TAR) element of human immunodeficiency virus. Proc Natl Acad Sci USA 1990;87:3624.
95. Sheline CT, Milocco LH, Jones KA. Two distinct nuclear transcription factors recognize loop and bulge residues of the HIV-1 TAR RNA hairpin. Genes Dev 1991;5:2508.
96. Wu F, Garcia J, Sigman D, Gaynor R. Tat regulates binding of the human immunodeficiency virus trans-activating region RNA loop-binding protein TRP-185. Genes Dev 1991;5:2128.
97. Hart CE, Saltarelli MJ, Galphin JC, Schochetman G. A human chromosome 12-—associated 83-kilodalton cellular protein specifically binds to the loop region of human immunodeficiency virus type 1 trans-activation response element RNA. J Virol 1995;69:6593.
98. Martin MA. The molecular and biological properties of the human immunodeficiency virus. Mol Basis Blood Dis 1993;863.
99. Gruss P, Lia CJ, Dhar R, Khoury G. Splicing as a requirement for biogenesis of functional 16S mRNA of simian virus 40. Proc Natl Acad Sci USA 1979;76:4317.
100. Gruss P. Rescue of a splicing defective mutant by insertion of an heterologous intron. Nature 1980;286:634.
101. Lai CJ, Khoury G. Deletion mutants of simian virus 40 defective in biosynthesis of late viral mRNA. Proc Natl Acad Sci USA 1979;76:71.
102. Feinberg MB, Jarrett RF, Aldovini A, Gallo RC, Wong-Staal F. HTLV-III expression and production involve complex regulation at the levels of splicing and translation of viral RNA. Cell 1986;46:807.
103. Sodroski J, Goh WC, Rosen C, Dayton A, Terwilliger E, Haseltine W. A second post-transcriptional trans-activator gene required for HTLV-III replication. Nature 1986;321:412.
104. Parslow TG. Post-transcriptional regulation of human retroviral gene expression. In: Cullen BR, ed. Human retroviruses. Oxford: Oxford University Press, 1993:101.
105. Malim MH, Tiley L, McCarn D, Rusche J, Hauber J, Cullen BR. HIV-1 structural gene expression requires binding of the Rev trans-activator to its RNA target sequence. Cell 1990;60:675.
106. Heaphy S, Finch JT, Gait MJ, Karn J, Singh M. Human immunodeficiency virus type 1 regulator of virion expression, rev, forms nucleoprotein filaments after binding to a purine-rich "bubble" located within the rev-responsive region of viral mRNAs. Proc Natl Acad Sci USA 1991;88:7366.
107. Wingfield PT, Stahl SJ, Payton MA, Venkatesan S, Misra M, Steven AC. HIV-1 Rev expressed in recombinant Escherichia coli: purification, polymerization, and conformational properties. Biochemistry 1991;30:7527.
108. Lazinski D, Grzadzielska E, Das A. Sequence-specific recognition of RNA hairpins by bacteriophage antiterminators requires a conserved arginine-rich motif. Cell 1989;59:207.
109. Malim MH, Bohnlein S, Hauber J, Cullen BR. Functional dissection of the HIV-1 rev trans-activator: derivation of a trans-dominant repressor of rev function. Cell 1989;58:205.
110. Venkatesh LK, Chinnadurai G. Mutants in a conserved region near the carboxy-terminus of HIVÄ1 Rev identify functionally important

residues and exhibit a dominant negative phenotype. Virology 1990;178:327.

111. Chang DD, Sharp PA. Regulation by HIV Rev depends upon recognition of splice sites. Cell 1989;59:789.

112. Malim MH, Hauber J, Le S-Y, Maizel JV, Cullen BR. The HIV-1 rev trans-activator acts through a structured target sequence to activate nuclear export of unspliced viral mRNA. Nature 1989;338:254.

113. Felber BK, Hadzopoulou-Cladaras M, Cladaras C, Copeland T, Pavlakis GN. Rev protein of human immunodeficiency virus type 1 affects the stability and transport of the viral mRNA. Proc Natl Acad Sci USA 1989;86:1495.

114. Pomerantz RJ, Seshamma T, Trono D. Efficient replication of human immunodeficiency virus type 1 requires a threshold level of Rev: potential implications for latency. J Virol 1992;66:1809.

115. Malim MH, Cullen BR. HIV-1 structural gene expression requires the binding of multiple Rev monomers to the viral RRE: implications for HIV-1 latency. Cell 1991;65:241.

116. Seshamma T, Bagasra O, Trono D, Baltimore D, Pomerantz RJ. Blocked early-stage latency in the peripheral blood cells of certain individuals infected with human immunodeficiency virus type 1. Proc Natl Acad Sci USA 1992;89:10663.

117. Saksela K, Stevens C, Rubinstein P, Baltimore D. Human immunodeficiency virus type 1 mRNA expression in peripheral blood cells predicts disease progression independently of the numbers of CD4+ lymphocytes. Proc Natl Acad Sci USA 1994;91:1104.

118. Michael NL, Mo T, Merzouki A, et al. Human immunodeficiency virus type 1 cellular RNA load and splicing patterns predict disease progression in a longitudinally studied cohort. J Virol 1995;69:1868.

119. Felsenstein KM, Goff SP. Expression of the gag-pol fusion protein of Moloney murine leukemia virus without gag protein does not induce virion formation or proteolytic processing. J Virol 1988;62:2179.

120. Jacks T, Power MD, Masiarz FR, Luciw PA, Barr PJ, Varmus HE. Characterization of ribosomal frameshifting in HIV-1 gag-pol expression. Nature 1988;331:280.

121. Parkin NT, Chamorro M, Varmus HE. Human immunodeficiency virus type 1 gag-pol frameshifting is dependent on downstream mRNA secondary structure: demonstration of expression in vivo. J Virol 1992;66:5147.

122. Schwartz S, Felber BK, Pavlakis GN. Mechanism of translation of monocistronic and multicistronic human immunodeficiency virus type 1 mRNAs. Mol Cell Biol 1992;12:207.

123. Kozak M. The scanning model for translation: an update. J Cell Biol 1989;108:229.

124. Schwartz S, Felber BK, Fenyo EM, Pavlakis GN. Env and Vpu proteins of human immunodeficiency virus type 1 are produced from multiple bicistronic mRNAs. J Virol 1990;64:5448.

125. Purcell DFJ, Martin MA. Alternative splicing of human immunodeficiency virus type 1 mRNA modulates viral protein expression, replication, and infectivity. J Virol 1993;67:6365.

126. Trono D, Feinberg MG, Baltimore D. HIV-1 Gag mutants can dominantly interfere with the replication of the wild-type virus. Cell 1989;59:113.

127. Schultz AM, Oroszian S. In vivo modifications of retroviral gag gene-encoded polyproteins by myristic acid. J Virol 1983;46:355.

128. Chazal N, Gay B, Carrier C, Tournier J, Boulanger P. Human immunodeficiency virus type 1 MA deletion mutants expressed in baculovirus-infected cells: cis and trans effects on the gag precursor assembly pathway. J Virol 1995;69:365.

129. South TL, Blake PR, Sowder RC, Arthur LO, Henderson LE, Summers MF. The nucleocapsid protein isolated from HIV-1 particles binds zinc and forms retroviral-type zinc fingers. Biochemistry 1990;29:7786.

130. Tirumalai RS, Modak MJ. Photoaffinity labeling of the primer binding domain in murine leukemia virus reverse transcriptase. Biochemistry 1991;30:6436.

131. Huang Y, Mk J, Cao Q, Li Z, Wainberg MA, Kleiman L. Incorporation of excess wild-type and mutant tRNA3Lys into human immunodeficiency virus type 1. J Virol 1994;68:7676.

132. Dorfman T, Burkovsky A, Ohagen A, Hoglund S, Gottlinger HG. Functional domains of the capsid protein of human immunodeficiency virus type 1. J Virol 1994;68:8180.

133. Kaplan AH, Manchester M, Swanstrom R. The activity of protease of human immunodeficiency virus type 1 is initiated at the membrane of infected cells before the release of viral protein and is required for release to occur with maximum efficiency. J Virol 1994;68:6782.

134. Pettit SC, Moody MD, Wehbie RS, et al. The p2 domain of human immunodeficiency virus type 1 gag regulates sequential proteolytic processing and is required to produce fully infectious virions. J Virol 1994;68:8017.

135. Erickson-Viitanen S, Manfredi J, Viitanen P, et al. Cleavage of HIV-1 gag polyprotein synthesized in vitro: sequential cleavage by the viral protease. AIDS Res Hum Retroviruses 1989;5:577.

136. Dewar RL, Vasudevachi MB, Natarajan V, Salzman NP. Biosynthesis and processing of human immunodeficiency virus type 1 envelope glycoproteins: effects of monensin on glycosylation and transport. J Virol 1989;63:2452.

137. Earl PL, Doms RW, Moss B. Oligomeric structure of the human immunodeficiency virus type 1 envelope glycoprotein. Proc Natl Acad Sci USA 1990;87:648.

138. Dubay JW, Dubay SR, Shin H-J, Hunter E. Analysis of the cleavage site of the human immunodeficiency virus type 1 glycoprotein: requirement of precursor cleavage for glycoprotein incorporation. J Virol 1995;69:4675.

139. Willey RL, Klimkait T, Frucht DM, Bonifacino JS, Martin MA. Mutations within the human immunodeficiency virus type 1 gp160 envelope glycoprotein alter its intracellular transport and processing. Virology 1991;184:319.

140. Rhee SS, Hunter E. Myristylation is required for intracellular transport but not for assembly of D-type retrovirus capsids. J Virol 1987;61:1045.

141. Bednarik DP, Folks TM. Mechanisms of HIV-1 latency. AIDS 1992;6:3.

142. Folks T, Kelly J, Benn S, et al. Susceptibility of normal human lymphocytes to infection with HTLV-III/LAV. J Immunol 1986;136:4049.

143. Gaynor R. Cellular transcription factors involved in the regulation of HIV-1 gene expression. AIDS 1992;6:347.

144. Margolick JB, Volkman DJ, Folks TM, Fauci AS. Amplification of HTLV-III/LAV infection by antigen-induced activation of T cells and direct suppression by virus of lymphocyte blastogenic responses. J Immunol 1987;138:1719.

145. Butera ST, Folks TM. HIV-1 latency and activation in the pathogenesis of AIDS. In: Montagnier L, Gougeon M-L, eds. New concepts in AIDS pathogenesis. New York: Marcel Dekker, 1993:1.

146. Bentwich Z, Kalinkovich A, Weisman Z. Immune activation is a dominant factor in the pathogenesis of African AIDS. Immunol Today 1995;16:187.

147. Clouse KA, Powell D, Washington I, et al. Monokine regulation of human immunodeficiency virus-1 expression in a chronically infected human T cell clone. J Immunol 1989;142:431.

148. Folks TM, Justement J, Kinter A, Dinarello CA, Fauci AS. Cytokine-induced expression of HIV-1 in a chronically infected promonocyte cell line. Science 1987;238:800.

149. Butera ST, Perez VL, Wu B-Y, Nabel GJ, Folks TM. Oscillation of the human immunodeficiency virus surface receptor is regulated by the state of viral activation in a CD4+ cell model of chronic infection. J Virol 1991;65:4645.

150. Perez VL, Rowe T, Justement JS, Butera ST, June CH, Folks TM. An HIV-1-infected T cell clone defective in IL-2 production and Ca2+ mobilization after CD3 stimulation. J Immunol 1991;147:3145.

151. Tong-Starksen S, Peterlin BM. Mechanism of retroviral transcriptional activation. Semin Virol 1990;1:215.

152. Butera ST. Cytokine involvement in viral permissiveness and the progression of HIV diseases. J Cell Biochem 1993;53:336.

153. Pantaleo G, Graziosi C, Fauci AS. The immunopathogenesis of human immunodeficiency virus infection. N Engl J Med 1993;328:327.

154. Embretson J, Zupancic M, Ribas JL, et al. Massive covert infection of helper T lymphocytes and macrophages by HIV during the incubation period of AIDS. Nature 1993;362:359.

155. Wei X, Ghosh SK, Taylor ME, et al. Viral dynamics in human immunodeficiency virus type 1 infection. Nature 1995;373:117.

156. Ho DD, Neumann AU, Perelson AS, Chen W, Leonard JM, Markowitz M. Rapid turnover of plasma virions and CD4 lymphocytes in HIV-1 infection. Nature 1995;373:123.

157. Butera ST, Roberts BD, Lam L, Hodge T, Folks TM. Human immunodeficiency virus type 1 RNA expression by four chronically infected cell lines indicates multiple mechanisms of latency. J Virol 1994;68:2726.

158. Coffin JM. HIV population dynamics in vivo: implications for genetic variation, pathogenesis, and therapy. Science 1995;267:483.

159. Butera ST, Folks TM. Application of latent HIV-1 infected cellular models to therapeutic intervention. AIDS Res Hum Retroviruses 1992;8:991.

160. Hoxie JA, Haggerty BS, Rackowski JL, Pilsbury N, Levy JA. Persistent noncytopathic infection of human lymphocytes with AIDS associated retrovirus (ARV). Science 1985;229:1400.

161. Chapel A, Bensussan A, Vilmer V, Dormont D. Differential human immunodeficiency virus expression in CD4+ cloned lymphocytes. J Virol 1992;66:3966.

162. Levy DN, Refaeli Y, McGregor RR, Weiner DB. Serum Vpr regulates productive infection and latency of human immunodeficiency virus type 1. Proc Natl Acad Sci USA 1994;91:10873.

163. Spina CA, Kwoh TJ, Chowers MY, Guatelli JC, Richman DD. The importance of nef in the induction of human immunodeficiency virus type 1 replication from primary quiescent CD4 lymphocytes. J Exp Med 1994;179:115.

164. Miller MD, Warmerdam MT, Gaston I, Greene WC, Feinberg MB. The human immunodeficiency virus-1 nef gene product: a positive factor for viral infection and replication in primary lymphocytes and macrophages. J Exp Med 1994;179:101.

165. Zogury D, Gallo RC. Cytopathic effect of HIV in T4 cells is linked to the last stage of virus infection. Proc Natl Acad Sci USA 1988;85:3570.

166. Kowalski M, Potz J, Basiripour L, et al. Functional regions of the envelope glycoprotein of human immunodeficiency virus type 1. Science 1987;237:1351.

167. Sodroski J, Goh WC, Rosen C, Campbell K, Haseltine WA. Role of the HTLV-III/LAV envelope in syncytium formation and cytopathicity. Nature 1986;322:470.

168. Miller MA, Garry RF, Jaynes JM, Montelaro RC. A structural correlation between lentivirus transmembrane proteins and natural cytolytic peptides. AIDS Res Hum Retroviruses 1991;7:511.

169. Tencza SB, Miller MA, Islam K, Mietzner TA, Montelaro RC. Effect of amino acid substitutions on calmodulin binding and cytolytic properties of the LLP-1 peptide segment of human immunodeficiency virus type 1 transmembrane protein. J Virol 1995;69:5199.

170. Groux H, Torpier G, Monte D, Mouton Y, Capron A, Ameisen JC. Activation-induced death by apoptosis in CD4+ T cells from human immunodeficiency virus-infected asymptomatic individuals. J Exp Med 1992;175:331.

171. Laurent-Crawford AG, Krust B, Muller S, et al. The cytopathic effect of HIV is associated with apoptosis. Virology 1991;185:829.

172. Banda NK, Bernier J, Kurahara DK, et al. Crosslinking CD4 by HIV gp120 primes T cells for activation-induced apoptosis. J Exp Med 1992;176:1099.

173. Westendorp MO, Frank R, Ochsenbauer C, et al. Sensitization of T cells to CD95-mediated apoptosis by HIV-1 Tat and gp120. Nature 1995;375:497.

174. Larder BA, Darby G, Richman DD. HIV with reduced sensitivity to zidovudine (AZT) isolated during prolonged therapy. Science 1989;243:1731.

175. Craig JC, Duncan IB, Hockley D, Grief C, Roberts NA, Mills JS. Antiviral properties of Ro 31-8959, an inhibitor of human immunodeficiency virus (HIV) proteinase. Antiviral Res 1991;16:295.

176. Li CJ, Dezube BJ, Biswas DK, Ahlers CM, Pardee AB. Inhibitors of HIV-1 transcription. Trends Microbiol 1994;2:164.

177. Hoglund S, Ohagen A, Lawrence K, Gabuzda D. Role of vif during packing of the core of HIV-1. Virology 1994;201:349.

178. Klimkait T, Strebel K, Hoggan D, Martin MA, Orenstein JM. The human immunodeficiency virus type 1-specific protein vpu is required for efficient virus maturation and release. J Virol 1990;64:621.

179. Willey RL, Maldarelli F, Martin MA, Strebel K. Human immunodeficiency virus type 1 Vpu protein induces rapid degradation of CD4. J Virol 1992;66:7193.

180. Strebel K, Saughtery D, Clouse K, Cohen D, Folks T, Martin MA. A novel gene of HIV-1, vpu, and its 16 kilodalton product. Science 1988;241:1221.

181. Aiken C, Konner J, Landau NR, Lenburg ME, Trono D. Nef induces CD4 endocytosis: requirement for a critical dileucine motif in the membrane-proximal CD4 cytoplasmic domain. Cell 1994;76:853.

182. Schwartz O, Dautry-Varsat A, Goud B, et al. Human immunodeficiency virus type 1 Nef induces accumulation of CD4 in early endosomes. J Virol 1995;69:528.

183. Sawai ET, Baur A, Struble H, Peterlin BM, Levy JA. Human immunodeficiency virus type 1 Nef associates with a cellular serine kinase in T-lymphocytes. Proc Natl Acad Sci U S A 1994;91:1539.

184. Aiken C, Trono D. Nef stimulates human immunodeficiency virus type 1 proviral DNA synthesis. J Virol 1995;69:5048.

AIDS: Biology, Diagnosis, Treatment and Prevention, fourth edition, edited by Vincent T. DeVita, Jr., Samuel Hellman, and Steven A. Rosenberg. Lippincott–Raven Publishers, © 1997

CHAPTER 3

The Molecular Biology of Human Immunodeficiency Virus Type 1

George N. Pavlakis

The causative agent of acquired immunodeficiency syndrome (AIDS), human immunodeficiency virus type 1 (HIV-1), is a retrovirus of the lentivirus subfamily. Although a lentivirus (ie, equine infectious anemia virus) was one of the first known viral agents,[1] the study of lentiviruses intensified after the discovery of HIV-1[2,3] and its similarity to other lentiviruses.[4,5]

The lentiviruses are exogenous, nononcogenic retroviruses causing persistent (ie, chronic/active) infections; the diseases have long incubation periods. These viruses usually infect cells of the immune system, such as macrophages and T cells, and have cytopathic effects in permissive cells, such as syncytia and cell death. Lentiviral infections are not cleared by the immune system, and their damage accumulates over many years. This important characteristic is reflected in the name of the subfamily; *lenti* means slow. Lentiviruses have a larger RNA genome (approximately 10 kilobases [kb]), which encodes additional proteins. They produce a large and heavily glycosylated envelope protein (Env) and, in the case of HIVs, a magnesium ion (Mg^{2+})-dependent reverse transcriptase. They encode essential regulatory and accessory genes that allow regulation of their own expression in the infected cell. Unlike other retroviruses, lentiviruses can infect nondividing cells.

Many lentiviruses affect the immune system, causing acquired immunodeficiency. The ovine and caprine lentiviruses primarily infect monocytes, and the viral DNA is integrated into the cellular DNA. The provirus remains silent until the monocyte matures into a macrophage.[6] Equine infectious anemia virus also infects macrophages, but the feline, simian, and human immunodeficiency viruses primarily infect T lymphocytes. Replication of the lentiviruses usually is toxic to the cell and leads to cell dysfunction and death. The structure and replication properties of the lentiviruses may be the reason that the immune system is unable to eliminate the infection.

Many structural and functional properties of HIV-1 are common to all retroviruses. Initial studies on the AIDS virus benefited greatly from the existing knowledge on oncoretroviruses. During the past decade, the discovery of the AIDS virus triggered detailed studies of its structure, replication, and pathogenic properties. As a result, HIV-1 is probably the most intensely studied virus. We have detailed knowledge of its molecular biology and thus it serves as the prototype retrovirus. Several conclusions about HIV-1 are applicable to other retroviruses and have increased our understanding of many other cellular and viral systems.

The vast literature about HIV-1 makes any attempt for comprehensive citation difficult. This chapter, which examines the molecular biology of HIV, focuses more intensely on new developments in the field. Many thorough reviews on general and specialized aspects of HIV biology exist and should be consulted for additional information and citations.

Because the continuous replication of HIV-1 is generally accepted as the underlying cause of the development of immunodeficiency, inhibition of HIV-1 replication should lead to inhibition or moderation of symptomatic disease. Understanding the biology of this virus has therefore become a priority. The detailed analysis of viral function at the molecular level may lead to opportunities for targeted antiviral intervention.

George N. Pavlakis: Human Retrovirus Section, ABL-Basic Research Program, Bldg. 539, Room 121, NCI-FCRDC, P.O. Box B, Frederick, MD 21702-1201.

By acceptance of this article, the publisher or recipient acknowledges the right of the U.S. Government and its agents and contractors to retain a nonexclusive, royalty-free license in and to any copyright covering the article.

GENOME AND VIRION STRUCTURE

Retroviruses are enveloped, positive-strand (ie, having as the genome the same strand as the mRNA) RNA viruses that rely on a unique enzyme, reverse transcriptase, to convert their RNA genome into a DNA "provirus," which is integrated into the cellular genome. The viral envelope is a lipid bilayer that is produced by the cellular plasma membrane and contains the protruding viral Env glycoprotein. The core viral particle is composed of the p24 capsid (CA) protein and contains the viral RNA and enzymes.

The genomic organization of HIV-1 is shown in Figure 3-1. All retroviruses have in common the three coding regions *gag*, *pol*, and *env*, which encode the capsid proteins (Gag), the viral enzymes necessary for replication (Pol), and the external glycoprotein (Env) that protrudes out of the lipid viral envelope and is responsible for the infectivity of the viral particle by means of attachment to specific cellular receptors. The viral enzymes encoded by *pol* are reverse transcriptase, integrase, and protease.

Retroviruses have one promoter and one polyadenylation site within the long terminal repeats (LTRs) and express one primary transcript. An exception to this rule has been detected by the identification of an internal promoter in spumaretroviruses.[7-9] The location of the polyadenylation signal and processing site are such that they allow efficient polyadenylation only at the 3' LTR. In some retroviruses, this is achieved by the localization of the AAUAAA polyadenylation signal within the U3 region, and in others a specific secondary structure is responsible for the formation of an efficient polyadenylation site. In HIV-1, U3 and U5 region elements appear to be responsible for polyadenylation at the 3' LTR.[10-13]

To produce many proteins from a single primary transcript, the retroviruses use different strategies: generation and proteolytic processing of precursor polyproteins; ribosomal frameshifting or suppression of translation termination; alternative splicing of the primary transcript; and bicistronic mRNAs producing two proteins.

The additional proteins expressed by HIV-1 (Table 3-1) are part of the viral particle (ie, Vif, Vpr, Vpx), regulate directly viral gene expression (ie, Tat, Rev), or interact with the cellular machinery to promote virus propagation (ie, Vpu, Nef). The additional proteins increase the complexity of the organization and expression of HIV and the other lentiviruses. It has been proposed that the lentiviruses be included in a subgroup of retroviruses named complex retroviruses, together with the human T-cell leukemia virus family of primate oncoretroviruses.[14,15] The distinguishing characteristic of the complex retroviruses is the ability to regulate their own expression through virally encoded protein factors. This property appears to be essential for the long-term association of the complex retroviruses with the host and generation of chronic active infections.

VIRAL LIFE CYCLE

The retroviral life cycle is depicted in Figure 3-2. After the virus attaches to the cell and penetrates the plasma mem-

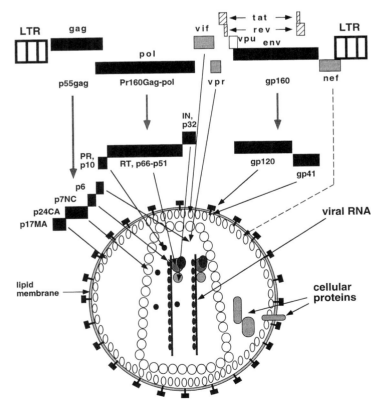

FIG. 3-1. Genomic organization and virion structure of HIV-1.

TABLE 3-1. *Human immunodeficiency virus and simian immunodeficiency virus proteins*

Name	Size	Function	Localization
Gag MA	p17	Membrane anchoring, Env interaction, nuclear transport of viral core (myristylated protein)	Virion
Gag CA	p24	Core capsid	Virion
Gag NC	p7	Nucleocapsid, binds RNA	Virion
	p6	Binds Vpr	Virion
Protease	p15	Gag-Pol cleavage and maturation	Virion
Reverse Transcriptase, RNase H	p66 p51 (heterodimer)	Reverse transcription, RNase H activity	Virion
Integrase		DNA provirus integration	Virion
Env	gp 120/gp41	External viral glycoproteins bind to CD4 receptor	Plasma membrane, virion envelope
Tat	p16/p14	Viral trancriptional transactivator	Primarily in nucleolus/ nucleus
Rev	p19	RNA transport, stability and factor (phosphoprotein)	Primarily in nucleolus/ nucleus use shuttling between nucleolus and cytoplasm
Vif	p23	Promotes virion maturation and infectivity	Cytoplasm (cytosol, membranes), virion
Vpr	p10–15	Promotes nuclear localization of preintegration complex, inhibits cell division, arrests infected cells at G_2/M	Virion, nucleus (nuclear membrane?)
Vpu	p16	Promotes extracellular release of viral particles, degrades CD4 in the endoplasmic reticulum (phosphoprotein); only in HIV-1 and SIVcpz	Integral membrane protein
Nef	p27/p25	CD4 downregulation (myristylated protein)	Plasma membrane, cytoplasm (virion?)
Vpx	p12–16	Virion protein, vpr homologue (not in HIV-1, only in HIV-2 and SIV)	Virion (nucleus?)
Tev	p28	Tripartite Tat–Env–Rev protein (also named Tnv)	Primarily in nucleolus/ nucleus

brane, reverse transcriptase converts the viral RNA to DNA. This DNA is transported to the nucleus and integrated into the cellular DNA by the viral integrase. Because of the replication characteristics of the retroviruses, the proviral DNA is flanked by tandemly repeated sequences, LTRs, that have important regulatory functions.

After integration, the retroviral DNA (provirus) uses the cellular transcription machinery to express viral RNA that has two essential roles: it serves as the genomic RNA that is incorporated in the virion and as the messenger RNA that produces all the viral proteins. The genomic RNA and the viral proteins are assembled into the viral particle, which buds out of the cell and infects new cells by attaching to specific cellular receptors.

Virus Entry

HIV-1 Env binds to the surface receptor CD4, a member of the Ig superfamily.[16–19] CD4 is found in T lymphocytes, monocytes, B lymphocytes, and other cells and is also the receptor for HIV-2 and simian immunodeficiency virus (SIV).[20] Expression of human CD4 in human CD4-negative (CD4−) cells by DNA transfection was necessary and sufficient for HIV-1 infection, while mouse cells expressing human CD4 were not infected by HIV-1.[18] Additional unidentified factors in human,

but not mouse, cells are necessary for infection. Although CD4 is the primary receptor for HIV-1, alternative receptors for HIV-1 entry in CD4− cells have also been identified; for instance, the sphingolipid galactosyl ceramide mediates infection of CD4− cells of neural or epithelial origin.[21]

CD4 is a transmembrane glycoprotein of 58 kd (Fig. 3-3). The Env-binding site on the CD4 glycoprotein has been mapped to amino acids 40 through 82. CD4 contributes to T-cell recognition of foreign antigens in the context of class II major histocompatibility complex (MHC) determinants. CD4 was shown to interact with MHC class II molecules and with the T-cell receptor. Specific activation of T cells by antigen presentation induces the CD4–T-cell receptor cointernalization. CD4 is associated with p56[lck], an internal membrane tyrosine protein kinase and a member of the Src family of tyrosine kinases.[22] Signal transduction through the CD4 receptor involves the activation of p56[lck]. CD4 interaction with Env is of paramount importance for HIV-1 and leads to infection and CD4 dysregulation. This affects the function of T cells and eventually leads to depletion of the CD4-positive (CD4+) subset of T cells and to immunodeficiency. The importance of the Env-CD4 interaction for HIV is further underscored by the multiple mechanisms that lead to CD4 modulation: Env, Vpu, and Nef interact with and affect CD4 at various stages.

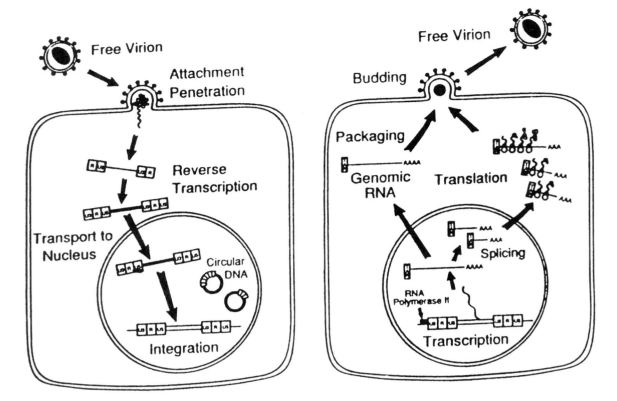

FIG. 3-2. Schematic diagram of the retrovirus life cycle. (Reproduced from Haseltine WA. Molecular biology of HIV-1. In: AIDS, etiology, diagnosis, treatment, and prevention. DeVita VT, Jr., Hellman S, Rosenberg SA, eds. Philadelphia: JB Lippincott, 1992:39.)

Virus entry requires fusion of the virus and cell membrane, which is mediated by the N-terminal hydrophobic region of the Env transmembrane subunit.[23–25] Unlike other retroviruses, HIV-1 Env promotes fusion at the near-neutral pH of the extracellular milieu. Env is also responsible for the formation of syncytia, which is the result of membrane fusion among many cells.

DNA Provirus Synthesis

After virus entry, the viral capsid is disrupted and the viral reverse transcriptase is fully activated. Experimental evidence suggests that reverse transcription of HIV-1 may be initiated within the virion.[26,27] A ribonucleoprotein complex (ie, preintegration complex) is formed in the cytoplasm of the infected cell and is responsible for reverse transcription and transport to the nucleus. This ribonucleoprotein complex contains the genomic RNA, the nucleocapsid (NC) and matrix (MA) proteins, and the viral enzymes reverse transcriptase and integrase.[28]

During reverse transcription, the two RNA molecules in the virion are converted to a linear double-stranded DNA.[29,30] The process of reverse transcription requires priming provided by tRNA^{lys3}, which is annealed to the primer-binding site (PBS) at the 5' part of the viral genome during particle formation. tRNA^{lys3} is selectively incorporated in the HIV-1

virion, which contains approximately eight molecules of tRNA^{lys3} per two copies of genomic RNA. The Pr160$^{gag-pol}$ precursor is involved in primer tRNA^{lys3} incorporation into virion. Viral particles containing only unprocessed Pr55^{gag} protein did not selectively incorporate tRNA^{lys3}, and virions containing unprocessed Pr55^{gag} and Pr160$^{gag-pol}$ proteins demonstrated selective tRNA^{lys3} packaging. The PBS is not required for the selective incorporation of tRNA^{lys3}.[31] Six base pairs at the ends of the PBS are sufficient for reverse transcription; mismatches in PBS can be tolerated.[32]

Elongation at the PBS generates a nascent DNA molecule of approximately 630 nucleotides (nt) (ie, minus-strand strong-stop DNA; Fig. 3-4, *step 1*), spanning the region from the PBS to the CAP site at the 5' end of the viral RNA. The RNA part of the RNA-DNA hybrid is specifically degraded by the ribonuclease H (RNase H) activity of reverse transcriptase, leaving the 3' end of the strong-stop DNA free to anneal to the R region of the second RNA molecule *(step 2)*. This template "jump" requires components of the viral capsid[33] and depends on the affinity of reverse transcriptase for its template. After this jump, elongation by reverse transcriptase results in a near-complete DNA copy terminating at the PBS *(step 3)*, because the R and U5 regions have been removed by the RNase H.

The synthesis of the complementary (plus-strand) DNA is initiated at the junction between the polypurine tract

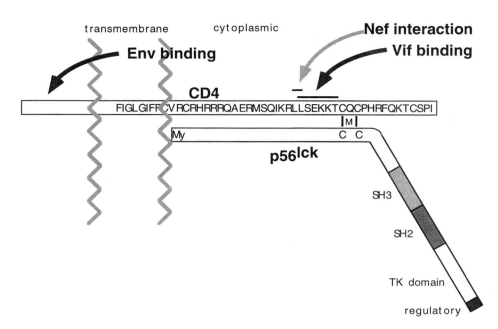

FIG. 3-3. CD4 interaction with cellular and viral components. In addition to Env binding, CD4 cytoplasmic domain binds Vpu and interacts directly or indirectly with Nef. Both of these interactions result in a decrease of CD4 protein. The cytoplasmic domain of CD4 interacts also with p56^{lck}, a Tyr-kinase that is responsible for signal transduction. The Src homology (SH2, SH3, tyrosine kinase (TK d), and regulatory domains of p56^{lck} are shown. *My*, myristyl residue; *M*, metal ion shared between Cys pairs on CD4 and p56^{lck}.

(PPT) and the U5 region of the LTR. The PPT is highly conserved among the known HIV-1 isolates. Specific cleavage of the RNA-DNA hybrid at this site *(step 4)* initiates the plus-strand DNA synthesis *(step 5)*, which terminates within the PBS. Copying of the PBS and removal of the RNA by RNase H generates a DNA molecule that can anneal to the 3′ end of the opposite DNA strand at the

minus-strand pbs *(step 6)*. This second template jump allows elongation of the plus-strand DNA to the end of a complete LTR. The completion of DNA synthesis *(step 7)* results in a linear molecule with one complete LTR at each end. This is the template for integration after transfer to the nucleus. Side products of this process are circular molecules containing one or two LTRs, which can be detected

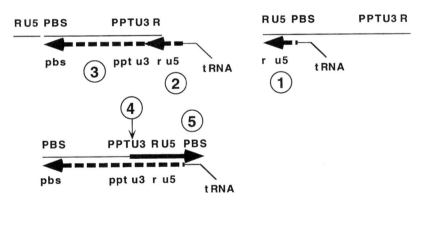

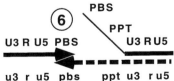

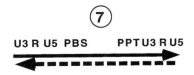

FIG. 3-4. Steps in retroviral reverse transcription. The thin lines represent RNA, and the thick lines represent DNA. Solid lines represent the plus-strand and dotted lines represent the minus-strand. *R*, repeat region on the viral mRNA and the LTR; *U5* and *U3*, unique 5′ and 3′ regions on the viral mRNA; *PBS*, primer binding site for tRNA binding; *PPT*, polypurine tract. Small letters indicate the same elements in the opposite strand.

after acute infection by HIV-1. These molecules are not able to integrate but may express proteins if transported into the nucleus.

In summary, HIV-1 uses two RNA priming sites (ie, PBS, PPT) to initiate the synthesis of the minus- and plus-strand strong-stop DNAs. These DNAs are involved in specific template jumps, allowing elongation of the DNA and completion of reverse transcription.

Nuclear Transport and Integration

The double-stranded proviral DNA complexed with proteins (ie, preintegration complex) is transported to the nucleus of the infected cell. The proviral DNA is integrated at random sites throughout the cellular genome by the action of viral integrase. Unlike oncoretroviruses, HIV-1 can enter the nucleus of nondividing cells such as differentiated macrophages. The two viral proteins important for nuclear transport are the phosphorylated MA protein and Vpr.[28,34-38]

Gene Expression

The integrated provirus flanked by the tandem LTRs (see Fig. 3-1) is organized as a eukaryotic transcriptional unit. The 5' LTR contains a strong enhancer-promoter and the 3' LTR contains an efficiently used polyadenylation site. Transcription of the provirus by the cellular RNA polymerase II results in a primary transcript that has two important functions: it serves as the genomic RNA that is incorporated into the virion, and it is processed to provide all the mRNAs encoding the viral proteins. The HIV-1 promoter is highly regulated by viral and cellular factors. Its activity varies greatly, depending on the cell status. In many infected cells in HIV-positive individuals, virus expression is undetectable. A state of viral latency exists in individual cells, although the infection is chronically active because of continuous expression of HIV in a fraction of cells.

The viral protein Tat greatly increases the expression of the HIV promoter. Tat function leads to high mRNA expression early after productive infection. Whereas Tat activation leads to mostly spliced HIV-1 mRNAs, the posttranscriptional regulatory Rev protein regulates the balance of spliced to unspliced and partially spliced mRNAs. Rev activation leads to the late stage of viral expression, in which the unspliced and partially spliced HIV-1 mRNAs predominate and efficiently express all the viral proteins. Rev function leads to a balanced expression of viral proteins through negative feedback, whereas Rev dysfunction leads to virus fixed in an early, nonproductive pattern of gene expression. Human cells with this pattern of expression have been identified.[39,40] In most cells, the transition from the early stage of viral expression (ie, Tat production and mostly spliced mRNAs) to the late stage (ie, Tat and Rev production and efficient expression of all the viral mRNAs) happens rapidly, within hours from the onset of expression. Although many cells containing the HIV genome but not expressing any

viral proteins can be detected, only a few cells appear to be blocked at the early stage of viral expression.[41]

Virion Assembly

The expressed structural proteins accumulate inside the plasma membrane. Pr55^{gag} associates with the plasma membrane through N-terminal myristic acid and possibly other sites within the MA protein. Gag also interacts with Env, which is embedded in the plasma membrane. Pr55^{gag} multimerization results in the initiation of particle formation. Together with the Pr55^{gag}, some Pr160$^{gag-pol}$ is incorporated into the virion. Two molecules of genomic RNA are also encapsidated with tRNA molecules, primarily tRNA^{lys3}. The integration of Pr160$^{gag-pol}$ into the particle leads to protease dimerization and activation. The orderly cleavage of Pr160$^{gag-pol}$ and Pr55^{gag} leads to particle maturation and budding. This is an essential step for production of infectious virions, because immature viral particles containing the precursor molecules are noninfectious. Cleavage also initiates the maturation and activation of the other viral enzymes. Reverse transcriptase is associated with the tRNA–viral RNA complex and initiates reverse transcription if nucleotide triphosphates are available. The accessory proteins Vif and Vpr (and possibly Nef) are incorporated into the virion along with cellular proteins. In some cases, these cellular proteins (eg, cyclophilin A) may be important for viral infectivity.

VIRAL PROMOTERS

In an arrangement similar to that of several inducible cellular promoters (eg, lymphokine promoters), the potent HIV-1 promoter contains a TATA box and binding sites for cellular DNA-binding transcriptional factors (Fig. 3-5), including sites for NF-kB and Sp1.[42-46] These transcriptional factors are essential for promoter function. There are two tandem NF-kB binding sites (positions −104 and −90) and three Sp1 binding sites (positions −78 to −47). Deletion of the Sp1 sites reduces the enhancer activity.[42,47] Deletion of both NF-kB sites also reduces activity, but retention of one NF-kB site is enough for full promoter activity.[48] The minimal promoter element must contain one NF-kB site, the Sp1 sites, a TATA box, the transcription initiation site, and the Tat-reponsive element (TAR).

The HIV-1 promoter is highly inducible and responds to the activation status of the infected cell. NF-kB is the major inducible activator. Binding sites for several other factors such as NFAT and AP1 have been identified within the U3 region. Functionally, only the Sp1, NF-kB, Ap2, and HIP-1 sites were shown to affect expression of the HIV-1 promoter in human cells.[49] These interactions link HIV-1 expression to the activation of T-cell–specific genes and contribute to the observed biologic properties of the virus. The cellular factors interacting with the promoter have been studied intensely and are the subject of several reviews.[50-52]

Many cells in the lymphoid tissue of infected individuals are latently infected by HIV-1,[53,54] although viral replication

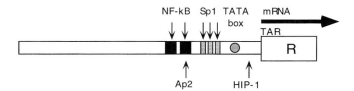

FIG. 3-5. HIV promoter. The sites for factors known to be essential for HIV-1 promoter activity are indicated.

in the body is always active. In resting T cells, the activity of the HIV-1 promoter is minimal, which is one of the important mechanisms leading to viral quiescence in most infected primary cells. Cell activation is associated with viral activation. Because of the low basal LTR activity in resting T lymphocytes, NF-kB–dependent transactivation is necessary for induction of the HIV-1 LTR and for virus propagation. CD4 T lymphocytes infected with a mutant HIV-1 carrying inactivating point mutations in the NF-kB–responsive elements did not show detectable transcriptional activity upon cell activation and prolonged culture in vitro.[55]

HIV-1 employs a second essential regulatory step provided by the viral Tat protein. Tat binds to the TAR RNA element at the beginning of the viral RNA transcript and greatly increases transcription. The fully activated HIV-1 promoter is one of the most potent promoters known in human cells.

REGULATORY SIGNALS ON VIRAL RNA

Many important sites have been identified on HIV-1 RNA that are essential in the life cycle of the virus (Fig. 3-6). They include positively acting RNA elements (ie, TAR and Rev-responsive element [RRE]) and negatively acting elements that inhibit HIV expression (ie, INS or CRS). These negative elements downregulate expression by interfering with the stability, transport, and translatability of the viral mRNAs. Rev function relieves this block, resulting in efficient structural protein expression. The polyadenylation signal site is found twice in the RNA within the R regions, but only the site at the 3' end of the mRNA is used efficiently for polyadenylation.

In addition to sites important for expression, the viral mRNA contains several sites necessary for other steps in the viral life cycle, such as genomic RNA dimerization and encapsidation (ie, psi site), and priming sites for reverse transcriptase (ie, PBS for minus-strand priming and PPT for plus-strand priming). PPT is found twice within the RNA: at the junction of U3 and within the *int* coding region.

The splice sites and exons identified within HIV-1 are shown in Figure 3-7. Like the other lentiviruses, HIV-1 contains many splice sites compared with oncoretroviruses. The precise control of splicing is essential for retroviruses, because they require the unspliced mRNA for encapsidation into the viral particle to be used as genomic RNA. Splicing of HIV-1 does not occur rapidly in vitro or in vivo,[56] allowing regulation at this level. Slow splicing allows the binding of nuclear factors to the unspliced and partially spliced mRNAs and their transport to the cytoplasm

by means of Rev, which cycles between the nucleolus and the cytoplasm.[57–60]

VIRAL MESSENGER RNAS

The HIV-1 primary transcript, produced by the cellular RNA polymerase II, is capped at the 5' end and polyadenylated at the 3' end. A portion of the RNA transcript is alternatively spliced to more than 30 different species producing viral proteins.[61–68]

Despite the great complexity in the HIV-1 mRNAs, for regulatory purposes two classes of these mRNAs can be differentiated (see Fig. 3-7). The first class, including the unspliced and intermediate-spliced mRNAs, contains the RRE and depends on Rev protein for efficient expression. These mRNAs encode Gag, Pol, Vif, Vpr, Vpu, Env, and Tat-1 (the one-exon Tat). The second class comprises the small multiply spliced mRNAs, which lack RRE and the sequences from the *gag/pol* and *env* regions. These mRNAs are expressed efficiently in the absence of Rev and encode Tat (Tat-2), Rev, and Nef proteins, as well as Vpr and other variant products such as Tev.

Detailed analyses of the mRNAs produced by HIV-1 and the expressed proteins have underscored the importance of regulation at the level of mRNA expression. The genomes of other lentiviruses, such as SIV, visna, caprine arthritis-encephalitis virus, and feline immunodeficiency virus, share this complex organization and regulation. Production of the differentially spliced mRNAs is governed by the interaction of the viral regulatory proteins Tat and Rev with *cis*-acting elements on the mRNAs (ie, TAR and RRE).

Monocistronic (eg, *gag-pol, tat, tat-1*) and bicistronic (eg, *rev/nef, vpu/env*) mRNAs have been identified. In general, each viral protein is produced by more than one mRNA. These mRNAs are alternatively spliced and encode one of the proteins as the first open reading frame (ORF), resulting in optimal expression. The exceptions to this general rule are that the Gag-Pol precursor is produced only by the single unspliced mRNA by ribosomal frameshifting, and Env is produced as the second ORF by bicistronic *vpu/env* mRNAs.[65,66,69] The arrangement for Env expression in HIV-1 is unexpected, because in general, retroviral Env proteins are abundant and are expressed by dedicated monocistronic mRNAs. This arrangement underlines the functional link between Vpu and Env and the need for coordinate expression of the two proteins. Vpu degrades CD4 and promotes Env trafficking from the Golgi to the plasma membrane.

LANDMARKS ON THE HIV-1 GENOMIC RNA

GENES

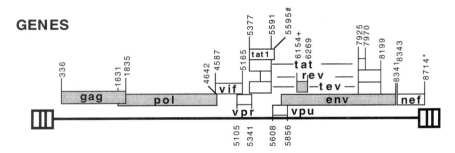

RNA SITES

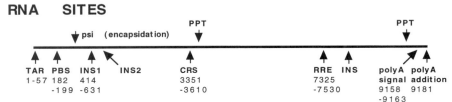

SPLICE SITES AND EXONS

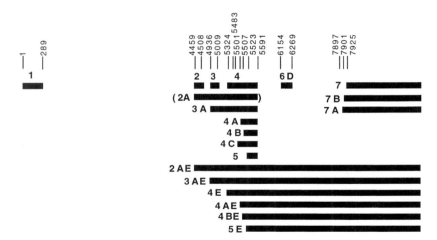

FIG. 3-6. Important functional sites on HIV-1 genomic RNA. Numbers indicate the location of the various genes and elements in the molecular HIV-1 clone HXB2R. This molecular clone has defective or variant *vpr, vpu,* and *nef* genes and expresses Tev, a "hybrid" Tat and Rev molecule with dual function. The splice sites known to be used in the production of the HIV mRNAs are shown.

In addition to mRNAs shown in Figure 3-7, several other minor species have been identified by cloning and sequencing.[63–68,70] Some of these mRNAs can encode variant proteins, such as the additional regulatory protein named Tev or Tnv that has Tat and Rev activities.[63,67] Tev is reminiscent of the regulatory proteins of some DNA viruses, which contain several independent functional domains.

Most of the studies of HIV-1 expression have been performed with laboratory isolates or molecular clones of HIV-1. The development of efficient RNA amplification methods using polymerase chain reaction (PCR) protocols has allowed the study of HIV-1 transcription directly in cells of infected individuals. Extensive splicing variation in the quantities and types of RNA species has been detected among the different HIV-1 strains and in infected individuals (M.J. Saltarelli, G.N. Pavlakis, unpublished data).[39,68,70] This variation suggests that virus production can take place within a broad range of mRNA levels.

The different HIV-1 isolates vary widely in their biologic characteristics such as tropism, levels of expression, and cytopathicity. Because of the extensive splicing variation of the primary isolates, it is conceivable that some of the variability in the biologic properties of different HIV-1 strains may be the result of splicing differences.

STRUCTURAL PROTEINS

Gag Proteins

The Gag precursor Pr55^{gag} forms the core viral particle and interacts with other viral and cellular components, including RNA, Pol and Env proteins, and the plasma membrane, to facilitate their incorporation into the budding viral particle. Pr55^{gag} is a self-associating protein capable of assembling into virion-like particles without the requirement of any other viral factors. In addition to Gag precursor, a Gag-Pol fusion protein (Pr160$^{gag-pol}$) is produced by ribosomal

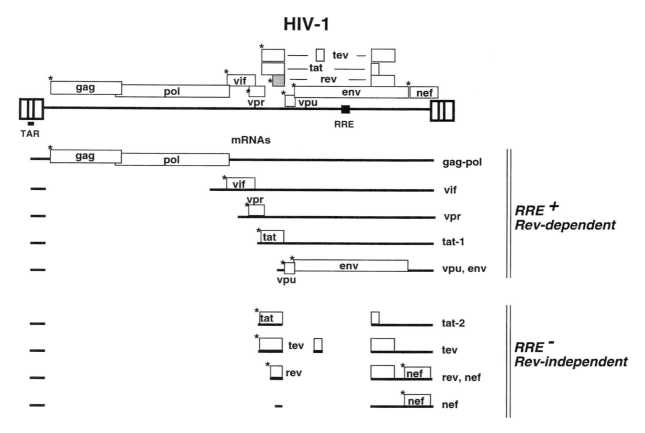

FIG. 3-7. Representative types of mRNAs produced by HIV-1. They are distinguished in three size classes (unspliced, partially spliced or intermediate, and multiply spliced), and two functional groups, Rev-dependent and Rev-independent.

frameshifting. The self-associating properties of the Gag portion also direct the incorporation of some molecules of the Gag-Pol fusion protein into the forming particle (Fig. 3-8). During or shortly after assembly, the protease is activated, and the Gag precursor is cleaved into four proteins (ie, matrix [p17^{MA}], capsid [p24^{CA}], nucleocapsid [p7^{NC}], and p6^{gag}) and two small peptides (ie, p1^{gag} and p2^{gag}; Fig. 3-9). The proteolytic cleavage products form the core of the mature virus. Pr160$^{gag-pol}$ polyprotein is also cleaved by protease into the Gag components and several active enzymes: protease, reverse transcriptase, and integrase.

Figure 3-9 indicates posttranslational modifications, proteolytic cleavages, and sites for various interactions of the HIV-1 Gag and Gag-Pol precursors. Proteolytic cleavage by cellular and viral enzymes, myristylation, and phosphorylation of the Gag precursor are essential steps in the viral life cycle. After translation of the Gag precursor, the initiator Met residue is removed, and a myristoyl group is attached to the amino group of Gly2 by cellular enzymes. The p17^{MA} and p24^{CA} proteins are phosphorylated by cellular kinases. The p7^{NC} protein binds two zinc ions to form the two zinc fingers of the NC domain, which are necessary for protein-RNA interactions.

Gag interacts with additional cellular factors, which are essential for formation of infectious virions. A region between residues 178 and 300 in the CA domain of the Gag precursor has been shown to bind cyclophilin A,[71] a peptidyl-prolyl *cis-trans* isomerase thought to play a role in immune regulation. This protein has been found in purified HIV-1 virions (L. Henderson, personal communication). Viral particles formed by Pr55^{gag}, in contrast to particles formed by the Gag polyproteins of other retroviruses, contain significant amounts of cyclophilin A. Mutation of the cyclophilin A–binding domain results in noninfectious viral particles.[72,73] Cyclosporine and cyclosporine analogs disrupt the binding of cyclophilin A to Gag and inhibit HIV-1 replication. In contrast, a cyclosporine analog was shown to be inactive against SIV$_{mac}$, which does not incorporate cyclophilin A.[73] Moreover, a cyclosporine analog (SDZ NIM 811) that is completely devoid of immunosuppressive capacity was found to have potent and selective anti-HIV-1 activity. SDZ NIM 811 may interfere with Gag–cyclophilin A interaction and affect the infectivity of the virions and early events of viral nuclear transport and integration.[74]

The arrangement of the Gag-Pol transcription and translation unit is essential for packaging the viral enzymes en-

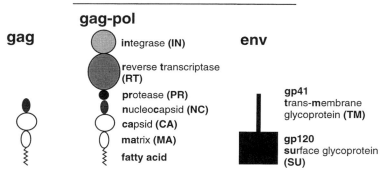

HIV-1 POLYPROTEINS

CAPSID FORMATION

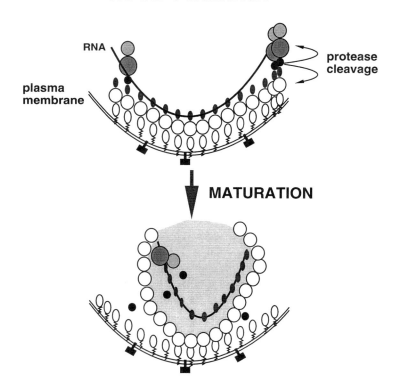

FIG. 3-8. HIV-1 capsid assembly and maturation. The involved precursor proteins Gag, Gag-Pol, and Env are schematically depicted at the top.

coded by *pol*. The *pol*-encoded products are expressed as a Gag-Pol fusion protein after a −1 ribosomal frameshifting, which happens at a frequency of approximately 5%. A stem-loop structure 3′ of the HIV-1 shift site is important for wild-type levels of frameshifting in vivo.[75] In vitro studies did not show the importance of the 3′ stem-loop structure for frameshifting.[76] The resulting fusion protein, the Gag-Pol precursor (Pr160[gag-pol]), contains the Gag proteins required for incorporation into the virion.

Mature Gag Proteins

Matrix Domain

The N-terminal myristoyl group and the 31 N-terminal amino acids of the MA domain are necessary for targeting the Gag precursor to the cell membrane.[77–81] The 100 N-terminal amino acids of the MA domain have also been implicated in the interaction with Env, resulting in the anchoring of Env to the viral particle.[82]

The mature MA protein remains associated with the inner side of the lipid envelope. In addition, MA plays a role in the transport of the preintegration complex to the nucleus.[34] A nuclear localization signal has been proposed within the MA protein, located between residues 14 through 36 and 107 through 116 of the HIV-1 p17[MA] protein.[35] In contrast to these results, other studies involving some of the same MA domain mutants concluded that infectivity in monocyte-derived macrophages was retained even when combined with a mutant Vpr.[83] The MA protein detected in the nucleus is phosphorylated, but the MA protein in the virion is not. The

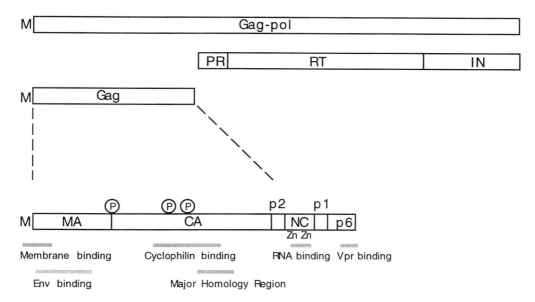

FIG. 3-9. Posttranslational modifications, proteolytic cleavages, and sites for various interactions on the HIV-1 Gag and Gag-Pol proteins. *P*, phosphorylation sites; *Zn,* the zinc finger domains within NC.

phosphorylation of MA at the C-terminal Tyr residue occurs during or after the viral infection and is a key regulator for the nuclear transport and integration of the viral genome.[38]

Several domains of the MA protein in which single amino acid substitutions dramatically reduce the efficiency of virion particle production were identified by mutagenesis. These domains include the six N-terminal residues of MA, the region between amino acids 55 and 59, and the region between amino acids 84 and 95.[84] Mutagenesis results also suggest the existence of a specific functional interaction between the MA protein and the gp41 cytoplasmic tail: virion incorporation of envelope glycoproteins with long, but not short, cytoplasmic tails was blocked by specific, single amino acid substitutions in the MA protein.[82,85]

Capsid Domain

In the CA domain of HIV-1, amino acids 240 through 430 are essential for self-association.[86,87] The CA domain of all retroviruses contains a major homology region (MHR) that is required for efficient viral replication and particle production. In the MHRs of all primate lentiviruses, several amino acids are completely conserved. The MHR of HIV-1 is located within residues 285 through 304. Deletions within the MHR or deletions C-terminal to this region blocked viral replication and significantly reduced the ability to form viral particles, whereas deletions N-terminal to the MHR prevented virus replication but resulted in abnormal particles.[88] Conservative substitution of two invariant residues within the MHR abolished viral replication and significantly reduced the particle-forming ability of the mutant *gag* gene products. Conservative substitution of a third invariant residue or of an invariably aromatic residue (Tyr) had only a moderate effect. However,

nonconservative substitutions of these amino acids with Ala prevented viral replication and affected virion morphogenesis. The results of these studies indicate that specific residues within the MHR are required for particle assembly and for the correct assembly of the viral core.[89]

Nucleocapsid Domain

The Gag precursor binds to and is responsible for the packaging of the viral genomic RNA. The NC domain of the Gag precursor is directly involved in this nucleic acid binding. Rich in basic residues (ie, Lys and Arg), the NC domain contains two copies of a zinc-binding sequence [$Cys(X)_2 Cys(X)_4 His(X)_4 Cys$], referred to as a retroviral CCHC zinc finger. The basic residues confer a nucleic acid binding property to the domain and the CCHC zinc fingers contribute to the specificity for the viral RNA. During viral assembly, the NC domain of the Gag precursor binds to the encapsidation site (ie, psi site) near the 5' end of the genomic RNA.

Disruption of either of the two zinc fingers in the NC domain resulted in noninfectious particles with reduced levels of packaged viral genome.[90–92] Deletion of the zinc fingers also eliminated virus particle formation.[80] Gag sequences up to and including the first zinc finger domain are necessary and sufficient for virion formation[93] (R. Schneider, G.N. Pavlakis, unpublished data). Mutants of the NC protein that still packaged RNA but had alterations within the zinc-finger structures, reduced infectivity. It has been suggested that the NC protein is involved in annealing of tRNA[lys3] to the PBS on the viral RNA. These activities may also have implications in strand-transfer reactions that occur after the first strong-stop synthesis of the proviral DNA to complete the synthesis of the provirus for subsequent integration.[33]

The NC protein also catalyzes the formation of the genomic RNA dimer found in virion particles.[94] HIV-1 encoding a defective protease incorporated RNA with a different dimer structure.[95] This indicates that dimer formation is probably catalyzed by the mature NC protein and not by the Gag precursor.

The selective encapsidation of retroviral RNA requires a *cis*-acting RNA packaging signal—the psi site—near the 5′ end of the genomic transcript. HIV-1 Gag polyprotein and processed NC protein bind specifically to viral RNA containing the encapsidation signal, as detected by RNA mobility shift assays.[93,96] A model for the psi RNA structure of HIV-1 has been developed. The psi site comprises four independent stem-loops spanning the major splice donor site and the *gag* start codon of HIV-1.[97] Other reports have suggested that the HIV-1 genome does not require sequences between the 5′ splice donor site and the *gag* start codon for efficient packaging.[98] Packaging of spliced, subgenomic RNAs has been observed,[99] suggesting recognition by Gag of psi elements upstream of the splice donor.

p6^gag^ Protein

The only established function of p6^gag^ is the interaction with Vpr, resulting in virion incorporation of this accessory protein. The p6^gag^ protein is necessary and sufficient for this incorporation.[100] The role of Vpr is not known exactly, but it appears to block cells in the G_2 or S phase of the cell cycle.

p1 and p2 Peptides

The role of the p1 peptide is unknown. The p2 sequences were shown to modulate the rates of Gag processing. The proteolytic processing sites of the Gag precursor are cleaved in a sequential manner by viral protease. The exact hierarchy of proteolytic processing may be important for capsid formation and viral infectivity. The presence of a C-terminal p2 tail on processing intermediates slows cleavage at the upstream CA/p2 site. Deletion of the p2 domain of Gag resulted in released virions that were less infectious despite the presence of the processed final products of Gag.[101,102]

Env Protein

The HIV-1 Env precursor gp160 is cleaved intracellularly into gp120 and gp41 by a cellular protease. The surface glycoprotein gp120 binds CD4 in the initial step of virus-cell interaction. This binding leads to conformational changes and membrane fusion assisted by the N terminus of gp41. The part of Env interacting with CD4 has been identified within four noncontiguous regions of gp120.[103] The overall structure of gp120 is important for virus-receptor interaction and virus entry. Several conserved disulfide bonds contribute to the folding of the Env.[104] Env is a heavily glycosylated protein. N-linked glycans are necessary for the creation, but not the maintenance, of a bioactive conformation, and drug-induced alteration of the glycosylation pattern can impair virus infectivity.[105]

The extensive glycosylation of gp120 has precluded definition of its structure by crystallographic methods. However, information about the surface topology of gp120, provided by studies using antibodies, is being used to model the structures of individual gp120 domains and the ways in which these domains interact in the folded protein.[106] It has been predicted that only a few areas of the polypeptide chain, such as the CD4 binding site and the V3 loop, are exposed. HIV Env also interacts with the viral core, but the details of this interaction are unknown. The p17^MA^ protein is most likely the site of interaction of HIV Env with the core virion particle.

The functional Env protein is a multimer (trimer?) that can be detected as spikes on the virion.[107] Multimerization appears to be essential for function and directs a different immune response. Multimerization of Env glycoproteins is mediated by the ectodomain of the transmembrane glycoprotein gp41. Deletion of gp41 residues 550 through 561 resulted in gp41 sedimenting as a monomer in sucrose gradients, while the gp160 precursor sedimented as a mixture of monomers and oligomers. Deletion of the nearby residues 571 through 582 did not affect the oligomeric structure of gp41 or gp160, but deletion of both sequences resulted in monomeric gp41 and predominantly monomeric gp160.[108] Residues 550 through 561 are therefore essential for maintaining the gp41 oligomeric structure; this sequence and additional sequences contribute to the maintenance of gp160 oligomers.

Comparison of the sequences of divergent HIV-1 isolates showed significant diversity concentrated primarily in the gp120 coding region of *env*, in five discreet regions named hypervariable regions (V1 through V5).[109–111] The regions between the variable regions are more conserved and were named constant (C1 through C5). Immunization with purified Env proteins leads to neutralizing antibodies binding to the V3 hypervariable region, a loop of 33 to 35 amino acids confined by a conserved disulfide bond (V3 loop). This region has been named the principal neutralizing determinant of HIV-1.[112,113] Immunization with oligomeric Env generates a large proportion of antibodies to conformational epitopes in gp120 and gp41, many of which may be absent from monomeric Env. Fewer than 7% of the monoclonal antibodies derived from mice immunized with oligomeric Env recognized the V3 loop. Monoclonal antibodies to linear epitopes in the C-terminal domain of gp120 were not obtained, suggesting that this region of the protein may be partially masked in the oligomeric molecule.[114,115]

Different isolates of HIV-1 vary in their cell tropism, that is the range of cell types in which they are able to establish a productive infection. The Env glycoprotein gp120 is responsible for the difference in cell tropism in many cases. The region of Env involved in the determination of cell tropism includes sequences that encode the V3 loop of gp120. Control of cell tropism by a part of Env including the V3 loop may be a general phenomenon that applies to many different HIV-1 isolates.[116] The overall conformation of gp120 appears to be strain specific and plays an important role in determining HIV-1 tissue tropism and sensitivity to soluble CD4 neutralization.[117]

A cellular protease processes gp160[env]. A membrane-bound processing protease for the gp160 precursor has been identified.[118] Most of the processing activity was found in the fractions of endoplasmic reticulum and Golgi. The cleavage site of gp160 is between Arg511 and Ala512. The enzyme activity was inhibited by trypsin-type protease inhibitors, but it was not affected by $CaCl_2$, $MgCl_2$, or chelating agents.

Interactions between gp120 and CD4 are responsible for the entry of HIV-1 into host cells in most cases. HIV-1 replication is commonly followed by the disappearance or down-modulation of cell-surface CD4. This process potentially renders cells nonsusceptible to subsequent infection by HIV-1 and other viruses that use CD4 as a receptor. Disappearance of CD4 from the cell surface is mediated by several different viral proteins that act at various stages through the course of the viral life cycle. At the cell surface, gp120 triggers cellular pathways leading to CD4 internalization. Vpu degrades CD4 intracellularly through the formation of intracellular Vpu-CD4 complexes. Nef is also able to internalize the membrane-bound CD4. These mechanisms contribute to the depletion of CD4 at the cell surface.

ENZYMES

Protease

HIV-1 protease is an aspartic protease containing the characteristic active center of such enzymes (ie, Asp-Thr-Gly). Protease is only active as a dimer, which is formed after Gag and Gag-Pol multimerization, and contains two identical subunits of approximately 10 kd.[119–121] In contrast, cellular aspartic proteases (eg, pepsinogen) are monomers containing two Asp-Thr-Gly domains that form the active center. Premature activation of protease does not occur before capsid formation at the plasma membrane, because the amount of Pr160[gag-pol] is limited. Several mutations prevented protease activation in the context of a Gag-protease polyprotein, perhaps by preventing polyprotein dimerization.[122] The appropriate activation of protease is essential for virus maturation, but excess protease activity is detrimental to the virus.[123,124]

Inhibition of HIV protease results in noninfectious particles and is an attractive target for therapy designed to block the progression of HIV infection.[121,125] Elucidation of the tertiary structure of HIV-1 protease[126–128] has aided the rational design and development of protease inhibitors. Inhibitors of HIV protease from a variety of chemical classes have been synthesized, and antiviral activity has been demonstrated in lymphocytes and cells of the monocyte-macrophage lineage. Several of these inhibitors have shown promise in clinical trials. Saquinavir (Invirase, Hoffman-La Roche) was the first protease inhibitor in clinical trials, and other protease inhibitors are under clinical evaluation, including MK-639 (Merck), ABT-538 (Abbott Laboratories), KNI-272 (Kyoto/National Cancer Institute), U-96988 and U-103107 (Upjohn), and AG-1343 (Agouron).

Reverse Transcriptase/Ribonuclease H

Active reverse transcriptase is a heterodimer produced by proteolytic processing of Pr160[gag-pol] by the viral protease.[129] The Gag-Pol precursor first produces p66, which presumably dimerizes. The p66 subunits in the homodimer are loosely associated, and the dimer has low enzymatic activity. During viral infection, the p66 homodimer is further cleaved at the C-terminal part of one p66 subunit to give a tightly associated p66-p51 heterodimer, which has full enzymatic activity.

Enzymatic Activities

Reverse transcriptase possesses three enzymatic activities: RNA-dependent DNA polymerase, DNA-dependent DNA polymerase, and ribonuclease H (RNase H). The polymerase activity of reverse transcriptase lies within the N-terminal portion of p66, and the RNase H activity lies within the C-terminal portion of p66. A "tether" region lies between the two domains. Reverse transcriptase also binds specifically to tRNA[lys3], which is preferentially encapsidated and subsequently hybridized to the PBS. When isolated from HIV virions, the tRNA is annealed to the RNA at the PBS.

The three-dimensional structure of HIV reverse transcriptase reveals an unprecedented degree of asymmetry within the heterodimer.[130,131] The p66 subunit has a large cleft similar to that of other polymerases, while the p51 subunit has a very different structure. The cleft of the p66 subunit resembles a right hand, with subdomains referred to as fingers, palm, and thumb.

Reverse transcriptase uses RNA primers with 3' OH ends to initiate DNA synthesis. The RNase H activity is responsible for the cleavage of the RNA strand in the RNA-DNA hybrid. The synthesis of the minus-strand starts at the PBS by the tRNA primer, while the synthesis of the plus-strand starts at the PPT, next to the U3 region (see Fig. 3-4).

The fidelity of the DNA polymerases is largely attributable to a two-step nucleotide binding mechanism. In the first step, binding contacts are initially made between the template and the incoming nucleotide triphosphates. In the second step, a change in protein conformation occurs, which leads to rapid incorporation of the nucleotide triphosphates into the growing polymer. The fidelity of polymerization due to these mechanisms approaches one error in 10^5 or 10^6 nt. The proofreading function of the DNA polymerases increases the fidelity by another 10^3 to 10^4, resulting in the extraordinary overall fidelity approaching one error in 10^{10} nt. Reverse transcriptase does not have a 3' exonuclease proofreading activity, which results in high error rates. During one replication cycle, the viral genetic information is copied twice, first by the reverse transcriptase to proviral DNA and second by the RNA polymerase II to RNA. The combined error rate results in about one error in 10^4 nt, which means that every genomic RNA molecule of approximately 10^4 nucleotides contains one misincorporation.

Inhibitors of Reverse Transcription

Reverse transcriptase has been the first and most successful target for anti-HIV-1 intervention.[132] Nucleoside analogs were found to be potent inhibitors of reverse transcriptase, resulting in widespread clinical utility. The nucleoside analogs that have been approved for clinical use or are at various stages of clinical development include AZT (zidovudine, Retrovir), ddI (didanosine, Videx), ddC (zalcitabine, Hivid), d4T (stavudine, Zerit), and 3TC (lamivudine). These nucleoside analogs act after phosphorylation to nucleotide triphosphates to inhibit elongation at the active site of reverse transcriptase.

The major problems with these drugs are their toxicity, caused in part by inhibition of cellular polymerases, and the rapid development of resistance to the drugs by HIV-1. Resistant viruses can be detected soon after treatment. Multiple reverse transcriptase mutations have been shown to confer resistance to AZT, including mutations at amino acids 41, 67, 70, 215, and 219. Accumulation of more than one mutation leads to higher resistance. Treatment with different nucleoside analogs may result in different mutations conferring resistance. Many mutations have been observed in vitro[133-135] and in vivo.[136-139] Ongoing clinical trials are testing combinations, with the hope that different inhibitors may prevent or delay the development of resistance.

Nonnucleoside analogs, such as nevirapine, TIBO, and L697661, that inhibit reverse transcriptase also have been developed.[140-142] These inhibitors are specific for HIV-1 reverse transcriptase and interact with the same region of the enzyme, YQYMDDLY, at amino acids 181 through 188, which is distinct from, but functionally and spatially related to, the substrate (dNTP) binding site. The Tyr residues at positions 181 and 188 play a crucial role in the interaction of TIBO and its congeners with the target site. High-level resistance against nonnucleoside inhibitors can be developed after single point mutations in reverse transcriptase.[143] A common position conferring resistance to all nonnucleoside HIV-1–specific reverse transcriptase inhibitors has been identified (Tyr181 to Cys).[143,144] The rapid emergence of drug-resistant escape mutants in vitro (ie, cell culture) and in vivo (ie, patients) is predominantly linked to this mutation.

Integrase

Integrase is the viral protein responsible for the integration of the proviral DNA into the host nuclear DNA. Integrase is a 31-kd protein produced from the C-terminal part of Pol after processing of Pr160$^{gag-pol}$. Integrase possesses the 3′-processing and DNA strand-transfer activities that are required to integrate HIV-1 DNA into a host chromosome. It cleaves the ends of the linear viral RNA, leaving 3′ recessed termini that may slow self-ligation and favor integration of the linear two-LTR DNA. Integrase also cleaves the cellular DNA randomly and joins the viral DNA to the host's chromosome. These activities have been reconstituted and studied extensively in vitro.

Biochemical analysis of HIV-1 integrase with purified protein and synthetic DNA substrates has revealed extensive information regarding the mechanism of action of the enzyme and identified critical residues and functional domains. In vitro, a stable complex containing only purified HIV integrase and a model viral DNA substrate processively executes the 3′-trimming and DNA-joining steps in the integration reaction. Purified integrase was also shown to promote the same reaction in reverse, a process called disintegration.[145] Integrase is an important component of the preintegration complex. Association of integrase, but not reverse transcriptase or MA proteins, with viral DNA was stable in the presence of detergents.[28] The domains involved in the integration of integrase with the viral DNA substrate have also been studied.[146,147]

HIV-1 integrase consists of domains similar to other retroviral integrases: an N-terminal HH-CC zinc finger, a centrally located region with the conserved D,D-35-E protein motif required for catalytic activity and oligomerization, and a DNA-binding domain implicated in the 3′-DNA-processing activity and integration.[148] Numerous mutagenesis studies have identified the amino acid residues and protein domains of HIV-1 integrase that are critical for in vitro activity.

Integrase acts as a multimer involving sequences that map to the catalytic center. A nonspecific DNA-binding domain has been detected at the C terminus of the protein. A stable complex of integrase and viral DNA is formed in the presence of Mn^{2+} and requires the complete integrase protein.[149,150] The crystal structure of the catalytically active integrase reveals the central feature of a five-stranded β-sheet flanked by helical regions. The structure shows that integrase belongs to a superfamily of polynucleotidyl transferases, including RNase H and the Holliday junction resolvase RuvC.[151,152]

Integration is an obligate step in productive HIV-1 infection of activated peripheral blood mononuclear cells (PBMCs) and primary human macrophages. Mutations introduced into infectious DNA clones of HIV-1 affect virus replication at a variety of steps. Mutations that altered virion morphology, levels of particle-associated integrase and reverse transcriptase, and viral DNA synthesis have been identified. Although none of the replication-defective mutants were able to integrate into the host genome, a subset of them with alterations in the catalytic triad were capable of Tat-mediated transactivation of an indicator gene linked to the viral LTR promoter. Although unintegrated viral DNA can serve as a template for Tat expression in infected indicator cells, this level of expression is insufficient to support a spreading viral infection in CD4-positive lymphocytes. Integration of the HIV-1 provirus is essential not only for productive infection of T cells but also for virus passage in cultured peripheral blood lymphocytes and macrophages.[153,154] Similarly, SIV$_{mac}$ attenuated by mutation of *int* established a transient infection of permissive cells, resulting in the expression of viral antigen from episomal viral DNA during a limited period.[155]

A temperature-sensitive mutant of integrase, K136A/E138A, has been constructed and introduced into a molecular HIV-1 clone. The defect responsible for the temperature-sensitive phenotype is localized to a step after provirus formation and integrase synthesis but before particle maturation. The temperature at which the temperature-sensitive virion is synthesized, not the temperature at which infection occurs, determines the ability of the virus to integrate.[156]

REGULATORY PROTEINS

The two essential regulatory proteins of HIV-1 are Tat and Rev. These are the two gene products for which there is direct proof of involvement in different steps of gene expression: transcription for Tat and posttranscriptional regulation for Rev. Because the other nonstructural gene products do not appear to be directly involved in gene expression control, they were named accessory to differentiate them from Tat and Rev, which act on gene expression. Tat and Rev appear to recognize specifically a limited number of functional groups in the major groove of an RNA double helix distorted by virtue of unpaired or non–Watson-Crick paired nucleotides.[157]

Tat

Tat is an essential regulatory protein for HIV-1 replication.[158,159] The 16-kd, two-exon Tat protein is encoded from two separate exons of multiply spliced mRNAs[48,160,161] whereas a one-exon, 14-kd form of Tat (Tat-1) is produced by singly spliced mRNAs (see Fig. 3-7). Tat varies in size among the different isolates (86 to 101 amino acids); truncated (58 to 72 amino acid) forms encoded by the first exon are also functional. Tat accumulates in the nucleolus and is responsible for the transcriptional activation of HIV expression.[48,162–166] It is the first characterized eukaryotic transcription factor that binds to a nascent leader RNA and affects the HIV enhancer-promoter.[167–170]

All HIV-1 mRNAs contain a region at the 5′ end named TAR, which has been mapped to nt +1 through 44.[167,171] This sequence is necessary for transactivation of viral gene expression by Tat. TAR is predicted to form a stable stem-loop structure, with a bulge in the stem (Fig. 3-10).[172] Results of mutational analyses indicate that the bulge and the stem are necessary for transactivation.[173–177] Tat binds directly to the bulge region of the TAR element.[166,169,170,177–183] The nucleotide sequence of the bulge, UCU, is critical for Tat binding.[166,170] Specific sequences are also required for Tat binding in the double-stranded region that flanks the bulge. These interactions are necessary but not sufficient for Tat function; cellular fac-

tors have also been shown to bind to TAR or to Tat and some cooperate with Tat in promoter activation.[184–190] Factors produced by the human chromosome 12 contribute to the binding of Tat to TAR.[191–194] In mouse cells, which lack these factors, the HIV promoter is significantly less activated in the presence of Tat. Understanding of the role of these factors in the transactivation process may provide insights into the mechanism by which Tat activates HIV-1 mRNA transcription.

Tat also interacts with factors binding to the enhancer-promoter elements located in the promoter region. The upstream enhancer elements and the composition of the TATA element have been suggested to be important for Tat function.[195,196] Factors that can downmodulate Tat function also were identified.[197,198] The LTR promoter can be rapidly downregulated by cellular factors, even in the presence of Tat.[199] Initially, Tat causes rapid and high activation of transcription from the HIV-1 LTR promoter and accumulation of viral mRNAs. Expression is downregulated within a short period (hours), even in the continuous presence of Tat. Experiments using hybrid equine infectious anemia virus/HIV-1 Tat proteins further suggested that cofactors necessary for transactivation are present in limited amounts.[200]

Various mechanisms for transactivation by Tat have been proposed: an increase in transcription initiation; an increase in elongation through increased processivity of the polymerase complex; and, increased elongation through suppression of specific termination events.[170,199,201–206] The inclusion of ribozyme-processing sites within the viral RNA suggested that the role of Tat is crucial for initiation, although it may not be needed for elongation.[207]

Several lentiviruses express Tat molecules acting through a mechanism similar to HIV-1 Tat, while others have transcriptional activators that are not RNA binding. Therefore although all known lentiviruses do contain transcriptional activators, the mechanism of transcriptional activation may vary. Comparisons of RNA-binding Tat proteins from different lentiviruses and numerous mutagenesis studies have shown that Tat contains distinct conserved functional domains. All RNA-binding Tat proteins contain an "activation domain" and an arginine-rich basic domain, which are necessary for activation of transcription, specific binding to TAR RNA, and nuclear localization. These domains constitute a minimal lentivirus Tat.[208]

The region of amino acids 40 through 48 contains a motif (RKGLGI) that is conserved between HIV-1, HIV-2, and SIV Tat and considered essential for activation. The RNA-binding domain (amino acids 49 through 72) contains a basic RKKRRQRRR motif. These amino acids are responsible for RNA binding and for nuclear localization of the protein. Amino acids outside of this domain also contribute to specific binding.[209,210]

In HIV-1 Tat, amino acids 22 through 37 contain seven highly conserved Cys residues between different isolates of HIV. Individual mutations in six of the seven Cys residues abolish Tat function. Although it was originally thought that Tat forms dimers by means of the conserved Cys residues, Tat

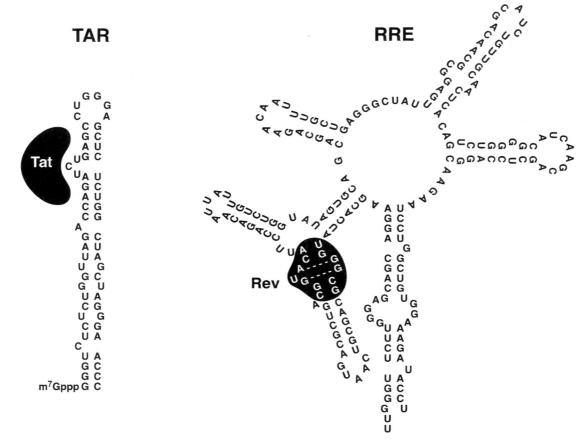

FIG. 3-10. Secondary structures of the RNA binding sites for Tat and Rev (TAR and RRE). The sites of Tat and Rev interaction are shown.

apparently acts as a monomer, and the Cys residues are important for the formation of intramolecular disulfide bonds.[211,212]

Viruses defective for Tat do not replicate, except in some in vitro cell lines after cytokine stimulation[213] (A. Valentin, M. Korneyeva, G. N. Pavlakis, unpublished data). UV irradiation can also activate expression of *tat−* integrated proviruses.[214] Tat-defective proviruses could easily be detected in patient tissues.[215] Transitions from *tat+* to *tat−* and back may be a mechanism for latency in human tissues. Tat has been found in the medium of infected cells, suggesting that it may have an extracellular role.[216–218] Tat has also been implicated as one of the cofactors in Kaposi's sarcoma induction.[216]

Tat is a potent and essential transactivation element acting through RNA binding. Its role in the virus life cycle is complex and has the potential to interact with multiple cellular components. It has been used as a reliable marker for HIV-1 infection[219–221] and as a target for development of antiviral strategies.

Rev

Rev is an essential regulatory viral protein[222,223] that accumulates in the nucleolus[224,225] and shuttles between the nucleolus

and the cytoplasm.[57–60] Rev is a small, positively charged protein of approximately 116 amino acids. The abnormal mobility of Rev on denaturing gels (19 kd) probably results from the structure of the protein. Rev is phosphorylated on Ser residues. Mutagenesis studies indicated that phosphorylation is not essential for Rev function in vitro.[226,227]

In the absence of Rev, most of the viral mRNAs are multiply spliced, the production of the structural proteins is very low, and no virions are formed.[222,228–231,238–240] Rev regulates expression of a subset of viral mRNAs at the posttranscriptional level by binding to RRE,[232–237] a unique RNA element located in the *env*-coding region of HIV-1.[225,228–240] This interaction promotes the transport, stability, and translation of unspliced and partially spliced HIV mRNAs responsible for the production of the viral structural proteins.[225,228,230,231,241–244] Rev can be replaced by cellular posttranscriptional control elements[245,246] during propagation of the virus in cultured cells. Rev is only required for the posttranscriptional regulation of the unspliced and partially spliced mRNAs.[246]

By promoting nucleocytoplasmic transport and the use of HIV RNA containing RRE, Rev antagonizes inhibitory/instability regions (ie, INS or CRS) that prevent RNA expression.[229,239,244,247] Multiple INS sequences that can act independently were found on the viral RNA.[229,247–250] Mutation of the INS sequences within *gag* resulted in Rev-independent expression[249] and viral particle formation in the absence of any HIV regulatory factors (R. Schneider, G.N. Pavlakis, unpublished data).

Rev Localization

Rev is localized primarily in the nucleolus[224,225,251] and is not found in the virion (E. Afonina, G.N. Pavlakis, unpublished data). Prevention of nuclear transport eliminates Rev function. The fusion of Rev to the glucocorticoid receptor remains inactive in the cytoplasm, while nuclear transport of Rev/glucocorticoid receptor results in Rev activation.[252] Mutations in the proposed RNA-binding motif eliminate nucleolar localization and function.

Rev can be tethered to a heterologous RNA binding site by the MS2 RNA-binding coat protein.[253] In this case, nucleolar accumulation probably is unnecessary for the biologic function of Rev.

Functional Domains of Rev

Rev has distinct functional domains identified by mutagenesis. Mutations in the region between amino acids 18 and 56 result in a recessive negative phenotype.[227,254,255] Mutations in the region 75 to 89 result in *trans*-dominant negative mutants.[227,256] The arginine-rich region of amino acids 35 through 50 (RQARRNRRRRWRERQR) is required for the nuclear-nucleolar localization and for RNA binding. The core sequence in this region is conserved among the *rev* genes of many HIV-1 isolates and is at least partially responsible for the RNA-binding specificity. Sequences outside of the core also contribute to the specificity of binding.[257]

It has been reported that a Rev peptide containing amino acids 34 through 50 binds specifically in vitro to RRE[258] and that the same peptide inhibits splicing in vitro.[259] Rev requires the effector domain (amino acids 75 through 89) for in vivo function. Additional sequences (amino acids 18 through 56) flanking the proposed core RNA binding site are necessary for function and may affect Rev multimerization. Therefore, the region of amino acids 18 through 56 has multiple and most likely overlapping functions of nuclear-nucleolar localization, RNA binding, and multimerization. It was proposed that amino acids 14 through 20 contain an essential domain for Rev function in vivo. These amino acids are involved in protein-protein interactions or form part of the RNA-binding domain.[255] One of the most evolutionarily conserved amino acid strings on Rev (LYQSNP), followed by additional prolines, is located in this region. This region of Rev is at the end of the first coding exon (amino acids 1 through 25), which under certain conditions may be dispensable for function. For example, the variant HIV-1 protein Tev[63] does not contain the first coding exon of Rev, but it has Rev activity. Other hybrid proteins containing the second exon of Rev (amino acids 26 through 116) are inactive,

and therefore, the nature of the sequences in the first exon is important for function.

The region of amino acids 75 through 84 (LPPLERLTLD) constitutes the core of the leucine-rich effector domain. Leu78, Leu81, and Leu83 are required for Rev function. Leu75 and Glu79 are also important for activity. Leu75 is not essential according to some reports,[254,260] whereas others[261] reported inactive Leu75 mutants.

A consensus sequence ZxxLJJLTLJ (ie, Z equals any hydrophobic and J equals any hydrophilic residue) was proposed for the core element of the effector region for all lentiviruses.[260] The effector domain may extend to Cys 89[254–256] and is the most C-terminal functional domain of Rev, because several C-terminal deletions of Rev (ie, Rev 1 through 102 and Rev 1 through 91) are fully active.[260] The effector domain is considered to be a signal for nuclear export after association with cellular factors.[58,262,263]

A dual function for the arginine-rich binding motif in oligomerization and RNA binding has been proposed.[264] Formation of the RNA-binding site may depend on Rev multimerization.[265] Rev tends to multimerize efficiently in vivo and in vitro. Chemical crosslinking[264] and gel filtration[266] indicated that Rev exists as a tetramer. Rev multimerization is essential for function and takes place regardless of the presence of RRE.[264,265,267] Purified Rev aggregates in solution. Other studies have suggested that Rev binds as a monomer and multimerizes on the template.[268] A high-affinity binding site for Rev on the RRE has been identified (see Fig. 3-10).[233] Binding of Rev-derived peptides to this RNA stem-loop is accompanied by a conformational change in the RNA, which results in the formation of additional base pairs not present in the free RNA. Two of these induced base pairs are purine-purine pairs within the internal loop of the RRE.[235,269] The formation of non–Watson-Crick base pairs, interactions in the major groove, and protein-induced conformational changes, which have been documented in the Rev-RRE binding studies, may prove to be common characteristics of RNA recognition of proteins.[269]

Several proteins have been proposed to bind to Rev in vivo. Rev may associate with nucleolar protein B23,[270] translation initiation factor 5A,[271] or other cellular components participating in intracellular trafficking such as nucleoporins.[221,272]

Transdominant Rev Mutants

Transdominant or dominant-negative mutants of Rev (TDRev) have been identified and may provide a potent and specific way to inhibit HIV-1 expression. Many mutants in the effector region have a dominant-negative phenotype; they inhibit the function of wild-type Rev in the same cell.[227,256,261,260] Multimerization and RNA binding are essential for the transdominant inhibition.[264,267,273] The mechanism of function of such mutants is the inhibition of nuclear export of Rev by formation of inactive multimers.[58,262,274,275] Like Rev, TDRev localizes to the nucleolus[227] and has been shown to bind specifically RRE RNA in vitro,[273] but TDRev fails to shuttle to the cytoplasm.[58,262,274,275]

Expression of the transdominant mutant TDRevM10 drastically reduces HIV-1 propagation in selected cell clones,[276,277] immortalized cell lines,[278] PBMCs,[279] and CD4+ T lymphocytes.[280] These studies showed that TDRev could be useful for the inhibition HIV-1 expression. The advantage of such an antiviral approach is that it is targeted specifically against the viral Rev protein. One potential problem is that excess TDRev is necessary to inhibit Rev function.[227,255,256,261] A gene therapy approach using TDRevM10 in a phase I clinical trial has been proposed and initiated.[281]

ACCESSORY PROTEINS

The accessory genes (ie, *vif, vpr, vpu,* and *nef*) and proteins of HIV-1 were so named because they were dispensable for virus replication in many cultured cells in vitro,[132] although their conservation in all virus isolates demonstrates that they are essential during the virus life cycle in the host. Most of the accessory proteins appear to enter the virion, and they interact with viral and cellular components to increase viral replication in the host. Two of the accessory genes, *vif* and *vpr*, have recognizable homologs in nonprimate lentiviruses.

The function of accessory proteins underscores the importance of Env-CD4 interactions for the life cycle of HIV-1. Unlike that of other retroviruses, CD4, the primary HIV-1 receptor, is an abundant surface protein in certain cells. As a result, many viral particles can potentially infect the same cell, which results in large numbers of unintegrated DNA molecules after in vitro infection. Other retroviruses may inhibit superinfection by engaging their surface receptor with the newly produced Env. In the case of HIV, this process may be problematic, because CD4 is abundant in lymphocytes. Another problem with the Env-CD4 interaction is that the intracellular binding of newly produced molecules may inhibit Env trafficking and virus production. Therefore, HIV-1 produces additional proteins that are able to engage and downregulate CD4. One of the functions of Nef is to downregulate CD4 at the cell surface, possibly resulting in less superinfection. In addition, Vpu affects CD4 in the endoplasmic reticulum, resulting in less CD4 transport in the plasma membrane and more free Env.

Three HIV proteins—Env, Nef, and Vpu—focus on modulating virus interactions with its receptor. Vpu and Nef are produced by ORFs at the beginning and the end of *env*, respectively. Vpu production is from the same *vpu/env* bicistronic mRNAs, a rare organization in retroviruses. These accessory proteins are localized in the membrane, which brings them in contact with Env. It seems reasonable to propose that the two proteins evolved from parts of Env with similar functions, which in the process of evolution became autonomous ORFs.

Vif

The viral infectivity factor Vif (previously named sor or Q) has been shown to influence the infectivity but not the production of virus particles. The *vif* ORF is located after the *pol* ORF and overlaps with the 3′ part of *pol*. Homologs of *vif* exist in all lentiviruses, with the one exception of equine infectious anemia virus.[282] Moreover, there is significant conservation among *vif* ORFs of the different lentiviruses.[5] The *vif* gene encodes a 23-kd protein, which is immunogenic in infected individuals.[283–285] Vif is expressed from partially spliced mRNAs; its expression is activated by Rev.[66,286] Vif is a cytoplasmic protein, existing in a soluble cytosolic form and a membrane-associated form. The latter form of Vif is a peripheral membrane protein that is tightly associated with the cytoplasmic side of cellular membranes.[287,288] This localization and other observations suggest that Vif is incorporated in the virion.

Vif is required for HIV-1 replication in the CD4-positive T-cell lines CEM and H9 and in peripheral blood T lymphocytes, but it is not required for replication in the SupT1, C8166, and Jurkat T-cell lines. As in HIV-1, Vif of HIV-2 is crucial for viral infectivity in primary cells.[287,289] Cell-free infection of a *vif*–mutant of HIV-2 was not impaired when the SupT1 cell line was used. However, differential degrees of impairment in viral replication were observed when other cell lines (eg, Molt-3, U-937) were used. In most cell lines, *vif*– mutant proviruses have lower replicating capacity. In PBMCs, they replicate at low levels only after cell-mediated infection; however, cell-free infection is not possible.[290]

The mechanism of function of Vif is not clear. Several studies agree with the conclusion that Vif affects late events in the viral life cycle, which result in lower infectivity. Vif may affect virus particle maturation. It was shown that nonhomogeneous packing of the core takes place in most *vif*– virions produced in CEM and Jurkat cells.[291] In the absence of Vif, the cone-shaped virus core contained dense material in its broad end, but in contrast to *vif*+ virions, the material inside its narrow end appeared transparent. Notably, *vif*– virions recovered from restrictive cells, but not from permissive cells, were abnormal in terms of morphology and viral protein content. They contained significantly reduced quantities of Env[292,293] and altered quantities of Gag and Pol, consistent with the conclusion that the processing of the capsid proteins was affected.[293] Although wild-type and *vif*– virions from restrictive cells contain similar quantities of viral RNA, no viral DNA synthesis was detectable after acute infection of target cells with phenotypically *vif*– virions.[293]

Vif is required for proper assembly of the virion and for efficient Env-mediated infection of target cells. Failure to infect target cells results from a defect in the formation of the viral particle in PBMCs or nonpermissive cell lines.[294,295] In a single round of infection, *vif*– virus is approximately 25 (from CEMx174 cells) to 100 (from H9 cells) times less infectious than wild-type virus produced from these cells or than the *vif*– mutant produced from HeLa cells.

The observation that *vif*– virions do not produce cDNA after infection led to an alternative proposal, suggesting that Vif stimulates efficient nucleocapsid internalization or activation of reverse transcription after infection.[296,297] The levels of viral DNA were examined by RNA-PCR during infection by *vif+* and *vif−* viruses of MT-2 and H9 cells, in which Vif is required for HIV-1 replication. Viral DNA was detected within hours of infection by both viruses, but the accumulation of *vif−* viral DNA was impeded in terms of extent and kinetics. Inefficient viral DNA synthesis correlated with restricted replication of the *vif−* virus.[296] Instead, *vif−* virions were severely impaired in their ability to complete the synthesis of viral DNA after they were internalized in the target cell.[297] The impaired reverse transcription may be the result of defects in virus maturation in the nonpermissive producer cell. This hypothesis is in agreement with the structural data, the expression pattern and localization of Vif, and the known requirements for the presence of Vif in the producing cell and not the recipient cell for appropriate function.[298]

The C terminus of Vif is required for the stable association of Vif with membranes and is essential for Vif function, suggesting that this association is likely to be important for its biologic activity. The highly conserved regions at residues 103 through 115 and 142 through 150 were important for Vif function but did not affect membrane association, indicating that these regions are likely to be important for other, unknown functions.[288] Mutant viruses containing substitutions in Cys114, Cys133, or both residues displayed a *vif−* infection phenotype.[299] A search for local sequence similarity revealed that a unifying feature of predicted lentiviral Vif proteins is the presence of at least one of two short, highly conserved sequence motifs, SL(I/V)X4YX9Y and SLQXLA. The latter was present in 34 of 38 lentiviruses examined, whereas SL(I/V)X4YX9Y was found only in primate lentiviruses and in bovine immunodeficiency-like virus.

Vpr

Vpr (viral protein R) is a 96–amino acid, 14-kd protein that is incorporated into the virion. It interacts with the p6^{gag} part of the Pr55^{gag} precursor.[300–303] Vpr detected in the cell is localized to the nucleus.[36,304] Proposed functions for Vpr include the nuclear import of preintegration complexes, cell growth arrest, transactivation of cellular genes, and induction of cellular differentiation.

For most retroviruses, the newly synthesized viral DNA in the preintegration complex is thought to gain access to the nucleus of the infected cell after the dissolution of the nuclear membrane during mitosis. Most retroviral integration requires cell division. In contrast, HIV-1 and the other lentiviruses can integrate their genomes in nondividing cells by transporting the preintegration complex into the nucleus. Vpr is one of the two identified nucleophilic components that promote nuclear localization of viral nucleic acids in nondividing cells. The other protein involved in this translocation is p17^{MA}. Introduction of p17^{MA} and Vpr mutations in HIV-1 attenuated nuclear localization of viral nucleic acids in nondividing cells and viral replication in monocyte-derived macrophages.[36] In contrast, infections of viruses containing mutations on Vpr or in the proposed p17^{MA} nuclear localization sequence were indistinguishable from those of wild-type HIV-1. These viruses retained the ability to replicate in dividing and nondividing host cells, including monocyte-derived macrophages. These studies indicated the presence of redundant nucleophilic determinants of HIV-1 that independently permit nuclear localization of viral nucleic acids and viral replication in nondividing cells. Other investigators reported only modest effects on virion production with some of the MA and Vpr mutants, while none of the mutants abolished infectivity in primary human monocyte-derived macrophages.[83]

Several observations raise the possibility that some aspects of HIV-1–induced pathologies are caused by a disturbance of cells by Vpr.[305,306] Although Vpr has no effect on the initial cytopathic effect of HIV-1, viruses that contain an intact *vpr* gene are unable to establish a chronic infection of T cells, whereas viruses with a mutated *vpr* gene can readily establish such long-term cultures.[306,307] The replication of a *vpr* mutant but not that of wild-type HIV-1 was compatible with cellular proliferation. Expression of Vpr alone affects the progression of cells in the cell cycle,[307] arresting the cells in G$_2$/M phase.[272] These results suggest that HIV-1 uses Vpr to modulate chronic infection of T cells. Vpr can directly inhibit cell proliferation and induce cell differentiation of the human rhabdomyosarcoma cell line TE671.[305] These results may be related to the ability of Vpr to block cell division, and link this protein with cellular proliferation pathways possibly relevant to the control of HIV-1 replication. Substantial amounts of Vpr were found in the medium of infected cultures and in the serum of infected patients. Serum Vpr was implicated in the activation of HIV replication in vivo and in the control of latency.[308]

The C-terminal third of the Vpr protein caused cell growth arrest and structural defects in yeast cells, indicated by osmotic sensitivity and gross cell enlargement.[309] Vpr shows some sequence similarity to Sac1p, a protein with functions relating to the yeast cytoskeleton.[310] Vpr's effect in yeast may be to disrupt normal Sac1p functions. In HIV-1, the function of Vpr may be to bring about cell growth arrest or cytoskeletal changes at an early step in viral infection.

The *vpr−* molecular clones were viable and did not have any obvious defects when grown in T cells, but their growth was severely delayed in macrophages.[311] Loss of *vpr* reduced viral antigen production in macrophages by up to 1000-fold but only marginally affected replication in lymphocytes. The *vpr* genes of HIV-2 and SIV$_{mac}$ also affect monocyte infection.[312] The block to infection in monocytes was identified at a step in the viral life cycle after entry and reverse transcription, but before or at the time of proviral transcription.[313] Infection of mononuclear phagocytes with virions that had been loaded with Vpr molecules in the producer cells by transcomplementation still showed a *vpr−* phenotype, suggesting a role for Vpr produced in newly infected cells in addition to its presumed function in the virion. In support of this theory, Vpr was found to be produced by multiply spliced (Rev-independent) and by singly spliced

(Rev-dependent) mRNAs,[70] suggesting that Vpr is present early after infection.

HIV-2 and SIV express another protein similar to Vpr, named Vpx, which is probably the result of a gene duplication. Vpx is also a virion protein, but its function and its relation to Vpr are not fully elucidated. In contrast to growth in the lymphoid cell lines, replication of *vpx−* viruses in macaque PBMCs was severely impaired, indicating that Vpx is necessary for efficient replication in these cells.[314] In contrast, the replication of the *vpr−* viruses was only slightly impaired in these cells. These studies indicate that Vpx and Vpr proteins may be functionally distinct.

Progression to AIDS and death in SIV-infected animals can occur in the absence of Vpr or Vpx.[315] Double-mutant virus lacking *vpr* and *vpx* was severely attenuated, with much lower virus burdens and no evidence of disease progression. The double-mutant affected SIV pathogenicity in vivo, suggesting a redundancy in the function of Vpr and Vpx related to virus pathogenicity. Additional evidence for an important role of Vpr in viral replication comes from experiments showing that a *vpr−* molecular clone reverted to wild-type in 3 of 5 animals, indicating that Vpr is important for replication in vivo.[316]

The minimal viral genetic information necessary for Vpr incorporation in the virion was mapped within the Pr55^{gag} polyprotein precursor. Incorporation of Vpr requires the expression but not the processing of Gag products and is independent of the presence of Pol and Env. Direct interaction of Vpr with the Pr55^{gag} precursor protein was indicated by coprecipitation experiments with Gag-specific antibodies.[303] Deletion analysis indicated that the association motif for Vpr is located within residues 1 through 46 of p6^{gag}.[100] Vpx protein of HIV-2 also recognizes a packaging signal within the C terminus of the HIV-2 Gag precursor protein.[317]

Vpr contains an amphipathic α-helical domain in the N terminus (residues 17 through 34) that is highly conserved among *vpr* sequences of different isolates. Acidic and hydrophobic residues and the helical structure in this region are critical for the stability of Vpr and its efficient incorporation into virions. Mutation of the highly conserved acidic residues in the N-terminal domain (residues 17 through 34) disrupted the α-helical structure and eliminated virion incorporation. In contrast, alterations of the conserved Gln65, Cys76, or the basic domain (ie, Arg87 and Lys95) did not impair the Gag-directed incorporation of Vpr into virions, suggesting that protein-protein interactions mediated through the putative helical domain of Vpr participate in its incorporation into the virion.[318,319] The single Cys near the C terminus was required for production of a stable protein, but the Arg was not important for incorporation or stability of tagged Vpr.

Experiments have identified a 41-kd cytosolic protein interacting with Vpr in vitro.[320] Vpr induced nuclear translocation of this protein, as did glucocorticoid receptor-II–stimulating steroids. Vpr and the Vpr-binding protein coimmunoprecipitated with the human glucocorticoid receptor as part of an activated receptor complex. A 200-kd protein

(RIP) also bound Vpr. Vpr nuclear localization seemed to correlate with Vpr interaction with RIP.[321]

Mutational analysis failed to identify in Vpr a typical nuclear localization signal rich in basic amino acid residues. Mutations in the C-terminal 20–amino acid region containing a provisional nuclear localization signal did not abolish Vpr nuclear localization or interaction with RIP, whereas point mutations in a leucine- or isoleucine-rich domain abolished Vpr interaction with RIP and rendered Vpr unstable during transient expression. Cells infected with HIV-1 strains with C-terminal truncations of Vpr manifested a different pattern of Vpr expression.[304] A mutant with an alteration of residues 79 through 85 exhibited a 23% reduction in the total level of Vpr expression but a marked accumulation of Vpr in intracellular rather than extracellular virions. A mutant with a deletion of the last 17 amino acids of Vpr expressed only 10% of wild-type level of Vpr.

Vpu

Vpu (viral protein U) is unique to HIV-1 and SIV$_{cpz}$, a close relative of HIV-1. There is no similar gene in HIV-2 or SIV. Vpu is produced by the bicistronic *vpu/env* mRNAs and is therefore a "late" product.[65] Vpu is a 16-kd, 81–amino acid, type I integral membrane protein[322] with at least two different biologic functions: degradation of CD4 in the endoplasmic reticulum and enhancement of virion release from the plasma membrane of HIV-1–infected cells. Vpu probably possesses an N-terminal hydrophobic membrane anchor and a hydrophilic moiety.[323] It is phosphorylated by casein kinase II at positions Ser52 and Ser56 within a predicted α-helix–turn–α-helix motif.[324,325]

CD4 Degradation

Intracellular complexing between Env and CD4 results in trapping of both molecules in the endoplasmic reticulum. The presence of Vpu releases Env from these complexes. In several systems, Vpu was shown to act on CD4 in the absence of Env or any other viral protein. Coexpression of Vpu and CD4 in HeLa cells resulted in the degradation of CD4 in the endoplasmic reticulum.[326–328] The sensitivity of CD4 to Vpu-mediated degradation depended on the presence of specific sequences located between amino acids 402 and 420 in the CD4 cytoplasmic domain. Degradation of CD4 by Vpu requires the two proteins to be present in the same membrane compartment. Immunoprecipitation experiments showed that Vpu specifically binds to the cytoplasmic tail of CD4.[328] The ability of CD8/CD4 chimeric molecules and various CD4 mutants to form complexes with Vpu correlates with their sensitivity to degradation, and amino acid residues in the CD4 cytoplasmic tail that are important for degradation are also necessary for Vpu binding.

Other studies showed that CD4 contains a determinant located within amino acids 418 through 425 that is critical for susceptibility to Vpu-induced degradation. Neither the phosphorylation sites in the cytoplasmic domain nor the p56[lck]-interaction region was required for binding to Vpu. Vpu-induced degradation was specific for CD4, because CD8, even when retained in the endoplasmic reticulum, was not degraded. CD4 degradation could be observed in the absence of gp160 or other means of retaining CD4 in the endoplasmic reticulum.[329] Stimulation of CD4 degradation also requires the transmembrane domain of CD4. This domain appears to provide critical sequence or structural elements through which the Vpu protein could access CD4 for degradation in the endoplasmic reticulum.[330,331]

Sequences on Vpu critical for CD4 downregulation were localized to the hydrophilic C-terminal domain.[332] A deletion mutant of Vpu and a phosphorylation mutant were biologically inactive in CD4 degradation but retained the capacity to interact with the CD4 cytoplasmic domain. Nonphosphorylated Vpu was unable to induce degradation of CD4, even when the proteins were artificially retained in the endoplasmic reticulum. Therefore, Vpu binding is necessary but not sufficient to trigger CD4 degradation. Binding is an early critical event triggering the multistep process leading to CD4 degradation.[333]

Virus Release

In addition to CD4 degradation, Vpu appears to have another function; it enhances the release of virions from the infected cells. This function of Vpu may be related to the multimerization of Vpu and potential ion channel–forming capacity.[322] A structural homology of Vpu with the influenza M2 membrane protein has been observed. M2 forms ion channels and may modulate the pH of intracellular compartments. This activity of Vpu is not restricted to HIV-1. It was reported that Vpu enhances the release of capsids produced by the *gag* genes of widely divergent retroviruses in CD4-negative cells.[334,335]

Vpu-mediated enhancement of virion release only partially depended on Vpu phosphorylation. Enhancement of virion release by wild-type Vpu was efficiently blocked when Vpu was artificially retained in the endoplasmic reticulum, suggesting that the two biologic functions of Vpu are independent, occur at different sites within the cell, and exhibit different sensitivities to phosphorylation.[336] Another reported consequence of *vpu* expression is the reduction of cytopathic effects by decreasing the rate of syncytia formation.[337]

Nef

Nef (previously named 3′ ORF) is an approximately 27-kd myristylated protein produced by an ORF located at the 3′ end of the primate lentiviruses. Other forms of Nef are known, including nonmyristylated variants. Nef is predominantly cytoplasmic and associated with the plasma membrane through the myristyl residue linked to the conserved second amino acid (Gly). Nef has also been identified in the nucleus and found associated with the cytoskeleton in some experiments. Its association with the virion is suspected but not proven. Nef is not

preferentially accumulated in the virion, but its membrane localization may result in virion incorporation.

Initially thought to be a negative factor, Nef was found to be important for viral replication in vivo. The *nef* genes of HIV and SIV are dispensable in vitro but are essential for efficient viral spread and disease progression in vivo. Nef was necessary for the maintenance of high virus loads and for the development of AIDS in macaques.[338] A *nef*– SIV replicated at lower levels, did not cause disease, and protected the animals from disease after superinfection with wild-type virus.[339] A *nef*+ HIV-1 molecular clone induced severe depletion of human thymocytes in immunodeficient (scid) mice containing human lymphoid tissues (scid-hu) within 6 weeks of infection, but a *nef*– HIV-1 did not.[340] Thus, HIV-1 Nef is required for efficient viral replication and pathogenicity in vivo.

Downregulation of Surface CD4

A well-established function of Nef is the downregulation of CD4, the primary viral receptor.[341,342] Nef acts by inducing CD4 endocytosis, resulting in its degradation in lysosomes.[343] CD4 downregulation is strongly enhanced by the association of Nef with cell membranes through myristylation. A study of chimeric molecules revealed that a region containing the 20 membrane-proximal residues of the CD4 cytoplasmic domain are sufficient to confer Nef sensitivity. Within this region, a leucine-leucine motif, reminiscent of an endocytosis and lysosomal targeting signal found in the CD3 γ and δ chains, is crucial for CD4 response to Nef.

The portion of the cytoplasmic domain required for the downregulation of CD4 by Nef overlaps with the binding site of p56[lck], but the cysteine residues that are essential for the association of CD4 with p56[lck] are not required. Others have reported that Nef or cellular factors recruited by Nef interact with this segment of CD4 to displace p56[lck] from the complex and induce CD4 endocytosis.[344] Several experiments indicated that the presence of p56[lck] is not essential for Nef function on CD4. Although a decrease in total CD4 was observed in lysates of cells expressing Nef, the levels of p56[lck] were not significantly affected.[345] CD4 downregulation was found in cells not producing p56[lck].

This function of Nef appears to be redundant with the function of Vpu, which degrades CD4 in the endoplasmic reticulum. For both proteins, membrane association is essential for CD4 degradation, which suggests that in both cases the mechanism of degradation involves binding to CD4. Binding has been demonstrated for Vpu; however, no direct evidence exists for an association between Nef and CD4, and attempts to demonstrate CD4-Nef complexes have failed. Whatever the mechanism, this function of Nef results in rapid CD4 downregulation and possible prevention of superinfection. In concert with the function of Vpu, these effects may result in higher levels of intact Env protein in the capsid and increased virus production.

CD4 downregulation is a property of *nef* alleles found in many primary HIV-1 isolates. It was proposed that CD4 downregulation is a conserved function of Nef, selected in vivo during human HIV-1 infection.[346]

Expression of the Nef protein in transgenic mice perturbs development of CD4+ T cells in the thymus and elicits depletion of peripheral CD4+ T cells. Downregulation of CD4 by Nef in human and transgenic murine T cells indicates that the relevant interactions are conserved in these two systems and suggests that the consequences of Nef expression on the host cell function can be analyzed in vivo in the murine system.[347,348] A possible complication of experiments with transgenic mice is that Nef also downregulates murine CD8 in murine cells, but it does not affect human CD8 in human cells.[342]

Thymic T cells expressing Nef of HIV-1$_{NL4-3}$ showed altered activation responses. In contrast, the Nef protein of the HIV-1$_{HXB3}$ isolate did not have an overt effect on T cells when expressed in transgenic animals. The differential effects of the two HIV-1 nef alleles in transgenic mice correlated with downregulation of CD4 expression on thymic T cells.[348] The analysis of Nef variants demonstrated the variability in sequence and function found in nef genes. This variability may reflect the different selection pressures operating in the host.

Nef-Induced Increase in Infectivity

Nef has also been shown to increase the infectivity of produced virions. The two functions of Nef may be related, in that downregulation of CD4 may promote the production of HIV-1 that has greater infectivity. Initial reports on the effect of Nef on the expression of molecular clones were variable. The demonstration of a positive effect of Nef on viral replication in animals led to intense examination of in vitro effects and the establishment of experimental conditions that also resulted in a positive effect of Nef. Such studies indicate that optimal infectivity of HIV-1 in vitro requires an intact nef gene.[349-354] Nef confers a positive growth advantage, which becomes readily discernible in the primary cell setting of virus induction through T-cell activation.[355]

One reason for the variable results concerning Nef function may be that Nef expression is toxic to the cell. A hybrid CD8-Nef protein expressed in Jurkat cells resulted in two opposite phenotypes, which depended on the intracellular localization of Nef. Expressed in the cytoplasm or on the cell surface, the chimera inhibited or activated early signaling events from the T-cell antigen receptor, respectively. Activated Jurkat cells died by apoptosis, and only cells with mutated nef genes expressing truncated Nef proteins survived. The effects of functionally variable Nef proteins may reconcile the different actions of Nef in different experimental settings.[356]

Nef is suspected to alter the activation status of the cells by interacting with cellular kinases. A serine kinase activity is associated with Nef expressed in human T lymphocytes.[357] Experiments show that proline-rich (PxxP) motifs in HIV-1 Nef bind to SH3 domains of a subset of Src kinases and are required for the enhanced growth of nef+ viruses but not for the downregulation of CD4. Nef PxxP motifs show specific binding to biotinylated SH3 domains of Hck and Lyn, although not to those of other tested Src family kinases or less related proteins. Endogenous Hck of monocytic U937 cells can be specifically precipitated by matrix-bound HIV-1 Nef but not by mutants lacking PxxP. These experiments suggest that CD4 downregulation and promotion of viral growth are two distinct functions of Nef, because intact Nef PxxP motifs are dispensable for Nef-induced CD4 downregulation but are required for the higher in vitro replicative potential of nef+ viruses.[358] An additional cellular protein interacting with Nef, human β-COP, has been detected. This protein is a major coat component of non–clathrin-coated vesicles. Nef and β-COP interacted in vitro and were found to be physically associated in HIV-1–infected cells by coimmunoprecipitation.[359]

Many other functions have been attributed to Nef, including involvement in abnormal hematopoiesis through inhibition of bone marrow progenitor cells,[360] B-cell activation that requires contact between T and B cells and induction of interleukin-6,[361] elimination by Nef of the proliferative response to bombesin and platelet-derived growth factor,[362] and inhibition of protein synthesis.[363]

HUMAN IMMUNODEFICIENCY VIRUS VARIABILITY

Nucleotide sequencing of HIV-1 isolates from different geographic locations have demonstrated extensive divergence.[364] HIV-1 can be subdivided into at least nine genetic subtypes (ie, clades): A through H and O. In Europe and the United States, there is an almost complete dominance of subtype B. In other parts of the world, other subtypes, alone or in combinations, predominate. The relation of the different HIV-1 genotypes to serotypes is unknown. This is an important consideration for vaccine development.

The development of appropriate assays for understanding the consequences of viral divergence is critical for combatting the worldwide epidemic. Some of the non-B genetic subtypes were proposed to be transmitted differently than subtype B and have the potential to cause epidemics with different characteristics. For example, subtypes A and E are thought to be more efficient in heterosexual transmission and may cause new and severe epidemics in developing and developed countries.

Generation of variability in HIV-1 is similar to the other retroviruses. Lack of proofreading by the viral and cellular enzymes involved in viral replication results in high error rates (10^{-4} per site per generation) and the continuous generation of variants. During chronic active infection, the continuous high-level propagation of the virus results in many rounds of replication and in generation of a huge number of variants, a swarm of quasispecies. Selection of antigenic variants and drug-resistant mutants is easily achieved in such conditions. The genomic diversity of HIV-1 is one of the major obstacles in the fight for the development of effective therapeutic and prophylactic regimens and will have to be addressed successfully to achieve progress in these fields.

ACKNOWLEDGMENTS

I thank B. K. Felber for suggestions and discussions and A. Arthur for editing. Research is sponsored by the National Cancer Institute, Department of Health and Human Services, under contract with ABL.

REFERENCES

1. Vallee K, Carre H. Sur l'anemie infectieuse du cheval. C R Acad Sci 1904;139:1239.
2. Barre-Sinoussi F, Cherman J-C, Rey F, et al. Isolation of a T-lymphotropic retrovirus from a patient at risk for acquired immune deficiency syndrome (AIDS). Science 1983;220:868.
3. Gallo RC, Salahuddin SZ, Popovic M, et al. Frequent detection and isolation of cytopathic retroviruses (HTLV-III) from patients with AIDS and at risk for AIDS. Science 1984;224:500.
4. Gonda MA, Wong-Staal F, Gallo RC, et al. Sequence homology and morphogenic similarity of HTLV-III and visna virus, a pathogenic lentivirus. Science 1985;227:173.
5. Sonigo P, Alizon M, Staskus K, et al. Nucleotide sequence of the visna lentivirus: relationship to the AIDS virus. Cell 1985;42:369.
6. Clements JE, Zink MC, Narayan O, Gabuzda DH. Lentivirus infection of macrophages. Immunol Ser 1994;60:589.
7. Lochelt M, Muranyi W, Flugel RM. Human foamy virus genome possesses an internal, Bel-1-dependent and functional promoter. Proc Natl Acad Sci USA 1993;90:7317.
8. Campbell M, Renshaw-Gegg L, Renne R, Luciw PA. Characterization of the internal promoter of simian foamy viruses. J Virol 1994;68:4811.
9. Lochelt M, Yu SF, Linial ML, Flugel RM. The human foamy virus internal promoter is required for efficient gene expression and infectivity. Virology 1995;206:601.
10. Böhnlein S, Hauber J, Cullen BR. Identification of a U5-specific sequence required for efficient polyadenylation within the human immunodeficiency virus long terminal repeat. J Virol 1989;63:421.
11. Brown PH, Tiley LS, Cullen BR. Efficient polyadenylation within the human immunodeficiency virus type 1 long terminal repeat requires flanking U3-specific sequences. J Virol 1991;65:3340.
12. Valsamakis A, Zeichner S, Carswell S, Alwine JC. The human immunodeficiency virus type-1 polyadenylation signal—a 3' long terminal repeat element upstream of the AAUAAA necessary for efficient polyadenylation. Proc Natl Acad Sci USA 1991;88:2108.
13. DeZazzo JD, Scott JM, Imperiale MJ. Relative roles of signals upstream of AAUAAA and promoter proximity in regulation of human immunodeficiency virus type 1 mRNA 3' end formation. Mol Cell Biol 1992;12:5555.
14. Cullen BR. Human immunodeficiency virus as a prototypic complex retrovirus. J Virol 1991;65:1053.
15. Myers G, Pavlakis GN. Evolutionary potential of complex retroviruses. In Levy J, ed. The retroviridae. New York: Plenum Press, 1992:1.
16. Dalgleish AG, Beverley PCL, Clapham PR, et al. The CD4 (T4) antigen is an essential component of the receptor for the AIDS virus. Nature 1984;312:763.
17. McDougal JS, Mawle A, Cort SP, et al. Cellular tropism of the human retrovirus HTLV-III/LAV. I. Role of T cell activation and expression of the T4 antigen. J Immunol 1985;135:3151.
18. Maddon PJ, Dalgleish, McDougal JS, et al. The T4 gene encodes the AIDS virus receptor and is expressed in the immune system and the brain. Cell 1986;47:333.
19. McDougal JS, Nicholson JK, Cross GD, et al. Binding of the human retrovirus HTLV-III/LAV/ARV/HIV to the CD4 (T4) molecule: conformation dependence, epitope mapping, antibody inhibition, and potential for idiotypic mimicry. J Immunol 1986;137:2937.
20. Sattentau QJ, Clapham PR, Weiss RA, Beverley PC, et al. The human and simian immunodeficiency viruses HIV-1, HIV-2 and SIV interact with similar epitopes on their cellular receptor, the CD4 molecule. AIDS 1988;2:101.
21. Harouse JM, Bhat S, Spitalnik SL, et al. Inhibition of entry of HIV-1 in neural cell lines by antibodies against galactosyl ceramide. Science 1991;253:320.
22. Veillette A, Bookman MA, Horak EM, Bolen JB. The CD4 and CD8 T cell surface antigens are associated with the internal membrane tyrosine protein kinase p56[lck]. Cell 1988;55:301.
23. Gallaher WR. Detection of a fusion peptide sequence in the transmembrane protein of HIV. Cell 1987;50:327.
24. Kowalski M, Potz J, Basiripour L, et al. Functional regions of the envelope glycoprotein of human immunodeficiency virus type 1. Science 1987;237:1351.
25. Freed EO, Myers DJ, Risser R. Characterization of the fusion domain of the human immunodeficiency virus type 1 envelope glycoprotein gp41. Proc Natl Acad Sci USA 1990;87:4650.
26. Lori F, di Marzo Veronese F, de Vico AL, et al. Viral DNA carried by human immunodeficiency virus type 1 virions. J Virol 1992;66:5067.
27. Trono D. Partial reverse transcripts in virions from human immunodeficiency and murine leukemia viruses. J Virol 1992;66:4893.
28. Bukrinsky MI, Sharova N, McDonald TL, et al. Association of integrase, matrix, and reverse transcriptase antigens of human immunodeficiency virus type 1 with viral nucleic acids following acute infection. Proc Natl Acad Sci USA 1993;90:6125.
29. Varmus HE, Swanstrom R. Replication of retroviruses. In: Weiss RA, Teich N, Varmus HE, Coffin JM, eds. RNA tumor viruses. Cold Spring Harbor, NY: Cold Spring Harbor Laboratory, 1985:75.
30. Varmus HE. Retroviruses. Science 1988;240:1427.
31. Mak J, Jiang M, Wainberg MA, et al. Role of Pr160[gag-pol] in mediating the selective incorporation of tRNA(Lys) into human immunodeficiency virus type 1 particles. J Virol 1994;68:2065.
32. Wakefield JK, Rhim H, Morrow CD. Minimal sequence requirements of a functional human immunodeficiency virus type 1 primer binding site. J Virol 1994;68:1605.
33. Darlix JL, Vincent A, Gabus C, et al. Trans-activation of the 5' to 3' viral DNA strand transfer by nucleocapsid protein during reverse transcription of HIV-1 RNA. C R Acad Sci III 1993;316:763.
34. Bukrinsky MI, Sharova N, Dempsey MP, et al. Active nuclear import of human immunodeficiency virus type 1 preintegration complexes. Proc Natl Acad Sci USA 1992;89:6580.
35. Bukrinsky MI, Haggerty S, Dempsey MP, et al. A nuclear localization signal within HIV-1 matrix protein that governs infection of non-dividing cells. Nature 1993;365:666.
36. Heinzinger NK, Bukrinsky MI, Haggerty SA, et al. The Vpr protein of human immunodeficiency virus type 1 influences nuclear localization of viral nucleic acids in nondividing host cells. Proc Natl Acad Sci USA 1994;91:7311.
37. Von Schwedler U, Kornbluth RS, Trono D. The nuclear localization signal of the matrix protein of human immunodeficiency virus type 1 allows the establishment of infection in macrophages and quiescent T lymphocytes. Proc Natl Acad Sci USA 1994;91:6992.
38. Gallay P, Swingler S, Aiken C, Trono D. HIV-1 infection of nondividing cells: C-terminal tyrosine phosphorylation of the viral matrix protein is a key regulator. Cell 1995;80:379.
39. Neumann M, Kleinschmidt A, Felber BK, Froese B, et al. Restriction of HIV-1 production in a human astrocytoma cell line is associated with a cellular block in Rev function. J Virol 1994;69:2159.
40. Tornatore C, Meyers K, Atwood W, et al. Temporal patterns of human immunodeficiency virus type 1 transcripts in human fetal astrocytes. J Virol 1994;68:93.
41. Saksela K, Stevens C, Rubinstein P, Baltimore D. Human immunodeficiency virus type 1 mRNA expression in peripheral blood cells predicts disease progression independently of the numbers of CD4+ lymphocytes. Proc Natl Acad Sci U S A 1994;91:1104.
42. Jones KA, Kadonaga JT, Luciw PA, Tjian R. Activation of the AIDS retrovirus promoter by the cellular transcription factor SP1. Science 1986;232:755.
43. Nabel G, Baltimore D. An inducible transcription factor activates expression of human immunodeficiency virus in T cells. Nature 1987;326:711.
44. Harrich D, Garcia J, Wu F, et al. Role of SP-1 binding domains in in vivo transcriptional regulation of the human immunodeficiency virus type 1 long terminal repeat. J Virol 1989;63:2585.
45. Parrot C, Seidner T, Duh E, et al. Variable role of the long terminal repeat Sp1-binding sites in human immunodeficiency virus replication in T lymphocytes. J Virol 1991;65:1414.
46. Ross EK, Buckler-White AJ, Rabson AB, et al. Contribution of NF-kB and Sp1 binding motifs to the replicative capacity of human immunodeficiency virus type 1: distinct patterns of viral growth are determined by T-cell types. J Virol 1991;65:4350.
47. Nabel GJ, Rice SA, Knipe DM, Baltimore D. Alternative mechanisms for activation of human immunodeficiency virus enhancer in T cells. Science 1988;239:1299.

48. Wright CM, Felber BK, Paskalis H, Pavlakis GN. Expression and characterization of the *trans*-activator of HTLV-III/LAV virus. Science 1986;234:988.

49. Nabel GJ. The role of cellular transcription factors in the regulation of human immunodeficiency virus gene expression. In: Cullen BR, ed. Human retroviruses. New York: Oxford University Press, 1993.

50. Jones KA. HIV *trans*-activation and transcription control mechanisms. New Biol 1989;1:127.

51. Haseltine WA, Wong-Staal F. Genetic structure and regulation of HIV. Gene regulation of human retroviruses. New York: Raven Press 1991;1:1.

52. Meyers GB, Korber BH, Hahn K-T, et al. Human retroviruses and AIDS. A compilation and analysis of nucleic acid and amino acid sequences. Los Alamos, NM: Los Alamos National Laboratory, 1995.

53. Embretson J, Zupancic M, Ribas JL, et al. Massive covert infection of helper T lymphocytes and macrophages by HIV during the incubation period of AIDS. Nature 1993;362:359.

54. Pantaleo G, Graziosi C, Demarest J, et al. HIV infection is active and progressive in lymphoid tissue during the clinically latent stage of disease. Nature 1993;362:355.

55. Alcami J, Lain de Lera T, Folgueira L, et al. Absolute dependence on kappa B responsive elements for initiation and Tat-mediated amplification of HIV transcription in blood CD4 T lymphocytes. EMBO J 1995;14:1552.

56. Staffa A, Cochrane A. The *tat/rev* intron of human immunodeficiency virus type 1 is inefficiently spliced because of suboptimal signals in the 3′ splice site. J Virol 1994;68:3071.

57. Kalland KH, Szilvay AM, Brokstad KA, et al. The human immunodeficiency virus type 1 Rev protein shuttles between the cytoplasm and nuclear compartments. Mol Cell Biol 1994;14:7436.

58. Meyer BE, Malim MH. The HIV-1 Rev *trans*-activator shuttles between the nucleus and the cytoplasm. Genes Dev 1994;8:1538.

59. Richard N, Iacampo S, Cochrane A. HIV-1 Rev is capable of shuttling between the nucleus and cytoplasm. Virology 1994;204:123.

60. D'Agostino DM, Ciminale V, Pavlakis GP, Chieco-Bianchi L. Intracellular trafficking of the human immunodeficiency virus type 1 Rev protein: involvement of continued rRNA synthesis in nuclear retention. AIDS Res Hum Retroviruses 1995;11:1063.

61. Muesing MA, Smith DH, Cabradilla CD, et al. Nucleic acid structure and expression of the human AIDS/lymphadenopathy retrovirus. Nature 1985;313:450.

62. Arya SK, Gallo RC. Three novel genes of human T-cell lymphotropic virus type III: immune reactivity of their products with sera from acquired immune deficiency syndrome patients. Proc Natl Acad Sci USA 1986;83:2209.

63. Benko DM, Schwartz S, Pavlakis GN, Felber BK. A novel human immunodeficiency virus type 1 protein, tev, shares sequences with tat, env, and rev proteins. J Virol 1990;64:2505.

64. Schwartz S, Felber BK, Benko DM, et al. Cloning and functional analysis of multiply spliced mRNA species of human immunodeficiency virus type 1. J Virol 1990;64:2519.

65. Schwartz S, Felber BK, Fenyö EM, Pavlakis GN. Env and Vpu proteins of human immunodeficiency virus type 1 are produced from multiple bicistronic mRNAs. J Virol 1990;64:5448.

66. Schwartz S, Felber BK, Pavlakis GN. Expression of human immunodeficiency virus type-1 vif and vpr mRNAs is Rev-dependent and regulated by splicing. Virology 1991;183:677.

67. Salfeld J, Gottlinger H, Sia R, et al. A tripartite HIV-1 tat-env-rev fusion protein. EMBO J 1990;9:965.

68. Purcell DFJ, Martin MA. Alternative splicing of human immunodeficiency virus type 1 mRNA modulates viral protein expression, replication, and infectivity. J Virol 1993;67:6365.

69. Pavlakis GN, Schwartz S, D'Agostino DM, Felber BK. Structure, splicing, and regulation of expression of HIV-1: a model for the general organization of lentiviruses and other complex retroviruses. In: Kennedy R, Wong-Staal F, Koff WC, eds. Annual Review of AIDS Research. New York: Marcel Dekker, 1991:41.

70. Neumann M, Saltarelli M, Harrison J, et al. Splicing variability in HIV-1 revealed by quantitative RNA-PCR. AIDS Res Hum Retroviruses 1994;10:1527.

71. Luban J, Bossolt KL, Franke EK, et al. Human immunodeficiency virus type 1 Gag protein binds to cyclophilins A and B. Cell 1993;73:1067.

72. Franke EK, En Hui Yuan H, Luban J. Specific incorporation of cyclophilin A into HIV-1 virions. Nature 1994;372:359.

73. Thali M, Bukovsky A, Kondo E, et al. Functional association of cyclophilin A with HIV-1 virions. Nature 1994;372:363.

74. Steinkasserer A, Harrison R, Billich A, et al. Mode of action of SDZ NIM 811, a nonimmunosuppressive cyclosporin A analog with activity against human immunodeficiency virus type 1 (HIV-1): interference with early and late events in HIV-1 replication. J Virol 1995;69:814.

75. Parkin NT, Chamorro M, Varmus HE. Human immunodeficiency virus type 1 gag-pol frameshifting is dependent on downstream mRNA secondary structure: demonstration by expression in vivo. J Virol 1992;66:5147.

76. Wilson W, Braddock M, Adams SE, et al. HIV expression strategies: ribosomal frameshifting is directed by a short sequence in both mammalian and yeast systems. Cell 1988;55:1159.

77. Schultz AM, Henderson LE, Oroszlan S. Fatty acylation of proteins. Annu Rev Cell Biol 1988;4:611.

78. Bryant M, Ratner L. Myristoylation-dependent replication and assembly of human immunodeficiency virus 1. Proc Natl Acad Sci USA 1990;87:523.

79. Yuan X, Yu X, Lee TH, Essex M. Mutations in the N-terminal region of human immunodeficiency virus type 1 matrix protein block intracellular transport of the Gag precursor. J Virol 1993;67:6387.

80. Spearman P, Wang JJ, Vander Heyden N, Ratner L. Identification of human immunodeficiency virus type 1 Gag protein domains essential to membrane binding and particle assembly. J Virol 1994;68:3232.

81. Zhou W, Parent LJ, Wills JW, Resh MD. Identification of a membrane-binding domain within the amino-terminal region of human immunodeficiency virus type 1 Gag protein which interacts with acidic phospholipids. J Virol 1994;68:2556.

82. Dorfman T, Mammano F, Haseltine WA, Gottlinger HG. Role of the matrix protein in the virion association of the human immunodeficiency virus type 1 envelope glycoprotein. J Virol 1994;68:1689.

83. Freed EO, Englund G, Martin MA. Role of the basic domain of human immunodeficiency virus type 1 matrix in macrophage infection. J Virol 1995;69:3949.

84. Freed EO, Orenstein JM, Buckler-White AJ, Martin MA. Single amino acid changes in the human immunodeficiency virus type 1 matrix protein block virus particle production. J Virol 1994;68:5311.

85. Freed EO, Martin MA. Virion incorporation of envelope glycoproteins with long but not short cytoplasmic tails is blocked by specific, single amino acid substitutions in the human immunodeficiency virus type 1 matrix. J Virol 1995;69:1984.

86. Luban J, Alin KB, Bossolt KL, Humaran T, et al. Genetic assay for multimerization of retroviral gag polyproteins. J Virol 1992;66:5157.

87. Reicin AS, Paik S, Berkowitz RD, et al. Linker insertion mutations in the human immunodeficiency virus type 1 *gag* gene: effects on virion particle assembly, release, and infectivity. J Virol 1995;69:642.

88. Dorfman T, Bukovsky A, Ohagen A, et al. Functional domains of the capsid protein of human immunodeficiency virus type 1. J Virol 1994;68:8180.

89. Mammano F, Ohagen A, Hoglund S, Gottlinger HG. Role of the major homology region of human immunodeficiency virus type 1 in virion morphogenesis. J Virol 1994;68:4927.

90. Aldovini A, Young RA. Mutations of RNA and protein sequences involved in human immunodeficiency virus type 1 packaging result in production of noninfectious virus. J Virol 1990;64:1920.

91. Gorelick RJ, Nigida SM, Bess JW, et al. Noninfectious human immunodeficiency virus type 1 mutants deficient in genomic RNA. J Virol 1990;64:3207.

92. Dorfman T, Luban J, Goff SP, et al. Mapping of functionally important residues of a cysteine-histidine box in the human immunodeficiency virus type 1 nucleocapsid protein. J Virol 1993;67:6159.

93. Dannull J, Surovoy A, Jung G, Moelling K. Specific binding of HIV-1 nucleocapsid protein to PSI RNA in vitro requires N-terminal zinc finger and flanking basic amino acid residues. EMBO J 1994;13:1525.

94. Darlix JL, Gabus C, Nugeyre MT, et al. *Cis* elements and *trans*-acting factors involved in the RNA dimerization of the human immunodeficiency virus HIV-1. J Mol Biol 1990;216:689.

95. Fu W, Gorelick RJ, Rein A. Characterization of human immunodeficiency virus type 1 dimeric RNA from wild-type and protease-defective virions. J Virol 1994;68:5013.

96. Berkowitz RD, Goff SP. Analysis of binding elements in the human immunodeficiency virus type 1 genomic RNA and nucleocapsid protein. Virology 1994;202:233.

97. Clever J, Sassetti C, Parslow TG. RNA secondary structure and binding sites for *gag* gene products in the 5′ packaging signal of human immunodeficiency virus type 1. J Virol 1995;69:2101.

98. Lee PP, Linial ML. Efficient particle formation can occur if the matrix domain of human immunodeficiency virus type 1 Gag is substituted by a myristylation signal. J Virol 1994;68:6644.

99. Luban J, Goff SP. Mutational analysis of cis-acting packaging signals in human immunodeficiency virus type 1 RNA. J Virol 1994;68:3784.

100. Kondo E, Mammano F, Cohen EA, Gottlinger HG. The p6^{gag} domain of human immunodeficiency virus type 1 is sufficient for the incorporation of Vpr into heterologous viral particles. J Virol 1995;69:2759.

101. Pettit SC, Moody MD, Wehbie RS, et al. The p2 domain of human immunodeficiency virus type 1 Gag regulates sequential proteolytic processing and is required to produce fully infectious virions. J Virol 1994;68:8017.

102. Krausslich HG, Facke M, Heuser AM, et al. The spacer peptide between human immunodeficiency virus capsid and nucleocapsid proteins is essential for ordered assembly and viral infectivity. J Virol 1995;69:3407.

103. Lasky LA, Nakamura G, Smith DH, et al. Delineation of a region of the human immunodeficiency virus type 1 gp120 glycoprotein critical for interaction with the CD4 receptor. Cell 1987;50:975.

104. Leonard CK, Spellman MW, Riddle L, et al. Assignment of intrachain disulfide bonds and characterization of potential glycosylation sites of the type 1 recombinant human immunodeficiency virus envelope glycoprotein (gp120) expressed in Chinese hamster ovary cells. J Biol Chem 1990;265:10373.

105. Fenouillet E, Gluckman JC, Jones IM. Functions of HIV envelope glycans. Trends Biochem Sci 1994;19:65.

106. Moore JP, Jameson BA, Sattentau QJ, et al. Towards a structure of the HIV-1 envelope glycoprotein gp120: an immunochemical approach. Philos Trans R Soc Lond B Biol Sci 1993;342:83.

107. Gelderblom HR. Assembly and morphology of HIV: potential effect of structure on viral function. AIDS 1991;5:617.

108. Poumbourios P, el Ahmar W, McPhee DA, Kemp BE. Determinants of human immunodeficiency virus type 1 envelope glycoprotein oligomeric structure. J Virol 1995;69:1209.

109. Wong-Staal F, Shaw GM, Hahn BH, et al. Genomic diversity of human T-lymphotropic virus type III (HTLV-III). Science 1985;229:759.

110. Modrow S, Hahn BH, Shaw GM, et al. Computer-assisted analysis of envelope protein sequences of seven human immunodeficiency virus isolates: prediction of antigenic epitopes in conserved and variable regions. J Virol 1987;61:570.

111. Meyerhans A, Cheynier R, Albert J, et al. Temporal fluctuations in HIV quasispecies in vivo are not reflected by sequential HIV isolations. Cell 1989;58:901.

112. Rusche JR, Javaherian K, McDanal C, et al. Antibodies that inhibit fusion of human immunodeficiency virus-infected cells bind a 24-amino acid sequence of the viral envelope, gp120. Proc Natl Acad Sci USA 1988;85:3198.

113. Javaherian K, Langlois AJ, McDanal C, et al. Principal neutralizing domain of the human immunodeficiency virus type 1 envelope protein. Proc Natl Acad Sci USA 1989;86:6768.

114. Earl PL, Doms RW, Moss B. Oligomeric structure of the human immunodeficiency virus type 1 envelope glycoprotein. Proc Natl Acad Sci USA 1990;87:648.

115. Earl PL, Broder CC, Long D, et al. Native oligomeric human immunodeficiency virus type 1 envelope glycoprotein elicits diverse monoclonal antibody reactivities. J Virol 1994;68:3015.

116. Cann AJ, Churcher MJ, Boyd M, et al. The region of the envelope gene of human immunodeficiency virus type 1 responsible for determination of cell tropism. J Virol 1992;66:305.

117. Koito A, Harrowe G, Levy JA, Cheng-Mayer C. Functional role of the V1/V2 region of human immunodeficiency virus type 1 envelope glycoprotein gp120 in infection of primary macrophages and soluble CD4 neutralization. J Virol 1994;68:2253.

118. Kido H, Kamoshita K, Fukutomi A, Katunuma N. Processing protease for gp160 human immunodeficiency virus type I envelope glycoprotein precursor in human T4+ lymphocytes. Purification and characterization. J Biol Chem 1993;268:13406.

119. Debouck C, Gorniak JG, Strickler JE, et al. Human immunodeficiency virus protease expressed in Escherichia coli exhibits autoprocessing and specific maturation of the gag precursor. Proc Natl Acad Sci USA 1987;84:8903.

120. Copeland TD, Oroszlan S. Genetic locus, primary structure, and chemical synthesis of human immunodeficiency virus protease. Gene Anal Tech 1988;5:109.

121. Kohl NE, Emini EA, Schleif WA, et al. Active human immunodeficiency virus protease is required for viral infectivity. Proc Natl Acad Sci U S A 1988;85:4686.

122. Luban J, Lee C, Goff SP. Effect of linker insertion mutations in the human immunodeficiency virus type 1 gag gene on activation of viral protease expressed in bacteria. J Virol 1993;67:3630.

123. Karacostas V, Wolffe EJ, Nagashima K, et al. Overexpression of the HIV-1 gag-pol polyprotein results in intracellular activation of HIV-1 protease and inhibition of assembly and budding of virus-like particles. Virology 1993;193:661.

124. Luukkonen BG, Fenyo EM, Schwartz S. Overexpression of human immunodeficiency virus type 1 protease increases intracellular cleavage of Gag and reduces virus infectivity. Virology 1995;206:854.

125. Kaplan AH, Manchester M, Swanstrom R. The activity of the protease of human immunodeficiency virus type 1 is initiated at the membrane of infected cells before the release of viral proteins and is required for release to occur with maximum efficiency. J Virol 1994;68:6782.

126. Navia M, Fitzgerald PM, McKeever BM, et al. Three-dimensional structure of aspartyl protease from HIV-1. Nature 1989;337:615.

127. Weber IT, Miller M, Jaskolski M, et al. Molecular modeling of the HIV-1 protease and its substrate binding site. Science 1989;243:928.

128. Wlodawer A, Miller M, Jaskolski M, et al. Conserved folding in retroviral proteases: crystal structure of a synthetic HIV-1 protease. Science 1989;245:616.

129. Di Marzo Veronese F, Copeland TD, DeVico AL, et al. Characterization of highly immunogenic p66/p51 as the reverse transcriptase of HTLV-III/LAV. Science 1986;231:1289.

130. Kohlstaedt LA, Wang J, Friedman JM, et al. Crystal structure at 3.5-A resolution of HIV-1 reverse transcriptase complexed with an inhibitor. Science 1992;256:1783.

131. Jacobo-Molina A, Ding J, Nanni RG, et al. Crystal structure of human immunodeficiency virus type 1 reverse transcriptase complexed with double-stranded DNA at 3.0-A resolution shows bent DNA. Proc Natl Acad Sci USA 1993;90:6320.

132. Broder S, Mitsuya H, Yarchoan R, Pavlakis GN. Antiretroviral therapy in AIDS. Ann Intern Med 1990;113:604.

133. Larder BA, Kellam P, Kemp SD. Convergent combination therapy can select viable multidrug-resistant HIV-1 in vitro. Nature 1993;365:451.

134. Gu Z, Gao Q, Fang H, et al. Identification of a mutation at codon 65 in the IKKK motif of reverse transcriptase that encodes human immunodeficiency virus resistance to 2',3'-dideoxycytidine and 2',3'-dideoxy-3'-thiacytidine. Antimicrob Agents Chemother 1994;38:275.

135. Larder BA. Interactions between drug resistance mutations in human immunodeficiency virus type 1 reverse transcriptase. J Gen Virol 1994;75:951.

136. Richman DD. Emergence of mutant HIV reverse transcriptase conferring resistance to AZT. J Enzym Inhib 1992;6:55.

137. Kellam P, Boucher CA, Tijnagel JM, Larder BA. Zidovudine treatment results in the selection of human immunodeficiency virus type 1 variants whose genotypes confer increasing levels of drug resistance. J Gen Virol 1994;75:341.

138. Najera I, Richman DD, Olivares I, et al. Natural occurrence of drug resistance mutations in the reverse transcriptase of human immunodeficiency virus type 1 isolates. AIDS Res Hum Retroviruses 1994;10:1479.

139. Kellam P, Larder BA. Retroviral recombination can lead to linkage of reverse transcriptase mutations that confer increased zidovudine resistance. J Virol 1995;69:669.

140. Debyser Z, Pauwels R, Andries K, De Clercq E. Specific HIV-1 reverse transcriptase inhibitors. J Enzym Inhib 1992;6:47.

141. De Clercq E. HIV-1-specific RT inhibitors: highly selective inhibitors of human immunodeficiency virus type 1 that are specifically targeted at the viral reverse transcriptase. Med Res Rev 1993;13:229.

142. De Clercq E. New developments in the chemotherapy of lentivirus (human immunodeficiency virus) infections: sensitivity/resistance of HIV-1 to non-nucleoside HIV-1-specific inhibitors. Ann N Y Acad Sci 1994;724:438.

143. Balzarini J, Karlsson A, Perez-Perez MJ, et al. HIV-1-specific reverse transcriptase inhibitors show differential activity against HIV-1 mutant strains containing different amino acid substitutions in the reverse transcriptase. Virology 1993;192:246.

144. Balzarini J, Karlsson A, Sardana VV, Emini EA, et al. Human immunodeficiency virus 1 (HIV-1)-specific reverse transcriptase (RT) inhibitors may suppress the replication of specific drug-resistant (E138K)RT HIV-1 mutants or select for highly resistant (Y181C → C181I)RT HIV-1 mutants. Proc Natl Acad Sci USA 1994;91:6599.

145. Chow SA, Vincent KA, Ellison V, Brown PO. Reversal of integration and DNA splicing mediated by integrase of human immunodeficiency virus. Science 1992;255:723.

146. Bushman FD, Craigie R. Integration of human immunodeficiency virus DNA: adduct interference analysis of required DNA sites. Proc Natl Acad Sci U S A 1992;89:3458.

147. Drelich M, Haenggi M, Mous J. Conserved residues Pro-109 and Asp-116 are required for interaction of the human immunodeficiency virus type 1 integrase protein with its viral DNA substrate. J Virol 1993;67:5041.

148. Engelman A, Bushman FD, Craigie R. Identification of discrete functional domains of HIV-1 integrase and their organization within an active multimeric complex. EMBO J 1993;12:3269.

149. Vink C, Oude Groeneger AM, Plasterk RH. Identification of the catalytic and DNA-binding region of the human immunodeficiency virus type I integrase protein. Nucleic Acids Res 1993;21:1419.

150. Vink C, Lutzke RA, Plasterk RH. Formation of a stable complex between the human immunodeficiency virus integrase protein and viral DNA. Nucleic Acids Res 1994;22:4103.

151. Dyda F, Hickman AB, Jenkins TM, et al. Crystal structure of the catalytic domain of HIV-1 integrase: similarity to other polynucleotidyl transferases. Science 1994;266:1981.

152. Yang W, Steitz TA. Recombining the structures of HIV integrase, RuvC and RNase H. Structure 1995;3:131.

153. Engelman A, Englund G, Orenstein JM, et al. Multiple effects of mutations in human immunodeficiency virus type 1 integrase on viral replication. J Virol 1995;69:2729.

154. Englund G, Theodore TS, Freed EO, et al. Integration is required for productive infection of monocyte-derived macrophages by human immunodeficiency virus type 1. J Virol 1995;69:3216.

155. Vogel M, Cichutek K, Norley S, Kurth R. Self-limiting infection by int/nef-double mutants of simian immunodeficiency virus. Virology 1993;193:115.

156. Wiskerchen M, Muesing MA. Identification and characterization of a temperature-sensitive mutant of human immunodeficiency virus type 1 by alanine scanning mutagenesis of the integrase gene. J Virol 1995;69:597.

157. Asseline U, Grasby J, Hamy F, et al. HIV gene regulatory proteins tat and rev and their interactions with synthetic RNA. Nucleic Acids Symp Ser 1993;1993:113.

158. Dayton AI, Sodroski JG, Rosen CA, et al. The trans-activator gene of the human T-cell lymphotrophic virus type III is required for replication. Cell 1986;44:941.

159. Fisher AG, Feinberg MB, Josephs SF, et al. The transactivator gene of HTLV-III is essential for virus replication. Nature 1986;320:367.

160. Arya SK, Guo C, Josephs SF, Wong-Staal F. Trans-activator gene of human T-lymphotrophic virus type III (HTLV-III). Science 1985;229:69.

161. Sodroski J, Patarca R, Rosen C, et al. Location of the trans-activating region on the genome of human T-cell lymphotrophic virus type III. Science 1985;229:74.

162. Cullen BR. Trans-activation of human immunodeficiency virus occurs via a bimodal mechanism. Cell 1986;46:973.

163. Peterlin BM, Luciw PA, Barr PJ, Walker MD. Elevated levels of mRNA can account for the trans-activation of human immunodeficiency virus. Proc Natl Acad Sci U S A 1986;83:9734.

164. Hauber J, Malim MH, Cullen BR. Mutational analysis of the conserved basic domain of human immunodeficiency virus tat protein. J Virol 1989;63:1181.

165. Ruben S, Perkins A, Purcell R, et al. Structural and functional characterization of human immunodeficiency virus tat protein. J Virol 1989;63:1.

166. Roy S, Delling U, Chen C-H, et al. A bulge structure in HIV-1 TAR RNA is required for tat binding and tat-mediated trans-activation. Genes Dev 1990;4:1365.

167. Rosen CA, Sodroski JG, Haseltine WA. The location of cis-acting regulatory sequences in the human T cell lymphotropic virus type III (HTLV-III/LAV) long terminal repeat. Cell 1985;41:813.

168. Berkhout B, Silverman RH, Jeang K-T. Tat trans-activates the human immunodeficiency virus through a nascent RNA target. Cell 1989;59:273.

169. Dingwall C, Ernberg I, Gait MJ, et al. Human immunodeficiency virus 1 tat protein binds trans-activation-responsive region (TAR) RNA in vitro. Proc Natl Acad Sci USA 1989;86:6925.

170. Dingwall C, Ernberg I, Gait M, et al. HIV-1 Tat protein stimulates transcription by binding to a U-rich bulge in the stem of the TAR RNA structure. EMBO J 1990;9:4145.

171. Hauber J, Cullen BR. Mutational analysis of the trans-activation-responsive region of the human immunodeficiency virus type 1 long terminal repeat. J Virol 1988;62:673.

172. Muesing MA, Smith DH, Capon DJ. Regulation of mRNA accumulation by a human immunodeficiency virus trans-activator protein. Cell 1987;48:691.

173. Feng S, Holland EC. HIV-1 tat trans-activation requires the loop sequence within tar. Nature 1988;334:165.

174. Berkhout B, Jeang K. Trans-activation of human immunodeficiency virus type I is sequence specific for both the single-stranded bulge and loop of the trans-acting responsive hairpin: a quantitative analysis. J Virol 1989;63:5501.

175. Garcia JA, Harrich D, Soultanakis E, et al. Human immunodeficiency virus type 1 LTR TATA and TAR region sequences required for transcriptional regulation. EMBO J 1989;8:765.

176. Selby MJ, Bain ES, Luciw PA, Peterlin BM. Structure, sequence, and position of the stem-loop structure in tar determine transcriptional elongation by tat through the HIV-1 long terminal repeat. Genes Dev 1989;3:547.

177. Roy S, Parkin NT, Rosen C, et al. Structural requirements for trans-activation of HIV-1 LTR-directed gene expression by Tat: importance of base pairing, loop sequence, and bulges in the TAR region. J Virol 1990;64:1402.

178. Harper JW, Logsdson NJ. Refolded HIV-1 tat protein protects both bulge and loop nucleotides in TAR RNA from ribonucleolytic cleavage. Biochemistry 1991;30:8060.

179. Weeks KM, Ampe C, Schultz SC, et al. Fragments of the HIV-1 tat protein specifically bind TAR RNA. Science 1990;249:1281.

180. Berkhout B, Jeang KT. Detailed mutational analysis of TAR RNA: critical spacing between the bulge and loop recognition domains. Nucleic Acids Res 1991;19:6169.

181. Calnan B, Tidor B, Biancalana S, et al. Arginine-mediated RNA recognition: the arginine fork. Science 1991;252:1167.

182. Karn J, Dingwall C, Finch J, et al. RNA binding by the tat and rev proteins of HIV-1. Biochimie 1991;73:9.

183. Puglisi J, Tan R, Calnan B, et al. Conformation of the TAR RNA-arginine complex by NMR spectroscopy. Science 1992;257:76.

184. Gatignol A, Kumar A, Rabson A, Jeang K-T. Identification of cellular proteins that bind to the human immunodeficiency virus type 1 trans-activation-responsive TAR element RNA. Proc Natl Acad Sci USA 1989;86:7828.

185. Gaynor R, Soultanakis E, Kuwabara M, et al. Specific binding of a HeLa cell nuclear protein to RNA sequences in the human immunodeficiency virus transactivating region. Proc Natl Acad Sci USA 1989;86:4858.

186. Marciniak RA, Garcia-Blanco MA, Sharp PA. Identification and characterization of a HeLa nuclear protein that specifically binds to the trans-activation-response (TAR) element of human immunodeficiency virus. Proc Natl Acad Sci USA 1990;87:3624.

187. Gatignol A, Buckler-White A, Berkhout B, Jeang K-T. Characterization of a human TAR-RNA-binding protein that activates the HIV-1 LTR. Science 1991;251:1597.

188. Sheline C, Milocco L, Jones K. Two distinct nuclear transcription factors recognize loop and bulge residues of the HIV-1 TAR RNA hairpin. Genes Dev 1991;5:2508.

189. Wu F, Garcia J, Sigman D, Gaynor R. Tat regulates binding of the human immunodeficiency virus trans-activating region RNA loop-binding protein TRP-185. Genes Dev 1991;5:2128.

190. Yu L, Zhang Z, Loewenstein PM, et al. Molecular cloning and characterization of a cellular protein that interacts with the human immunodeficiency virus type 1 Tat transactivator and encodes a strong transcriptional activation domain. J Virol 1995;69:3007.

191. Hart CE, Ou CY, Galphin JC, et al. Human chromosome 12 is required for elevated HIV-1 expression in human-hamster hybrid cells. Science 1989;246:488.

192. Newstein M, Stanbridge J, Casey G, Shank PR. Human chromosome 12 encodes a species-specific factor which increases human immunodeficiency virus type 1 tat-mediated trans activation in rodent cells. J Virol 1990;64:4565.

193. Alonso A, Derse D, Peterlin B. Human chromosome 12 is required for optimal interactions between Tat and TAR of human immunodeficiency virus type 1 in rodent cells. J Virol 1992;66:4617.

194. Alonso A, Cujec TP, Peterlin BM. Effects of human chromosome 12 on interactions between Tat and TAR of human immunodeficiency virus type 1. J Virol 1994;68:6505.

195. Berkhout B, Jeang KT. Functional roles for the TATA promoter and enhancers in basal and Tat-induced expression of the human immunodeficiency virus type 1 long terminal repeat. J Virol 1992;66:139.

196. Olsen H, Rosen C. Contribution of the TATA motif to Tat-mediated transcriptional activation of human immunodeficiency virus gene expression. J Virol 1992;66:5594.

197. Kato H, Horikoshi M, Roeder RG. Repression of HIV-1 transcription by a cellular protein. Science 1991;251:1476.

198. Garcia JA, Ou S-HI, Wu F, et al. Cloning and chromosomal mapping of a human immunodeficiency virus 1 "TATA" element modulator factor. Proc Natl Acad Sci USA 1992;89:9372.

199. Drysdale CM, Pavlakis GN. Rapid activation and subsequent down-regulation of the human immunodeficiency virus type 1 promotor in the presence of Tat: possible mechanisms contributing to latency. J Virol 1991;65:3044.

200. Carroll R, Peterlin B, Derse D. Inhibition of human immunodeficiency virus type 1 Tat activity by coexpression of heterologous trans activators. J Virol 1992;66:2000.

201. Rice AP, Mathews MB. Transcriptional but not translational regulation of HIV-1 by the tat gene product. Nature 1988;332:551.

202. Laspia M, Rice A, Mathews M. HIV-1 tat protein increases transcriptional initiation and stabilizes elongation. Cell 1989;59:283.

203. Marciniak RA, Calnan BJ, Frankel AD, Sharp PA. HIV-1 tat protein trans-activates transcription in vitro. Cell 1990;63:791.

204. Feinberg M, Baltimore D, Frankel A. The role of Tat in the human immunodeficiency virus life cycle indicates a primary effect on transcriptional elongation. Proc Natl Acad Sci USA 1991;88:4045.

205. Kato H, Sumimoto H, Pognonec P, Chen C, et al. HIV-1 Tat acts as a processivity factor in vitro in conjunction with cellular elongation factors. Genes Dev 1992;6:655.

206. Kessler M, Mathews M. Premature termination and processing of human immunodeficiency virus type 1-promoted transcripts. J Virol 1992;66:4488.

207. Jeang KT, Berkhout B. Kinetics of HIV-1 long terminal repeat trans-activation. Use of intragenic ribozyme to assess rate-limiting steps. J Biol Chem 1992;267:17891.

208. Derse D, Carvalho M, Carroll R, Peterlin BM. A minimal lentivirus Tat. J Virol 1991;65:7012.

209. Churcher MJ, Lamont C, Hamy F, et al. High affinity binding of TAR RNA by the human immunodeficiency virus type-1 tat protein requires base-pairs in the RNA stem and amino acid residues flanking the basic region. J Mol Biol 1993;230:90.

210. Luo Y, Madore SJ, Parslow TG, et al. Functional analysis of interactions between Tat and the trans-activation response element of human immunodeficiency virus type 1 in cells. J Virol 1993;67:5617.

211. Rice AP, Chan F. Tat protein of human immunodeficiency virus type 1 is a monomer when expressed in mammalian cells. Virology 1991;185:451.

212. Koken SE, Greijer AE, Verhoef K, et al. Intracellular analysis of in vitro modified HIV Tat protein. J Biol Chem 1994;269:8366.

213. Luznik L, Kraus G, Guatelli J, et al. Tat-independent replication of human immunodeficiency viruses. J Clin Invest 1995;95:328.

214. Sadaie MR, Tschachler E, Valerie K, et al. Activation of tat-defective human immunodeficiency virus by ultraviolet light. New Biol 1990;2:479.

215. Wain-Hobson S. HIV genome variability in vivo. AIDS 1989;.

216. Ensoli B, Barillari G, Salahuddin SZ, et al. Tat protein of HIV-1 stimulates growth of cells derived from Kaposi's sarcoma lesions of AIDS patients. Proc Natl Acad Sci USA 1990;87:3479.

217. Buonaguro L, Barillari G, Chang HK, et al. Effects of the human immunodeficiency virus type 1 Tat protein on the expression of inflammatory cytokines. J Virol 1992;66:7159.

218. Ensoli B, Buonaguro L, Barillari G, et al. Release, uptake, and effects of extracellular human immunodeficiency virus type 1 Tat protein on cell growth and viral transactivation. J Virol 1993;67:277.

219. Felber BK, Pavlakis GN. A quantitative bioassay for HIV-1 based on trans-activation. Science 1988;239:184.

220. Ciminale V, Felber BK, Campbell M, Pavlakis GN. A bioassay for HIV-1 based on Env-CD4 interaction. AIDS Res Hum Retroviruses 1990;6:1281.

221. Bogerd HP, Fridell RA, Madore S, Cullen BR. A novel cellular co-factor for HIV-1 Rev. Cell 1995;82:485.

222. Feinberg MB, Jarrett RF, Aldovini A, et al. HTLV-III expression and production involve complex regulation at the levels of splicing and translation of viral RNA. Cell 1986;46:807.

223. Sodroski J, Goh WC, Rosen C, Dayton A, et al. A second post-transcriptional trans-activator gene required for HTLV-III replication. Nature 1986;321:412.

224. Cullen BR, Hauber J, Campbell K, Sodroski JG, et al. Subcellular localization of the human immunodeficiency virus trans-acting art gene product. J Virol 1988;62:2498.

225. Felber BK, Hadzopoulou-Cladaras M, Cladaras C, et al. rev protein of human immunodeficiency virus type 1 affects the stability and transport of the viral mRNA. Proc Natl Acad Sci U S A 1989;86:1495.

226. Cochrane AW, Golub E, Volsky D, Ruben S, et al. Functional significance of phosphorylation to the human immunodeficiency virus Rev protein. J Virol 1989;63:4438.

227. Malim MH, Böhnlein S, Hauber J, Cullen BR. Functional dissection of the HIV-1 Rev trans-activator derivation of a trans-dominant repressor of Rev function. Cell 1989;58:205.

228. Emerman M, Vazeux R, Peden K. The rev gene product of the human immunodeficiency virus affects envelope-specific RNA localization. Cell 1989;57:1155.

229. Hadzopoulou-Cladaras M, Felber BK, Cladaras C, et al. The rev (trs/art) protein of human immunodeficiency virus type 1 affects viral mRNA and protein expression via a cis-acting sequence in the env region. J Virol 1989;63:1265.

230. Hammarskjöld ML, Heimer J, Hammarskjöld B, et al. Regulation of human immunodeficiency virus env expression by the rev gene product. J Virol 1989;63:1959.

231. Malim MH, Hauber J, Le S-Y, et al. The HIV-1 rev trans-activator acts through a structured target sequence to activate nuclear export of unspliced viral mRNA. Nature 1989;338:254.

232. Daly TJ, Cook KS, Gray GS, et al. Specific binding of HIV-1 recombinant Rev protein to the Rev-responsive element in vitro. Nature 1989;342:816.

233. Heaphy S, Dingwall C, Ernberg I, et al. HIV-1 regulator of virion expression (Rev) protein binds to an RNA stem-loop structure located within the Rev response element region. Cell 1990;60:685.

234. Holland SM, Ahmad N, Maitra RK, et al. Human immunodeficiency virus Rev protein recognizes a target sequence in Rev-responsive element RNA within the context of RNA secondary structure. J Virol 1990;64:5966.

235. Bartel D, Zapp M, Green M, Szostak J. HIV-1 Rev regulation involves recognition of non-Watson-Crick base pairs in viral RNA. Cell 1991;67:529.

236. Cook KS, Fisk GJ, Hauber J, et al. Characterization of HIV-1 REV protein: binding stoichiometry and minimal RNA substrate. Nucleic Acids Res 1991;19:1577.

237. Holland SM, Chavez M, Gerstberger S, Venkatesan S. A specific sequence with a bulged guanosine residue(s) in a stem-bulge-stem structure of Rev-responsive element RNA is required for trans activation by human immunodeficiency virus type 1 Rev. J Virol 1992;66:3699.

238. Dayton AI, Terwilliger EF, Potz J, Kowalski M, et al. Cis-acting sequences responsive to the rev gene product of the human immunodeficiency virus. J Acquir Immune Defic Syndr 1988;1:441.

239. Rosen CA, Terwilliger E, Dayton A, et al. Intragenic cis-acting art gene-responsive sequences of the human immunodeficiency virus. Proc Natl Acad Sci USA 1988;85:2071.

240. Cochrane A, Chen C-H, Rosen CA. Specific interaction of the human immunodeficiency virus Rev protein with a structured region in the env mRNA. Proc Natl Acad Sci USA 1990;87:1198.

241. Arrigo SJ, Chen ISY. Rev is necessary for translation but not cytoplasmic accumulation of HIV-1 vif, vpr, and env/vpu 2 RNAs. Genes Dev 1991;5:808.

242. Lawrence JB, Cochrane AW, Johnson CV, et al. The HIV-1 Rev protein: a model system for coupled RNA transport and translation. New Biol 1991;3:1220.

243. D'Agostino DM, Felber BK, Harrison JE, Pavlakis GN. The Rev protein of human immunodeficiency virus type 1 promotes polysomal association and translation of gag/pol and vpu/env mRNA. Mol Cell Biol 1992;12:1375.

244. Schwartz S, Felber BK, Pavlakis GN. Distinct RNA sequences in the *gag* region of human immunodeficiency virus type 1 decrease RNA stability and inhibit expression in the absence of Rev protein. J Virol 1992;66:150.

245. Bray M, Prasad S, Dubay JW, et al. A small element from the Mason-Pfizer monkey virus genome makes human immunodeficiency virus type 1 expression and replication Rev-independent. Proc Natl Acad Sci USA 1994;91:1256.

246. Zolotukhin AS, Valentin A, Pavlakis GN, Felber BK. Continuous propagation of RRE(-) and Rev(-)RRE(-) human immunodeficiency virus type 1 molecular clones containing a *cis*-acting element of simian retrovirus type 1 in human peripheral blood lymphocytes. J Virol 1994;68:7944.

247. Cochrane AW, Jones KS, Beidas S, et al. Identification and characterization of intragenic sequences which repress human immunodeficiency virus structural gene expression. J Virol 1991;65:5305.

248. Maldarelli F, Martin MA, Strebel K. Identification of posttranscriptionally active inhibitory sequences in human immunodeficiency virus type 1 RNA: Novel level of gene regulation. J Virol 1991;65:5732.

249. Schwartz S, Campbell M, Nasioulas G, et al. Mutational inactivation of an inhibitory sequence in human immunodeficiency virus type-1 results in Rev-independent *gag* expression. J Virol 1992;66:7176.

250. Nasioulas G, Zolotukhin AS, Tabernero C, et al. Elements distinct from the human immunodeficiency virus type 1 splice sites are responsible for the Rev dependence of the env mRNA. J Virol 1994;68:2986.

251. Cochrane A, Kramer R, Ruben S, et al. The human immunodeficiency virus *rev* protein is a nuclear phosphoprotein. Virology 1989;171:264.

252. Hope TJ, Huang X, McDonald D, Parslow TG. Steroid-receptor fusion of the human immunodeficiency virus type 1 Rev transactivator: mapping cryptic functions of the arginine-rich motif. Proc Natl Acad Sci USA 1990;87:7787.

253. McDonald D, Hope TJ, Parslow TG. Posttranscriptional regulation by the human immunodeficiency virus type-1 Rev and human T-cell leukemia virus type-I Rex proteins through a heterologous RNA binding site. J Virol 1992;66:7232.

254. Perkins A, Cochrane AW, Ruben SM, Rosen CA. Structural and functional characterization of the human immunodeficiency virus *rev* protein. J Acquir Immune Defic Syndr 1989;2:256.

255. Hope TJ, McDonald D, Huang XJ, et al. Mutational analysis of the human immunodeficiency virus type 1 Rev transactivator: essential residues near the amino terminus. J Virol 1990;64:5360.

256. Mermer B, Felber BK, Campbell M, Pavlakis GN. Identification of *trans*-dominant HIV-1 rev protein mutants by direct transfer of bacterially produced proteins into human cells. Nucleic Acids Res 1990;18:2037.

257. Solomin L, Felber BK, Pavlakis GN. Different sites of interaction for Rev, Tev, and Rex proteins within the Rev responsive element of human immunodeficiency virus type 1. J Virol 1990;64:6010.

258. Kjems J, Calnan BJ, Frankel AD, Sharp PA. Specific binding of a basic peptide from HIV-1 Rev. EMBO J 1992;11:1119.

259. Kjems J, Frankel AD, Sharp PA. Specific regulation of mRNA splicing in vitro by a peptide from HIV-1 rev. Cell 1991;67:169.

260. Malim MH, McCarn DF, Tiley LS, Cullen BR. Mutational definition of the human immunodeficiency virus type 1 Rev activation domain. J Virol 1991;65:4248.

261. Venkatesh LK, Chinnadurai G. Mutants in a conserved region near the carboxy-terminus of HIV-1 Rev identify functionally important residues and exhibit a dominant negative phenotype. Virology 1990;178:327.

262. Stauber R, Gaitanaris AS, Pavlakis GN. Analysis of trafficking of Rev and transdominant Rev proteins in living cells using green fluorescent protein fusions: transdominant Rev blocks the export of Rev from the nucleus to the cytoplasm. 1995;213:439.

263. Wen W, Meinkoth JL, Tsien RY, Taylor SS. Identification of a signal for rapid export of proteins from the nucleus. Cell 1995;82:463.

264. Zapp ML, Hope TJ, Parslow TG, Green MR. Oligomerization and RNA binding domains of the type 1 human immunodeficiency virus Rev protein: a dual function for an arginine-rich binding motif. Proc Natl Acad Sci USA 1991;88:7734.

265. Olsen HS, Cochrane AW, Dillon PJ, et al. Interaction of the human immunodeficiency virus type 1 Rev protein with a structured region in *env* mRNA is dependent on multimer formation mediated through a basic stretch of amino acids. Genes Dev 1990;4:1357.

266. Nalin CM, Purcell RD, Antelman D, et al. Purification and characterization of recombinant Rev protein of human immunodeficiency virus type 1. Proc Natl Acad Sci USA 1990;87:7593.

267. Hope TJ, Klein NP, Elder ME, Parslow TG. *Trans*-dominant inhibition of human immunodeficiency virus type 1 Rev occurs through formation of inactive protein complexes. J Virol 1992;66:1849.

268. Malim MH, Cullen BR. HIV-1 structural gene expression requires the binding of multiple Rev monomers to the viral RRE: implications for HIV-1 latency. Cell 1991;65:241.

269. Battiste JL, Tan R, Frankel AD, Williamson JR. Binding of an HIV Rev peptide to Rev responsive element RNA induces formation of purine-purine base pairs. Biochemistry 1994;33:2741.

270. Fankhauser C, Izaurralde E, Adachi Y, et al. Specific complex of human immunodeficiency virus type 1 rev and nucleolar B23 proteins: dissociation by the Rev response element. Mol Cell Biol 1991;11:2567.

271. Ruhl M, Himmelspach M, Bahr G, et al. Eukaryotic initiation factor 5A is a cellular target of the human immunodeficiency virus type 1 Rev activation domain mediating trans-activation. J Cell Biol 1993;123:1309.

272. Fritz CC, Zapp ML, Green MR. A human nucleoporin-like protein that specifically interacts with HIV Rev. Nature 1995;376:530.

273. Benko DM, Robinson R, Solomin L, et al. Binding of trans-dominant mutant rev protein of human immunodeficiency virus type 1 to the *cis*-acting rev responsive element does not affect the fate of viral mRNA. New Biol 1990;2:1111.

274. Szilvay AM, Brokstad KA, Kopperud R, et al. Nuclear export of the human immunodeficiency virus type 1 nucleocytoplasmic shuttle protein Rev is mediated by its activation domain and is blocked by transdominant negative mutants. J Virol 1995;69:3315.

275. Wolff B, Cohen G, Hauber J, et al. Nucleocytoplasmic transport of the Rev protein of human immunodeficiency virus type 1 is dependent on the activation domain of the protein. Exp Cell Res 1995;217:31.

276. Bevec D, Dobrovnik M, Hauber J, Böhnlein E. Inhibition of human immunodeficiency virus type 1 replication in human T cells by retroviral-mediated gene transfer of a dominant-negative Rev trans-activator. Proc Natl Acad Sci USA 1992;89:9870.

277. Malim MH, Freimuth WW, Liu J, et al. Stable expression of transdominant Rev protein in human T cells inhibits human immunodeficiency virus replication. J Exp Med 1992;176:1197.

278. Bahner I, Zhou C, Yu X-J, et al. Comparison of *trans*-dominant inhibitory mutant human immunodeficiency virus type 1 genes expressed by retroviral vectors in human T lymphocytes. J Virol 1993;67:3199.

279. Woffendin C, Yang Z-Y, Udaykumar, et al. Nonviral and viral delivery of a human immunodeficiency virus protective gene into primary human T cells. Proc Natl Acad Sci USA 1994;91:11581.

280. Vandendriessche T, Chuah MKL, Chiang L, et al. Inhibition of clinical human immunodeficiency virus (HIV) type 1 isolates in primary CD4+ T lymphocytes by retroviral vectors expressing anti-HIV genes. J Virol 1995;69:4045.

281. Nabel GJ, Fox BA, Post L, et al. A molecular genetic intervention for AIDS—effects of a transdominant negative form of Rev. Hum Gene Ther 1994;5:79.

282. Oberste MS, Gonda MA. Conservation of amino-acid sequence motifs in lentivirus Vif proteins. Virus Genes 1992;6:95.

283. Rabson AB, Daugherty DF, Venkatesan S, et al. Transcription of novel open reading frames of AIDS retrovirus during infection of lymphocytes. Science 1985;229:1388.

284. Kan NC, Franchini G, Wong-Staal F, et al. Identification of HTLV-III/LAV sor gene product and detection of antibodies in human sera. Science 1986;231:1553.

285. Lee TH, Coligan JE, Allan JS, et al. A new HTLV-III/LAV protein encoded by a gene found in cytopathic retroviruses. Science 1986;231:1546.

286. Garrett ED, Tiley LS, Cullen BR. Rev activates expression of the human immunodeficiency virus type 1 vif and vpr gene products. J Virol 1991;65:1653.

287. Michaels FH, Hattori N, Gallo RC, Franchini G. The human immunodeficiency virus type 1 (HIV-1) vif protein is located in the cytoplasm of infected cells and its effect on viral replication is equivalent in HIV-2. Aids Res Hum Retroviruses 1993;9:1025.

288. Goncalves J, Jallepalli P, Gabuzda DH. Subcellular localization of the Vif protein of human immunodeficiency virus type 1. J Virol 1994;68:704.

289. Reddy TR, Kraus G, Yamada O, et al. Comparative analyses of human immunodeficiency virus type 1 (HIV-1) and HIV-2 Vif mutants. J Virol 1995;69:3549.

290. Fan L, Peden K. Cell-free transmission of Vif mutants of HIV-1. Virology 1992;190:19.

291. Hoglund S, Ohagen A, Lawrence K, Gabuzda D. Role of vif during packing of the core of HIV-1. Virology 1994;201:349.

292. Sakai H, Shibata R, Sakuragi J, et al. Cell-dependent requirement of human immunodeficiency virus type 1 Vif protein for maturation of virus particles. J Virol 1993;67:1663.

293. Borman AM, Quillent C, Charneau P, et al. Human immunodeficiency virus type 1 Vif- mutant particles from restrictive cells: role of Vif in correct particle assembly and infectivity. J Virol 1995;69:2058.

294. Blanc D, Patience C, Schulz TF, et al. Transcomplementation of VIF-HIV-1 mutants in CEM cells suggests that VIF affects late steps of the viral life cycle. Virology 1993;193:186.

295. Courcoul M, Patience C, Rey F, et al. Peripheral blood mononuclear cells produce normal amounts of defective Vif− human immunodeficiency virus type 1 particles which are restricted for the preretrotranscription steps. J Virol 1995;69:2068.

296. Sova P, Volsky DJ. Efficiency of viral DNA synthesis during infection of permissive and nonpermissive cells with vif-negative human immunodeficiency virus type 1. J Virol 1993;67:6322.

297. Von Schwedler U, Song J, Aiken C, Trono D. Vif is crucial for human immunodeficiency virus type 1 proviral DNA synthesis in infected cells. J Virol 1993;67:4945.

298. Gabuzda DH, Lawrence K, Langhoff E, et al. Role of vif in replication of human immunodeficiency virus type 1 in CD4+ T lymphocytes. J Virol 1992;66:6489.

299. Ma XY, Sova P, Chao W, Volsky DJ. Cysteine residues in the Vif protein of human immunodeficiency virus type 1 are essential for viral infectivity. J Virol 1994;68:1714.

300. Cohen EA, Dehni G, Sodroski JG, Haseltine WA. Human immunodeficiency virus vpr product is a virion-associated regulatory protein. J Virol 1990;64:3097.

301. Yuan X, Matsuda Z, Matsuda M, et al. Human immunodeficiency virus vpr gene encodes a virion-associated protein. AIDS Res Hum Retroviruses 1990;6:1265.

302. Paxton W, Connor RI, Landau NR. Incorporation of Vpr into human immunodeficiency virus type 1 virions: requirement for the p6 region of gag and mutational analysis. J Virol 1993;67:7229.

303. Lavallee C, Yao XJ, Ladha A, et al. Requirement of the Pr55gag precursor for incorporation of the Vpr product into human immunodeficiency virus type 1 viral particles. J Virol 1994;68:1926.

304. Wang JJ, Lu Y, Ratner L. Particle assembly and Vpr expression in human immunodeficiency virus type 1-infected cells demonstrated by immunoelectron microscopy. J Gen Virol 1994;75:2607.

305. Levy DN, Fernandes LS, Williams WV, Weiner DB. Induction of cell differentiation by human immunodeficiency virus 1 vpr. Cell 1993;72:541.

306. Levy DN, Refaeli Y, Weiner DB. Extracellular Vpr protein increases cellular permissiveness to human immunodeficiency virus replication and reactivates virus from latency. J Virol 1995;69:1243.

307. Rogel ME, Wu LI, Emerman M. The human immunodeficiency virus type 1 vpr gene prevents cell proliferation during chronic infection. J Virol 1995;69:882.

308. Levy DN, Refaeli Y, MacGregor RR, Weiner DB. Serum Vpr regulates productive infection and latency of human immunodeficiency virus type 1. Proc Natl Acad Sci USA 1994;91:1083.

309. Macreadie IG, Castelli LA, Hewish DR, et al. A domain of human immunodeficiency virus type 1 Vpr containing repeated H(S/F)RIG amino acid motifs causes cell growth arrest and structural defects. Proc Natl Acad Sci USA 1995;92:2770.

310. Cleves AE, Novick PJ, Bankaitis VA. Mutations in the SAC1 gene suppress defects in yeast Golgi and yeast actin function. J Cell Biol 1989;109:2939.

311. Balliet JW, Kolson DL, Eiger G, et al. Distinct effects in primary macrophages and lymphocytes of the human immunodeficiency virus type 1 accessory genes vpr, vpu, and nef: mutational analysis of a primary HIV-1 isolate. Virology 1994;200:623.

312. Hattori N, Michaels F, Fargnoli K, et al. The human immunodeficiency virus type 2 vpr gene is essential for productive infection of human macrophages. Proc Natl Acad Sci U S A 1990;87:8080.

313. Connor RI, Chen BK, Choe S, Landau NR. Vpr is required for efficient replication of human immunodeficiency virus type-1 in mononuclear phagocytes. Virology 1995;206:935.

314. Park IW, Sodroski J. Functional analysis of the vpx, vpr, and nef genes of simian immunodeficiency virus. J Acquir Immune Defic Syndr Hum Retrovirol 1995;8:335.

315. Gibbs JS, Lackner AA, Lang SM, et al. Progression to AIDS in the absence of a gene for vpr or vpx. J Virol 1995;69:2378.

316. Lang SM, Weeger M, Stahl HC, et al. Importance of vpr for infection of rhesus monkeys with simian immunodeficiency virus. J Virol 1993;67:902.

317. Wu X, Conway JA, Kim J, Kappes JC. Localization of the Vpx packaging signal within the C terminus of the human immunodeficiency virus type 2 Gag precursor protein. J Virol 1994;68:6161.

318. Mahalingam S, Khan SA, Jabbar MA, et al. Identification of residues in the N-terminal acidic domain of HIV-1 Vpr essential for virion incorporation. Virology 1995;207:297.

319. Mahalingam S, Khan SA, Murali R, et al. Mutagenesis of the putative alpha-helical domain of the Vpr protein of human immunodeficiency virus type 1: effect on stability and virion incorporation. Proc Natl Acad Sci U S A 1995;92:3794.

320. Refaeli Y, Levy DN, Weiner DB. The glucocorticoid receptor type II complex is a target of the HIV-1 vpr gene product. Proc Natl Acad Sci USA 1995;92:3621.

321. Zhao LJ, Mukherjee S, Narayan O. Biochemical mechanism of HIV-I Vpr function. Specific interaction with a cellular protein. J Biol Chem 1994;269:15577.

322. Maldarelli F, Chen MY, Willey RL, Strebel K. Human immunodeficiency virus type 1 Vpu protein is an oligomeric type I integral membrane protein. J Virol 1993;67:5056.

323. Henklein P, Schubert U, Kunert O, et al. Synthesis and characterization of the hydrophilic C-terminal domain of the human immunodeficiency virus type 1-encoded virus protein U (Vpu). Pept Res 1993;6:79.

324. Schubert U, Schneider T, Henklein P, et al. Human immunodeficiency-virus-type-1-encoded Vpu protein is phosphorylated by casein kinase II. Eur J Biochem 1992;204:875.

325. Schubert U, Henklein P, Boldyreff B, et al. The human immunodeficiency virus type 1 encoded Vpu protein is phosphorylated by casein kinase-2 (CK-2) at positions Ser^{52} and Ser^{56} within a predicted alpha-helix-turn-alpha-helix-motif. J Mol Biol 1994;236:16.

326. Willey RL, Maldarelli F, Martin MA, Strebel K. Human immunodeficiency virus type 1 Vpu protein regulates the formation of intracellular gp160-CD4 complexes. J Virol 1992;66:226.

327. Willey RL, Maldarelli F, Martin MA, Strebel K. Human immunodeficiency virus type 1 Vpu protein induces rapid degradation of CD4. J Virol 1992;66:7193.

328. Willey RL, Buckler-White A, Strebel K. Sequences present in the cytoplasmic domain of CD4 are necessary and sufficient to confer sensitivity to the human immunodeficiency virus type 1 Vpu protein. J Virol 1994;68:1207.

329. Lenburg ME, Landau NR. Vpu-induced degradation of CD4: requirement for specific amino acid residues in the cytoplasmic domain of CD4. J Virol 1993;67:7238.

330. Buonocore L, Turi TG, Crise B, Rose JK. Stimulation of heterologous protein degradation by the Vpu protein of HIV-1 requires the transmembrane and cytoplasmic domains of CD4. Virology 1994;204:482.

331. Raja NU, Vincent MJ, abdul Jabbar M. Vpu-mediated proteolysis of gp160/CD4 chimeric envelope glycoproteins in the endoplasmic reticulum: requirement of both the anchor and cytoplasmic domains of CD4. Virology 1994;204:357.

332. Chen MY, Maldarelli F, Karczewski MK, et al. Human immunodeficiency virus type 1 Vpu protein induces degradation of CD4 in vitro: the cytoplasmic domain of CD4 contributes to Vpu sensitivity. J Virol 1993;67:3877.

333. Bour S, Schubert U, Strebel K. The human immunodeficiency virus type 1 Vpu protein specifically binds to the cytoplasmic domain of CD4: implications for the mechanism of degradation. J Virol 1995;69:1510.

334. Geraghty RJ, Panganiban AT. Human immunodeficiency virus type 1 Vpu has a CD4- and an envelope glycoprotein-independent function. J Virol 1993;67:4190.

335. Gottlinger HG, Dorfman T, Cohen EA, Haseltine WA. Vpu protein of human immunodeficiency virus type 1 enhances the release of capsids produced by gag gene constructs of widely divergent retroviruses. Proc Natl Acad Sci USA 1993;90:7381.

336. Schubert U, Strebel K. Differential activities of the human immunodeficiency virus type 1-encoded Vpu protein are regulated by phosphorylation and occur in different cellular compartments. J Virol 1994;68:2260.

337. Yao XJ, Garzon S, Boisvert F, et al. The effect of vpu on HIV-1-induced syncytia formation. J Acquir Immune Defic Syndr 1993;6:135.

338. Kestler HW, Ringler DJ, Mori K, et al. Importance of the nef gene for maintenance of high virus loads and for development of AIDS. Cell 1991;65:651.

339. Daniel MD, Kirchoff F, Czajak SC, et al. Protective effects of a live-attenuated SIV vaccine with a deletion in the *nef* gene. Science 1992;258:1938.

340. Jamieson BD, Aldrovandi GM, Planelles V, et al. Requirement of human immunodeficiency virus type 1 nef for in vivo replication and pathogenicity. J Virol 1994;68:3478.

341. Garcia JV, Miller AD. Serine phosphorylation-independent downregulation of cell-surface CD4 by nef. Nature 1991;350:508.

342. Garcia JV, Alfano J, Miller AD. The negative effect of human immunodeficiency virus type 1 Nef on cell surface CD4 expression is not species specific and requires the cytoplasmic domain of CD4. J Virol 1993;67:1511.

343. Aiken C, Konner J, Landau NR, et al. Nef induces CD4 endocytosis: requirement for a critical dileucine motif in the membrane-proximal CD4 cytoplasmic domain. Cell 1994;76:853.

344. Salghetti S, Mariani R, Skowronski J. Human immunodeficiency virus type 1 Nef and p56lck protein-tyrosine kinase interact with a common element in CD4 cytoplasmic tail. Proc Natl Acad Sci USA 1995;92:349.

345. Anderson SJ, Lenburg M, Landau NR, Garcia JV. The cytoplasmic domain of CD4 is sufficient for its down-regulation from the cell surface by human immunodeficiency virus type 1 Nef. [Published erratum appears in J Virol 1994;68:4705]. J Virol 1994;68:3092.

346. Mariani R, Skowronski J. CD4 down-regulation by nef alleles isolated from human immunodeficiency virus type 1-infected individuals. Proc Natl Acad Sci U S A 1993;90:5549.

347. Brady HJ, Pennington DJ, Miles CG, Dzierzak EA. CD4 cell surface downregulation in HIV-1 Nef transgenic mice is a consequence of intracellular sequestration. EMBO J 1993;12:4923.

348. Skowronski J, Parks D, Mariani R. Altered T cell activation and development in transgenic mice expressing the HIV-1 *nef* gene. EMBO J 1993;12:703.

349. De Ronde A, Klaver B, Keulen W, et al. Natural HIV-1 NEF accelerates virus replication in primary human lymphocytes. Virology 1992;188:391.

350. Zazopoulos E, Haseltine WA. Mutational analysis of the human immunodeficiency virus type 1 Eli Nef function. Proc Natl Acad Sci USA 1992;89:6634.

351. Zazopoulos E, Haseltine WA. Effect of *nef* alleles on replication of human immunodeficiency virus type 1. Virology 1993;194:20.

352. Chowers MY, Spina CA, Kwoh TJ, et al. Optimal infectivity in vitro of human immunodeficiency virus type 1 requires an intact *nef* gene. J Virol 1994;68:2906.

353. Miller MD, Warmerdam MT, Gaston I, et al. The human immunodeficiency virus-1 *nef* gene product: a positive factor for viral infection and replication in primary lymphocytes and macrophages. J Exp Med 1994;179:101.

354. Miller MD, Warmerdam MT, Page KA, et al. Expression of the human immunodeficiency virus type 1 (HIV-1) *nef* gene during HIV-1 production increases progeny particle infectivity independently of gp160 or viral entry. J Virol 1955;69:579.

355. Spina CA, Kwoh TJ, Chowers MY, et al. The importance of nef in the induction of human immunodeficiency virus type 1 replication from primary quiescent CD4 lymphocytes. J Exp Med 1994; 179:115.

356. Baur AS, Sawai ET, Dazin P, et al. HIV-1 Nef leads to inhibition or activation of T cells depending on its intracellular localization. Immunity 1994;1:373.

357. Sawai ET, Baur A, Struble H, et al. Human immunodeficiency virus type 1 Nef associates with a cellular serine kinase in T lymphocytes. Proc Natl Acad Sci USA 1994;91:1539.

358. Saksela K, Cheng G, Baltimore D. Proline-rich (PxxP) motifs in HIV-1 Nef bind to SH3 domains of a subset of Src kinases and are required for the enhanced growth of Nef+ viruses but not for down-regulation of CD4. EMBO J 1995;14:484.

359. Benichou S, Bomsel M, Bodeus M, et al. Physical interaction of the HIV-1 Nef protein with beta-COP, a component of non-clathrin-coated vesicles essential for membrane traffic. J Biol Chem 1994;269:30073.

360. Calenda V, Graber P, Delamarter JF, Chermann JC. Involvement of HIV nef protein in abnormal hematopoiesis in AIDS: in vitro study on bone marrow progenitor cells. Eur J Haematol 1994;52:103.

361. Chirmule N, Oyaizu N, Saxinger C, Pahwa S. Nef protein of HIV-1 has B-cell stimulatory activity. AIDS 1994;8:733.

362. De SK, Marsh JW. HIV-1 Nef inhibits a common activation pathway in NIH-3T3 cells. J Biol Chem 1994;269:6656.

363. Poulin L, Fauchon M, Darveau A, Levy JA. Inhibition of protein synthesis by the human immunodeficiency virus type 1 *nef* gene product. J Gen Virol 1994;75:2977.

364. Myers G, Korber B, Berzofsky JA, et al. Human retroviruses and AIDS. A compilation and analysis of nucleic acid and amino acid sequences. Los Alamos, NM: Los Alamos National Laboratory, 1994.

AIDS: Biology, Diagnosis, Treatment and Prevention, fourth edition, edited by Vincent T. DeVita, Jr., Samuel Hellman, and Steven A. Rosenberg. Lippincott–Raven Publishers, © 1997

CHAPTER 4

Immunopathogenesis of Human Immunodeficiency Virus Infection

Giuseppe Pantaleo, Oren Cohen, Cecilia Graziosi, Mauro Vaccarezza, Stephania Paolucci, James F. Demarest, and Anthony S. Fauci

The immunopathogenesis of human immunodeficiency virus (HIV) infection is extremely complex. A variety of virologic and immunologic mechanisms contribute to the progressive deterioration of immune function and to progression of HIV disease to the acquired immunodeficiency syndrome (AIDS).[1] Because of the multifactorial and multiphasic nature of HIV infection, these mechanisms may vary according to the different phases of infection.[2] Among the multiple pathogenic mechanisms that have been proposed, four are critical for the establishment and propagation of HIV infection over time and for the progression of HIV disease: (1) lack of elimination of HIV after primary infection; (2) persistent virus replication in lymphoid organs throughout the course of HIV infection; (3) chronic stimulation of the immune system, which may cause inappropriate immune activation and progressive exhaustion of the immune response; and (4) destruction of lymphoid tissue, which results in severe impairment of the ability to maintain over time an effective HIV-specific immune response and to generate immune responses against new pathogens. Identification of these pathogenic mechanisms has resulted from recent advances in the delineation of the virologic and immunologic events associated with primary infection[3-13] and of the anatomic compartments that serve as reservoirs for HIV and the sites at which virus replication primarily occurs.[14-17] These observations represent a fundamental

advance in our understanding of the pathogenesis of HIV infection. However, a series of important mechanisms, such as those allowing HIV to elude the immune response, those determining the effectiveness of the HIV-specific immune response, and those leading to the destruction of the lymphoid tissue, have not yet been fully delineated. Recent studies on the kinetics of virus turnover[18,19] have supported previous findings that virus replication is continuous in all stages of HIV infection[14,20] and have provided a precise determination of the number of virions produced every day. In the same studies, a mathematic model has been used to calculate the potential number of CD4+ T lymphocytes that are depleted and replenished every day, and it has been proposed that there is a very high turnover of CD4+ T cells (a mean of 1.8×10^9 cells per day). With regard to CD4+ T cells, it has been debated whether these mathematical calculations truly reflect changes in the numbers of CD4+ T cells resulting from de novo proliferation or whether there is an important contribution from redistribution of CD4+ T cells from the lymphoid tissue to the peripheral blood.

The clinical course of HIV infection has been well studied. Although progression to AIDS occurs in most HIV-infected individuals, in a small percentage, HIV disease does not progress for an extended period of time. This latter finding, together with the observations that HIV-specific immune responses may be detected in individuals who are multiply exposed to HIV despite the fact that they are seronegative, supports the concept that HIV infection can be effectively controlled or even prevented by the immune response. In this review, we analyze the different patterns of the clinical course of HIV disease, the kinetics of virologic and immunologic events in the different stages of infection, and the variety of mechanisms that directly or indirectly contribute to the quantitative and qualitative defects of CD4+ T lymphocytes.

Giuseppe Pantaleo, Oren Cohen, Cecilia Graziosi, Mauro Vaccarezza, Stephania Paolucci, James F. Demarest, and Anthony S. Fauci: Laboratory of Immunoregulation, National Institute of Allergy and Infectious Diseases, National Institutes of Health, Bethesda, Maryland.

Corresponding author: Dr. Giuseppe Pantaleo, National Institute of Allergy and Infectious Diseases, National Institutes of Health, Bldg 10, Rm 11B-13, 10 Center Dr MSC 1876, Bethesda, MD 20892-1876, phone 301-496-5508, fax 301-402-0070.

THE COURSE OF HIV INFECTION

On the basis of the duration of HIV infection and the kinetics of virologic and immunologic events observed throughout HIV disease, three dominant patterns of evolution of HIV disease have been described: (1) 80% to 90% of HIV-infected persons are "typical progressors" and experience a course of HIV disease with a median survival time of approximately 10 years[1] (Fig. 4-1A); (2) 5% to 10% of HIV-infected persons are "rapid progressors" and experience an unusually rapid (3 to 4 years) course of HIV disease[21,22] (Fig. 4-1B); (3) about 5% of HIV-infected persons do not experience disease progression for an extended period of time (at least 7 years) and are termed "long-term nonprogressors" (LTNP)[23–31] (Fig. 4-1C).

Typical Progressors

The typical course of HIV infection includes three phases: primary infection, clinical latency, and clinically apparent disease. The diagnosis of primary HIV infection is made in only a minor percentage of cases. Difficulties reside in the variable severity and nonspecificity of the clinical syndrome, which is characterized by mononucleosis- or flu-like symptoms such as fever, lethargy, sore throat, malaise, macupapular rash, lymphadenopathy, arthralgias, myalgias, headaches, retroorbital pain, photophobia, and, rarely, meningitis.[3–5] Hospital-ization is required in only a minority (10% to 15%) of individuals, and this phase therefore usually goes unnoticed. Furthermore, during the initial period of primary infection the laboratory blood test that is widely used for the diagnosis of HIV infection (ie, detection of HIV antibody specific for various viral proteins) may be negative. On the basis of the clinical history, however, it is thought that an acute clinical syndrome of variable severity may occur in a relatively large proportion (50% to 70%) of HIV-infected individuals, and although HIV-specific antibodies may not be detected, the initial period of primary infection is characterized by high levels of virus in the circulation (ie, viremia).[3–6] Determination of plasma viremia or p24 antigenemia represents the only valid laboratory approach for the diagnosis of primary infection. Appearance of symptoms during acute primary infection usually occurs within 3 to 6 weeks of infection, together with the high levels of viremia. In most patients, both resolution of symptoms and downregulation of viremia occur within 9 to 12 weeks after the onset of symptoms; both of these events are associated with the appearance of HIV-specific immune responses (see later discussion).[4–6]

The phase of primary infection is followed by the long, clinically latent period of HIV infection. In typical progressors, this phase of infection may last for years (median, 8 to 10 years).[23,24,32] During the initial years of the AIDS epidemic, the absence of symptoms together with the technical difficulties in

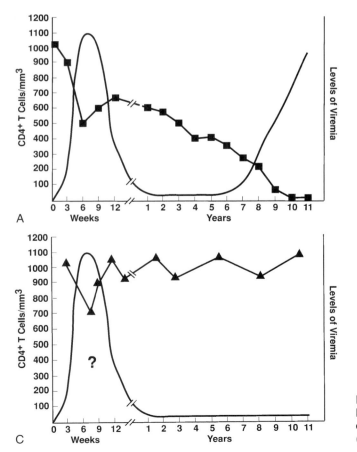

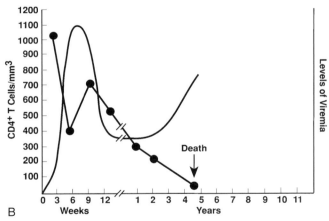

FIG. 4-1. Schematic representation of the decline in CD4+T lymphocytes and the kinetics of viremia during the various courses of HIV infection observed in: (**A**) typical progressors; (**B**) rapid progressors, and (**C**) long term non-progressors.

detecting active virus replication in peripheral blood generated a series of misconceptions. It is now clear that this long period of clinical latency does not reflect microbiologic latency, as was previously thought. The observations that active replication of HIV is continuous and occurs primarily in the lymphoid organs throughout the entire course of infection,[14] together with the development of highly sensitive and quantitative polymerase chain reaction techniques for the determination of viremia,[20,33] have clearly demonstrated that HIV disease is active and progressive even during this prolonged asymptomatic phase. These findings have helped to explain the discrepancy between the absence of clinical signs of active disease and the progressive decline of CD4+ T lymphocytes that invariably accompanies the clinically latent period.[32]

Progression to AIDS and clinically apparent disease occurs within 8 to 10 years in typical progressors. The progression to AIDS results from the continuous replication of virus in the lymphoid tissue, which is associated with progressive destruction of this tissue (see later discussion) and severe impairment of immune function. This advanced phase of infection is characterized by severe and persistent constitutional signs and symptoms or by opportunistic infections or neoplasms, or both.[34] In those persons who develop generalized lymphadenopathy or the AIDS-defining conditions of Kaposi's sarcoma or neurologic disease,[34] clinical disease may be apparent before the progression to advanced-stage disease.

Rapid Progressors

In a minor percentage (5% to 10%) of HIV-infected persons, rapid progression to AIDS occurs within 2 to 3 years after seroconversion.[21,22] Immune responses are usually defective in these rapid progressors. Levels of antibodies against HIV proteins and neutralizing antibody are low to absent.[35–39] Although it is unclear whether HIV-specific cytotoxicity is defective in rapid progressors,[40,41] it has been shown that the CD8+ T-cell–mediated suppression of HIV replication (ie, mediated by a soluble factor) is severely impaired.[42,43] A series of immunologic abnormalities typical of HIV-infected individuals in late-stage disease are usually observed in rapid progressors, including high percentages of activated CD8+ T cells expressing CD38 and HLA-DR[40,44] and elevated serum levels of β_2-microglobulin, neopterin, soluble CD8, and soluble interleukin-2 (IL-2) receptors.[45–47] The levels of viral load are usually very high in rapid progressors. In particular, it has been reported that rapid progressors have elevated levels of unspliced HIV mRNA compared with typical progressors[48–53] and that HIV isolates from rapid progressors are more homogeneous than those from typical progressors and LTNPs.[54]

Long-Term Nonprogressors

Now that considerable experience has accumulated in prospective studies of HIV-infected individuals, it has become clear that a small percentage of infected persons (5%) do not experience clinical progression of HIV infection and have stable CD4+ T-cell counts for many years (7 or more years) despite lack of therapy.[23–31] The criteria we have used for nonprogression include documented HIV infection for more than 7 years, stable CD4+ T-cell counts higher than 600 cells/µL, absence of symptoms, and no antiretroviral therapy. From an immunologic standpoint, immune functions are conserved in LTNPs, and both HIV-specific humoral and cell-mediated immune responses are very strong.[23–31] In addition to normal and stable CD4+ T-cell counts, the absolute number of CD8+ T lymphocytes is significantly and consistently higher in most LTNPs.[23–31] In addition, quantitative differences in the distribution of certain surface markers on CD8+ T cells, which have been associated with either a favorable or a severe prognosis in HIV infection, have been observed in LTNPs. For example, the presence of an increased percentage of CD8+CD38+ T cells is associated with a severe prognosis in typical progressors; the percentage of CD8+CD38+ T cells in LTNPs is significantly lower than in typical progressors. Similarly, other immunologic parameters such as serum levels of β_2-microglobulin, elevated levels of which have been associated with an unfavorable prognosis in HIV infection,[45–47] are within the normal range in LTNPs. Furthermore, in contrast to typical progressors, LTNPs exhibit preserved proliferative responses to mitogens (eg, phytohemagglutinin, pokeweed mitogen), alloantigens, and soluble antigens (eg, tetanus toxoid).

HIV-specific cytotoxic T lymphocytes (CTLs) against various HIV proteins, including Env and Gag, can readily be detected in LTNPs, either in freshly isolated peripheral blood mononuclear cells or after in vitro stimulation.[29,55] In contrast to typical progressors,[56] who experience a decline over time of HIV-specific activity, this activity remains stable in LTNPs.[55] Although these differences are clearly observed if LTNPs are compared with typical progressors who have been infected for a comparable period of time, no differences in HIV-specific cytotoxicity may be observed between LTNPs and HIV-infected individuals in early-stage disease who have high CD4+ T-cell counts (ie, >600 cells/µL).[55] Therefore, the contribution of persistent cytotoxic activity to the maintenance of the status of nonprogression remains to be clarified. In this regard, it may be important to determine whether the fine epitopes in the different HIV proteins recognized by CTLs are similar in LTNPs and in typical progressors. It is conceivable that qualitative differences (ie, CTL recognition of different epitopes) in the cytotoxic responses of LTNPs compared with typical progressors may be associated with a more effective immune response. As with HIV-specific cytotoxicity, significant differences in the CD8+ T-cell–mediated suppressor function are observed between LTNPs and typical progressors only if the former are compared with individuals in late-stage disease.[26,31] With regard to the humoral immune response, recent studies have shown higher titers of neutralizing antibodies in LTNPs compared with typical progressors. In addition, a wide breadth of cross-reactive neutralizing antibodies was observed in LTNPs in one study,[31] although these data were not confirmed in another study.[29] Furthermore, HIV isolated from LTNPs was not usually neutralized by autologous serum obtained at the time of virus isolation.[57] Therefore, the contribution of neutralizing antibodies in preventing disease progression in LTNPs still remains still to be determined.

From a virologic standpoint, levels of viral load, including frequency of HIV DNA–containing cells and virus replication in both peripheral blood and lymph node mononuclear cells as well as plasma viremia, are fourfold to 20-fold lower in LTNPs than in typical progressors.[29,31] Despite this very low viral load, virus replication is persistent in LTNPs, as indicated by a retrospective analysis of plasma viremia in specimens collected over a period of 5 years.[29] Furthermore, virus was consistently isolated from lymph node mononuclear cells,[29] indicating that it was replication-competent and infectious; however, very little information is available concerning the pathogenicity of HIV in LTNPs. In this regard, a *nef*-deleted HIV has been isolated from a LTNP.[30] This, together with the lack of pathogenicity of *nef*-deleted simian immunodeficiency virus (SIV) in rhesus monkeys,[30] has led to speculation that LTNPs may be infected with low-pathogenic or nonpathogenic viruses. Of particular interest is the fact that lymph node architecture is preserved, the degree of lymphoid tissue activation (ie, formation of germinal centers) is significantly lower, and tissue involution is rarely observed in LTNPs[29] (see later discussion). These data are consistent with the low levels of viral load and the intact immune function that are observed in LTNPs. Furthermore, involvement of genetic factors (ie, major histocompatibility complex [MHC] class I and II molecules) has been proposed as an explanation for the lack of disease progression in LTNPs.[58] However, at the present time, the relative contributions of immunologic, genetic, and virologic factors in determining progression of HIV infection remain unclear.

ANALYSIS OF VIROLOGIC AND IMMUNOLOGIC EVENTS ASSOCIATED WITH HIV INFECTION IN PERIPHERAL BLOOD AND LYMPH NODES

Primary HIV Infection

The sequelae of virologic and immunologic events associated with primary HIV infection in peripheral blood and lymph nodes have only recently been delineated (Fig. 4-2). The SIV model of acute infection has been an ideal experimental system to determine the initial anatomic site of virus localization and spread. For this purpose, sequential lymph node biopsies were performed in monkeys, and analysis of virus distribution demonstrated that virus may be detected in lymph nodes as early as 1 week after inoculation.[12,13,59] Significant changes in virus distribution occurred after primary infection and during the transition from the acute to the

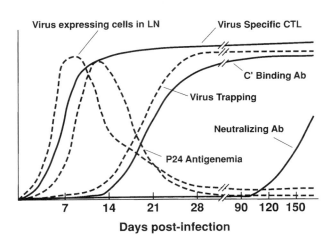

FIG. 4-2. Virologic and immunologic events associated with primary HIV infection. The kinetics represented were extrapolated from information available in humans and in the SIV experimental model of acute infection. HIV/SIV initially localizes in lymphoid organs as determined by the detection of virus-expressing cells very early following infection. The peak in virus-expressing cells and spread of virus throughout the lymphoid tissue precedes the increase in plasma viremia. The appearance of virus-specific cytotoxic T lymphocytes (CTL) coincides with a rapid clearance of virus-expressing cells in the lymph nodes. Production of complement (C′) binding antibodies (Abs) facilitates trapping of virions in the follicular dendritic cell network of the lymph node germinal centers. Both the CTL response and production of C′ binding Abs contribute to the dramatic decrease in viremia. Neutralizing Abs are detectable at the transition from the acute to the chronic stage of infection. (Adapted from Annu. Rev. Immunol. 13, 487–512, 1995)

chronic phase of HIV infection. Virus that is detected in lymph nodes early after inoculation (ie, day 7) is exclusively cell-associated, and a peak in numbers of individual virus-expressing cells is detected at this time. Rapid changes in virus distribution occur during the 2 to 3 weeks after inoculation. The number of virus-expressing cells is dramatically reduced by day 14; this event is probably the result of the emergence of virus-specific immune responses (see later discussion). By 3 to 4 weeks after inoculation, virus particles trapped in the follicular dendritic cell (FDC) network in the germinal centers represent the predominant form of virus detected in the lymph nodes. Definitive evidence that the initial replication and spread of virus in lymph nodes may account for systemic virus dissemination was obtained by comparing the kinetics of virus replication in lymph nodes with that in the circulation (ie, p26 antigenemia).[13] This analysis revealed that the peak in numbers of virus-expressing cells in lymph nodes precedes the peak in p26 antigenemia. These phenomena are usually observed during the first 2 weeks of primary infection, and this early period, during which intense virus spreading occurs, has been designated the stage of virus dissemination.[17]

Subsequent to the stage of virus dissemination, the course of primary infection is characterized by a dramatic downregulation of viremia. During this latter period, levels of virus replication are significantly reduced in both peripheral blood and lymph nodes; in addition, in lymph nodes there is a switch in predominance from cell-associated virus (ie, virus-expressing cells) to extracellular virus trapped in the FDC network.[13,17] In addition to the elimination of virus-expressing cells by HIV-specific CTLs (see later discussion), the trapping of virus particles in the FDC network represents an important mechanism for the decrease of virus in the circulation. In this regard, virus particles complexed with antibody and complement (C′) may be trapped either in the lymphoid tissue, by virtue of the C′ receptors expressed on the FDCs, or in the reticuloendothelial system. In favor of this hypothesis, the transition from cell-associated to trapped virus in lymph nodes is associated with the formation of germinal centers, and these events coincide with a decrease in plasma viremia.[13] For obvious reasons, longitudinal studies on the kinetics of virus distribution cannot be performed in lymphoid tissue in individual human subjects. However, cross-sectional studies (ie, analyses of virus distribution in lymph nodes and peripheral blood obtained from different individuals within 10 months of the onset of symptoms) indicate that the kinetics observed in the SIV models are comparable to those obtained in humans (Pantaleo and Fauci, unpublished observations).

The major decrease in virologic parameters observed during the first weeks of infection are predominantly limited to those that reflect active replication, such as number of virus-expressing cells, viremia, p26 in SIV and p24 in HIV, and titers of infectious virus[13,4–6]; changes in the number of HIV proviral DNA copies have not consistently been observed.[5,6] During the acute phase of SIV or HIV infection, in addition to the systemic dissemination of the virus, other crucial pathogenic events may significantly influence the propagation of the infection over time; these include the generation of a large pool of HIV latently infected cells (ie, cells containing proviral DNA) and the large number of trapped virus particles that may represent a source of virus for de novo infection of target cells that reside in or migrate through the lymphoid organs.[1,17]

With regard to HIV-specific immune responses, robust cell-mediated and humoral responses are readily detected during primary infection.[4,5] Usually, virus-specific CTLs can be detected within 2 to 4 weeks from the onset of symptoms, and their appearance coincides with the dramatic decrease in viremia[7,9,12] in both humans and monkeys. HIV-specific CTLs play a major role in the initial downregulation of viremia by killing virus-expressing cells that are responsible for the high level of virion production. In the SIV model of acute infection, it has been shown that the appearance of virus-specific CTLs coincides with a dramatic decrease in the number of virus-expressing cells in lymph nodes.[12] HIV-specific CTLs have been detected against both structural (eg, Env, Gag-Pol) and regulatory (eg, Nef, Tat) viral proteins. Variable frequencies and specificities of HIV-specific CTLs have been observed among different individuals.

However, it is unclear whether these quantitative and qualitative differences in HIV-specific cytotoxicity significantly influence the initial downregulation of viremia and the ability to control virus replication and spread over time. In addition to typical HIV-specific cytotoxicity, CD8+ T cells may also potentially mediate suppression of virus replication by release of a soluble factor; this CD8+ T-cell–mediated suppressor activity has been detected during primary infection.[10] Taken together these observations strongly support an important role for CD8+ T cells in the primary immune response to HIV infection.

With regard to the virus-specific humoral immune response, neutralizing antibodies, which represent the protective component of this response, are usually detected after the phase of downregulation of viremia,[7] when the transition from the acute to the chronic phase of infection has already occurred. Although these findings suggest that neutralizing antibodies may have little effect in the control of the initial spread of HIV, they do not rule out the involvement of nonneutralizing antibodies in the initial downregulation of viremia.[11,13,17] In the SIV model of acute infection, it has been observed that the decrease in viremia coincides with a rise in the level of virus-specific C′-binding antibodies,[13,17] suggesting that complexes formed by virus particles, immunoglobulin (Ig), and C′ may be trapped by FDCs that express C′ receptors on their surface or may be cleared in the reticuloendothelial system. Therefore, although the humoral immune response may have little effect on the initial spread of virus, it may contribute mechanically to the downregulation of viremia by trapping virus particles in lymphoid tissue. In addition to antibody and cytotoxic mechanisms of suppression of HIV replication, cytokines may play an important role in the initial regulation of virus expression. High levels of expression of certain cytokines, such as interferon-γ (IFN-γ), tumor necrosis factor-α (TNF-α), and IL-10, have been observed during primary infection (Graziosi and colleagues, unpublished observations); the role of these cytokines in the primary immune response to HIV is the subject of ongoing investigation.

Although the immune system is capable of downregulating virus replication dramatically, HIV is almost never completely eliminated, and progression to the chronic phase of infection occurs in most cases. Failure of the immune response to completely clear HIV may be related to certain pathogenic mechanisms such as viral latency and trapping of virus; both mechanisms may be critical to the ability of the virus to evade specific immune responses. It is also conceivable that certain components of the virus-specific primary immune response may favor the establishment of chronic infection. In this regard, it is important to understand why individual patients experience different clinical outcomes despite apparently qualitatively and quantitatively similar immune responses. Recent studies of the T-cell receptor (TCR) repertoire during primary infection have shown striking qualitative differences in the primary immune response to HIV that are not appreciated by standard measures of immune response.[9,13] Analysis of the TCR repertoire was performed with the use of sequential peripheral blood mononuclear cell samples collected during the first 12 weeks after primary infection. Major perturbations (ie, expansions followed by declines) were observed involving cells that express a restricted number of variable domains of the β chain (Vβ) of the TCR.[9] If present, these expansions may be major (with a relative percentage of expanded Vβ >20%), involving a single Vβ family; moderate (relative percentage <20%), involving two families; or minimal (relative percentage <10%), involving multiple families. The cells involved in these expansions are CD8+ T cells that are activated as indicated by the expression of HLA-DR antigen. More importantly, they contain HIV-specific CTLs.[9] Molecular analysis of the expanded CD8+ Vβ cell subsets has demonstrated that these expansions are oligoclonal in nature.[9] These different patterns of Vβ expansion seem to be associated with favorable or non-favorable clinical outcomes. Qualitative differences in the virus-specific immune response may thus reflect the effectiveness of the immune response, which directly influences the progression of HIV disease.

The Clinically Latent Period

Transition from the acute to the chronic phase of HIV infection is marked by the downregulation of viremia and resolution of symptoms.[4-6] All virologic parameters, including viremia, virus expression, and titers of infectious virus in peripheral blood mononuclear cells, as well as frequency of cells containing HIV DNA, are usually very low in peripheral blood during this clinically latent period.[1] However, determinations of viral load in lymphoid tissue have demonstrated that the frequency of cells containing HIV DNA and the levels of virus expression in mononuclear cells are 1 to 3 logs higher in lymph nodes than in peripheral blood.[14,16] These observations indicate that virus replication is continuous throughout the entire course of infection, including the asymptomatic period. This concept has been further supported by the detection of viremia during the clinically latent period with the use of a highly sensitive polymerase chain reaction assay,[20,33] and by recent studies that have shown that not only is viral replication continuous but the turnover of virus is very high (up to 10^9 virus particles every 1.5 to 2 days).[18,19]

Another important pathogenic event associated with the early stage of infection is the trapping of virus particles in the FDC network of the lymph node germinal centers.[14,15,60-64] The trapping of virus is related to the histopathologic changes associated with the early stage of HIV disease, when CD4+ T-cell counts are higher than 500 cells/μL (Figs. 4-3A and B). The typical histopathologic abnormality of this stage of HIV infection is follicular hyperplasia (see Fig. 4-3A), which is a reflection of the state of immune activation of the lymphoid tissue and of the ongoing immune response to HIV or other pathogens.[1,17,61] These histopathologic changes are not unique to people with HIV infection but rather represent normal events that occur after generation of an immune response. However, certain features of the follicular hyperplasia associated with HIV infection are characteristic and perhaps unique. These include irregular shape and larger size of germinal centers, tendency of germinal centers to fuse, and abnormal location (ie, germinal centers that are not limited to the cortex of the lymph node but invade the medulla).[61] These histopathologic abnormalities, together with increased cellular activation, which is critical for effective virus replication (see later discussion), may contribute to the dichotomy of viral load between peripheral blood and lymph nodes by promoting trapping of virus particles in the FDC network (see Fig. 4-3B) and by creating environmental conditions (ie, close cellular contact, high concentration of HIV, and abnormal retrafficking of lymphocytes) that favor the sequestration of HIV in the tissue.

With the progression of HIV disease from the early to the intermediate stage (ie, CD4+ T-cell counts between 200 and 500 cells/μL), levels of viral load increase in peripheral blood, and the differences in viral load between peripheral blood and lymph nodes tend to minimize.[14] The increase of viral load in peripheral blood reflects in part a progressive deterioration of the immune system, which in turn results in defective control of virus replication. However, this increase is also the result of important histopathologic changes that occur in lymphoid tissue as disease progresses. Increasing proportions of lymphoid tissue show signs of disruption of tissue architecture, including abnormal location of germinal centers in the medulla, greater numbers of germinal centers undergoing follicular involution, and increased vascularity and fibrosis (see Fig. 4-3C). The disruption of lymph node architecture leads to a progressive loss of the ability of lymphoid tissue to trap virus[1,14,17] (see Fig. 4-3D); this, together with the accelerated replication of virus as disease progresses, probably contributes to the increase in viremia observed in patients in the intermediate stage of disease.[1,14,17] In support of the hypothesis that virus replication and trapping in lymph nodes may significantly influence the levels of viremia, it has recently been shown that decreases in plasma viremia during antiretroviral therapy reflect downregulation of virus replication in the lymphoid tissue.[65] In contrast to the diminution in the ability to trap virus, the number of individual cells that express HIV increases during this stage of infection. Therefore, as disease progresses there is a major change in virus distribution in lymph nodes, which is characterized by a decrease in virus trapping together with an increase in the number of virus-expressing cells.[1,14,17]

With regard to cell-mediated immunity, both HIV-specific CD4+ and CD8+ T-cell–mediated immune responses to a variety of HIV proteins are usually detected in early-stage disease.[66-68] In addition, in vitro proliferative responses to mitogens, alloantigens, and soluble antigens such as tetanus toxoid are conserved in most individuals in early-stage disease. With regard to humoral immunity, a variety of antibodies against HIV structural and regulatory proteins are generated during HIV infection. Among these are neutralizing antibodies that are directed against the V3 loop of the gp120 envelope protein. They inhibit the infectivity of free HIV virions, but they

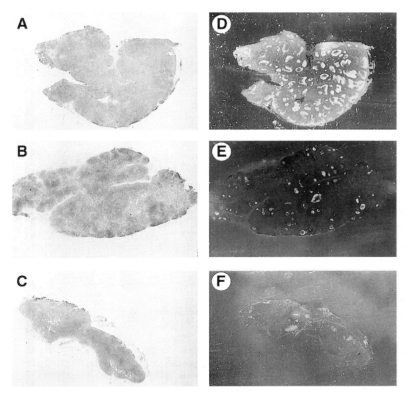

FIG. 4-3. Excisional lymph node biopsies from HIV-infected individuals at various stages of disease. (**A**) Lymph node from a subject in early-stage disease with numerous large germinal centers invading the medulla, having irregular shapes, and a tendency to fuse. (**B**) Lymph node from a subject in intermediate-stage disease with large areas of tissue involution and focal fibrosis. (**C**) Lymph node from a subject in advanced stage disease. Most of the lymphoid tissue has been replaced by fibrotic tissue and fatty infiltration. (**D–F**) Dark-field images of in situ hybridization of the same lymph nodes shown in **A** through **C**. The location of HIV RNA is indicated by the silver grains, which appears as white dots. (**D**) The hybridization signal is mostly localized in the germinal centers, and HIV RNA corresponds to extracellular virions trapped in the FDC network; virus trapping is very efficient in this hyperplastic lymph node. (**E**) Reduction of trapping of virus is associated with follicular involution. (**F**) The trapping ability of the lymph node tissue virtually is lost completely in this lymph node that manifests lymphocyte depletion and follicular involution. Also see Color Figure 4.3.

seem to be less effective in blocking cell-to-cell transmission.[69–76] These antibodies represent the protective component of the humoral response. In contrast, antibodies against the gp41 may represent the detrimental component of the humoral immune response because they have been shown to enhance HIV infectivity in vitro.[77–79] Impairment of HIV-specific and nonspecific cell-mediated and humoral immune responses is usually observed during the progression from early to intermediate stages of disease.[68]

Advanced Stages of HIV Infection

From a virologic standpoint, the advanced stage of HIV infection (ie, CD4+ T-cell counts <200 cells/μL) is characterized by a substantial increase in all virologic parameters in both peripheral blood and lymph nodes.[14,17] In advanced-stage disease, the levels of viral load equilibrate between peripheral blood and lymph nodes.[14,17] Lymphoid tissue has for the most part been destroyed and replaced by fibrotic tissue (see Fig. 4-3E); most of the virus is cell-associated, and virus trapping is minimal or absent[14,17] (see Fig. 4-3F). The obvious consequence of the destruction of lymphoid tissue is the severe impairment of immune function and profound immune suppression.

LYMPH NODES IN LONG-TERM NONPROGRESSORS

Three major histopathologic patterns have been observed in lymph nodes of LTNPs.[29] These include (1) lymph nodes with typical follicular hyperplasia (Fig. 4-4A); (2) lymph nodes

with follicular hyperplasia mixed with diffuse, nonorganized lymphoid tissue (Fig. 4-4C); and (3) lymph nodes with minimal or absent follicular hyperplasia and predominantly nonorganized lymphoid tissue (Fig. 4-4E). With regard to the follicular hyperplasia observed in LTNPs, germinal centers usually have a smaller size, regular shape, intact structure, and normal location in the cortex. In essence, the follicular hyperplasia observed in LTNPs is very similar to that observed in reactive lymph nodes of HIV-negative individuals, and the areas of nonorganized lymphoid tissue do not show signs of tissue involution such as fibrosis or fatty infiltration. Furthermore, morphometric analysis has demonstrated that the area occupied by germinal centers in lymph nodes in LTNPs is significantly smaller than in typical progressors.[29] These analyses indicate that lymph node tissue architecture is preserved in LTNPs, and the degree of tissue activation is much less than in typical progressors.[29] As in typical progressors, virus trapping in the lymph nodes of LTNPs, if detected, is dependent on the presence of germinal centers (see Figs. 4B, D, and F). However, the relative paucity of virus trapping in lymph nodes of LTNPs is not the result of destruction of lymphoid tissue, as it is in typical progressors; rather, it probably results from a very low level of virus replication together with a low level of tissue activation. Individual virus-expressing cells are rarely observed in lymph nodes of LTNPs.[8]

INDUCTION OF HIV EXPRESSION

Several factors have been proposed as being involved in the regulation of HIV expression and the potentiation and modu-

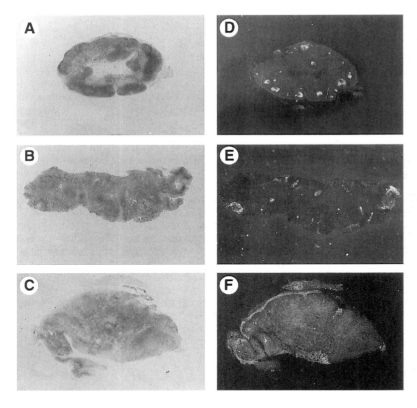

FIG. 4-4. Lymph nodes from HIV-infected individuals who are long term non-progressors (LTNP). **(A)** Lymph node from a LTNP with numerous small germinal centers having regular shape. **(B)** Lymph node from a LTNP in which germinal centers are seen in half of the tissue section, whereas the other half contains non-organized lymphoid tissue. **(C)** Lymph node from a LTNP in which most of the tissue section is occupied by non-organized lymphoid tissue, whereas germinal center formation is minimal or absent. **(D–F)** in situ hybridization of the same lymph nodes shown in **A–C**. The location of HIV RNA is indicated by silver grains that appear as white dots. There are variable degrees of virus trapping, which in general is minimal and far lower than the degree of trapping noted in typical progressors early in the course of their disease. (Adapted from Schrager LK, Young JM, Fowler MG, Mathieson BJ, Vermund SH. Long-term survivors of HIV-1 infection: definition and research challenges. AIDS 1994; 8:895) See also Color Figure 4-4.

lation of virus replication. These include endogenous viral regulatory proteins such Tat and Rev, cellular transcription factors acting at the level of the proviral long terminal repeat (LTR), the state of immune activation, other pathogens, and cytokines.

Both Tat and Rev are crucial for efficient virus replication.[80–83] Tat protein acts at both the transcriptional and post-transcriptional levels; Rev protein plays an important role in the export of unspliced and incompletely spliced viral messages from the nucleus to the cytoplasm of the infected cell. Because these messages encode for structural proteins, optimal Rev function is essential for production of infectious virions.

It has been demonstrated that certain cellular transcription factors that bind to consensus sequences on the proviral LTR, including Sp1, TATA, TAR, and NF-kB, activate HIV RNA synthesis and thus exert positive regulation on viral transcription.[80–84]

A general state of immune activation is associated with all stages of HIV infection.[44,56,85–90] The inability to eliminate HIV after primary infection and the continuous replication of virus throughout the entire course of HIV disease represent the primary mechanisms responsible for the chronic state of immune activation. Both individual virus-expressing cells and trapped virus in lymphoid tissue represent the source of antigen responsible for maintaining chronic stimulation of the immune system over time. Although a state of immune activation is necessary in order to maintain HIV-specific immune responses, at the same time it may indirectly

enhance virus replication, either by leading to the secretion of HIV-inducing cytokines (see later discussion) or by generating a large pool of activated target cells that efficiently support virus replication. HIV in vitro can infect both resting and activated CD4+ T lymphocytes with equal efficiency; however, it replicates only in activated T cells.[91,92] As in CD4+ T cells, efficient virus replication in monocytes or macrophages depends on the state of cellular activation and differentiation.[93]

Several pathogens, including cytomegalovirus, herpes simplex virus, hepatitis B virus, human herpesvirus 6, human T-cell lymphotropic virus type I, and microbes such as *Mycoplasma,* have been shown to enhance HIV expression in several experimental in vitro systems.[93] It is not certain whether these pathogens mediate a similar effect in vivo.

Since the initial observation that certain cytokines induce HIV expression from a state of latent or chronic infection to that of active virus expression,[94] the effects of several cytokines on virus expression and replication have been extensively investigated. On the basis of their ability to modulate virus expression and replication, they may be divided into three groups[95]: inducers of virus expression, suppressors of virus expression, and bifunctional modulators (which can mediate either induction or suppression of virus replication, depending on the experimental system). Cytokines that induce HIV expression include IL-1, IL-2, IL-3, IL-6, IL-12, granulocyte-macrophage colony-stimulating factor (GM-CSF), macrophage colony-stimulating factor (M-CSF), TNF-α, and TNF-β. Of these, IL-2 and IL-12 induce virus expression only in T cells, TNF-α and TNF-β induce expression in both T cells and macrophages, and the remaining cytokines induce expression only in macrophages. Among the suppressors of HIV expression, IFN-α, IFN-β, and IL-10 act on both T cells and macrophages. Finally, the bifunctional cytokines include IFN-γ, IL-4, and TGF-β; of these, IL-4 is active only on macrophages, and the other two are active on both T cells and macrophages. Most cytokines induce HIV expression by mechanisms acting at both the transcriptional and post-transcriptional levels; TNF-α, TNF-β, and IL-1 induce HIV expression by activation of the transcription factor NF-kB. Although the regulatory effect of cytokines on HIV replication is limited to in vitro observations, the fact that several of these cytokines may be found at increased levels in plasma, cerebrospinal fluid, and lymphoid tissue of HIV-infected individuals suggests that they probably mediate similar effects in vivo. It is possible that cytokines play an important role in maintaining the constant levels of virus expression and replication, particularly in lymphoid tissue.

In addition to the potential direct modulation by cytokines of HIV expression in vivo, particular attention has recently been given to the possibility that cytokines may play a major role in the progression of HIV disease through other mechanisms.[96] Different patterns of cytokines have been found to be associated with protective or nonprotective immune responses in several pathologic conditions in animal models.[97,98] In general, the T_{H1} pattern of cytokine secretion (ie, IL-2, IFN-γ, TNF-α, and TNF-β) is associated with protective immune responses, whereas the T_{H2} pattern of cytokine secretion (ie, IL-4, IL-5, and IL-10) is associated with nonprotective immune responses. This distinction is based on the expression of these cytokine patterns by CD4+ T-cell clones; however, in humans these distinctions are not as clear-cut as they are in mice.[99–101] CD4+ T cells that produce both T_{H1} and T_{H2} cytokines have been designated T_{H0}. On the basis of these observations, an imbalance in the pattern of cytokine production may induce a nonprotective immune response, resulting in defective control of virus replication and disease progression. It was initially proposed that a predominance of the T_{H2} pattern of cytokine secretion was associated with HIV infection and that the expression of this pattern was a critical step in the progression of HIV disease.[96] This hypothesis has been tested in several studies by analysis of either cytokine secretion or cytokine expression in peripheral blood and lymph nodes of HIV-infected individuals at different stages of HIV disease. Both cross-sectional and longitudinal analyses have failed to demonstrate a "switch" from the T_{H1} to T_{H2} cytokine pattern as disease progresses.[102–105] Constitutive expression of IL-2 and IL-4 was rarely observed throughout the entire course of HIV infection. In contrast, high levels of constitutive expression of IFN-γ and IL-10 were found at all stages of disease; CD8+ T cells were predominantly responsible for the expression of IFN-γ and at least a portion of IL-10 was expressed by non–T-cell subsets (ie, macrophages).[102] In studies that have analyzed cytokine secretion, a tendency toward a T_{H0} cytokine phenotype has been observed during the progression of HIV disease.[103–105]

Mechanisms of CD4+ T-Cell Depletion and Dysfunction

CD4+ T lymphocytes are the primary targets of HIV infection.[106–107] The progressive depletion of CD4+ T lymphocytes is characteristic of every stage of HIV infection, and CD4+ T-cell counts represent a valid surrogate marker to monitor the progression of HIV disease. For these reasons, the potential mechanisms responsible for the depletion of CD4+ T lymphocytes have been studied extensively, and several mechanisms have been proposed. These can be divided into two groups: direct virologic mechanisms that result from an HIV-mediated cytopathic effect, and indirect, nonvirologic mechanisms that include predominantly immunologic phenomena triggered during the course of HIV infection.

With regard to direct virologic mechanisms, HIV-mediated cytopathic effects may occur through either single-cell killing or HIV-induced syncytia formation.[108] However, that the evidence that HIV mediates direct killing of CD4+ T cells rests on the in vitro observation that cell death can be detected in cultures of cells that are acutely inoculated with virus even in absence of syncytia formation. It has been proposed that HIV may mediate single-cell killing by both accumulation of unintegrated viral DNA and inhibition of cellular protein synthesis.[108] The other primary mechanism of cell depletion observed after acute inoculation of virus in vitro in both peripheral blood and various CD4+ T-cell lines is syncytia formation.[108] This process involves multiple steps of cell membrane fusion between HIV-expressing cells and uninfected CD4+ T cells; in the fusion process, one infected cell could potentially be responsible for the elimination of up several hundred uninfected cells. Although the interaction of gp120 with the CD4 molecule represents a necessary step in this process, it has been demonstrated that the adhesion molecule leukocyte function–associated antigen 1 (LFA-1) plays a fundamental role in the regulation of syncytia formation of peripheral blood CD4+ T lymphocytes. Experiments performed with a panel of antibodies directed against the α and β chains of LFA-1 molecules and the intracellular adhesion molecules-1, -2, and -3 (the natural ligands for the LFA-1 molecule) have provided evidence that the process of HIV-mediated syncytia formation is regulated by the LFA-1/ICAM-1/-2/-3 pathway of cell-to-cell adhesion.[109–113]

Despite these in vitro data, it is still not entirely clear whether syncytia formation is an important mechanism of CD4+ T-cell depletion in vivo. Although syncytia formation in vivo in human tissue has been observed rarely, extensive formation of multinucleated giant cells in lymphoid tissue has been observed in monkeys inoculated with the highly pathogenic SIV molecular clone PBj.[114] Furthermore, in favor of the hypothesis that syncytia may play a role in vivo in humans are recent studies that have clearly demonstrated a relation between the appearance of primary virus isolates with the syncytium-inducing phenotype and the rapid decline of CD4+ T cells and progression of HIV disease.[115–122] Although these results do not demonstrate that syncytia formation occurs in vivo, they do indicate that the switch from a non–syncytium-inducing to a syncytium-inducing phenotype of certain primary isolates studied in vitro is associated with a rapid progression of HIV disease.

The group of indirect nonvirologic mechanisms include autoimmune mechanisms, anergy, superantigens, apoptosis, and virus-specific immune responses. With regard to the autoimmune hypothesis, it has been demonstrated that non-polymorphic determinants of MHC class I and II molecules share some degree of homology with the gp120 and gp41 proteins of HIV-1.[123,124] It is possible that both cellular and humoral immune responses directed against these HIV-1 proteins may cross-react with self-HLA class I and II molecules. Antibodies that react with class I and II molecules have been detected in the sera of patients with HIV infection.[125,126] In particular, antibodies against class II molecules could react with the class II molecules expressed on antigen-presenting cells, causing abnormal antigen presentation or suppressing antigen-specific helper CD4+ T-cell–mediated functions.[123,125] It is unclear whether class I reacting antibodies have a pathogenic (ie, nonprotective) role or whether their presence is beneficial. The hypothesis that gp120 can function as an "alloepitope"[127] is based on the homology between HLA-DR/HLA-DQ molecules and HIV-1 envelope glycoprotein. In favor of this hypothesis, it has been recently shown that gp120 is bound to the CD4 molecule of T cells in HIV-infected individuals.[128] This CD4-bound gp120 may trigger a long-term allogeneic immune response.

With regard to the induction of anergy in HIV infection, it has been shown that after binding of gp120-antibody complexes to the CD4 molecule, CD4+ T cells become refractory to further in vitro stimulation.[128,129] These observations have led to the hypothesis that gp120 or gp120–anti-gp120 complexes may deliver a negative signal to CD4+ T cells. Anti-gp120 antibodies have been detected on CD4+ T lymphocytes in patients with AIDS,[130] suggesting that gp120 is bound to the surface of these cells by the CD4 molecule. In this context, it has been proposed that gp120 bound to CD4+ T cells may mediate a pathogenic role by being presented to other CD4+ T cells[131]; this abnormal presentation of gp120 by other CD4+ T cells could induce anergy in already activated CD4+ T cells and could generate CD4+ cytotoxic T cells from the pool of resting T cells.

The hypothesis that HIV proteins may function as super-antigens or that superantigens unrelated to HIV may play an important role in the pathogenesis of HIV infection[132] is still the subject of active investigation. Microbial antigens of various types can potentially function as superantigens by binding to virtually all T cells that display a specific variable (V) region of the β chain of the T-cell antigen receptor.[133–147] Endogenous or exogenous murine retroviral superantigens stimulate in vivo a large proportion of CD4+ T cells and induce anergy or deletion of those stimulated CD4+ T-cell sub-

sets that display the specific Vβ regions.[133–147] Massive deletion of a large number of Vβ families[148] has not been confirmed in other studies.[149–151] These latter studies have shown perturbations (reductions or expansions, or both) of a limited set of Vβ families; however, there is no evidence that these perturbations were the result of an HIV-associated superantigen.

It has been demonstrated that a large proportion of CD4+ T lymphocytes from HIV-infected individuals undergo apoptosis after in vitro stimulation,[152–157] and it has been hypothesized that apoptosis represents the primary mechanism of CD4+ T-cell death in HIV infection. The fact that this phenomenon was observed in the majority of these cells after in vitro stimulation suggests that a large percentage of CD4+ T lymphocytes had been already primed in vivo to undergo apoptosis. The apoptosis hypothesis is particularly attractive because it would help to explain the depletion of CD4+ T cells without requiring that infection with HIV be responsible for each and every depleted cell. It has been shown that in HIV-infected patients apoptosis also occurs in substantial numbers of CD8+ T lymphocytes, which are not a target of HIV infection.[158] The obvious question arises regarding the role of apoptosis in the death of cells that are actually infected with HIV. A recent study has questioned the role of apoptosis as a mechanism of death in HIV- or SIV-infected cells; in this study, DNA fragmentation (the hallmark of apoptosis) was rarely observed in productively infected cells, suggesting that other mechanisms may be responsible for the death of HIV-infected cells.[159] In addition, although apoptosis is greatly increased in HIV infection, recent studies performed in both peripheral blood and lymphoid tissue have failed to show a relation between the level of apoptosis and clinical stage of HIV disease.[160,161] These findings have raised a series of questions regarding the significance of increased apoptosis and the precise role of apoptosis in the pathogenesis of HIV disease.

With regard to the physiologic role of apoptosis in the immune system, it is the primary mechanism leading to the elimination of autoreactive T cells (negative selection), and it may be involved in the regulation of the termination of antigen-specific immune responses by causing death of those cells that have been stimulated repetitively with a specific antigen.[162,163] These observations indicate that the phenomenon of apoptosis is directly dependent on the state of cellular activation, which would explain why, in addition to CD4+ T cells, different effector cells involved in the normal immune response, including those not permissive to HIV infection (ie, B cells and CD8+ T cells), may undergo apoptosis in HIV-infected individuals. The increased apoptosis observed in HIV infection may reflect, at least in part, an amplification of the normal mechanism of elimination of activated effector cells that have been involved in specific immune responses to HIV or other pathogens.[164] This latter interpretation, however, does not exclude the possibility that induction of apoptosis can occur in several other conditions, such as abnormal signaling after gp120-CD4 interaction,[157] inappropriate stimulation in both CD4+ and CD8+ T cells caused by abnormal antigen-presenting cell function,[165] and deficiencies in certain growth factors such as IL-2 or abnormal patterns of cytokine expression (high IFN-γ versus low IL-2).[102,166] A number of molecular mechanisms that may be responsible for apoptosis in HIV infection are currently being investigated, including involvement of *BCL2* gene expression,[167] increased sensitivity to reactive oxygen species,[168] the role of cell cycle and mitotic arrest,[169] and Fas/Apo1 antigen expression.[170]

Finally, HIV-specific immune responses, including humoral and cell-mediated immunity, play an important role in the control of HIV replication and spread in vivo. These phenomena may contribute significantly to the elimination of HIV-infected cells, including CD4+ T cells, macrophages, and FDCs, either by HIV-specific CTLs or by antibody-dependent cellular cytotoxicity. It has been hypothesized that HIV may cause immunosuppression and disease progression by virus-specific cytotoxic T cell–mediated immunopathology.[171] Therefore, although in the initial phase of infection effective immune responses may be critical for the containment of virus, it is possible that during the chronic phase of infection these virus-specific immune responses may have a pathogenic role.

CONCLUSIONS

Major advances have been made over the past few years in the delineation of the complex pathogenic mechanisms leading to the propagation of HIV infection over time and to the progression of HIV disease. Lymphoid organs are the primary anatomic sites for the initial establishment of HIV infection; after establishment of chronic infection, active virus replication and propagation of HIV infection over time occurs in the lymphoid organs. Active virus replication and high virus turnover are continuous throughout the entire course of HIV infection; these processes include multiple phases and are characterized by multiple pathogenic mechanisms. In most patients, progression to AIDS occurs over a period of 10 to 12 years; however, a small percentage of HIV-infected persons do not show any clinical or immunologic signs of progression of HIV disease for an extended period of time, indicating that virus replication may be effectively kept at a very low level in these patients. A vigorous immune response is detected very early during primary HIV infection, and it is able to effect a dramatic downregulation of virus replication; however, this immune response is rarely able to completely eliminate the virus. Striking qualitative differences have been observed in the primary immune response to HIV infection among different individuals, and these differences seem to correlate with favorable or nonfavorable clinical outcomes.

The delineation of the complexities of the virus-specific immune responses and of the pathogenic mechanisms of HIV disease are critical for the development of vaccine and therapeutic strategies. Although suppression of HIV replication with antiretroviral drugs remains the primary therapeutic approach to HIV disease, other strategies that have as their objective the modulation of the immune response to HIV are appropriate to consider for use in combination with antiretroviral therapy during certain stages of HIV disease.

REFERENCES

1. Pantaleo G, Graziosi C, Fauci AS. The immunopathogenesis of human immunodeficiency virus infection. N Engl J Med 1993;328:327.
2. Fauci AS. The human immunodeficiency virus: infectivity and mechanisms of pathogenesis. Science 1988;239:617.
3. Tindall B, Cooper DA. Primary HIV infection: host responses and intervention strategies. AIDS 1991;5:1.
4. Clark SJ, Saag MS, Decker WD, et al. High titers of cytopathic virus in plasma of patients with symptomatic primary HIV-1 infection. N Engl J Med 1991;324:954.
5. Daar ES, Moudgil T, Meyer RD, Ho DD. Transient high levels of viremia in patients with primary human immunodeficiency virus type 1 infection. N Engl J Med 1991;324:961.
6. Graziosi C, Pantaleo G, Butini L, et al. Kinetics of HIV DNA and RNA synthesis during primary HIV-1 infection. Proc Natl Acad Sci USA 1993;90:6505.
7. Koup RA, Safrit JT, Cao Y, et al. Temporal association of cellular immune response with the initial control of viremia in primary human immunodeficiency virus type 1 syndrome. J Virol 1994;68:4650.
8. Borrow P, Lewicki H, Hahn BH, Shaw GM, Oldstone MB. CTL activity associated with control of viremia in primary HIV-1 infection. J Virol 1994;68:6103.
9. Pantaleo G, Demarest JF, Soudeyns H, et al. Major expansion of CD8+ T cells with a predominant Vβ usage during the primary immune response to HIV. Nature 1994;370:463.
10. Mackewicz CE, Yang LC, Lifson JD, Levy JA. Non-cytolytic CD8 T-cell anti-HIV responses in primary HIV-1 infection. Lancet 1994;344:1671.
11. Moore JP, Cao Y, Ho DD, Koup RA. Development of the anti-gp120 antibody responses during seroconversion to human immunodeficiency virus type 1. J Virol 1994;68:5142.
12. Reimann KA, Tenner-Racz K, Racz P, et al. Immunopathogenic events in acute infection of rhesus monkeys with simian immunodeficiency virus of macaques. J Virol 1994;68:2362.
13. Pantaleo G, Fauci AS. New concepts in the immunopathogenesis of HIV infection. Ann Rev Immunol 1995;13:487.
14. Pantaleo G, Graziosi C, Demarest JF, et al. HIV infection is active and progressive in lymphoid tissue during the clinically latent stage of disease. Nature 1993;362:355.
15. Embretson J, Zupancic M, Ribas JL, Burke A, Tenner-Racz K, Haase AT. Massive covert infection of helper T lymphocytes and macrophages by HIV during the incubation period of AIDS. Nature 1993;362:359.
16. Pantaleo G, Graziosi C, Butini L, et al. Lymphoid organs function as major reservoirs for human immunodeficiency virus. Proc Natl Acad Sci USA 1991;88:9838.
17. Pantaleo G, Graziosi C, Demarest JF, et al. Role of lymphoid organs in the pathogenesis of human immunodeficiency virus (HIV) infection. Immunol Rev 1994;140:105.
18. Wei X, Chosh SK, Taylor ME, et al. Viral dynamics in human immunodeficiency virus type 1 infection. Nature 1995;373:117.
19. Ho DD, Neumann AU, Perelson AS, Chen W, Leonard JM, Markowitz M. Rapid turnover of plasma virions and CD4 lymphocytes in HIV-1 infection. Nature 1995;373:123.
20. Piatak M, Saag MS, Yang LC, et al. High levels of HIV-1 in plasma during all stages of infection determined by competitive PCR. Science 1993;259:1749.
21. Sheppard HW. Characterization of long-term HIV-1 infection without CD4+T-cell loss (non-progressors), abstract. Ninth International Conference on AIDS, Berlin, June 6–11, 1993;WS-BO3-1.
22. Phair JP. Keynote address: variations in the natural history of HIV infection. AIDS Res Human Retroviruses 1994;10:883.
23. Lifson AR, Buchbinder SP, Sheppard HW, et al. Long-term human immunodeficiency virus infection in asymptomatic homosexual and bisexual men with normal CD4+ lymphocyte counts: immunologic and virologic characteristics. J Infect Dis 1991;163:959.
24. Buchbinder SP, Katz MH, Hessol NA, O'Malley PM, Holmberg SD. Long-term HIV-1 infection without immunologic progression. AIDS 1994;8:1123.

25. Sheppard HW, Lang W, Ascher MS, Vittinghoff E, Winkelstein W. The characterization of non-progressors: long-term HIV-1 infection with stable CD4+ T-cell levels. AIDS 1993;7:1159.
26. Levy JA. HIV pathogenesis and long-term survival. AIDS 1993;7:1401.
27. Easterbrook PJ. Non-progression in HIV infection. AIDS 1994;8:1179.
28. Schrager LK, Young JM, Fowler MG, Mathieson BJ, Vermund SH. Long-term survivors of HIV-1 infection: definitions and research challenges. AIDS 1994;8:S95.
29. Pantaleo G, Menzo S, Vaccarezza M, et al. Studies in subjects with long-term nonprogressive human immunodeficiency virus infection. N Engl J Med 1995;332:209.
30. Korchhoff F, Greenough TC, Brettler DB, Sullivan L, Desrosiers RC. Brief report: absence of intact nef sequences in a long-term survivor with nonprogressive HIV-1 infection. N Engl J Med 1995;332:228.
31. Cao Y, Quin L, Zhang L, Safrit J, Ho DD. Virologic and immunologic characterization of long-term survivors of human immunodeficiency virus type 1 infection. N Engl J Med 1995;26:201.
32. Fauci AS, Schnittman SM, Poli G, Koenig S, Pantaleo G. Immunopathogenic mechanisms in human immunodeficiency virus (HIV) infection. Ann Intern Med 1991;114:678.
33. Bagnarelli P, Menzo S, Valenza A, et al. Molecular profile of HIV type 1 infection in symptomless patients with AIDS. J Virol 1992;66:7328.
34. Fauci AS, Lane HC. The acquired immunodeficiency syndrome (AIDS). In: Wilson JD, Braunwald E, Isselbacher KJ, ed. Harrison's principles of internal medicine, vol 2. New York: McGraw-Hill, 1991: 1402.
35. Raska K Jr, Kim HC, Raskall K, et al. Human immunodeficiency virus (HIV) infection in hemophiliacs: long-term prognostic significance of the HIV serologic pattern. Clin Exp Immunol 1989;77:1.
36. Janvier B, Mallet F, Cheynet V, et al. Prevalence and persistence of antibody titers to recombinant HIV-1 core and matrix proteins in HIV-1 infection. J Acquir Immune Defic Syndr 1993;6:898.
37. Kozlowski PA, Chen D, Eldridge JH, Jackson S. Contrasting IgA and IgG neutralization capacities and responses to HIV type 1 gp120 V3 loop in HIV-infected individuals. AIDS Res Hum Retroviruses 1994;10:813.
38. Pincus SH, Messer KG, Nara PL, Blattner WA, Colebugh G, Reitz M. Temporal analysis of the antibody response to HIV envelope protein in HIV-infected individuals. J Clin Invest 1994;93:2505.
39. Cavacini LA, Emes CL, Power J, et al. Loss of serum antibodies to a conformational epitope of HIV-1/gp120 identified by a human monoclonal antibody is associated with disease progression. J Aquir Immune Defic Syndr 1993;6:1093.
40. Giorgi JV, Liu Z, Hultin LE, et al. Elevated levels of CD38+ T cells in HIV infection add to the prognostic value of low CD4+ T cell levels: results of 6 years of follow-up. The Los Angeles Center, Multicenter AIDS Cohort Study. J Aquir Immune Defic Syndr 1993;6:904.
41. Ho HN, Hultin LE, Mitsuyasu RT, Matud JL. Circulating HIV-specific CD8+ cytotoxic T cells express CD38 and HLA-DR antigens. J Immunol 1993;150:3070.
42. Mackewicz CF, Ortega HW, Levy JA. CD8+ cell anti-HIV activity correlates with the clinical state of the infected individuals. J Clin Invest 1991;87:1462.
43. Landay AL, Mackewicz CE, Levy JA. An activated CD8+ T cell phenotype correlates with anti-HIV activity and asymptomatic clinical status. Clin Immunol Immunopathol 1993;69:106.
44. Pantaleo G, Koenig S, Baseler M, Lane HC, Fauci AS. Defective clonogenic potential of CD8+ T lymphocytes in patients with AIDS. J Immunol 1990;144:1696.
45. Lifson AR, Hessol NA, Buchbinder SP, Holmberg SD. The association of clinical conditions and serologic tests with CD4+ lymphocyte counts in HIV-infected subjects without AIDS. AIDS 1991;5:1209.
46. Fahey J, Taylor J, Detels R, et al. The prognostic value of cellular and serologic markers in infection with human immunodeficiency virus type 1. N Engl J Med 1990;322:166.
47. Munoz A, Vlahov D, Solomon L, et al. Prognostic indicators for development of AIDS among intravenous drug users. J Acquir Immune Defic Syndr 1992;5:694.
48. Gupta P, Kingsley L, Armstrong J, Ding M. Enhanced expression of human immunodeficiency virus type 1 correlates with development of AIDS. Virology 1993;196:586.
49. DeMartino M. The Italian Register for HIV Infection in Children: Features of children perinatally infected with HIV-1 surviving longer than 5 years. Lancet 1994;343:191.
50. Schnittman SM, Greenhouse JJ, Lane HC, Pierce PF, Fauci AS. Frequent detection of HIV-1-specific mRNAs in infected individuals suggests ongoing active viral expression in all stages of disease. AIDS Res Hum Retroviruses 1991;7:361.
51. Seshamma T, Bagasra O, Trono D, Baltimore D, Pomerantz RJ. Blocked early-stage latency in the peripheral blood cells of certain individuals infected with human immunodeficiency virus type 1. Proc Natl Acad Sci USA 1992;89:10663.
52. Arens M, Joseph T, Nag S, Miller JP. Alterations in spliced and unspliced HIV-1–specific RNA detection in peripheral blood mononuclear cells of individuals with varying CD4-positive lymphocyte counts. AIDS Res Hum Retroviruses 1993;9:1257.
53. Saksela K, Stevens C, Rubinstein P, Baltimore D. Human immunodeficiency virus type 1 mRNA expression in peripheral blood cells predicts disease progression independently of the numbers of CD4+ lymphocytes. Proc Natl Acad Sci USA 1994;91:1104.
54. Delwart EL, Sheppard HW, Walker BD, Goudsmit J, Mullins JI. Human immunodeficiency virus type 1 evolution in vivo tracked by DNA heteroduplex mobility assays. J Virol 1994;68:6672.
55. Klein MR, van Ballen CA, Holwerda AM, et al. Kinetics of gag-specific cytotoxic T lymphocyte responses during the clinical course of HIV-1 infection: a longitudinal analysis of rapid progressors and long-term asymptomatics. J Exp Med 1995;181:1365.
56. Pantaleo G, De Maria A, Koenig S, et al. CD8+ T lymphocytes of patients with AIDS maintain normal broad cytolytic function despite the loss of human immunodeficiency virus–specific cytotoxicity. Proc Natl Acad Sci USA 1990;87:4818.
57. Montefiori DC, Pantaleo G, Fink LM, et al. Neutralizing and infection-enhancing antibody responses to human immunodeficiency virus type 1 in long term non-progressors. J Infect Dis 1996;173:60.
58. Kaslow RA, Mann DL. The role of the major histocompatibility complex in human immunodeficiency virus infection: ever more complex? J Infect Dis 1994;169:1332.
59. Chakrabarti L, Isola P, Cumont M-C, et al. Early stages of simian immunodeficiency virus infection in lymph nodes. Am J Pathol 1994;144:1226.
60. Tenner-Racz K, Racz P, Bofill M, et al. HTLV-III/LAV viral antigens in lymph nodes of homosexual men with persistent generalized lymphadenopathy and AIDS. Am J Pathol 1986;123:9.
61. Biberfeld P, Ost A, Porwit A, et al. Histopathology and immunohistology of HTLV-III/LAV related lymphadenopathy and AIDS. Acta Pathol Microbiol Immunol Scand 1987;95:47.
62. Emilie D, Peuchmaur M, Maillot M, et al. Production of interleukins in human immunodeficiency virus-1––replicating lymph nodes. J Clin Invest 1990;86:148.
63. Fox CH, Tenner-Racz K, Racz P, Firpo A, Pizzo PA, Fauci AS. Lymphoid germinal centers are reservoirs of human immunodeficiency virus type 1 RNA. J Infect Dis 1991;164:1051.
64. Spiegel H, Herbst H, Niedobitek G, Foss HD, Stein H. Follicular dendritic cells are a major reservoir for human immunodeficiency virus type 1 in lymphoid tissues facilitating infection of CD4+ T-helper cells. Am J Pathol 1992;140:15.
65. Cohen OJ, Pantaleo G, Holodniy M, et al. Decreased human immunodeficiency virus type 1 plasma viremia during antiretroviral therapy reflects downregulation of viral replication in lymphoid tissue. Proc Natl Acad Sci U S A 1995;92:6017.
66. Clerici M, Stocks NI, Zajac RA, et al. Interleukin-2 production used to detect antigenic peptide recognition by T-helper lymphocytes from asymptomatic HIV-seropositive individuals. Nature 1989;339:383.
67. Torseth JW, Berman PW, Merigan TC. Recombinant HIV structural proteins detect specific cellular immunity in vitro in infected individuals. AIDS Res Hum Retrovirses 1988;4:23.
68. Haynes BF. Immune responses to HIV infection. In: AIDS etiology, diagnosis, treatment and prevention. Philadelphia: JB Lippincott, 1992;77.
69. Berman PW, Gregory TJ, Riddle L, et al. Protection of chimpanzees from infection by HIV-1 after vaccination with recombinant glycoprotein gp120 but not gp160. Nature 1994;345:622.
70. Emini EA, Nara PL, Schleif WA, et al. Antibody-mediated in vitro neutralization of human immunodeficiency virus type 1 abolishes infectivity for chimpanzees. J Virol 1990;64:3674.
71. Girard M, Kieny M-P, Pinter A, et al. Immunization of chimpanzees confers protection against challenge with human immunodeficiency virus. Proc Natl Acad Sci USA 1991;88:542.
72. Matthews TJ, Langlois AJ, Robey WG, et al. Restricted neutralization of divergent human T-lymphotropic virus type III isolates by antibodies to the major envelope glycoprotein. Proc Natl Acad Sci USA 1986;83:9709.

73. Weiss RA, Clapham RP, Cheingsong-Popov R, et al. Neutralization of human T-lymphotropic virus type III by sera of AIDS and AIDS-risk patients. Nature 1985;316:69.

74. Robert-Guroff M, Brown M, Gallo RC, et al. HTLV-III-neutralizing antibodies in patients with AIDS and AIDS-related complex. Nature 1985;316:72.

75. Weiss RA, Clapham R, Weber JN, et al. Variable and conserved neutralization antigens of human immunodeficiency virus. Nature 1986;324:572.

76. Pantaleo G, Demarest JF, Vaccarezza M, et al. Effect of anti-V3 antibodies on cell-free and cell-to-cell human immunodeficiency virus transmission. Eur J Immunol 1995;25:226.

77. Robinson WE, Montefiori DC, Mitchell WM, et al. Antibody-dependent enhancement of human immunodeficiency virus type 1 (HIV-1) infection in vitro by serum from HIV-1 infected and passively immunized chimpanzees. Proc Natl Acad Sci USA 1989;86:4710.

78. Robinson WE, Kawamura T, Gorny MK, et al. Human monoclonal antibodies to the human immunodeficiency virus type 1 (HIV-1) transmembrane glycoprotein gp41 enhance HIV-1 infection in vitro. Proc Natl Acad Sci USA 1990;87:3815.

79. Homsy J, Meyer M, Levy J. Serum enhancement of human immunodeficiency virus (HIV) infection correlates with disease in HIV- infected individuals. J Virol 1990;64:1437.

80. Cullen BR. Regulation of human immunodeficiency virus replication. Annu Rev Microbiol 1991;45:219.

81. Felber BK, Pavlakis GN. Molecular biology of HIV-1: positive and negative regulatory elements important for virus expression. AIDS 1993;7:S51.

82. Vaishnav YN, Wong-Staal F. The biochemistry of AIDS. Annu Rev Biochem 1991;60:577.

83. Pavlakis GN, Schwartz S, D'Agostino DM, Felber BK. Structure, splicing, and regulation of expression of HIV-1: a model for the general organization of lentiviruses and other complex retroviruses. In: Koff WC, Wong-Staal F, Kennedy RC, ed. AIDS research review. New York: Marcel Dekker, 1992:41.

84. Gaynor R. Cellular transcription factors involved in the regulation of HIV-1 gene expression. AIDS 1992;6:347.

85. Ascher MS, Sheppard HW. AIDS as immune system activation: a model for pathogenesis. Clin Exp Immunol 1988;73:165.

86. Ascher MS, Sheppard HW. AIDS as immune system activation: II. The panergic imnesia hypothesis. J Acquir Immune Defic Syndr 1990;3:177.

87. Bass HZ, Nishanian P, Hardy WD, et al. Immune changes in HIV infection: significant correlations and differences in serum markers and lymphoid phenotypic antigens. Clin Immunol Immunopathol 1992;64:63.

88. Lang JM, Coumaros G, Levy S, et al. Elevated serum levels of soluble IL-2 receptor in HIV infection: correlation studies with markers of cell activation. Immunol Lett 1988;19:99.

89. Sheppard HW, Ascher MS, McRae B, Anderson RE, Lang W, Allain JP. The initial immune response to HIV and immune system activation determine the outcome of HIV disease. J Acquir Immune Defic Syndr 1991;4:704.

90. Pantaleo G, Fauci AS. Tracking HIV during disease progression. Curr Opin Immunol 1994;6:600.

91. Zack JA, Arrigo SJ, Weitsman SR, Go AS, Haislip A, Chen IS. HIV-1 entry into quiescent primary lymphocytes: molecular analysis reveals a labile, latent viral structure. Cell 1990;61:213.

92. Bukrinsky MI, Stanwick TL, Dempsey MP, Stevenson M. Quiescent T lymphocytes as an inducible virus reservoir in HIV-1 infection. Science 1991;18:423.

93. Rosenberg ZF, Fauci AS. Immunopathogenesis of HIV infection. FASEB J 1991;5:2382.

94. Poli G, Fauci AS. The effect of cytokines and pharmacologic agents on chronic HIV infection. AIDS Res Hum Retroviruses 1992;8:191.

95. Poli G, Pantaleo G, Fauci AS. Immunopathogenesis of human immunodeficiency virus infection. Clin Infect Dis 1993; Suppl 1:S224.

96. Clerici M, Shearer GM. A TH1-TH2 switch is a critical step in the etiology of HIV infection. Immunol Today 1993;14:107.

97. Urban JJ, Katona IM, Paul WE, Finkelman FD. Interleukin-4 is important in protective immunity to a gastrointestinal nematode infection in mice. Proc Natl Acad Sci U S A 1991;88:5513.

98. Salgame P, Abrams JS, Clayberger C, et al. Differing lymphokine profiles of functional subsets of human CD4 and CD8 T cell clones. Science 1991;254:279.

99. Mosmann T, Cherwinski H, Bond M, Giedlin M, Coffman R. Two types of murine helper T cell clones: I. Definition according to profiles of lymphokine activities and secreted proteins. J Immunol 1986;136:2348.

100. Romagnani S. Human TH1 and TH2 subsets: doubt no more. Immunol Today 1991;12:256.

101. DelPrete G, DeCarli M, Almerigogna F, GraziaGiudizi M, Biagiotti R, Romagnani S. Human IL-10 is produced by both type 1 helper (Th1) and type 2 helper (Th2) T cell clones and inhibits their antigen-specific proliferation and cytokine production. J Immunol 1993;150:353.

102. Graziosi C, Pantaleo G, Gantt KR, et al. Lack of evidence for dichotomy of Th1 and Th2 predominance in HIV-infected individuals. Science 1994;265:248.

103. Maggi E, Mazzetti M, Ravina A, et al. Ability of HIV to promote a TH11 to TH0 shift and to replicate preferentially in TH2 and TH0 cells. Science 1994;265:244.

104. Meyaard L, Otto SA, Keet IP, van Lier RAW, Miedema F. Changes in cytokine secretion patterns of CD4+ T-cell clones in human immunodeficiency virus infection. Blood 1994;84:4262.

105. Autran B, Leqac E, Blanc C, Debre P. A Tho/Th2-like function of CD4+ CD7– T helper cells from normal donors and HIV infected patients. J Immunol 1995;154:1408.

106. Dalgleish AG, Beverley PCL, Clapham PR, Crawford DH, Greaves MF, Weiss RA. The CD4 (T4) antigen is an essential component of the receptor for the AIDS retrovirus. Nature 1984;312:763.

107. Klatzmann D, Champagne E, Chamaret S, et al. T-lymphocyte T4 molecule behaves as the receptor for human retrovirus LAV. Nature 1984;312:767.

108. Garry RF. Potential mechanisms for the cytopathic properties of HIV. AIDS 1989;3:683-694.

109. Hildreth JEK, Orentas RJ. Involvement of a leukocyte adhesion receptor (LFA-1) in HIV-induced syncytium formation. Science 1989;244:1075.

110. Valentin A, Lundin K, Patarroyo M, Asjo B. The leukocyte adhesion glycoprotein CD18 participates in HIV-1–induced syncytia formation in monocytoid and T cells. J Immunol 1990;144:934.

111. Pantaleo G, Butini L, Graziosi C, et al. Human immunodeficiency virus (HIV) infection in CD4+ T lymphocytes genetically deficient in LFA-1: LFA-1 is required for HIV-mediated cell fusion but not for viral transmission. J Exp Med 1991;173:511.

112. Pantaleo G, Poli G, Butini L, Fox C, et al. Dissociation between syncytia formation and HIV spreading: suppression of syncytia formation does not necessarily reflect inhibition of HIV infection. Eur J Immunol 1991;21:1771.

113. Butini L, DeFougerolles AR, Vaccarezza M, et al. Intercellular adhesion molecules (ICAM)-1 ICAM-2 and ICAM-3 function as counter-receptors for lymphocyte function-associated molecule 1 in human immunodeficiency virus-mediated syncytia formation. Eur J Immunol 1994;24:2191.

114. Rosenberg YJ, Zack PM, White BD, et al. Decline in the CD4+ lymphocyte population in the blood of SIV-infected macaques is not reflected in the lymph node. AIDS Res Human Retroviruses 1992;9:639.

115. Schuitemaker H, Koot M, Kootstra NA, et al. Biological phenotype of human immunodeficiency virus type 1 clones at different stages of infection: progression of disease is associated with a shift from monocytotropic to T-cell–tropic virus population. J Virol 1992;66:1354.

116. Tersmette M, deGoede RE, Al BJ, et al. Differential syncytium-inducing capacity of human immunodeficiency virus isolates: frequent detection of syncytium-inducing isolates in patients with acquired immunodeficiency syndrome (AIDS) and AIDS-related complex. J Virol 1988;62:2026.

117. Tersmette M, Gruters RA, deWolf F, et al. Evidence for a role of virulent human immunodeficiency virus (HIV) variants in the pathogenesis of acquired immunodeficiency syndrome: studies on sequential HIV isolates. J Virol 1989;63:2118.

118. Asjo B, Sharma UK, Morfeldt-Manson L, et al. Naturally occurring HIV-1 isolates with differences in replicative capacity are distinguished by in situ hybridization of infected cells. AIDS Res Hum Retroviruses 1990;6:1177.

119. Cheng-Mayer Homsy J, Evans LA, Levy JA. Identification of HIV subtypes with distinct patterns of sensitivity to serum neutralization. Proc Natl Acad Sci USA 1988;85:2815.

120. Schellekens PT, Tersmette M, Roos MT, et al. Biphasic rate of CD4+ cell count decline during progression to AIDS correlates with HIV-1 phenotype. AIDS 1992;6:665.

121. Koot M, Keet IP, Vos AH, et al. Prognostic value of HIV-1 syncytium-inducing phenotype for rate of CD4+ cell depletion and progression to AIDS. Ann Intern Med 1993;118:681.

122. Connors M, Giese NA, Kulkarni AB, Firestone CY, Morese III HC, Murphy BR. Enhanced pulmonary histopathology induced by respiratory syncytial virus (RSV) challenge of formalin-inactivated RSV-immunized BALB/c mice is abrogated by depletion of interleukin-4 (IL-4) and IL- 10. J Virol 1994;68:5321.

123. Golding H, Robey FA, Gates FT, et al. Identification of homologous regions in human immunodeficiency virus I gp41 and human MHC class II β1 domain: I. Monoclonal antibodies against the gp41-derived peptide and patients' sera react with native HLA class II antigens, suggesting a role for autoimmunity in the pathogenesis of acquired immune deficiency syndrome. J Exp Med 1988;167:914.

124. Golding H, Shearer GM, Hillman K, et al. Common epitope in human immunodeficiency virus (HIV)1 I-GP41 and HLA class II elicits immunosuppressive autoantibodies capable of contributing to immune dysfunction in HIV-1 infected individuals. J Clin Invest 1989;83:1430.

125. Grassi F, Meneveri R, Gullberg M, et al. Human immunodeficiency virus (HIV)-1 gp120 mimics a hidden epitope borne to major histocompatibility complex class I heavy chain. J Exp Med 1991;174:53.

126. Beretta, Grassi F, Pelagi M, et al. HIV env glycoprotein shares a cross-reacting epitope with a surface protein present on activated human monocytes and involved in antigen presentation. Eur J Immunol 1987;17:71793.

127. Habeshaw JA, Dalgleish AG, Bountiff L. AIDS pathogenesis: HIV envelope and its interaction with cell proteins. Immunol Today 1990;11:418.

128. Mittler RS, Hoffman MK. Synergism between HIV gp120 and gp120-specific antibody in blocking human T cell activation. Science 1989;245:1380.

129. Linette GP, Hartzman RJ, Ledbetter JA, June CH. HIV-I–infected T cells show a selective signaling defect after perturbation of CD3/antigen receptor. Science 1988;241:573.

130. Amadori A, Silvestro G, Zamarchi R, et al. CD4 epitope masking by gp120/anti-gp12 antibody complexes: a potential mechanism for CD4+ cell function down-regulation in AIDS patients. J Immunol 1992;148:2709.

131. Pichler WJ, Wyss-Coray T. T cells as antigen-presenting cells. Immunol Today 1994;15:312.

132. Janeway C. Mls: makes a little sense. Nature 1991;349:459.

133. Kappler JW, Staerz U, White J, Marrack PC. Self-tolerance eliminates T cells specific for Mls-modified products of the major histocompatibility complex. Nature 1988;332:35.

134. MacDonald HR, Schneider R, Less RK. T-cell receptor Vβ use predicts reactivity and tolerance to Mls-encoded antigens. Nature 1988;332:40.

135. Woodland D, Happ MP, Bill J, Palmer E. Requirement for cotolerogenic gene products in the clonal deletion of I-E reactive T cells. Science 1990;247:964.

136. Abe R, Foo-Philips M, Hodes RJ. Analysis of Mls genetics: a novel instance of genetic redundancy. J Exp Med 1989;170:1059.

137. Bill J, Kanagawa O, Woodland DL, Palmer E. The MHC molecule I-E is necessary but not sufficient for the clonal deletion of Vβ11-bearing T cells. J Exp Med 1989;169:1405.

138. Rammensee H-G, Kroschewski R, Frangoulis B. Clonal anergy induced in mature Vβ6+ T lymphocytes on immunizing Mls16 mice with Mls-1a expressing cells. Nature 1989;339:541.

139. Webb S, Morris C, Sprent J. Extrathymic tolerance of mature T cells: clonal elimination as a consequence of immunity. Cell 1990;63:1249.

140. Marrack P, Kushnir E, Kappler J. A maternally inherited superantigen encoded by a mammary tumour virus. Nature 1991;349:542.

141. Frankel WN, Rudy C, Coffin JM, Huber BT. Linkage of Mls genes to endogenous mammary tumour viruses of inbred mice. Nature 1991;349:526.

142. Woodland DL, Happ MP, Gollob KJ, Palmer E. An endogenous retrovirus mediating deletion of αβ T cells? Nature 1991;349:529.

143. Dyson PJ, Knight AM, Fairchild S, Simpson E, Tomonari K. Genes encoding ligands for deletion of Vβ11 T cells cosegreate with mammary tumour virus genomes. Nature 1991;349:531.

144. Choi Y, Kappler JW, Marrack P. A superantigen encoded in the open reading frame of the 3' long terminal repeat of mouse mammary tumour virus. Nature 1991;350:203.

145. Acha-Orbea H, Shakov AN, Scarpellino L, et al. Clonal deletion of Vβ14-bearing T cells in mice transgenic for mammary tumour virus. Nature 1991;350:207.

146. Paliard X, West SG, Lafferty JA. Evidence for the effects of a superantigen in rheumatoid arthritis. Science 1991;253:325.

147. Cole BC, Atkin CL. The mycoplasma arthritidis T-cell mitogen, MAM: a model superantigen. Immunol Today 1991;12:271.

148. Imberti L, Sottini A, Bettinardi A, Pouti M, Primi D. Selective depletion in HIV infection of T cells that bear specific T cell receptor Vβ sequences. Science 1991;254:860.

149. Rebai N, Pantaleo G, Demarest JF, et al. Analysis of the T-cell receptor beta-chain variable-region (Vbeta) repertoire in monozygotic twins discordant for human immunodeficiency virus evidence for perturbations. Proc Natl Acad Sci USA 1994;91:1529.

150. Hodara V, Jeddi-Tehrani M, Grunewald J, et al. HIV infection leads to differential expression of T-cell receptor Vbeta genes in CD4+ and CD8+ T cells. AIDS 1993;7:633.

151. Posnett DN, Kabak SK, Hodtsev AS, et al. T-cell antigen receptor Vbeta subsets are not preferentially deleted in AIDS. AIDS 1992;7:625.

152. Ameisen JC, Capron A. Cell dysfunction and depletion in AIDS: the programmed cell death hypothesis. Immunol Today 1991;12:102.

153. Gougeon ML, Olivier R, Garcia S, et al. Mise en evidence d'un procesus d'engagment vers la mort cellulaire par apoptose dans less lymphocytes de patients infectes par le VIH. C R Acad Sci III 1991;312:529.

154. Groux H, Torpier G, Monte D, Mouton Y, Capron A, Ameisen JC. Activation-induced death by apoptosis in CD4+ T cells from human immunodeficiency virus-infected asymptomatic individuals. J Exp Med 1992;175:331.

155. Laurent-Crawford AG, Krust B, et al. The cytopathic effect of HIV is associated with apoptosis. Virology 1991;185:829.

156. Terai C, Kornbluth RS, Pauza CD, Richman DD, Carson DA. Apoptosis as a mechanism of cell death in cultured T lymphoblasts acutely infected with HIV-1. J Clin Invest 1991;87:1710.

157. Banda NK, Bernier J, Kurahara DK, et al. Crosslinking CD4 by human immunodeficiency virus gp120 primes T cells for activation-induced apoptosis. J Exp Med 1992;176:1099.

158. Meyaard L, Otto SA, Jonker RR, Mijnster MJ, Keet RPM, Miedema F. Programmed death of T cells in HIV-1 infection. Science 1992;257:217.

159. Finkel TH, Tudor-Williams G, Banda NK, et al. Apoptosis occurs predominantly in bystander cells and not in productively infected cells of HIV- and SIV-infected lymph nodes. Nature Med 1995;1:129.

160. Meyaard L, Otto SA, Hooibrink B, et al. Quantitative analysis of CD4+ T cell function in the course of human immunodeficiency virus infection: gradual decline of both naive and memory alloreactive T cells. J Clin Invest 1994;94:1947.

161. Muro-Cacho C, Pantaleo G, Fauci AS. Analysis of apoptosis in lymph nodes of HIV-infected individuals: intensity of apoptosis correlates with the general state of activation of the lymphoid tissue and not with stage of disease or viral burden. J Immunol 154:5555.

162. Cohen JJ, Duke RC, Fadok VA, Sellins KS. Apoptosis and programmed cell death in immunity. Ann Rev Immunol 1992;10:267.

163. Lenardo MJ. Interleukin-2 programs mouse alphabeta T lymphocytes for apoptosis. Nature 1991;353:858.

164. Pantaleo G, Fauci AS. Apoptosis in HIV infection. Nature Med 1995;1:118.

165. Meyaard L, Schuitemaker H, Miedema F. T-cell dysfunction in HIV infection: anergy due to defective antigen-presenting cell function? Immunol Today 1993;14:163.

166. Fan J, Bass HZ, Fahey JL. Elevated IFN-gamma and decreased IL-2 gene expression are associated with HIV infection. J Immunol 1993;151:5031.

167. Akbar AN, Borthwick N, Salmon M, et al. The significance of low bcl-2 expression by CD45RO T cells in normal individuals and patients with acute viral infections: The role of apoptosis in T cell memory. J Exp Med 1993;178:427.

168. Sandstrom PA, Roberts B, Folks TM, Buttke TM. HIV gene expression enhances T cell susceptibility to hydrogen peroxide–induced apoptosis. AIDS Res Hum Retroviruses 1993;9:1107.

169. Cohen D, Tani Y, Tian H, Boone E, Samelson LE, Lane C. Participation of thyrosine phosphorylation in the cytopathic effect of human immunodeficiency virus-1. Science 1992;256:542.

170. Itoh N, Yonehara S, Ishi A, et al. The polypeptide encoded by the cDNA for human cell surface antigen Fas can mediate apoptosis. Cell 1991;66:233.

171. Zinkernagel RM, Hengartner H. T-cell–mediated immunopathology versus direct cytolysis by virus: implications for HIV and AIDS. Immunol Today 1994;15:262.

AIDS: Biology, Diagnosis, Treatment and Prevention, fourth edition, edited by Vincent T. DeVita, Jr., Samuel Hellman, and Steven A. Rosenberg. Lippincott–Raven Publishers, © 1997

CHAPTER 5

Immune Responses To Human Immunodeficiency Virus Infection

Barton F. Haynes

The immune response to the human immunodeficiency virus (HIV) is determined by many complex factors. First, the extraordinary host-virus interactions that lead to the pathogenesis of acquired immunodeficiency syndrome (AIDS) induce profound functional host immune defects, beginning soon after infection with HIV (see Chap. 2).[1] Prominent forms of HIV-induced immune dysfunction include defects in T- and B-cell responses to specific antigens, polyclonal hypergammaglobulinemia, enhanced autoantibody and immune complex formation, dysregulated cytokine production, decreased natural killer cell activity, and defective monocyte and dendritic cell function.[1–4] At the time when the host immune system begins to mount an anti-HIV immune response designed to neutralize free HIV and eliminate HIV-infected cells, many of the cellular components of the immune responses are being adversely affected by HIV. Second, evidence suggests that the route of HIV infection,[5] the amount of HIV in the inoculum, the pathogenic potential of a given HIV strain,[6] and host genetic factors[7] may modify the host response to HIV. Third, evidence suggest that some components of an immune response to HIV may enhance HIV infectivity or may be directly responsible for clinical manifestations of the disease.[8–11] Fourth, the remarkable ability of HIV to mutate genome sequences and change the primary amino acid sequence of HIV proteins effectively allows HIV to evade otherwise effective antiviral immune responses.[12–15]

In individuals with advanced HIV disease, as many as 10^9 new HIV virions are produced each day and as many as 2×10^9 CD4-positive (CD4+) T cells turn over per day, with a half-life of HIV and CD4+ T cells of approximately 2 days.[16,17] Studies suggest that CD4+ T-cell depletion in HIV infection result from the high replicative capacity of HIV

and direct viral cell killing,[16,17] although CD4+ cell loss could in part be caused by immune mediated cell killing or to T-cell apoptosis, or both.[18] The complexities of HIV-host interactions create myriad obstacles to an effective immune response to HIV.

Research has focused on long-term follow-up of cohorts of those at risk for infection with HIV. This work has documented that approximately 10% of those infected with HIV progress to AIDS within the first 2 or 3 years of HIV infection (ie, rapid progressors)[19] and that approximately 5% to 10% of HIV-infected patients are clinically asymptomatic after 7 to 10 years and have stable peripheral blood CD4+ T-cell levels; these are called nonprogressors.[19–22] The remaining HIV-infected persons are projected to develop AIDS within a median time of 10 years from initial infection; these are called typical progressors (Fig. 5-1).[19–22] It has been suggested that 10% to 17% of HIV-infected individuals will be AIDS-free 20 years after HIV infection.[23] Evidence suggests there is a group of 10% to 20% of infected persons in whom natural anti-HIV immune responses, alone or in concert with host and viral factors, protects them from developing AIDS (see Fig. 5-1).[24,25]

In this chapter, the spectrum of anti-HIV humoral and cellular immune responses that occur in HIV infection are discussed, and the types of immune responses that occur in rapid progressors and nonprogressors to AIDS are reviewed.

ANTIBODY RESPONSES TO HIV

Studies have documented the immunologic and virologic events that occur during acute HIV infection.[6,26–35] Acute HIV infection frequently presents as an influenza or mononucleosis-like syndrome, with fever, adenopathy, pharyngitis, rash, myalgias, and arthralgias as common symptoms. Abnormal liver function test results, hepatosplenomegaly, encephalopathy, and neuropathy occur less commonly.[6]

Barton F. Haynes, Box 3258, Duke Hospital, Durham, North Carolina 27710.

Between 5 and 10 days after HIV infection, serum p24 protein levels rise rapidly, serum infectious HIV levels rise, the numbers of circulating HIV-infected CD4+ T cells rise, and the total number of circulating CD4+ T cells transiently decreases.[6,35] Circulating infectious virus levels peak from 10 to 20 days after HIV infection and precipitously fall coincident with an increase in anti-HIV cytotoxic T-cell (CTL) activity and usually, resolution of initial clinical symptoms.[6,36,37] However, the initial fall in plasma viremia may also reflect trapping of HIV in the spleen and lymph nodes (see Fig. 5-1).

HIV-Neutralizing Antibodies

Neutralizing (anti-HIV) antibodies inhibit the infectivity of free HIV or HIV-infected cells and have been proposed to be one component of a salutary or protective anti-HIV immune response.[38–43] Human serum anti-HIV antibodies are isolate (ie, type) specific (ie, each neutralizes only one isolate or related isolates)[40,44–47] or are group specific (ie, each neutralizes many types of HIV isolates, regardless of the degree of primary sequence diversity).[43,48,49] The epitopes to which most anti-HIV antibodies bind have been located on envelope glycoproteins gp120 or gp41 (Tables 5-1 and 5-2).[40–47,50–52] Animal studies have suggested neutralizing epitopes may be present on HIV core proteins as well,[53] although most naturally occurring HIV-neutralizing antibodies have activity against envelope proteins.[52]

Type-specific HIV-neutralizing antibodies bind to the third hypervariable region (V3) of HIV Env gp120.[44–47,52,54,55] Because the region to which the predominant species of type-specific neutralizing antibodies bind (ie, gp120 Env amino acids 303 through 338) are flanked by cysteine residues that join in a disulfide bond to form a loop structure, this region is called the gp120 V3 loop.[52,55] Antibodies against the V3 loop region have been postulated to inhibit HIV infection by pre-

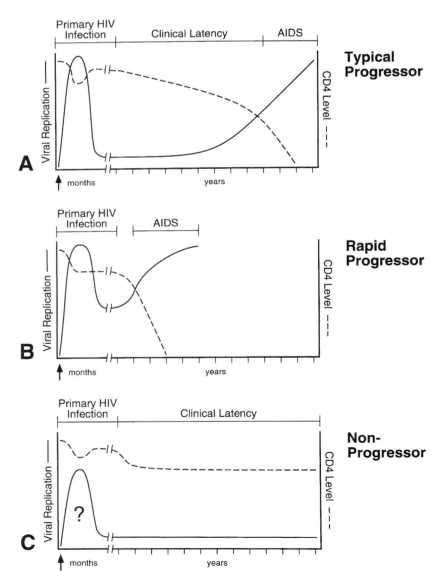

FIG. 5-1. Representative courses of progression to acquired immunodeficiency syndrome (AIDS) in a typical progressor. (A) Rapid progressor. (B) Nonprogressor. (C) HIV-infected patients. The question mark in C indicates that few long-term nonprogressors to AIDS have been studied during the primary stages of human immunodeficiency (HIV) infection. (Haynes BF, Panteleo G, Fauci AS. Towards an understanding of the correlates of protective immunity to AIDS. 1995 [in press].)

TABLE 5-1. *Antibody responses to human immunodeficiency virus infection*

Antibody Specificity	Comment	References
Anti-HIV (neutralizing) antibody	Isolate-specific antibodies against V3 loop of gp120, aa 303–37; group-specific (cross neutralize many isolates) antibodies against carbohydrate or conformational determinants; onset 2–4 weeks after primary HIV infection; present throughout course of HIV infection; found in serum, CSF, urine. Antibodies against the V3 loop do not efficiently neutralize HIV primary isolates grown in PB mononuclear cells. Conformational Env neutralization determinants possibly related to Env oligomerization or glycosylation, and gp41 determinants are candidates for biologically relevant epitopes to which neutralizing antibody responses are made that neutralize HIV primary isolates grown in PBMC	38,39,40–58,59–63
Antibodies that bind to NK cells and monocytes by FcR and sensitize FcR+ cells to kill gp120+ cells through ADCC	ADCC anti-HIV antibodies bind to multiple epitopes of gp120 anf pg41 HIV Env protein; present in the highest levels in early stages of HIV infection; levels decrease as AIDS develops; found in serum and CSF	80–92
Anti-p24 HIV Gag antibodies	Rise after initial HIV antigenemia of acute HIV infection decrease; stays elevated until ARC/AIDS develop; fall in anti-p24 antibody levels heralds rise in HIV antigenemia and onset of AIDS	6,29,33,35,65
Anti-Nef HIV antibodies	Rise before antibodies to other structural proteins after seroconversion; decrease before onset of AIDS	94,98
Anti-Rev, Vpr, Vpu protease and Tat HIV antibodies	Present in variable numbers of patients; decrease before development of AIDS in some studies	93,95–97
HIV-enhancing antibodies	Antibodies against epitopes of HIV gp41 that promote HIV infectivity in vitro; presence has been correlated with progression to AIDS	8–10

aa, amino acids; ADCC, antibody-dependent cellular cytotoxicity; AIDS, acquired immunodeficiency syndrome; ARC, AIDS-related complex; CSF, cerebrospinal fluid; FcR, receptor for the Fc portion of immunoglobulin G; Mc, mononuclear cells; NK, natural killer; PB, peripheral blood.

venting cleavage of gp120, preventing a necessary conformational change in gp120 required for entry of HIV into the cell or required for infected cell fusion.[56–58]

Regions of HIV proteins to which relatively group-specific HIV-neutralizing antibodies bind are conformational epitopes around the CD4-binding site on gp120[59,60] or are carbohydrate in nature.[61] After HIV infection, type-specific neutralizing antibodies appear in serum, followed by broader-reactive group-specific anti-HIV antibodies.[48,49]

The HIV V3 loop and CD4-binding site on gp120 is well exposed on the surface of HIV strains grown in vitro in T-cell lines, but they are poorly available on HIV primary isolates grown in peripheral blood mononuclear cells.[62,63] Most antibodies against the HIV gp120 V3 loop and the CD4-binding site efficiently neutralize laboratory-adapted HIV strains grown in T-cell lines, but they only weakly neutralize HIV primary isolates grown in peripheral blood mononuclear cells.[62,63] It is likely that the assay for determining the presence of biologically relevant neutralizing antibodies requires the use of HIV primary isolates grown in vitro in peripheral blood

mononuclear cells.[63] Serum levels of neutralizing antibody begin to rise 2 to 4 weeks after primary HIV infection[15,48,49] and peak during the asymptomatic phase of HIV infection.[41–43,64–66] Most studies have demonstrated that anti-HIV antibodies are present in the symptomatic stages of AIDS-related complex and AIDS, although frequently at lower levels than in the asymptomatic stages of HIV infection.[41,43,64–69]

Although HIV-neutralizing antibodies are measurable later in primary HIV infection than CTLs, antibodies are detected in patients in the primary and later stages of HIV infection that neutralize autologous HIV isolates grown in vitro in peripheral blood mononuclear cells.[15,60,70] Neutralizing antibodies are probably one component, in addition to anti-HIV CTLs, of an immune responses that initially partially controls HIV replication, but over time, new HIV variants emerge in most patients that are not neutralized by autologous sera. Table 5-2 summarizes select major neutralizing epitopes of HIV.[40–49,59,60,62,63,71–76]

The specificity of neutralizing antibodies in HIV-positive patient sera that neutralize HIV primary isolates is

TABLE 5-2. *Major HIV-neutralizing antibody specificities*

Antibody Specificity	Comment	References
gp120 V3 loop	Anti-V3 HIV antibodies are type- or strain-specific neutralizing antibodies that neutralize laboratory-adapted HIV strains well, but poorly neutralize HIV primary isolates grown in peripheral blood mononuclear cells; arise early on in HIV infection and decrease with progression to AIDS	40–49
gp120 V1 region	Antibodies against the gp120 V1 loop region are type-specific neutralizing antibodies found primarily in laboratory workers accidently infected with HIVLAI/IIIB and chimpanzees challenged with HIVLAI/IIIB	71
gp120 V2 region	Antibodies against gp120 V2 region are conformationally determined anti-HIV neutralizing antibodies that in some cases neutralize HIV primary isolates. Some anti-V2 neutralizing antibodies depend on envelope gp120 carbohydrates	72,73
gp41 region (ELDKWA)	Antibodies against gp41 ELDKWA sequences bind to and neutralize HIV primary isolates grown in peripheral blood mononuclear cells. However, this region is poorly immunogenic in HIV-infected patients. Antibodies against the homologous region in SIV gp32 neutralize simian immunodeficiency virus (SIV) and protect rhesus monkeys from SIV challenge	74,75,79
gp41 region (RILAVERY)	Mutations at the alanine of this region have protected HIV variants from being neutralized by neutralizing antibodies in vitro. The ability of antibodies against this region to neutralize HIV primary isolates is unknown	76
CD4-binding site antibodies	Conformational determinants centered around the C4 region of gp120 that neutralize laboratory-adapted HIV strains well but usually poorly neutralize HIV primary isolates grown in peripheral blood mononuclear cells.	51,60,63

unknown, although anti-V3 gp120 antibodies have neither protected against developing AIDS nor prevented maternofetal HIV transmission.[77,78] In rhesus monkeys, antibodies against a membrane-proximal region of gp32 correlated with protection from a simian immunodeficiency virus (SIV) challenge,[79] and antibodies against the homologous HIV gp41 region neutralized in vitro HIV primary isolates.[75]

Antibodies That Promote Antibody-Dependent Cellular Cytotoxicity of HIV-Infected Cells

Anti-gp160 antibodies in the serum and cerebrospinal fluid of HIV-infected persons bind to IgG Fc receptor (R)–bearing natural killer (NK) cells by means of the antibody Fc region and sensitize IgG FcR-positive cells to kill HIV gp160-expressing, or gp120-coated, target cells.[80–87] Peripheral blood monocytes from AIDS patients can also mediate antibody-dependent cellular cytotoxicity (ADCC) of HIV-infected cells.[88]

Although ADCC antibodies against p24 Gag proteins have been described, most studies have found serum anti-HIV ADCC antibodies to react with HIV gp120 or gp41 envelope proteins.[82–85,89,90] Anti-HIV antibodies that mediate ADCC of gp120 or gp41-expressing target cells arise soon after infection with HIV, are predominantly of the IgG1 subclass, and are detected throughout all stages of HIV infection, although ADCC antibody levels decrease somewhat with the onset of AIDS.[80–84,91,92]

Anti-Gag Antibodies

Anti-p24 antibodies appear within the first 2 weeks of acute HIV infection.[6,29,33,35,65] Rises in p24 antibody levels correlate well with the precipitous fall in infectious HIV antigenemia that occurs as the symptoms of acute HIV infection subside.[6,35] Antibodies to HIV p24 Gag proteins rise to their highest levels during the asymptomatic seropositive stage and then fall to usually undetectable levels with the onset of AIDS.[6,29,33,35] Antibodies against the p17 Gag protein of HIV have been reported to neutralize HIV and to cross-react with the thymic hormone thymosin α_1.[53]

Antibodies to Other HIV Proteins

Antibodies to HIV Rev, Nef, Tat, Vpu, Vpr, and HIV protease proteins have been reported in various percentages of HIV patients.[93–97] Antibodies to Nef proteins have been found in HIV-infected persons who were otherwise HIV seronegative.[98] In general, antibody levels to all of these HIV proteins decrease as HIV infection progresses to AIDS.[93–97]

HIV-Enhancing Antibodies

Robinson and colleagues described antibodies in AIDS patient sera that augment rather than inhibit HIV infectivity in vitro.[8,9] HIV-enhancing antibodies bind to epitopes of Env gp41.[9] The presence of HIV-enhancing antibodies has been correlated with progression of HIV infection to AIDS.[10] As new HIV variants emerge over time, new HIV variants are not neutralized by autologous sera, and in some cases, antibodies against newly emerged HIV variants may enhance HIV replication in vitro, although the significance in vivo of enhancing antibodies is controversial.

T-LYMPHOCYTE RESPONSES TO HIV

Cellular T-lymphocyte responses are essential for the control of numerous viral infections. CD4+ helper T-cell responses are required for induction of B-cell antibody production and for induction of other T-cell responses. In patients with HIV infection, anti-HIV helper T-cell responses, major histocompatibility complex (MHC) class I and MHC class II anti-HIV CTLs, and non-MHC–restricted CD8-positive (CD8+) T-cell anti-HIV activities have been identified (Table 5-3).

Helper T-Cell Epitopes of HIV Proteins

Several MHC class II–restricted helper T-cell epitopes of HIV proteins are recognized by HIV-infected humans and immunized animals.[99–101] Although helper T-cell epitopes have been found in many HIV proteins, including Env, Gag, and Pol,[99–101] a few of these epitopes are immunodominant in that they are frequently recognized by T cells of infected humans or immunized animals.[99] Although these epitopes are clearly presented to CD4+ helper T cells in the context of polymorphic MHC class II molecules, many of the HIV helper T-cell epitopes can be presented by more than one MHC class II type.[99,100] For example, Cease and colleagues identified two immunodominant T-cell epitopes, called T_1 and T_2, on the gp120 molecule.[102] T cells of 85% of HIV-infected persons recognize and secrete interleukin-2 in response to one of the two peptides in vitro.[100] Proliferative responses to HIV gp120 in vitro are highest in asymptomatic seropositive persons and decrease with the onset of AIDS.[103]

Anti-HIV Major Histocompatibility Complex–Restricted Cytotoxic T Lymphocytes

MHC class I–restricted CTLs have been demonstrated against Gag, Env, Nef, and Pol HIV proteins.[11,104–111] Remarkably, anti-HIV class I–restricted CTLs in asymptomatic HIV seropositive persons circulate in extraordinary frequency, on the order of 10 to 20 CTL precursors per 10^4 peripheral blood mononuclear cells.[112] This level is sufficiently high to frequently allow the detection of anti-HIV CTLs in suspensions of fresh peripheral blood T cells—a measurement not routinely possible when measuring CTLs against other infectious agents such an influenza virus.[11,104,105] In influenza and other human infectious diseases, the CTL precursor frequency is a lower than that for HIV, and in vitro expansion of CTL precursors in the presence of HIV antigen has been necessary to detect CTLs.[113] Class I–restricted anti-HIV CTLs are most concentrated in frequency in peripheral blood during the asymptomatic seropositive stage and fall to low or nondetectable levels in AIDS.[112]

In primary HIV infection, the initial fall in viremia correlates best with the appearance in peripheral blood of anti-HIV MHC class I–restricted CD8+ CTLs.[36,37] CD8+ CTLs are also thought to be important in the immune response to HIV during the chronic phase of HIV infection for the elimination of productively infected cells and for control of the viral load.[114] HIV-specific CD8+ CTLs may also play a role in the immunopathogenesis of HIV infection by contributing to depletion of HIV-infected antigen-presenting cells or through tissue damage after the release from CTLs of certain cytokines (eg, tumor necrosis factor-α, interferon-β) during the process of cytolysis.[115]

Nowak and coworkers described a model of HIV mutations that continually escape anti-HIV CTLs,[116] which might explain the observations in patients of new HIV variants resistant to anti-HIV CTLs.[117] Data suggest that CTL responses that use many T-cell receptor types (ie, are polyclonal)[118] and that are targeted to a few or one select immunodominant CTL epitope[116] are the most effective anti-HIV CTL responses.

TABLE 5-3. *T-Lymphocyte responses to human immunodeficiency virus infection*

Type of T Lymphocyte Response	Comment	References
T-cell proliferative response to HIV Env gp120	High in asymptomatic seropositive subjects; decreases with onset of AIDS	99,100,103
Class I–restricted anti-HIV CTL	High in asymptomatic seropositive subjects; decreases with onset of AIDS; likely participate in control of primary HIV infection	104–112
Class II–restricted anti-HIV CTL	Precursors present in noninfected, infected, and gp160-immunized subjects	104,119,120
CD8+ anti-HIV T cells that suppress HIV reverse transcriptase in vitro	CD8+ T-cell suppressor of HIV reverse transcriptase production and infection mediated by a secreted factor from CD8 cells; non-MHC restricted; activity decreases with progression to AIDS	123,124

AIDS, acquired immunodeficiency syndrome; CTL, cytotoxic T cells; MHC, major histocompatibility complex.

Precursors of MHC class II–restricted CTLs have been identified in peripheral blood of HIV-infected persons[119] and in noninfected persons who have been immunized with recombinant HIV gp160.[120] The in vivo relevance of MHC class II–restricted CTLs in the control of HIV infection is unknown.

As HIV infection progresses to AIDS, the number of MHC class I–restricted CTLs decreases.[11,104,121] Reasons for the loss of MHC-restricted anti-HIV CTL effector function in AIDS patients are unknown. It has been proposed that a combination of factors, such as a decrease in CD4 T-cell function and interleukin-2 production, HIV infection of antigen-presenting cells leading to immune system dysfunction and destruction, and HIV infection of generative hematopoietic microenvironments, may contribute to the decrease in HIV-specific CTLs.[11,104,121] The effector cytolytic mechanisms of CD8+ CTLs in AIDS patients are intact, but there is a defect in the ability of clonal expansion of anti-HIV CTL precursors.[121] One study demonstrated that HIV-infected humans have CD8+ CTLs that are capable of killing *uninfected* CD4+ target cells in an MHC-restricted manner.[122]

Cytotoxic T Cells That Suppress HIV Replication By Secretion of Soluble Factors

CD8+ T lymphocytes from HIV-infected individuals have inhibited HIV replication in naturally infected CD4+ cells in vitro.[123] This antiviral activity is not mediated by NK cells, is not HLA restricted, and depends on the number of CD8+ cells present.[123,124] This type of anti-HIV activity is not mediated though target cell killing but is mediated through CD8+ cell secretion of undelineated soluble anti-HIV factors.[124–126] Studies by Mackewicz and colleagues demonstrated that the gradual decrease of CD8+ T-cell antiviral activity over time may be related to progression to AIDS in HIV-infected individuals.[124]

NON–T-CELL–MEDIATED ANTI-HIV CELLULAR IMMUNE RESPONSES

Non–T-cell–mediated immunity, as is mediated by NK and other FcR-positive cells that directly kill virally infected cells or that mediate ADCC, is potentially important as an anti-HIV immune response, because these forms of immunity can eliminate virally infected cells in a non-MHC–restricted fashion and do not require a memory T-cell response for effector cell induction (Table 5-4).[31,104] Devising ways of augmenting or inducing NK responses against HIV-infected allogeneic cells or against malignant cells that arise in the context of AIDS are important areas of research. The roles that anti-HIV NK and ADCC activation play in the maintenance of the asymptomatic HIV seropositive state are unknown, but data demonstrate decreases in anti-HIV ADCC and NK effector cell function with progression to AIDS, suggesting a pathophysiologic link to the development of AIDS.[80–91] The discovery that the level of MHC class I expression on virus-infected cells regulates susceptibility of the target cells to NK-mediated lysis provides a new area

of investigation into the role of MHC genes in regulating anti-HIV NK responses.[127]

Although monocytes in AIDS patients have a chemotactic defect,[128] monocytes from asymptomatic seropositive persons mediate ADCC against HIV-coated target cells[88] and mediate monocyte tumoricidal activity in vitro—a potential mechanism of immune response against Kaposi's sarcoma and other tumors that occur in AIDS.[129]

IMMUNE RESPONSES TO HIV IN CHILDREN

Most HIV infections in children in the United States occur perinatally.[130] Most infants born to HIV-positive mothers passively acquire maternal anti-HIV antibody in utero, which may persist for 15 to 18 months postnatally.[130] In this situation, the polymerase chain reaction (PCR) assay for HIV proviral DNA sequences has been used to detect HIV infection and differentiate the truly infected infant from the uninfected infant with passively acquired HIV antibody.[131] In children younger than 12 months of age, AIDS frequently occurs in the presence of higher T-cell levels (500 to 1000 cells/mm^3) than are seen in adults with AIDS.[2] However, in older infants and children, anti-HIV immune responses and progressive immune defects that develop over the course of HIV infection are similar to those seen in adults.[2] The types of immune responses that may be protective in children born to mothers with HIV infection are unknown, but data suggest CTLs may be important.[132,133]

PATHOGENIC VERSUS SALUTARY ANTI-HIV IMMUNE RESPONSES

Because of the observations that CD4+ T cells, human monocytes, macrophages, dendritic cells, and Langerhans' cells are all capable of infection by HIV in vivo, numerous investigators have suggested that one component of the pathogenesis of immune dysfunction in HIV might be immune-mediated damage to HIV-infected T cells and antigen-presenting cells.[11,134–138] Moreover, gp120 Env protein exists in a cell-free soluble form, and it has been proposed that anti-HIV antibody and cellular responses can damage uninfected CD4+ cells that have soluble gp120 bound to the cell surface.[139,140] The presence of enhancing antibody against HIV Env gp41 has been associated with progressive HIV infection.[8–10]

It is difficult to determine if anti-HIV immune responses are salutary, destructive, or both. There is reason to speculate that, at least in the case of anti-HIV CTLs, salutary and destructive anti-HIV immune responses occur.[11,104] That HIV-specific antibody responses and anti-HIV CTL responses decrease in the wake of progression to AIDS suggests that these immune responses promote the asymptomatic HIV seropositive state. However, there is increasing evidence for the involvement of HIV-specific CTLs in HIV-induced pulmonary inflammatory disease, central nervous system disease, and lymphadenitis.[11,104] For example, high numbers of anti-HIV CTLs have been isolated from the lung

TABLE 5-4. *Non–T-cell anti-HIV cellular immune responses*

Type of Cellular Responses	Comment	References
ADCC mediated by NK cells	Antibodies capable of sensitizing IgG FcR-positive NK cells present in high levels in asymptomatic HIV seropositive subjects; decreased ADCC activity in AIDS due to decrease in NK function and decrease in level of anti-HIV ADCC antibodies	80–92,111
Monocyte-mediated ADCC against HIV-infected cells	Present in peripheral blood monocytes of HIV-infected subjects	88
Monocyte-mediated tumorcidal activity	Present in AIDS patients; may be relevant to control of Kaposi's sarcoma in AIDS	129
NK cell cytotoxic activity for HIV-infected cells	Present early in HIV infection; decreases as AIDS develops; decrease in NK activity related in part to lack of IL2 production needed for NK cell activation	111,155,156

ADCC, antibody-dependent cellular cytotoxicity; AIDS, acquired immunodeficiency syndrome; FcR, receptor for the Fc portion of immunoglobulin G; HIV, human immunodeficiency virus; IL2, interleukin-2; NK, natural killer.

of HIV-infected patients with lymphocytic alveolitis that are capable of killing HIV-infected macrophages.[141,142] Moreover, the presence of anti-HIV CTLs capable of killing a variety of types of HIV-infected antigen-presenting cells in lymph nodes, bone marrow, and thymus support to the notion that, over time, anti-HIV CTLs that originally keep HIV infection in check by killing virally infected cells, by continued killing of antigen-presenting cells and other immune types could gradually promote progressive immune system dysfunction.[11,104,115,138]

Anti-HIV Immune Responses in Rapid Progressors and Nonprogressors to Acquired Immunodeficiency Syndrome

Rapid progressors to AIDS have a profound decline in CD4+ T-cell levels, usually within 2 to 3 years after primary HIV infection (Table 5-5).[19–22] Rapid progressors have lower levels of anti-HIV antibodies[19,143,144] and low or absent HIV-neutralizing antibodies that neutralize autologous HIV primary isolates grown in peripheral blood mononuclear cells.[143,144] High levels of HIV-enhancing antibodies have been reported in rapid progressors.[10] Levy and associates found CD8+ noncytolytic T-cell responses that suppress

HIV replication are decreased or absent in rapid progressors.[124,125,145] Rinaldo and colleagues found low levels of memory CD8+ CTLs by precursor frequency analysis in rapid progressors compared with nonprogressors, although anti-HIV CTL effector cell activity was present in fresh peripheral blood cells from rapid progressors that compared with CTL activity in nonprogressors (C. Rinaldo, personal communication, 1995). Rapid progressors to AIDS have elevated numbers of CD8+, CD38+, and DR+ T cells,[146,147] elevated levels of serum neopterin, and β_2-microglobulin levels that signify chronic immune system activation.[148]

Nonprogressors to AIDS have strong peripheral blood CD8+ class I–restricted anti-HIV CTL levels that do not fall over time,[143,144] strong CD8+ non-MHC–restricted HIV suppressor activity,[149] and high levels of anti-HIV antibodies.[143,144] Increased HIV-neutralizing antibodies or a wide breadth of cross-reactive neutralizing antibodies have been reported in nonprogressors to AIDS.[143,144] Neutralizing antibodies may contribute along with cellular anti-HIV responses to control of HIV in nonprogressors, although the specificity of such antibodies is unknown.

There appear to be quantitative and qualitative differences in anti-HIV immune responses among nonprogressors and rapid progressors.[24,143,144] It is unknown if nonprogressors

TABLE 5-5. *Comparison in immune responses in rapid progressors and nonprogressors to AIDS*

Characteristics	Rapid Progressors	Nonprogressors
Peripheral blood CD4+ T-cell levels	Rapid decline over 2–3 years	No or minimal decline
Neutralizing antibodies	Low levels or absent antibodies that neutralize autologous HIV isolates	Present or high levels of antibodies that neutralize autologous HIV variants
Noncytolytic CD8+ suppresor T-cell activity of HIV replication	Initially present; then declines with onset of AIDS	Persistent
CD8+ MHC-restricted CTL	Present, with low numbers of memory CD8+ CTL; oligoclonal TCR usage	Robust CD8+ CTL responses; polyclonal TCR usage; targets conserved immunodominant CTL epitopes

AIDS, acquired immunodeficiency syndrome; CTL, cytotoxic T lymphocytes; HIV, human immunodeficiency virus; TCR, T-cell receptor.

only have higher levels of neutralizing antibodies and CD8+ CTL responses than rapid progressors or if nonprogressors have only salutary anti-HIV immune responses while rapid progressors have a preponderance of pathologic immune responses to HIV that damage lymphoid tissue cells.[24]

Immunologic Characteristics of HIV-Exposed, Seronegative Individuals

Studies of exposed and persistently HIV-seronegative persons have suggested that rare individuals may be resistant to HIV or may have cleared the infection without making anti-HIV antibodies. CD8+ CTLs have been found in seronegative sexual contacts of HIV-infected patients[150] and found in seronegative infants born to HIV-infected mothers.[132]

Bryson and coworkers reported an HIV-infected neonate who initially had serum anti-HIV antibodies and positive peripheral blood cell and plasma HIV cultures, but the infant eventually became HIV antibody and viral culture negative, having apparently cleared HIV infection.[133] Clerici and colleagues found peripheral blood T-cell proliferative responses to HIV envelope peptides in seronegative homosexual persons with multiple exposures to HIV through sexual contacts.[151] Multiply exposed prostitutes in Africa have been reported who are HIV negative by serology and PCR for viral DNA and who have HIV specific CTLs.[152]

TRENDS AND FUTURE STUDIES

With HIV infection rates increasing in underdeveloped countries, the development of an effective HIV vaccine remains a top priority of HIV investigators. Understanding the correlates of protective immunity to HIV would facilitate HIV vaccine development by targeting the specific salutary immune responses that need to be induced by an immunogen. Many nonprogressors to AIDS have anti-HIV immune responses that are quantitatively and probably qualitatively superior to anti-HIV immune responses that occur in HIV-infected individuals who rapidly progress to AIDS.

A key issue that must be resolved is the role of the host genetic background in determining the rate of progression of HIV infection.[24] It is important to know if MHC-encoded or other host proteins are responsible for a qualitatively more effective anti-HIV immune responses in nonprogressors. That there are MHC genes that appear to be associated with rapid progression to AIDS suggests that this might be the case.[24]

The types of anti-HIV immune responses that are generated by HIV infection through the genital mucosa are also critical to understand. Studies are necessary that profile mucosal and systemic immune responses to HIV after systemic or mucosal infection.

Because attenuated SIV strains protect rhesus monkeys from infection with SIV[153] and primary infection with HIV-2 may confer some protection against HIV-1 in humans,[154] it is critical to study and understand the correlates of protective immunity in these settings. There do appear to be correlates

of protective immunity to HIV in some patients and animal models of immunodeficiency-causing retrovirus infections, and this has provided investigators with guarded optimism for the prospects of eventually controlling HIV infection.

REFERENCES

1. Fauci AS. The human immunodeficiency virus: Infectivity and mechanisms of pathogenesis. Science 1988;239:617.
2. Stiehm ER, Wara DW. Immunology of HIV. In: Pizzo PA, Wilfert CM, eds. Pediatric AIDS: the challenge of HIV infection in infants, children, and adolescents. Baltimore: Williams & Wilkins, 1991;95.
3. Edelman AS, Zolla-Pazner S. AIDS: a syndrome of immune dysregulation, dysfunction, and deficiency. FASEB J 1989;3:22.
4. Sattentau QJ. HIV infection and the immune system. Biochem Biophys Acta 1989;989:255.
5. Weiss SH, Goedert JJ, Gartner S, et al. Risk of human immunodeficiency virus (HIV-1) infection among laboratory workers. Science 1988;239:68.
6. Clark SJ, Saag MS, Decker WD, et al. High titers of cytopathic virus in plasma of patients with symptomatic primary HIV-1 infection. N Engl J Med 1991;324:954.
7. Itescu S, Brancato LJ, Buxbaum J, et al. A diffuse infiltrative CD8 lymphocytosis syndrome in human immunodeficiency virus (HIV) infection: a host immune response associated with HLA-DR5. Ann Intern Med 1990;112:3.
8. Robinson WE, Montefiori DC, Mitchell WM, et al. Antibody-dependent enhancement of human immunodeficiency virus type 1 (HIV-1) infection in vitro by serum from HIV-1 infected and passively immunized chimpanzees. Proc Natl Acad Sci USA 1989;86:4710.
9. Robinson WE, Kawamura T, Gorny MK, et al. Human monoclonal antibodies to the human immunodeficiency virus type I (HIV-1) transmembrane glycoprotein gp41 enhance HIV-1 infection in vitro. Proc Natl Acad Sci USA 1990;87:3815.
10. Homsy J, Meyer M, Levy JA. Serum enhancement of human immunodeficiency virus (HIV) infection correlates with disease in HIV-infected individuals. J Virol 1990;64:1437.
11. Plata, F, Dadaglio G, Chenciner N, et al. Cytotoxic T lymphocytes in HIV-induced disease: implications for therapy and vaccination. Immunodefic Rev 1989;1:227.
12. Reitz MS, Wilson C, Naugle C, Gallo RC, Robert-Guroff M. Generation of a neutralization-resistant variant of HIV-1 is due to selection for a point mutation in the envelope gene. Cell 1988;54:57.
13. McKeating JA, Gow J, Goutsmit J, Pearl LH, Mulder C, Weiss RA. Characterization of HIV-1 neutralization escape mutants. AIDS 1989;3:777.
14. Masuda T, Matsushita S, Kuroda MJ, Kannagi M, Takatsuki K, and Harada S. Generation of neutralization-resistant HIV-1 in vitro due to amino acid interchanges of third hypervariable env region. J Immunol 1990;145:3240.
15. Albert J, Abrahamsson B, Nagy K, Aurelius E, Gaines H, Nystrom G, Fenyo EM. Rapid development of isolate-specific neutralizing antibodies after primary HIV-1 infection and consequent emergence of virus variants which resist neutralization by autologous sera. AIDS 1990;4:107.
16. Wei X, Ghosh SK, Taylor ME, et al. Viral dynamics in human immunodeficiency virus type 1 infection. Nature 1995;373:117.
17. Ho DD, Neumann AU, Perelson AS, et al. Rapid turnover of plasma virions and CD4 lymphocytes in HIV-1 infection. Nature 1995;373:123.
18. Li CJ, Friedman DJ, Wang C, et al. Induction of apoptosis in uninfected lymphocytes by HIV-1 Tat protein. Science 1995;268:429.
19. Phair J, Jacobson L, Detals R, et al. Acquired immune deficiency syndrome occurring within 5 years of infection with human immunodeficiency virus type-1: the multicenter AIDS cohort study. J Acquir Immune Defic Syndr 1995;5:490..
20. Sheppard HW, Ascher MS, McRae B, et al. The initial immune response to HIV and immune system activation determine the outcome of HIV disease. J Acquir Immune Defic Syndr 1991;4:704.
21. Sheppard HW, Lang W, Ascher MS, et al. The characterization of nonprogressors: long-term HIV-1 infection with stable CD4+ T-cell levels. AIDS 1993;7:1159.

22. Munoz A, Wang M-C, Bass S, et al. Acquired immunodeficiency syndrome (AIDS)—free time after human immunodeficiency virus type 1 (HIV-1) seroconversion in homosexual men. Am J Epidemiol 1989;130:530.

23. Phair J. Variations in the natural history of HIV infection. AIDS Res Hum Retroviruses 1994;10:883.

24. Haynes BF, Panteleo G, Fauci AS. Towards and understanding of the correlates of protective and immunity to HIV infection. Science 1996; 271:324.

25. Paul WE. Can the immune response control HIV infection? Cell 1995;82:177.

26. Cooper DA, Gold J, MacLean P, et al. Acute AIDS retrovirus infection. Lancet 1985;1:537.

27. Ho DD, Sarngadharan MG, Resnick L, DiMarzo-Veronese F, Rota TR, Hirsch MS. Primary human T lymphotropic virus type III infection. Ann Intern Med 1985;103:880.

28. Goudsmit J, de Wolf F, Paul DA, et al. Expression of human immunodeficiency virus antigen (HIV-Ag) in serum and cerebrospinal fluid during acute and chronic infection. Lancet 1986;2:177.

29. Allain J-P, Lauvian Y, Paul DA, Senn D, Serological markers in early stages of human immunodeficiency virus infection in hemophiliacs. Lancet 1986;2:1233.

30. Gaines H, Albert J, von Sydow M, et al. HIV antigenemia and virus isolation from plasma during primary HIV infection. Lancet 1987;1:1317.

31. Albert J, Gaines H, Sonnerborg A, et al. Isolation of human immunodeficiency virus (HIV) from plasma during primary HIV infection. J Med Virol 1987;23:67.

32. Wall RA, Denning DW, Amos A. HIV antigenemia in acute HIV infection. Lancet 1987;1:566.

33. Paul DA, Falk LA, Kessler HA, et al. Correlation of serum HIV antigen and antibody with clinical status in HIV-infected patients. J Med Virol 1987;22:357.

34. Von Sydow M, Gaines H, Sonnerborg A, Forsgren M, Pehrson PO, Strannegard O. Antigen detection in primary HIV infection. Br Med J 1988;296:238.

35. Daar ES, Moudgil T, Meyer RD, Ho DD. Transient high levels of viremia in patients with primary human immunodeficiency virus type I infection. N Engl J Med 1991;324:961.

36. Koup RA, Safrit JT, Cao Y, et al. Temporal association of cellular immune responses with the initial control of viremia in primary human immunodeficiency virus type 1 syndrome. J Virol 1994;68:4650.

37. Borrow P, Lewicki H, Hahn BH, et al. Virus-specific CD8+ cytotoxic T-lymphocyte activity associated with control of viremia in primary human immunodeficiency virus type 1 infection. J Virol 1994;68:6103.

38. Berman PW, Gregory TJ, Riddle L, et al. Protection of chimpanzees from infection by HIV-1 after vaccination with recombinant glycoprotein gp120 but not gp160. Nature 1990;345:622.

39. Girard M, Kieny MP, Pinter A, et al. Immunization of chimpanzees confers protection against challenge with human immunodeficiency virus. Proc Natl Acad Sci U S A 1991;88:542.

40. Matthews TJ, Langlois AJ, Robey WG, et al. Restricted neutralization of divergent human T-lymphotropic virus type III isolates by antibodies to the major envelope glycoprotein. Proc Natl Acad Sci U S A 1986;83:9709.

41. Weiss RA, Clapham RP, Cheingsong-Popov R, et al. Neutralization of human T-lymphotropic virus type III by sera of AIDS and AIDS-risk patients. Nature 1985;316:69.

42. Robert-Guroff M, Brown M, Gallo RC. HTLV-III-neutralizing antibodies in patients with AIDS and AIDS-related complex. Nature 1985;316:72.

43. Weiss RA, Clapham PR, Weber JN, Dalgleish AG, Lasky LA, Berman PW. Variable and conserved neutralization antigens of human immunodeficiency virus. Nature 1986;324:572.

44. Putney SD, Matthews TJ, Robey WG, et al. HTLV-III/LAV-neutralization antibodies to an E. coli-produced fragment of the virus envelope. Science 1986;234:1392.

45. Palker TJ, Clark ME, Langlois AJ, et al. Type-specific neutralization of the human immunodeficiency virus with antibodies to env-encoded synthetic peptides. Proc Natl Acad Sci USA 1988;85:1932.

46. Rusche JR, Javaherian K, McDanal C, et al. Antibodies that inhibit fusion of human immunodeficiency virus-infected cells bind a 24 amino acid sequence of the viral envelope gp120. Proc Natl Acad Sci USA 1988;85:3198.

47. Goudsmit J, Debouck C, MeLeon RH, et al. Human immunodeficiency virus type I neutralization with conserved architecture elicits early type-specific antibodies in experimentally infected chimpanzees. Proc Natl Acad Sci USA 1988;85:4478.

48. Nara PL, Robey WG, Arthur LV, et al. Persistent infection of chimpanzees with human immunodeficiency virus: serological responses and properties of reisolated viruses. J Virol 1987;61:3173.

49. Goudsmit J, Thiriart C, Smit L, Bruck C, Gibbs CJ. Temporal development of cross-neutralization between HTLV-IIIB and HTLV-IIIRF in experimentally infected chimpanzees. Vaccine 1986;6:229.

50. Ho DD, Sarngadharan MG, Hirsh MS, et al. Human immunodeficiency virus neutralizing antibodies recognize several conserved domains on the envelope glycoproteins. J Virol 1987;61:2024,

51. Weiss RA, Clapham PR, McClure MO, et al. Human immunodeficiency viruses: neutralization and receptors. J Acquir Immune Defic Syndr 1988;1:536.

52. Putney SD, Javaherin K, Rusche J, Matthews TJ, Bolognesi DP. Features of the HIV envelope and development of a subunit vaccine. In: Putney SD, Bolognesi DP, eds. AIDS vaccine: basic research and clinical trials. New York: Marcel Dekker, 1989:3.

53. Sarin PS, Sun DK, Thornton AH, Naylor PH, Goldstein AL. Neutralization of HTLV-III/LAV replication by antiserum to thymosin α1. Science 1986;232:1135.

54. Palker TJ, Matthews TJ, Langlois AJ, et al. Polyvalent human immunodeficiency virus synthetic immunogen comprised of envelope gp120 T helper cell sites and B cell neutralization epitopes. J Immunol 1989;142:3612.

55. Javaherian K, Langlois AJ, McDanal C, et al. Principal neutralizing domain of the human immunodeficiency virus type I envelope protein. Proc Natl Acad Sci U S A. 86:6768.

56. Hattori T, Koito A, Takasuki K, Kido H, Katanuma N. Involvement of tryptase-related cellular protease(s) in human immunodeficiency virus type I infection. FEBS Lett 1989;248:48.

57. Kido H, Fukutomi A, Katanuma N. A novel membrane-bound serine esterase in human T4+ lymphocytes immunologically reactive with antibody inhibiting syncytia induced by HIV-1. J Biol Chem 1990;265:21979.

58. Clements GJ, Price-Jones MJ, Stephens PE, et al. The V3 loops of the HIV-1 and HIV-2 surface glycoproteins contain proteolytic cleavage sites: a possible function in viral fusion? AIDS Res Hum Retroviruses 1991;7:3.

59. Back NKT, Thiriart C, Delers A, Ramautarsing C, Bruck C, Goudsmit J. Association of antibodies blocking HIV-1 gp160-sCD4 attachment with virus neutralizing activity in human sera. J Med Virol 1990;31:200.

60. Moore JP, Cao Y, Ho DD, et al. Development of the anti-gp120 antibody response during seroconversion to human immunodeficiency virus type 1. J Virol 1994;68:5142.

61. Hansen JS, Clausen H, Nielsen C, et al. Inhibition of HIV infection in vitro by anti-carbohydrate monoclonal antibodies: peripheral glycosylation of HIV envelope glycoprotein gp120 may be a target for virus neutralization. J Virol 1990;64:2833.

62. Sullivan N, Sun Y, Li J, et al. Replicative function and neutralization sensitivity of envelope glycoproteins from primary and T-cell line-passaged human immunodeficiency virus type 1 isolates. J Virol 1995;69:4413.

63. Moore JP. Back to primary school. Nature 1995;376:115.

64. Weber JN, Weiss RA, Robert C, et al. Human immunodeficiency virus infection in two cohorts of homosexual men: neutralizing sera and association of anti-gag antibody with prognosis. Lancet 1987;1: 119.

65. Sei Y, Tsang PH, Chu FN, et al. Inverse relationship between HIV-1 p24 antigenemia, anti-p24 antibody and neutralizing antibody response in all stages of HIV-1 infection. Immunol Lett 1989;20:223.

66. Alesi DR, Ajello D, Lupo G, Vitale F, et al. Neutralizing antibody and clinical status of human immunodeficiency virus (HIV)-infected individuals. J Med Virol 1989;27:7.

67. Boucher CAB, de Wolf F, Houweling JTM, et al. Antibody response to a synthetic peptide covering a LAV-I/HTLV-IIIB neutralization epitope and disease progression. AIDS 1989;3:71.

68. Berkower I, Smith GE, Giri C, Murphey D. Human immunodeficiency virus I. Predominance of a group-specific neutralizing epitope that persists despite genetic variation. J Exp Med 1989;170:1681.

69. Katzenstein DA, Vujcil LK, Latif A, et al. Human immunodeficiency virus neutralizing antibodies in sera from North Americans and Africans. J Acquir Immune Defic Syndr 1990;3:810.

70. Von Gegerfelt A, Albert J, Morfeld-Manson L, et al Isolate-specific neutralizing antibodies in patients with progressive HIV-1 related diseases. Virology 1991;185:162.

71. Pincus SH, Messer KG, Nara PL, et al. Temporal analysis of the antibody response to HIV envelop protein in HIV-infected laboratory workers. J Clin Invest 1994;93:2502.
72. Warrier SV, Pinter A, Honnen WJ, et al. A novel, glycan-dependent epitope in the V2 domain of human immunodeficiency virus type 1 gp120 is recognized by a highly potent, neutralizing chimpanzee monoclonal antibody. J Virol 1994;68:4636.
73. Gorny MK, Moore JP, Conley AJ, et al. Human anti-V2 monoclonal antibody that neutralizes primary but not laboratory isolates of human immunodeficiency virus type 1. J Virol 1994;68:8312.
74. Muster T, Steindl F, Purtscher M, et al. A conserved neutralizing epitope on gp41 of HIV-1. J Virol 1993;67:6642.
75. Conley AJ, Kessler JA, Boots LJ, et al. Neutralization of divergent HIV-1 variants and primary isolates by IAM-41-2F5, an anti-gp41 human monoclonal antibody. Proc Natl Acad Sci U S A 1994;91:3348.
76. Reitz MS, Wilson C, Naugle C, et al. Generation of a neutralization-resistant variant of HIV-1 is due to selection for a point mutation in the envelope gene. Cell 1988;54:57.
77. Hogervorst E, Jurriaans S, de Wolff F, et al. Predictors for non- and slow progression in human immunodeficiency virus (HIV) type 1 infection: low viral RNA copy numbers in serum and maintenance of high HIV-1 p24 specific but not V3-specific antibody levels. J Infect Dis 1995;171:811.
78. Markham RB, Coberly J, Ruff AJ, Hoover D, et al. Maternal IgG1 and IgA antibody to V3 loop consensus sequence and maternal-infant HIV-1 transmission. Lancet 1994;343:390.
79. Shafferman A, Jahrling PB, Benveniste RE, et al. Protection of macaques with a simian immunodeficiency virus envelope peptide vaccine based on conserved human immunodeficiency virus type 1 sequences. Proc Natl Acad Sci USA 1991;88:7126.
80. Lyerly HK, Matthews TJ, Langlois AJ, Bolognesi DP, Weinhold KJ. Human T-cell lymphotropic virus IIIB glycoprotein (gp120) bound to CD4 determinants on normal lymphocytes and expressed by infected cells serves as a target for immune attack. Proc Natl Acad Sci USA 1987;84:4601.
81. Ojo-Amaize EA, Nishanian P, Keith DE, et al. Antibodies to human immunodeficiency virus in human sera induce cell-mediated lysis of human immunodeficiency virus-infected cells. J Immunol 1987;139:2458.
82. Weinhold KJ, Lyerly HK, Matthews TJ, et al. Cellular anti-gp120 reactivities in HIV-1 seropositive individuals. Lancet 1988;1:902.
83. Tyler DS, Lyerly HK, Weinhold KJ. Anti-HIV-1 ADCC. AIDS Res Hum Retroviruses 1989;5:557.
84. Tyler DS, Stanley SD, Nastala CA, et al. Alterations in antibody-dependent cellular cytotoxicity during the course of HIV infection. J Immunol 1990;144:3375.
85. Tyler DS, Stanley SD, Zolla-Pazner S, et al. Identification of sites within gp41 that serve as target for antibody-dependent cellular cytotoxicity by using human monoclonal antibodies. J Immunol 1990;145:3276.
86. Ljunggren K, Chiodi F, Broliden PA, et al. HIV-1 specific antibodies in cerebral spinal fluid mediate cellular cytotoxicity and neutralization. AIDS Res Hum Retroviruses 1989;5:629.
87. Emskoetter T, Laer DV, Veismann S, Ermer M. HIV-specific antibodies, neutralizing activity and ADCC in the cerebrospinal fluid of HIV-infected patients. J Neuroimmunol 1989;24:61.
88. Jewett A, Giorgi JV, Bonavida B. Antibody dependent cellular cytotoxicity against HIV-coated target cells by peripheral blood monocytes from HIV seropositive asymptomatic patients. J Immunol 1990;145:4065.
89. Koup RA, Sullivan JL, Levine PH, et al. Antigenic specificity of antibody-dependent cell-mediated cytotoxicity directed against human immunodeficiency virus in antibody positive sera. J Virol 1989;63:584.
90. Tanneau F, McChesney M, Lopez O, Sansonetti P, Montagnier L, Rivieri Y. Primary cytotoxicity against the envelope glycoprotein of human immunodeficiency virus-1: evidence for antibody dependent cellular cytotoxicity in vivo. J Infect Dis 1990;162:837.
91. Ljunggren K, Karlson A, Fenyo EM, Jondal M. Natural and antibody-dependent cytotoxicity in different clinical stages of human immunodeficiency virus type I infection. Clin Exp Immunol 1989;75:184.
92. Ojo-Amaize E, Nishanian PG, Heitjan DF, et al. Serum and effector-cell antibody-dependent cellular cytotoxicity (ADCC) activity remains high during human immunodeficiency virus (HIV) disease progression. J Clin Immunol 1989;9:454.
93. Reiss P, DeRonde A, Lange JMA, et al. Low antigenicity of HIV-1 rev: rev-specific antibody response of limited value as correlate of rev gene expression and disease progression. AIDS Res Hum Retroviruses 1989;5:621.
94. Reiss P, de Ronde A, Lange JMA, et al. Antibody response to the viral negative factor (nef) in HIV-1 infection: a correlates of levels of HIV-1 expression. AIDS 1989;3:227.
95. Boucher CAB, DeJager MH, Debouck C, et al. Antibody response to human immunodeficiency virus type I protease according to risk group and disease stage. J Clin. Microbiol 1989;27:1577.
96. Reiss P, Lange JMA, de Ronde A, et al. Antibody response to viral proteins U (vpu) and R (vpr) in HIV-1-infected individuals. J Acquir Immune Defic Syndr 1990;3:115.
97. Reiss P, Lange JMA, de Ronde A, et al. Speed of progression to AIDS and degree of antibody response to accessory gene products of HIV-1. J Med Virol 1990;30:163.
98. Ameisen JC, Guy B,. Lecocq JP, et al. Persistent antibody response to the HIV-1 negative regulatory factor in HIV-1 infected seronegative persons. N Engl J Med 1989;320:251.
99. Clerici M, Stocks NI, Zajac RA, et al. Interleukin-2 production used to detect antigenic peptide recognition by T-helper lymphocytes from asymptomatic HIV-seropositive individuals. Nature 1989;339:383.
100. Schrier RD, Gnann JW, Landes R, et al. T cell recognition of HIV synthetic peptides in a natural infection. J Immunol 1989;142:1166.
101. Korber B. Los Alamos National Database 1995: CTL and T helper epitopes of HIV proteins. Los Alamos, NM: Los Alamos National Laboratory, 1995.
102. Cease KB, Margaut H, Cornette JL, et al. Helper T cell antigenic site identification in the acquired immunodeficiency syndrome virus gp120 envelope protein and induction of immunity in mice to the native protein using a 16-residue synthetic peptide. Proc Natl Acad Sci USA 1987;84:4249.
103. Torseth JW, Berman PW, Merigan TC. Recombinant HIV structural proteins detect specific cellular immunity in vitro in infected individuals. AIDS Res Hum Retroviruses 1988;4:23.
104. Walker BD, Plata F. Cytotoxic T lymphocytes against HIV. AIDS 1990;4:177.
105. Walker BD, Chakrabarti S, Moss B, et al. HIV-specific cytotoxic T lymphocytes in seropositive individuals. Nature 1987;328:345.
106. Nixon DF, Townsend ARM, Elvin JG, et al. HIV-1 gag-specific cytotoxic T lymphocytes defined with recombinant vaccinia virus and synthetic peptides. Nature 1988;336:484.
107. Clerici M, Lucey DR, Zajac RA, et al. Detection of cytotoxic T lymphocytes specific for synthetic peptides of gp160 in HIV-seropositive individuals. J Immunol 1991;146:2214.
108. Hosmalin A, Cleric M, Houghten R, et al. An epitope in human immunodeficiency virus I reverse transcriptase recognized by both mouse and human cytotoxic T lymphocytes. Proc Natl Acad Sci USA 1990;87:2344.
109. Koenig S, Fuerst TR, Wood LV, et al. Mapping the fine specificity of a cytolytic T cell response to HIV-1 nef protein. J Immunol 1990;145:127.
110. Koup RA, Sullivan JL, Levine PH, et al. Detection of major histocompatibility complex class I restricted HIV-specific cytotoxic T lymphocytes in the blood of infected hemophiliacs. Blood 1989;73:1909.
111. Riviere P, Tanneau-Salvadori F, Regnault A, et al. Human immunodeficiency virus-specific cytotoxic responses of seropositive individuals. Distinct types of effector cells mediate killing of targets expressing gag and env proteins. J Virol 1989;63:2270.
112. Hoffenbach A, Langlade-Demoyen P, Dadaglio G, et al. Unusually high frequencies of HIV-specific cytotoxic T lymphocytes in humans. J Immunol 1989;142:452.
113. Morrison LA, Braciale VL, Braciale TJ. Distinguishable pathways of viral antigen presentation to T lymphocytes. Immunol Res 1986;5:294.
114. Walker BD, Plata, F. Cytotoxic T lymphocytes against HIV. AIDS 1990;4:177.
115. Zinkernagel RM, Hengartner H. T-cell-mediated immunopathology versus direct cytolysis by virus:implications for HIV and AIDS. Immunol Today 1994;15:262.
116. Nowak MA, May RM, Phillips RE, et al. Antigenic oscillations and shifting immunodominance in HIV-1 infections. Nature 1995;373:606.
117. Phillips RE, Rowland-Jones S, Nixon DF, et al. Human immunodeficiency virus genetic variation that can escape cytotoxic T cell recognition. Nature 1991;354:453.

118. Pantaleo G, Demarest JF, Soudeyns H, et al. Major expansion of CD8+ T cells with a predominant Vb usage during the primary immune response to HIV. Nature 1994;370:463.

119. Sethi KK, Naher H, Strehmann I. Phenotypic heterogeneity of cerebrospinal fluid-derived HIV-specific and HLA-restricted cytotoxic T cell clones. Nature 1988;335:178.

120. Orentas RJ, Hildreth JEK, Obah E, et al. Induction of CD4+ human cytolytic T cell specific for HIV infected cells by a gp160 subunit vaccine. Science 1990;248:1234.

121. Pantaleo G, DeMaria A, Koenig S, et al. CD8+ T lymphocytes of patients with AIDS maintain normal broad cytolytic function despite the loss of human immunodeficiency virus-specific cytotoxicity. Proc Natl Acad Sci USA 1990;87:4818.

122. Zarling JM, Ledbetter JA, Sias J, Fultz P, Eichberg J, Gjerset G, Moran PA. HIV-infected humans, but not chimpanzees, have circulating cytotoxic T lymphocytes that lyse uninfected CD4+ cells. J Immunol 1990;144:2992.

123. Walker CM, Moody DJ, Stites DP, Levy JA. CD8+ lymphocytes can control HIV infection in vitro by suppressing virus replication. Science 1986;234:1563.

124. Mackewicz CE, Ortega HW, Levy JA. CD8+ cell anti-HIV activity correlates with the clinical state of the infected individual. J Clin Invest 1991;87:1462.

125. Laurence J, Gottlieb AB, Kunkel HG. Soluble suppressor factors in patients with acquired immune deficiency syndrome and its prodrome J Clin Invest 1983;12:2072.

126. Siegel JP, Djeu JY, Stocks NI, Masur H, Gelmann EP, Quinnan GV. Sera from patients with the acquired immunodeficiency syndrome inhibit production of interleukin-2 by normal lymphocytes. J Clin Invest 1985;75:1957.

127. Brutkiewicz RR, Welsch RM. Major histocompatibility complex class I antigens and the control of viral infections by natural killer cells. J Virol 1995;69:3967.

128. Smith PD, Ohura K, Masur H, Lane HC, Fauci AS, Wahl SM. Monocyte function in the acquired immune deficiency syndrome: defective chemotaxis. J Clin Invest 1984;74:2121.

129. Kleinerman ES, Ceccorulli LM, Zwelling LA, et al. Activation of monocyte-mediated tumoricidal activity in patients with acquired immunodeficiency syndrome. J Clin Oncol 1985;3:1005.

130. Rogers MF, Ou CY, Kilbourne B, Schochet MAN. Advances and problems in the diagnosis of HIV infection in infants. In: Pizzo PA, Wilfert CM, eds. Pediatric AIDS: the challenge of HIV infection in infants, children and Adolescents. Baltimore: William & Wilkins, 1991:159.

131. Rogers MF, Ou CY, Rayfield M, et al. Use of the polymerase chain reaction for early detection of the proviral sequences of human immunodeficiency virus in infants born of seropositive mothers. N Engl J Med 1989;320:1649.

132. Rowland-Jones S, Nixon DF, Aldhous MC. HIV-specific cytotoxic T-cell activity in an HIV-exposed but uninfected infant. Lancet 1993;341:860.

133. Bryson YJ, Pang S, Wei LS, et al. Clearance of HIV infection in a perinatally infected infant. N Engl J Med 1995;332:833.

134. Siliciano RF, Lawton T, Knall C, Karr RW, et al. Analysis of host-virus interactions in AIDS with anti-gp120 T cell clones: effect of HIV sequence variation and an mechanism for CD4+ cell depletion. Cell 1988;54:561.

135. Tschachler E, Groh V, Popovic M, et al. Epidermal Langerhans' cells—a target for HTLV-III/LAV infection. J Invest Dermatol 1987;88:233.

136. Macatonia SE, Patterson S, Knight SC. Suppression of immune responses by dendritic cells infected with HIV. Immunology 1989;67:285.

137. Laman JD, Claassen E, Von Rooijen N, Boersma WMJ. Immune complexes on follicular dendritic cells as a target for cytotoxic cells in AIDS. AIDS 1989;3:543.

138. Macatonia SE, Lau R, Patterson S, Pinching AJ, Knight SC. Dendritic cell infection, depletion and dysfunction in HIV infected individuals. Immunology 1990;71:38.

139. Weinhold KJ, Lyerly HK, Stanley SD, Austin AA, Matthews TJ, Bolognesi DP. HIV-1-mediated immune suppression and lymphocyte destruction in the absence of viral infection. J Immunol 1989;142:3091.

140. Manca F, Habeshaw JA, Dalgleish AG. HIV envelope glycoprotein, antigens specific T-cell responses and soluble CD4. Lancet 1990;335:811.

141. Guillon JM, Autran B, Devis M, et al. HIV-related lymphocytic alveolitis. Chest 1988;94:1264.

142. Autran B, Joly P, Guillon JM, Qevis M, Mayard LM, Debre P. T cell mediated cytotoxicity against HIV in seropositive patients: a physicopathological approach. Res Immunol 1989;140:103.

143. Cao Y, Qin L, Zhang L. Virologic and immunologic characterization of long-term survivors of human immunodeficiency virus type I infections. N Engl J Med 1995;332:201.

144. Pantaleo G, Menzo S, Vaccarezza M, et al. Studies in subjects with long-term nonprogressive human immunodeficiency virus infection. N Engl J Med 1995;332:209.

145. Landay AL, Mackewicz CE, Levy JA. An activated CD8+ T cell phenotype correlates with anti-HIV activity and asymptomatic clinical status. Clin Immunol Immunopathol 1993;69:106.

146. Giorgi JV, Liu Z, Hultin LE, et al. Elevated levels of CD38+ CD8+ T cells in HIV infection add to the prognostic value of low CD4+ T cell levels of 6 years of follow-up. J Acquir Immune Defic Syndr 1993;6:904.

147. Ho, H-N, Hultin LE, Mitsuyasu RT, et al. Circulating HIV-specific CD8+ cytotoxic T cells express cD38 and HLA-DR antigens. J Immunol 1993;150:3070.

148. Munoz A, Vlahov D, Solomon L, et al. Prognostic indicators for development of AIDS among intravenous drug users. J Acquir Immune Defic Syndr 1992;5:694.

149. Levy JA. Features of human immunodeficiency virus infection and disease. Pediatr Res 1993;33:S63.

150. Langlade-Demoyen P, Ngo-Giang-Huong N, Ferchal F, et al. Human immunodeficiency virus (HIV) nef-specific cytotoxic T lymphocytes in non-infected heterosexual contact of HIV-infected patients. J Clin Invest 1994;93:1293.

151. Clerici M, Giorgi JV, Chou C-C, et al. Cell-mediated immune response to human immunodeficiency virus (HIV) type 1 in seronegative homosexual men with recent sexual exposure to HIV-1. J Infect Dis 1992;165:1012.

152. Rowland-Jones S, Sutton J, Ariyoshi K, et al. HIV-specific CTL in HIV-exposed but uninfected Gambian women. Nature Med 1995;1:59.

153. Daniel MD, Kirchhoff F, Czajak SC, et al. Protective effects of a live attenuated SIV vaccine with a deletion in the nef gene. Science 1992;258:1938.

154. Travers K, Mboup S, Marlink R, et al. Natural protection against HIV-1 infection provided by HIV-2. Science 1995;268:1612.

155. Bonavida B, Katz J, Gottlieb M. Mechanism of defective NK cell activity in patients with acquired immunodeficiency syndrome (AIDS) and AIDS-related complex. J Immunol 1986;137:1157.

156. Mansour I, Doinel C, Rouger P. CD16+ NK cells decrease in all stages of HIV infection through a selective depletion of the CD16+ CD8+ CD3+ subset. AIDS Res Hum Retroviruses 1990;6:1451.

PART II

Epidemiology

AIDS: Biology, Diagnosis, Treatment and Prevention, fourth edition, edited by Vincent T. DeVita, Jr., Samuel Hellman, and Steven A. Rosenberg. Lippincott–Raven Publishers, © 1997

CHAPTER **6**

Global Aspects of Human Immunodeficiency Virus Epidemiology: General Considerations

Thierry Mertens and Peter Piot

The epidemic of human immunodeficiency virus (HIV) infection and acquired immunodeficiency syndrome (AIDS) emerged in the last quarter of the 20th century, and within less than two decades has affected over 190 countries.[1] HIV distribution is characterized by a marked heterogeneity among continents and countries or even within a single country, with geographic areas of HIV prevalence of up to 30% of the adult population contiguous with areas of much lower prevalence.[2] These differences are producing a checkered pattern of visible impact, with AIDS the leading cause of adult deaths in some populations and HIV effects not yet detectable in others.

The study of trends in HIV spread has contributed to a better understanding of the dynamics and impact of the epidemic in various parts of the world. The data indicate the emergence of new epidemic foci and shifts in transmission patterns in established epidemics and suggest that prevention efforts may be influencing the overall course of the pandemic. This chapter discusses the distribution and transmission patterns of HIV and considers some implications of the estimates and projections made by the World Health Organization (WHO).

TYPES OF HUMAN IMMUNODEFICIENCY VIRUSES

HIV infection can be caused by HIV-1 and HIV-2, the two main types of the virus. Globally, HIV-1 accounts for most HIV infections, and HIV-2 appears largely confined to West Africa, with foci in Angola and Mozambique and some cases reported in Europe, the Americas, and India.[3-5] The prevalence of HIV-2 is lower than that of HIV-1 where the

two types coexist, with the exception of Guinea-Bissau, where HIV-2 predominates.[6] Compared with HIV-1, HIV-2 appears less transmissible through sexual intercourse, its spread is slower,[7] and the disease it causes progresses more slowly.[8] In contrast to HIV-1, HIV-2 prevalence increases steadily with age.[6] Throughout this chapter, the abbreviation HIV refers to HIV-1.

Throughout the world, HIV infection is characterized by a wide genetic diversity of viral strains.[9] Figure 6-1 presents the main geographic distribution of various genetic subtypes of HIV-1. In vitro studies have found important differences in the biologic properties of HIV-1 subtypes,[10] but little is known about possible differences in transmissibility of the different subtypes. The detection in West Africa of a grossly divergent genetic subtype of HIV-1, named subtype O, raised concerns that some standard serologic tests do not detect antibodies directed to viruses of this subtype.[11-13] These commercial tests have been removed from the market or amended by including subtype O–specific epitopes. There is concern that other major variants of HIV-1 may emerge or remain to be identified.[14]

MODES OF TRANSMISSION OF HIV-1

An understanding of the ways in which HIV can be transmitted is central to an understanding of the epidemiology of the global epidemic. HIV can be transmitted in three ways: through sexual intercourse, through blood, and from mother to child.[15]

Sexual Transmission

Transmission as a result of sexual intercourse accounts for about three fourths of all HIV infections worldwide.[15] This means that HIV infection is mainly a sexually transmitted disease (STD). Initially, men in developed countries were

Thierry Mertens, World Health Organization, and Peter Piot, UNAIDS, 20 Av. Appia, 1211 Geneva 27, Switzerland.

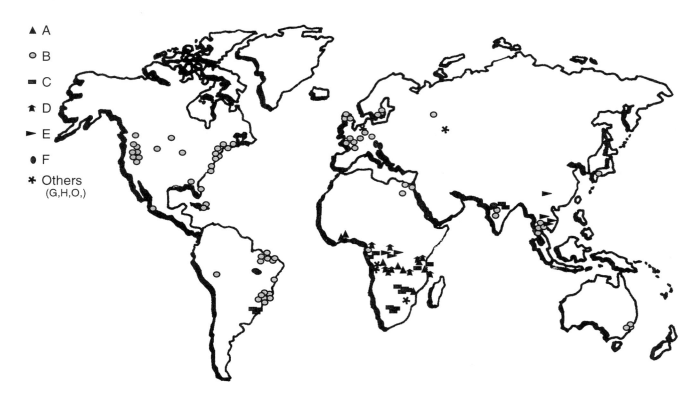

FIG 6-1. Worldwide distribution of main HIV-1 subtypes.

more exposed to HIV than women, primarily as a result of sexual intercourse between men or from injecting drug use, but the difference between the numbers of men and women infected with HIV has been slowly narrowing as heterosexual transmission is becoming more common. In other parts of the world, where heterosexual transmission predominated from the outset, the male to female ratio of persons infected with HIV is close to 1, and in some parts of Africa, infected women may even outnumber men for some periods.[16]

Because the main transmission mode of HIV is through heterosexual intercourse, the probability of HIV infection during a single heterosexual exposure to an infected partner is an important parameter determining the rate of HIV spread. If, as reported in the United States, this probability is less than 0.003 in the absence of any cofactor and independent of the time elapsed since infection,[17,18] extensive spread of infections may take many years. However, modeling in Thailand suggests that this probability may be 10 times higher for male to female and female to male transmission in some other settings.[19] This high variation in the transmission probability per sexual act may reflect a combination of factors, including the inherently heterogeneous nature of sex (eg, frequency and types of sexual partnerships, patterns of sexual mixing, types of sexual practices), variation in viral strains, concomitant risk factors (eg, other

STDs),[20-24] the use of vaginal desiccants, and having sex during menses,[25] or to variation in average infectiousness at the community level in different phases of the epidemic. The latter can be explained by the fact that newly infected persons are generally more infectious than persons infected for a long time, and persons progressing to AIDS regain infectiousness.[3,26,27] Figure 6-2 shows levels of viremia during the course of asymptomatic HIV infection and when HIV-infected persons start developing AIDS.[28]

Vertical Transmission

Mother-to-child transmission of HIV includes transmission during pregnancy, during delivery, and through breast-feeding.[29] Unlike HIV-2, which is uncommonly transmitted from mother to child,[30] HIV-1 is transmitted to the fetus or infant by 13% to 48% of infected mothers.[31-37] The wide variation of rates of transmission in different studies may reflect differences in the distribution of determinants of transmission, such as the degree of maternal immune deficiency, the presence of chorioamnionitis, maternal vitamin A deficiency, or exposure to infected breast milk.[32,38-41] In populations with a low rate of breast-feeding, as in most industrialized countries, most mother-to-child transmission occurs during pregnancy and delivery. Data from various countries suggest that

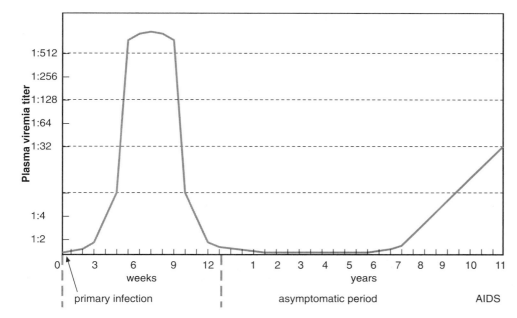

FIG 6-2. A schematic representation of the time course of the level of HIV viremia during HIV infection. (Adapted from Pantaleo G, Graziosi C, Fauci AS. The immunopathogenesis of human immunodeficiency virus infection. N Engl J Med 1993; 328:327)

as many as 15% of babies breast-fed by HIV-infected mothers may become infected through breast-feeding.[31] As is the case for heterosexual transmission, these transmission rates appear to be strongly influenced by the level of maternal viremia, with higher levels producing higher infectiousness.[32]

Transmission by Blood Products and Contaminated Equipment

As with certain other STDs, HIV infection can be transmitted through blood. In industrialized countries, the blood supply has been made safe, but in some parts of the developing world, blood safety is still problematic, although steadily improving.[42–44] Less commonly, HIV is transmitted through the use of nonsterile instruments in health facilities (ie, nosocomial transmission) and outside the health care setting.[45–47] Localized outbreaks of HIV transmission have occurred among infants and young children as a result of unsafe medical practices, such as using shared syringes contaminated with HIV-infected blood in the Russian Federation (ie, Kalmykia and Elista outbreaks)[48] and through transfusions of unscreened blood and improperly sterilized needles in Romania.[49] Although such infections undoubtedly occur, specifically designed epidemiologic studies conducted in developing countries, particularly in Africa,[47] and the virtual absence of infection in the group 10 to 15 years of age suggest that this route is not contributing substantially to overall transmission.

A major problem in the developed and developing world is HIV transmission resulting from the use of contaminated injection equipment by drug users. Although prevention programs, particularly needle exchange programs, are being implemented in several parts of the industrialized world, major epidemics continue to occur among populations of injecting drug users (IDUs). In western Europe, this trans-

mission route accounts for 44% of recent AIDS cases, up from about 16% of AIDS cases in 1985.[50] IDUs constitute two thirds or more of AIDS cases reported from Italy and Spain.[50] In Australia, home to one of the most dynamic prevention programs, transmission among IDUs appears to be decreasing.[51] Sharing equipment among IDUs is also a major route of HIV transmission in parts of Asia. Although the epidemics among IDUs have been well described in Thailand[52] and in Manipur, northeast India,[53] substantial rates of HIV infection have recently been detected in such populations in Ho Chi Minh City, Vietnam, Myanmar (Burma), peninsular Malaysia, and Yunnan province, China.[3] In Latin America, HIV infection rates among selected urban populations of IDUs are greater than 30% in Argentina and well over 20% in selected cities of Brazil.[1]

Laboratory and epidemiologic studies have shown that HIV is not transmitted by mosquitoes and other biting insects.[54,55] Table 6-1 summarizes the relative proportions of worldwide HIV infections by transmission categories estimated by the WHO as of the end of 1994.

INTERACTION BETWEEN HIV-1 AND TUBERCULOSIS

An alarming increase in cases of tuberculosis has been reported simultaneously with the emerging AIDS epidemic in many countries, particularly in Africa.[56–59] HIV infection has become a strong risk factor for the development of active tuberculosis in developing countries with a high prevalence of HIV.[58–61] Between 5% and 10% of persons with HIV and *Mycobacterium tuberculosis* may develop active tuberculosis each year.[56] Conversely, it has been suggested that tuberculosis may worsen HIV-induced immunodeficiency[62] and may accelerate the course of HIV disease.[63,64] Data from the United States indicate that some of the

TABLE 6-1. *Transmission or risk*
of human immunodeficiency infection

Route of Transmission	Percentage*
Sexual	70–80
Perinatal	5–10
Sharing injection equipment	5–10
Blood transfusion	5–10

Percentage of global population, 1994.

increase in active tuberculosis cases is attributable to new infections—rather than reactivation of old infections—among those with HIV infection, who may have increased susceptibility to tuberculosis for a given exposure.[65,66] The advent and continuing spread of HIV infection significantly complicates tuberculosis control programs in countries heavily affected by the AIDS epidemic, and the clinical complications for patients with HIV during antituberculosis therapy, including thiacetazone, raises further concern.[67]

DETERMINANTS OF THE SPREAD OF HIV-1

Behavioral and Demographic Determinants

The risk of acquiring HIV infection by sexual contact is a function of the number of HIV-infected sexual partners to which an individual is exposed, the extent of exposure to each partner (ie, duration and type of exposure), and the degree of infectiousness of each partner, which probably varies over time. Accurate information on each of these parameters is difficult to collect. Moreover, a measure such as the mean number of sexual partners may not be absolutely relevant, because heterogeneity inherent to sexual behavior at the population level is extensive and may be a more important determinant of the spread of HIV. Figure 6-3 shows the proportion of men and women reporting nonregular and commercial sex in the last 12 months in 15 countries.[68] Mathematical modeling has demonstrated the importance of sexual mixing patterns according to age and social classes, of concomitant sexual relationships, and of "core" groups with a high incidence and transmission rate of

STD.[69–71] In general, populations most vulnerable to HIV infection are affected first. For example, in Thailand, a first wave appeared among IDUs, a second wave occurred among sex workers and their clients, and then spread in the general population took place within a few years.[72]

Sexual activity does not occur in a social vacuum. There is increasing evidence that HIV infection and AIDS is associated with various socioeconomic determinants[73,74] and that the social context is one of the main driving forces behind "risk." Policies that ignore the social and economic constraints on behavioral changes may be counterproductive and stigmatizing, because personal failure is blamed when behavioral changes do not come about.

As with other STDs, young age is an important determinant of HIV transmission because, in general, young persons have higher rates of sexual partner change and young women may be biologically more susceptible to genital infection.[2,3] As the HIV epidemic ages in some parts of the world and the pool of noninfected sexually active adults at risk of HIV infection decreases, the large numbers of young persons becoming sexually active will replenish the pool of susceptible persons, especially in developing countries, where the base of the age pyramid is broad. Figure 6-4 shows the pyramid of ages in France in 1990 compared with the pyramid of ages in Ethiopia in 1990. Approximately 38% of the population is between 10 and 24 years of age in France, compared with 55% in Ethiopia. If there is substantial sexual mixing between age groups, the new cohorts of adolescents will rapidly become infected by their older partners and will then contribute greatly to a sustained epidemic over many years. Moreover, the proportion of new infections accounted for by youth is likely to increase with time.[3] Evidence of high incidences in young age groups compared with older cohorts is already emerging in Zaire (Fig. 6-5).[75]

Biologic Factors

Infectiousness varies over time in individuals with HIV infection (see Fig. 6-2). Given similar levels of sexual behavior and mixing patterns, variable infectiousness may be the driving force behind the rapid expansion phase

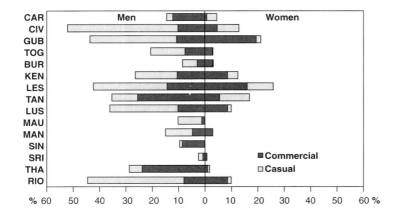

FIG 6-3. Percentage of 15–49-year-old men and women, who reported nonregular and commercial sex in the 12 months before June 1994.

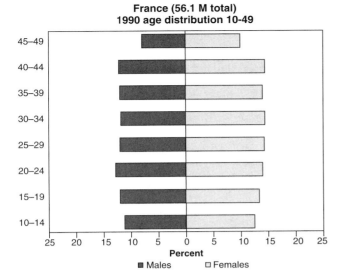

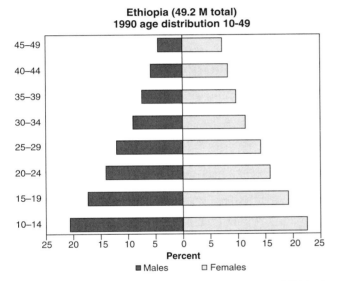

FIG 6-4. Comparative age pyramids in France and Ethiopia.

observed in many epidemics[3,26] and may contribute to the decreased overall HIV incidence later in the course of a given epidemic as the overall transmission efficacy decreases.[1] It is still unclear whether the considerable genetic variability of HIV-1 has any implications for viral spread.[9,10]

Genital ulcers and some nonulcerative STDs, such as gonorrheal and chlamydial infections, facilitate transmission of HIV by increasing the infectiousness of infected individuals and the susceptibility to HIV of noninfected sex partners.[21,24,76] The magnitude of the attributable risk of STD in the transmission of HIV can be assessed by community-based randomized trials.[22] The results of the first such trial showed an important impact of improved treatment of STD on HIV incidence; about 40% of HIV incidence was reduced

in rural communities of Tanzania, East Africa.[76] The role of other biologic factors possibly influencing the transmission of HIV, such as oral contraceptive use[77] or male circumcision, are far from being elucidated.[78–83]

Socioeconomic Factors and Geographic Variability

In addition to the heterogeneity observed in the spread of HIV between countries, an important feature of the dynamics of the epidemic has been much higher infection levels in urban than rural populations in most countries. Because the degree to which HIV spreads from urban to rural populations is a major uncertainty in forecasting the future magnitude of the epidemic, particularly in Africa and Asia, urban-rural variations are increasingly under scrutiny.

There are some notable exceptions to the rule of a large urban-rural differential. As early as 1989, data from Côte d'Ivoire[84] suggested that the urban-rural differential in HIV prevalence level was less pronounced than in most other countries. Zimbabwe is another country with high urban-rural mobility, involving circular migration. By 1992, infection rates of 15% to 20% in the sexually active urban population and 5% to 10% in rural areas were seen.[15] High levels of seroprevalence in some areas may reflect longer exposure to the virus rather than higher risk behaviors. Countries with a well-developed transportation infrastructure may experience more rapid spread of HIV infection to rural areas, as seen in Zimbabwe and Côte d'Ivoire. In contrast, in a remote rural area of Zaire where travel is restricted by a poor infrastructure, the seroprevalence rates among the general population remained stable at about 1% over a 10-year period between the late 1970s and the late 1980s.[85]

Stereotypical dichotomies of urbanization, individualism, and modernity versus village, community, and tradition obscure the fact that new urban residents often adapt their cultural norms to the constraints of a new environment.[3] One study found that the longer the duration of postpartum sexual abstinence imposed on men in Ibadan, Nigeria, the more common were STDs acquired by these men, because they would seek nonregular sexual partners for that period.[86] Sexual networks typical of urban environments can also be found in areas where migrant labor is concentrated, such as mining areas and industrial plantations. Analyses of multi-site surveys of sexual behavior in developing countries sponsored by the Global Programme on AIDS suggest that some of the observed differences in sexual behaviors may result from the diverse compositions of urban and rural populations in terms of age, education, and marital status.[68]

Less attention has been given to migration patterns that create unbalanced sex ratios in "exporting" and "recipient" geographic areas. In such circumstances, marriage patterns and sexual behavior may be permanently affected. Seasonal migration was the only social factor associated with STDs and HIV seropositivity in rural populations of Casamance, Senegal.[87] In many parts of Southeast Asia, adolescents of both sexes migrate from rural areas to neighboring cities

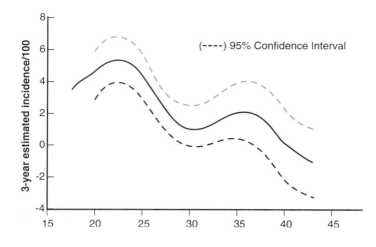

FIG 6-5. Cumulative HIV-1 incidence from 1986 to 1989 among childbearing women in Kinshasa. (Batter V, Matela M, Nsuami M, et al. High HIV-1 incidence in young women marked by stable overall seroprevalence among childbearing women in Kinshasa, Zaïre: estimating incidence from serial seroprevalence data. AIDS 1994;8:811.)

with appealing economic opportunities and return to their rural homes to marry. HIV and other STDs are often contracted in the city through commercial or casual sex and then introduced to the rural populations.[3] Sudden, large migration flows and economic crises—events that rupture social structures and break norms—are often associated with an increase in sexually transmitted diseases.[88] War or the long presence of an army may also place rural populations at higher risk of HIV infection.

SUBCONTINENTAL EPIDEMICS

One of the distinguishing features of the AIDS epidemic has been its global spread within the last 20 years. However, the spread of HIV presents distinct characteristics in different societies, requiring descriptions by epidemiologic regions.

Western Europe, North America, Australia, and New Zealand

In Western Europe, North America, Australia, and New Zealand, more than 1.8 million cumulative HIV infections in adults were estimated to have occurred as of end-1995, with about two thirds, or 1.2 million infections, in the United States. In total, more than 700,000 AIDS cases are

estimated by the WHO to have occurred in adults alone as of end-1995 (Fig. 6-6).

The persons predominantly affected have been men who have sex with men and IDUs,[1,89] together with their sex partners, with the proportion of heterosexually acquired infections slowly increasing over the past decade.[73,90] Marked differences continue to exist between and even within these countries in the distribution of AIDS cases among homosexual men and IDUs, reflecting the variability in HIV transmission patterns. For a discussion of the situation in the United States, the reader is referred to Chapter 9. Most AIDS cases in Scandinavia and England are homosexual men, and IDUs constitute two thirds or more of the AIDS cases reported from Italy and Spain.[50]

During the last few years, the proportion of AIDS cases attributable solely to sexual transmission between men has decreased. In Western Europe, the proportion of AIDS cases attributable to homosexual transmission fell from 62% in 1985 to 35% in 1992.[50] However, caution should be used in comparing proportions of cases infected through different modes of transmission across countries, because such proportions do not necessarily reflect the magnitude of the problem attributable to these different modes of transmission. For example, in 1994, the proportion of AIDS cases infected through homosexual contact was much lower in

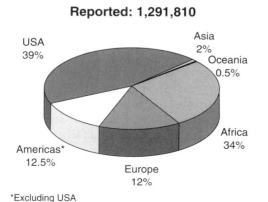

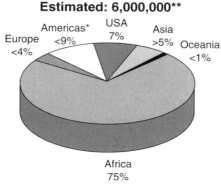

FIG 6-6. Total cumulative number of reported and estimated AIDS cases in adults and children at the end of 1995. (Mertens TE, Burton A. Estimates and trends of the HIV/AIDS epidemic. AIDS 1996; 10(A):S221.)

Spain (15%) than in Germany (69%), but the number of AIDS cases per million members of the total population attributable to homosexual contact was higher in Spain (20.6%) than in Germany (14.8%).[91] Substantial numbers of new HIV infections have been documented in younger homosexual men, with a prevalence rate of HIV of 9.4% in a San Francisco survey,[89] and there is concern that HIV incidence may increase again among men who have sex with men in other places of the industrialized world.

The proportion of transmission solely attributable to injecting drug use continues to grow in many places. In the European Union, this transmission route accounts for 44% of recent AIDS cases, up from about 16% of AIDS cases in 1985,[50] and in the United States, it rose from 17% in 1985 to 25% in 1992.[92]

Transmission of HIV through heterosexual intercourse increased during the latter half of the 1980s and the early 1990s, with especially noticeable increases in urban populations with high rates of injecting drug use,[1] crack (cocaine base) use in the United States,[93] or STDs. In the United Kingdom, HIV prevalence among heterosexuals attending STD clinics overall was 4.6 per 1000 in 1991.[94] Among pregnant women in London, the rate was 2.6 per 1000 in 1993, a significant increase from 1990, and it was 5.5 per 1000 in Paris, without significant changes between 1990 and 1993.[91] In the region surrounding Rome, the prevalence decreased between 1990 and 1992 from 2.8 to 1.5 per 1000.[91] In Australia, the number of HIV infections reported to the WHO has decreased since 1988, and reported AIDS cases have decreased since 1991 (WHO, unpublished data).

Latin America and the Caribbean

As of end-1995, the WHO estimated that over 1.7 million cumulative adult HIV/AIDS infections had occurred in Latin America and the Caribbean and that the adult HIV/AIDS prevalence was close to 1.5 million (Fig. 6-7).[1] As of end-1995, more than 140,000 adult and pediatric AIDS cases had been reported.[1] The number and the rate of AIDS cases per population are highest in Brazil, which had over 70,000 reported cases as of end-1995.

Data from the national AIDS programs and the Pan American Health Organization indicate that most infections in Latin America were initially among homosexual or bisexual men. Since then, there has been increasing heterosexual transmission, principally among bisexual men and their female sex partners, and among female sex workers and their clients. For example, in Brazil, the percentage of reported AIDS cases attributable to heterosexual transmission increased from 7.5% in 1987 to 26% in 1993 and 1994. Although AIDS case data suggest a predominance of HIV infection in the southeastern states of Brazil, data on HIV prevalence among selected male STD clinic attenders indicate that the geographic distribution is more extensive.[95] In 1992 through 1994, the prevalence among antenatal clinic attenders was 0.5% in São Paulo state and 2.2% in Itajai, southern Brazil.[95] HIV infections among IDUs are also a growing problem across the subcontinent. In Argentina, for example, the prevalence of HIV infection among IDUs ranges from 30% to 50%, and in Brazil it ranges from 20% to 60%.[1]

In most of the Caribbean, heterosexual transmission has been the predominant mode of transmission for at least a decade.[1] Studies from national programs among pregnant women attending antenatal clinics in 1990 and 1991 found HIV prevalences close to 3% in the Bahamas and more than 1% in Santo Domingo, Dominican Republic. In Haiti, HIV prevalence among antenatal clinic attenders was 7.5% in urban areas and 5.5% in rural areas in 1993, with the highest rate of seropositivity in the young age groups.[96]

Estimated distribution of adult HIV/AIDS prevalence as of late 1995

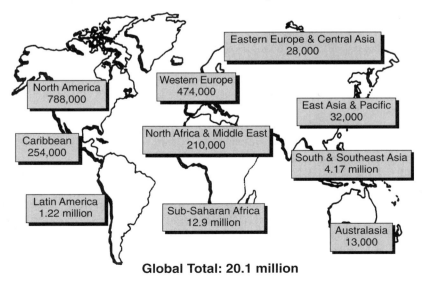

Global Total: 20.1 million

FIG 6-7. Estimated global distribution of HIV and AIDS prevalence in adults by continent or region at the end of 1995.

Sub-Saharan Africa

As of end-1995, the WHO estimated that 4.5 million AIDS cases have occurred in sub-Saharan Africa, constituting 75% of the global total (see Fig. 6-6). As of end-1995, land following an extensive country-by-country review of HIV/AIDS data, WHO also estimated that 16 million adult HIV infections had occurred in sub-Saharan Africa, with 12.9 million of these adults still alive with HIV or AIDS (see Fig. 6-7). Epidemiologic evidence indicates that heterosexual intercourse is the predominant mode of transmission in this region.

East and Central Africa total 50% to 60% of the HIV infections that have occurred in sub-Saharan Africa, despite accounting for only about 15% of the total population of the region.[1] Data on HIV incidence collected in the last few years reflect most directly the trends of infection in this major epicenter. In the general population cohort in the Kagera region, northwest Tanzania, where HIV prevalence among antenatal clinic attenders is about 8% to 10% in rural areas and 17% in urban areas (WHO, unpublished data), the HIV incidence was 0.8 per 100 person-years in rural and 4.8 in urban areas in 1992.[97] During 1992 and 1993, the crude annual mortality rates for urban factory workers in northwest Tanzania were 4.9% per 100 person-years in those with and 0.3% in those without HIV infection, giving an age- and sex-adjusted mortality ratio of 12.9. Of all deaths, 62% were attributable to HIV infection.[98] Data from urban sentinel surveillance sites in Uganda suggest HIV prevalence rates of well above 20% among pregnant women. In some rural areas of southern Uganda, seroprevalence rates have been estimated to be higher than 10% for the general population (WHO, unpublished data). However, studies of HIV incidence indicate that in a rural district of southwest Uganda the annual incidence for those 13 years of age and older declined from 7.5% in 1989 through 1990 to 4.6% in 1993. Rates were highest in those 25 to 34 years of age.[99] In two rural areas of the Rakai district, the annual incidence was 2.1% in 1991 and 1992 for those 13 years of age and older.[100]

Epidemiologic analysis of AIDS case surveillance in combination with HIV prevalence data from East Africa and mathematical modeling suggest a substantial shift of HIV incidence to younger age groups of males and females as the epidemic matures (R.L. Stoneburner, D. Low-Beer, G. Tembo, G. Asiimwe-Okiror, T.E. Mertens, unpublished data). In rural areas of northwest Tanzania, a survey revealed trends in sexual behaviors where men and women from earlier generation were older at first intercourse and had fewer lifetime partners than participants from younger cohorts,[101] pointing to the high risk of HIV infection among young generations.

Serologic data from national programs in sub-Saharan Africa indicate that the epidemic continues to evolve in western and southern Africa. In West Africa, extensive spread is estimated to have begun in the late 1980s. Among pregnant women in one state of Nigeria, HIV prevalence was estimated to be 6% in 1992.[1] Among antenatal clinic attenders in Abidjan, Côte d'Ivoire, HIV prevalence was 10% to 15% in 1994.[1] Similar HIV levels to those in West Africa are emerging in southern Africa. HIV prevalence rates of more than 20% to 30% have been observed among adults in the major urban areas of Botswana. Aggregated data collected in antenatal clinics across the Republic of South Africa indicated an overall HIV prevalence of 2.4% as of 1992. Two serial cross-sectional surveys conducted in March 1992 and December 1993 in a rural district in the northeast of South Africa among antenatal clinic attenders showed an increase in seroprevalence from 4.2% to 7.9%. The highest prevalence rates were in the 20- to 24-year-old group (6.4% and 12.3% in 1992 and 1993, respectively).[102] Figure 6-8 shows trends in HIV prevalence among antenatal clinic attenders in different cities of sub-Saharan Africa between 1986 and 1993.[1,103]

Despite the grim picture prevailing in most of sub-Saharan Africa, there are indications that HIV prevalence may still be relatively low among the general population in selected countries (see Fig. 6-8). For example, in Cameroon and Benin, the prevalence among antenatal clinic attenders appeared to be less than 5% for several years between 1989 and 1993 (WHO, unpublished data). The reasons for the disparities in the spread of the epidemic across the subcontinent need to be understood by examining in a standardized way sexual mixing patterns in various parts of the world. However, assessing the contribution of HIV genetic variability to infectiousness and transmission, accounting for the time of virus introduction, and quantifying differences in behaviors related to various situations or prevention efforts are likely to be difficult.

South and Southeast Asia

Although the extensive spread of HIV in South and Southeast Asia began only in the mid-1980s, the progression of the pandemic in this region has been rapid in several populations. As of end-1995, the WHO estimated that over 4.25 million HIV infections had cumulatively occurred in adults, with over 4.15 million prevalent infections (see Fig. 6-7). An estimated 300,000 cumulative adult AIDS cases are thought to have occurred, but only 25,090 adult and pediatric cases have been reported.

In Thailand, HIV has been described as spreading in waves among IDUs, commercial sex workers, their clients, and regular partners of clients.[72] Rapidly rising seroconversion rates toward the end of the 1980s, followed by a relative decline and stabilization around 1991 to 1992, have been described for IDUs in Bangkok.[52] Data from the national AIDS program indicate that HIV prevalence among antenatal clinic attenders is about 8% in Chiang Mai and Chiang Rai in the northern part of the country, and the median prevalence nationwide was 1.7% by mid-1994.[1] Among female sex workers in northern Thailand, the preva-

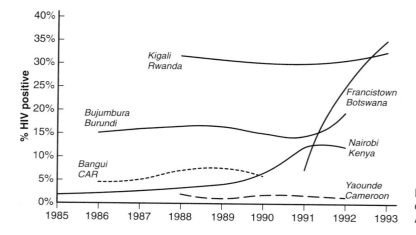

FIG 6-8. Trends in HIV prevalence among antenatal clinic attenders in selected cities of sub-Saharan Africa.

lence is above 30%, and the prevalence among army conscripts was more than 7% in 1993 (WHO, unpublished data). A decline in the incidence appears to have occurred among selected female sex workers[104] and among Royal Thai Army conscripts in northern Thailand, where an incidence of 0.87 per 100 person-years compares favorably with a previous annual incidence of about 3.4%.[105] In the latter part of the 1990s, Thailand is facing the terrible exponential rise in AIDS cases and associated deaths due to a previous very high incidence of HIV infections.

Rapid HIV spread probably continues in India, home to 16% of the world's population.[53,106–108] Gaining an accurate picture of HIV spread across different parts of India is difficult because of the variability of the epidemiologic environments, the multitude of urban and semiurban areas and the lack of consistency in serologic surveys regarding the period and population tested. Convenience sampling is likely to overestimate, and period prevalence data are likely to underestimate the real prevalence.[3] Nevertheless, because of its population size, gauging the extent of the epidemic and assessing trends in India are key to forecasting the future dimensions of the pandemic.

The most complete longitudinal seroprevalence studies are from South India, reporting data for patients seeking STD treatment and sex workers. In Madras, seroprevalence among STD patients increased from about 1% from 1986 through 1989 to 8.5% from 1991 through 1992.[109,110] In Madurai, the prevalence in the STD population was 6.5% in 1991.[111] In the State of Maharashtra, west India, with close to 100 million inhabitants and an urban population of more than 23 million, the epidemic is well established, with 2.5% of antenatal clinic attenders in Bombay infected in 1994.[1] Farther north, in Jaipur, Rajasthan, HIV prevalence was 3.3% and 0.8% in 1994 among STD patients and antenatal clinic attenders, respectively.[1] In north, central and east India (except for the northeastern state of Manipur, where there is an important epidemic related to injecting drug use),[53] available data suggest that the epidemic has not yet taken off, although the scarcity of rigorously conducted serosurveys preclude any conclusion.[1]

Rapid spread of HIV into the general population has occurred in some parts of urban and rural Myanmar, contiguous to Thailand. In Cambodia, the epidemic is spreading mainly through heterosexual contact, with a prevalence among blood donors of 3.5% in Phnom Penh by mid-1994.[1] Figure 6-9 illustrates the parallel increases, albeit with a few years' lag, of seroprevalence rates among blood donors in Chiang Mai, Thailand, and in Phnom Penh, Cambodia. In Vietnam, predictably rapid increases in seroprevalence were observed among IDUs in 1992 and 1993, with more than a tenfold increase from 2% to 30%,[3] and there is concern that heterosexual transmission of HIV will follow a pattern similar to that in Thailand.[51] The extent of the epidemic is less clear in Bangladesh, Pakistan, and Indonesia.

East Asia and Western Pacific

The WHO estimated that there were 32,000 adult HIV infections in East Asia and the Western Pacific region by end-1995. A large proportion of the reported AIDS cases in Japan have been among persons with hemophilia who were transfused with HIV-infected blood products in the early to mid-1980s.[112] There is diversity in transmission modes across the region. For example, in Papua New Guinea, more than 70% of those with known exposure were infected through heterosexual transmission. In Yunnan Province, China, which is geographically contiguous with Southeast Asia, there is an outbreak of HIV infections among IDUs. Further spread into the adjoining Guangxi and Guangdong Provinces of China is likely. If the epidemic gains a foothold in China, the potential for a large increase in the numbers of HIV infections in the world's most populous country, even with a low incidence, is of serious concern.[1] An important increase in reported STDs (WHO, unpublished data) concomitant to the economic boom in many parts of China contributes to this concern.

Eastern Europe and Central Asia

The magnitude of the HIV and AIDS problem in Eastern Europe and Central Asia remains poorly defined. Data from

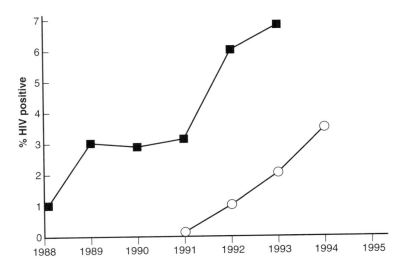

FIG 6-9. Trend in HIV prevalence among blood donors of Chiang Mai, Thailand, and Phnom Penh, Cambodia, 1988–1994. (Mertens TE, Belsey E, Stoneburner RL, et al. Global estimates of HIV infections and AIDS: further heterogeneity in spread and impact. AIDS 1995;9[suppl 1]:S251.)

St Petersburg, Russia, indicate that the 1993 incidence of newly detected persons with HIV infection by mass screening was twice the yearly mean for the previous 5 years and that most infections were attributed to heterosexual transmission.[113]

In two countries, localized outbreaks of HIV transmission have occurred in infants and young children as a result of unsafe medical practices. In the Kalmykia (Russian Federation) outbreak in 1988, several hundred children were infected through injections of medicines using shared syringes that had been contaminated with HIV-infected blood.[1] In the 1989 Romanian outbreak, in which it is believed that several thousands of children were involved, transmission occurred through transfusions of unscreened blood and possibly as a result of the use of needles and syringes that had not been properly disinfected or sterilized.[49] However, there is no reason to think these are the main routes of HIV transmission in this region.

In some Eastern European countries, injecting drug use is associated with very high rates of HIV infection; a cross-sectional study conducted in Warsaw, Poland, in 1993 found a seroprevalence of 46% among IDUs attending treatment centers.[114] Social and structural changes likely to increase the risk of HIV transmission are taking place throughout much of the region.

North Africa and the Middle East

The spread of HIV began in some parts of North Africa and the Middle East in the late 1980s. As of end-1995, the WHO estimated that about 210,000 adult HIV infections in the whole region, which includes Sudan, contiguous to sub-Saharan Africa. Only 3474 AIDS cases have been reported (see Fig. 6-6). Most available data come from North Africa. In Morocco, HIV prevalence among blood donors was 0.01% in 1993.[115] In Nouakchott, Mauritania, the period prevalence between 1988 and 1992 among blood donors was 0.4%.[116] In Eritrea, data from national serosurveillance from 1994 indi-cated a prevalence of 25% among sex workers, 2.7% among blood donors, and 3% among antenatal clinic attenders.[1] Contiguous to North Africa is Niger, where a study conducted in 1993 of antenatal clinic attenders, truck drivers, and STD patients in Niamey revealed prevalences of 1.3%, 3.4%, and 15.4%, respectively.[117]

Only limited and indirect information is available regarding the extent of high-risk behaviors in the Middle East. HIV prevalence data are practically nonexistent; of the approximately 1500 HIV infections among resident and immigrant expatriates—one of the few populations for which data are available—reported over the past 7 years in one Gulf state, one third were thought to have occurred during 1992 alone.[1]

GLOBAL ESTIMATES AND PROJECTIONS OF HIV-1 INFECTIONS

Global Estimates

By December 15, 1995, a total of 1,291,810 AIDS cases had been reported to the WHO, but the organization estimates that as of mid-1995, allowing for underdiagnosis, underreporting, and delays in reporting and based on the estimated number of HIV infections, there have been 6 million cumulative AIDS cases worldwide (see Fig. 6-6).

Figure 6-7 shows the global distribution of prevalent adult HIV infections (including AIDS cases alive). For a chronic infection such as HIV, cumulative incidence estimates were close to prevalence estimates early in the epidemic. As persons infected with HIV early in the epidemic die of AIDS, the gap between the two measurements is widening. As the global epidemic progresses, the gap will widen further, particularly in regions that are furthest into the epidemic: Australasia, Latin America and the Caribbean, North America, sub-Saharan Africa, and Western Europe. It is therefore important to focus on HIV prevalence rather than cumulative incidence.

Globally, there are 3 men infected for every 2 infected women, and by the year 2000, the number of new infections among women may be closer to that among men.[1] Figure 6-10 shows the trends in the proportion of AIDS cases in females in selected countries. In sub-Saharan Africa, the male to female ratio is close to 1, and in the rest of the world, a steady increase in female AIDS cases is observed.[118] The rising infection rates among women are accompanied by a corresponding rise in the number of children born with HIV infection. It is estimated that over 1.5 million children have been infected with HIV through mother-to-child transmission. These children rapidly develop AIDS and die, usually before the age of 5, although in the United States and Europe the survival period is longer.

These figures are the testimony of the tragedy unfolding for the last 15 years and point to the fact that HIV is still spreading very fast across continents. There is, however, evidence to suggest that a stabilization and perhaps a decline in the prevalence of HIV infection may be taking place in certain areas and populations of the industrialized regions of Australia, New Zealand, North America, and Western Europe, as well as in the high-prevalence areas of East and Central Africa.[1,3,75,119,120] Stabilization occurs when the number of deaths from AIDS over a period equals the number of new HIV infections. However, this change may result from a series of factors and is not easy to interpret accurately. For example, in some countries, particularly in sub-Saharan Africa, the apparent stabilization may result from an increase in the number of deaths, paralleling or following a decrease in HIV incidence. Even if stabilization is caused by a decrease in the incidence of HIV infection, an equilibrium may indicate saturation—a condition in which most persons engaging in any kind of high-risk behavior are already infected with HIV or dead from AIDS—and may not be a result of prevention efforts. Stabilization may also mask increases in particular modes of HIV transmission,[3] such as an increase in heterosexually transmitted HIV hidden by a increase in general mortality and a decrease in the incidence of HIV infections acquired through other transmission modes or disproportionate increases in new HIV infections among young persons. Evidence of high incidences for young age groups compared with older cohorts is emerging from various countries (WHO, unpublished data).[83]

Such phenomena are evidence of the transition from epidemic to endemic HIV infection and AIDS and constitute one more facet of the ever-changing pandemic. Effective identification and response to these changing patterns of the pandemic is particularly pressing, because epidemiologic studies have shown the effectiveness of specific prevention activities in some populations.[121,122]

At the population level, changes in HIV incidences over time may be explained by a variety of factors. These factors include saturation of susceptible populations, possible behavioral changes, potential changes in the virulence of HIV-1 or in the natural immunity, or change in infectiousness of persons infected with HIV over time.[1,3,26,123]

Notwithstanding the fact that stabilization or decline in HIV prevalence may occur independently of prevention efforts, as a result of the intrinsic dynamic of the epidemic, the decreases in incidence observed among sex workers and Royal Thai Army conscripts in northern Thailand or those observed in parts of East Africa may genuinely reflect prevention efforts. These declines possibly reflect a reduction in the number of commercial sex contacts, the success of the Thai government's "100% condom" policy in brothels, or behavioral changes resulting from a variety of factors, including the death of relatives or friends. Consistent with these observations are declining trends in reported STDs in several countries. Figure 6-11 shows trends for the total number of all STD cases treated at government clinics in Thailand, all STDs reported from primary health care clinics in Harare, Zimbabwe, and male and female reported gonorrhea rates per 10,000 members of the population in Costa Rica.[1] These trends may be related to a number of causes, including increasing clinic fees and a shift from public health facilities to other sources of treatment, but they may also reflect prevention efforts, resulting in behavioral changes and increased condom use.

Projections of HIV and AIDS Cases

As a result of HIV infection rates, the number of new AIDS cases is expected to stabilize in large parts of the industrialized world by the mid-1990s, while continuing to increase in most parts of the developing world where the health care infrastructure is already overwhelmed by other causes of morbidity. Around 700 000 and close to half a million new AIDS cases are projected to occur annually by the year 2000 in Africa and Asia, respectively. The longer-term dimensions of the HIV/AIDS pandemic cannot be forecasted with confidence. However, on the basis of available data on the current global status of the pandemic and recent trends in its spread, WHO has generated a plausible range of projected new HIV infections during the 1990s. In making projections of the future magnitude of the pandemic, the lower limit of the estimated range of HIV prevalence for each region was used. The results of HIV/AIDS forecasting by WHO should be considered conservative.

For the year 2000, WHO currently projects a cumulative total of close to 40 million HIV infections in men, women and children, of whom more than 90% will live in the developing countries. The projected cumulative total of adult AIDS cases for the year 2000 is well over 10 million. Cumulatively, as many as 5 million children under age 5 will be HIV-infected through their mothers, the majority of them in sub-Saharan Africa. Table 6-2 shows WHO estimates, by region, of the number of adults infected with HIV and alive as of the end of 1995, and its projections of the number who will be living with HIV infection in the year 2000.

Projections of the number of AIDS cases in infants and children are based on perinatal transmission rates of about

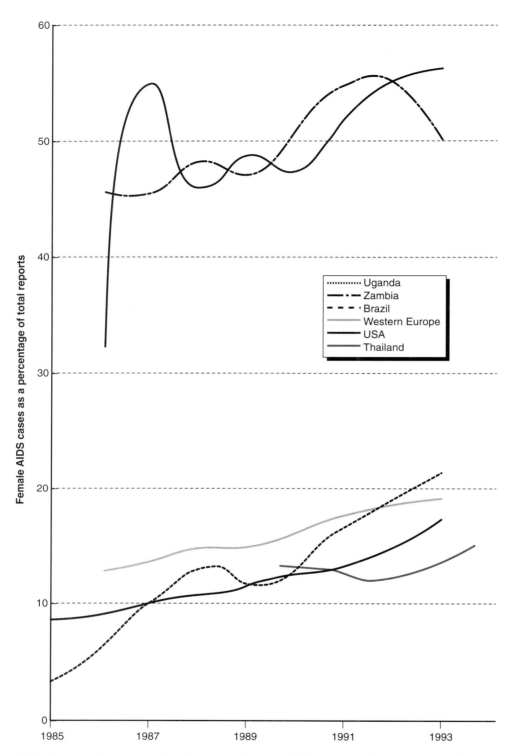

FIG 6-10. Trends in the proportion of reported AIDS cases in females in selected countries (Low-Beer D, Stoneburner RL, Mertens TE, Berkley S, Burton A. The global burden of HIV. In: Murray C, Lopez A, eds. The global burden of diseases. 1996 [in press].)

30%. However, because their infected mothers are likely to die of AIDS within 5 to 10 years of their birth, the uninfected infants will constitute a growing population of orphans. WHO estimates that close to 5 million children under 10 years of age will be orphaned by the end of the 1990s as a result of the HIV-related deaths of their mothers. The number of maternal orphans will increase further in the early years of the next century as a result of the death of

those mothers who were infected with HIV in the 1990s. These forecasts of HIV and AIDS are based on country and regional estimates, as well as scenarios of HIV incidence reflecting our current understanding of HIV transmission. With a better understanding of the transmission dynamics of HIV in different parts of the world, new scenarios are being developed, allowing for more accurate and longer term projections.

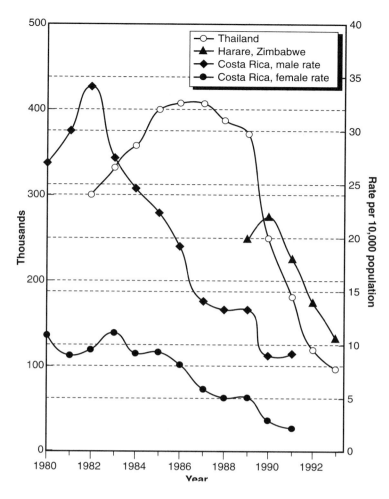

FIG 6-11. Trends in reports and rates of various sexually transmitted disease by country as reported by the Venereal Disease Division of the Ministry of Health of Thailand, the Statistics Department of the Ministry of Health of Costa Rica, and the Harare City Health Department of Zimbabwe. (Mertens TE, Belsey E, Stoneburner RL, et al. Global estimates of HIV infections and AIDS: further heterogeneity in spread and impact. AIDS 1995; 9[Suppl 1]:S251.)

IMPACT OF THE HIV PANDEMIC

The epidemic of illness and death associated with HIV is only starting. In 1990, about one-half million persons required care for AIDS worldwide; in the year 2000, this figure will quadruple. The suffering and loneliness related to illness and fear of death are immense, albeit unquantifiable. The factors that determine how HIV is likely to influence the demography of different regions include the present and future AIDS-specific mortality rates for adults and children, the effect of maternal HIV infection on the mortality of HIV-negative children, and the effect of adult HIV infection on fertility.

HIV is already causing enormous increases in adult mortality. In some countries that are furthest into the epidemic in Africa, more than one half of adult mortality is now attributable to HIV infection.[98,124] In Zambia, the crude mortality rate for employees of 33 factories and other businesses soared from 2.5 deaths per 1000 persons in 1987 to 183 in 1993, an increase virtually wholly attributable to HIV-related disease.[125] In many large cities of Australia, North America, and Western Europe, AIDS has become a leading cause of death for young adults. A variety of simulations for Sub-Saharan Africa suggests that changes in population growth are unlikely to be detected in the early decades of the

TABLE 6-2. *Estimated and projected regional prevalence of human immunodeficiency virus infection among adults*

Region	Late 1995 Estimated HIV Prevalence*	2000 Projected HIV Prevalence†
Australia, Oceania, Europe & North America	>1.2 million	1 million
Latin America & Caribbean	1.5 million	>2 million
Africa	>13 million	>14 million
Asia	>4 million	8 million
Global total	20 million	>25 million

*Total number of HIV-infected adults currently alive.
†Total number of HIV-infected adults alive in the year 2000.

epidemic.[126,127] However, the loss of a substantial proportion of the active work force is likely to have a serious socioeconomic impact, potentially impeding development.

The economic impact of HIV infection is likely to be more important than for most other diseases, because AIDS is a 100% fatal disease, it affects primarily adults in their most productive years, and a large number of persons have already been infected. The costs of production loss are thought to be 10 to 20 times greater than direct medical costs. Together with the loss of income-earning opportunities and of productive labor time, the diversion of cash to medical expenses has been the main problem observed at the household level in sub-Saharan Africa.[128]

REFERENCES

1. Mertens TE, Belsey E, Stoneburner RL, et al. Global estimates of HIV infections and AIDS: further heterogeneity in spread and impact. AIDS 1995;9(Suppl 1):S251.
2. Piot P, Laga M, Ryder R, et al. The global epidemiology of HIV infection: continuity, heterogeneity, and change. J Acquir Immune Defic Syndr 1990;3:403.
3. Mertens TE, Burton A, Stoneburner R, et al. Global estimates and epidemiology of HIV infections and AIDS. AIDS 1994;8(Suppl 1):S361.
4. De Cock KM, Adjorlolo G, Ekpni E, et al. Epidemiology of HIV-2. Why there is no HIV-2 pandemic. JAMA 1993;270:2083.
5. Kanki PJ. West African human retroviruses related to STLV III. AIDS 1987;1:141.
6. Poulsen AG, Kvinesval B, Aaby P, et al. Prevalence of and morbidity from human immunodeficiency virus type 2 in Bissau, West Africa. Lancet 1989;1:827.
7. Kanki PJ, Travers KU, Mboup S, et al. Slower heterosexual spread of HIV-2 than HIV-1. Lancet 1994;343:943.
8. Marlink R, Kanki P, Thior I, et al. Reduced rate of disease development after HIV-2 infection as compared to HIV-1. Science 1994;265:1587.
9. Sharp PM, Robertson DL, Gao F, Hahu B. Origins and diversity of human immunodeficiency viruses. AIDS 1994;8(Suppl 1):S27.
10. Kuiken CL, Korber BTM. Epidemiological significance of intra- and inter-person variation of HIV-1. AIDS 1994;8(Suppl 1):S73.
11. De Leys R, Vanderborght B, Vanden Haesevelde M, et al. Isolation and partial characterization of an unusual human immunodeficiency retrovirus from two persons of west-central African origin. J Virol 1990;64:1207.
12. Gürtler LG, Hauser PH, Eberle J, et al. A new subtype of human immunodeficiency virus type 1 (MVP-5180) from Cameroon. J Virol 1994;68:1581.
13. Loussert-Ajaka I, Ly TD, Chaix ML, et al. HIV-1/HIV-2 seronegativity in HIV-1 subtype O infected patients. Lancet 1994;343:1393.
14. Dondero TJ, Hu DJ, George JR. HIV-1 variants: yet another challenge to public health. Lancet 1994;343:1376.
15. World Health Organization, Global Programme on AIDS. The HIV/AIDS pandemic: 1993 overview. Geneva: World Health Organization, 1994.
16. Berkley S, Naamara W, Okware S, et al. AIDS and HIV infection in Uganda—are women more infected than men? AIDS 1990;4:1237.
17. Peterman TA, Stoneburner RL, Allen JR, et al. Risk of HIV transmission from heterosexual adults with transfusion-associated injections. JAMA 1988;259:55.
18. Holmberg SD, Horsburgh CR Jr, Ward JW, Jaffe HW. Biological factors in the sexual transmission of human immunodeficiency virus. J Infect Dis 1989;160:116.
19. Mastro TD, Satten GA, Nopkesorn T, Sangkharomya S, Longini IM. Probability of female-to-male transmission of HIV-1 in Thailand. Lancet 1994;343:204.
20. European Study Group. Risk factors for male to female transmission of HIV. Br Med J 1989;298:411.
21. Cameron DW, D'Costa LJ, Maitha GM, et al. Female to male transmission of human immunodeficiency virus type 1: risk factors for seroconversion in men. Lancet 1989;2:403.
22. Mertens TE, Hayes RJ, Smith PG. Epidemiological methods to study the interaction between HIV infection and other sexually transmitted diseases. AIDS 1990;4:57.
23. Laga M, Nzila N, Goeman J. The inter-relationship of sexually transmitted disease and HIV infections: implications for the control of both epidemics in Africa. AIDS 1991;5(Suppl):S55.
24. Laga M, Manoka A, Kivuvu M, et al. Non ulcerative sexually transmitted diseases as risk factors for HIV-1 transmission in women. Results from a cohort study. AIDS 1993;7:95.
25. Padian N, Marquis L, Francis DP, et al. Male-to-female transmission of human immunodeficiency virus. JAMA 1987;258:788.
26. Jacquez JA, Koopman JS, Simon CP, Longini IM. Role of the primary infection in epidemics of HIV infection in gay cohorts. J Acquir Immune Defic Syndr 1994;7:1169.
27. Laga M, Taelman H, Van der Stuyft P, Bonneux L, Vercauteren G, Piot P. Advanced immunodeficiency as a risk factor for heterosexual transmission of HIV. AIDS 1989;3:361.
28. Pantaleo G, Graziosi C, Fauci AS. The immunopathogenesis of human immunodeficiency virus infection. N Engl J Med 1993;328:327.
29. Pizzo PA, Butler KM. In the vertical transmission of HIV, timing may be everything. N Engl J Med 1991;325:652.
30. Adjorlolo-Johnson G, De Cock KM, Ekpini E, et al. Prospective comparison of mother-to-child transmission of HIV-1 and HIV-2 in Abidjan, Côte d'Ivoire. JAMA 1994;272:462.
31. Dunn DT, Newell ML, Ades AA, Peckham CS. Risk of human immunodeficiency virus 1 transmission through breastfeeding. Lancet 1992;340:585.
32. Van de Perre P, Meda N. Interventions to reduce mother to child transmission of HIV. AIDS 1995;9(Suppl 1):559.
33. The Working Group on Mother-to-Child Transmission of HIV. Rates of mother-to-child transmission of HIV in Africa, America and Europe: results from 13 perinatal studies. J Acquir Immune Def Syndr 1995;8:506.
34. Ryder RW, Nsa W, Hassig SE, et al. Perinatal transmission of the human immunodeficiency virus type 1 to infants of seropositive women in Zaire. N Engl J Med 1988;320:1637.
35. Lallemant M, Lallemant-Le Coeur S, Cheynier E, et al. Mother-child transmission of HIV-1 and infant survival in Brazzaville, Congo. AIDS 1989;3:643.
36. Hira SK, Kamanga J, Bhat GJ, et al. Perinatal transmission of HIV-1 in Zambia. Br Med J 1989;299:1250.
37. Lepage P, Hitimana DG. Natural history and clinical presentation of HIV-1 infection in children. AIDS 1991;5(Suppl 1):S117.
38. Van de Perre P, Simonon A, Msellati P, et al. Postnatal transmission of human immunodeficiency virus type 1 from mother to infant. A prospective cohort study in Kigala, Rwanda. N Engl J Med 1991; 325:593.
39. Bove F, Pons JC, Keros L, et al. Risk for HIV-1 perinatal transmission varies with the mother's stage of HIV infection. Sixth international conference on AIDS. Abstract ThC44. San Francisco, June 1990.
40. Semba RD, Miotti PG, Chiphangwi JD, et al. Maternal vitamin A deficiency and mother-to-child transmission of HIV-1. Lancet 1994;343:1593.
41. Bridbord K, Willoughby A. Vitamin A and mother-to-child HIV-1 transmission. Lancet 1994;343:1585.
42. Piot P, Goeman J, Laga M. The epidemiology of HIV and AIDS in Africa. In: Essex M, Mboup S, Kanki PJ, Kalengayi MR, eds. AIDS in Africa. New York: Raven Press, 1994:157.
43. Jäger H, Nseka K, Goussard B, et al. Voluntary blood donor recruitment: a strategy to reduce transmission of HIV-1, hepatitis B and syphilis in Kinshasa, Zaire. Infusionsther Transfusionsmed 1990;17:224.
44. Mhalu FS, Ryder RW. Blood transfusion and AIDS in the tropics. Ballieres Clin Trop Med Commun Dis 1988;1:551.
45. Berkley S. Parenteral transmission of HIV in Africa AIDS 1991;5(Suppl 1):S87.
46. Vincent-Ballereau F, Lafaix C, Haroche G. Incidence of intramuscular injections in rural dispensaries in developing countries. Trans R Soc Trop Med Hyg 1989;83:106.
47. Lepage P, Van de Perre P. Nosocomial transmission of HIV in Africa: what tribute is paid to contaminated blood transfusions and medical injections? Infect Control Hosp Epidemiol 1988;9:200.
48. Pokrovsky VV, Eramova EU. Nosocomial outbreak of HIV infection in Elista, USSR. Abstract WA05. Fifth international conference on AIDS. Montreal, June 1989.
49. Patrascu IV, Constantinescu SN, Dublanchet A. HIV-1 infection in Romanian children. [Letter] Lancet 1990;335:672.

50. European Centre for the Epidemiological Monitoring of AIDS. AIDS surveillance in the European community and cost countries. Report No. 27. St Maurice: Hôpital National de St Maurice, June 30, 1994.
51. Kaldor JM, Effler P, Sarda R, et al. HIV and AIDS in Asia and the Pacific: an epidemiological overview. AIDS 1994;8(Suppl 2):S165.
52. Kitayaporn D, Uneklabh C, Weniger BG, et al. HIV-1 incidence determined retrospectively among drug users in Bangkok, Thailand. AIDS 1994;8:1443.
53. Sarkar S, Panda S, Das N, et al. Rapid spread of HIV among injecting drug users in north-eastern states of India. Centre AIDS Res Control 1993;6:23.
54. Piot P, Schofield CJ. No evidence for arthropod transmission of AIDS. Parasitol Today 1986;2:294.
55. Webb PA, Happ CM, Maupin GO, Johnson BJB, Ou C-Y, Monath TP. Potential for insect transmission of HIV: experimental exposure of *Cimex hemipterus* and *Toxorhynchites amboirensis* to human immunodeficiency virus. J Infect Dis 1989;160:970.
56. Horsburgh CR, Poznick A. Epidemiology of tuberculosis in the era of HIV. AIDS 1993;17(Suppl 1):S109.
57. Snider DE, Roper WL. The new tuberculosis. N Engl J Med 1992;326:703.
58. Perriëns JH, Mukadi Y, Nunn P. Tuberculosis and HIV infection: implications for Africa. AIDS 1991;5(Suppl 1):S127.
59. Nunn P, Kibuga D, Elliott A, Gathua S. Impact of human immunodeficiency virus on transmission and severity of tuberculosis. Trans R Soc Trop Med Hyg 1990;84(Suppl 1):9.
60. De Cock KM, Gnaore E, Adjololo G, et al. Risk of tuberculosis in patients with HIV-1 and HIV-2 infections in Abidjan, Ivory Coast. Br Med J 1991;302:1103.
61. Daley CL, Small PM, Schecter GF, et al. An outbreak of tuberculosis with accelerated progression among persons infected with human immunodeficiency virus: an analysis using restriction fragment length with polymorphisms. N Engl J Med 1992;326:231.
62. Mukadi Y, Perriëns JH, St Louis ME, et al. Spectrum of immunodeficiency in HIV-1-infected patients with pulmonary tuberculosis in Zaire. Lancet 1993;342:143.
63. Brindle RJ, Nunn P, Batchelor BI, et al. Infection and morbidity in patients with tuberculosis in Nairobi, Kenya. AIDS 1993;7:1469.
64. Wallis RS, Vjecha M, Amir-Tahmasseb M, et al. Influence of tuberculosis on human immunodeficiency virus (HIV-1): enhanced cytokine expression and elevated beta-microglobulin in HIV-1-associated tuberculosis. J Infect Dis 1993;167:43.
65. Alland D, Kalkert GE, Moss AR, et al. Transmission of tuberculosis in New York City. An analysis by DNA fingerprinting and conventional epidemiologic methods. N Engl J Med 1994;330:1710.
66. Small PM, Hoperwell PC, Singh SP, et al. The epidemiology of tuberculosis in San Francisco. A population-based study using conventional and molecular methods. N Engl J Med 1994;330:1703.
67. Perriëns JH, Colebunders R, Karahunga C, et al. Increased mortality and tuberculosis treatment failure rate among HIV-seropositive patients compared to HIV-seronegative patients with pulmonary tuberculosis treated with "standard" chemotherapy in Kinshasa, Zaire. Am Rev Respir Dis 1991;144:750.
68. Carael M. Sexual behaviour. In: Cleland J, Ferry B, eds. Sexual behaviour and knowledge about AIDS in the developing world. London: Taylor & Francis, 1995.
69. Gupta S, Anderson R, May R. Networks of sexual contacts: implications for the pattern of spread of HIV. AIDS 1989;3:807.
70. Watts C, May R. The influence of concurrent partnerships on the dynamics of HIV/AIDS. Math Biosci 1992;108:89.
71. Hethcote HW, Yorke JA. Gonorrhoeae transmission dynamics and control. Lect Notes Biomath 1984;56:105.
72. Weniger BG, Limpakrnjanarat K, Ungchusak K, et al. The epidemiology of HIV infection and AIDS in Thailand. AIDS 1991;5(Suppl 2):S71.
73. Holmes KK, Karon JM, Kreiss J. The increasing frequency of heterosexually acquired AIDS in the United States, 1983–1988. Am J Public Health 1990;80:858.
74. Simon PA, Hu DJ, Diaz T, Kerndt PR. Income and AIDS rates in Los Angeles County. AIDS 1995;9:281.
75. Batter V, Matela M, Nsuami M, et al. High HIV incidence in young women marked by stable overall seroprevalence among childbearing women in Kinshasa, Zaïre: estimating incidence for serial seroprevalence data. AIDS 1994;8:811.
76. Grosskurth H, Mosha F, Todd J, et al. Impact of randomised controlled trial. Lancet 1995;346:530.
77. Plummer F, Simonsen J, Cameron D, et al. Co-factors in male-female sexual transmission of human immunodeficiency virus type 1. J Infect Dis 1991;163:233.
78. Bongaarts J, Reining P, Way P, Conant F. The relationship between male circumcision and HIV infection in African populations. AIDS 1989;3:373.
79. De Vincenzi I, Mertens T. Male circumcision: a role in HIV prevention? AIDS 1994;8:153.
80. Cook LS, Koutsky LA, Holmes KK. Circumcision and sexually transmitted diseases. Am J Public Health 1994;84:197.
81. Mertens TE. Estimating the effects of misclassification. Lancet 1993;342:418.
82. Seed J, Allen S, Mertens T, et al. Male circumcision, sexually transmitted diseases, and risk of HIV. J Acquir Immune Defic Syndr Hum Retrovirol 1995;8:83.
83. Mertens TE, Carael M. Sexually transmitted diseases, genital hygiene and male circumcision may be associated: a working hypothesis for HIV prevention. Health Transit Rev 1995;5:104.
84. Soro BN, Gershy-Damet GM, Coulibaly A, et al. Seroprevalence of HIV infection among the general population of the Ivory Coast, West Africa. J Acquir Immune Defic Syndr 1989;3:1193.
85. Nzila N, De Cock KM, Forthal DN, et al. The prevalence of infection with HIV over a 10-year period in rural Zaire. N Engl J Med 1988;318:276.
86. Caldwell P, Caldwell JC. The function of child-spacing in traditional societies, and the direction of change. In: Page HJ, Lesthaeghe R, eds. Child-spacing in tropical Africa: tradition and change. London: Academic Press, 1981.
87. Pison G, Le Guenno B, Lagarde E, et al. Seasonal migration: a risk factor for HIV infection in rural Senegal. J Acquir Immune Defic Syndr 1993;6:196.
88. Brandt AM. No magic bullet. A social history of venereal disease in the United States since 1880. New York: Oxford University Press, 1987.
89. Lemp GF, Hirozawa AM, Givertz D, et al. Sero-prevalence of HIV and risk behaviours among young homosexual and bisexual men. JAMA 1994;272:449.
90. Prevots DR, Ancelle-Park R, Neal JJ, Remis RS. The epidemiology of heterosexually acquired HIV infections and AIDS in western industrialized countries. AIDS 1994;(Suppl 1):S109.
91. European Centre for the Epidemiological Monitoring of AIDS. AIDS surveillance in the European community and cost countries. Quarterly report No. 44. St Maurice: Hôpital National de St Maurice, December 1994.
92. Centers for Disease Control and Prevention. HIV/AIDS surveillance report. Atlanta: Centers for Disease Control and Prevention, October 1993.
93. Edlin B, Irwin KI, Faruque S, et al. Intersecting epidemics—crack cocaine use and HIV infection among inner-city young adults. N Engl J Med 1994;331:1422.
94. European Centre for the Epidemiological monitoring of AIDS. AIDS surveillance in Europe. Quarterly report No. 40. St Maurice: Hôpital National de St Maurice, December 31, 1993.
95. Rodrigues L, Lauria L, Berro O, Ferreia J, Sereno A, Loures L. HIV sero surveillance in Brazil: a new epidemic emerges. Tenth international conference on AIDS/international conference on STD. Abstract 072C. Yokohama, Japan, August 7–12, 1994.
96. Bernard YM Camara B, Ferrus A, et al. Résultats d'une étude de surveillance sérosentinelle: prévalence du VIH du VHB et de la syphilis chez les femmes enceintes dans 5 sites serosentinelles en Haiti. Haiti Epidemiol 1994;1:30.
97. Killewo JZJ, Sandstrom A, Bredberg Raden U, Mhalu FS, Biberfeld G, Wall S. Incidence of HIV-1 infection among adults in the Kagera region of Tanzania. Int J Epidemiol 1993;22:528.
98. Borgdorff MW, Barongo NR, Klokke AH, et al. HIV-1 incidence and HIV-1 associated mortality and morbidity in a cohort of urban factory workers in Tanzania. In: Epidemiology of HIV-1 infection in Monza region, Tanzania (Borgdorff M, Ph.D. thesis). Amsterdam: Royal Tropical Institute, 1994.
99. Kengeya-Kayondo J, Kamali A, Nunn AJ, Malamba S, Wagner HV, Mulder DW. HIV-1 incidence in adults and risk factors for seroversion in a rural population in Uganda: 3 years of follow up. Abstract 068C. Tenth international conference on AIDS/international conference on STD. Yokohama, Japan, August 7–12, 1994.

100. Wawer MJ, Sewankambo NK, Berkley S, et al. Incidence of HIV-1 infection in a rural region of Uganda. Br Med J 1994;308:171.

101. Konings E, Blattner WA, Levin A, et al. Sexual behaviour survey in a rural area of north-west Tanzania. AIDS 1994;8:987.

102. Wilkinson D. Anonymous antenatal HIV seroprevalence surveys in rural South Africa. Tenth international conference on AIDS/international conference on STD. Abstract O70C. Yokohama, Japan, August 7–12, 1994.

103. Mertens TE, Low-Beer D. HIV and AIDS: where is the epidemic going? Bull World Health Organ 1996:74.

104. Sawanpanyalert P, Ungchusak K, Thanprasertsuk S, Akarasewi P. HIV-1 seroconversion rates among female commercial sex workers, Chang Mai, Thailand: a multi cross-sectional study. AIDS 1994;8:825.

105. Khamboonruang C, Beyrer C, Natpatan C, Eiumtrakol S, Selentano D, Nelson KE. HIV incidence in adults in northern Thailand. Tenth international conference on AIDS/international conference on STD. Abstract 038C. Yokohama, Japan, August 7–12, 1994.

106. United States Bureau of the Census, Centre for International Research. AIDS/HIV surveillance database. Washington, DC: United States Bureau of the Census, 1990–1994.

107. Ramalingaswami V. India: national plan for AIDS control. Lancet 1992;339:1162.

108. Jain MK, John JT, Keusch GT. Epidemiology of HIV and AIDS in India. AIDS 1994;8(Suppl 2):S61.

109. Jayapaul K, Mdneeran M, Ravinathrin R, et al. Sero-epidemiological study of HIV infection in and around Madras. Sixth international conference on AIDS. Poster FC613. San Francisco, June 1990.

110. Solomon S, Jagadeeswari T, Anuoradha K. Sentinel surveillance for HIV infection. Eighth international conference on AIDS. Abstract POC4086. Amsterdam, July 1992.

111. Parkajalakshimi VV, Uma A, Sethuranan R, et al. HIV seropositivity among STD patients. Second international conference on AIDS in Asia and the Pacific. Poster B704. New Delhi, India, November 1992.

112. Shiokawa Y, Soda K. Current status of HIV/AIDS epidemic in Japan. Second international conference on AIDS/Third World STD Congress. Abstract POC4085. Amsterdam, July 1992.

113. Kozlov AP, Volkova GV, Verevochkin SV, et al. New features of HIV/AIDS epidemic in Russia. Tenth international conference on AIDS/international conference on STD. Abstract 126C. Yokohama, Japan, August 7–12, 1994.

114. Stark K, Wirth D. High HIV seroprevalence in injecting drug users in Warsaw, Poland. [Letter] J Acquir Immune Defic Syndr 1994;7:877.

115. El Alaqui AM, El Makil K, Joundy S, Khamrich M, Benchemsi N. Prévalence des anticorps anti-HIV chez les donneurs de sang. Eighth international conference on AIDS/African conference on STD. Abstract MPC079. Marrakesh, December 12–16, 1993.

116. Baidy BL, Adimourty M, Sow A, Fatimata C. Evolution et projection de l'infection VIH en Mauritanie. Eighth international conference on AIDS/African conference on STD. Abstract TPC094. Marrakesh, December 12–16, 1993.

117. Hassane A, Paradis R, Moukaila A, et al. Estimation rapide de prévalence des MST/VIH à Niamey, Niger. Eighth international conference on AIDS/African conference on STD. Abstract ThPC087. Marrakesh, December 12–16, 1993.

118. Low-Beer D, Stoneburner RL, Mertens TE, Berkeley S, Burton A. The global burden of HIV. In: Murray C, Lopez A, eds. The global burden of diseases. Cambridge, MA: Harvard University Press, 1996 (in press).

119. Magazani K, Laleman G, Perriens JH, et al. Low and stable HIV seroprevalence in pregnant women in Shaba province, Zaïre. J Acquir Immune Defic Syndr 1993;6:419.

120. Stoneburner R, Lessner L, Fordyce EJ, Bevier P, Chiasson MA. Insight into the infection dynamics of the AIDS epidemic: a birth cohort analysis of New York City AIDS mortality. Am J Epidemiol 1993;138:1093.

121. Choi KH, Coates TJ. Prevention of HIV infection. AIDS 1994; 8:1371.

122. Mertens T, Caraël M, Sato P, et al. Prevention indicators to evaluate the progress of national AIDS programmes. AIDS 1994;8:1359.

123. Seitz ST, Mueller GE. Viral load and sexual risk. Epidemiologic and policy implications for HIV/AIDS. In: Kaplan EH, Brandeau ML, eds. Modelling the AIDS epidemic: planning, policy and prediction. New York: Raven Press, 1994:461.

124. Mulder DW, Nunn AJ, Kamali A, Nakiyingi J, Wagner HU, Kenggeya-Kayondo JF. Two-year HIV-1 associated mortality in a Ugandan rural population. Lancet 1994;343:1021.

125. Baggaley R, Godfrey-Faussett P, Msiska R, et al. Impact of HIV infection on Zambian businesses. Br Med J 1994;309:1549.

126. Gregson S, Garnett GP, Anderson RM. Is HIV-1 likely to become a leading cause of adult mortality in sub-Saharan Africa? J Acquir Immune Defic Syndr 1994;7:839.

127. Mertens TE, Burton A. Estimates and trends of the HIV/AIDS epidemic. AIDS 1996; 10(A):S221.

128. Barnett T, Blaikie P. AIDS in Africa: its present and future impact. London: Belhaven Press, 1992.

AIDS: Biology, Diagnosis, Treatment and Prevention, fourth edition, edited by Vincent T. DeVita, Jr., Samuel Hellman, and Steven A. Rosenberg. Lippincott–Raven Publishers, © 1997

CHAPTER 7

Global Distribution of Human Immunodeficiency Virus-1 Clades

Donald S. Burke and Francine E. McCutchan

The global spread of human immunodeficiency virus (HIV) has been swift and relentless; no country has been spared. Worldwide, 10 million human beings are infected, and the global toll is projected to rise to 40 million by the year 2000.[1-2] Genetic analyses of stains collected from around the world have disclosed substantial diversity.[3-9] At least eight distinct HIV-1 genotypes, or *clades,* are recognized. When the distributions of clades defined by molecular genetics are analyzed from an epidemiologic perspective, clear patterns become discernible.

We review here the global molecular epidemiology of HIV-1, focusing on viral divergence and phylogenetic relationships, geographic and temporal dispersion patterns, and ongoing ecologic adaptation to the human host. Our main conclusion is that the HIV epidemic is still in an unpredictable stage.

DIVERGENCE

Phylogenetic Relationships of Mammalian Lentiviruses

The genetic relationships of lentiviruses follow their host range; the main branches of the lentivirus family tree correspond to those of mammalian phylogeny. Five major lineages of simian immunodeficiency virus (SIV) have been discerned among primate lentiviruses,[10,11] each in a different nonhuman primate species native to Africa: African green monkeys (SIV_{agm}), mandrills (SIV_{mnd}), Sykes' monkeys (SIV_{syk}), sooty mangabeys (SIV_{sm}), and chimpanzees (SIV_{cpz}). The human lentivirus HIV-2 violates this neat host-related viral phylogeny and clusters genetically with the SIV_{sm}.

Donald S. Burke, Walter Reed Army Institute of Research, 1600 East Gude Drive, Rockville, Maryland 20850.

Francine E. McCutchan, Henry M. Jackson Foundation for the Advancement of Military Medicine, 1600 East Gude Drive, Rockville, Maryland 20850.

Some unusual human isolates, called HIV-1 O for outlier strains, are similar to SIV viruses isolated from common chimpanzees, but the exact primate species harboring the progenitors of HIV-1 has not been established.[12-15]

Phylogenetic Relationships Among HIV-1 Strains

Nucleotide sequences have been deduced from hundreds of HIV-1 strains from around the world and fitted into phylogenetic organizations. Various research teams have selected different regions of the HIV-1 genome for analysis. With a few important exceptions, the phylogenetic relationships deduced from analysis of different regions of the HIV-1 genome, such as *gag* or *env,* are closely congruent.[16]

Recognized clades are commonly referred to by the letter designations, A through H, a scheme that roughly reflects the order in which they were recognized. Maximum HIV-1 intragenotype strain to strain variation is typically less than 15%, but intergenotypic *env* variations are 20% to 30%. Remarkably, there is no apparent linear descent relationship between genotypes. In unrooted trees, all genotypes are essentially equidistant and appear to have radiated from a hypothetical central common progenitor.

Approximately 50% of all strains reported belong to clade B, the prototype of which is the original HIV-1 LAV/IIIB isolate. Clades A (16%), C (9%), D (10%), and E (10%) together account for another 45% of all reported strains, and clades F, G, and H and the genetic outliers account for only 5% of the global total. However, these relative frequencies almost certainly do not accurately reflect the true worldwide prevalence proportions because of gross underinvestigation of HIV-1 strains from less developed countries.

None of the several hundred strains sequenced is a candidate HIV-1 "protovirus." The oldest known HIV-1 strain, Z321, which was isolated from a stored serum specimen obtained in Zaire in 1976, is a rather unremarkable A genotype strain.[17-19]

Recombination

HIV may evolve by mechanisms other than the gradual accumulation of point mutations. Retroviruses contain two complete RNA genome strands per virion, and recombination occurs frequently during reverse transcription (Fig. 7-1).[20]

Naturally recombinant HIV-1 strains appear to be common. The entire E clade—which has a unique E *env* gene but a *gag* gene that clusters with the A viruses—appears to be derived from one such recombinant.[8] We and others have identified five additional strains that also appear to be *gag/env* recombinants[6]: MAL (Zaire), K124 (Kenya), and UG266 (Uganda) are all apparent D*env*/A*gag* recombinants; VI191 (Zaire) is an A*env*/G*gag* recombinant; and VI525 (Gabon) is a G*env*/H*gag* recombinant.

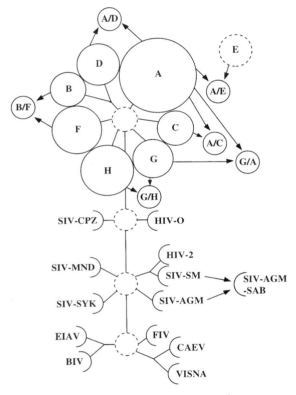

FIG. 7-1. Schematic of entire lentivirus phylogenetic tree, showing relationships between major groups, human **A** through **H** and **O** clades and simian immunodeficiency viruses (**SIV**) from African green monkeys (**AGM**), mandrils (**MND**), Sykes' monkeys (**SYK**), sooty mangabeys (**SM**), and chimpanzees (**CPZ**). For viruses other than HIV-1, the size and length of the branches do not reflect genetic distances nor group diversity. For the HIV-1 clades, the distances from the cluster centers are roughly proportional to interclade genetic distances, and clade circle sizes are proportional to intraclade diversity. Known recombinant viruses are shown. The E virus clade is shown as a hypothetical, because all known E are probably E/A recombinants. BIV, bovine immunodeficiency virus; CAEV, caprine arthritis-encephalitis virus; FIV, feline immunodeficiency virus; VISNA, Visna retrovirus. (Data from references 2, 5, and 6.)

The exact genomic location of recombination in these viruses is under study. HIV-1 isolates that appear to be intra-*env* B/F recombinants have also been described.[21]

Mutation, Molecular Clocks, and Dating of Emergence

Replication of HIV, like that of all RNA viruses that lack enzymes for editing of freshly replicated nucleotide strands, is error prone.[22,23] HIV-1 generates, on average, 1 error per 10^4 nucleotides, which is also the size of its genome. Potentially, each provirus is a new mutant strain, unique at least one base site. Mutations accumulate over successive replication cycles, leading to a swarm of closely related but nonidentical viruses in each infected individual. The blood and lymphoid tissue of a human adult contains 10^{11} CD4-positive lymphocytes, of which between 10^9 and 10^{10} can be shown to harbor viral DNA in HIV-infected patients.[24,25] With 10^7 HIV-infected patients worldwide, there may be as many as 10^{17} HIV genetically unique strain variants in circulation. This vast reservoir of genetic variants may increase the potential for successful adaptation.

HIV-1 clade B genotype mutation rates were directly measured among isolates obtained in Amsterdam in a 10-year period, from 1981 to 1990.[26] Overall strain diversity increased from 6% to 9%, but the consensus sequence for later isolates was exactly the same as that for earlier isolates; there was no net directional change. Comparable measurements on divergence rates are not available for other genotypes.

When did HIV-1 enter humans, and when did the current phylogeny of HIV-1 genotypes arise? Estimates vary widely. Myers and colleagues, using linear distance-time correlations estimated that HIV-1 first diverged from HIV-2 around 1950 and then diverged to its current phylogeny over the past 40 years.[27–29] Gojobori and colleagues estimated that the HIV-1/HIV-2 divergence node occurred in the early 1800s.[30] Eigen and Nieselt-Struwe calculated that the oldest node linking all human and simian viruses dated back 600 to 1200 years, and the HIV-1 strains causing AIDS were estimated to be 50 to 100 years old.[31]

DISPERSION

Early Abortive HIV-1 Epidemics

Sporadic AIDS cases in humans occurred long before the current pandemic was recognized in 1980. Eight early cases of HIV-1 infection have been well documented by serology or by detection of HIV-1 genome in clinical samples. Two African cases were asymptomatic persons from whom a specimen had been obtained for other reasons and fortuitously saved: a male blood donor in Kinshasa in 1959[32] and an adult woman in a serosurvey for Ebola virus antibodies in northern Zaire in 1976.[17–19] Six European and American cases were patients who had been ill with puzzling AIDS-like diseases and from whom stored blood or tissue specimens were available for analysis: a 26-year-old British sailor in 1958[33-35]; a 32-year-old Norwegian sailor, his wife, and daughter between 1966 and 1976[36]; a 15-year-old boy in St. Louis, Missouri, in 1968[37,38]; and a 39-year-old Portuguese man living in London in 1974.[39]

Virus or virus genes were obtained only from the Zaire 1976 case, which yielded the Z321 (A clade) strain, although six others were identified as HIV-1 without further genotyping. The 1958 British case was shown to be artifactual, caused by specimen cross-contamination. The 1974 Portuguese case was shown to be caused by HIV-2 by serologic analysis. Of the five legitimate index cases here, only one (the Norwegian sailor) is known or even thought to have transmitted the infection to others.

Global Dispersion of HIV-1 Genotypes

The clade distributions of the 669 HIV-1 strains of known genotype[4,6,7,9,21,40-59] are displayed by country of specimen origin in Table 7-1. Global dispersion patterns are strikingly nonuniform:

Every one of more than 250 strains from the United States, Haiti, and Western Europe has been clade B.
Clade B also predominates in Brazil, but clade F is not uncommon (10%), and at least one C clade strain has been detected.
Western Europe harbors clade B virtually exclusively, but almost one half of the strains from Eastern Europe have been other than clade B, including clades A, D, C, F, and G.
Clades A and D predominate in most of sub-Saharan Africa, but in Central Africa, six other clades are also recovered.
Clade C predominates in Southern Africa, the Horn of Africa, and in West Asia (Bombay).
Clade B predominates in most of East Asia.
Clade E predominates in Thailand.

Extreme caution must be used when drawing inferences about global dispersion patterns from these data. Global sampling can at best be regarded as patchy; only 39 countries were sampled at all, and only 16 countries were assessed with at least 10 specimens. Because the techniques for detecting, amplifying, and analyzing gene sequences were initially developed and standardized on clade B viruses, they may be biased toward detection of viruses of that clade.

The clear predominance of distinctive genotypes in particular countries does permit some inferences about the global spread of HIV-1. The HIV-1 epidemics in Latin America, Europe, and East Asia may have originated in the United States,[60-62] because clade B predominates in all these regions. However, it is highly unlikely that the HIV-1 epidemic in India (C genotype) originated in the United States or Europe.[45] A more likely source is one of the C clade epidemics in Southern Africa or the Horn of Africa. The E clade epidemic in Thailand and Southeast Asia may have originated in the equatorial Africa, where clade E viruses are also found.[46]

Genotype E: A Case Study

During the past 7 years, an epidemic of the HIV-1 clade E virus has erupted in Southeast Asia.[63,64] A reconstruction of the molecular epidemiology of this genotype is presented here.

Recombination in Africa

Although the *env* gene of E viruses is distinct from that of all other clades, the *gag* genes from the African E strains and the Asian E strains cluster phylogenetically with *gag* genes of the A clade. There are two possible accounts for this genetic dislinkage. A hypothetical E*env*/E*gag* may have recombined in nature with a conventional A*env*/A*gag* strain to produce an E*env*/A*gag* strain. Conventional A strains are abundant in central Africa, but no E*env*/E*gag* strains have been detected. Alternatively, the *env* gene of a conventional A strain rapidly mutated into a new type E while the *gag* remained unchanged as a typical A. This latter scenario seems unlikely because *env* and *gag* have co-evolved in all other HIV-1 clades and in related lentiviruses.

Dispersion to Thailand

In the mid-1980s, while the HIV epidemic raged in North America, Europe, and Africa, Thailand and the rest of Asia appeared to be spared. HIV surveillance studies in populations of female sex workers found no evidence of infection.[65] Epidemic HIV in Thailand was first detected in the Bangkok area in late 1987, with explosive spread in populations of intravenous drug users (IDUs).[66,67] Nucleotide sequencing of the first Bangkok isolates in 1989 showed them to be clade B viruses similar to those found in the United States and Europe.[8] Subsequent serologic surveys using genotype specific peptides confirmed that this initial outbreak among IDUs was exclusively genotype B.[64]

An abrupt rise in the HIV-1 prevalence of asymptomatic blood donors in northern Thailand in 1989 was the first clue of a new epidemiologic twist. In 1990, we obtained HIV-1 isolates from young male military conscripts in northern Thailand found to be seropositive at the time of voluntary blood donation, whose only exposure was heterosexual contact with female sex workers[68-70]; 12 of 13 of these initial northern Thailand isolates belonged to a new genotype, now called E. Although the recruits had lived in different provinces in northern Thailand, their virus isolates were phylogenetically remarkably homogeneous. The serologic evidence of recent introduction, coupled with the genetic evidence of limited divergence, strongly suggested a recent point source for the epidemic—an epidemiologic cloning.

Exactly how HIV entered northern Thailand is not certain. During the late 1980s, Thailand experienced considerable difficulty with an influx of foreign drug smugglers, including some from Africa, who transported illegal opiates from the Golden Triangle to the United States and Europe.[71] Although logical, this linkage is speculative.

TABLE 7-1. *Geographic distribution of human immunodeficiency virus type 1 clades for all viruses typed by genetic analysis*

Country		Total	B	A	D	C	E	F	G	H
						Number of Strains in Each Clade				
Americas	USA	79	78	0	1*	0	0	0	0	0
	HTI	26	26	0	0	0	0	0	0	0
	BRA	58	52	0	0	1	0	5	0	0
	PER	1	1	0	0	0	0	0	0	0
Europe										
West	NLD	91	91	0	0	0	0	0	0	0
	GBR	8	8	0	0	0	0	0	0	0
	DEU	2	2	0	0	0	0	0	0	0
	FRA	2	1	0	1	0	0	0	0	0
	SWE	5	5	0	0	0	0	0	0	0
East	FIN	23	16	1*	0	3*	0	3*	0	0
	EST	6	6	0	0	0	0	0	0	0
	RUS	8	1	0	0	0	0	0	0	7*
	BLR	7	3	1	1*	2*	0	0	0	0
	ROM	9	0	0	0	0	0	9	0	0
Africa										
Northwest	EGY	4	4	0	0	0	0	0	0	0
	SEN	1	0	0	1	0	0	0	0	0
	CIV	28	1	26	1	0	0	0	0	0
	GHA	1	0	1	0	0	0	0	0	0
Central	NIG	5	0	1	0	0	0	0	4	0
	GAB	10	1	5	1	0	0	0	1	2
	ZAR	30	0	16	11	0	0	1	1	1
	CAR	25	0	11	1	3	9	0	0	1
	UGA	62	1	23	37	1	0	0	0	0
	RWA	12	0	11	0	0	0	1	0	0
	BDI	1	0	1	0	0	0	0	0	0
East	TZA	14	0	4	10	0	0	0	0	0
	KEN	8	0	7	1	0	0	0	0	0
South	ZMB	3	0	0	0	3	0	0	0	0
	MIW	15	0	0	0	15	0	0	0	0
	ZAF	3	0	0	0	3	0	0	0	0
Horn	ETH	9	0	0	0	9	0	0	0	0
	SOM	1	0	0	0	1	0	0	0	0
	DJI	2	0	1	0	1	0	0	0	0
Asia	IND	20	4	0	0	16	0	0	0	0
	THA	74	14	0	0	0	60	0	0	0
	TWN	2	0	0	0	0	0	0	2	0
	PHL	2	2	0	0	0	0	0	0	0
	CHN	10	10	0	0	0	0	0	0	0
	JPN	2	2	0	0	0	0	0	0	0
Totals		669	329	109	66	58	69	19	8	11

*Strains from each of 39 countries (shown by three-letter standard abbreviations) with one or more typed HIV-1 strains are shown. Incompletely studied, nontypable, HIV-1 O strains and HIV-2 strains are excluded. Countries are grouped into arbitrary regions to emphasize geographic clade patterns, which are outlined by dark boxes. Cases or groups of cases known to be imported are shown by asterisks. The clustering of C, E, F, G, and H clade viruses in equatorial Africa is outlined by a light box.

Association of Clade and Transmission Route: Two Simultaneous Epidemics

The E genotype has overtaken and overwhelmed genotype B as the predominant genotype throughout Thailand. Approximately 95% of heterosexually acquired cases in Thailand are E genotype, although the B genotype continues to be the most common (80%) genotype among IDUs.[64,72]

Thailand is experiencing two simultaneous epidemics, one relatively slow and relatively confined to IDUs that is caused by genotype B and the other rampant, heterosexually transmitted, and caused by genotype E. The burgeoning case load of clinical AIDS patients in northern Thailand, where most AIDS patients have been shown to be E virus infected, is evidence that E clade is no less virulent than the more familiar B clade.[41]

Regional and International Dispersion From Asia

Rising HIV prevalences have been reported in Burma and Cambodia, suggesting that the E variant may have spread extensively throughout Southeast Asia.[73] Serologic evidence for E clade infections also has been found for Japanese men who contacted female sex workers in Southeast Asia.[74] Male military personnel from several countries who participated in United Nations peace-keeping operations in Cambodia have been found to be infected with E clade strains.[75]

Clonal Epidemics

The salient features of the clade E epidemic are probably shared by several other component epidemics contributing to the global pandemic; the HIV-1 strains in the new India (clade C) and to some extent the Brazilian (clade F) epidemics are also remarkable for their genetic homogeneity.[1,2,76–79] It appears that each of these epidemics represents outgrowth of a single epidemiologic clone on a massive scale. In each case, more heterogeneous clusters of genetically related viruses are known to exist in Africa, and it is likely the strains were dispersed from Africa to a new continent, with a bottleneck reduction in diversity.

Early in the U.S. epidemic, a single patient was thought to have seeded the virus throughout North America and was therefore identified as "patient zero."[80] However, this patient must have been infected with genotype B and therefore could have been patient zero for only that genotype. There may have been as many as eight patient zeros, one for each genotype.

Global Projections

The World Health Organization (WHO) projects that the incidence of new HIV infections in the epidemic in Asia will overtake and exceed the incidence of new infections on other continents by the end of this decade.[1] We have multiplied the incidence estimates from the WHO by the proportions of cases in each continent known to be caused by each clade and thereby projected the future global burden of incident HIV cases caused by each clade. By the end of the 1990s, clades E and C will probably account for more infections worldwide than all other clades combined (Fig. 7-2).

ADAPTATION

Transmissibility of HIV-1

HIV-1 is transmitted more efficiently and is more virulent than HIV-2.[81,82] Preliminary data suggest that among HIV-1 viruses some clades may differ in their transmissibility and perhaps virulence properties as well.

Distinctive HIV transmission patterns have been recognized from the earliest days of the epidemic. In 1986, the WHO categorized countries as displaying pattern I (ie,

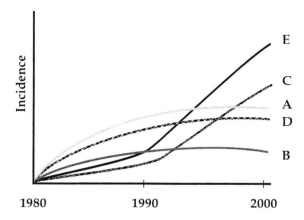

FIG. 7-2. Estimated global incidences of HIV-1 clades A through E for 1980 through 2000.

homosexual and IDU transmission), pattern II (ie, heterosexual transmission), or pattern III (ie, mixed or no transmission).[83] A global map of these patterns, defined before HIV-1 genotypes were known to exist, shows a close congruence between pattern I and those countries where the B clade predominates.

More compelling are the observations from Thailand, where the B clade predominates among IDUs, but the E clade predominates among heterosexually acquired cases.[84] The E virus may be more heterosexually transmissible than the B virus. In Thailand, the risk of infection to a male per sexual encounter with an infected female is 10-fold higher than it is the United States (3% versus 0.3%).[85] These differences in transmissibility are quantitative, not qualitative; blood-to-blood transmissible viruses can probably be transmitted heterosexually and vice versa, although with lower efficiency. As Anderson and May underscored, in any epidemic, the pathogen and the host population are dynamic, not static, variables.[86]

Virulence of HIV-1 Clades

Rates of disease progression from infection to symptoms to death can vary dramatically from person to person. Disease progression has been best studied in the United States and Western Europe, where the mean interval from infection to death is 11 years, but the range is 1 to 15+ years.[87–89] These earlier opinions were based almost entirely on observations of clade B viruses. No natural history studies have been done in populations infected with a virus of a non-B genotype.

Immunology of HIV-1 Clades

Cross-neutralization studies of primary isolates of viruses from clades B, C, and E have shown that polyclonal sera from infected patients do preferentially neutralize virus strains of the homologous clade.[90] Although the congruences are clear, they are not inviolate; some sera do show low-level cross-neutralization of viruses of heterologous clades, and some viruses are more easily neutralized than others. Studies of monoclonal antibody binding to oligomeric HIV-1 proteins on the surface of infected cells have identified group- and clade-restricted antigens. Like the cross-neutralization data, these studies suggest that genotypic and immunologic analyses of HIV-1 will give rise to congruent classification schemes.[91]

EVOLUTIONARY CONSIDERATIONS: THE CHAOTIC MODEL

HIV, with its high replication error frequency (ie, 1 million–fold greater than the human DNA genome) and high replication rate (ie, measured in hours rather than years), compresses evolution and affords a singular opportunity to prospectively examine evolutionary theory against unfolding contemporary events.

The evidence presented in this paper challenges the conventional gradualistic view of the global HIV pandemic, which posits that the epidemic began with a single emergence of an SIV into humans some years ago and that the virus gradually mutated and smoothly spread worldwide.

Notions of chance and chaos have only recently been assimilated into evolutionary biology theory. Gould and Feldriges's theory of punctuated equilibrium holds that the tempo of evolution may accelerate rapidly, particularly during encounters with new ecologic settings, only to then decelerate and return to a pattern of gradualism and predictability.[92]

We think that the global HIV epidemic can best be understood by a variation of punctuated equilibrium theory that we refer to as the chaotic model:

- *Divergence:* The current global HIV pandemic is composed of at least five major virologically and geographically distinct sustained subepidemics.
- *Dispersion:* International HIV-1 dispersions are commonplace, but only some become sustained regional epidemics.
- *Adaptation:* In each of the five subepidemics, HIV-1 independently continues to adapt to local host populations.

Implicit in this model are the likelihood that new variants are being continually generated through random mutation and recombination; any minor clade (ie, F, G, H, or a new recombinant) could become the next major epidemic clade; and any clade, major or minor, could develop new virulence or transmission properties.

CONCLUSION

The global HIV pandemic is still in an unstable and unpredictable phase. New variants with a range of transmission or virulence properties are arising and dispersing around the globe in a chaotic manner. Virologic surveillance for HIV-1 should be intensified, and clade and strain transmission patterns should be urgently evaluated throughout the world. HIV-1 clade variation may be a dominant factor in the global effort to develop vaccines and other epidemic interventions.

ACKNOWLEDGMENTS

We thank G. Meyers of the Los Alamos National Laboratory and members of our own laboratory, especially J. Louwagie and J. McNeil for useful discussions; A. Salvado and J. Lowe for encouragement; P. Bell for library assistance; and M. Hall for manuscript preparation. This effort was supported by a Cooperative Agreement between the U.S. Army Medical Research Development and Material Command and the Henry M. Jackson Foundation for the Advancement of Military Medicine and a grant from the World Health Organization. The views expressed here do not necessarily reflect those of the U.S. Department of the Army nor the Department of Defense.

REFERENCES

1. Merson MH. Slowing the spread of HIV: agenda for the 1990s. Science 1993;260:1266.
2. Berkley S. AIDS in the developing world: an epidemiologic overview. Clin Infect Dis 1993;17(Suppl 2):S329.
3. Louwagie J, McCutchan FE, Peeters M, et al. Phylogenetic analysis of *gag* genes from 70 international HIV-1 isolates provides evidence for multiple genotypes. AIDS 1993;7:769.
4. Delwart EL, Shpaer EG, Louwagie J, et al. Genetic relationships determined by a DNA heteroduplex mobility assay: analysis of HIV-1 *env* genes. Science 1993;262:1257.
5. McCutchan FE, Sanders-Buell E, Oster CW, et al. Genetic comparison of human immunodeficiency virus (HIV) isolates by polymerase chain reaction. J AIDS 1991;4:1241.
6. Louwagie J, Janssens W, Mascola J, et al. Genetic diversity of the envelope glycoprotein from HIV-1 isolates of African origin. J Virol 1995; 69:263.
7. McCutchan FE, Ungar BLP, Hegerich P, et al. Genetic analysis of HIV-1 isolates from Zambia and and expanded phylogenetic tree for HIV-1. J Acquir Immune Defic Syndr 1992;5:441.
8. McCutchan FE, Hegerich PA, Brennan TP, et al. Genetic variants of HIV-1 in Thailand. AIDS Res Hum Retrovirus 1992;8:1887.
9. Louwagie J, Delwart EL, Mullins JI, McCutchan FE, Eddy G, Burke DS. Genetic analysis of HIV-1 isolates from Brazil reveals the presence of two distinct genotypes. AIDS Res Hum Retrovirus 1994;10:561.
10. Sharp PM, Robertson DL, Gao F, Hahn BH. Origins and diversity of human immunodeficiency viruses. AIDS 1994;8(Suppl 1):S27.
11. Hirsch VM, Dapolito GA, Goldstein S, et al. A distinct African lentivirus from Sykes' monkeys. J Virol 1993;67:1517.
12. Huet T, Cheynier R, Meyerhans A, Roelants G, Wain-Hobson S. Genetic organization of a chimpanzee lentivirus related to HIV-1. Nature 1990;345:356.
13. Gurtler LG, Hauser PH, Eberle J, et al. A new subtype of human immunodeficiency virus type 1 (MVP-5180) from Cameroon. J Virol 1994;68:1581.
14. Vanden Haesevelde M, DeCourt J-L, De Leys RJ, et al. Genomic cloning and complete sequence analysis of a highly divergent African human immunodeficiency virus isolate. J Virol 1994;68:1586.
15. Janssens W, Nkengasong JN, Heyndrickx L, et al. Further evidence of the presence of genetically aberrant HIV-1 strains in Cameroon and Gabon. AIDS 1994;8:1012.
16. Myers G, Korber B, Wain-Hobson S, Smith RF, Pavlakis GN. Human retroviruses and AIDS, 1993. Los Alamos, NM: Los Alamos National Laboratory, 1993.
17. Srinivasan A, York D, Butler D, et al. Molecular characterization of HIV-1 isolated from a serum collected in 1976: nucleotide sequence comparison to recent isolates and generation of hybrid HIV. AIDS Res Hum Retrovirus 1989;5:121.
18. Nzilambi N, De Cock KM, Forthal DN, et al. The prevalence of infection with human immunodeficiency virus over a 10-year period in rural Zaire. N Engl J Med 1988;318:276.

19. Getchell JP, Hicks DR, Svinivasan A, et al. Human immunodeficiency virus isolated from a serum sample collected in 1976 in Central Africa. J Infect Dis 1987;156:833.

20. Hu W-S, Temin HM. Genetic consequences of packaging two RNA genomes in one retroviral particle: pseudodiploidy and high rate of genetic recombination. Proc Natl Acad Sci USA 1990; 87:1556.

21. Sabino EC, Shpaer EG, Morgado MG, et al. Identification of human immunodeficiency virus type 1 envelope genes recombinant between subtypes B and F in two epidemiologically linked individuals from Brazil. J Virol 1994;68:6340.

22. Holland J. Replication error, quasispecies populations, and extreme evolution rates of RNA viruses. In: Morse S, ed. Emerging viruses. Oxford: Oxford University Press, 1993:203.

23. Vartanian J-P, Meyerhans A, Asjo B, Wain-Hobson S. Selection, Recombination, and G→A Hypermutation of human immunodeficiency virus type 1 Genomes. J Virol 1991;65:1779.

24. Embretson J, Zupancic M, Ribas JL, et al. Massive covert infection of helper T lymphocytes and macrophages by HIV during the incubation period of AIDS. Nature 1993;362:359.

25. Pantaleo G, Graziosi C, Demarest JF, et al. HIV infection is active and progressive in lymphoid tissue during the clinically latent stage of disease. Nature 1993;362:355.

26. Kuiken CL, Zwart G, Baan E, Coutinho RA, van den Hoek AR, Goudsmit J. Increasing antigenic and genetic diversity of the V3 variable domain of the human immunodeficiency virus envelope protein in the course of the AIDS epidemic. Proc Natl Acad Sci USA 1993;90:9061.

27. Smith TF, Srinivasan A, Schochetman G, Marcus M, Myers G. The phylogenetic history of immunodeficiency viruses. Nature 1988;333:573.

28. Myers G, MacInnes K, Korber B. The emergence of simian/human immunodeficiency viruses. AIDS Res Hum Retroviruses 1992;8:373.

29. Myers G, MacInnes K, Myers L. Phylogenetic moments in the AIDS epidemic. In: Morse S, ed. Emerging viruses. Oxford: Oxford University Press, 1993:120.

30. Gojobori T, Moriyama EN, Ina Y, et al. Evolutionary origin of human and simian immune deficiency viruses. Proc Natl Acad Sci USA 1990;87:4108.

31. Eigen M, Nieselt-Struwe K. How old is the immunodeficiency virus? AIDS 1990;4(Suppl 1):S85.

32. Nahmias AJ, Weiss J, Yao X, et al. Evidence for human infection with an HTLV III/LAV-like virus in Central Africa, 1959. Lancet 1986;1:1279.

33. Corbitt G, Bailey AS, Williams G. HIV infection in Manchester, 1959. Lancet 1990;336:51.

34. Williams G, Stretton TB, Leonard JC. AIDS in 1959? Lancet 1983;2:1136.

35. Williams G, Stretton TB, Leonard JC. Cytomegalic inclusion disease and *Pneumocystis carinii* infection in an adult. Lancet 1960; 2:951.

36. Froland SS, Jenum P, Lindboe CF, Wefring KW, Linnestad PJ, Bohmer T. HIV-1 Infection in Norwegian Family Before 1970. Lancet 1988;1:1344.

37. Witte MH, Witte CL, Mennich LL, Finley PR, Drake WL Jr. AIDS in 1968. JAMA 1984;251:2657.

38. Garry RF, Witte MH, Gottlieb AA, et al. Documentation of an AIDS virus infection in the United States in 1968. JAMA 1988;260:2085.

39. Bryceson A, Tomkins A, Ridley D, et al. HIV-2-associated AIDS in the 1970s. Lancet 1988;2:221.

40. Kuiken CL, Korber BTM. Epidemiological significance of intra- and inter-person variation of HIV-1. AIDS 1994;8(Suppl 1):S73.

41. Yu X-F, Wang Z, Beyrer C, Celentano DD, Khamboonruang C, Nelson K. Phenotypic and genotypic characteristics of HIV-1 from AIDS patients in northern Thailand. J Virol 1995;69:4649.

42. Louwagie J, McCutchan F, Van der Groen G, et al. Genetic comparison of HIV-1 isolates from Africa, Europe, and North America. AIDS Res Hum Retrovirus 1992;8:1467.

43. Bruce C, Clegg C, Featherstone A, Smith J, Oram J. Sequence analysis of the gp120 region of the *env* gene of Ugandan human immunodeficiency proviruses from a single individual. AIDS Res Hum Retrovirus 1993;9:357.

44. Oram JD, Downing RG, Roff M, et al. Sequence analysis of the V3 loop regions of the *env* genes of Ugandan human immunodeficiency proviruses. AIDS Res Hum Retrovirus 1991;7:605.

45. Dietrich U, Grez M, von Briesen H, et al. HIV-1 Strains from India are highly divergent from prototypic African and US/European strains, but are linked to a South African isolate. AIDS 1993;7:23.

46. Murphy E, Korber B, Georges-Courbot M-C, et al. Diversity of V3 region sequences of human immunodeficiency virus type 1 from the Central African Republic. AIDS Res Hum Retrovirus 1993;9:997.

47. Orloff GM, Kalish ML, Chiphangwi J, et al. V3 loops of HIV-1 specimens from pregnant women in Malawi uniformly lack a potential N-linked glycosylation site. AIDS Res Hum Retrovirus 1993;9:705.

48. Potts KE, Kalish ML, Lott T, et al. Genetic heterogeneity of the V3 region of the HIV-1 envelope glycoprotein in Brazil. AIDS 1993;7:1191.

49. WHO Network for HIV isolation and characterization. HIV type 1 variation in World Health Organization-sponsored vaccine evaluation sites: genetic screening, sequence analysis, and preliminary biological characterization of selected viral strains. AIDS Res Hum Retrovirus 1994; 10:1327.

50. Huet T, Dazza M-C, Brun-Vezinet F, Roelants GE, Wain-Hobson S. A highly defective HIV-1 strain isolated from a healthy Gabonese individual presenting an atypical Western blot. AIDS 1989;3:707.

51. Louwagie J, McCutchan F, Mascola J, et al. Technical challenges and scientific issues. AIDS Res Hum Retrovirus 1993;9(Suppl 1):S147.

52. Salminen M, Nykanen A, Brummer-Korvenkontio H, Kantanen ML, Liitsola K, Leinikki P. Molecular epidemiology of HIV-1 based on phylogenetic analysis of in vivo gag p7/p9 direct sequences. Virology 1993;195:185.

53. Janssens W, Heyndrickx L, Van de Peer Y, et al. Molecular phylogeny of part of the *env* gene of HIV-1 strains isolated in Cote d'Ivoire. AIDS 1994;8:21.

54. Bobkov A, Cheingsong-Popov R, Garaev M, et al. Identification of a new *env* G subtype and heterogeneity of HIV-1 strains in the Russian federation and Belarez. AIDS 1994;8:1649.

55. Dumitrescu O, Kalish ML, Kliks SC, Bandea CI, Levy JA. Characterization of human immunodeficiency virus type 1 isolates from children in Romania: identification of a new envelope subtype. J Infect Dis 1994;169:281.

56. Guo H-G, Reitz MS, Gallo RC, Ko YC, Chang KSS. A new subtype of HIV-1 gag sequence detected in Taiwan. AIDS Res Hum Retrovirus 1993;9:925.

57. Grez M, Dietrich U, Balfe P, et al. Genetic analysis of human immunodeficiency virus type 1 and 2 (HIV-1 and HIV-2) mixed infections in India reveals a recent spread of HIV-1 and HIV-2 from a single ancestor for each of these viruses. J Virol 1994;68:2161.

58. Ichimura H, Kliks SC, Visrutaratna S, Ou C-Y, Kalish M, Levy JA. Biological, serological, and genetic characterization of HIV-1 subtype E isolates from northern Thailand. AIDS Res Hum Retrovirus 1994;10:263.

59. Alizon M, Wain-Hobson S, Montagnier L, Sonigo P. Genetic variability of the AIDS virus: nucleotide sequence analysis of two isolates from African patients. Cell 1986;46:63.

60. Hattori T, Shiozaki K, Eda Y, et al. Characteristics of the principal neutralizing determinant of HIV-1 prevalent in Japan. AIDS Res Hum Retrovirus 1991;7:825.

61. Kroner BL, Rosenberg PS, Aledort LM, Alvord WG, Goedert JJ. HIV-1 infection incidence among persons with hemophilia in the United States and Western Europe, 1978–1990. J Acquir Immune Defic Syndr 1994;7:279.

62. Reeves WC, Cuevas M, Arosemena JR, et al. Human immunodeficiency virus infection in the Republic of Panama. Am J Trop Med Hyg 1988;39:398.

63. Weniger BG, Limpakarnjanarat K, Ungchusak K, et al. The epidemiology of HIV infection and AIDS in Thailand. AIDS 1991;5(Suppl 2):S71.

64. Weniger BG, Takebe Y, Ou C-Y, Yamazaki S. The molecular epidemiology of HIV in Asia. AIDS 1994;8(Suppl 2):S1.

65. Traisupa A, Wongba C, Taylor DN. AIDS and prevalence of antibody to human immunodeficiency virus (HIV) in high risk groups in Thailand. Genitourin Med 1987;63:106.

66. Wright NH, Vanichseni S, Akarasewi P, Wasi C, Choopanya K. Was the 1988 HIV epidemic among Bangkok's injecting drug users: a common source outbreak? AIDS 1994;8:529.

67. Poshyachinda V. Drugs and AIDS in Southeast Asia. Forensic Sci Int 1993;62:15.

68. VanLandingham MJ, Suprasert S, Sittitrai W, Vaddhanaphuti C, Grandjean N. Sexual activity among never-married men in northern Thailand. Demography 1993;30:297.

69. Nelson KE, Celentano DD, Suprasert S, et al. Risk factors for HIV infection among young adult men in northern Thailand. JAMA 1993;270:955.
70. Nopkesorn T, Mastro TD, Sangkharomya S, et al. HIV-1 infection in young men in northern Thailand. AIDS 1993;7:1233.
71. Kramer R. Nigerian drug trade taints U.S. relations. The Washington Post 1994;May 25:A16.
72. Chotpitayasunondh T, Chearskul S, Siriwasin W, Roongpisuthipong A, Young N, Shaffer N. HIV-1 vertical transmission in Bangkok, Thailand. Abstract for the Tenth International Conference on AIDS. Yokohama, Japan, August 7–12, 1994.
73. Global AIDS News. Cambodia faces new threat of AIDS. Newslett World Health Organ Global Programme IDS 1993;2:8.
74. Takebe Y, Pau C-P, Oka S, Ou C-Y, Weniger BG, Yamazaki S, et al. Identification of Thailand HIV-1 subtypes in Japan. Ninth international conference on AIDS. Abstract PO-A11-0178. Berlin, Germany, June 6–11, 1993.
75. Artenstein AA, Coppola J, Brown AE, et al. Multiple introductions of HIV-1 subtype E into the western hemisphere. Lancet 2:1197.
76. Potts M, Anderson R, Boily MC. Slowing the spread of human immunodeficiency virus in developing countries. Lancet 1991;338:608.
77. Santos BR, Beck EJ, Peixoto MF, Kitchen V, Weber J. Changing patterns of HIV-1 transmission in southern Brazil 1985–1991. J STD AIDS 1994;5:202.
78. Li PC, Yeoh EK. Current epidemiological trends of HIV infection in Asia. AIDS Clin Rev 1992;1:1.
79. Mertens TE, Burton A, Stoneburner R, et al. Global estimates and epidemiology of HIV infections and AIDS. AIDS 1994;8(Suppl 1);S361.
80. Shilts R. And the band played on. New York: St. Martin's Press, 1987.
81. Markovitz DM. Infection with the human immunodeficiency virus type 2. Ann Intern Med 1993;118:211.
82. De Cock KM, Adjorlolo G, Ekpini E, et al. Epidemiology and transmission of HIV-2. JAMA 1993;270:2083.
83. Mann JM, Chin J, Piot P, Quinn T. The international epidemiology of AIDS. Sci Am 1988;259:82.
84. Ou C-Y, Takebe Y, Weniger BG, et al. Independent introduction of two major HIV-1 genotypes into distinct high-risk populations in Thailand. Lancet 1993;341:1171.
85. Mastro TD, Satten GA, Nopkesorn T, Sangkharomya S, Longini IM Jr. Probability of female-to-male transmission of HIV-1 in Thailand. Lancet 1994;343:204.
86. Anderson RM, May RM. Population biology of infectious diseases: part I. Nature 1979;280:361.
87. Kramer A, Biggar RJ, Hampl H, et al. Immunologic markers of progression to acquired immunodeficiency syndrome are time-dependent and illness-specific. Am J Epidemiol 1992;136:71.
88. MacDonell KB, Chmiel JS, Poggensee L, Wu S, Phair JP. Predicting progression to AIDS: combined usefulness of CD4 lymphocyte counts and p24 antigenemia. Am J Med 1990;89:706.
89. Easterbrook PJ, Margolick J, Saah AJ, et al. Racial differences in rate of CD4 decline in HIV-1 infected homosexual men. Eighth international conference in AIDS. Abstract MOCOO64, Amsterdam, July 1992.
90. Mascola JR, Louwagie J, McCutchan FE, et al. Two antigenically distinct subtypes of HIV-1: viral genotype predicts neutralization immunotype. J Infect Dis 1994;169:48.
91. Zolla-Pazner S, O'Leary J, Burda S, Gorny MK, Mascola J, McCutchan F. Serotyping of primary human immunodeficiency virus type I isolates from diverse geographic locations by flow cytometry. J Virol 1995; 69:3807.
92. Gould SJ, Eldredge N. Punctuated equilibrium comes of age. Nature 1993;366:223.

AIDS: Biology, Diagnosis, Treatment and
Prevention, fourth edition, edited by Vincent T.
DeVita, Jr., Samuel Hellman, and Steven A.
Rosenberg. Lippincott–Raven Publishers, © 1997

CHAPTER 8

Epidemiology and Natural History of Human Immunodeficiency Virus Type 2

Phyllis Kanki

Human immunodeficiency virus type 2 (HIV-2) was first described in Senegal, West Africa, in 1985.[1] Subsequent characterization of the virus and reports of related AIDS cases suggested to some researchers that HIV-2 biology could be readily predicted from studies of HIV-1 and that a second acquired immunodeficiency syndrome (AIDS) epidemic was imminent.[2] During the past decade, research has further elucidated the virologic similarities and differences between HIV-2 and HIV-1.[3,4] Epidemiologic and natural history studies of HIV-2 have provided the foundation for our appreciation of the unique characteristics of this second HIV. The study of HIV-2 has been important for public health in endemic areas and for the HIV and AIDS research field overall. Through comparative studies of HIV-2 and HIV-1, we have had the opportunity to better appreciate the spectrum of HIV epidemiology and pathogenesis.

HIV-2 DIAGNOSIS

Studies of HIV-2 epidemiology and natural history depend on accurate HIV-2 viral diagnoses. The same procedures for serologic testing, virus culture, and genetic diagnostics such as the polymerase chain reaction (PCR) that were developed for HIV-1 have been modified for HIV-2 diagnosis and improved over the years. The similarity of HIV-2 to HIV-1 on genetic and antigenic levels has necessitated the development and implementation of type-specific diagnostic assays.

The initial HIV antibody tests in the middle to late 1980s were developed for HIV-1 diagnosis using HIV-1 antigens, and the degree of cross-reactivity and specificity for HIV-2 was variable. The extensive cross-reactivity in antibodies directed at conserved antigens such as Gag and Pol was responsible for the capability of the original enzyme-linked immunoabsorbent assay (ELISA) HIV-1 tests to detect 75% to 90% of HIV-2–positive sera.[5-7] In June 1992, the U.S. Food and Drug Administration recommended that all blood donations be screened with serologic assays for HIV-1 and HIV-2.[8] Combination HIV-1 and HIV-2 ELISA screening tests are employed in all U.S. blood banks and most other clinical diagnostic settings. Because the combination screening assays are incapable of differentiating HIV types, HIV-1 and HIV-2 confirmatory assays must be performed on all ELISA-positive samples to obtain a type-specific diagnosis.

Immunoblots demonstrating a profile of major structural gene product recognition are typically used for HIV-1 and HIV-2 diagnoses, and standard criteria for HIV-2 blot diagnosis has been established by the World Health Organization.[9] HIV-2–specific diagnosis by immunoblot requires antibody reactivity to Env, Gag, and Pol antigens. In the absence of reactivity to Gag or Pol antigens, the presence of reactivity to two envelope antigens (ie, gp120 and gp32, transmembrane protein) is required.[9]

Various investigations have focused on identifying type-specific antigens, forming the basis of confirmatory tests that differentiate HIV-1 from HIV-2. These have included envelope-based synthetic peptides[10-13] or larger, bacterially expressed peptides assays.[14-16] The tests varied in sensitivity and specificity, and because most were selected for specificity, sensitivity often was compromised. In Senegal, my colleagues and I used semipurified, recombinant-expressed HIV-1 (566) and HIV-2 (996) Env proteins, homologous with the N-terminal region of gp41 (HIV-1) and gp35 (HIV-2) for HIV type-specific screening.[14,15] These antigens were evaluated in an immunoblot assay and then adapted to a dot-blot miniblotter technique. The relative cost of this assay was 10-fold lower than conventional commercial assays, and the test

Phyllis J. Kanki, Associate Professor of Pathobiology, Harvard AIDS Institute, Harvard School of Public Health, 655 Huntington Avenue, Boston, MA 02115.

could be easily performed in less than 2 hours. When the two Env peptides were used together, there was virtually 100% specificity and sensitivity for detecting and typing HIV-positive sera in immunoblot and dot-blot formats.[14]

Since 1986, several West African countries have reported significant rates of HIV-1 and HIV-2 infections, and individuals with dual HIV serologic profiles have been described.[17–20] The dual antibody profile is characterized by antibodies with equally strong reactivity to the Env antigens of HIV-1 and HIV-2, demonstrated by immunoblot and/or radioimmunoprecipitation analysis (RIPA). Several explanations for this type of dual HIV serologic reactivity must be entertained, including extensive cross-reactivity by either of the HIV types, dual infection, infection by one type and exposure to a second type, or infection with an intermediate virus.

Isolation of HIV-1 and HIV-2 has been reported from selected dual HIV cases,[21] and PCR evidence for both viruses has been reported in similar populations.[22–24] Two studies were reported from the Ivory Coast in which 21 (61.7%) of 34 serologically diagnosed HIV-infected persons with dual reactivity were confirmed by PCR.[22] A second report confirmed dual reactivity in 12 (33.3%) of 36 persons.[23] In Senegal, with an HIV-1 prevalence of 4.7% and an HIV-2 prevalence of 10.8% in a cohort of 1354 registered prostitutes,[25] theory would predict about 0.51% dual reactivity if the viruses were behaving independently. My colleagues and I used a panel of HIV-2 and HIV-1 assays, including immunoblot, RIPA, recombinant Env peptides, and Vpx/Vpu testing, yielding a 0.7% rate of dual reactivity, compatible with the expected estimate. This rate was further confirmed by PCR analysis, demonstrating HIV-1– and HIV-2–specific sequences in all peripheral blood mononuclear cell DNA of individuals with the dual HIV serologic profile (Kanki P, unpublished observations).

The dual infection measured by DNA-PCR occurs in populations with significant prevalence rates of both virus types. Although the existence of an intermediate virus in these populations cannot be ruled out, it is apparent that rates of dual HIV reactivity have been inflated in the past because of suboptimal specificity of the serologic methods employed. Because of improvement of serologic assays and newer genetic methods for differentiating the two viruses, current seroprevalence rates for dual HIV reactivity should be considered more reliable.

GLOBAL DISTRIBUTION OF HIV-2

The discovery of HIV-2 in West Africa prompted numerous serologic surveys to further identify its geographic distribution. Direct comparisons of prevalence rates in diverse countries are difficult because of differences in study design and diagnostic methodologies; this is particularly pertinent in comparing rates of dual HIV infection. Nonetheless, during the past decade, significant HIV-2 infection has been well documented in most West African countries (Fig. 8-1). A second epidemiologic pattern of

HIV-2 infection has been suggested from reports of HIV-2 in Portugal and in Mozambique, Angola, southwestern India, and Brazil, all areas with former ties to Portugal. Case reports or exceedingly low HIV-2 prevalence rates have been documented in other parts of Africa, Europe, the Americas, the Middle East, and Asia, but its spread has been quite limited. This estimate is further supported by the reduced sexual and perinatal transmission rate of the virus.[26] The data suggest that HIV-2 has been present in certain populations long enough to establish endemic infection and that its spread outside of these endemic areas is limited by a low transmission potential.

The prevalence of HIV-2 infection in West Africa varies greatly among different countries and groups (Table 8-1).[6,17,18,20,25–28] The highest rates of HIV-2 infection in the general population have been found in Guinea-Bissau, where seroprevalence levels as high as 13.4% have been demonstrated in asymptomatic men.[29] In Guinea-Bissau, Gambia, Cape Verde, and Senegal, the prevalence of HIV-2 infection exceeds that of infection with HIV-1, but HIV-1 infection appears to be increasing.[3,6,25,29,30–34] Evidence from cross-sectional prevalence studies has been presented from Guinea-Bissau,[29] Ivory Coast,[35] and Senegal,[25,36] where a disproportionate increase in HIV-1 prevalence compared with HIV-2 infection has been described.

In most other countries of West Africa, including Burkina Faso, Ghana, Ivory Coast, Nigeria, and Mali, HIV-1 infection is 3- to 24-fold more prevalent than HIV-2 infection.[6,26,37–40] The rapid spread of HIV-1 in West Africa has been documented, and prevalence and incidence trends indicate that this will become the predominant HIV type in much of the region.[41] The existence of significant rates of HIV-1 and HIV-2 in many of these countries begs the question of what will be the outcome of these related viruses as they interact at a population level.

Angola and Mozambique, two African countries outside of West Africa have exhibited significant rates of HIV-2 in the past, but more recent data are not available.[28,34,42] These former Portuguese colonies maintain ties with other former colonies such as Guinea-Bissau and Cape Verde, both HIV-2 endemic regions. Aside from these two exceptions, HIV-2 has been virtually absent from various at-risk populations and AIDS patients in Central and East Africa, where significant HIV-1 infection exists.[28,43,44]

In the late 1980s, serologic survey data from Portugal coupled with data from Mozambique and Angola suggested that former colonial ties might play a role in the unusual distribution of HIV-2. Although data are still accumulating in support of this hypothesis, the rates of HIV-2 infection in Portugal and perhaps neighboring Spain are distinctly higher than other European countries. In Portugal, HIV-2 accounted for 10% to 12% of HIV infections,[45,46] and 48% of HIV-2–infected persons had some link with West Africa or Angola. In the HIV-2–infected persons for whom no link with Africa was established, presumed risk factors were transfusion of blood or blood products (74% of cases), het-

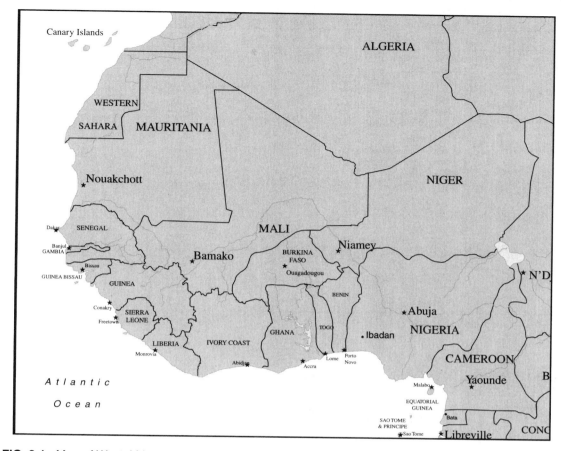

FIG. 8-1. Map of West Africa.

erosexual contact (21% of cases), and injecting drug use (4% of cases).[45] In Portugal, a greater number of cases of HIV-2 than HIV-1 infection are associated with ties to Africa, blood transfusion, and heterosexual contact, and a lower proportion are associated with male-to-male sex and injecting drug use.[45,46] Of the 34 cases of HIV-2 infection recognized in neighboring Spain, 31 were in African immigrants, and 3 were Spanish seamen with histories of possible heterosexual exposure to HIV-2–infected persons in Africa.[47]

The detection and reporting of HIV-2 infection in other European countries has depended somewhat on when HIV-2 testing was instituted as a public health measure and when research studies demonstrated significant rates. France was one of the first countries to institute HIV-2 testing of blood donors, and several HIV-2 cases were identified.[48] Of 75 HIV-2–infected persons studied in Paris, 58 were of African origin, 12 were European, and 5 were Caribbean.[49] In a 1988 to 1993 survey of 15,611 individuals attending an anonymous test site in Paris, a 0.07% rate of HIV-2 infection was found, compared with a rate of 0.23% for HIV-1 infection.[50] To a lesser degree, other European countries have reported sporadic cases of HIV-2 infection in large serosurveys; the cases usually had links to West Africa.[28,44,51] The relatively high rates of HIV-2 infection

reported in France may reflect significant ties with former colonies in French West Africa.

In North America, only sporadic cases of HIV-2 infection have been reported.[52] Of the 17 HIV-2–infected persons detected through case reports by the Centers for Disease Control and Prevention (CDC), 13 were West Africans.[52] Another 15 infections were recognized in United States through serologic surveillance, but the origins of the infected persons were not determined. Only one HIV-2–infected blood donor has been identified in the United States, indicating that HIV-2 infection is extremely rare in the U.S. blood donor population.[53] A 1993 study of sexually transmitted disease (STD) centers, intravenous drug users, and clients at HIV testing sites found 2 HIV-2–positive results among the 31,533 sera tested; both HIV-2–positive persons were from STD centers in the Northeast.[54] Out understanding of HIV-2 epidemiology indicates that select groups in the United States with ties to West Africa or Portugal may be important groups for HIV-2 surveillance.

Elsewhere in the Americas, HIV-2 infection has been documented in persons originating from the Caribbean, including Cuba.[55] Although comprehensive surveillance data have not been published, some HIV-2 infections were identified in Cuban soldiers returning from campaigns in Africa. The epidemiologic status of HIV-2 infection in

TABLE 8-1. *Prevalence of HIV-1 and HIV-2 infections in selected populations*

Site	Group	HIV-1 (%)	HIV-2 (%)	Dual (%)	Year (Ref)
Dakar, Senegal	Blood donors	0.5	0.2	0	1993 (98)
	Male STD paitents	1.4	1.1	0	1993 (98)
	Pregnant women	0.3	0.5	0	1994 (27)
	Prostitutes	4.7	10.8	0.7	1993 (25)
Gambia	General population	0.1	1.6		1988 (33)
	Pregnant women	0.8	0		1992 (30)
	Prostitutes	0.6	25		1988 (32)
Abidjan, Ivory Coast	Pregnant women	14.0	1.0	1.0	1993 (35)
	Male STD patients	14.0	2.0	4.0	1993 (35)
	Prostitutes	41.7	6.9	20.8	1993 (41)
Maiduguri, Lagos, Nigeria	Pregnant women	1.9	0.1	0.24	1994 (99)
	Prostitutes	12.3	2.1	0.7	1993 (39)
	Blood donors	3.8	3.2		1993 (38)
	Male STD patients	6.6	6.9		1993 (38)
Kumasi, Ghana	Hospital admissions	6.0	0.8	5.8	1994 (37)
Bissau, Guinea-Bissau	Police officers	0.3	13.4	0.3	1992 (29)
	Prostitutes	0	16.7	0	1987 (100)
Goa, Bombay, India	STD patients	9.8	4.9		1994 (63)
	STD patients & prostitutes	30.9	1.6	6.7	1991 (61)
	Homosexual risk	12.7	4.8	3.2	1994 (62)

STD, sexually transmitted disease.

Brazil, which has important links with West Africa and Portugal, has been confusing. Early reports of dual serologic reactivity in residents of Brazil were interpreted as indicative of HIV-2 infection,[56,57] but subsequent studies showed no evidence of HIV-2 infection in high-risk Brazilian populations.[58] A more recent report of hospitalized patients found monotypic HIV-2 and dual HIV infections demonstrated by PCR.[59]

The rate of HIV-2 is significant in the southwestern Maharashtra state of India.[60] Of the HIV-positive serum samples from patients with STDs or other conditions in Bombay, 76% were reactive to HIV-1, 4% to HIV-2, and 20% to both viruses.[61] A later study of Bombay men attending an STD clinic with a history of homosexual behavior reported a 4.8% rate of HIV-2 infection, 12.7% rate of HIV-1 infection, and 3.2% rate of dual HIV infection.[62] Goa, a former Portuguese colony situated south of Bombay on the western coast of India, reported a 4.9% rate of HIV-2 infection among STD patients and 9.8% rate of HIV-1 infection.[63] Epidemiologic data on the prevalence and distribution of HIV-1 and HIV-2 infections in other parts of India are still being collected and analyzed. As of 1995, significant HIV-2 infection has not been reported in other parts of Asia.

HIV-2 infection is well established in West Africa, and based on survey data from the past decade, epidemic spread of HIV-2 outside of West Africa seems unlikely. The potential association of HIV-2 geographic distribution with historic colonial ties and current links between diverse parts of the world is intriguing.[51,64] Studies have shown that areas of the world with significant migration of individuals from HIV-2 endemic areas should be high-priority areas for further surveillance efforts.

TRANSMISSION OF HIV-2

Data suggest that HIV-2 can be transmitted by the same modes as HIV-1, but the rates of HIV-2 transmission are significantly lower. Case reports of HIV-2 transmitted by blood and blood products have been published, but widespread HIV testing in blood bank settings has limited the risk of this mode of transmission.[8,65] The most common modes of HIV transmission in HIV-2 endemic areas are perinatal and heterosexual transmission. Because most West African countries have been afflicted with HIV-1 and HIV-2 infections, direct comparison of transmission rates between the two viruses has been possible.

Perinatal Transmission

Reported rates of perinatal transmission of HIV-1 have ranged from 13% to 32% in industrialized countries and from 25% to 48% in developing countries.[66] Although investigation of HIV-2 perinatal transmission has been more limited, numerous studies indicate that perinatal transmission of HIV-2 can occur but that this is much less frequent than observed with HIV-1 infection. Cruder indications that perinatal transmission can occur come from virologic and epidemiologic studies. HIV-2 has been isolated from infants of HIV-2–infected mothers.[67] A family cluster has been reported in which a mother and two of her children were infected with HIV-2,[68] and other mother-child couples have been described in which both were HIV-2 positive.[69] Serologic concordance between HIV-2–positive women and their children was rare, and cross-sectional surveys in different West African countries have shown pediatric HIV-2 infection to be extremely uncommon.[30,70,71]

TABLE 8-2. *Perinatal transmission rates of HIV-2 and HIV-1*

Study Site	HIV-2		HIV-1		
	n	% Transmitted	n	% Transmitted	Reference
Guinea Bissau	53	0			72
France	41	0	260	21	73
Ivory Coast	93	1.2	138	25	74
Senegal	29	3.4	29	34	75

Prospective studies of HIV-2 perinatal transmission have been conducted in Guinea-Bissau, Ivory Coast, France, and Senegal, and all have demonstrated extremely low rates of perinatal transmission of HIV-2 compared with HIV-1 (Table 8-2).[27,72–75] In studies that compared HIV-2 and HIV-1 transmission, the rate of HIV-1 transmission was 10- to 20-fold higher than that of HIV-2. No information is available concerning HIV-2 transmission by breast milk. Because all available data show HIV-2 infection to be uncommon in children, transmission of HIV-2 by breast milk must be extremely rare.

Heterosexual Transmission

Population groups that are followed prospectively with sequential HIV serology allow direct measurement of HIV incidence. HIV-1 and HIV-2 incidence trends have been reported for registered female prostitutes in Dakar, Senegal, who were followed for 9 years (Kanki PJ, unpublished data).[36] Between 1985 and 1994, the overall incidence of HIV-2 was 0.92 per 100 person-years of observation (PYO) and was 1.15 per 100 PYO for HIV-1. Over the 9-year period, the annual incidence of HIV-1 dramatically increased, with a 1.4-fold increased risk per year and a 12- to 17-fold increase in risk over the entire study period. The incidence of HIV-2 remained stable despite higher HIV-2 prevalence. In this high-risk group, the heterosexual transmission of HIV-2 was significantly slower than that of HIV-1, which strongly suggests differences in the infectivity potentials of these two related immunodeficiency viruses.

Using mathematical modeling techniques, the efficiency of heterosexual transmission of HIV-2 has been estimated to be five to nine times less than that of HIV-1 per sexual act with an infected partner.[76] Prospective studies of discordant couples would be useful in further assessing rates of heterosexual transmission of HIV-1 and HIV-2, particularly in determining the relation of viral load and immunodeficiency in the index case to the transmission event.

DISEASES ASSOCIATED WITH HIV-2 INFECTION

Many case reports and cross-sectional studies of hospitalized patients have described AIDS associated with HIV-2 infection.[2,77] Similar opportunistic conditions, including tuberculosis and AIDS associated with HIV-2 infection,

were described in these studies.[33,77–80] In West African HIV-2 AIDS cases, disease characteristics have included tuberculosis, chronic diarrhea, and *Candida* infections similar to HIV-1–associated AIDS. Central nervous system involvement has also been described in HIV-2–infected persons.[81,82]

In an autopsy study of 294 HIV-infected patients in the Ivory Coast, tuberculosis, bacteremia with a predominance of gram-negative rods, and cerebral toxoplasmosis were responsible for a significant proportion of all HIV-positive deaths.[83] Forty-three cadavers were HIV-2 positive, and 40 (93%) of 43 had died of HIV-related disease. The pathologies in HIV-2–positive cadavers were similar to HIV-1–positive cadavers, except for three conditions, including severe multiorgan cytomegalovirus infection, multinucleated giant cell encephalitis, and intrahepatic or extrahepatic cholangitis. All three lesions were associated with extreme immunosuppression, suggesting a prolonged survival with HIV-2 infection. These data suggest a modified natural history for HIV-2; patients may survive longer in the terminal stage of HIV-2 infection.

NATURAL HISTORY OF HIV-2

Studies of HIV-infected, asymptomatic individuals followed over time have been critical to our understanding of HIV pathogenesis. The long latency period of the HIV viruses has made such prospective studies lengthy and logistically difficult. Natural history studies of HIV in heterosexually exposed individuals are rare, particularly in Africa, where HIV infection is so prevalent.[84–87] However, from the time that HIV-2 was discovered, it was critical to determine if the disease progression and natural history of this virus would differ from that of HIV-1.

Studies from Dakar, Senegal, have described the natural history of HIV-2 and HIV-1 during a 9-year period. These studies are unique because the presence of HIV-2 and HIV-1 in Senegal allowed the measurement and comparison of disease development for both viruses.[87] Among the 103 HIV-2–infected women followed, one AIDS case was observed after 435 PYO, yielding an AIDS incidence of 0.23 per 100 PYO (95% confidence interval [CI] = 0.01–1.28). The rate of AIDS development for 33 seroincident HIV-2–infected women was 0 (95% CI = 0–3.30). Among the 46 seroprevalent HIV-1–infected women, 1 AIDS case yielded an AIDS incidence of 0.94 per 100 PYO (95% CI = 0.02–5.23), and

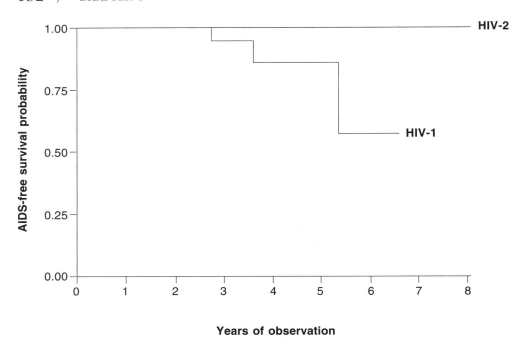

FIG. 8-2. AIDS-free survival in seroincident women according to serostatus.

for 32 seroincident HIV-1–infected women, the rate was 4.85 per 100 PYO (95% CI = 1.32–12.4). Kaplan-Meier analysis comparing HIV-2 and HIV-1 seroincident women (Fig. 8-2), showed a 60% rate of AIDS-free survival for HIV-1 incident women at 5 years after infection. In contrast, none of the HIV-2 seroincident women developed AIDS, who therefore exhibited a 100% probability of AIDS-free survival after 5 years, a statistically significant difference (log rank test; $P = 0.01$; Kanki PJ, unpublished data). These differences in survival probabilities between HIV-2 and HIV-1 were also seen for CDC stage IV disease and CD4+ lymphocyte counts below 400 cells/mm^3 as outcomes (Kanki PJ, unpublished data).[87]

Differences in the rate of HIV-2 transmission and disease development may reflect characteristics of the virus or elicited host responses that result in a lower virus burden. Immunologic studies have also supported the clinical observations of HIV-related disease: CD4+ lymphocyte counts and CD4 to CD8 ratios appear reduced in HIV-2–infected healthy carriers, although less dramatically than in HIV-1–infected carriers.[32,83–88] This has been true in subset values evaluated cross-sectionally and over time. Similar results were observed with evaluation of delayed-type hypersensitivity measured by skin test anergy to tuberculin antigen (ie, PPD skin test).[86,87] Neopterin and β_2-microglobulin levels were elevated in HIV-2–infected individuals, although less so than in HIV-1–infected persons.[89,90] Lymphocyte proliferative responses to mitogens and antigens were also less pronounced in HIV-2 infection.[32] Lower and stable plasma tumor necrosis factor-α levels have been found in HIV-2–infected patients with lower viral loads and higher CD4+ lymphocyte counts, suggesting a more efficient and appropriate immune response in HIV-2 infection.[91]

Evidence for a lower viral burden in HIV-2–infected individuals has been reported from virus isolation and PCR studies.[92–94] The isolation rate of HIV-2 from peripheral blood mononuclear cells or plasma of asymptomatic HIV-2–infected individuals was lower than the isolation rate for HIV-1.[92] At lower CD4+ lymphocyte counts, virus isolation was equally efficient in both infections. Quantitative PCR provides a more reliable measurement of viral burden or load. Studies in Gambia and Senegal suggest that proviral HIV-2 copies increase with disease development and with the drop of CD4+ lymphocytes.[93,94] When compared with HIV-1–infected individuals, the proviral copy number was significantly lower throughout most of the course of HIV-2 infection.[93,95]

HIV-2 is known to exhibit genetic variation, similar to HIV-1, although less well studied. Interpatient variation in the HIV-2 V3 loop was comparable to that seen in HIV-1.[96] Evaluation of intrapatient variation in the V3 region of HIV-2 in asymptomatic and symptomatic individuals followed over time has shown a lower variation than for HIV-1.[95] This lower intrapatient variation appears to be a distinct feature of HIV-2 infection that may result from decreased viral burden and that may contribute to lower rates of transmission and disease development.

HIV-2 PROTECTION FROM HIV-1 INFECTION

The low transmissibility and long AIDS-free survival time of HIV-2 infection has suggested the possibility that this virus might protect against subsequent infection by HIV-1. During a 9-year period in Dakar, Senegal, the seroincidence of both HIVs was measured in a cohort of female prostitutes.[97] For the 618 women initially HIV seronegative, 61 seroconverted to HIV-1; the overall HIV-1 incidence was 2.53 per 100 PYO. Among 187 women seropositive for HIV-2, 7 women seroconverted to a dual HIV reactive status. All 7 women were PCR positive for both viruses, and all demonstrated seroconversion to both recombinant Env type-specific proteins. The HIV-1 incidence in the HIV-2 positive group was 1.07 per 100 PYO, lower than the incidence among the HIV-seronegative group. A multivariate Poisson regression analysis included age, nationality, age at registration, incident gonorrhea, incident HIV-1 infection, and calendar year. The multivariate analysis indicated a decrease in the risk of HIV-1 infection was associated with prior HIV-2 infection, with an adjusted relative risk of 0.32 ($P = 0.008$). In the reverse analysis, HIV-1 did not protect against subsequent HIV-2 infection. Further studies are needed to understand the cross-protective mechanisms that may be involved in this interaction, but the data suggest a novel mode of inducing HIV-1 immunity.

CONCLUSIONS

Epidemiologic and natural history studies of HIV-2 infection conducted in large part by West African researchers have amply demonstrated the unique biologic properties of this virus. The data suggest differences between HIV-2 and HIV-1 in virologic features, geographic distribution, risk determinants for prevalent and incident infection, distinct temporal trends in incidence, and differences in perinatal transmission rates and incubation periods to the development of AIDS. The worldwide distribution of HIV-2 poses intriguing questions regarding the longevity of this virus in human populations and how former colonialist relationships have appeared to spread the virus within and outside of Africa. The epidemiologic differences in the rates of transmission and disease progression are striking and worthy of further study. The data indicating protection of HIV-2–infected individuals from subsequent HIV-1 suggest that further understanding of HIV-2 immunity and cross-immunity may be useful for HIV vaccine development. Additional comparative studies of HIV-2 and HIV-1 infection should continue to provide new insights into the pathogenesis of HIV and its ultimate control and prevention.

REFERENCES

1. Barin F, MBoup S, Denis F, et al. Serological evidence for virus related to simian T-lymphotropic retrovirus III in residents of West Africa. Lancet 1985;2:1387.
2. Clavel F, Guetard D, Brun-Vezinet F, et al. Isolation of a new human retrovirus from West African patients with AIDS. Science 1986;233:343.
3. Marlink R. The biology and epidemiology of HIV-2. In: Essex M, MBoup S, Kanki P, Kalengayi M, eds. AIDS in Africa. New York: Raven Press, 1994:47.
4. Markovitz DM. Infection with the human immunodeficiency virus type 2. Ann Intern Med 1993;118:211.
5. Denis F, Leonard G, Sangare A, et al. Comparison of 10 enzyme immunoassays for the detection of HIV-1 antibody to human immunodeficiency virus type 2 in West African sera. J Clin Microbiol 1988;26:1000.
6. Kanki PJ. West African human retroviruses related to STLV-III. AIDS 1987;1:408.
7. George R, Rayfield M, Phillips S, et al. Efficacies of U.S. food and drug administration-licensed HIV-1 screening enzyme immunoassays for detecting antibodies to HIV-2. AIDS 1990;4:321.
8. Parkman PD. Recommendations for the prevention of human immunodeficiency virus (HIV) transmission by blood and blood products (Memorandum to all registered blood establishments. Bethesda, MD: Food and Drug Administration, Center for Biologics Evaluation and Research, 1990.
9. Anonymous. Recommendations for interpretation of HIV-2 Western blot results. Wkly Epidemiol Rec 1990;10:74.
10. Gnann JW Jr, McCormick JB, Mitchell S, Nelson JA, Oldstone MBA. Synthetic peptides immunoassay distinguishes HIV type 1 and HIV type 2 infections. Science 1987;237:1346.
11. Norrby E, Biberfeld G, Chiodi F, et al. Discrimination between antibodies to HIV and to related retroviruses using site-directed serology. Nature 1987;329:248.
12. Baillou A, Barin F, Leonard G, et al. Competitive enzyme-immunoassays using native viral antigens to discriminate between HIV-1 and HIV-2 infections. J Virol Methods 1990;29:81.
13. Broliden PA, Ruden U, Ouattara AS, et al. Specific synthetic peptides for detection of and discrimination between HIV-1 and HIV-2 infection. J Acquir Immune Defic Syndr 1991;4:952.
14. Gueye-NDiaye A, Clark RJ, Samuel KP, et al. Cost-effective diagnosis of HIV-1 and HIV-2 by recombinant-expressed env peptide (566/966) dot blot analysis. AIDS 1993;7:475.
15. Zuber M, Samuel KP, Lautenberger JA, Kanki PJ, Papas TS. Bacterially produced HIV-2 env polypeptides specific for distinguishing HIV-2 from HIV-1 infections. AIDS Res Hum Retroviruses 1990;6:525.
16. Berry N, Pepin J, Gaye I, et al. Competitive EIA for anti-HIV-2 detection in The Gambia: use as a screening assay and to identify possible dual infections. J Med Virol 1993;39:101.
17. Kanki PJ, MBoup S, Ricard D, et al. Human T-lymphotropic virus type 4 and the human immunodeficiency virus in West Africa. Science 1987;236:827.
18. Denis F, Barin F, Gershey-Damet G, et al. Prevalence of human T-lymphotropic retroviruses type III (HIV) and type IV in Ivory Coast. Lancet 1987;1:408.
19. Tedder RS, O'Connor T, Hughs A, N'Hjie H, Corrah T, Whittle H. Envelope cross-reactivity in Western blot for HIV-1 and HIV-2 may not indicate dual infection. Lancet 1988;2:927.
20. De Cock KM, Porter A, Odehouri K, et al. Rapid emergence of AIDS in Abidjan, Ivory Coast. Lancet 1989;2:408.
21. Evans LA, Moreau J, Odehouri K, et al. Simultaneous isolation of HIV-1 and HIV-2 from an AIDS patient. Lancet 1988;2:1389.
22. George R, Ou CY, Parekh B, et al. Prevalence of HIV-1 and HIV-2 mixed infections in Cote d'Ivoire. Lancet 1992;340:337.
23. Peeters M, Gershy-Damet GM, Fransen K, et al. Virological and polymerase chain reaction studies of HIV-1/HIV-2 dual infection in Cote d'Ivoire. Lancet 1992;340:339.
24. Rayfield M, De Cock K, Heyward W, et al. Mixed human immunodeficiency virus (HIV) infection in an individual: demonstration of both HIV type 1 and type 2 proviral sequence by using polymerase chain reaction. J Infect Dis 1988;158:1170.
25. Kanki P, MBoup S, Marlink R, et al. Prevalence and risk determinants of human immunodeficiency virus type 2 (HIV-2) and human immunodeficiency virus type 1 (HIV-1) in West African female prostitutes. Am J Epidemiol 1992;136:895.
26. Kanki PJ, De Cock KM. Epidemiology and natural history of HIV-2. AIDS 1994;8:S1.
27. Abbott RC, Ndour-Sarr A, Diouf A, et al. Risk determinants for HIV infection and adverse obstetrical outcomes in pregnant women in Dakar, Senegal. J Acquir Immune Defic Syndr 1994;7:711.
28. De Cock KM, Brun-Vezinet F. Epidemiology of HIV-2. AIDS 1989;3:S89.
29. Naucler A, Anderson B, Norrgren H, Dias F, Johansson I, Biberfeld G. Prevalence and incidence of HIV-1, HIV-2, HTLV, and *Treponema pallidum* infections among police officers in Guinea-Bissau. Eighth International Conference on AIDS in Africa. Abstract. Yaounde, December 1992.
30. Del Mistro A, Chotard J, Mali AJ, Whittle H, De Rossi A, Chieco-Bianchi L. HIV-1 and HIV-2 seroprevalence rates in mother-child pairs living in The Gambia, West Africa. J Acquir Immune Defic Syndr 1992;5:19.

31. Harrison L, Da Silva APJ, Gayle H, et al. Risk factors for HIV-2 infection in Guinea-Bissau. J Acquir Immune Defic Syndr 1991;4:1155.
32. Pepin J, Dunn D, Gaye I, et al. HIV-2 infection among prostitutes working in The Gambia: association with serological evidence of genital ulcer diseases and generalized lymphadenopathy AIDS 1991;5:69.
33. Mabey DC, Tedder RS, Hughes AS, et al. Human retroviral infections in The Gambia: prevalence and clinical features. Br Med J 1988;296:83.
34. Saal F, Sidibe S, Alves-Cardoso E, et al. Anti-HIV-2 serological screening in Portuguese populations native from or having had close contact with Africa. AIDS Res Hum Retroviruses 1987;3:341.
35. De Cock KM, Adjorlolo G, Ekpino E, et al. Epidemiology and transmission of HIV-2: why there is no HIV-2 pandemic. JAMA 1993;270:2083.
36. Kanki PJ, Travers K, MBoup S, et al. Slower heterosexual spread of HIV-2 than HIV-1. Lancet 1994;343:943.
37. Ankrah TC, Roberts MA, Antwi P, et al. The African AIDS case definition and HIV serology in medical in-patients at Komfo Anokye Teaching Hospital, Kumasi, Ghana. West Afr J Med 1994;13:98.
38. Olaleye OD, Bernstein L, Ekweozor CC, et al. Prevalence of human immunodeficiency virus types 1 and 2 infections in Nigeria. J Infect Dis 1993;167:710.
39. Kline RL, Dada A, Blattner W, Quinn TC. Diagnosis and differentiation of HIV-1 and HIV-2 infection by two rapid assays in Nigeria. J Acquir Immune Defic Syndr 1994;7:623.
40. Maiga YI, Sissoko Z, Maiga MA. Etude de la seroprevalence de l'infection a VIH dans les 7 regions economiques du Mali. Eighth International Conference on AIDS in Africa and Eighth African Conference on Sexually Transmitted Diseases. Abstract. Marrakesh, December 1993.
41. Koffi K, Gershey-Damet GM, Peeters M, Soro B, Rey J-L, Delaporte E. Rapid spread of HIV infections in Abidjan, Ivory Coast, 1987–1990. Eur J Clin Microbiol Infect Dis 1992;11:271.
42. Santos-Ferreira MO, Cohen T, Lourenco MH, Matos Almedia MJ, Camaret S, Montagnier L. A study of seroprevalence of HIV-1 and HIV-2 in six provinces of People's Republic of Angola: clues to the spread of HIV infection. J Acquir Immune Defic Syndr 1990;3:780.
43. Kanki P, Allan J, Barin F, et al. Absence of antibodies to HIV-2/HTLV-4 in six Central African nations. AIDS Res Hum Retroviruses 1987;3:317.
44. Kanki P, Marlink R, Siby T, Essex M, Mboup S. Biology of HIV-2 infection in West Africa. In: Papas TS, ed. Gene regulation and AIDS. Houston: Portfolio Publishing Company of Texas, 1990:255.
45. Mota-Miranda A, Gomes MH, Sarmento R, et al. HIV-2 infection in the north of Portugal. Ninth International Conference on AIDS. Abstract. Berlin, June 1993.
46. Centro de vigilancia epidemioloca das doencas transmissiveis sindrome de immunodeficiencia adquirida. A situacao em Portugal em 30 de Junho de 1992. In: Machado Caetano J, Bandeira Costa J, Champalimaud J, Almeida Goncalves J, Terrinha A, Paixao MT, eds. Lisbon, Portugal: Instituto Nacional de Saude, 1992.
47. Soriano V, Gutierrez M, Fernandez JL, Aguilera A, Gonsalez A, Bernal A, and the HIV-2 Spanish Study Group. HIV-2 infection in Spain: report of the first 34 cases. AIDS 1992;6:1222.
48. Courouce A-M, the Retrovirus Study Group of the French Society of Blood Transfusion. HIV-2 infection among blood donors and other subjects in France. Transfusion 1989;29:368.
49. Matheron S, Simon F, Sassi G, et al. Infection HIV-2 chez l'adulte; etude de cohorte; Paris: 1986–1993. Eighth International Conference on AIDS in Africa and Eighth African Conference on Sexually Transmitted Diseases. Abstract. Marrakesh, December 1993.
50. Mazeron MC, Cerboni J, Alain S, et al. Prevalence of HIV infections among patients attending a Parisian anonymous testing center between 1988 and 1993. Pathol Biol (Paris) 1994;42:520.
51. Smallman-Raynor M, Cliff A. The spread of human immunodeficiency virus type 2 into Europe: a geographical analysis. Int J Epidemiol 1991;20:480.
52. O'Brien TR, George JR, Holmberg SD. Human immunodeficiency virus type 2 infection in the United States: epidemiology, diagnosis, and public health implications. JAMA 1992;267:2775.
53. Centers for Disease Control. Surveillance for HIV-2 infection in blood donors—United States, 1987–1989. MMWR 1990;39:829.
54. Onorato IM, O'Brien TR, Schable CA, Spruill C, Holmberg SD. HIV-2 surveillance in hgh-risk populations. Am J Public Health 1993;83:515.

55. Martin R, Machedo F, Menedez J, Zamora F. Study for the detection of antibodies and follow-up of seropositive subjects to HIV and AIDS patients. Sixth International Conference on AIDS. Abstract. San Francisco, June 1990.
56. Veronesi R, Mazza CC, Santos Ferreira MO, Lourenco MH. HIV-2 in Brazil. Lancet 1987;2:402.
57. Cortes E, Detels R, Aboulafia D, et al. HIV-1, HIV-2, and HTLV-1 infection in high-risk groups in Brazil. N Engl J Med 1989;320:953.
58. Hendry RM, Parks DE, Campos Mello DLA, Quinnan GV, Balao Castro B. Lack of evidence for HIV-2 infection among at-risk individuals in Brazil. J Acquir Immune Defic Syndr 1991;4:623.
59. Pieniazek D, Peralta JM, Ferreira JA, et al. Identification of mixed HIV-1/HIV-2 infections in Brazil by polymerase chain reaction. AIDS 1991;5:1293.
60. Rubsamen-Waigmann H, Briesen HV, Maniar JK, Rao PK, Scholz C, Pfutzner A. Spread of HIV-2 in India. Lancet 1991;337:550.
61. Pfutzner A, Dietrich U, Von Eichel U, et al. HIV-1 and HIV-2 infections in a high-risk population in Bombay, India: evidence for the spread of HIV-2 and presence of a divergent HIV-1 subtype. J Acquir Immune Defic Syndr 1992;5:972.
62. Nandi J, Kamat H, Bhavalkar V, Banerjee K. Detection of human immunodeficiency virus antibody among homosexual men from Bombay. Sex Transm Dis 1994;21:235.
63. Rubsamen-Waigmann H, Maniar J, Gerte S, et al. High proportion of HIV-2 and HIV-1/2 double-reactive sera in two Indian states, Maharashtra and Goa: first appearance of an HIV-2 epidemic along with an HIV-1 epidemic outside of Africa. Int J Med Microbiol Virol Parasitol Infect Dis 1994;280:398.
64. Quinn TC. Population migration and the spread of types 1 and 2 human immunodeficiency viruses. Proc Natl Acad Sci U S A 1994;94:2407.
65. Dufoort G, Courouce A-M, Ancelle-Park R, Beltry O. No clinical signs 14 years after HIV-2 transmission via blood transfusion. Lancet 1988;2:510.
66. Mofenson LM, Epidemiology and determinants of vertical HIV transmission. Semin Pediatr Infect Dis 1994;5:252.
67. Matheron S, Courpotin C, Simon F, et al. Vertical transmission of HIV-2. Lancet 1990;335:1103.
68. Gnaore E, De Cock KM, Gayle H, et al. Prevalence mortality from HIV type 2 in Guinea-Bissau, West Africa. Lancet 1989;2:408.
69. Morgan G, Wilkins HA, Pepin J, Jobo O, Brewster D, Whittle H. AIDS following mother-to-child transmission of HIV-2. AIDS 1990;4:879.
70. Poulsen AG, Kvinesdal BB, Aaby P, et al. Lack of evidence of vertical transmission of human immunodeficiency virus type 2 in a sample of the general population in Bissau. J Acquir Immune Defic Syndr 1992;5:25.
71. Gayle H, Gnaore E, Adjorlolo G, et al. HIV-1 and HIV-2 infection in children in Abidjan, Cote D'Ivoire. J Acquir Immune Defic Syndr 1992;5:513.
72. Andreasson PA, Dias F, Naucler A, Anderson S, Biberfeld G. A prospective study of vertical transmission of HIV-2 in Bissau, Guinea-Bissau. AIDS 1993;7:989.
73. Adjorlolo-Johnson G, DeCock KM, Ekpini E, et al. Prospective comparison of mother-to-child transmission of HIV-1 and HIV-2 in Abidjan, Ivory Coast. JAMA 1994;272:462.
74. Anonymous. Comparison of vertical human immunodeficiency virus type 2 and human immunodeficiency virus type 1 transmission in the French prospective cohort. The HIV Infection in Newborns French Collaborative Study Group. Pediatr Infect Dis J. 1994;13:502.
75. Ngagne-MBaye, Diouf A, Kebe F, et al. Histoire naturelle de la transmission verticale VIH1 et VIH 2 a Dakar. Ninth International Conference on AIDS and Associated Cancers in Africa. Abstract. Kampala, Uganda, December 1995.
76. Donnelly C, Leisenring W, Kanki P, Awerbach T, Sandberg S. Comparison of transmission rates of HIV-1 and HIV-2 in a cohort of prostitutes in Senegal. Bull Math Biol 1993;55:731.
77. Romieu I, Marlink R, Kanki P, MBoup S, Essex M. HIV-2 link to AIDS in West Africa. J Acquir Immune Defic Syndr 1990;3:220.
78. Saimot AG, Coulaud JP, Mechali D, et al. HIV-2/LAV-2 in Portuguese man with AIDS (Paris, 1978) who had served in Angola in 1968–74. Lancet 1987;1:688.
79. Naucler A, Albino P, Da Silva AP, Andreasson PA, Andersson S, Biberfeld G. HIV-2 infection in hospitalized patients in Bissau, Guinea-Bissau. AIDS 1991;5:301.

80. De Cock KM, Odehouri K, Colebunders R, Adjorlolo G, Lafontaine MF, Porter A, et al. A comparison of HIV-1 and HIV-2 infections in hospitalized patients in Abidjan, Cote d'Ivoire. AIDS 1990;4:443.
81. Schneider J, Luke W, Kirchhoff F, et al. Isolation and characterization of HIV-2 obtained from a patient with predominantly neurological defects. AIDS 1990;4:455.
82. Dwyer DE, Matheron S, Bakchine S, Bechet JM, Montagnier L, Vazeux R. Detection of human immunodeficiency virus type 2 in brain tissue. J Infect Dis 1992;166:888.
83. Lucas SB, Hounnou A, Peacock A, et al. The mortality and pathology of HIV infection in a West African city. AIDS 1993;7:1569.
84. Nagelkerke N, Plummer F, Holton D, et al. Transition dynamics of HIV disease in a cohort of African prostitutes: a Markov model approach. AIDS 1990;4:743.
85. Ngaly B, Ryder RW, Bila K, et al. Human immunodeficiency virus infection among hospital employees in an African hospital. N Engl J Med 1988;319:1123.
86. Marlink R, Ricard D, MBoup S, et al. Clinical, hematologic, and immunologic cross-sectional evaluation of individuals exposed to human immunodeficiency virus type 2 (HIV-2). AIDS Res Hum Retroviruses 1988;4:137.
87. Marlink R, Thior I, Travers K, et al. Reduced virulence of HIV-2 compared to HIV-1. Science 1994;265:1587.
88. Lisse IM, Poulsen AG, Aaby P, et al. Immunodeficiency in HIV-2 infection: a community study from Guinea-Bissau. AIDS 1990;4:1263.
89. Kestens L, Brattegaard K, Adjorlolo G, et al. Immunological comparison of HIV-1-, HIV-2-, and dually reactive women delivering in Abidjan, Cote d'Ivoire. AIDS 1992;6:803.
90. Whittle H, Egboga A, Todd J, et al. Clinical and laboratory predictors of survival in Gambian patients with symptomatic HIV-1 or HIV-2 infection. AIDS 1992;6:685.
91. Chollet-Martin S, Simon F, Matheron S, Joseph CA, Elbim C, Gougerot-Pocidalo MA. Comparison of plasma cytokine levels in African patients with HIV-1 and HIV-2 infection. AIDS 1994;8:879.
92. Simon F, Matheron S, Tamalet C, et al. Cellular and plasma viral load in patients infected with HIV-2. AIDS 1993;7:1411.
93. Korber B, Kanki P, Barin F, MBoup S, Travers K, Essex M. Genetic and antigenic variability in different HIV-2 viral isolates. Fourth International Conference on AIDS and Associated Cancers in Africa. Abstract. Marseilles, October 1989.
94. Berry N, Ariyoshi K, Jobe O, et al. HIV type 2 proviral load measured by quantitative polymerase chain reaction correlates with CD4+ lymphopenia in HIV type 2–infected individuals. AIDS Res Hum Retroviruses 1994;10:1031.
95. Sankalé J-L, Sallier de la Tour R, Renjifo B, et al. Intra-patient variability of the human immunodeficiency virus type-2 (HIV-2) envelope V3 loop. AIDS Res Hum Retroviruses 1995;11:617.
96. Boeri E, Giri A, Lillo F, et al. In vivo genetic variability of the human immunodeficiency virus type 2 V3 region. J Virol 1992;66:4546.
97. Travers K, MBoup S, Marlink R, et al. Natural protections against HIV-1 infection provided by HIV-2. Science 1995;268:1612.
98. Wade A, Dieng-Sarr A, Diallo A, et al. Infection HIV-1 and HIV-2 in Senegal. Eighth International Conference on AIDS in Africa and Eighth African Conference on Sexually Transmitted Diseases. Abstract. Marrakesh, December 1993.
99. Harry TO, Bukbuk DN, Idrisa A, Akoa MB. HIV infection among pregnant women. A worsening situation in Maiduguri, Nigeria. Trop Geogr Med 1994;46:46.
100. Nauclér A, Andreasson P-A, Mendes Costa C, Thorstensson R, Biberfeld G. HIV-2 Associated AIDS and HIV-2 seroprevalence in Bissau, Guinea-Bissau. J Acquire Immune Defic Syndr 1989;2:88.

AIDS: Biology, Diagnosis, Treatment and Prevention, fourth edition, edited by Vincent T. DeVita, Jr., Samuel Hellman, and Steven A. Rosenberg. Lippincott–Raven Publishers, © 1997

CHAPTER 9

Epidemiology of Human Immunodeficiency Virus Infection in the United States

Susan Y. Chu and James W. Curran

In 1981, the first cases of acquired immunodeficiency syndrome (AIDS) were reported from Los Angeles in five young homosexual men; by the end of 1994, more than 440,000 cases of AIDS had been reported in the United States.[1] In this country, human immunodeficiency virus (HIV) infection is having a startling effect on mortality among young adults. In 1993, HIV or AIDS was the leading cause of death among men 25 to 44 years of age and the fourth leading cause of death among women 25 to 44 years of age (Figs. 9-1 and 9-2).[2]

The impact of HIV and AIDS on mortality is particularly devastating in certain areas. For example, in 1992, HIV infection was the leading cause of death among men 25 to 44 years of age in 99 cities; the proportion of deaths caused by HIV among men in this age group ranged from 15% in Las Vegas, Nevada, to 65% in Fort Lauderdale, Florida, with a median of 25% in Fort Worth, Texas. Although many of these cities are densely clustered around major urban centers of the HIV epidemic, others are widely scattered throughout the Midwest and the South: Omaha, Nebraska; Akron, Ohio; Springfield, Missouri; Charlotte, North Carolina; and Columbia, South Carolina.[3]

The HIV epidemic in the United States has changed in magnitude and in character; the current epidemiology has become more complex, having developed into a series of subepidemics with different times of onset and patterns of spread. For example, although the number of cases among men who have sex with men (MSMs) is not increasing as rapidly as before, new infections are occurring at high rates among young MSMs in urban centers and among black MSMs in the South.[4] Moreover, risk groups are not homogeneous; a single exposure category may include several diverse social and cultural groups.[5] The diversity means that no single prevention strategy can address all persons in a particular risk group. For example, MSMs may self-identify as homosexual, bisexual, or heterosexual; different strategies are required to reach these men who identify and probably affiliate with different social groups. Specific behaviors in a particular risk group also vary widely by geographic location. For example, interviews of HIV-infected injecting drug users (IDUs) from 1990 through 1993 showed that 94% of IDUs in Detroit most often injected heroin, but 56% of IDUs in Atlanta and 46% in Denver reported primarily injecting cocaine. In Washington state, 56% of IDUs said they injected amphetamines more often than other drugs.[6]

Strategies for prevention and intervention must understand these subtle differences to assess risk behavior and to comprehend how gender, race, class, and religion affect a person's perception of personal risk, lifestyle choices, and ability to make those choices. For example, the social and economic status of women often limits their ability to negotiate a partner's condom use, especially in cultures where having children is a critical part of a woman's role.[7] Gender can affect other risks; a study of heterosexual couples who both injected drugs found that women more often used injection equipment after men.[8] Cultural differences between different racial or ethnic groups can also influence risk behavior. For example, black MSMs are more likely than white MSMs to report also having sex with women.[9,10] The factors underlying this difference may make these men harder to reach while indicating prevention needs for their female as well as male partners. Some have suggested that

Susan Y. Chu and James W. Curran, Division of HIV/AIDS Prevention, Centers for Disease Control and Prevention, Public Health Service, U.S. Department of Health and Human Services, Atlanta, GA 30333.

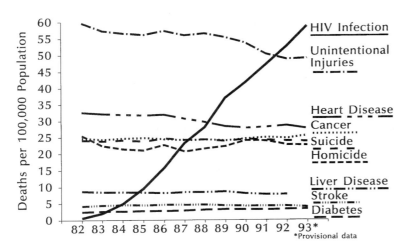

FIG. 9-1. Leading causes of death among men 25 to 44 years of age in the United States from 1981 through 1992. (Data from National Center for Health Statistics. Annual summary of births, marriages, divorces, and deaths: United States, 1993. Monthly vital statistics report, vol 42, no 13. Hyattsville, MD: Public Health Service, 1994.).

being identified as homosexual is more stigmatized in the black community and that affiliation with the gay white community is seen as a betrayal of the black community.[11]

One pattern has remained consistent throughout the epidemic: the disproportionately high rates of HIV infection and AIDS among black and Hispanic men, women, and children, who are overrepresented in almost every transmission category.[12] This disproportion in rates primarily reflects the much higher rates of AIDS among black and Hispanic IDUs and their sex partners and infants; however, AIDS rates among MSMs are also higher among black and Hispanic men than among white men. The increase in the number of persons with AIDS has greatly affected death rates among racial and ethnic minorities, particularly young adults. Since 1991, HIV infection has been the leading cause of death among black and Hispanic men between 25 and 44 years of age.[13] However, these national statistics do not necessarily reflect differences in various communities of the same race or ethnicity. For example, AIDS rates and modes of HIV exposure vary greatly among minority populations by place of birth, especially among Hispanics, Asians, and Pacific Islanders.[14] These differences relate in part to different social, economic, and cultural influences and emphasize that prevention strategies must increasingly be targeted at the specific local community.

SURVEILLANCE IN THE UNITED STATES

From 1981 through December 1994, 441,528 cases of AIDS in the United States were reported to the Centers for Disease Control and Prevention (CDC); 270,870 (61%) of these persons with AIDS were reported to have died. All 50 states require reporting of AIDS to state health departments, which report these cases, without names, to the CDC. The surveillance case definition was initially developed before the cause of AIDS was known. Revisions of the definition in 1985, 1987, and 1993 broadened the list of conditions reportable as AIDS, including presumptively diagnosed diseases (eg, *Pneumocystis carinii* pneumonia [PCP] and Kaposi's sarcoma) and conditions more common among IDUS (eg, recurrent bacterial pneumonia), and they placed greater emphasis on HIV testing and CD4+ lymphocyte criteria as components of diagnosis.[15–17] The 1987 revision significantly increased the number of reported cases, particularly among women, blacks, Hispanics, and IDUs.[18] The 1993 revision expanded the case definition to include all HIV-infected persons with less than 200 CD4+ T lymphocytes/μL or a CD4+ T-lymphocyte percentage less than 14% (ie, severe immunosuppression) and added to the 23 conditions in the 1987 AIDS case definition three clinical

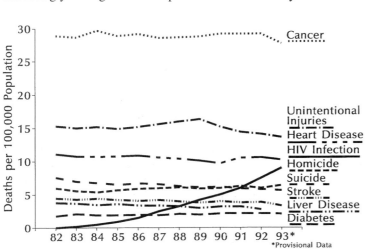

FIG. 9-2. Leading causes of death among women 25 to 44 years of age in the United States from 1981 through 1992. (Data from National Center for Health Statistics. Annual summary of births, marriages, divorces, and deaths: United States, 1993. Monthly vital statistics report, vol 42, no 13. Hyattsville, MD: Public Health Service, 1994.).

conditions: pulmonary tuberculosis, recurrent pneumonia, and invasive cervical cancer. The 1993 expansion was instituted so that AIDS surveillance would more accurately reflect the number of persons with severe HIV-related immunosuppression and those at highest risk for HIV-related morbidity. A substantial increase in the number of reported AIDS cases occurred after the expansion, predominantly reflecting HIV-infected persons reported because of a CD4+ count of less than 200 cells/μL or CD4+ percentage of less than 14%, which typically occurs before the onset of AIDS-defining opportunistic illnesses.[19]

Because AIDS develops years after a person is infected with HIV, the epidemiology of reported AIDS cases reflects the pattern of HIV infections that occurred several years earlier. Surveys of HIV seroprevalence can give a more current picture of the pattern of HIV infection rates. For example, a study of MSMs recruited from public venues in San Francisco and Berkeley, California, during 1992 and 1993 found that 4% of those between 17 and 19 years of age and 12% of those between 18 and 22 years of age were infected with HIV.[20] Such high prevalence rates among young men suggest substantial recent infection rates.

Data from HIV seroprevalence surveys,[21] along with data from AIDS case surveillance and the Third National Health and Nutrition Examination Survey,[22] can be used to estimate the number of persons infected with HIV in the United States.[23] These data suggest that 650,000 to 900,000 persons in the United States were infected with HIV in 1992 and that one fifth to one sixth of these persons were women. Statistical models based on AIDS cases indicate that HIV prevalence increased from 1987 to 1992, with greater relative increases among women than among men.

Men Who Have Sex With Men

MSMs have represented the largest number of persons reported with AIDS in the United States; 228,954 cases had been reported among MSMs without a history of injecting drug use and 28,521 among MSM IDUs by the end of 1994 (Table 9-1). Although most MSMs reported with AIDS are white (72%), the

rate of AIDS among exclusively homosexual men is 1.3 and 1.7 times higher among black and Hispanic men, respectively, than among white men; among bisexual men with AIDS, the differential is greater, 3.6 and 2.5 times higher among black and Hispanic men, respectively, than among white men.[24] This racial or ethnic disparity has widened recently: between 1989 and 1994, rates increased 79% among black and 62% among Hispanic MSMs, but rates increased only 11% among white MSMs.

Although the increase in AIDS is not as dramatic as it was early in the epidemic[25] and declines in syphilis, gonorrhea, and amebiasis among MSMs in the early 1980s suggest that reductions in high-risk sexual behavior have occurred,[26-28] large numbers of cases of AIDS in MSMs continue to be reported each year (eg, 34,974 in 1994). Although AIDS incidences are rising faster among black and Hispanic MSMs than among white MSMs, the AIDS incidence is increasing among MSMs in all racial and ethnic groups in many areas across the country, including Atlanta, Dallas, and Detroit. A survey of men who patronized gay bars in 16 small and moderate-sized cities found that high-risk behavior patterns were still common and suggested that the new "front line" for prevention among MSMs has shifted to the country's smaller cities.[29] This shift may be reflected in the differences in increase in AIDS among MSMs by population size; in rural areas (<50,000 persons), AIDS rates among MSMs increased 71% between 1989 and 1994, and in large urban centers (>2.5 million persons), rates increased only 19% during that period.[30,31] and many young homosexual men continue to engage in high-risk sexual behavior and have high seroconversion rates.[-34] A study of young MSMs men 18 to 24 years of age in New York City found that the proportion who engaged in anal intercourse and the median number of sex partners increased significantly from 1990 to 1991. HIV prevalence was much higher among blacks (40%) and Hispanics (30%) than among whites and other ethnic groups (2%), suggesting that prevention efforts have been less successful in reaching black and Hispanic MSMs than other racial or ethnic groups. A 1990 survey in the San Francisco Bay area had similar find-

TABLE 9-1. *AIDS cases among adults and adolescents by exposure category and sex, reported through December 1994 in the United States*

Exposure Category	Men Number	(%)	Women Number	(%)	Total Number	(%)
Men who have sex with men	228,954	(61)			228,954	(53)
Injecting drug use (heterosexual)	81,491	(22)	27,902	(48)	109,393	(25)
Men who have sex with men and inject drugs	28,521	(8)			28,521	(7)
Hemophilia or coagulation disorder	3,545	(1)	97	(0)	3,642	(1)
Heterosexual contact	10,641	(3)	21,021	(36)	31,663	(7)
Receipt of blood transfusion, blood components, or tissue	4,047	(1)	2,819	(5)	6,866	(2)
Other or undetermined	19,690	(5)	6,589	(11)	26,280	(6)
Total	376,889	(100)	58,428	(100)	435,319	(100)

ings: black MSMs reported a substantially higher prevalence of unprotected anal intercourse during the past 6 months (52%) than did white MSMs (15% to 20%).[35]

Efforts to prevent further expansion of the epidemic of HIV among MSMs must focus on developing programs in smaller communities and instituting interventions that effectively reach those who remain at greatest risk, including adolescent and minority MSMs. These efforts must consider the social and cultural factors that will affect MSMs' ability to access these interventions. For example, black MSMs may have less contact with the visible gay community and its network of HIV support services, less social support for behavior change, and greater prevalence of other HIV-related behaviors, such as alcohol and drug use.[36] In addition, MSMs who belong to racial or ethnic minorities do not concentrate as often as white MSMs in a particular neighborhood; they instead live more widely dispersed, often in areas where their racial or ethnic group is more highly concentrated. Prevention services should be expanded into neighborhoods where MSMs of color live and incorporate greater understanding of the cultural differences and norms of different groups of MSMs.

Behaviorally bisexual men may be particularly hard to reach. Bisexual men in general may be less likely to identify with gay communities or to view themselves as at risk for HIV infection.[37] Behaviors associated with HIV risk may vary by sexual self-identification; one study found that behaviorally bisexual men who identified as heterosexual used condoms at lower rates than men who identified as homosexual or bisexual.[38] Behaviorally bisexual men who identify as heterosexual, especially those who are married, may not feel able to disclose their HIV status or risk behavior to their sexual partners.[39] More black and Hispanic MSMs with AIDS report bisexual behavior than white MSMs with AIDS. The interaction between race or ethnicity and bisexual behavior is affected by several factors, including acculturation,[40] social norms, and economics, including prostitution.[41] For example, the Hispanic population in the United States is diverse in country of origin and degree of acculturation. Unless bisexual Hispanic men are highly acculturated, their behavior patterns may be more similar to those in their country of origin. Studies in Mexico found that behaviorally bisexual men who took the insertive role in male-to-male sex viewed themselves as heterosexual, a potentially difficult group to reach.[42] Increased understanding of the interaction between sexual self-identification, sexual behavior, and race or ethnicity is critical to the development of effective HIV prevention programs for MSMs.

Injecting Drug Users

Almost one quarter of all persons with AIDS in the United States were infected through injecting drug use; among women, the proportion of those so infected is almost one half. The epidemiology of drug abuse and HIV are critically linked and influences seroprevalence of HIV among IDUs, their sex partners, and their children. For example, one change during the past decade has had a major influence on HIV transmission among IDUs. Heroin is no longer the primary injected drug in many areas, and increasingly, cocaine, amphetamines, and other drugs are injected.[43] These drugs are often injected more frequently than heroin, and they have been associated with increased needle sharing.[44] An important consequence of this change is that most interventions to reduce high-risk behaviors among IDUs have primarily targeted opiate users through methadone programs, but these interventions may not reach or effectively address the needs of persons who primarily or additionally inject other drugs such as amphetamines and cocaine.

Through December 1994, 172,953 AIDS cases reported in the United States were associated directly or indirectly with injecting drug use. Of these cases, 109,393 were women and heterosexual men reported as injecting drug users, 31,663 were heterosexual partners of IDUs, 28,521 were MSMs who were also IDUs, and 3376 were children whose mothers were IDUs or sex partners of IDUs. Rates of IDU-associated AIDS vary considerably by race or ethnicity. In 1990, the incidence of AIDS cases associated with IDU was 11 times higher among black men (37.4 per 100,000) and eight times higher among Hispanic men (28.7 per 100,000) than among white men (3.5 per 100,000).[45] The racial or ethnic disparity was even greater among women with IDU-associated AIDS. The rates among black (16.0 per 100,000) and Hispanic women (9.5 per 100,000) were 18 and 11 times higher, respectively, than the rate among white women (0.9 per 100,000). IDU-associated AIDS cases accounted for 17% of all AIDS cases in whites, 52% in blacks, 52% in Hispanics, 8% in Asians and Pacific Islanders, and 35% in American Indians and Alaskan Natives. Among Hispanics, IDU-associated AIDS rates were highest among those born in Puerto Rico.[46] Except for the West, where rates among whites, blacks, and Hispanics were similar, this difference by race or ethnicity was observed in all regions of the country and was greatest in the Northeast.

Rates also vary widely by geographic location. For example, seroprevalence studies of IDUs in 114 drug treatment programs in 40 U.S. cities reported HIV seroprevalence rates ranging from 1% to 53% (median, 8%) in 1991 and 1992. To what extent clients entering drug treatment represent all IDUs is unknown, and differences in infection rates remain incompletely explained but may be related to differences in access to drug treatment;[47,48] differences in access to sterile needles and injection equipment, including needle exchange programs;[49,50] differences in needle-sharing practices; increasing use of intranasal heroin; or other factors.

In most cities, HIV seroprevalence rates among IDUs are remaining fairly constant, though some rates are very high. For example, in New York City, seroprevalence among IDUs entering detoxification programs remained stable between

1984 through 1992 at slightly more than 50%.[51] Stable seroprevalence rates over time, however, do not mean that new infections did not occur. For example, approximately 5% to 10% of HIV-infected IDUs are estimated to die each year; a similar number of IDUs must become infected each year for observed seroprevalence rates to remain unchanged. The explosive HIV epidemics among IDUs in other countries (eg, Thailand, Italy, Scotland) indicate the serious potential for HIV to spread rapidly into low-prevalence areas.[52]

Drug use behaviors among IDUs also varies considerably by geographic location. For example, IDUs with AIDS in South Carolina and in Atlanta, Georgia, most commonly inject cocaine (64% and 56%, respectively), but IDUs with AIDS in Seattle, Washington, most commonly inject amphetamines (56%). Within regions, drug use patterns vary between subgroups; for example, although more persons with AIDS in the North injected heroin, a substantial proportion of Puerto Ricans with AIDS in the North injected cocaine. Determining the most effective interventions for drug users requires careful assessment of drug use behavior, including types of drugs used, and the availability of treatment services and access to sterile injection equipment within each community.

Heterosexual Transmission

Worldwide, heterosexual intercourse is the predominant mode of HIV transmission. In the United States, heterosexual contact is the third most common mode of HIV transmission, accounting for 7% of all AIDS cases. However, that proportion is changing, and heterosexual contact is the transmission category currently increasing most rapidly in the United States; the number of heterosexual contact cases increased an average of 30% between 1988 and 1992.[53] In 1993, 42% of heterosexually acquired AIDS cases were attributed to heterosexual contact with an IDU.[54] Reducing heterosexual transmission of HIV requires that intervention programs targeted at IDUs specifically address risky sexual behavior in addition to drug injection practices.[55]

Data other than AIDS case surveillance can provide information on trends in heterosexual transmission of HIV. For example, the primary and secondary syphilis rates remain high in the South, the U.S. region also reporting the highest proportion of AIDS cases associated with heterosexual contact (42%) during 1993. Moreover, certain sexually transmitted diseases (STDs), such as those causing genital ulcers (eg, chancroid, syphilis, genital herpes), facilitate transmission or acquisition of HIV;[56] some other more common STDs such as chlamydial and gonorrheal infections also have been associated with increased HIV transmission rates in some studies.[57,58] For these reasons, prevention of other STDs is primarily important and because this approach may decrease HIV transmission.

Trends in rates of STDs can also indicate changes in sex behavior. For example, rates of gonorrheal infection, the most frequently reported STD in the United States,[59] decreased 65% between 1975 and 1993. Although this decrease primarily reflected decreases among older age groups, smaller decreases (13% to 20%) also occurred among adolescents 15 to 19 years of age. This trend mirrors recent changes in sexual behavior among adolescents; after the substantial increase in the proportion of high school students who had reported premarital sexual intercourse during the 1980s, the trend stabilized, with the proportion of students who reported being sexually experienced remaining constant (53% to 54%) between 1990 and 1993.[60] A survey of high school students in all 50 states found evidence that condom use is increasing among adolescents; the percentage of students who reported condom use at last sexual intercourse increased from 46% in 1991 to 53% in 1993.[61]

The epidemic of smokable freebase cocaine (ie, crack) abuse has had a substantial effect on the syphilis and HIV epidemics among heterosexuals, especially women.[62] Crack cocaine first appeared on the streets of New York City in late 1985, and because of its low cost and high addictive potential, its abuse quickly became widespread.[63] Although crack use itself does not transmit HIV, those who use crack tend to engage in unsafe sexual activity with multiple partners, including exchanging sex for money or drugs, that increases the potential for sexual transmission of HIV and other infections.[64–66] Without effective interventions that address crack addiction and risky sexual behavior among crack users, crack use is likely to facilitate continued heterosexual transmission of HIV.

In the United States, heterosexual contact is the one transmission category in which reported cases among women outnumber those among men; in 1994, 62% of reported heterosexual AIDS cases were among women. In the first decade of the HIV epidemic, most cases of AIDS in women were attributed to injection drug use. However, this trend is gradually changing. The proportion of AIDS cases in women attributed to heterosexual contact increased from 15% in 1983 to 43% in 1994. This trend differed notably by region; injecting drug use remained the predominant mode of transmission among women in the Northeast, but heterosexual contact became the predominant mode of transmission among women in the South, especially in smaller communities and rural areas.[67,68]

Many societal factors influence risky sexual behavior, and these affect women and men differently. For example, in an interview study of 497 persons with heterosexually acquired HIV, 49% of the men reported having paid women for sex, and 83% reported having had multiple partners in the past 5 years.[69] Although 60% of women also reported having multiple sex partners, 35% reported having had only one sex partner in the past 5 years. Monogamous women may not be aware of or may deny their risk due to their partner's sexual or drug-using behavior with others. Acknowledging risk could involve confronting a partner's sexual activity with others and possibly losing the partner; for women with few personal and social resources, this possibility may be overwhelming.[70] Counseling that emphasizes a reduction in the number of sexual partners would not effectively reduce these women's risk of HIV infection.

Among women reported with heterosexually acquired AIDS, 9% were infected from sexual contact with a bisexual man. For many reasons, including the stigma of homosexuality and infidelity, a bisexual man may be reluctant to inform his female partner of his male sexual contacts. The female partner also may be the bisexual man's primary sex partner or his spouse. Data linking AIDS surveillance and death certificates have shown that 3% of men with AIDS who reported sex with men only were married at death, compared with 24% of men with AIDS who reported sex with both male and female partners.[71] Mutual dependency and lack of awareness of risk often complicate prevention efforts. Moreover, awareness may differ by racial or ethnic group. Among 52 female partners of HIV-seropositive bisexual men enrolled in the California Partners' Study, 80% (28 of 35) of white, 20% (1 of 5) of black, and 22% (2 of 9) of Latino women were aware of their partner's bisexuality at entry into the study.[72] Similar findings were reported from Chicago.[73] Rates for AIDS due to sexual contact with bisexual men are highest among black and Hispanic women, those women who may be the ones least aware of their risk.

Perinatal Transmission

Through 1994, 6209 children younger than 13 years of age were reported with AIDS (Table 9-2); 89% of these children were infected perinatally, and 70% were younger than 3 years of age when AIDS was diagnosed. Because most children acquired HIV infection from their mothers, the racial or ethnic and geographic distribution of children with AIDS parallels that of women with AIDS. Fifty-nine percent of perinatally acquired AIDS cases are black children, and 26% are Hispanic children; black and Hispanic children have cumulative AIDS incidences 17 and 7 times higher, respec-

tively, than those among white children.[74] Of the mothers, 43% were reported to be IDUs, and 32% were sex partners of infected men, 58% of whom were IDUs. Although perinatal cases have been reported from all states, most have been reported from New York, Florida, New Jersey, Puerto Rico, California, and Washington, DC.

Seroprevalence data have provided estimates of the number of infected infants in the United States. A national survey measuring seroprevalence of HIV among women giving birth in the United States[75] found that approximately 7000 women with HIV infection gave birth in 1993.[76] Assuming a perinatal transmission rate of 15% to 30%, approximately 1000 to 2000 infants were born with HIV infection that year. From 1989 through 1993, the annual prevalence of HIV infection among childbearing women remained relatively stable (1.6 to 1.7 per 1000), although prevalence varied regionally; in the Northeast, prevalence decreased from 4.1 to 3.4 per 1000; in the South, prevalence increased from 1.6 in 1989 to 2.0 in 1991 and remained stable through 1993. In 1994, a regimen of zidovudine given to asymptomatic HIV-infected mothers before and at the time of birth and to infants following birth was shown to reduce the risk of perinatal transmission by two thirds.[77] Given that approximately 7000 infants are born to HIV-infected women in the United States each year, these findings emphasize the need for women to know their HIV-infection status.[78] The CDC has issued guidelines for routine counseling and voluntary HIV testing for all pregnant women in the United States.[79] If these guidelines are widely implemented and if use of zidovudine is widely adopted by HIV-infected pregnant women, cases of perinatally acquired HIV should begin to decline during the late 1990s.

BLOOD AND BLOOD PRODUCTS

Through December 1994, 11,086 persons (10,508 adults; 578 infants and children) were reported with AIDS acquired through receipt of blood or blood products in the United States. Of these, 35% had a history of hemophilia or another coagulation disorder, and 65% were transfusion-associated cases. Most of these persons were infected before 1985. HIV antibody screening of all blood donations, instituted in 1985, and heat treatment of clotting factor concentrates, begun in 1984, have vastly reduced HIV transmission through blood components and virtually eliminated transmission from clotting factors.[80]

Because routinely used HIV screening tests cannot detect antibody in infected persons until about 45 days after infection (ie, the "window" period),[81] a small but finite risk of HIV infection from a blood transfusion remains; this risk will decrease as the quality of test and donor deferral methods improves.[82] Very few cases of AIDS have been attributed to blood testing negative for HIV antibody during the window period between infection and seroconversion. From 1985 to the end of 1994, only 29 of the 6866 cumulative transfusion-associated AIDS were attributed to blood screened negative for HIV antibody.

TABLE 9-2. *AIDS cases among children younger than 13 years of age by exposure category and sex, reported through December 1994 in the United States*

Exposure Category	Number	Percentage of Total
Hemophilia or coagulation disorder	221	4
Perinatally acquired (mother's exposure):	5,541	89
Injecting drug use	2,338	
Sex with IDU	1,038	
Sex with bisexual male	107	
Sex with a person with hemophilia	2	
Sex with transfusion recipient	5	
Sex with HIV-infected person, risk unspecified	583	
Receipt of blood transfusion, blood components, or tissue	357	6
Risk not report or identified	90	1
Total	6,209	100

Female-to-female Sexual Contact

A review of 164 AIDS cases among women who reported sexual contact only with other women found that 152 (93%) injected drugs and that 12 (7%) had a history of a blood transfusion before March 1985; no cases were attributed to female-to-female sexual transmission of HIV.[83] However, at least five instances of female-to-female sexual transmission of HIV have been reported in the medical literature.[84–88] These data suggest that, as with other sexually transmitted infections, female-to-female HIV transmission does occur but is much less common than male-to-female transmission; however, the actual risk of female-to-female transmission is unknown.[89]

Donor Insemination

HIV transmission through intravaginal insemination with unprocessed and processed donor semen has been reported,[90–93] although data regarding the magnitude of the risk are conflicting.[94] Because no procedures to remove HIV from semen have been proven effective, insemination with semen from HIV-infected men is not recommended under any circumstances. All semen donors should be screened for HIV infection, and the semen should not be used until the donor has been tested again 6 months after donation to ensure that the semen was not collected from a recently infected donor who had no detectable antibody.[95] Use of "fresh" donor semen is discouraged, because the use of frozen specimens allows for more thorough evaluation of the donor for HIV and other infections.[96]

Health Care Workers

Although HIV infection in health care workers results primarily from HIV-related risk behavior outside the health care setting, exposure to HIV-infected blood poses an occupational risk for health care and laboratory workers.[97,98] HIV transmission in the health care setting generally is caused by blood contacts resulting from needle-stick injuries, although other exposures to HIV-infected blood or blood products pose a risk. As of December 1994, the CDC received reports of 42 health care workers in the United States who seroconverted to HIV after a documented occupational exposure to HIV-infected blood, and another 91 reports delineated health care workers in whom HIV infection was thought to be occupationally acquired, but seroconversion after a specific incident could not be documented.

HUMAN IMMUNODEFICIENCY VIRUS TYPE 2

A second human immunodeficiency virus (HIV-2) was first described in 1986 in West Africans with AIDS (see Chap. 8).[99] HIV-2 is closely related to HIV-1, and the spectrum of disease and modes of transmission are thought to be similar.[100] Most cases of HIV-2 have been reported among persons born in West Africa, although well-documented cases have been reported from Europe and North America. Seventeen persons with HIV-2 infection in the United States have been reported to the CDC; all of the 15 with historical information available had recently immigrated from West Africa, had sexual contact with West Africans, or traveled to West Africa.[101,102] Several large surveys of blood donors in the United States have detected no donors with HIV-2 infection. These data collectively suggest that HIV-2 infection is still rare in the United States and is unlikely to have a major impact on HIV-associated morbidity or mortality in the near future.

CONCLUSION

Since the initial case reports of AIDS in homosexual and bisexual men in 1981, the number of persons reported with HIV infection and AIDS has grown rapidly, and as of December 1994, 441,528 persons had been reported with AIDS in the United States. The characteristics of the epidemic have changed and become more complex, moving into different populations and into more diverse geographic locations.[103] Prevention strategies must be compatible with the social and cultural norms of each local community and be sufficiently flexible to accommodate differences in each population. Because AIDS is a social and medical disease, understanding the patterns and determinants of risk behavior as well as the environment and contexts in which behavioral choices are made will require a long-term commitment by scientists and society to prevent HIV infection in future generations.

REFERENCES

1. Centers for Disease Control and Prevention. HIV/AIDS surveillance report. 1995;6:1.
2. National Center for Health Statistics. Annual summary of births, marriages, divorces, and deaths: United States, 1993. Monthly vital statistics report, vol 42, no 13. Hyattsville, MD: Public Health Service, 1994.
3. Selik RM. Written communication. Atlanta: Centers for Disease Control and Prevention, 1995.
4. Centers for Disease Control and Prevention. Update: trends in acquired immunodeficiency syndrome among men who have sex with men—United States, 1989–1994. MMWR 1995;44:401.
5. Fee E, Krieger N. Understanding AIDS: historical interpretations and the limits of biomedical individualism. Am J Public Health 1993;83:1477.
6. Diaz T, Chu SY, Byers RH, et al. The types of drugs used by HIV-infected injection drug users in a multistate surveillance project: implications for intervention. Am J Public Health 1994;84:1971.
7. McCauley AP, Robey B, Blanc AK, Geller JS. Opportunities for women through reproductive choice. Population reports, series M, No. 12. Baltimore: John Hopkins School of Public Health, 1994.
8. Clark LL, Calsyn DA, Saxon AJ, Jackson TR, Wrede IAF. HIV risk behaviors of heterosexual couples in methadone maintenance. Presented at the 8th International Conference on AIDS, Amsterdam, July 1992.
9. Lever J, Kanouse DE, Rogers WH, Carson S, Hertz R. Behavior patterns and sexual identity of bisexual men. J Sex Res 1992;29:141.
10. Diaz T, Chu SY, Frederick M, et al. Sociodemographics and HIV risk behaviors of bisexual men with AIDS: results from a multistate interview project. AIDS 1993;7:1227.
11. Doll LS, Peterson J, Magana JR, Carrier JM. Male bisexuality and AIDS in the United States. In: Tielman R, Carballo M, Hendriks A, eds. Bisexuality and HIV/AIDS. Buffalo, NY: Prometheus Books, 1991.
12. Centers for Disease Control and Prevention. AIDS among racial/ethnic minorities—United States, 1993. MMWR 1994;43:644.

13. Centers for Disease Control and Prevention. Update: mortality attributable to HIV infection among persons aged 25–44 years—United States, 1991 and 1992. MMWR 1993;42:869.
14. Diaz T, Buehler JW, Castro KG, Ward JW. AIDS trends among Hispanics in the United States. Am J Public Health 1993;83:504.
15. Centers for Disease Control and Prevention. Revision of the case definition of acquired immunodeficiency syndrome for national reporting—United States. MMWR 1985;34:373.
16. Centers for Disease Control and Prevention. Revision of the CDC surveillance case definition of acquired immunodeficiency syndrome. MMWR 1987;36(Suppl 1):1S.
17. Centers for Disease Control and Prevention. 1993 revised classification system for HIV infection and expanded surveillance case definition for AIDS among adolescents and adults. MMWR 1992;41:608.
18. Selik RM, Buehler JW, Karon JM, Chamberland ME, Berkelman RL. Impact of the 1987 revision of the case definition of acquired immunodeficiency syndrome in the United States. J Acquir Immune Defic Syndr 1990;3:73.
19. Centers for Disease Control and Prevention. Update: trends in AIDS diagnosis and reporting under the expanded surveillance definition for adolescents and adults—United States, 1993. MMWR 1994;43:826.
20. Lemp G, Hirozawa AM, Givertz D, et al. Seroprevalence of HIV and risk behaviors among young homosexual and bisexual men: the San Francisco/Berkeley Young Men's Survey. JAMA 1994;272:449.
21. Centers for Disease Control and Prevention. National HIV serosurveillance summary: results through 1993, update for vol 3. Atlanta: Public Health Service, U.S. Department of Health and Human Services, 1994.
22. McQuillan GM, Khare M, Ezzati-Rice TM, et al. The seroepidemiology of human immunodeficiency virus in the United States household population: NHANESIII, 1988–1991. J Acquir Immune Defic Syndr 1994;7:1195.
23. Karon JM. Written communication. Atlanta: Centers for Disease Control and Prevention, 1995.
24. Selik RM, Castro KG, Pappaioanou M. Racial/ethnic differences in the risk of AIDS in the United States. Am J Public Health 1988;78:1539.
25. Karon JM, Berkelman RL. The geographic and ethnic diversity of AIDS incidence in homosexual/bisexual men in the United States. J Acquir Immune Defic Syndr 1991;4:1179.
26. Centers for Disease Control and Prevention. Declining rates of rectal and pharyngeal gonorrhea in males—New York City. MMWR 1984;33:295.
27. Sorvillo FJ, Lieb L, Mascola L, Waterman SH. Declining rates of amebiasis in Los Angeles County: a sentinel for decreasing immunodeficiency incidence? Am J Public Health 1989;79:1563.
28. Aral SO, Holmes KK. Sexually transmitted diseases in the AIDS era. Sci Am 1991;264:62.
29. Kelly JA, Murphy DA, Roffman RA, et al. Acquired immunodeficiency syndrome/human immunodeficiency virus risk behavior among gay men in small cities. Arch Intern Med 1992;152:2293.
30. O'Reilly KR, Higgins DL, Galavotti C, et al. Relapse from safer sex among homosexual men: evidence from four cohorts in the AIDS Community Demonstration Projects. Presented at the 6th International Conference on AIDS, San Francisco, June 1990.
31. Stall R, Ekstrand M, Pollack L, et al. Relapse from safer sex: the next challenge for AIDS prevention efforts. J Acquir Immune Defic Syndr 1990;3:1181.
32. Hays Rb, Kegeles SM, Coates TJ. High HIV risk-taking among young gay men. AIDS 1990;4:901.
33. Osmond DH, Page K, Wiley J, et al. HIV infection in homosexual and bisexual men 18 to 29 years of age: the San Francisco Young Men's Health Study. Am J Public Health 1994;84:1933.
34. Dean L, Meyer I. HIV prevalence and sexual behavior in a cohort of New York City gay men (aged 18–24). J Acquir Immune Defic Syndr 1995;8:208.
35. Peterson JL, Coates TJ, Catania JA, Middleton L, Hilliard B, Hearst N. High-risk sexual behavior and condom use among gay and bisexual African-American men. Am J Public Health 1992;82:1490.
36. Tagle R, Gerald G, Patermaster M, Haywood M. Assessing the HIV-prevention needs of gay and bisexual men of color. Presented at the United States Conference of Mayors; United States Conference of Local Health Officers, Washington, DC, 1993.
37. Doll LS, Peterson LR, White C, Johnson ES, Ward JW. Homosexually and non-homosexually identified men who have sex with men: a behavioral comparison. J Sex Res 1992;29:1.
38. Centers for Disease Control and Prevention. Condom use and sexual identity among men who have sex with men, Dallas, 1991. MMWR 1993;42:7.
39. Earl WL. Married men and same sex activity: a field study of HIV risk among men who do not identify as gay or bisexual. J Sex Marital Ther 1990;16:251.
40. Carrier JM. Mexican male bisexuality. In: Klein F, Wolf TJ, eds. Bisexualities: theory and research. New York: Hayworth Press, 1985.
41. Morse EV, Simon PA, Osofsky H, Balson PM, Gaumer HR. The male street prostitute: a vector for transmission of HIV infection into the heterosexual world. Soc Sci Med 1991;32:535.
42. Hernandez M, Uribe P, Gortmaker S, et al. Sexual behavior and status for human immunodeficiency virus type 1 among homosexual and bisexual males in Mexico City. Am J Epidemiol 1992;135:883.
43. Miller HG, Turner CF, Moses LE, eds. AIDS—the second decade. Washington DC: National Academy Press, 1990.
44. Chaisson RE, Bacchetti P, Osmond D, Brodie B, Sande MA, Moss AR. Cocaine use and HIV infection in intravenous drug users in San Francisco. JAMA 1989;261:561.
45. Nwanyanwu OC, Chu SY, Green TA, Buehler JW, Berkelman RL. Acquired immunodeficiency syndrome in the United States associated with injecting drug use, 1981–1991. Am J Drug Alcohol Abuse 1993;19:399.
46. Menendez BS, Drucker E, Vermund SH, et al. AIDS mortality among Puerto Ricans and other Hispanics in New York City, 1981–1987. J Acquir Immune Defic Syndr 1990;3:644.
47. Watters JK, Lewis DK. HIV infection, race, and drug-treatment history. (Letter) AIDS 1990;4:697.
48. Centers for Disease Control and Prevention. Risk behaviors for HIV transmission among IVDUs not in drug treatment—U.S., 1987–1989. MMWR 1990;39:273.
49. Lurie P, Reingold AL. The public health impact of needle exchange programs in the United States and abroad: summary, conclusions, and recommendations. Rockville, MD: CDC National AIDS Clearinghouse, 1993.
50. Kaplan EH, Khoshnood R, Heimer R. A decline in HIV-infected needles returned to New Haven's needle exchange program: client shift or needle exchange? Am J Public Health 1994;84:1991.
51. Des Jarlais DC, Friedman SR, Sotheran JL, et al. Continuity and change within an HIV epidemic: injecting drug users in New York City, 1984 through 1992. JAMA 1994;271:121.
52. Mann JM, Tarantola DJM, Netter TW, eds. AIDS in the world. Cambridge: Harvard University Press, 1992.
53. Prevots DR, Ancelle-Park RA, Neal JJ, Remis RS. The epidemiology of heterosexually acquired HIV infection and AIDS in Western industrialized countries. AIDS 1994;8(Suppl 1):S109.
54. Centers for Disease Control and Prevention. Heterosexually acquired AIDS—United States, 1993. MMWR 1994;43:155.
55. Kim MY, Marmor M, Dubin N, Wolfe H. HIV risk-related behaviors among heterosexuals in New York City: associations with race, sex, and intravenous drug use. AIDS 1993;7:409.
56. Aral SO. Heterosexual transmission of HIV: the role of other sexually transmitted infections and behavior in its epidemiology, prevention, and control. Annu Rev Public Health 1993;14:451.
57. Laga M, Manoka A, Kivuvu M, et al. Non-ulcerative sexually transmitted diseases as risk factors for HIV-1 transmission in women: results from a cohort study. AIDS 1993;7:95.
58. Wasserheit JN. Epidemiological synergy: interrelationships between human immunodeficiency virus infection and other sexually transmitted diseases. Sex Transm Dis 1992;19:61.
59. Webster LA, Berman SM, Greenspan JR. Surveillance for gonorrhea and primary and secondary syphilis among adolescents, United States, 1981–1991. In: CDC surveillance summaries, August 13, 1993. MMWR 1993;42:1.
60. Centers for Disease Control and Prevention. Pregnancy, sexually transmitted diseases, and related risk behaviors among U.S. adolescents. Adolescent health: state of the nation monograph series, No. 2. CDC publication No. 099-4630. Atlanta: U.S. Department of Health and Human Services, 1994.
61. Centers for Disease Control and Prevention. Trends in sexual risk behaviors among high school students—United States, 1990, 1991, and 1993. MMWR 1995;44:124.
62. Marx R, Aral SO, Rolfs RT, et al. Crack, sex, and STD. Sex Transm Dis 1991;18:92.

63. Chiasson MA, Stoneburner RL, Hildebrandt DS, Ewing WE, Telzak EE, Jaffe HW. Heterosexual transmission of HIV-1 associated with the use of smokable freebase cocaine (crack). AIDS 1991;5:1121.

64. Chirgwin K, DeHovitz JA, Dillon S, McCormack WM. HIV infection, genital ulcer disease, and crack cocaine use among patients attending a clinic for sexually transmitted diseases. Am J Public Health 1991;81:1576.

65. Edlin BR, Irwin KL, Faruque S, et al. Intersecting epidemics—crack cocaine use and HIV infection among inner-city young adults. N Engl J Med 1994;331:1422.

66. Minkoff HL, McCalla S, Delke I, et al. The relationship of cocaine use to syphilis and human immunodeficiency virus infections among inner city parturient women. Am J Obstet Gynecol 1990;163:521.

67. Ellerbrock TV, Bush TJ, Chamberland ME, Oxtoby MJ. Epidemiology of women with AIDS in the United States, 1981 through 1990. JAMA 1991;265:2971.

68. Wasser SC, Gwinn M, Fleming P. Urban-nonurban distribution of HIV infection in childbearing women in the United States. J Acquir Immune Defic Syndr 1993;6:1035.

69. Diaz T, Chu SY, Conti L, et al. Risk behaviors of persons with heterosexually acquired HIV infection in the United States: results of a multistate surveillance project. J Acquir Immune Defic Syndr 1994; 7:958.

70. Moore JS, Harrison JS, Doll LS. Interventions for sexually active, heterosexual women in the United States. In: DiClemente RJ, Peterson JL, eds. Preventing AIDS: theories and methods of behavioral interventions. New York: Plenum Press, 1994.

71. Chu SY, Peterman TA, Doll LS, Buehler JW, Curran JW. AIDS in bisexual men in the United States. Am J Public Health 1992;82:220.

72. Padian NS. Female partners of bisexual men. Presented at the CDC Workshop in Bisexuality and AIDS, Atlanta, GA, October 1989.

73. McKirnan D, Burzette R, Stokes J. Differences in AIDS risk behavior among black and white bisexual men. Presented at the 7th International Conference on AIDS, Florence, Italy, June 1991.

74. Oxtoby MJ. Vertically acquired HIV infection in the United States. In: Pizzo PA, Wilfert CM, eds. Pediatric AIDS. 2nd ed. Baltimore: Williams & Wilkins, 1994.

75. Gwinn M, Pappaioanou M, George JR, et al. Prevalence of HIV infection in childbearing women in the United States. JAMA 1991;265:1704.

76. Gwinn M. Written communication. Atlanta: Centers for Disease Control and Prevention, 1995.

77. Connor EM, Sperling RS, Gelber R, et al. Reduction of maternal-infant transmission of human immunodeficiency virus type 1 with zidovudine treatment. N Engl J Med 1994;331:1173.

78. Centers for Disease Control and Prevention. U.S. Public Health Service recommendations for HIV counseling and testing for pregnant women. MMWR 1995;44:1.

79. Centers for Disease Control and Prevention. Recommendations of the U.S. Public Health Service Task Force on the use of zidovudine to reduce perinatal transmission of human immunodeficiency virus. MMWR 1994;43:1.

80. Ward JW, Holmberg SD, Allen JR, et al. Transmission of human immunodeficiency virus (HIV) by blood transfusions screened as negative for HIV antibody. N Engl J Med 1988;318:473.

81. Petersen LR, Satten GA, Busch M, et al. Duration of time from onset of human immunodeficiency virus infectiousness to development of detectable antibody. Transfusion 1994;34:283.

82. Busch MP, Lee LL, Satten GA, et al. Time course of detection of viral and serologic markers preceding human immunodeficiency virus type 1 seroconversion: implications for screening of blood and tissue donors. Transfusion 1995;35:91.

83. Chu SY, Hammett TA, Buehler JW. Update: epidemiology of reported cases of AIDS in women who report sex only with other women, United States, 1980–1991. AIDS 1992;6:518.

84. Sabatini MT, Patel K, Hirschman R. Kaposi's sarcoma and T-cell lymphoma in an immunodeficient woman: a case report. AIDS Res 1984;1:135.

85. Marmor M, Weiss LR, Lyden M, et al. Possible female-to-female transmission of human immunodeficiency virus. (Letter) Ann Intern Med 1986;105:969.

86. Monzon OT, Capellan JMB. Female-to-female transmission of HIV. (Letter) Lancet 1987;2:40.

87. Perry S, Jacobsberg L, Fogel K. Orogenital transmission of HIV. Ann Intern Med 1989;111:951.

88. Rich JD, Buck A, Tuomala RE, et al. Transmission of human immunodeficiency virus presumed to have occurred via female homosexual contact. Clin Infect Dis 1993;17:1003.

89. Kennedy MB, Scarlett MI, Duerr AC, Chu SY. Assessing HIV risk among women who have sex with women: scientific and communication issues. JAMWA 1995;50:103.

90. Stewart GJ, Tyler JP, Cunningham AL, et al. Transmission of human T-cell lymphotropic virus type III (HTLV-III) by artificial insemination by donor. Lancet 1985;2:581.

91. Chiasson MA, Stoneburner RL, Joseph SC. Human immunodeficiency virus transmission through artificial insemination. J Acquir Immune Defic Syndr 1990;3:69.

92. Centers for Disease Control and Prevention. HIV-1 infection and artificial insemination with processed semen. MMWR 1990;39:249.

93. Araneta MRG, Mascola L, Eller A, et al. HIV transmission through donor artificial insemination. JAMA 1995;273:854.

94. Eskenazi B, Pies C, Newstetter A, Shepard C, Pearson K. HIV serology in artificially inseminated lesbians. J Acquir Immune Defic Syndr 1989;2:187.

95. Centers for Disease Control and Prevention. Semen banking, organ and tissue transplantation, and HIV antibody testing. MMWR 1988;37:57.

96. Guinan ME. Artificial insemination by donor: safety and secrecy. JAMA 1995;273:890.

97. Henderson DK. HIV-1 in the health-care setting. In: Mandell GL, Douglas RG Jr, Bennett JE, eds. Principles and practice of infectious disease. 4th ed. New York: Churchill Livingstone, 1995:2632.

98. Gerberding JL. Incidence and prevalence of human immunodeficiency virus, hepatitis B virus, hepatitis C virus, and cytomegalovirus among health care personnel at risk for blood exposure: final report from a longitudinal study. J Infect Dis 1994;170:1410.

99. Clavel F, Guetard D, Brun-Vezinet F, et al. Isolation of a new human retrovirus from West Africa patients with AIDS. Science 1986;233:343.

100. De Cock KM, Adjorlolo G, Ekpini E, et al. Epidemiology and transmission of HIV-2: why there is no HIV-2 pandemic. JAMA 1993;270:2083.

101. O'Brien TR, George JR, Holmberg SD. Human immunodeficiency virus type 2 infection in the United States. JAMA 1992;267:2775.

102. Centers for Disease Control and Prevention. Surveillance for HIV-2 infection in blood donors—United States, 1987–1989. MMWR 1990;39:829.

103. Hu DJ, Fleming Pl, Mays MA, Ward JW. The expanding regional diversity of the acquired immunodeficiency syndrome epidemic in the United States. Arch Intern Med 1994;154:654.

AIDS: Biology, Diagnosis, Treatment and Prevention, fourth edition, edited by Vincent T. DeVita, Jr., Samuel Hellman, and Steven A. Rosenberg. Lippincott–Raven Publishers, © 1997

CHAPTER 10 Transmission of the HIV

10.1 Transmission of HIV-1 Among Adolescents and Adults

Sten H. Vermund

The first reports of a previously unrecognized acquired immunodeficiency syndrome (AIDS) were made in 1981.[1-4] *Pneumocystis carinii* pneumonia in homosexual men with multiple sexual partners suggested a sexual origin of an infectious agent that suppressed a normal immune response; cytomegalovirus was the first suspect etiologic agent.[3,5] By 1982, AIDS cases had been reported among men and women who injected drugs, recent Haitian immigrants to the United States, and persons with hemophilia.[6,7] Reports soon followed of apparent acquired immune deficiencies among infants born to injection drug users (IDUs), women who did not inject drugs but whose sexual partners injected drugs, and infants born to female sexual partners of IDUs.[8–10] Blood transfusion recipients, including those who were elderly, were reported with AIDS, adding to the transmission patterns reminiscent of hepatitis B.[11,12] The clinical presentation among infants was distinct from known congenital immune deficiencies.[8,13] Bisexual men may have been at special risk and served as a bridge population for the human immunodeficiency virus (HIV) into the female population.[14–17]

The appearance of AIDS in diverse populations implicated several routes of transmission: contaminated needles or injection equipment; clotting factor concentrates, blood, and selected other blood products; transplacental and intrapartum and breast-feeding; anal and vaginal sex.[18,19] Although the major routes of transmission were delineated by clever clinicians and epidemiologists in the first 2 years of the recognized pandemic,[20,21] the subsequent decade unraveled key cofactors for transmission and introduced new conundrums that continue to challenge our quest for control of HIV spread (Fig. 10.1-1).[22]

SEXUAL TRANSMISSION

Worldwide, more than 90% of HIV infections are associated with heterosexual transmission.[3] In the United States, cumulative 1981 through 1994 AIDS surveillance reports received through April 14, 1995 to the Centers for Disease Control and Prevention (CDC) indicate that 60% of adult cases of AIDS are linked to either male-to-male sexual (53%) or heterosexual (7.3%) exposure categories, with an additional 6.6% reporting both male-to-male sexual and IDU activity.[24] The World Health Organization (WHO) highlighted an epidemiologic distinction between countries in which there was a predominance of male homosexual and IDU (ie, pattern I) or heterosexual (ie, pattern II) transmission.[25,26] Many countries have experienced a shift from pattern I to II types of transmission, particularly in Latin America.[27–30] The largest epidemics in Africa and Asia have been based in the pattern II mode.[31–34] Pattern III countries (ie, sporadic, imported cases only) have become fewer as the worldwide pandemic has spread; vigilance in preventing extension of the epidemic to relatively unaffected countries is needed.

Infectiousness

The risk factors and cofactors associated with HIV transmission through sexual contact are often amenable to intervention (Table 10.1-1). Virus load may be the key unifying feature of transmission risk.[35–37] Because the dominant HIV binding affinity is for immunologic cells expressing the CD4 molecule, any physical or physiologic facilitator of this

Sten H. Vermund, Department of Epidemiology and Division of Geographic Medicine, Department of Medicine, University of Alabama at Birmingham, 720 20th Street South (TH203), Birmingham, AL 35294-0008.

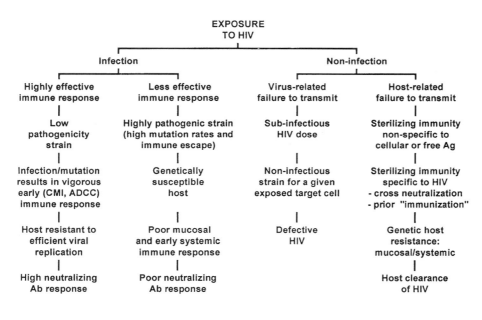

FIG. 10.1-1. Possible virologic and immunologic events related to HIV transmission through sexual and parenteral routes. Ab, antibody; ADCC, antibody-dependent cellular cytotoxicity; Ag, antigen; CMI, cell mediated immunity.

contact may be expected to increase transmission risk. The complex associations that may exist between sexual risk factors and the difficulties in measuring these factors make it challenging to identify consistently the same significant factors in all populations at all times.[38–40] Risk of sexual transmission is greatest when the infected partner has a high circulating virus load, because this may correlate well with genital tract virus load. When an HIV-infected individual is in the "window period" between infection and seroconversion, the virus load is very high.[41,42] The seroconversion event marks the vigorous immune response, with cell-mediated activity recognizable weeks before humoral immunity is evident. Viral clearance from the peripheral circulation probably correlates with a period of substantially lower infectiousness. However, not all viral predictors are quantitative; viral phenotype and cellular tropism (eg, macrophages versus lymphocytes) are probably relevant to infectiousness.[43,44]

A second, more prolonged period of higher infectiousness occurs when the HIV-infected person becomes increasingly immunosuppressed.[45–48] This is likely to be a consequence of high viremia and increased free and cell-associated virus load in cervicovaginal secretions, rectal fluids, and ejaculate, consequent to the deterioration of the immunologic gauntlet and the structural disruptions of the lymph node architecture that traps circulating virus for presentation to lymph node–based humoral and cellular defenses.[49–51]

Although it has been apparent that higher transmission rates have been associated with depleted CD4+ cells among HIV-infected sexual partners,[46,48,52–54] causality is hard to establish because higher transmission rates in late stage disease may also reflect longer duration of exposure to an infected partner.[49–51] Longitudinal studies that simultaneously monitor sexual behavior and the clinical progression and evolving immunologic status of discordant sexual partners are in

progress to address this issue.[55–60] U.S. studies have failed to address this issue because of the low seroconversion rates, probably an incidental "study effect" of enrollment into a cohort that offers education and counseling, sexually transmitted disease (STD) screening and treatment, and condom distribution.[55,58,61,62] Ethical concerns and the need to intervene in encouraging prevention of transmission between discordant couples (ie, one seropositive and the other seronegative) make human studies challenging.

Further contributions to infectiousness are those that recruit more CD4+ cells into the genital tract of the infected individual.[63] Sexually transmitted infections that result in frank genital ulcers may include chancroid, herpes, syphilis, and other diseases. Infections and conditions resulting in inflammation and exudation include chlamydial infection, gonorrhea, trichomoniasis, bacterial vaginosis, and candidiasis. Recruitment of infectious lymphocytes, macrophages, or other cells into seminal or vaginal secretions may increase transmissibility, as occurs with sexually transmitted infections and their inflammatory urethral, prostatic, cervical, vaginal, and anal responses.[64–68] Mucosal ulceration, inflammation, exudation, or trauma to protective epithelial surfaces, as occurs with infection or "dry sex," is likely to increase the efficiency of viral release and viral entry.[69–73] STD patients commonly report other high-risk activities and high-risk partners.[74]

Although hypothesized, it is unknown whether systemic coinfections in the HIV-infected person increase infectiousness. Coinfections such as cytomegalovirus, Epstein-Barr virus, human T-cell lymphotropic virus types I or II, human herpesviruses type 6 or 7, *Mycoplasma fermentans*,[75,76] and others may increase viral expression in vitro and could increase in vivo viremia and infectiousness. Human studies have not been strongly confirmatory of these laboratory observations, although the negative data do not disprove the hypotheses.

TABLE 10.1-1. *Factors of interest in the sexual transmission of HIV*

Number of sexual partners
Number of sexual exposures
Likelihood sexual partner is infected
  Gay or bisexual man
  Injection drug users
  Commercial sex worker (prostitute)
  HIV prevalence in geographic area of residence
  Hemophiliac or recipient of multiple blood transfusions or products
Probability of transmission during sexual activity
  Viral variations in tropism and infectivity
  Host factors
    Other infectious diseases (STD, systemic viral infections)
    Stage of infection (window period, advanced immunosuppression)
    Immunogenetic profile
    Blood during sex (menses, first coitus)
    Youthful age
    Lack of circumcision in men
    Presence of female circumcision
    Contraceptives (oral, condoms, intrauterine device, spermicides)
    Behavioral and biologic interactions
      Nature of sexual contact; insertive most infectious versus receptive most susceptible
    Penile-vaginal (common)
    Penile-anal (common)
    Penile-oral (rare)
    Oral-vaginal (unknown)
    Oral-anal (unknown)
    Oral-oral (if blood contact, saliva to saliva unknown)
    Manual-anal (if traumatic and followed by exposure)
    Manual-vaginal (if traumatic and followed by exposure)
  Noninjecting drug use (cocaine, alcohol, nitrites) through facilitation of high-risk sexual contact
  Vaginal douches, astringents, abrasives, or trauma
  Anal douches or trauma

The uncircumcised male may have a higher intraurethral and subprepucal load of potentially infectious cells than the uncircumcised man, explaining the data suggesting this as a risk factor for transmission to a sexual partner.[7,77–79] It is plausible, but unknown, that a woman who has been circumcised with an infundibulectomy would be more infectious if infected because of the trauma to the unnatural postsurgical genital anatomy.[80–86]

Host genetics may influence natural history and viral load.[87] Some persons may be more infectious as a consequence of their greater genetic susceptibility to rapid progression.

The antiretroviral experience of the infectious individual is important, but we are not sure whether this increases through longevity[88] or decreases through lower viral load[37] the person's lifetime infectiousness. The drug-naive, HIV-infected recipient of antiretroviral chemotherapy usually experiences a decline in viral load and a rise in CD4+ cell count.[89] This is transient. Although patients are less infectious early in the course of chemotherapy, the prolonged survival and AIDS-free state[90–92] may permit longer duration of high-risk sexual

activity, if educational messages and personal experience do not combine to influence safer sexual practices of the infected individual. What the population consequences are of widespread antiviral chemoprophylaxis and chemotherapy—net benefits to society in reduced transmission from reduced infectiousness or net increased transmission because of longer lifespan of infected individuals—is unknown.[93] The issue highlights the urgency of effective behavior change programs focussed on HIV-infected persons.[94]

Susceptibility

Factors that probably facilitate transmission include those that increase contact with blood and infectious genital secretions during sexual acts and increase virus-cell contact with vulnerable cells in the mucosal epithelia of the rectum, cervix, vagina, or oral cavity. Increased contact time with infectious secretions that are kept warm and moist is likely to increase transmissibility, suggesting why male-to-female transmission rates are more efficient than female-to-male and why uncircumcised men may be at increased risk for heterosexual transmission from vaginal sex.[56,67,79,95] Rates of female-to-male transmission in Thailand are much higher than noted in United State and European studies, suggesting at least one reason for the rapid expansion of the heterosexual epidemic in developing countries.[96]

Risk of infection is related to specific sexual behaviors rather than to sexual orientation or preference.[97] The risk of becoming infected through sexual transmission is associated with several well-documented factors:

The number of different partners, increasing the likelihood of encountering an HIV-infected person[98,99]
The likelihood of a person's sexual partners being infected, which depends on risk factors associated with the partner's behavior or previous exposure[8,100]
The number of sexual exposures from an infected partner, which may increase the likelihood of successful infection[101,102]
The integrity of the epithelial mucosa of the exposed sexual, oral, or rectal-anal orifice, as determined by cofactors for transmission such as STDs or traumatic abrasions[68,103]
The use of barriers to block HIV, especially the correct use of latex condoms[56,60,61,104–107]
The infectiousness of the partner.

Less well documented, but highly plausible, are other susceptibility variables:

Anal sex, because of the trauma that can be associated with insertion into a nonepithelialized orifice[108]
The activation status of the exposed, uninfected individual's immune system from coinfections or other antigenic challenges, resulting in the priming of cellular targets for HIV-CD4 molecular linkages
Genetic susceptibility to HIV infection with certain human leukocyte antigen (HLA) and transporter associated with antigen processing (TAP) profiles[109–115]

Exocervical exposure of the endocervical columnar epithelium with a large, exposed transformation zone susceptible to STD or HIV infection (ie, cervical ectopy)[116]

Abnormal vaginal colonization after antibiotic use, douching, or other non-STD trauma.[117,118]

More speculative are the following possible risk or protective factors:

Oral contraceptive use that may be associated with increased cervical ectopy and risk of infection or that may result in lower risk because of salutary hormonal influences and pregnancy prevention[109,119,120]

Prior exposure to HIV or cellular antigens without infection, possibly resulting in protection (or in sensitization) with a vaccine-like effect[121,122]

Genital anatomic variations that result in increased or decreased contact time with infectious genital secretions after intercourse

Cultural differences in clothing and dressing patterns, particularly tighter and looser clothing that may affect postcoital genital friction among men such that genital fluid contact time may be affected

Female circumcision, as practiced widely in Sudan and in parts of east and west Africa, because of the original trauma and subsequent unnatural genital anatomy that may facilitate coital bleeding.

Although there is considerable interest in teasing out additional cofactors that facilitate or inhibit HIV transmission, the knowledge base since 1982 has been adequate to state that unprotected sex with a high-risk partner is the principal risk factor for sexual acquisition of HIV. The difficulty inherent in changing human sexual behavior gives incentive to further delineate possible points of intervention through a more detailed appreciation of the cofactors for transmission.

Nutritional status, particularly vitamin A deficiency, has emerged as a likely cofactor for perinatal transmission.[123] It will be important to assess whether sexual transmission occurs more easily in vitamin A deficient adults, because this introduces a potential intervention method for developing countries.[124,125]

Sexually transmitted infections

Although it is widely appreciated that STDs are associated with HIV risk, only recently has it been documented that a reduction in STDs can reduce HIV transmission.[61,126] Ulcerative STDs disrupt the integrity of the epithelial mucosa and facilitate HIV contact with the lymphatic and circulatory systems, as well as recruiting CD4+ lymphocytes and macrophages to the site of injury or infection.[127] Genital ulcers have had the highest relative risk estimates, with a 5-fold to 10-fold excess risk demonstrated in cross-sectional studies.[58,64,67,70,77,103,109,128-135] Inflammatory and exudative STDs are less disruptive of the epithelial tissues, but the exudate

may recruit large volumes of cervical or urethral discharge filled with susceptible cells, and inflammation may result in microulcerations and superficialization of capillaries, facilitating contact with HIV with more easily infectable cells. Relative risk estimates for excess risk for HIV with nonulcerogenic STDs may be in the 2-fold to 5-fold range.[104,130,136-140]

This may suggest that ulcerogenic STDs should be the target of intervention. However, inflammatory and exudative STDs such as chlamydial infection, gonorrhea, and trichomoniasis are far more common than ulcerogenic STDs such as herpes, syphilis, and chancroid. The risk within a given population attributable to STDs is greater, therefore, for inflammatory and exudative STDs than for ulcerogenic STDs, suggesting the strong need to target all STDs.

Risk and Age, Race or Ethnicity, and Gender

Cumulative 1981 through 1994 surveillance data in the United States have revealed that 48.5% of AIDS cases have occurred among non-Hispanic whites. African-Americans and Hispanics or Latinos account for 50.4% of cases, representing more than 75% of heterosexual men, women, and children.[24] Sociologic and behavioral characteristics, such as higher prevalence of IDU and poorer educational backgrounds, are the roots of drug abuse frequencies and high sexual risk behaviors in some minority populations.[141]

Crack house sex-for-drugs exchanges, most prevalent in eastern U.S. inner-city and southeastern U.S. rural minority communities, is a powerful multiplier for HIV transmission, analogous to the bathhouse environments prevalent in San Francisco, New York City, Los Angeles, and elsewhere from 1977 to 1984.[58,132,142-144] The bathhouse catering to homosexual and bisexual men, "swinging singles" clubs for heterosexuals, and crack house environments for drug addicts and their sexual partners are perfect for HIV transmission when a highly infectious individual is introduced into the arena of multiple, unprotected sexual encounters. The efficient multiplier is a classic feature of STDs with a "core" transmitter group, but rarely is there a more rapid spread than when the core transmitters combine expanded social networks with high frequency of infectious contacts.[145-151]

Black women in Alabama have HIV and AIDS rates approximately 20 times that of white women, a frequency that may be related to higher rates of HIV in African-American heterosexual men in Alabama and to higher efficiency of transmission because of the relative rarity of condom use and frequency of STDs.[52] This pattern in the rural and urban southeast United States is reminiscent of well-established patterns in the urban northeast and in south Florida. Nor can old stereotypes of a "gay, white" epidemic be sustained into the 21st century. Male-to-male high-risk sex is prevalent in minority communities as diverse as rural Alabama and Washington, DC.[152,153] Drug abuse is prevalent in many racial and ethnic groups. However, IDU is far more common among U.S.-born African-American and Puerto Rican populations than among whites, Caribbean-born blacks, and other Hispanic or Latino groups.[58,154–157] The heterosexual and drug-related epidemics therefore are more prevalent in these groups.

The origin of racial and gender differences in sexual risk may be multifactorial.[158] Biologic factors such as HLA types may play a currently unknown role. Differential STD rates are highly relevant, perhaps explaining the differential heterosexual epidemic in Asia and Africa compared with North America and Europe. Douching practices that lower the *Lactobacillus* rates in otherwise healthy women may differ by race and ethnic tradition, resulting in higher bacterial vaginosis and genital tract inflammation in one group compared with another.[117]

Sexual risk taking can differ in different populations. In more than 2000 men screened anonymously in a Baltimore STD clinic, HIV infection was independently associated with black race in multiple regression analysis, presumably because of a racial correlation with unmeasured behavioral variables.[159–162] A New York City study found a similar result and postulated an unmeasured behavioral origin.[163,164] Among married men in the National AIDS Behavioral Survey (1991–1993), high-risk sexual activity did not differ among white, black, and Hispanic or Latino men. However, unmarried minority men had higher reported risk than whites.[22,165] Young, unmarried, African-American males have the highest risk in U.S. Army studies.[98,166] Racial and ethnic differences in HIV transmission will require investigation to help facilitate culturally sensitive prevention strategies.[156,167–170] Biologic differences that may have ethnic correlations also need exploration, sensitive to how such topics have been abused in past discussions of eugenics and racist ideologies.[171,172]

Young and postmenopausal women may be at comparatively higher risk of HIV infection for a given number of exposures.[173–175] Immature vaginal mucosa in adolescents, with large cervical ectopy zones may be more susceptible to trauma during sex and may be especially prone to infection with STDs because of the large transformation zone and exposed columnar epithelia.[116,176–178] HIV transmission may be facilitated by sexual activity at times in which there is expected to be blood exposure, as during menses,[179] rape,[180–184] or first coital experience.[176] Improved understanding of mucosal immunity is needed to appreciate the relative importance of physical and immunochemical barriers to transmission.[73,185–189]

A few studies of the correlation of HIV infection with circumcision have demonstrated higher infection rates for uncircumcised men.[67,77–79,133,190,191] Several potential cofactors for this association have been proposed, including retention of viable virus under the prepuce of the uncircumcised male.[49,192] Bleeding during intercourse for the circumcised female is an important gender-related concern where it is practiced; female circumcision is a common practice in parts of east and west Africa where HIV is endemic, but little has been documented about any relation between HIV

risk and female infundibulectomy. Because this practice is unsafe for women and girls for a host of other genitourinary and infectious reasons, its reduction is indicated even before AIDS control becomes a documented motive.[80–86]

Anal sex may facilitate HIV transmission better than vaginal sex, as suggested by its independent risk association among heterosexuals.[108,160,193,194] This would be biologically plausible because of the abundance of infectable cells in the distal large intestine.[195,196] Similarly, oral sex is probably less infectious, although epidemiologic studies are weak in divining causal associations because of the congruence of oral sexual risk with anal or vaginal sexual activity.[197,198] Animal studies may prove useful in assessing human risk through vaginal and anal viral challenges, microbicide screening, and the role of trauma as a facilitator of transmission. Given the species specificity of STDs, the animal models are not now well developed to test features of STDs as HIV transmission cofactors.

Lesbian sexual practices are rarely traumatic or blood contaminated, and they rely on safer sexual activities, such as mutual masturbation and oral sex. The sexual activities may be considered far safer than heterosexual or male homosexual activity.[199] However, lesbian women may choose gay male partners for bisexual activity or insemination in childbearing efforts, may chose artificial insemination with attendant risks, may engage in heterosexual activity with a false sense of security based on their primary homosexual orientation, and may inject drugs.[200–202] Behavioral and educational attention therefore must be focussed on lesbian women in ways somewhat distinct from from the messages suitable for heterosexual women or homosexual men.

Older persons are less likely to practice high-risk behaviors, but those who do have high-risk sexual behavior are less likely to take precautions.[203,204] Hence, attention to risk beyond the adolescent and young adult populations is needed.

Monitoring Sexual Transmission

Limitations exist in tracking the heterosexual component of the epidemic using surveillance data. Worldwide reporting of AIDS is poor outside of the industrialized countries of Europe, Australia, and North America. A few tropical or developing countries have excellent reporting, but most resource-poor settings rely on samples of convenience and modeled estimates of HIV.[25,205,206] The proportion of the epidemic burden attributed to heterosexual transmission is especially unreliable. In the United States, for example, reported AIDS cases are grouped by risk exposure according to a hierarchical risk assignment. An individual with AIDS who had reported a single IDU episode would be categorized as IDU-related risk, even if he or she had experienced thousands of unprotected sexual encounters with an infected partner, underestimating the proportion of AIDS cases due to heterosexual transmission. Some cases with no identifiable risk are likely to have been infected through heterosexual contact, perhaps without appreciating the risk status of a given partner. Also distorting the accuracy of AIDS risk reporting are persons not wishing to reveal potentially stigmatizing behavior who may report heterosexual risk to avoid being identified as bisexual, homosexual, or injecting drugs.[207,208]

The rapidly changing clinical profile due to therapy has made surveillance of AIDS less useful than in the pretreatment era. The 1993 CDC surveillance case definition revisions tried to equate severe HIV disease with the AIDS surveillance definition by including CD4+ cell count under 200/μL as AIDS-defining alongside the slightly expanded list of AIDS-defining clinical diagnoses.[209] Even as CDC surveillance efforts are cut to accommodate budgetary restrictions, wider HIV screening efforts motivated by the clinical need to identify persons needing prophylactic therapy, such as pregnant women, may give us a better idea of the extent of the sexual epidemic in the United States

PARENTERAL TRANSMISSION: INJECTION DRUG USERS

Even before the first report associating AIDS and use of injectable drugs in 1983,[6] the epidemic among IDUs had spread worldwide. The number of IDUs infected with HIV in the United States may be between 200,000 and 320,000, which is more than 25% of all IDUs.[210,211] IDU-associated AIDS cases constitute the second largest risk exposure category in CDC surveillance statistics.[24,212] In newly reported cases, IDU and heterosexual cases exceed male-to-male sex as the reported risk in many parts of the United States.[93,153,210,213] Through 1994, 32% of the 435,319 adult and adolescent AIDS cases reported in the United States and its territories were associated with IDU. This included 81,491 male heterosexual IDUs, 27,902 female IDUs, and 28,521 male homosexual or bisexual IDUs. Thousands of infected women and men whose heterosexual partners were IDUs, children whose mothers were IDUs, and children whose mothers were sex partners of IDUs may attribute their infections indirectly to the use of injectable drugs.

Secondary spread of HIV infection through heterosexual activity from the ever-increasing reservoir of IDUs continues to rise.[153,214–217] This is in dramatic contrast to the situation within the male homosexual and bisexual community, in which incident HIV infection has fallen since 1983 among older men,[218] largely because of rapid and dramatic alterations in sexual behavior. Rates among young men and gay or bisexual men of minority background have not declined as notably.[219]

Infectiousness

Viral load, as with sexual exposure, may be the major factor predicting the infectiousness of an HIV-infected IDU. Viral load is highest shortly after infection, before the host immune system has time to marshal its defenses, and late in

the course of disease at the time of systemic immune collapse.[41,42] Low CD4+ cell counts are thought to be associated with increased infectiousness, although this is much harder to ascertain in needle sharing partners than among sexual couples. Behaviors related to drug use that increase cross-contamination activities in the window period and late in disease would be expected to increase risk. However, given the parenteral nature of the inoculation, it is known that HIV can be transmitted at just about any time in the course of infection. An infected IDU in open member sharing groups for drug use, as is common in "shooting galleries," are expected to be an especially dangerous vector for widespread transmission.[155,163] Similarly, the non-IDU who is exchanging crack cocaine for sex can be in a highly efficient transmission environment in which IDUs are among the sexual clients and STD prevalence is substantial.

Continued injection of drugs after HIV infection may be a cofactor in the development of AIDS through increased immune activation and viral expression.[220] In vitro immunologic stimulation of infected T cells leads to greater viral replication and cell death, and injection is known to stimulate T-cell activation, suggesting a possible mechanism for this association.[221] It is plausible that infectiousness could be increased in such circumstances, giving yet more incentive to ensure that all drug users, especially those who are HIV infected, have maximum access to treatment assistance. Coinfection with STDs and with systemic viruses may activate the immune system and stimulate higher HIV production, resulting in a higher probability for successful HIV infection. However plausible this seems, the data for such a risk are not convincing, and ongoing injection could result in a paradoxical slowing of clinical progression, perhaps through a therapeutic vaccine-like effect.[40] Of course, IDUs are infectious through sexual routes.[222,223] An IDU who rarely injects or never shares needles or syringes but is a frequent crack cocaine smoker may transmit the virus through sex, sometimes exchanging sex for drugs or money.

Susceptibility

Needle-sharing networks and the "human bridges" that connect them are critical in predicting the efficiency of transmission. Drug users tend to share in groups. Most dangerous is promiscuous sharing in a shooting gallery environment, where anonymous sharing occurs. Social sharing with a more defined needle-sharing group is of intermediate risk. Appreciation of bridging behaviors and individuals across groups can be valuable in trying to reduce HIV risk in active needle users. Syringes and needles that appear to be clean or do not have visible blood may nonetheless harbor HIV.[224] In south Florida shooting galleries, 20% of needles or syringes with visible blood were positive for HIV antibodies, although 5% were HIV positive without visible blood. Needles and syringes without visible blood but identified as "dirty" by drug users were equally likely to be HIV seropositive as those identified as "clean" (4.7% versus 5.5%).[225]

A sterile needle that is used by a single user and is never shared can remain HIV free, which is the underlying principle behind education and wider availability of clean needles and syringes. One of the great tragedies of the HIV epidemic is society's reluctance to ensure that the addicted drug user has access to clean needles, syringes, and other "works."[155,163,226–240]

Reduction in the IDU epidemic would result in a marked reduction in the epidemic among women and children in North America and Europe.[241] Cases associated with IDU accounted for 47.8% of all female AIDS cases reported through 1994 in the United States.[24] Almost 36% of the 58,428 adult female AIDS cases reported in 1981 through 1994 are attributed to heterosexual contact, many of these with an intravenous drug user.[24] Drug injection by male sexual partners is an important factor for HIV infection in women in the United States. Extension of the HIV epidemic among drug users in Asia will predictably increase drug-related heterosexual transmission.[240] Male drug users commonly have female sexual partners who do not use drugs.[155,242] Heterosexual HIV transmission is more frequent among women than men, partly because of the greater numbers of infected heterosexual men who tend to be greater users of intravenous drugs. There is a greater likelihood of a woman encountering an infected male sexual partner in a locale with prevalent HIV and IDU than for a man to encounter an HIV-infected woman.[43] Moreover, sexual transmission appears to be more biologically efficient from male to female. Women who overcome addictions may continue to be at risk of HIV transmission through sexual encounters.[223]

Female former IDUs whose sexual partners currently inject drugs display a higher HIV seroprevalence than do female IDUs whose sexual partners do not inject drugs. Most women who inject drugs are in their prime childbearing years; of the 6209 AIDS cases in children, 5541 were attributed to perinatal acquisition of HIV from 1981 through 1994, most from mothers who were IDUs or were sexual partners of IDUs.[24] IDU-associated AIDS cases represents over one half of all AIDS cases in Hispanics and African-Americans reported from 1981 through 1994 in the United States[24]

In addition to sharing needles, attendance at shooting galleries as important risk factors.[155,163,243–252] IDUs may purchase drugs and rent needles and syringes at these clandestine establishments, resulting in the repetitive use of drug paraphernalia by strangers. "Booting," or priming the syringe by pulling blood back into the syringe before injection, increases blood admixture between needle sharers. These activities add to the mystique of using drugs in certain settings; exact practices vary by neighborhood and region.[53]

Heroin and cocaine are the drugs commonly associated with seropositivity among intravenous drug users. There may be an estimated 400,000 to 600,000 IDUs in the United States, where the peak age group of users is persons in their thirties. The U.S. cocaine epidemic in the 1980s appears to involve many persons who have been heavy marijuana users[254] and has included adolescents.[255,256] Although the crack epidemic is abating somewhat, there remains a large problem in the 1990s.[58,129,216] Illustrative of the wider problem of multiple drug use, 83% of a sample of heroin users in New York City and 81% in Seattle also used parenteral cocaine.[257,258]

Cocaine can effect a "high" by smoking (ie, freebasing), intranasal use, injection alone, or in combination with heroin (ie, speedballing). Studies suggest cocaine to be more strongly associated with HIV acquisition than heroin or other drugs,[259] probably owing to the greater frequency of its use.[260] Non-IDU crack use is HIV associated because of exchange of sex for drugs and other high-risk sexual activity.[261,262] Given the resurgence of heroin use in cities such as New York and its purity and low cost, some addicts are shifted toward sniffing or smoking heroin. Because of the sedation associated with heroin and the lower usage frequency, the rate of associated HIV transmission through sexual routes may not be as high as among crack abusers.[16]

High-risk sexual practices and drug use are related behaviors.[263] Participants in a methadone treatment program reported a history of syphilis and gonorrhea, 6% and 36% respectively, in one study, probably a minimum estimate of true cumulative incidence.[245] One half of 835 prostitutes interviewed in various cities across the United States admitted to using intravenous drugs, and only 4% reported frequent condom use.[264] IDUs are less likely to incorporate safe sex behaviors than to use safer needle-sharing practices.[265–268] Male IDUs with steady female sexual partners reveal a high frequency of multiple sexual partners and low rates of condom use.[215,217,223,269,270] In an effort to evaluate the risks of simultaneous IDU and heterosexual activity, 58% of a sample of IDU prostitutes were found to be HIV seropositive, compared with 0% of a non-IDU prostitution group in Northeastern Italy in 1984, suggesting the relatively greater risk of IDU early in the AIDS epidemic.[271]

HIV-Contaminated Instruments

Use of HIV-contaminated instruments used for puncture or injection in other nontraditional ways may transmit HIV. A 6-week period of acupuncture therapy was implicated in the seroconversion of a previously healthy 17-year-old boy without any known risk factors.[272] Two persons may have contracted HIV from tattoos administered in prison with unsterilized tattoo needles.[273] Adolescent brothers may have transmitted HIV through sharing shaving equipment contaminated with with blood from cuts.[274]

Even professionally administered needle sticks or injections may cause HIV infection if proper sterilization techniques are not used. The pressure to reuse equipment when funds for replenishment of medical supplies are short could explain the occurrence of some HIV without the classic risk factors.[275] Epidemics in Romania and the former Soviet Union have been documented among hospitalized children with HIV-seronegative mothers. Shortages of medical supplies have resulted in reuse of needles presumably contaminated with HIV.[276,277]

In resource-poor areas of Africa, Asia, and Latin America, the potential exists for transmission of HIV through unsanitary use of needles.[278] A possible role for medical injections in the transmission of HIV in seropositive children of seronegative mothers was postulated in Zaire.[276] Data from Central Africa have suggested that HIV is associated with an increased number of medical injections,[279] although another study found no such association.[280]

Various cultural practices may result in exposure of individuals to HIV include medicinal bloodletting, blood brotherhood, ritual and medicinal enemas, and the use of shared instruments for ritual scarification or group circumcision of males or females.[190] One investigator has suggested that voodoo rituals and using powders with HIV-infected remains could facilitate infection.[281] Other areas of reported concern for parenteral transmission include tuberculosis screening,[282] jet injections,[283] medical waste disposal,[284] neurologic pins,[236] electroencephalographic testing,[285] earlobe sampling by stylet,[275] and prenatal diagnostic tests on seropositive mothers.[286]

Occupational Exposure

Occupational exposure among health care workers has been the topic of recent review; deep punctures with large-bore needles are the highest-risk event.[287] Nonparenteral exposures such as splash exposures carry much smaller risks. Nurses are most commonly exposed.[288,289] Zidovudine use has been associated with partial protection in an observational analysis performed by CDC, but it has not been demonstrated to protect all exposed health care workers.[290]

Tuberculosis

Although susceptibility to HIV infection is the topic of this chapter, transmission of tuberculosis commonly occurs among drug users, facilitated by poor housing and other social conditions.[220,291] Pneumonias are also more common among drug users, but these do not carry the community risk inherent in tuberculosis.[292–294] An epidemic within an epidemic is apparent, particularly in developing countries and among IDUs in the United States: the expanded tuberculosis problem facilitated by HIV-related immunosuppression.[295] In this way, the worldwide HIV epidemic becomes truly a threat to everyone because of the lack of personal control over aerosolized exposure compared with sexual or drug use exposure. It adds the need for chronic, directly observed chemotherapy and chemoprophylaxis among drug users with tuberculosis.[296,297] In developing nations, isoniazid prophylaxis for HIV-infected patients to prevent tuberculosis has proven efficacious.[298] Although not the focus of this

chapter, the special relationship of HIV and increased tuberculosis risk is an important issue, giving added incentive to prevent transmission of the former to inhibit transmission of the latter.

PARENTERAL TRANSMISSION: BLOOD AND BLOOD PRODUCTS

In July, 1982, three recipients of factor VIII concentrates for treatment of hemophilia were reported to have developed *P carinii* pneumonia, which suggested that transfusion of blood and blood products was a plausible mechanism for transmission.[299] In December, 1982, a newborn who had received multiple blood transfusions for erythroblastosis fetalis was reported to have become progressively immunocompromised and developed opportunistic infections, including *Mycobacterium avium* complex (formerly called *M avium-intracelluare*).[300] Investigation of the 19 blood donors revealed that one was later diagnosed with AIDS.[11,301]

Many early studies, including experiments with animals, confirmed the biologic plausibility of bloodborne transmission, finding evidence for passage of the virus in donor-recipient transfusion pairs.[302–306] Epidemiologic analyses of transfusion-associated AIDS cases have made unique contributions to the understanding of HIV transmission and the natural history of the disease. Table 10.1-2 summarizes these important observations.[12,225,302,304–322]

The risk of acquiring HIV infection through blood transfusion has varied by region, depending on the area's seroprevalence among blood donors, and the sensitivity of the screening strategies.[323,324] Before testing was available, 90% of 124 persons transfused with HIV-infected blood were infected.[325] The risk of contracting HIV infection from a seronegative blood donor has been estimated to be from 1.47 to 3.72 infections per 100,000 units in the United States in the postscreening era of 1985 through 1988.[326–329] Further analysis of annual blood supply data suggests that the num-

TABLE 10.1-2. *Contributions of transfusion-associated AIDS studies*

- Established that AIDS had an infectious cause and identified HIV-1 as the primary causal agent[12,302,305,306]
- Established the bloodborne nature of AIDS, and contributed to the rationale for hepatitis B–like transmission[225,304,308]
- Allowed estimations of the incubation period and precise date of seroconversion known for many persons[309–313]
- Evidence of a prolonged asymptomatic and infectious carrier state, based on studies of infected blood donor-recipient pairs and on studies of sexual partners of blood and blood product recipients[02,307,312,314–318]
- Blood infected with HIV poses a substantial risk to recipients; estimates of infectivity are 38% to 100%.[314,319–322]

Adapted from Friedland GH, Klein RS. Transmission of the human immunodeficiency virus. N Engl J Med 1987;317:1125.

ber of HIV-positive units entering the United States' blood supply has declined approximately 30% per year since April 1985.[330] At the initiation of serologic donor testing (1985), positive donations were identified at a rate of approximately 38 per 100,000 donations. The number has dropped to 10 per 100,000 donations, 40 times lower than would be expected for a random sample of the U.S. population.[331]

Circumstances in many developing countries remain more urgent. Transmission can occur from unscreened blood given for medical purposes, use of unclean needles in medical or traditional health care settings, unsterile surgical procedures and births, anabolic steroid use, suboptimal hemodialysis, and scarification and tattooing.[332] Resources are inadequate to guarantee a safe blood supply worldwide, a sad reminder that even when our knowledge base is complete and our plan for control is straightforward, HIV prevention programs may not ensue.

When untreated, whole blood, fresh-frozen platelets, packed cells, and clotting factors have been demonstrated to carry HIV. Hepatitis B vaccines derived from human or recombinant sources, albumin and immune globulin (including $Rh_o(D)$ immune globulin) have not been found to transmit HIV because of the purification processes which inactivates all known viruses.[307,333-335]

Other related retroviruses are spread through donated blood and plasma, including HTLV-I and HTLV-II associated with adult T-cell leukemia and HTLV-I myelopathy.[336,337] HTLV-II has been associated with hairy cell leukemia, but no disease has been definitively shown to be caused by HTLV-II.[338] Although the risk of acquiring HIV-1 infection in one large study was 3 per 100,000 units of blood product, the risk of acquiring HTLV-I infection was 24 per 100,000, suggesting the need to screen the blood supply for HTLV-I. In 1988, the U.S. Food and Drug Administration recommended that donated units be screened for HTLV-I. As of 1989, no cases of transfusion-related acute T-cell leukemia were documented, although causality will be very difficult to demonstrate because of the long viral latency.[326] Hepatitis B and C risk may presage HIV risk for blood and transplantation recipients.[339]

Hemophilia

A person with hemophilia was diagnosed with *P carinii* pneumonia at the end of 1981 in the United States, suggesting that transmission of an AIDS-related infectious agent could be spread through blood products.[7] Retrospective studies indicate that HIV antibodies were present in serum samples as early as 1978[340] and 1979, and fully 50% of one population had seroconverted by 1982.[341] By the end of December 1994,[342] adults and adolescents and 221 children (<13 years) with hemophilia or one of the rarer coagulation disorders had been reported with AIDS. Although the adult AIDS cases attributable to hemophilia represent 0.8% of all U.S. adult AIDS cases, children with hemophilia or other coagulation disorders account for 3.6% of all pediatric AIDS cases.[4]

Among individuals with coagulopathies, persons with hemophilia A and B experienced the impact of the AIDS epidemic the most severely. According to CDC estimates in the late 1980s, 33% to 92% of persons with hemophilia A and 14% to 52% of persons with hemophilia B were infected with HIV, depending on their geographic region of origin in the United States.[343] They require the use of factor VIII and IX concentrates in larger and more frequent doses than persons with milder clotting disorders. A typical vial of factor VIII concentrate contained clotting factors, alloantigenic compounds, and possibly, infectious agents from between 2000 to 20,000 blood and plasma donors.[40] Exclusion of risky donors, modifications in the application of heat treatment (ie, increased temperature and longer exposure times), and the addition of detergent treatment and monoclonal antibody–purified products have now virtually eliminated the risk of HIV transmission from the blood products of industrialized countries.[344,345]

Allograft and Organ Transplantation

Transmission of HIV through allograft transplantation has been uncommon and represents a minute proportion of all AIDS cases.[346] HIV or genomic fragments can be isolated from all bodily fluids and organs of an infected individual, including various blood compartments, tears, conjunctival epithelium, corneal tissue, saliva, semen, urine, sweat, vaginal secretions, breast milk, cerebrospinal fluid, alveolar fluid, and major organs.[42,127,195,347-351] Every organ in a seropositive individual is likely to be infected with HIV. Donated kidneys have been the most frequently associated with HIV transmission.[352-361] Several liver allograft recipients have been infected with HIV through transplantation.[362,363] HIV transmission has also been documented through bone[364] and bone marrow transplantations.[365,366] Skin allografts can transmit HIV from an infected donor.[367,368] In Australia, 4 of 8 women exposed to HIV transmission from a single infected semen donor seroconverted in 1985.[369] Isolation of HIV from tears, conjunctival epithelium, and corneal tissue has been successful, but despite inadvertent transplantation of corneas from a seropositive donor, no seroconversion in recipients has been reported.[357,370,371] Otologic homografts have also been identified as a potential vehicle of transmission, although no cases have been reported.[372] Blood transfusion, common during the peritransplantation period, may have contributed its own risk for acquiring HIV, thereby overestimating the already small risks from transplantation.[373,374]

Such episodes became exceedingly rare after institution of HIV testing in 1985 in the United States and after 1986 in Europe. Organ donors, including semen and ova donors, undergo routine screening, including HIV antibody testing.[362,375] The CDC and the American Fertility Society recommend that semen samples intended for artificial insemination should be frozen for at least 6 months, followed by another HIV-antibody test from the donor before sample use.[376,377]

RARE OR PUTATIVE MODES OF TRANSMISSION

Insects

There is no evidence of transmission of HIV through inoculation of HIV-infected blood by insect vectors. Biologic transmission does not seem to occur, because HIV is unable to multiply inside insects, and infection of mosquito cells in vitro has not been consistently successful.[378–380] North American and European mosquitoes feed typically only once in 3 days, decreasing the probability that an infected lymphocyte on the mosquito mouthparts would be viably inoculated to a second host. Even mosquitoes that feed daily (eg, certain subspecies of *Anopheles gambiae* in Africa) do not feed on a second person immediately after feeding on the first. Small mouthparts limit the amount of potentially infective material that could be transferred.[381] Mechanical vector studies of HIV and mosquitoes and bedbugs mimicking natural conditions have not demonstrated transmission through blood transfer from person to person.[382]

In the early 1980s, it was suggested by Florida physicians that arthropod transmission explained the high HIV rates in Belle Glade, Florida. Epidemiologic investigations by CDC did not support mosquito-borne transmission.[144,383,384] Perhaps the strongest argument against insect-borne transmission emerges from the epidemiology of HIV in tropical and temperate climates. If an insect such as a mosquito were to transmit HIV, infection would be seen in all age groups, especially in children who typically sustain scores of insect bites in their play and work outdoors, and the elderly, who tend to be more sedentary and may have difficulty avoiding insects. Consistent with the currently known routes of transmission, these two age groups are the lowest likelihood populations for HIV seropositivity.

Nonparenteral Bloodborne Transmission

Nonparenteral transmission of blood in nonoccupational settings deserves consideration. In boxing, forceful blows often cause broken skin and bleeding, which could result in mixing of blood from an HIV-infected competitor into his opponent's wounds,[385] a noteworthy concern given IDU problems reported among several boxers.[386] One case of a bloody soccer accident suggested on-field transmission, but no molecular evidence of HIV-1 strain similarity was offered.[387]

One young traveller was infected in Rwanda after sustaining substantial lacerations in a bus accident. Blood dripped into the traveller's wounds from other injured passengers who tended to him. In this highly endemic area, with seroprevalence rates in blood donors from Rwanda approaching 18%, it was postulated that this resulted in HIV transmission, because no other risk factors were apparent and the traveller had tested negative for HIV antibody when donating blood a few months before the accident.[388]

Saliva and Human Bites

Transmission depends on many factors, including the concentration and viability of the agent within a given fluid or tissue, access to a port of entry for the fluid or medium, the presence of CD4+ cells or other target cells at the site of HIV entry, and natural host defenses near the site of entry.[389] Although transmission through saliva is unlikely because of the extremely low viral load, transmission is conceivable by means of saliva through a bite wound, although longitudinal studies and published reports involving cases of bites do not offer this possibility much support. The medicolegal debates around exceedingly rare transmission possibilities include whether human bites are a form of assault with a deadly weapon.[390]

In 1990, the CDC reported preliminary results of a study, including 89 household members living with 25 HIV-infected children, mostly toddlers, who were infected through transfusion. No evidence of casual transmission among toddlers biting one another has been shown. None of the household members have tested positive for the virus, despite months of close contact before and after the child's diagnosis. Testing of 78 individuals household members with polymerase chain reaction methods revealed negative results.[391]

HIV transmission through a bite has been suspected. A 26-year-old health care worker with no other known risk factors was HIV seronegative in 1983, before a 1985 fight she had with her IDU sister. The subject had knocked out some of her sister's teeth, causing bleeding from the mouth, and was subsequently bitten by her sister, whose mouth was still bleeding. Transmission in this case was very likely through blood, not saliva.[392] In the second case, a 6-year-old boy without known risk factors for HIV was bitten by his younger brother, who had transfusion-acquired AIDS. It was assumed, but never confirmed, that the bite may have resulted in the transmission of the virus.[393] The younger brother had neurologic complications of AIDS. In another study of one particularly aggressive toddler who bit five of his cousins, all of the exposed children have remained uninfected.[394] A study of 198 health care workers included 30 who were traumatized through bites or scratches from an AIDS patient. None of the bitten personnel tested positive for HIV.[395] These cases, without molecular analyses to document viral genotypes, are not well documented.[396] Future studies of this kind should use molecular techniques to judge whether the transmitted virus truly came from the person doing the biting.

Casual Contact

There have been a few studies to assess the risk of transmission of HIV through casual household contacts, as occur between family members. These studies failed to demonstrate a HIV infection in household members who did not have additional exposure to HIV through blood, sexual activity, or perinatal transmission.[397–400] Sharing of common household facilities such as beds, towels, toilets, baths, showers, kitchen utensils, dishes, dishwashers, and clothes washers and dryers was documented. Personal interactions included hugging and kissing of the cheek and lips, wiping of fecal matter of infants and children by parents, and other family casual fluid contact. Many of the infected children were infected up to 2 years before becoming symptomatic with AIDS, and no specific precautions were taken before the HIV infection was recognized.[39] It has been stated correctly that these studies remain too small to definitively rule out small risk from casual contact.[401] There are two well-documented cases of household transmission suggesting the need for infection control counseling for families caring for or living with HIV-infected persons.[402,403] Nonetheless, the dearth of reported cases where such casual transmission has been even suspected is reassuring after almost 20 years of the epidemic.

Swimming pool concerns are insubstantial when the antiviral effects of chlorine are considered. Even unchlorinated pools have a huge dilutional effect. Food handlers would not be expected to be a public risk because of the transmission patterns of HIV. Fomites, such as bed clothes or dirty laundry, would be a risk if they were bloodied but would not otherwise be considered dangerous.

Health Care Worker to Patient Transmission

The greatest mystery in the topic of casual transmission of HIV is the "Florida dentist" case. Well studied and documented with elegant epidemiology and molecular virology, it is clear that a dentist transmitted to five of his patients through an unknown route.[404,405] Deliberate criminal inoculation, contaminated instrumentation, drooling or bleeding from the infected dentist into the mouths of the infected patients, sexual contact, or blood contamination all seem unlikely. It is unknown how these patients were infected. In subsequent look-back studies of over 22,000 patients from 51 HIV-infected health care workers, all 113 HIV seropositive patients had identified risk factors or strong molecular virologic evidence that the health care worker was not the source of the patient's infection.[406–408] The Florida dentist remains an isolated event, suggesting that spread from health care worker to patient is rare. This issue has implications for the day care industry and educational systems, as well as the rights and treatment of HIV-infected individuals, and it can be expected to periodically reemerge in the press and the mind of the public.[409]

PREVENTION

Successful behavioral and community-based educational and cofactor reduction efforts have been made around the world. In Thailand, condom promotion has shown some promise.[104] In Tanzania, STD control has achieved short-term reductions in HIV seroincidence.[126] In Zaire, STD and condom services for sex workers reduced HIV risk in proportion to the frequency with which the services were used.[1] In the United States, peer counseling among gay men and intensive counseling among run-away adolescents have proven effective in reducing high-risk behavior.[410–415] In the Netherlands, comprehensive services for drug users have reduced risk.[239] In the United States, needle-exchange programs to reduce contaminated injections among IDUs suggest efficacy and can be expected to affect sexual transmission from IDUs to their sexual partners and offspring.[226–234,237,416]

It is encouraging to see the success of pilot projects and progress where public health policy has overcome political objections to "all modality" efforts to reduce transmission by all reasonable and feasible routes. However, translating isolated successes into worldwide disease control efforts is elusive.[417–419] Given the rapid recognition of the mode of transmission of HIV, the failure of subsequent control activities to stem the pandemic is a discouraging reminder of the difficulties of translating knowledge into practice.[22,420] Cure-oriented health care systems must invest money for prevention, targeting the highest-risk groups in programs convenient for these populations rather than convenient for the health care system. Bold policy has been rare in confronting the epidemics in North America, Asia, Africa, South America, and southern Europe. In the realm of public policy and behavior change for "taboo" subjects, the AIDS epidemic requires political and community leaders to take risks with their leadership positions to advocate for effective, but controversial, strategies for control of HIV transmission.

REFERENCES

1. Centers for Disease Control. Kaposi's sarcoma and *Pneumocystis* pneumonia among homosexual men—New York City and California. MMWR 1981;30:305.
2. Centers for Disease Control. *Pneumocystis* pneumonia—Los Angeles. MMWR 1981;30:250.
3. Gottlieb MS, Schroff R, Schanker HM, et al. *Pneumocystis carinii* pneumonia and mucosal candidiasis in previously healthy homosexual men. N Engl J Med 1981;305:1425.
4. Masur H, Michelis MA, Greene JB, et al. An outbreak of community-acquired *Pneumocystis carinii* pneumonia: initial manifestation of cellular immune dysfunction. N Engl J Med 1981;305:1431.
5. Sonnabend JA, Saadoun S. The acquired immunodeficiency syndrome: a discussion of etiologic hypotheses. AIDS Res 1983;1:107.
6. Small CB, Klein RS, Friedland GH, Moll B, Emeson EE, Spigland I. Community-acquired opportunistic infections and defective cellular immunity in heterosexual drug abusers and homosexual men. Am J Med 1983;74:433.
7. Centers for Disease Control. Update on acquired immune deficiency syndrome (AIDS) among patients with hemophilia A. MMWR 1982;31:644.
8. Rubinstein A, Sicklick M, Gupta A, et al. Acquired immunodeficiency with reversed T4/T8 ratios in infants born to promiscuous and drug-addicted mothers. JAMA 1983;249:2350.
9. Rubinstein A. Pediatric AIDS. Curr Probl Pediatr 1986;16:361.
10. Nanda D, Minkoff HL. HIV in pregnancy—transmission and immune effects. Clin Obstet Gynecol 1989;32:456.
11. Francis DP, Curran JW, Essex M. Epidemic acquired immune deficiency syndrome: epidemiologic evidence for a transmissible agent. J Natl Cancer Inst 1983;71:1.

12. Jaffe HW, Francis DP, McLane MF, et al. Transfusion-associated AIDS: serologic evidence of human T-cell leukemia virus infection of donors. Science 1984;223:1309.
13. Oleske J, Minnefor A, Cooper R Jr, et al. Immune deficiency syndrome in children. JAMA 1983;249:2345.
14. Boulton M, Hart G, Fitzpatrick R. The sexual behaviour of bisexual men in relation to HIV transmission. AIDS Care 1992;4:165.
15. Diaz T, Chu SY, Frederick M, et al. Sociodemographics and HIV risk behaviors of bisexual men with AIDS: results from a multistate interview project. AIDS 1993;7:1227.
16. Wood RW, Krueger LE, Pearlman TC, Goldbaum G. HIV transmission: women's risk from bisexual men. Am J Public Health 1993;83:1757.
17. Chu SY, Peterman TA, Doll LS, Buehler JW, Curran JW. AIDS in bisexual men in the United States: epidemiology and transmission to women. Am J Public Health 1992;82:220.
18. Berkelman RL, Curran JW. Epidemiology of HIV infection and AIDS. Epidemiol Rev 1989;11:222.
19. Curran JW, Jaffe HW, Hardy AM, Morgan WM, Selik RM, Dondero TJ. Epidemiology of HIV infection and AIDS in the United States. Science 1988;239:610.
20. Jaffe HW, Bregman DJ, Selik RM. Acquired immune deficiency syndrome in the United States: the first 1,000 cases. J Infect Dis 1983;148:339.
21. Jaffe HW, Choi K, Thomas PA, et al. National case-control study of Kaposi's sarcoma and *Pneumocystis carinii* pneumonia in homosexual men: Part 1. Epidemiologic results. Ann Intern Med 1983;99:145.
22. Vermund SH. Casual sex and HIV transmission. Am J Public Health 1995;(In Press)
23. Mann JM. AIDS—the second decade: a global perspective. J Infect Dis 1992;165:245.
24. Centers for Disease Control and Prevention. 1994 HIV/AIDS surveillance report. (Abstract) MMWR CDC Surveill Summ 1995;CDC document #320201.
25. Chin J, Mann J. Global surveillance and forecasting of AIDS. Bull World Health Organ 1989;67:1.
26. Mann JM, Chin J, Piot P, Quinn T. The international epidemiology of AIDS. Sci Am 1988;259:82.
27. Garris I, Rodriguez EM, de Moya EA, et al. AIDS heterosexual predominance in the Dominican Republic. J Acquir Immune Defic Syndr 1991;4:1173.
28. Murillo J, Castro KG. HIV infection and AIDS in Latin America. Epidemiologic features and clinical manifestations. (Review) Infect Dis Clin North Am 1994;8:1.
29. Quinn TC, Narain JP, Zacarias FR. AIDS in the Americas: a public health priority for the region. AIDS 1990;4:709.
30. Pape J, Johnson WD Jr. AIDS in Haiti: 1982–1992. Clin Infect Dis 1993;17(Suppl 2):S341.
31. Quinn TC, Mann JM, Curran JW, Piot P. AIDS in Africa: an epidemiologic paradigm. Science 1986;234:955.
32. Weniger BG, Limpakarnjanarat K, Ungchusak K, et al. The epidemiology of HIV infection and AIDS in Thailand. [Published erratum appears in AIDS 1993;Jan 7:148] (Review) AIDS 1991;5(Suppl 2):S71.
33. Bollinger RC, Tripathy SP, Quinn TC. The human immunodeficiency virus epidemic in India. Medicine 1995;74:97.
34. Weniger BG, Takebe Y, Ou CY, Yamazaki S. The molecular epidemiology of HIV in Asia. AIDS 1994;8(Suppl 2):S13.
35. Piatak M Jr, Saag MS, Yang LC, et al. High levels of HIV-1 in plasma during all stages of infection determined by competitive PCR. Science 1993;259:1749.
36. Ho DD, Neumann AU, Perelson AS, Chen W, Leonard JM, Markowitz M. Rapid turnover of plasma virions and CD4 lymphocytes in HIV-1 infection [see comments]. Nature 1995;373:123.
37. Anderson DJ, O'Brien TR, Politch JA, et al. Effects of disease stage and zidovudine therapy on the detection of human immunodeficiency virus type 1 in semen. JAMA 1992;267:2769.
38. Allen JR. Heterosexual transmission of human immunodeficiency virus (HIV) in the United States. Bull N Y Acad Med 1988;64:464.
39. Friedland GH, Klein RS. Transmission of the human immunodeficiency virus: an updated review. Int Nurs Rev 1988;35:44, 54.
40. Holmberg SD, Horsburgh CR Jr, Ward JW, Jaffe HW. Biologic factors in the sexual transmission of human immunodeficiency virus. J Infect Dis 1989;160:116.

41. Pantaleo G, Graziosi C, Fauci AS. New concepts in the immunopathogenesis of human immunodeficiency virus infection. N Engl J Med 1993;328:327.
42. Levy JA. Pathogenesis of human immunodeficiency virus infection. Microbiol Rev 1993;57:183.
43. Koot M, Keet IPM, Vos AH, et al. Prognostic value of HIV-1 syncytium-inducing phenotype for rate of CD4+ cell depletion and progression to AIDS [see comments]. Ann Intern Med 1993;118:681.
44. Jehuda-Cohen T. A new look at HIV transmission from seropositive mothers to their infants: the facts beyond serology. (Review) Isr J Med Sci 1994;30:364.
45. Hopkins W. Needle sharing and street behavior in response to AIDS in New York City. Natl Inst Drug Abuse Res Monogr Ser 1988;80:18.
46. Goedert J, Eyster ME, Biggar RJ, Blattner WA. Heterosexual transmission of human immunodeficiency virus: association with severe depletion of T-helper lymphocytes in men with hemophilia. AIDS Res Hum Retroviruses 1987;3:355.
47. Johnson AM, Petherick A, Davidson SJ, et al. Transmission of HIV to heterosexual partners of infected men and women. AIDS 1989;3:367.
48. Laga M, Taelman H, van der Stuyft P, Bonneux L, Vercauteren G, Piot P. Advanced immunodeficiency as a risk factor for heterosexual transmission of HIV. AIDS 1989;3:361.
49. Holmes KK, Kreiss J. Heterosexual transmission of human immunodeficiency virus: overview of a neglected aspect of the AIDS epidemic. J Acquir Immune Defic Syndr 1988;1:602.
50. Andes WA, Rangan SR, Wulff KM. Exposure of heterosexuals to human immunodeficiency virus and viremia: evidence for continuing risks in spouses of hemophiliacs. Sex Transm Dis 1989;16:68.
51. Lawrence DN, Jason JM, Holman RC, Heine P, Evatt BL. Sex practice correlates of human immunodeficiency virus transmission and acquired immunodeficiency syndrome incidence in heterosexual. Am J Hematol 1989;30:68.
52. Goedert J, Biggar RJ, Winn DM, et al. Decreased helper T lymphocytes in homosexual men. II. Sexual practices. Am J Epidemiol 1985;121:637.
53. Goedert J, Biggar RJ, Winn DM, et al. Decreased helper T lymphocytes in homosexual men. I. Sexual contact in high-incidence areas for the acquired immunodeficiency syndrome. Am J Epidemiol 1985;121:629.
54. Jason JM, McDougal JS, Dixon G, et al. HTLV-III/LAV antibody and immune status of household contacts and sexual partners of persons with hemophilia. JAMA 1986;255:212.
55. de Gruttola V, Seage GR, III, Mayer KH, Horsburgh CR Jr. Infectiousness of HIV between male homosexual partners. J Clin Epidemiol 1989;42:849.
56. de Vincenzi I. A longitudinal study of human immunodeficiency virus transmission by heterosexual partners. European Study Group on Heterosexual Transmission of HIV [see comments]. N Engl J Med 1994;331:341.
57. Allen S, Tice J, Van De Perre P, et al. Effect of serotesting with counseling on condom use and seroconversion among HIV discordant couples in Africa. Br Med J 1992;304:1605.
58. Dehovitz JA, Kelly P, Feldman J, et al. Sexually transmitted diseases, sexual behavior, and cocaine use in inner city women. Am J Epidemiol 1994;140:1125.
59. Nicolosi A, Leite ML, Musicco M, Molinari S, Lazzarin A. Parenteral and sexual transmission of human immunodeficiency virus in intravenous drug users: a study of seroconversion. The Northern Italian Seronegative Drug Addicts (NISDA) study. Am J Epidemiol 1992;135:225.
60. Saracco A, Musicco M, Nicolosi A, et al. Man-to-woman sexual transmission of HIV: longitudinal study of 343 steady partners of infected men. J Acquir Immune Defic Syndr 1993;6:497.
61. Laga M, Alary M, Nzila N, et al. Condom promotion, sexually transmitted diseases treatment, and declining incidence of HIV-1 infection in female sex workers. Lancet 1994;344:246.
62. Padian NS, O'Brien TR, Chang Y, Glass S, Francis DP. Prevention of heterosexual transmission of human immunodeficiency virus through couple counseling. J Acquir Immune Defic Syndr 1993;6:1043.
63. Ilaria G, Jacobs JL, Polsky B, et al. Detection HIV-1 DNA sequences in pre-ejaculatory fluid. Lancet 1992;340:1469.
64. Rodriguez EM, de Moya EA, Guerrero E, et al. HIV-1 and HTLV-I in sexually transmitted disease clinics in the Dominican Republic. J Acquir Immune Defic Syndr 1993;6:313.

65. Berkley SF, Widy-Wirski R, Okware SI, et al. Risk factors associated with HIV infection in Uganda. J Infect Dis 1989;160:22.
66. Boulos R, Halsey H, Holt E, et al. HIV-1 in Haitian Women 1982-1988. The Cite Soleil/JHU AIDS Project Team. J Acquir Immune Defic Syndr 1990;3:721.
67. Hira SK, Kamanga J, Macuacua R, Mwansa N, Cruess DF, Perine PL. Genital ulcers and male circumcision as risk factors for acquiring HIV-1 in Zambia. J Infect Dis 1990;161:584.
68. Wasserheit JN. Epidemiological synergy. Interrelationships between human immunodeficiency virus infection and other sexually transmitted diseases. Sex Transm Dis 1992;19:61.
69. Gerberding JL. Transmission of HIV to health care workers: risk and risk reduction. Bull N Y Acad Med 1988;64:491.
70. Latif AS, Katzenstein DA, Bassett MT, Houston S, Emmanuel JC, Marowa E. Genital ulcers and transmission of HIV among couples in Zimbabwe. AIDS 1989;3:519.
71. Bassett MT, Mhloyi M. Women and AIDS in Zimbabwe: the making of an epidemic. Int J Health Serv 1991;21:143.
72. Green EC. The anthropology of sexually transmitted disease in Liberia. Soc Sci Med 1992;35:1457.
73. Miller CJ, McGhee JR, Gardner MB. Mucosal immunity, HIV transmission, and AIDS. (Review) Lab Invest 1993;68:129.
74. Beck EJ, Donegan C, Cohen CS, et al. Risk factors for HIV-1 infection in a British population: lessons from a London sexually transmitted diseases clinic. AIDS 1989;3:533.
75. Hawkins RE, Rickman LS, Vermund SH, Carl M. Association of mycoplasma and human immunodeficiency virus infection: detection of amplified *Mycoplasma fermentans* DNA in blood. J Infect Dis 1992;165:581.
76. Lo SC, Tsai S, Benish JR, Shih JWK, Wear DJ, Wong DM. Enhancement of HIV-1 cytocidal effects in CD4+ lymphocytes by the AIDS-associated mycoplasma. Science 1991;251:1074.
77. Cameron DW, Simonsen JN, d'Costa L, et al. Female to male transmission of human immunodeficiency virus type 1 risk factors for seroconversion in men. Lancet 1989;2:403.
78. Simonsen JN, Cameron DW, Gakinya MN, et al. Human immunodeficiency virus infection among men with sexually transmitted diseases. N Engl J Med 1988;319:274.
79. Moses S, Bradley JE, Nagelkerke NJ, Ronald AR, Ndinya-Achola JO, Plummer FA. Geographical patterns of male circumcision practices in Africa: association with HIV seroprevalence. Int J Epidemiol 1990;19:693.
80. Dirie MA, Lindmark G. The risk of medical complications after female circumcision. East Afr Med J 1992;69:479.
81. Dirie MA, Lindmark G. Female circumcision in Somalia and women's motives. Acta Obstet Gynecol Scand 1991;70:581.
82. Ozumba BC. Acquired gynetresia in eastern Nigeria. Int J Gynaecol Obstet 1992;37:105.
83. Dirie MA, Lindmark G. A hospital study of the complications of female circumcision. Trop Doct 1991;21:146.
84. Lightfoot-Klein H, Shaw E. Special needs of ritually circumcised women patients. J Obstet Gynecol Neonat Nurs 1991;20:102.
85. el-Dareer AA. Complications of female circumcision in the Sudan. Trop Doct 1983;13:131.
86. el-Dareer AA. Epidemiology of female circumcision in the Sudan. Trop Doct 1983;13:41.
87. Kaslow RA, Duquesnoy R, van Raden M, et al. A1, Cw7, B8, DR3 HLA antigen combinations associated with rapid decline of T-helper lymphocytes in HIV-1 infection. Lancet 1990;1:927.
88. Graham NM, Zeger SL, Park LP, et al. The effects on survival of early treatment of human immunodeficiency virus infection [see comments]. N Engl J Med 1992;326:1037.
89. Stein DS, Korvick JA, Vermund SH. CD4+ lymphocyte cell enumeration for prediction of clinical course of human immunodeficiency virus disease: a review. J Infect Dis 1992;165:352.
90. Graham NMH, Zeger SL, Park LP, et al. Effect of zidovudine and *Pneumocystis carinii* pneumonia prophylaxis on progression of HIV-1 infection to AIDS. The Multicenter AIDS Cohort Study. Lancet 1991;338:265.
91. Graham NMH, Zeger SL, Park LP, et al. The effects on survival of early treatment of human immunodeficiency virus infection. N Engl J Med 1992;326:1037.
92. Moore RD, Hidalgo J, Sugland BW, Chaisson RE. Zidovudine and the natural history of the acquired immunodeficiency syndrome. N Engl J Med 1991;324:1412.
93. Rosenberg PS, Gail MH, Schrager LK, et al. National AIDS incidence trends and the extent of zidovudine therapy in selected demographic and transmission groups. J Acquir Immune Defic Syndr 1991;4:392.
94. Oakley A, Fullerton D, Holland J. Behavioural interventions for HIV/AIDS prevention. AIDS 1995;9:479.
95. Marx JL. Circumcision may protect against the AIDS virus. (News) Science 1989;245:470.
96. Mastro TD, Satten GA, Nopkesorn T, Sangkharomya S, Longini IM. Probability of female-to-male transmission of HIV-1 in Thailand [see comments]. Lancet 1994;343:204.
97. Lorian V. AIDS, anal sex, and heterosexuals. (Letter) Lancet 1988;1:1111.
98. Levin LI, Peterman TA, Renzullo PO, et al. Risk behaviors associated with recent HIV-1 seroconversion among young men in the United States Army. Am J Public Health 1995;85:1500.
99. Chmiel JS, Detels R, Kaslow RA, van Raden M, Kingsley LA, Brookmeyer R. Factors associated with prevalent human immunodeficiency virus (HIV) infection in the Multicenter AIDS Cohort Study. Am J Epidemiol 1987;126:568.
100. Blower SM, Hartel D, Dowlatabadi H, Anderson RM, May RM. Drugs, sex and HIV. A mathematical model for New York City. Philos Trans R Soc Lond Biol 1991;331:171.
101. Blower SM, Boe C. Sex acts, sex partners, and sex budgets: implications for risk factor analysis and estimation of HIV transmission probabilities [see comments]. J Acquir Immune Defic Syndr 1993;6:1347.
102. Padian NS, Shiboski SC, Jewell NP. The effect of number of exposures on the risk of heterosexual HIV transmission. J Infect Dis 1990;161:883.
103. Stamm WE, Handsfield HH, Rompalo AM, Ashley RL, Roberts PL, Corey L. The association between genital ulcer disease and acquisition of HIV infection in homosexual men. JAMA 1988;260:1429.
104. Hanenberg RS, Rojanapithayakorn W, Kunasol P, Sokal DC. Impact of Thailand's HIV-control programme as indicated by the decline of sexually transmitted diseases. Lancet 1994;344:243.
105. Johnson AM. Condoms and HIV transmission. (Editorial; comment) N Engl J Med 1994;331:391.
106. Weller SC. A meta-analysis of condom effectiveness in reducing sexually transmitted HIV [see comments]. Soc Sci Med 1993;36:1635.
107. Stratton P, Alexander NJ. Prevention of sexually transmitted infections. Physical and chemical barrier methods. (Review) Infect Dis Clin North Am 1993;7:841.
108. Agnew J. Some anatomical and physiological aspects of anal sexual practices. J Homosex 1985;12:75.
109. Plourde PJ, Plummer FA, Pepin J, et al. Human immunodeficiency virus type 1 infection in women attending a sexually transmitted diseases clinic in Kenya. J Infect Dis 1992;166:86.
110. Greggio NA, Cameran M, Giaquinto C, et al. DNA HLA-DRB1 analysis in children of positive mothers and estimated risk of vertical HIV transmission. Dis Markers 1993;11:29.
111. Kaslow RA, Carrington M, Apple R, et al. Influence of combinations of human major histocompatibility complex genes on the course of HIV-1 infection. Nat Med 1996;2:405.
112. Kroner BL, Goedert JJ, Blattner WA, Wilson SE, Carrington MN, Mann DL. Concordance of human leukocyte antigen haplotype-sharing, CD4 decline and AIDS in hemophilic siblings. AIDS 1995;9:275.
113. Louie LG. Are human genes risk factors for AIDS? Nat Gen 1994;7:456.
114. Mann DL, Carrington M, O'Donnell M, Miller T, Goedert J. HLA phenotype is a factor in determining rate of disease progression and outcome in HIV-1 infected individuals. AIDS Res Hum Retrovir 1992;8:1345.
115. Itescu S, Mathur-Wagh U, Skovron ML, et al. HLA-B35 is associated with accelerated progression to AIDS. J Acquir Immune Defic Syndr 1992;5:37.
116. Moss GB, Clemetson D, d'Costa L, et al. Association of cervical ectopy with heterosexual transmission of human immunodeficiency virus: results of a study of couples in Nairobi, Kenya. J Infect Dis 1991;164:588.
117. Voeller B, Anderson DJ. Heterosexual transmission of HIV. JAMA 1992;267:1917.
118. Dallabetta G, Miotti P, Chiphangwi J, Liomba G, Saah AJ. Vaginal tightening agents as risk factors for acquisition of HIV. Presented at the Sixth International Conference on AIDS. San Francisco, CA, June, 1990.
119. Morrison CS, Schwingl PJ. Oral contraceptive use and infectivity of HIV-seropositive women. (Letter) JAMA 1993;270:2298.

120. Simonsen JN, Plummer FA, Ngugi EN, et al. HIV infection among lower socioeconomic strata prostitutes in Nairobi. AIDS 1990;4:139.
121. Arthur LO, Bess JW Jr, Urban RG, et al. Macaques immunized with HLA-DR are protected from challenge with simian immunodeficiency virus. J Virol 1995;69:3117.
122. Stott EJ, Mills KHG, Chan WL, et al. Significance of anti cell immunity in protection against SIV. AIDS Res Hum Retroviruses 1993;9(Suppl 1):S108.
123. Semba RD, Miotti PG, Chiphangwi JD, et al. Maternal vitamin A deficiency and mother-to-child transmission of HIV-1 [see comments]. Lancet 1994;343:1593.
124. Semba RD. Vitamin A, immunity, and infection. (Review) Clinical Infectious Diseases 1994;19:489.
125. Semba RD, Graham NM, Caiaffa WT, Margolick JB, Clement L, Vlahov D. Increased mortality associated with vitamin A deficiency during human immunodeficiency virus type 1 infection. Arch Intern Med 1993;153:2149.
126. Grosskurth H, Mosha F, Todd J, et al. Impact of improved treatment of sexually transmitted diseases on HIV infection in rural Tanzania: randomised controlled trial. Lancet 1995;346:530.
127. Clemetson DB, Moss GB, Willerford DM, et al. Detection of HIV DNA in cervical and vaginal secretions. Prevalence and correlates among women in Nairobi, Kenya. JAMA 1993;269:2860.
128. Jessamine PG, Ronald AR. Chancroid and the role of genital ulcer disease in the spread of human retroviruses. Med Clin North Am 1990;74:1417.
129. Martin DH, DiCarlo RP. Recent changes in the epidemiology of genital ulcer disease in the United States. The crack cocaine connection. (Review) Sex Transm Dis 1994;21:S76.
130. Otten MW Jr, Zaidi AA, Peterman TA, Rolfs RT, Witte JJ. High rate of HIV seroconversion among patients attending urban sexually transmitted disease clinics. AIDS 1994;8:549.
131. Piot P, Laga M. Genital ulcers, other sexually transmitted diseases, and the sexual transmission of HIV. Br Med J 1989;298:623.
132. Telzak EE, Chiasson MA, Bevier PJ, Stoneburner RL, Castro KG, Jaffe HW. HIV-1 seroconversion in patients with and without genital ulcer disease. A prospective study. Ann Intern Med 1993;119:1181.
133. Greenblatt RM, Lukehart SA, Plummer FA, et al. Genital ulceration as a risk factor for human immunodeficiency virus infection. AIDS 1988;2:47.
134. Chirgwin K, Dehovitz JA, Dillon S, McCormack WM. HIV infection, genital ulcer disease, and crack cocaine use among patients attending a clinic for sexually transmitted diseases. Am J Public Health 1991;81:1576.
135. Cameron DW, Ngugi EN, Ronald AR, et al. Condom use prevents genital ulcers in women working as prostitutes. Influence of human immunodeficiency virus infection. Sex Transm Dis 1991;18:188.
136. Karita E, Martinez W, Van De Perre P, et al. HIV infection among STD patients—Kigali, Rwanda, 1988 to 1991. Int J STD AIDS 1993;4:211.
137. Estebanez P, Fitch K, Najera R. HIV and female sex workers. (Review) Bull World Health Organ 1993;71:397.
138. ter Meulen J, Mgaya HN, Chang-Claude J, et al. Risk factors for HIV infection in gynaecological inpatients in Dar es Salaam, Tanzania, 1988-1990. East Afr Med J 1992;69:688.
139. Martin PM, Gresenguet G, Massanga M, Georges A, Testa J. Association between HIV1 infection and sexually transmitted disease among men in Central Africa. Res Virol 1992;143:205.
140. Mientjes GH, van Ameijden EJ, van den Hoek AJ, Goudsmit J, Miedema F, Coutinho RA. Progression of HIV infection among injecting drug users: indications for a lower rate of progression among those who have frequently borrowed injecting equipment. AIDS 1993;7:1363.
141. Fineberg HV. The social dimensions of AIDS. Sci Am 1988;259:128.
142. Edlin BR, Irwin KL, Faruque S, et al. Intersecting epidemics—crack cocaine use and HIV infection among inner-city young adults. Multicenter Crack Cocaine and HIV Infection Study Team [see comments]. N Engl J Med 1994;331:1422.
143. Weatherby NL, Shultz JM, Chitwood DD, et al. Crack cocaine use and sexual activity in Miami, Florida. J Psychoactive Drugs 1992;24:373.
144. Ellerbrock TV, Lieb S, Harrington PE, et al. Heterosexually transmitted human immunodeficiency virus infection among pregnant women in a rural Florida community. N Engl J Med 1992;327:1704.
145. Peto J. AIDS and promiscuity. (Letter) Lancet 1986;2:979.
146. Clumeck N, Taelman H, Hermans P, Piot P, Schoumacher M, de Wit S. A cluster of HIV infection among heterosexual people without apparent risk factors. N Engl J Med 1989;321:1460.
147. Leads from the MMWR. Positive HTLV-III/LAV antibody results for sexually active female members of social/sexual clubs—Minnesota (January 16, 1987). JAMA 1987;257:293.
148. Anderson RM, Gupta S, Ng W. The significance of sexual partner contact networks for the transmission dynamics of HIV. J Acquir Immune Defic Syndr 1990;3:417.
149. Saxon AJ, Calsyn DA, Whittaker S, Freeman G Jr. Sexual behaviors of intravenous drug users in treatment. J Acquir Immune Defic Syndr 1991;4:938.
150. Heterosexual AIDS: pessimism, pandemics, and plain hard facts (editorial). Lancet 1993;341:863.
151. Kane S. HIV, heroin and heterosexual relations. Soc Sci Med 1991;32:1037.
152. Holmes R, Fawal H, Moon T, et al. Acquired immunodeficiency syndrome in Alabama: special concerns for African-American women. Am J Public Health 1996;(in review).
153. Rosenberg PS, Levy ME, Brundage JF, et al. Population-based monitoring of an urban HIV/AIDS epidemic. Magnitude and trends in the District of Columbia. JAMA 1992;268:495.
154. Drucker E. AIDS and addiction in New York City. Am J Drug Alcohol Abuse 1986;12:165.
155. Alcabes P, Friedland G. Injection drug use and human immunodeficiency virus infection. J Infect Dis 1995;20:1467.
156. Menendez BS, Blum S, Singh TP, Drucker E. Trends in AIDS mortality among residents of Puerto Rico and among Puerto Rican immigrants and other Hispanic residents of New York City, 1981-1989. N Y State J Med 1993;93:12.
157. Vermund SH, Hein K, Gayle HD, Cary JM, Thomas PA, Drucker E. Acquired immunodeficiency syndrome among adolescents. Case surveillance profiles in New York City and the rest of the United States. Am J Dis Child 1989;143:1220.
158. Berkley SF, Naamara W, Okware SI, et al. AIDS and HIV infection in Uganda—are more women infected than men?. AIDS 1990;4:1237.
159. Quinn TC, Glasser D, Cannon RO, et al. Human immunodeficiency virus infection among patients attending clinics for sexually transmitted diseases. N Engl J Med 1988;318:197.
160. Quinn TC, Cannon RO, Glasser D, et al. The association of syphilis with risk of human immunodeficiency virus infection in patients attending sexually transmitted disease clinics. Arch Intern Med 1990;150:1297.
161. Quinn TC, Groseclose SL, Spence M, Provost V, Hook EW. Evolution of the Human Immunodeficiency Virus epidemic among patients attending sexually transmitted disease clinics: a decade of experience. J Infect Dis 1992;165:541.
162. Hook EW, Cannon RO, Nahmias AJ, et al. Herpes simplex virus infection as a risk factor for human immunodeficiency virus infection in heterosexuals. J Infect Dis 1992;165:251.
163. Schoenbaum EE, Hartel D, Selwyn PA, et al. Risk factors for human immunodeficiency virus infection in intravenous drug users. N Engl J Med 1989;321:874.
164. Schoenbaum EE, Hartel D. HIV in intravenous drug users. N Engl J Med 1990;322:632.
165. Catania JA, Binson D, Dolcini MM, et al. Changes in HIV/STD risk factors and prevention practices among heterosexual adults in the United States. Am J Public Health 1995;85:1492.
166. Brundage JF, Burke DS, Gardner LI Jr, et al. Tracking the spread of the HIV infection epidemic among young adults in the United States: results of the first four years of screening among civilian applicants for U.S. military service. J Acquir Immune Defic Syndr 1990;3:1168.
167. Smith KW, McGraw SA, Crawford SL, Costa LA, McKinlay JB. HIV risk among Latino adolescents in two New England cities. Am J Public Health 1993;83:1395.
168. Menendez BS, Drucker E, Vermund SH, et al. AIDS mortality among Puerto Ricans and other Hispanics in New York City, 1981–1987. J Acquir Immune Defic Syndr 1990;3:644.
169. Selik RM, Castro KG, Pappaioanou M. Racial/ethnic differences in the risk of AIDS in the United States. Am J Public Health 1988;78:1539.
170. Selik RM, Castro KG, Pappaioanou M, Buehler JW. Birthplace and the risk of AIDS among Hispanics in the United States. Am J Public Health 1989;79:836.

171. Jones JH. The Tuskegee legacy. AIDS and the black community. Hastings Cent Rep 1992;22:38.
172. Dawson JA. HIV in intravenous drug users. N Engl J Med 1990;322:632.
173. Melbye M, Njelesani EK, Bayley A, et al. Evidence for heterosexual transmission and clinical manifestations of human immunodeficiency virus infection and related conditions in Lusaka, Zambia. Lancet 1986;2:1113.
174. Peterman TA, Stoneburner RL, Allen JR, Jaffe HW, Curran JW. Risk of human immunodeficiency virus transmission from heterosexual adults with transfusion-associated infections. JAMA 1988;259:55.
175. Bowler S, Sheon AR, d'Angelo LJ, Vermund SH. HIV and AIDS among adolescents in the United States: increasing risk in the 1990s. J Adolesc 1992;15:345.
176. Bouvet E, de Vincenzi I, Ancelle-Park RA, Vachon F. Defloration as risk factor for heterosexual HIV transmission. (Letter) Lancet 1989;1:615.
177. Lehner T, Hussain L, Wilson J, Chapman M. Mucosal transmission of HIV. (Letter) Nature 1991;353:709.
178. Schwarcz SK, Bolan GA, Fullilove M, et al. Crack cocaine and the exchange of sex for money or drugs. Risk factors for gonorrhea among black adolescents in San Francisco. Sex Transm Dis 1992;19:7.
179. Meniscectomy in the patient with AIDS (editorial). Orthop Nurs 1988;7:12.
180. Irwin KL, Edlin BR, Wong L, et al. Urban rape survivors: characteristics and prevalence of human immunodeficiency virus and other sexually transmitted infections. Multicenter Crack Cocaine and HIV Infection Study Team. Obstet Gynecol 1995;85:330.
181. Zierler S, Feingold L, Laufer D, Velentgas P, Kantrowitz-Gordon I, Mayer K. Adult survivors of childhood sexual abuse and subsequent risk of HIV infection. Am J Public Health 1991;81:572.
182. Glaser JB, Hammerschlag MR, McCormack WM. Epidemiology of sexually transmitted diseases in rape victims. Rev Infect Dis 1989;11:246.
183. Murphy SM. Rape, sexually transmitted diseases and human immunodeficiency virus infection [editorial]. Int J STD AIDS 1990;1:79.
184. Vermund SH, Alexander-Rodriguez T, MacLeod S, Kelley KF. History of sexual abuse in incarcerated adolescents with gonorrhea or syphilis. J Adolesc Health Care 1990;11:449.
185. Forrest BD. Women, HIV, and mucosal immunity. Lancet 1991;337:835.
186. McGhee JR, Mestecky J, Dertzbaugh MT, Eldridge JH, Hirasawa M, Kiyono H. The mucosal immune system: from fundamental concepts to vaccine development. Vaccine 1992;10:75.
187. Mestecky J, Kutteh WH, Jackson S. Mucosal immunity in the female genital tract: relevance to vaccination efforts against the human immunodeficiency virus. (Review) AIDS Res Hum Retroviruses 1994;10(Suppl 2):S11.
188. Mestecky J, Jackson S. Reassessment of the impact of mucosal immunity in infection with the human immunodeficiency virus (HIV) and design of relevant vaccines. (Review) J Clin Immunol 1994;14:259.
189. Smith PD, Mai UE. Immunopathophysiology of gastrointestinal disease in HIV infection. (Review) Gastroenterol Clin North Am 1992;21:331.
190. Hrdy DB. Cultural practices contributing to the transmission of human immunodeficiency virus in Africa. Rev Infect Dis 1987;9:1109.
191. Fischl MA, Dickinson GM, Scott GB, Klimas N, Fletcher MA, Parks W. Evaluation of heterosexual partners, children, and household contacts of adults with AIDS. JAMA 1987;257:640.
192. Fink AJ. A possible explanation for heterosexual male infection with AIDS. (Letter) N Engl J Med 1986;315:1167.
193. Rosenblum L, Darrow W, Witte J, et al. Sexual practices in the transmission of hepatitis B virus and prevalence of hepatitis delta virus infection in female prostitutes in the United States. JAMA 1992;267:2477.
194. Melbye M, Ingerslev J, Biggar RJ, et al. Anal intercourse as a possible factor in heterosexual transmission of HTLV-III to spouses of hemophiliacs. (Letter) N Engl J Med 1985;312:857.
195. Fantini J, Yahi N, Baghdiguian S, Chermann JC. Human colon epithelial cells productively infected with human immunodeficiency virus show impaired differentiation and altered secretion. J Virol 1992;66:580.
196. Wexner SD. Sexually transmitted diseases of the colon, rectum, and anus. The challenge of the nineties. Dis Colon Rectum 1990;33:1048.
197. Spitzer PG, Weiner NJ. Transmission of HIV infection from a woman to a man by oral sex. (Letter) N Engl J Med 1989;320:251.
198. Rozenbaum W, Gharakhanian S, Cardon B, Duval E, Coulaud JP. HIV transmission by oral sex. (Letter) Lancet 1988;1:1395.
199. Petersen LR, Doll L, White C, Chu S. No evidence for female-to-female HIV transmission among 960,000 female blood donors. The HIV Blood Donor Study Group. J Acquir Immune Defic Syndr 1992;5:853.
200. Eskenazi B, Pies C, Newstetter A, Shepard C, Pearson K. HIV serology in artificially inseminated lesbians. J Acquir Immune Defic Syndr 1989;2:187.
201. Chu SY, Conti L, Schable BA, Diaz T. Female-to-female sexual contact and HIV transmission. (Letter) JAMA 1994;272:433.
202. Rich JD, Buck A, Tuomala RE, Kazanjian PH. Transmission of human immunodeficiency virus infection presumed to have occurred via female homosexual contact. (Review) Clin Infect Dis 1993;17:1003.
203. Stall R, Catania J. AIDS risk behaviors among late middle-aged and elderly Americans. The National AIDS Behavioral Surveys. Arch Intern Med 1994;154:57.
204. Feldman MD. Sex, AIDS, and the elderly. Arch Intern Med 1994;154:19.
205. Chin J. Current and future dimensions of the HIV/AIDS pandemic in women and children. Lancet 1990;336:221.
206. Chin J, Remenyi MA, Morrison F, Bulatao R. The global epidemiology of the HIV/AIDS pandemic and its projected demographic impact in Africa. World Health Stat Q 1992;45:220.
207. Greenberg AE, Hindin R, Nicholas AG, Bryan EL, Thomas PA. The completeness of AIDS case reporting in New York City. JAMA 1993;269:2995.
208. Thomas PA, Weisfuse IB, Greenberg AE, Bernard GA, Tytun A, Stellman SD. Trends in the first ten years of AIDS in New York City. The New York City Department of Health AIDS Surveillance Team. Am J Epidemiol 1993;137:121.
209. Centers for Disease Control. 1993 Revised classification system for HIV infection and expanded surveillance case definition for AIDS among adolescents and adults. JAMA 1993;269:729.
210. Brookmeyer R. Reconstruction and future trends of the AIDS epidemic in the United States. Science 1991;253:37.
211. Drucker E, Vermund SH. Estimating population prevalence of human immunodeficiency virus infection in urban areas with high rates of intravenous drug use: a model of the Bronx in 1988. Am J Epidemiol 1989;130:133.
212. DesJarlais DC, Friedman SR, Novick DM, et al. HIV-1 infection among intravenous drug users in Manhattan, New York City, from 1977 through 1987. JAMA 1989;261:1008.
213. Rosenberg PS. Backcalculation model of age-specific HIV incidence rates. Stat Med 1994;13:1975.
214. Weiss SH, Weston CB, Quirinale J. Safe sex? Misconceptions, gender differences and barriers among injection drug users: a focus group approach. AIDS Educ Prev 1993;5:279.
215. Singh BK, Koman JJ, 3d, Catan VM, et al. Sexual risk behavior among injection drug-using human immunodeficiency virus positive clients. Int J Addict 1993;28:735.
216. Booth RE, Watters JK, Chitwood DD. HIV risk-related sex behaviors among injection drug users, crack smokers, and injection drug users who smoke crack. Am J Public Health 1993;83:1144.
217. Battjes RJ, Pickens RW, Amsel Z, Brown LS Jr. Heterosexual transmission of human immunodeficiency virus among intravenous drug users. J Infect Dis 1990;162:1007.
218. Hoover DR, Munoz A, Carey V, et al. Estimating the 1978-1990 and future spread of human immunodeficiency virus type 1 in subgroups of homosexual men. Am J Epidemiol 1991;134:1190.
219. Lemp GF, Hirozawa AM, Givertz D, et al. Seroprevalence of HIV and risk behaviors among young homosexual and bisexual men. The San Francisco/Berkeley Young Men's Survey. JAMA 1994;272:449.
220. DesJarlais DC, Friedman SR, Stoneburner RL. HIV infection and intravenous drug use: critical issues in transmission dynamics, infection outcomes, and prevention. Rev Infect Dis 1988;10:151.
221. Purdy BD, Plaisance KI. Infection with the human immunodeficiency virus: epidemiology, pathogenesis, transmission, diagnosis, and manifestations. Am J Hosp Pharm 1989;46:1185.

222. Glaser JB, Strange TJ, Rosati D. Heterosexual human immunodeficiency virus transmission among the middle class. Arch Intern Med 1989;149:645.

223. Freeman RC, Rodriguez GM, French JF. A comparison of male and female intravenous drug users' risk behaviors for HIV infection. Am J Drug Alcohol Abuse 1994;20:129.

224. Raineri I, Senn HP, Scheideggar C, Hornung R, Luthy R, Vogt M. Detection of HIV-1 from needles discarded by IV drug users in Zurich and Basel using polymerase chain reaction assessment of in vitro infectivity. Abstract ThAP111. Fifth International Conference on AIDS. Montreal, Canada, 1989:159.

225. Chitwood DD, McCoy CB, Inciardi JA, et al. HIV seropositivity of needles from shooting galleries in south Florida. Am J Public Health 1990;80:150.

226. Kaplan EH, Khoshnood K, Heimer R. A decline in HIV-infected needles returned to New Haven's needle exchange program: client shift or needle exchange [see comments]? Am J Public Health 1994;84:1991.

227. Kaplan EH. A method for evaluating needle exchange programmes. Stat Med 1994;13:2179.

228. Kaplan EH, Heimer R. HIV incidence among needle exchange participants: estimates from syringe tracking and testing data. J Acquir Immune Defic Syndr 1994;7:182.

229. Vlahov D, Brookmeyer RS. The evaluation of needle exchange programs. (Editorial; comment) Am J Public Health 1994;84:1889.

230. Watters JK, Estilo MJ, Clark GL, Lorvick J. Syringe and needle exchange as HIV/AIDS prevention for injection drug users [see comments]. JAMA 1994;271:115.

231. Heimer R, Kaplan EH, Khoshnood K, Jariwala B, Cadman EC. Needle exchange decreases the prevalence of HIV-1 proviral DNA in returned syringes in New Haven, Connecticut. Am J Med 1993;95:214.

232. Lurie P, Reingold AL, et al. The public health impact of needle exchange programs in the United States and abroad—executive summary. Berkeley, CA: University of California, 1993.

233. Schwartz RH. Syringe and needle exchange programs: Part I. South Med J 1993;86:318.

234. Schwartz RH. Syringe and needle exchange programs worldwide: Part II. (Review) South Med J 1993;86:323.

235. Information and testing sites. Wis Med J 1989;88:156.

236. Cox J, Hodgson L. Hepatitis B, AIDS and the neurological pin. (Letter) Med Educ 1988;22:83.

237. Kaplan EH, Heimer R. HIV prevalence among intravenous drug users: model-based estimates from New Haven's legal needle exchange. J Acquir Immune Defic Syndr 1992;5:163.

238. Hart GJ, Sonnex C, Petherick A, Johnson AM, Feinmann C, Adler MW. Risk behaviours for HIV infection among injecting drug users attending a drug dependency clinic. Br Med J 1989;298:1081.

239. Coutinho RA. Epidemiology and prevention of AIDS among intravenous drug users. J Acquir Immune Defic Syndr 1990;3:413.

240. Sarkar S, Mookerjee P, Roy A, et al. Descriptive epidemiology of intravenous heroin users—a new risk group for transmission of HIV in India. J Infect 1991;23:201.

241. Ellerbrock TV, Rogers MF. Epidemiology of human immunodeficiency virus infection in women in the United States. Obstet Gynecol Clin North Am 1990;17:523.

242. Murphy DL. Heterosexual contacts of intravenous drug abusers: implications for the next spread of the AIDS epidemic. Adv Alcohol Subst Abuse 1987;7:89.

243. Friedland GH, Harris C, Butkus-Small C, et al. Intravenous drug abusers and the acquired immunodeficiency syndrome (AIDS). Arch Intern Med 1985;145:1413.

244. Marmor M, DesJarlais DC, Cohen H, et al. Risk factors for infection with human immunodeficiency virus among intravenous drug abusers in New York City. AIDS 1987;1:39.

245. Chaisson RE, Bacchetti P, Osmond D, Brodie B, Sande MA, Moss AR. Cocaine Use and HIV Infection in Intravenous Drug Users in San Francisco. JAMA 1989;261:561.

246. Kaplan EH. Needles that kill: modeling human immunodeficiency virus transmission via shared drug injection equipment in shooting galleries. Rev Infect Dis 1989;11:289.

247. Chandrasekar PH, Molinari JA, Kruse JA. Risk factors for human immunodeficiency virus infection among parenteral drug abusers in a low-prevalence area. South Med J 1990;83:996.

248. Vlahov D, Munoz A, Anthony JC, Cohn S, Celentano DD, Nelson KE. Association of drug injection patterns with antibody to human immunodeficiency virus type 1 among intravenous drug users in Baltimore, Maryland. Am J Epidemiol 1990;132:847.

249. Neaigus A, Friedman SR, Curtis R, et al. The relevance of drug injectors' social and risk networks for understanding and preventing HIV infection. Soc Sci Med 1994;38:67.

250. DesJarlais DC, Friedman SR. Shooting galleries and AIDS: infection probabilities and "tough" policies. Am J Public Health 1990;80:142.

251. Robles RR, Colon HM, Sahai H, Matos TD, Marrero CA, Reyes JC. Behavioral risk factors and Human Immunodeficiency Virus (HIV) prevalence among intravenous drug users in Puerto Rico. Am J Epidemiol 1992;135:531.

252. Metzger DS, Woody GE, McLellan AT, et al. Human immunodeficiency virus seroconversion among intravenous drug users in- and out-of-treatment: an 18-month prospective follow-up. J Acquir Immune Defic Syndr 1993;6:1049.

253. Friedman SR, Des Jarlais DC, Sterk CE. AIDS and the social relations of intravenous drug users. Milbank Q 1990;68(Suppl 1):85.

254. Kozel NJ, Adams EH. Epidemiology of drug abuse: an overview. Science 1986;234:970.

255. Goldsmith MF. Sex tied to drugs = STD spread. (News) JAMA 1988;260:2009.

256. Fullilove RE, Fullilove MT, Bowser B, Gross S. Crack users: the new AIDS risk group? Cancer Detect Prev 1990;14:363.

257. DesJarlais DC, Friedman SR. Intravenous cocaine, crack, and HIV infection. (Letter) JAMA 1988;259:1945.

258. Hopkins W. Needle sharing and street behavior in response to AIDS in New York City. NIDA Res Managr 1988;80:18.

259. Chitwood DD, McCoy CB, Comerford M, Trapido EJ. Risk behaviors of IV cocaine users: implications for intervention. Abstract WAP89. Fifth International Conference on AIDS, Montreal, Canada, 1989:134.

260. Raymond CA. Study of I.V. drug users and AIDS finds differing infection rate, risk behaviors. (News) JAMA 1988;260:3105.

261. Fullilove RE, Fullilove MT, Bowser BP, Gross SA. Risk of sexually transmitted disease among black adolescent crack users in Oakland and San Francisco, California. JAMA 1990;263:851.

262. Bourgois P, Dunlap E. Exorcising sex-for-crack: an ethnographic perspective from Harlem. In: Ratner MS, ed. Crack pipe as pimp: an ethnographic investigation of sex-for-crack exchanges. New York: Lexington Books, 1993:97.

263. Mandell W, Vlahov D, Latkin C, Oziemkowska M, Cohn S. Correlates of needle sharing among injection drug users. Am J Public Health 1994;84:920.

264. Centers for Disease Control. Antibody to human immunodeficiency virus in female prostitutes. MMWR 1987;36:157.

265. Delfraissy JF, Levy A, Abelhauser A, et al. Ineffectiveness of education in intravenous drug users to prevent HIV sexual transmission. Abstract WAP88. Fifth International Conference on AIDS, Montreal, Canada, 1989:134.

266. Skidmore CA, Robertson JR, Robertson AA, Elton RA. After the epidemic: follow up study of HIV seroprevalence and changing patterns of drug use. BMJ 1990;300:219.

267. Ronald AR, Ndinya-Achola JO, Plummer FA, et al. A review of HIV-1 in Africa. Bull N Y Acad Med 1988;64:480.

268. Friedman SR, DesJarlais DC, Sotheran JL. AIDS health education for intravenous drug users. Health Educ Q 1986;13:383.

269. Rhodes F, Corby NH, Wolitski RJ, et al. Risk behaviors and perceptions of AIDS among street injection drug users. J Drug Educ 1990;20:271.

270. Calsyn DA, Saxon AJ, Wells EA, Greenberg DM. Longitudinal sexual behavior changes in injecting drug users. AIDS 1992;6:1207.

271. Tirelli U, Vaccher E, Carbone A, et al. HTLV-III infection among 315 intravenous drug abusers: seroepidemiological, clinical, and pathological findings. AIDS Res 1986;2:325.

272. Vittecoq D, Mettetal JF, Rouzioux C, Bach JF, Bouchon JP. Acute HIV infection after acupuncture treatments. (Letter) N Engl J Med 1989;320:250.

273. Doll DC. Tattooing in prison and HIV infection. Lancet 1988;1:66.

274. Centers for Disease Control. HIV transmission between two adolescent brothers with hemophilia. MMWR 1993;42:948.

275. Singer DR, Almdal TP. Potential route of transmission of HTLV-III. (Letter) J Infect 1986;12:86.

276. Bohlen C. Romania's AIDS babies—a legacy of neglect. N Y Times 1990;139:A1.

277. Seale JR, Medvedev ZA. Origin and transmission of AIDS. Multi-use hypodermics and the threat to the Soviet Union: discussion paper. J R Soc Med 1987;80:301.

278. O'Farrell N. AIDS and the witch doctor. (Letter) Lancet 1987;2:166.

279. Roberts DJ, Harries AD. Tuberculosis and HIV infection in Africa. (Letter) Br Med J 1989;298:751.

280. Lepage P, Van De Perre P, Carael M, Butzler JP. Are medical injections a risk factor for HIV infection in children. (Letter) Lancet 1986;2:1103.

281. Greenfield WR. Night of the living dead II: slow virus encephalopathies and AIDS: do necromantic zombiists transmit HTLV-III/LAV during voodooistic rituals?. (Letter) JAMA 1986;256:2199.

282. Watkins J. Screening for tuberculosis—a possible transmission route of HIV. (Letter) J R Coll Gen Pract 1987;37:273.

283. Zachoval R, Deinhardt F, Gurtler L, Eisenburg J, Korger G. Risk of virus transmission by jet injection. (Letter) Lancet 1988;1:189

284. Bennett NM. Disposal of medical waste. Med J Aust 1988;149:400.

285. Shukla D. Preventing possible HTLV-III contamination from EEG electrodes. (Letter) N Engl J Med 1986;315:1167.

286. Ziegler JB, Robertson PW, Campbell P. Lack of transmission of the human immunodeficiency virus by unusual "needlestick" injuries. (Letter) Med J Aust 1988;149:161.

287. Robert LM, Bell DM. HIV transmission in the health-care setting. Risks to health-care workers and patients. (Review) Infect Dis Clin North Am 1994;8:319.

288. Becker CE, Cone JE, Gerberding J. Occupational infection with human immunodeficiency virus (HIV). Risks and risk reduction. Ann Intern Med 1989;110:653.

289. Gerberding JL, Henderson DK. Design of rational infection control policies for human immunodeficiency virus infection. J Infect Dis 1987;156:861.

290. Gerberding JL. Management of occupational exposures to bloodborne viruses. N Engl J Med 1995;332:444.

291. Stoneburner RL, DesJarlais DC, Benezra D, et al. A larger spectrum of severe HIV-1–related disease in intravenous drug users in New York City. Science 1988;242:916.

292. Selwyn PA, Feingold AR, Hartel D, et al. Increased risk of bacterial pneumonia in HIV infected intravenous drug users without AIDS. AIDS 1988;2:267.

293. Selwyn PA, Hartel D, Lewis VA, et al. A prospective study of the risk of tuberculosis among intravenous drug users with human immunodeficiency virus infection. N Engl J Med 1989;320:545.

294. Drucker E, Webber MP, McMaster P, Vermund SH. Increasing rate of pneumonia hospitalizations in the Bronx: a sentinel indicator for human immunodeficiency virus. Int J Epidemiol 1989;18:926.

295. de Cock KM, Grant A, Porter JD. Preventive therapy for tuberculosis in HIV-infected persons: international recommendations, research, and practice. (Review) Lancet 1995;345:833.

296. Frieden TR, Fujiwara PI, Washko RM, Hamburg MA. Tuberculosis in New York City—turning the tide. N Engl J Med 1995;333:229.

297. Bayer R, Wilkinson D. Directly observed therapy for tuberculosis: history of an idea. (Review) Lancet 1995;345:1545.

298. Pape JW, Jean SS, Ho JL, Hafner A, Johnson WD Jr. Effect of isoniazid prophylaxis on incidence of active tuberculosis and progression of HIV infection. Lancet 1993;342:268.

299. Centers for Disease Control. *Pneumocystis carinii* pneumonia among persons with hemophilia A. MMWR 1982;31:365.

300. Ammann AJ, Cowan MJ, Wara DW, et al. Acquired immunodeficiency in an infant: possible transmission by means of blood products. Lancet 1983;1:956.

301. Centers for Disease Control. Possible transfusion-associated acquired immune deficiency syndrome (AIDS)—California. MMWR 1982;31:652.

302. Groopman JE, Salahuddin SZ, Sarngadharan MG, et al. Virologic studies in a case of transfusion-associated AIDS. N Engl J Med 1984;311:1419.

303. Centers for Disease Control. Experimental infection of chimpanzees with lymphadenopathy-associated virus. MMWR 1984;33:442.

304. Sarngadharan MG, de Vico AL, Bruch L, Schupbach J, Gallo RC Jr. HTLV-III: the etiologic agent of AIDS. Symposium Princess Takamatsu 1984;15:301.

305. Feorino PM, Kalyanaraman VS, Haverkos HW, et al. Lymphadenopathy associated virus infection of a blood donor—recipient pair with acquired immunodeficiency syndrome. Science 1984;225:69.

306. Jaffe HW, Sarngadharan MG, de Vico AL, et al. Infection with HTLV-III/LAV and transfusion-associated acquired immunodeficiency syndrome. Serologic evidence of an association. JAMA 1985;254:770.

307. Friedland GH, Klein RS. Transmission of the human immunodeficiency virus. N Engl J Med 1987;317:1125.

308. Seage GR, III, Horsburgh CR Jr, Hardy AM, et al. Increased suppressor T cells in probable transmitters of human immunodeficiency virus infection. Am J Public Health 1989;79:1638.

309. Lagakos SW, de Gruttola V. The conditional latency distribution of AIDS for persons infected by blood transfusion. J Acquir Immune Defic Syndr 1989;2:84.

310. Lui KJ, Lawrence DN, Morgan WM, Peterman TA, Haverkos HW, Bregman DJ. A model-based approach for estimating the mean incubation period of transfusion-associated acquired immunodeficiency syndrome. Proc Natl Acad Sci U S A 1986;83:3051.

311. Medley GF, Anderson RM, Cox DR, Billard L. Incubation period of AIDS in patients infected via blood transfusion. Nature 1987;328:719.

312. Peterman TA, Jaffe HW, Feorino PM, et al. Transfusion-associated acquired immunodeficiency syndrome in the United States. JAMA 1985;254:2913.

313. Costagliola D, Mary JY, Brouard N, Laporte A, Valleron AJ. Incubation time for AIDS from French transfusion-associated cases. Nature 1989;338:768.

314. Ward JW, Bush TJ, Perkins HA, et al. The natural history of transfusion-associated infection with human immunodeficiency virus. Factors influencing the rate of progression to disease. N Engl J Med 1989;321:947.

315. Redfield RR. The researcher's initiative. Del Med J 1988;60:16.

316. Ward JW, Deppe DA, Samson S, et al. Risk of human immunodeficiency virus infection from blood donors who later developed the acquired immunodeficiency syndrome. Ann Intern Med 1987;106:61.

317. Laurence J, Brun-Vezinet F, Schutzer SE, et al. Lymphadenopathy-associated viral antibody in AIDS: immune correlations and definition of a carrier state. N Engl J Med 1984;311:1269.

318. Feorino PM, Jaffe HW, Palmer E, et al. Transfusion-associated acquired immunodeficiency syndrome. Evidence for persistent infection in blood donors. N Engl J Med 1985;312:1293.

319. Menitove JE. The decreasing risk of transfusion-associated AIDS. (Editorial) N Engl J Med 1989;321:966.

320. Peterman TA. Transfusion-associated acquired immunodeficiency syndrome. World J Surg 1987;11:37.

321. Kakaiya RM, Cable RG, Keltonic J. Look back: the status of recipients of blood from donors subsequently found to have antibody to HIV. JAMA 1987;257:1176.

322. Menitove JE. Status of recipients of blood from donors subsequently found to have antibody to HIV. (Letter) N Engl J Med 1986;315:1095.

323. Peterman TA, Lui KJ, Lawrence DN, Allen JR. Estimating the risks of transfusion-associated acquired immune deficiency syndrome and human immunodeficiency virus infection. Transfusion 1987;27:371.

324. Lefrere JJ, Girot R. Risk of HIV infection in polytransfused thalassaemia patients. (Letter) Lancet 1989;2:813.

325. Donegan E, Stuart M, Niland JC, et al. Infection with human immunodeficiency virus type 1 (HIV-1) among recipients of antibody-positive blood donations. Ann Intern Med 1990;113:733.

326. Cohen ND, Munoz A, Reitz BA, et al. Transmission of retroviruses by transfusion of screened blood in patients undergoing cardiac surgery. N Engl J Med 1989;320:1172.

327. Kleinman S, Secord K. Risk of human immunodeficiency virus (HIV) transmission by anti-HIV negative blood. Estimates using the look-back methodology. Transfusion 1988;28:499.

328. Ward JW, Holmberg SD, Allen JR, et al. Transmission of human immunodeficiency virus (HIV) by blood transfusions screened as negative for HIV antibody. N Engl J Med 1988;318:473.

329. Busch MP, Eble BE, Khayam-Bashi H, et al. Evaluation of screened blood donations for human immunodeficiency virus type 1 infection by culture and DNA amplification of pooled cells. N Engl J Med 1991;325:1.

330. Cumming PD, Wallace EL, Schorr JB, Dodd RY. Exposure of patients to human immunodeficiency virus through the transfusion of blood components that test antibody-negative. N Engl J Med 1989;321:941.
331. Dodd RY. Transfusion and AIDS. Int Ophthalmol Clin 1989;29:83.
332. Anabolic steroid use among male high school seniors. (Letter) JAMA 1989;261:2639.
333. Centers for Disease Control. Safety of therapeutic immune globulin preparations with respect to transmission of human T-lymphotropic virus type III/lymphadenopathy-associated virus infection. MMWR 1986;35:231.
334. Centers for Disease Control. Lack of transmission of human immunodeficiency virus through Rho(D) immune globulin (human). MMWR 1987;36:728.
335. Centers for Disease Control. Hepatitis B vaccine: evidence confirming lack of AIDS transmission. MMWR 1984;33:685.
336. Osame M, Matsumoto M, Usuku K, et al. Chronic progressive myelopathy associated with elevated antibodies to human T-lymphotropic virus type I and adult T-cell leukemialike cells. Ann Neurol 1987;21:117.
337. Osame M, Usuku K, Izumo S, et al. HTLV-I-associated myelopathy, a new clinical entity. Lancet 1986;1:1031.
338. Goldmann DA, Zuck TF. AIDS: understanding the pathogenesis of HIV infection. Infect Control Hosp Epidemiol 1989;10:248.
339. Sumethkul V, Suchirachato K, Iamsilp V, Pairoj W, Bodhiphala P, Chiewsilp P. Current status of viral hepatitis and HIV transmission in renal transplant recipients: a study in Southeast Asia. Transplant Proc 1994;26:2176.
340. Evatt BL, Stein SF, Francis DP, et al. Antibodies to human T cell leukaemia virus-associated membrane antigens in haemophiliacs: evidence for infection before 1980. Lancet 1983;2:698.
341. Eyster ME, Goedert J, Sarngadharan MG, Weiss SH, Gallo RC Jr, Blattner WA. Development and early natural history of HTLV-III antibodies in persons with hemophilia. JAMA 1985;253:2219.
342. Recommendations for preventing transmission of infection with human T-lymphotropic virus type III/lymphadenopathy-associated virus during invasive procedures. MMWR 1986;35:221.
343. HIV infection and pregnancies in sexual partners of HIV-seropositive hemophilic men—United States. MMWR 1987;36:593.
344. Gomperts ED. Procedures for the inactivation of viruses in clotting factor concentrates. Am J Hematol 1986;23:295.
345. Pierce GF, Lusher JM, Brownstein AP, Goldsmith JC, Kessler CM. The use of purified clotting factor concentrates in hemophilia Influence of viral safety, cost, and supply on therapy. JAMA 1989;261:3434.
346. Simonds RJ. HIV transmission by organ and tissue transplantation. (Review) AIDS 1993;7(Suppl 2):S35-8.
347. Centers for Disease Control. Recommendations for prevention of HIV transmission in health-care settings. MMWR 1987;36:1S.
348. Lu XS, Belec L, Pillot J. Anti-gp160 IgG and IgA antibodies associated with a large increase in total IgG in cervicovaginal secretions from human immunodeficiency virus type 1-infected women. J Infect Dis 1993;167:1189.
349. Yolken RH, Li S, Perman J, Viscidi R. Persistent diarrhea and fecal shedding of retroviral nucleic acids in children infected with human immunodeficiency virus. J Infect Dis 1991;164:61.
350. Pearce-Pratt R, Phillips DM. Studies of adhesion of lymphocytic cells: implications for sexual transmission of human immunodeficiency virus. Biol Reprod 1993;48:431.
351. Malamud D, Friedman HM. HIV in the oral cavity: virus, viral inhibitory activity, and antiviral antibodies: a review. (Review) Crit Rev Oral Biol Med 1993;4:461.
352. Perez G, Ortiz-Interian C, Bourgoignie JJ, et al. HIV-1 and HTLV-I infection in renal transplant recipients. J Acquir Immune Defic Syndr 1990;3:35.
353. Zaleski C, Burke G, Nery J, et al. Risk of AIDS (HIV) transmission in 581 renal transplants. Transplant Proc 1993;25:1483.
354. Quarto M, Germinario C, Fontana A, Barbuti S. HIV transmission through kidney transplantation from a living related donor. (Letter) N Engl J Med 1989;320:1754.
355. al-Sulaiman M, al-Khader AA, al-Hasani MK, Dhar JM. Impact of HIV infection on dialysis and renal transplantation. Transplant Proc 1989;21:1970.
356. Imbasciati E, de Cristofaro V, Sama F, Pagliari B, Baretta A. Acquired immunodeficiency syndrome transmitted by transplanted kidney: clinical course during maintenance haemodialysis. Nephrol Dial Transplant 1988;3:681.
357. Schwarz A, Hoffmann F, L'Age-Stehr J, Tegzess AM, Offermann G. Human immunodeficiency virus transmission by organ donation. Outcome in cornea and kidney recipients. Transplantation 1987;44:21.
358. Kumar P, Pearson JE, Martin DH, et al. Transmission of human immunodeficiency virus by transplantation of a renal allograft, with development of the acquired immunodeficiency syndrome. Ann Intern Med 1987;106:244.
359. L'Age-Stehr J, Schwarz A, Offermann G, et al. HTLV-III infection in kidney transplant recipients. (Letter) Lancet 1985;2:1361.
360. Kerman RH, Flechner SM, van Buren CT, et al. Investigation of human T-lymphocytic virus III serology in a renal transplant population. Transplant Proc 1987;19:2172.
361. Prompt CA, Reis MM, Grillo FM, et al. Transmission of AIDS virus at renal transplantation. (Letter) Lancet 1985;2:672.
362. Centers for Disease Control. Human immunodeficiency virus infection transmitted from an organ donor screened for HIV antibody—North Carolina. MMWR 1987;36:306.
363. Samuel D, Castaing D, Adam R, et al. Fatal acute HIV infection with aplastic anaemia, transmitted by liver graft. (Letter) Lancet 1988;1:1221.
364. Centers for Disease Control. Transmission of HIV through bone transplantation: case report and public health recommendations. MMWR 1988;37:597.
365. Furlini G, Re MC, Bandini G, Albertazzi L, La Placa M. Antibody response to human immunodeficiency virus after infected bone marrow transplant. Eur J Clin Microbiol Infect Dis 1988;7:664.
366. Atkinson K, Dodds AJ, Concannon AJ, Biggs JC. The development of the acquired immunodeficiency syndrome after bone-marrow transplantation. Med J Aust 1987;147:510.
367. Clarke JA. HIV transmission and skin grafts. (Letter) Lancet 1987;1:983.
368. Lawrence JC. Allografts as vectors of infection. (Letter) Lancet 1987;1:1318.
369. Stewart GJ, Tyler JP, Cunningham AL, et al. Transmission of human T-cell lymphotropic virus type III (HTLV-III) by artificial insemination by donor. Lancet 1985;2:581.
370. Scheiffarth OF, Stefani FH, Gabriel N, Lund OE. T lymphocytes of the normal human cornea. Br J Ophthalmol 1987;71:384.
371. Salahuddin SZ, Palestine AG, Heck E, et al. Isolation of the human T-cell leukemia/lymphotropic virus type III from the cornea. Am J Ophthalmol 1986;101:149.
372. Glasscock ME, III, Jackson CG, Knox GW. Can acquired immunodeficiency syndrome and Creutzfeldt-Jakob disease be transmitted via otologic homografts. Arch Otolaryngol Head Neck Surg 1988;114:1252.
373. Antin JH, Smith BR, Ewenstein BM, et al. HTLV-III infection after bone marrow transplantation. Blood 1986;67:160.
374. O'Connell PJ, Mahony JF, Sheil AG. AIDS after renal transplantation. (Letter) Med J Aust 1985;143:631.
375. Centers for Disease Control. Testing donors of organs, tissues, and semen for antibody to human T-lymphotropic virus type III/lymphadenopathy-associated virus. MMWR 1985;34:294.
376. Revised new guidelines for the use of semen-donor insemination. The American Fertility Society. Fertil Steril 1988;49:211.
377. Semen Banking, Organ and Tissue Transplantation, and HIV Antibody Testing. MMWR 1988;37:57.
378. Yaxley RP. The acquired immunodeficiency syndrome and mosquitoes. (Letter) Med J Aust 1989;150:665.
379. Istre GR. What about mosquitoes and saliva? Or, is the human immunodeficiency virus transmitted in other ways? J Okla State Med Assoc 1988;81:399.
380. Becker JL, Hazan U, Nugeyre MT, et al. [Infection of insect cell lines by the HIV virus, an agent of AIDS, and a demonstration of insects of African origin infected by this virus]. C R Acad Sci [III] 1986;303:303.
381. Transmission of AIDS by insects. J Med Assoc Ga 1987;76:492.
382. Jupp PG, Lyons SF. Experimental assessment of bedbugs (Cimex lectularius and Cimex hemipterus) and mosquitoes (Aedes aegypti formosus) as vectors of human immunodeficiency virus. AIDS 1987;1:171.
383. Lifson AR. Do alternate modes for transmission of human immunodeficiency virus exist? A review. JAMA 1988;259:1353.

384. Castro KG, Lieb S, Jaffe HW, et al. Transmission of HIV in Belle Glade, Florida: lessons for other communities in the United States. Science 1988;239:193.
385. Gunby P. Boxing: AIDS? (News) JAMA 1988;259:1613.
386. Alcena V. Boxing and the transmission of HIV. (Letter) N Y State J Med 1988;88:392.
387. Torre D, Sampietro C, Ferraro G, Zeroli C, Speranza F. Transmission of HIV-1 infection via sports injury. (Letter) Lancet 1990;335:1105.
388. Hill DR. HIV infection following motor vehicle trauma in central Africa. JAMA 1989;261:3282.
389. Schechter MT, Boyko WJ, Douglas B, et al. Can HTLV-III be transmitted orally? (Letter) Lancet 1986;1:379.
390. Human bite is a deadly weapon. N J Med 1989;86:338.
391. Okie S. Children with AIDS virus seen as no risk to family: bites did not spread infection, study finds. Washington Post 1990;Feb. 11:A7.
392. Transmission of HIV by human bite. (News) Lancet 1987;2:522.
393. Wahn V, Kramer HH, Voit T, Bruster HT, Scrampical B, Scheid A. Horizontal transmission of HIV infection between two siblings. (Letter) Lancet 1986;2:694.
394. Shirley LR, Ross SA. Risk of transmission of human immunodeficiency virus by bite of an infected toddler. J Pediatr 1989;114:425.
395. Tsoukas CM, Hadjis T, Shuster J, Theberge L, Feorino P, O'Shaughnessy M. Lack of transmission of HIV through human bites and scratches. J Acquir Immune Defic Syndr 1988;1:505.
396. Richman KM, Rickman LS. The potential for transmission of human immunodeficiency virus through human bites. J Acquir Immune Defic Syndr 1993;6:402.
397. Friedland GH, Saltzman BR, Rogers MF, et al. Lack of transmission of HTLV-III/LAV infection to household contacts of patients with AIDS or AIDS-related complex with oral candidiasis. N Engl J Med 1986;314:344.
398. Friedland G, Kahl P, Saltzman B, et al. Additional evidence for lack of transmission of HIV infection by close interpersonal (casual) contact. AIDS 1990;4:639.
399. Sande MA. Transmission of AIDS. The case against casual contagion. (Editorial) N Engl J Med 1986;314:380.
400. Thomison JB. HIV infection from casual contact (Editorial) South Med J 1989;82:1071.
401. Tessman I. Limited significance of null results. Lancet 1989;2:982.
402. HIV transmission in household settings. (News) Am Fam Physician 1994;50:855.
403. Centers for Disease Control and Prevention. Human immunodeficiency virus transmission in household settings-United States. MMWR 1994;43:347,353.
404. Ou CY, Ciesielski CA, Myers G, et al. Molecular epidemiology of HIV transmission in a dental practice [see comments]. Science 1992;256:1165.
405. Ciesielski CA, Marianos D, Ou CY, et al. Transmission of human immunodeficiency virus in a dental practice. Ann Intern Med 1992;116:798.
406. von Reyn CF, Gilbert TT, Shaw FE Jr, Parsonnet KC, Abramson JE, Smith MG. Absence of HIV transmission from an infected orthopedic surgeon. A 13-year look-back study. JAMA 1993;269:1807.
407. Robert LM, Chamberland ME, Cleveland JL, et al. Investigations of patients of health care workers infected with HIV. Ann Intern Med 1995;122:653.
408. Dickinson GM, Morhart RE, Klimas NG, Bandea CI, Laracuente JM, Bisno AL. Absence of HIV transmission from an infected dentist to his patients. An epidemiologic and DNA sequence analysis. JAMA 1993;269:1802.
409. Ciesielski CA, Bell DM, Marianos DW. Transmission of HIV from infected health-care workers to patients. AIDS 1991;5(Suppl 2):S93.
410. Kelly JA, St.Lawrence JS, Stevenson LY, et al. Community AIDS/HIV risk reduction: the effects of endorsements by popular people in three cities [see comments]. Am J Public Health 1992;82:1483.
411. Kelly JA, Murphy DA, Washington CD, et al. The effects of HIV/AIDS intervention groups for high-risk women in urban clinics. Am J Public Health 1994;84:1918.
412. Kelly JA, Murphy DA, Sikkema KJ, Kalichman SC. Psychological interventions to prevent HIV infection are urgently needed. New priorities for behavioral research in the second decade of AIDS. (Review) Am Psychol 1993;48:1023.
413. Rotheram-Borus MJ, Koopman C, Haignere C, Davies M. Reducing HIV sexual risk behaviors among runaway adolescents. JAMA 1991;266:1237.
414. Rotheram-Borus MJ, Koopman C, Ehrhardt AA. Homeless youths and HIV infection. Am Psychol 1991;46:1188.
415. Samuel MC, Guydish J, Ekstrand ML, Coates TJ, Winkelstein W Jr. Changes in sexual practices over 5 years of follow-up among heterosexual men in San Francisco. J Acquir Immune Defic Syndr 1991;4:896.
416. Kaplan EH. Needle exchange or needless exchange? The state of the debate. Infect Agents Dis 1992;1:92.
417. Leigh BC, Temple MT, Trocki KF. The sexual behavior of US adults: results from a national survey. Am J Public Health 1993;83:1400.
418. Wallace R. Traveling waves of HIV infection on a low dimensional 'socio-geographic' network. Soc Sci Med 1991;32:847.
419. Wallace R. Urban desertification, public health and public order: "planned shrinkage," violent death, substance abuse and AIDS in the Bronx. Soc Sci Med 1990;31:801.
420. Francis DP, Chin J. The prevention of acquired immunodeficiency syndrome in the United States. An objective strategy for medicine, public health, business, and the community. JAMA 1987;257:1357.

AIDS: Biology, Diagnosis, Treatment and Prevention, fourth edition, edited by Vincent T. DeVita, Jr., Samuel Hellman, and Steven A. Rosenberg. Lippincott–Raven Publishers, © 1997

10.2

Transmission of the Human Immunodeficiency Virus From Mother to the Fetus and Infant

K. Luzuriaga and J.L. Sullivan

EPIDEMIOLOGY

The World Health Organization estimates that by early 1993, a cumulative total of 12 million adults and 1 million children were infected worldwide with human immunodeficiency virus type 1 (HIV-1).[1] Approximately 90% of HIV-1–infected children in the United States and most HIV-1–infected children elsewhere acquired the infection from their mothers (ie, vertical transmission). Surveys indicate that 6% to 30% of pregnant women in sub-Saharan Africa are seropositive for HIV-1.[2] In the United States, 0.17% of all childbearing women are HIV-1 seropositive.[3] The seropositivity rates vary by geography and are highest in inner-city areas of New York City (1.25%) and the District of Columbia (0.9%) and the metropolitan areas of Puerto Rico (0.7%), New Jersey (0.56%), and Florida (0.54%).

One half of new infections worldwide occur in women of childbearing age.[1] The rising prevalence of HIV-1 infection in women of childbearing age, particularly in Africa, Asia, and Latin America, is expected to lead to a marked increase in vertical HIV-1 infection, such that an estimated 4 to 5 million children will have been born infected with HIV-1 by the year 2000. In developing nations, the HIV-1 epidemic has begun to reverse gains in infant and childhood morbidity and mortality previously realized through nutrition and vaccine programs.

Katherine Luzuriaga, Department of Pediatrics, University of Massachusetts Medical School, Room 318, Biotech 2, 373 Plantation Street, Worcester, MA 01605.

John L. Sullivan, Department of Pediatrics, University of Massachusetts Medical School, Room 318, Biotech 2, 373 Plantation Street, Worcester, MA 01605.

The lack of a cure and the rapidly increasing incidence of pediatric HIV-1 infection mandates the development of strategies to prevent vertical HIV-1 transmission. Advances in our understanding of the timing of vertical HIV-1 transmission, factors important in transmission, and events early in the infection process have contributed to the development of strategies for the prevention or management of vertical HIV-1 infection.

TIMING, MECHANISMS, AND RISK FACTORS FOR THE VERTICAL TRANSMISSION OF HIV-1

Direct evidence for the timing of the vertical transmission of HIV-1 is difficult to obtain, but it appears that HIV-1 may be transmitted from an infected woman to her infant during gestation (in utero), during delivery (intrapartum), or postpartum through breast feeding. The isolation of HIV-1 from or the detection of HIV-1 provirus in aborted fetal tissues as early as 10 weeks of gestation has been reported,[4-6] but potential contamination with maternal blood was not always excluded, particularly in first-trimester fetuses. The intrauterine transmission of HIV-1 also is suggested by the isolation of HIV-1 from amniotic fluid and cells and by detection of p24 antigen in fetal blood obtained at 16 to 24 weeks by cordocentesis.[7,8] The isolation of HIV-1 or the detection of HIV-1 genome in blood samples obtained at birth from 30% to 55% of HIV-1–infected infants also suggests the intrauterine transmission of HIV-1.[9-12]

The proportion of infants infected in each trimester of pregnancy is unknown, as are the routes or mechanisms of intrauterine infection. Potential routes of infection include admixture of maternal-fetal blood or infection across the placenta. Although HIV-1 has been detected in amniotic fluid,[7] placental trophoblasts, and Hofbauer cells, the detection of HIV-1 in placental tissues has not correlated with transmission. The importance of the placenta as a barrier to infection is suggested, however, by an increased risk of transmission from women with placentitis (eg, syphilitic) or women with illicit drug use (particularly vasoactive drugs, such as cocaine) during pregnancy.[13]

Indirect evidence suggests that the vertical transmission of HIV-1 can occur during the intrapartum period. Studies of twins born to HIV-1 seropositive women[14,15] have demonstrated a higher risk of infection for the first-born twin. In these studies, the risk of transmission increased after prolonged labor, suggesting that extensive mucocutaneous exposure to maternal blood and vaginal secretions may result in intrapartum infection. Negative diagnostic studies in the first 2 days of life followed by detection of infection at 1 to 3 months of age also suggests intrapartum transmission.[10–12,16] An increase in viral load has been observed between 3 and 16 weeks of age in infants with negative results in the first 2 days of life, which is frequently accompanied by transient lowering of the CD4 count and inversion of the CD4:CD8 ratio.[17] These T-cell changes, along with the burst of viremia, are similar to those observed in adults experiencing primary infection and suggest intrapartum infection. The routes and mechanisms of intrapartum transmission are unknown but probably include the admixture of maternal and fetal blood or mucocutaneous (eg, ocular, gastrointestinal tract) exposure of the infant to maternal blood and vaginal secretions. The importance of the mucocutaneous route of infection is suggested by the work of Baba and colleagues,[18] in which they demonstrated the establishment of infection after the inoculation of cell-free simian immunodeficiency virus into the conjunctival sac or oropharynx of newborn macaques.

Several cases of the transmission of HIV-1 through breast-feeding have been reported. HIV-1 has been detected by culture and by the polymerase chain reaction (PCR) method in the cellular and acellular components of breast milk; the colostral viral load appears to be particularly high.[19] Data from two large, prospective cohort studies suggest an increased risk of transmission associated with breast-feeding.[20,21] In a metanalysis, Dunn and colleagues[22] estimated that the proportion of transmission attributable to breast-feeding from a mother with established infection (ie, antibody positive before pregnancy) is 14% (95% confidence interval [CI], 7% to 22%). The risk of breast milk transmission appears to be especially high during maternal primary infection, particularly if maternal primary infection occurs in the first few months after delivery.[23,24] For these reasons, the guidelines recommend that women infected with or at risk of infection with HIV-1 abstain from breast-feeding their infants if local sanitary conditions and access to infant formulas are good. However, because studies in developing nations have demonstrated decreased morbidity and mortality in breast-fed infants of HIV-1–infected women, the benefits of breast-feeding are thought to out-

weigh the risks of vertical HIV-1 transmission in those settings, and breast-feeding is currently recommended.[25]

Based on the previous data, working definitions regarding the timing of infection have been proposed for non–breast-fed populations.[26] Infants are regarded as infected in utero if HIV-1 is cultured from or HIV-1 DNA is detected in peripheral blood lymphocytes within 48 hours of birth. Infants are regarded as infected during delivery (intrapartum) if HIV-1 culture and DNA PCR results are negative for blood samples obtained within the first week of life and positive thereafter. The application of these definitions to small cohort studies of non–breast-fed populations suggests that 45% to 70% of vertically infected infants are infected in utero, and the remainder are infected at delivery.[10–12]

Reported vertical HIV-1 transmission rates range from 14% to 40% in prospective cohort studies.[27] Differences in methodologies, most importantly the definition of infection, were probably responsible for the variability in vertical transmission rates reported early in the epidemic among different cohorts. With advances in techniques for the early diagnosis of vertical HIV-1 infection, the observed variability in transmission rates less likely reflects uncertainties regarding infection status and more likely reflects the multiple factors that influence vertical transmission. Several studies suggest that maternal blood viral load may be an important factor in transmission. A threefold increase in transmission was observed in the multicenter European Collaborative Study[20] when HIV-1 p24 antigen was detected in maternal serum, suggesting an increased risk of vertical transmission with higher blood viral load. Weiser and colleagues[28] reported higher peripheral blood mononuclear cell HIV-1 culture titers in women who transmitted than in women who did not transmit HIV-1 to their infants. Similarly, Borkowsky and colleagues[29] reported higher frequencies of HIV-1–infected peripheral blood mononuclear cells by culture and higher levels of plasma HIV-1 RNA in mothers of infected infants than in mothers of uninfected infants; higher frequencies of HIV-1–infected peripheral blood mononuclear cells were measured in mothers of infants with evidence of infection at birth than in mothers of infants with evidence of intrapartum infection. In studies by Dickover and colleagues,[30] higher peripheral blood mononuclear cell–associated HIV-1 proviral copy numbers and plasma HIV-1 RNA levels were associated with a higher risk of transmission; a significantly higher transmission rate was observed for women with HIV-1 RNA levels greater than 50,000 copies per milliliter of plasma (89%) than for women with HIV-1 RNA levels of less than 50,000 per milliliter of plasma (8%).

None of the preceding studies matched transmitting and nontransmitting mothers for variables such as CD4 cell counts, clinical disease status, or antiretroviral therapy. In a small cohort study reported by Husson and colleagues[31] in which transmitting and nontransmitting women were matched for CD4 counts, high maternal peripheral blood viral load (measured by quantitative plasma RNA PCR, acid-dissociated plasma 24 antigen concentration, and quantitative peripheral blood mononuclear cell cultures) did not appear to be associated with an increased risk of transmission.

Qualitative properties of maternal virus may be as important as viral load. At least two groups[32,33] have reported that analysis of the envelope variable region (V3) sequences from early vertically transmitted HIV-1 strains suggests limited transmission or posttransmission amplification of maternal viral strains. Others, however, have reported greater heterogeneity in other HIV-1 envelope-variable regions.[34] Variability in mechanisms and timing of infection may explain these conflicting observations. For example, the intrapartum acquisition of infection through ocular or gastrointestinal mucosal exposure may favor the passage or amplification of limited viral genotypes, as has been reported after the sexual transmission of HIV-1.[35] The acquisition of vertical infection through the admixture of maternal-fetal blood also may allow the transmission of multiple viral strains. Further work is ongoing to characterize the genotypic and phenotypic properties of vertically transmitted viruses and to compare them with those found in maternal blood and genital tract secretions.

Impaired maternal immunologic status appears to correlate with vertical HIV-1 transmission. In several cohort studies, an increased risk of vertical transmission was observed with maternal AIDS.[27] In the European Collaborative Study,[20] rates of transmission increased markedly when the maternal CD4 count was less than 700 per mm^3 or the CD4:CD8 ratio was less than 0.6. In the ongoing Women and Infants Transmission Study in the United States, transmission rates of 30% have been documented when maternal CD4 lymphocytes counts are less than 20%, but 5% of infants born to women with CD4 percentages higher than 35 are infected.

Although immunocompetence may be an important factor in vertical transmission, maternal HIV-1–specific immunity may be especially important. Scarlatti and colleagues[36] reported that mothers with high titers of serum antibodies capable of neutralizing their own viral strains in vitro are less likely to transmit HIV-1 to their infants. Others, however, reported low titers of maternal serum antibodies capable of neutralizing maternal blood isolates in most women studied and therefore did not find an association between neutralizing antibody titers and transmission.[31]

Because specificity for certain regions of the HIV-1 envelope appears to correlate with the ability of antibodies to neutralize HIV-1, there has been much interest in assessing titers and affinities of antibodies to these envelope regions in transmitters and nontransmitters, with conflicting results.[27] High titers of serum antibody titers capable of mediating antibody-dependent, cell-mediated cytotoxicity (ADCC) have been measured in most HIV-1–infected pregnant women and do not appear to protect against transmission.[37] Little is known about the potential role of maternal HIV-1 cell-mediated immunity (eg, HIV-1–specific cytotoxic T lymphocytes) in the protection from virus transmission.

NATURAL HISTORY OF VERTICAL HIV-1 INFECTION

The tempo of disease progression after vertical HIV-1 infection is highly variable. As a group, however, vertically infected children experience more rapid disease progression than children infected at an older age or adults.[38,39] More than 80% of vertically infected children manifest HIV-1–related symptoms or CD4 T-cell depletion by 2 years of age. In a study of 200 vertically infected Italian infants who were followed from birth,[38] the median age of onset of any HIV-1 related sign or symptom was 5.2 months (range, 0.03 to 56 months); the probability of remaining asymptomatic was 19% (95% CI, 14 to 25.1) at 12 months and 6.1% (95% CI, 2.6 to 11.7) at 5 years. In another large prospective cohort study,[39] approximately 23% and 40% of vertically infected infants developed an AIDS-defining condition by 1 and 4 years of age, respectively.

Improvements in our ability to detect, quantitate, and characterize early isolates have advanced our understanding of the infection process. Viral and host factors appear to contribute to the variability in the natural history of vertical HIV-1 infection. Virus-host dynamics in early infancy appear to be important determinants of infection outcome and may account for the particularly rapid disease progression observed after vertical HIV-1 infection.

Virologic evaluation may differentiate infants infected in utero from those infected during delivery. Within the framework of the proposed definitions regarding the timing of infection, several investigators have begun to examine the relation between timing of infection and clinical outcome. Dickover and colleagues[40] reported an association between in utero infection, high early blood load of HIV-1, and rapid disease progression. However, data from our laboratory and others[12,41] demonstrate a rapid increase in viral load over the first month of life in most infants, whether infected in utero or during the intrapartum period.

Other viral factors that may be important in the pathogenesis of vertical infection are the genotypic and phenotypic variability of vertically transmitted viruses. Phenotypic differences in growth characteristics, the ability of different viral strains to infect cells of the immune system (eg, T cells versus macrophages), and the ability to cause cell death have been described among HIV-1 strains in vitro. Most first infant isolates grow in macrophage as well as T-cell lines and do not form syncytia in MT-2 cells in vitro. Evidence of replication (ie, p24 antigen production and HIV-1 RNA detection by in situ hybridization) without syncytia formation has been described in MT-2 cells infected with isolates from vertically infected infants and children.[42] De Rossi and colleagues[43] reported an association between rapid in vitro growth kinetics and expanded cell tropism (ie, growth in macrophage and T cell lines) of early isolates with rapid disease progression. Although disease progression in older children and adults is often associated with a switch from the non–syncytium-inducing to syncytium-inducing phenotype, disease progression in infants usually occurs without this switch.[44] Further characterization of vertically transmitted viruses is necessary to determine whether the transmission and evolution of selected viral phenotypes are favored in vertical HIV-1 infection.

Host factors that may be particularly important in the pathogenesis of vertical HIV-1 infection include host genotype, the ability of host cells to support viral replication, and virus-specific immune responses. Data from adult studies of long-term survivors of vertical infection and studies of African prostitutes seemingly resistant to HIV-1 infection suggest correlations between certain human leukocyte antigen types and protection from infection or disease progression, but there are no data regarding the importance of host genotype in vertical infection.

Human and animal models of viral infection suggest that the ability of neonatal cells to support viral replication may render the neonate particularly susceptible to persistent viral infections or more severe sequelae of viral infections. For example, the administration of a simian immunodeficiency virus variant with deletions in the *nef, vpr,* and *ltr* genes that demonstrates attenuated replication kinetics and pathogenic potential when administered intravenously to adult macaques[45] results in rapid replication to high titers and destruction of the immune system when administered to juvenile macaques.[46] This may result from an increased permissiveness of neonatal cells for the replication of certain viruses; increased susceptibility of human neonatal mononuclear cells to measles virus[47] and HIV-1[48] infection have been reported.

Alternatively, infection at a time of reduced ability to generate virus-specific immune responses may affect infection outcome. Viral infections in the fetal or newborn periods commonly result in persistent infections. Deficient cell-mediated immune responses are thought to account for the increased severity and incidence of reactivation disease after human neonatal herpesvirus infections.[49] A deficit in the ability of human neonatal lymphocytes to proliferate and produce interferon-γ in response to specific antigenic stimulation has been described.[50] Jenkins and colleagues[51] demonstrated a diminished capability of neonatal natural killer cells to mediate ADCC of HIV-1–infected target cells. Studies in our laboratory indicate that after the decline of passively acquired maternal ADCC antibodies over the first 6 months of life, HIV-1–infected infants appear unable to generate ADCC antibodies until approximately 2 years of age (Pugatch D, Luzuriaga K, Sullivan JL, unpublished observations, 1995).

Virus-specific cytotoxic T lymphocytes (CTL) are important for the clearance of acute viral infections and suppression of viral replication in chronic infections. The capability of the young human infant to generate virus-specific CTL has not been well-defined. Vigorous HIV-1–specific CTL responses can be detected in most HIV-1–infected adults and children who are infected after the age of 2 years.[17] HIV-1–specific CTL responses in vertically infected infants are less vigorous and appear later in primary infection than in adults.[52,53] These deficiencies in HIV-1 specific cellular immunity may preclude effective containment of viral replication early in infection and contribute to the more rapid disease progression often observed after vertical infection.

EXPOSED BUT UNINFECTED INFANTS

Until recently, it was assumed that infection occurred or did not occur after exposure to HIV-1, and if infection occurred, it almost always resulted in eventual disease. The persistent detection of HIV-1 proviral DNA in high-risk individuals without other evidence of infection has been reported.[54] The detection of HIV-1 DNA in first- and second-trimester aborted fetuses in excess of the proportion of infected infants born to HIV-1–infected women[6] led to the proposal that HIV-1 infection may be cleared by some fetuses in utero. Bryson and associates[55] documented at least one case in which HIV-1 genome and infectious HIV-1 were transiently detected in the peripheral blood of an infant; genetic relatedness of infant viruses with maternal viruses was not proven, however.

Several investigators detected cellular immune responses, including lymphocyte proliferation, to HIV-1 peptides or HIV-1–specific CTL in exposed, apparently uninfected individuals and suggested that these responses are markers or perhaps even responsible for clearance of infection. However, HIV-1–specific CTL have also been detected in low-risk, uninfected individuals,[56] suggesting that the documented responses were not virus-specific but rather cross-reactive (eg, alloreactive CTL). The strongest data in support of the concept of exposure with resistance to or clearance of infection come from Rowland-Jones and collaborators,[57] who reported the detection of HIV-1–specific CTL that often shared cross-reactivity with HIV-2 epitopes in a cohort of highly exposed but apparently HIV-1– and HIV-2–uninfected Gambian female prostitutes. They were unable to demonstrate similar responses in a cohort of 19 uninfected, low-risk controls.

At least two groups[58,59] have detected HIV-1–specific CTL in the absence of in vitro stimulation in exposed, uninfected children, suggesting the maintenance of a vigorous CTL response in the absence of continued antigenic stimulation. Other groups, including our own, have not detected these responses, even after in vitro stimulation.[17,53,60] Using virus-specific stimulation, Rowland-Jones and coworkers[61] detected HIV-1–specific CTL of unspecified phenotype in an apparently uninfected infant. Further analyses of exposed but uninfected infants and children are necessary to determine whether clearance of infection occurs. The examination of viral properties and virus-specific immune responses that may aid in viral clearance is particularly important. If apparently protective responses are detected, documentation of virus specificity and characterization of the responses would have important implications for neonatal vaccine development.

STRATEGIES TO PREVENT THE VERTICAL TRANSMISSION OF HIV-1

Based on advances in our understanding of the timing and pathogenesis of vertical HIV-1 infection, a variety of strategies to prevent the vertical transmission of HIV-1 have been proposed. These strategies include the prevention or therapy of venereal infections, maternal nutritional intervention, bypassing the route of exposure, the reduction of viral load in maternal blood or vaginal secretions, and maternal or neonatal immunotherapy.

Although development of an effective antiretroviral or vaccine strategy for the prevention of vertical HIV-1 infection remains the ultimate goal, the tempo of the epidemic mandates that all other interventional strategies be considered. Of particular importance are strategies easily implemented in developing countries. Attention must be given to concomitant infections and factors such as nutritional status that may affect vertical HIV-1 transmission. Because concomitant maternal venereal infections may increase the risk of vertical HIV-1 transmission, efforts to prevent or treat these infections are important.

A study from Malawi[62] reported an increased risk of vertical HIV-1 transmission with maternal vitamin A deficiency. Potential explanations for the protective activity of vitamin A would include its role in the maintenance of mucosal surfaces, its role in B- and T-cell immunity, and the potential role of retinoids in the regulation of viral replication. Further evaluation of this association is important, because vitamin A supplementation would offer an inexpensive and easily feasible intervention for developing countries.

Data supporting the intrapartum route of transmission have prompted the development of techniques that may reduce the exposure of the neonate to HIV-1–infected vaginal secretions. Cell-free HIV-1 may be detected in cervical and vaginal secretions of 30% to 40% of HIV-1–infected pregnant women. The topical application of chlorhexidine reduces the vertical transmission of group B streptococcal infections. Although chlorhexidine is relatively ineffective against HIV-1, benzalkonium chloride is active in vitro, is not absorbed through the mucosa, and appears to be tolerated well for short periods of exposure. Protocols using benzalkonium chloride to disinfect the vagina of HIV-1–infected pregnant women during labor and delivery are in progress. Consideration is being given to bathing the neonate as well with the solution immediately after the delivery. The vaginal lavage protocols are simple and inexpensive enough to be implemented in developing countries if efficacy is demonstrated.

Because as many as 75% of infants may acquire HIV-1 infection at delivery through mucosal exposure to maternal blood or vaginal secretions, it has been suggested that cesarian section may reduce the risk of exposure, particularly if performed before the rupture of membranes. A metanalysis of published data suggests a significant (14% versus 20%, P <.05) reduction in transmission to infants delivered by cesarean section compared with vaginal delivery.[63] The enthu-siasm for cesarian section is tempered by the potential morbidity of the procedure, high cost, and lack of availability in developing nations.

Perinatal antiretroviral therapy protocols have been developed in an effort to reduce maternal blood or vaginal HIV-1 load. Zidovudine was the first antiretroviral to be given to HIV-1–infected pregnant women and their infants to evaluate its effects on vertical HIV-1 transmission (pediatric AIDS Clinical Trials Group Protocol [ACTG] 076).[64] Maternal participants were limited to nucleoside-naive women with peripheral blood absolute CD4 counts greater than 200/mm^3 who were identified before 34 weeks of pregnancy. Zidovudine or placebo was administered antenatally and during delivery to women and 6 weeks postnatally to their infants. The analysis of data from this study demonstrated a profound (67%) and significant reduction in the vertical transmission of HIV-1 in mother-infant pairs treated with zidovudine compared with those who received placebo. The only observed short-term toxic effect was anemia, which was not clinically significant. It is recommended that all pregnant women be offered HIV-1 counseling and testing, and recommendations for the management of women identified as seropositive have been developed.[65]

Although the outcome of ACTG 076 was encouraging, the continued evaluation of antiretroviral regimens must continue. First, the cost and logistic intensity of the ACTG 076 protocol make it impractical for use in developing nations, where most pediatric infections occur. Several ongoing studies are attempting to determine which component of the protocol may be responsible for its success. Second, only women with absolute CD4 counts greater than 200/mm^3 who did not require zidovudine for their own clinical indications and who did not breast-feed were eligible for participation in ACTG 076. The results of ACTG 076 may therefore not apply to women of more advanced status or to women who have received prolonged therapy with zidovudine before their pregnancy. The latter groups of women are likely to have high peripheral blood viral load. Women on prolonged ZDV therapy may harbor ZDV resistant viruses. The development of combination regimens that would potently inhibit viral replication and maintain activity in the face of antiretroviral resistance is therefore of high priority.

The detection of low titers of broadly neutralizing antibodies in the sera of most pregnant HIV-1–positive women sparked interest in the evaluation of the passive administration of monoclonal or polyclonal antibody preparations to mothers and their infants for the prevention of vertical HIV-1 transmission. Studies to evaluate various monoclonal or polyclonal antibody preparations are in progress and planned for the near future.

Neonatal active-passive immunization has proven to be extremely effective in preventing chronic hepatitis B infection in infants born to mothers who are chronic carriers. Based on this model, phase I studies evaluating potential active products are underway.

BIBLIOGRAPHY

Centers for Disease Control. Recommendations of the U.S. Public Health Task Force on the use of zidovudine to reduce perinatal transmission of human immunodeficiency virus. MMWR 1994;43:1.

Connor EM, Sperling RS, Gelber R, the ACTG 076 Study Group. Reduction of maternal-infant transmission of human immunodeficiency virus type 1 with zidovudine treatment. N Engl J Med 1994;331:1173.

Luzuriaga K, Sullivan JL. Pathogenesis of vertical HIV-1 infection: implications for intervention and management. Pediatr Ann 1994;23:159.

Peckham C, Gibb D. Mother to child transmission of the human immunodeficiency virus. N Engl J Med 1995;333:298.

Wilfert CM, Wilson C, Luzuriaga K, Epstein L. Pathogenesis of pediatric human immunodeficiency type 1 infection. J Infect Dis 1994;170:286.

REFERENCES

1. Stoneburner R, Sato P, Burton A, Mertens T. The global HIV pandemic. Acta Pediatr 1994;(Suppl 400):1.
2. Nicoll A, Timaeus I, Kigadye RM, Walraven G, Killewo J. The impact of HIV-1 infection on mortality in children under 5 years of age in sub-Saharan Africa: a demographic and epidemiologic analysis. AIDS 1994;8:995.
3. Rogers MF, Caldwell MB, Gwinn ML, Simonds RJ. Epidemiology of pediatric Human Immunodeficiency Virus infection in the United States. Int J Pediatr 1994;400:5.
4. Sprecher S, Soumenkoff G, Puissant F, Gueldre MD. Vertical transmission of HIV in 15 week fetus. Lancet 1985;2:288.
5. Jovaisas E, Koch MA, Schafer A. LAV/HTLV III in 20-week fetus. Lancet 1985;2:1129.
6. Courgnaud V, Laure F, Brossard A, et al. Frequent and early in utero HIV-1 infection. AIDS Res Hum Retroviruses 1991;7:337.
7. Viscarello R, Cullen MT, DeGennaro NJ, Hobbins JC. Fetal blood sampling in HIV-seropositive pregnancies before elective midtrimester termination of pregnancy. Am J Obstet Gynecol 1992;167:1075.
8. Mundy D, Schinazi RF, Gerver AR, et al. Human immunodeficiency virus isolated from amniotic fluid. Lancet 1987;2:459.
9. Rogers M, Ou CY, Rayfield M, et al. Use of the polymerase chain reaction for early detection of proviral sequences of human immunodeficiency virus in infants born to seropositive mothers. N Engl J Med 1989;320:1649.
10. Ehrnst A, Lindgren S, Dictor M, et al. HIV in pregnant women and their offspring: evidence for late transmission. Lancet 1991;338:203.
11. Krivine A, Firtion G, Cao L, et al. HIV replication during the first weeks of life. Lancet 1992;339:1187.
12. Luzuriaga K, McQuilken P, Alimenti A, et al. Early viremia and immune responses in vertical human immunodeficiency virus type 1 infection. J Infect Dis 1993;167:1008.
13. Nair P, Alger L, Hines S, et al. Maternal and neonatal characteristics associated with HIV infection in infants of seropositive women. J Acquir Immune Defic Syndr 1993;6:298.
14. Goedert JJ, Duliege A-M, Amos CI. The International Registry of HIV-exposed twins. High risk of HIV-1 infection for first-born twins. Lancet 1991;338:1471.
15. Duliege A, Amos CI, Felton S, Biggar RJ, Goedert JJ. Birth order, delivery route, and concordance in the transmission of human immunodeficiency virus type 1 from mothers to twins. International Registry of HIV-Exposed Twins. J Pediatr 1995;126:625.
16. Alimenti A, Luzuriaga K, Stechenberg B, Sullivan JL. Quantitation of human immunodeficiency virus in vertically infected infants and children. J Pediatr 1991;119:225.
17. Luzuriaga K, Koup RA, Pikora CA, Brettler DB, Sullivan JL. Deficient human immunodeficiency virus type 1-specific cytotoxic T cell responses in vertically infected children. J Pediatr 1991;119:230.
18. Baba T, Koch J, Stewart Mittler E, et al. Mucosal infection of neonatal rhesus monkeys with cell-free SIV. AIDS Res Hum Retroviruses 1994;10:351.
19. Ruff A, Yolken R, Desormeaux J, et al. HIV-1 and HIV-1 inhibitory activity in breast milk. Abstract. International Conference on AIDS. Berlin, Germany, 1993.
20. European Collaborative Study. Risk factors for mother-to-child transmission of HIV-1. Lancet 1992;339:1007.
21. The HIV Infection in Newborns French Collaborative Study Group. Comparison of vertical human immunodeficiency virus type 2 and human immunodeficiency virus type 1 transmission in the French prospective cohort. Pediatr Infect Dis J 1994;13:502.
22. Dunn D, Newell M-L, Ades AE, Peckham C. Risk of human immunodeficiency virus type 1 transmission through breastfeeding. Lancet 1992;340:585.
23. Van de Perre P, Simonon A, Mselatti P, et al. Postnatal transmission of human immunodeficiency virus type I from mother to infant. N Engl J Med 1991;325:593.
24. Palasinthran P, Ziegler JB, Stewart GJ, et al. Breastfeeding during primary human immunodeficiency virus infection and risk of transmission from mother to infant. J Infect Dis 1993;167:441.
25. World Health Organization. Consensus statement from the WHO/UNICEF consultation of HIV transmission and breastfeeding. Geneva: World Health Organization, 1992.
26. Bryson YJ, Luzuriaga K, Sullivan JL, Wara DW. Proposed definitions for in utero versus intrapartum transmission of HIV-1. (Letter) N Engl J Med 1992;327:1246.
27. Report of a consensus workshop. Maternal factors involved in mother-to-child transmission of HIV-1. J Acquir Immune Defic Syndr 1992;5:1019.
28. Weiser B, Nachman S, Tropper P, et al. Quantitation of human immunodeficiency virus type 1 during pregnancy: relationship of viral titer to mother-to-child transmission and stability of viral load. Proc Natl Acad Sci USA 1994;91:8037.
29. Borkowsky W, Krasinski K, Cao Y, et al. Correlation of perinatal transmission of human immunodeficiency virus type 1 with maternal viremia and lymphocyte phenotypes. J Pediatr 1994;125:345.
30. Dickover R, Herman S, Garratty E, von Seidlein L, Boyer P, Bryson Y. Maternal HIV RNA levels are directly related to perinatal transmission risk and significantly reduced by ZDV treatment. Abstract D4-410. Keystone Symposia. Keystone, CO, March, 1995.
31. Husson RN, Lan Y, Kojima E, et al. Vertical transmission of human immunodeficiency virus type 1: autologous neutralizing antibody, virus load, and virus phenotype. J Pediatr 1995;126:865.
32. Scarlatti G, Leitner T, Halapi E, et al. Comparison of variable region 3 sequences of human immunodeficiency virus type 1 from infected children with the RNA and DNA sequences of the virus populations of their mothers. Proc Natl Acad Sci USA 1993;90:1721.
33. Wolinsky SM, Wike CM, Korber BTM, et al. Selective transmission of human immunodeficiency virus type-1 variants from mothers to infants. Science 1992;255:1134.
34. Lammers S, Sleasman JW, She JX, et al. Independent variation and positive selection in env V1 and V2 domains within maternal-infant strains of human immunodeficiency virus type 1 in vivo. J Virol 1993;67:3957.
35. Zhu T, Mo H, Wang N, et al. Genotypic and phenotypic characterization of HIV-1 in patients with primary infection. Science 1993;261:1179.
36. Scarlatti G, Albert J, Rossi P, et al. Mother-to-child transmission of human immunodeficiency virus type 1: correlation with neutralizing antibodies against primary isolates. J Infect Dis 1993;168:207.
37. Broliden K, Sievers E, Tovo PA, et al. Antibody-dependent cellular cytotoxicity and neutralizing activity in sera of HIV-1 infected mothers and their children. Clin Exp Immunol 1993;93:56.
38. Galli L, deMartino M, Tovo PA, et al. Onset of clinical signs in children with HIV-1 perinatal infection. AIDS 1995;9:455.
39. Newell M-L, Peckham C, Dunn D, Ades T, Giaquinto C. Natural history of vertically acquired human immunodeficiency virus-1 infection. The European Collaborative Study. Pediatrics 1994;94:815.
40. Dickover R, Dillon M, Gillette S, et al. Rapid increases in load of human immunodeficiency virus correlate with early disease progression and loss of CD4 cells in vertically infected infants. J Infect Dis 1994;170:1279.
41. Palumbo P, Kwok S, Waters S, et al. Viral measurement by polymerase chain reaction-based assays in human immunodeficiency virus-infected infants. J Pediatr 1995;126:592.
42. Forte SE, Byron KS, Sullivan JL, Somasundaran M. Non-syncytium inducing HIV-1 isolated from infected individuals replicate in MT-2 cells. AIDS Res Hum Retroviruses 1994;10:1613.
43. De Rossi A, Giaquinto C, Ometto L, et al. Replication and tropism of human immunodeficiency virus type 1 as predictors of disease outcome in infants with vertically-acquired infection. J Pediatr 1993;123:929.
44. Spencer LT, Ogino MT, Dankner WM, Spector SA. Clinical significance of human immunodeficiency virus type 1 phenotype in infected children. J Infect Dis 1994;169:491.

45. Daniel MD, Kirchoff F, Czajak SC, Sehgal PK, Desrosiers RC. Protective effects of a live-attenuated SIV vaccine with a deletion in the nef gene. Science 1992;258:1938.
46. Baba T, Jeong YS, Penninck D, et al. Pathogenicity of live, attenuated SIV after mucosal infection of neonatal macaques. Science 1994;267:1820.
47. Sullivan JL, Barry DW, Lucas SJ, Albrecht P. Measles infection of human mononuclear cells I. Acute infection of peripheral blood lymphocytes and monocytes. J Exp Med 1975;142:773.
48. Sperduto A, Bryson YJ, Chen I. Increased susceptibility of neonatal macrophages to HIV-1 infection. AIDS Res Hum Retroviruses 1993;9:1277.
49. Brunell PA, Kotchmar GS. Zoster in infancy: failure to maintain virus latency following intrauterine infection. J Pediatr 1981;98:71.
50. Wilson CB, Westall J, Johnston L, et al. Decreased production of interferon gamma by human neonatal cells: intrinsic and regulatory deficiencies. J Clin Invest 1986;77:860.
51. Jenkins M, Mills J, Kohl S. Natural killer cytotoxicity and antibody-dependent cellular cytotoxicity of human immune deficiency virus-infected cells by leukocytes from human neonates and adults. Pediatr Res 1993;33:469.
52. Luzuriaga K, Holmes D, Hereema A, et al. HIV-1-Specific cytotoxic T lymphocyte responses in the first year of life. J Immunol 1995;154:433.
53. McFarland EJ, Harding PA, Luckey D, et al. High frequency of gag- and env-specific cytotoxic T lymphocyte precursors in children with vertically-acquired human immunodeficiency virus type 1 infection. J Infect Dis 1994;170:766.
54. Imagawa D, Lee MH, Wolinsky SM, et al. Human immunodeficiency virus type 1 infection in homosexual men who remain seronegative for prolonged periods. N Engl J Med 1989;320:1458.
55. Bryson YJ, Pang S, Wei LS, Dickover R, Diagne Y, Chen ISY. Clearance of HIV Infection in a perinatally infected infant. N Engl J Med 1995;332:833.
56. Langlade-Demoyen P, Hong NNG, Ferchal F, Oksenhendler E. Human immunodeficiency virus (HIV) nef-specific cytotoxic T lymphocytes in noninfected sexual contacts of HIV-infected patients. J Clin Invest 1994;93:1293.
57. Rowland-Jones S, Sutton J, Ariyoshi K, et al. HIV-1 specific cytotoxic T cells in HIV-exposed but uninfected Gambian women. Nature Med 1995;1:59.
58. Cheynier R, Langlade-Demoyen P, Marescot MR, et al. Cytotoxic T lymphocyte responses in the peripheral blood of children born to human immunodeficiency virus-1 infected mothers. Eur J Immunol 1992;22:2211.
59. De Maria A, Cirillo C, Moretta L. Occurrence of human immunodeficiency virus type 1 (HIV-1)-specific cytolytic T cell activity in apparently uninfected children born to HIV-1-infected mothers. J Infect Dis 1994;170:1296.
60. Buseyne F, Blanche S, Schmitt D, Griscelli C, Riviere Y. Detection of HIV-specific cell-mediated cytotoxicity in the peripheral blood from infected children. J Immunol 1993;150:3569.
61. Rowland-Jones SL, Nixon, DF, Aldhous M, et al. HIV-specific cytotoxic T-cell activity in an HIV-exposed but uninfected infant. Lancet 1993;341:860.
62. Semba R, Miotti P, Chiphangwi JD, et al. Maternal vitamin A deficiency and mother-to-child transmission of HIV-1. Lancet 1994;343:1593.
63. Villari P, Spino C, Chalmers TC, Lau J, Sacks S. Caesarean section to reduce perinatal transmission of human immunodeficiency virus. Online J Curr Clin Trials 1993;2:document 74.
64. Connor EM, Sperling RS, Gelber R, the ACTG 076 Study Group. Reduction of maternal-infant transmission of human immunodeficiency virus type 1 with zidovudine treatment. N Engl J Med 1994;331:1173.
65. Centers for Disease Control. Recommendations of the U.S. Public Health Task Force on the use of zidovudine to reduce perinatal transmission of human immunodeficiency virus. MMWR 1994;43:1.

PART III

Diagnosis of HIV Infection

AIDS: Biology, Diagnosis, Treatment and
Prevention, fourth edition, edited by Vincent T.
DeVita, Jr., Samuel Hellman, and Steven A.
Rosenberg. Lippincott–Raven Publishers, © 1997

CHAPTER 11

Acquired Immunodeficiency Syndrome: Serologic and Virologic Tests

Julia A. Metcalf, Richard T. Davey Jr., and H. Clifford Lane

Although the first published reports about acquired immunodeficiency syndrome (AIDS) appeared in 1981,[1,2] several years of intense investigation were required to isolate and confirm the causative agent and to develop reliable, sensitive screening methods of determining exposure to this agent. Before development of these tests, a presumptive diagnosis of AIDS could only be based on a distinct set of clinical illnesses occurring in the absence of other known causes of immunosuppression. The illnesses were primarily opportunistic infections and unusual malignancies that previously occurred almost exclusively in persons with profound immunosuppression. Within this framework, a comprehensive case definition was constructed that attempted to group presumptive cases of AIDS on the basis of common clinical and immunologic parameters even before the identification of the viral agent.[3,4]

After the isolation and identification of human immunodeficiency virus type 1 (HIV-1) as the cause of AIDS,[5,6] considerable emphasis was placed on the development and testing of serologic methods for detecting HIV infection. Using existing methods, solid-phase assays were developed, and when used properly and according to established guidelines, they proved to be highly sensitive and specific. Commercial production of these assays in relatively inexpensive kit forms allowed them to be adopted for wide-scale use.

The development of increasingly sophisticated virologic and immunologic techniques has further enhanced our ability to diagnose HIV-1 infection early and accurately. These methods, especially the assays for viral RNA, have also been adapted for use in the longitudinal monitoring of patients with known infection. However, despite the potential value of these newer techniques, various modifications of the original solid-phase serologic methods have remained the standard means by which most HIV-1 infections continue to be diagnosed in the United States and in many developed nations. The first part of this chapter reviews some of these standard serologic methods as they pertain to the laboratory diagnosis of HIV infection. In the second half, some of the direct viral detection methods used clinically or in research are reviewed.

HIV-1 ENZYME IMMUNOASSAYS

A strong impetus existed in the mid-1980s for the development of rapid serologic screening methods for HIV-1. Uncertainty about the epidemiologic pattern of the disease spurred the demand to have available a rapid, reliable, and inexpensive means of screening the nation's blood supply for the possibility of occult infection, and a sensitive method of screening patients for HIV-1 infection even in the absence of overt clinical disease. Before the commercial availability of solid-phase screening methods, the safety of donated blood, clotting factor concentrates, or other transfusion products could not be guaranteed.

In March of 1985, the routine testing of donated blood by a rapid solid-phase approach became available through the development, testing, and licensure of the first enzyme-linked immunoassay (ELISA) kit. It soon became evident that separate access to a system of testing at-risk individuals for infection with HIV-1 would also be required if deliberate blood donation as a means of determining HIV-1 serostatus was to be avoided. Given the relative ease with which standardized microtiter assays could be manufactured, at least eight different commercial ELISA tests had been

Julia A. Metcalf, Clinical and Molecular Retrovirology Section, Laboratory of Immunoregulation, Building 10 Room 8C306, National Institutes of Health, Bethesda, MD 20892.

Richard T. Davey, Jr., and H. Clifford Lane: Clinical and Molecular Retrovirology Section, Laboratory of Immunoregulation, National Institute of Allergy and Infectious Disease, National Institutes of Health, Bethesda, MD 20892.

licensed by the Food and Drug Administration (FDA) by 1987.[7,8] It was in this milieu that the HIV-1 ELISA was rapidly established as a primary diagnostic screening tool.[9,10] So-called alternate test sites that were established nationwide in government-sponsored clinics to allow confidential or anonymous testing of at-risk individuals were soon supplemented by wide-scale availability of these relatively inexpensive assays through other means, such as hospital-based or commercial laboratories.

An important principle underlying the successful development of these early serologic assays for HIV-1 infection was that most infected individuals produced a detectable antibody response to various protein components of the virus within a brief period after exposure (Fig. 11-1B).[11,12] Although exceptional individuals or small cohorts appear to have significant lag periods (≥3 years) between the time of presumed viral infection and the development of a measurable antibody response,[13,14] such persons continue to be quite uncommon.[15] Most individuals develop antibody against the virus within a few weeks to a few months after viral infection.

Wide-scale serologic testing of infected individuals has revealed that the major antigens against which antibodies are produced remain fairly consistent within the population, although the exact timing of appearance and relative intensity of individual antibody responses may vary from person to person. The genome of HIV-1 (see Fig. 11-1) codes for several structural and regulatory proteins. The three major protein groups of HIV-1 are the targets for most of the circulating antibody-like substances directed against the virus:[16]

Envelope (*Env*) proteins: the outer envelope glycoprotein gp120, the transmembrane glycoprotein gp41, and the gp160 precursor glycoprotein

Polymerase (*Pol*) proteins: the reverse transcriptase p66 and the endonuclease/integrase p31

Core (*Gag*) proteins: the major structural proteins p24 and p18, the internal structural protein p7, and the p55 precursor protein

Within 4 to 8 weeks (although a duration as short as 8 days has been described) after exposure to the virus,

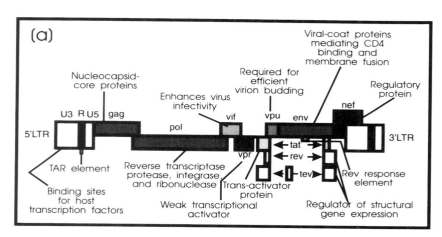

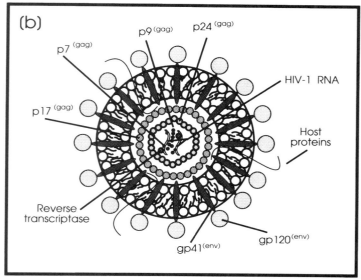

FIG. 11-1. Diagram of the HIV-1 viral genome (**A**) and the HIV-1 virion structure (**B**).

infected individuals usually experience a brief period of constitutional illness (eg, fever, fatigue, myalgias, rash, gastrointestinal complaints, neurologic symptoms) that has been likened to an influenza-like viral illness.[12] This period lasts for a few days to a few weeks and is accompanied by a burst of active viral replication in the host, as documented by high levels of circulating virus in plasma and measurable p24 antigen expression. With subsidence of the acute symptoms, increasing levels of virus-specific antibody begin to appear and can be quantified by a variety of serologic detection methods. Antibodies against p24 and against the viral envelope proteins, especially gp160 and gp41, are among the first detectable HIV-1–specific immunoglobulins produced during this period of acute seroconversion. The ELISA appears to be especially sensitive for early detection of anti-p24 antibody under these circumstances, and other tests such as the radioimmunoprecipitation assay (RIPA) may show early reactivity because of antibody directed against the higher-molecular-weight antigens such as gp160.[11]

The ELISA test is the standard screening test for HIV-1 infection. Individuals with indeterminate or positive ELISA results should undergo confirmation testing (usually with Western blot testing) to determine if the reactivity is secondary to HIV-1 infection or secondary to cross-reacting antibodies.

Enzyme-Linked Immunoassay Method

Like many diagnostic assays of this type, enzyme immunoassays for the detection of a serologic response to HIV-1 infection were developed in a series of stages, called generations. The first generation of enzyme immunoassays licensed as diagnostic kits was based on the use of viral lysates derived from strains of HIV-1 propagated in infected cells, particularly those employing the lymphoid leukemia cell lines H9 and CEM.[7] The basis for most assay kits is a solid-phase indirect antibody detector system; microtiter plate wells are commonly used, although polystyrene or latex beads are also used (Fig. 11-2). According to the method employed by most commercial manufacturers, viral lysate is prepared from common laboratory strains of virus (eg, HIV-1 LA1) that have been passaged in tissue culture and then bound to the solid phase of the particular assay system. The relative amounts of each of the major structural and expressed proteins of HIV-1 may differ significantly among commercial preparations. The external envelope glycoproteins (ie, gp120 and its precursor, gp160) and the *gag*-encoded products (especially p24 and p17 antigens) are well represented in the bound material.

As with most conventional ELISA kits, patients' sera (often tested in duplicates or triplicates to reduce error) are allowed to react with antigens bound on the solid phase for a specified period, after which unbound antibody is washed away in a rinse step. With some kits, care must be taken to minimize the use of heat-inactivated sera, because a higher

rate of false positivity has been reported when sera are treated in this fashion before testing.[17] If a patient's serum contains specific anti–HIV-1 antibody or cross-reacting immunoglobulin, these antibodies remain adherent to the viral preparation linked to the solid phase. Enzymatically labeled anti-human immunoglobulin is then added to the solid phase, it is allowed to incubate for a set period, and then the reaction mixture is washed as described previously. If human immunoglobulin has bound to the solid-phase antigen in the first step, the enzyme-labeled anti-human immunoglobulin binds to it in this step. Most assays employ alkaline phosphatase or horseradish peroxidase as the enzyme label. The substrate for the enzyme is then added to the reaction well. In the presence of the bound enzyme, the substrate is converted to a colored product.

The speed and intensity of the colorimetric reaction that follows is directly proportional to the amount of bound enzyme, which depends on the quantity of anti–HIV-1 antibody bound to viral lysate on the solid phase. The intensity of the reaction, which is recorded as the optical density (OD) of the reaction mixture, is easily quantitated by means of a spectrophotometer calibrated to read at the optimal wavelength of the substrate material. A specific OD can then be assigned to each test well in a panel; in a typical microtiter plate assay, up to 96 wells can be read from a single plate. Using a series of known positive and negative samples as controls, a standard curve for the colorimetric reaction is generated against which the OD of test samples can be compared. A cutoff value for the lowest OD still regarded as consistent with a positive determination can be calculated by a statistical comparison of the intensity of a panel of positive control samples with a panel of negative sera. Although test sera with OD values well above the cutoff point can be recorded as unequivocally positive, the scoring of samples with OD readings skirting the cutoff range can be more problematic. The propensity of test results to fall close to the cutoff range can vary among manufacturers' kits. Kits that produce positive readings closer to the cutoff range may exhibit slightly greater sensitivity than those requiring higher OD readings for a positive determination, but they may also be more prone to false-positive findings as a consequence of this narrow margin.

In accord with its planned role as an initial screening device, it should not be surprising that the HIV-1 ELISA was designed to optimize sensitivity at the expense of specificity. Because of the availability of backup or confirmatory assays to validate positive findings and the potentially serious consequences of undiagnosed infections, a reduction in the number of false negatives, even at the expense of a slightly higher rate of false positives, is generally regarded as a reasonable tradeoff. The ELISA test, although an excellent test for screening, should not be used alone for diagnosis of HIV-1 infection without a positive confirmatory test. Most of the commercially marketed ELISA preparations have had a sensitivity of at least 99.5% and a specificity of greater than 99.8% in large-scale testing of individuals with high-

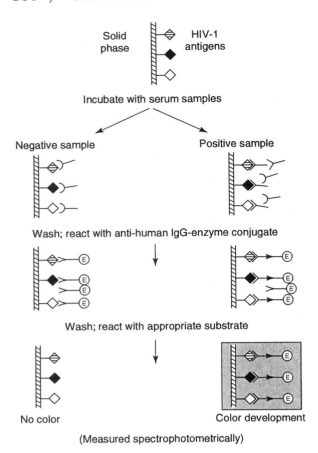

Solid phase — HIV-1 antigens

Incubate with serum samples

Negative sample   Positive sample

Wash; react with anti-human IgG-enzyme conjugate

Wash; react with appropriate substrate

No color   Color development
(Measured spectrophotometrically)

FIG. 11-2. Diagram of the standard commercial HIV-1 or HIV-1/HIV-2 ELISA technique.

risk behavior for HIV-1 acquisition.[16,18] However, the positive predictive value of the standard HIV-1 ELISA may fluctuate widely, depending on the population being screened.[19] For example, the false-positive rate for low-risk populations is substantially higher than that for high-risk populations, an observation that must be taken into account in the interpretation of preliminary test results. In a large study by the American Red Cross of a low-risk pool of volunteer blood donors, only 13% of those with a repeatedly reactive HIV-1 ELISA results were confirmed to be HIV-1 infected by means of a confirmatory Western blot test.[10] Such data have obvious implications for wide-scale screening of blood product donors, for whom the majority of positive ELISA reactions may be expected to be false-positive readings based on samples from uninfected donors. In contrast, the rate of false-negative results with conventional ELISA assays remains quite small, affecting no more than 1 in every 40,000 samples.[20] As continued refinements in solid-phase technology lead to development of even more sensitive probes, this rate should continue to drop.

As with any assay capable of processing large numbers of test sera at any one time, ELISA methodology is subject to several technical drawbacks that may diminish the significance of any single positive result. These problems range from frank procedural errors in the handling of samples, such

as mislabeling of specimens, to deficiencies in the manual or automated performance of sample processing, such as well-to-well carryover during pipetting and resultant contamination of neighboring wells. Apart from these purely technical considerations, the causes of false-positive ELISA results may be varied and obscure. In some cases, common elements have been identified that may provide an explanation for these findings. Chief among these is the presence of cross-reactive antibodies against certain common human leukocyte antigens (ie, HLA-DR and other class II antigens in particular) that may be in some patients' sera. These antibodies presumably recognize and bind to cellular contaminants within the viral lysates used in these kits. The use of the CEM cell line to propagate virus in tissue culture has reduced or eliminated this particular cause of cross-reactivity.[21]

Other causes of false-positive ELISA readings that have been identified include the presence of autoreactive antibodies (eg, antinuclear antibody, antimitochondrial antibody), heat inactivation of sera before testing, repetitive freeze-thaw cycles before assaying, severe hepatic disease, passive immunoglobulin administration (ie, isolated cases of transient "seroconversion" have been reported for patients receiving passive IgG injections), recent exposure to certain vaccine preparations (eg, influenza vaccine), and certain malignancies. Cross-reactivity of sera from patients with HIV-2 also occurs. In contrast, cross-reactivity of HIV-1 in ELISA testing generally does not occur with sera from patients with HTLV-I infection.

False-negative ELISA findings can result from improper handling of reagents in individual test kits. Other causes include performance of the assay too early in the period after HIV-1 exposure (ie, before seroconversion) and conditions that cause B-cell dysfunction and defective antibody synthesis, such as severe hypogammaglobulinemia.

A significant advance in the efforts to improve the sensitivity and specificity of existing solid-phase immunoassays came with the introduction of viral antigens produced through recombinant DNA technology to supplement or replace the crude mixtures of proteins derived from lysates. The former can be produced with considerably more purity and in higher amounts than protein derived from lysates, and they can also be bound to solid-phase surfaces with much tighter control over protein ratios and concentrations. A potential drawback of such recombinant proteins is that they may afford a more limited repertoire of antigenic sites. This appeared to have clinical significance in the failure of several of the commercial preparations used in Europe and Africa to detect infection with the subtype O strain of HIV-1. They may also differ somewhat from native proteins by virtue of altered patterns of glycosylation. Nonetheless, the avidity between these antigens and anti–HIV-1 antibodies appears to be quite high. In addition to diagnostic utility in the screening of individuals and blood products, the newer-generation immunoassays have proven especially valuable in the research setting. For example, immunoassays enriched in external envelope antigen such as gp 160 have been used in the detection of anti-envelope antibody responses in individuals immunized with candidate anti–HIV-1 vaccines, particularly those employing recombinant gp 160 or gp 120 protein as immunogen.[22,23] These assays have provided significantly enhanced sensitivity to early antibody responses over that afforded by a more conventional ELISA.

Most ELISA kits use enzyme-tagged anti-human IgG as the probe to detect the presence of bound HIV-1–specific antibody within a test well. Another refinement that may help to improve the sensitivity of existing immunoassays and that may lead to earlier detection of seroconversion involves the addition or substitution of enzyme-labeled anti-human IgM for anti-human immunoglobulin at this stage of the assay.

Interpretation of Enzyme-Linked Immunoassay Results

Sera from an individual infected with HIV-1 should routinely test positive by commercial HIV-1 ELISA within a few months of exposure. Because these assays are variously enriched in *gag*-derived proteins and envelope glycoproteins, antigens against which the humoral response in the host is characteristically brisk, the ELISA is usually quite sensitive to early detection of seroconversion. Given the uniformly high sensitivity of most commercial preparations,

a negative ELISA reading at an appropriate interval after exposure strongly militates against the likelihood of infection in most cases.

Barring procedural errors in the performance of the assay, there is usually no reason to require that a person with a negative ELISA result be immediately retested. However, if the interval between testing and presumed exposure is unknown and there is the possibility that the original test was performed relatively soon after a possible infection, it may be advisable to repeat the test on a new sample within a few months of the initial assay. Repeated ELISA testing also may be warranted if the initial results showed borderline reactivity according to the internal OD standards generated within each test kit. The OD readings falling slightly under (ie, less than one standard deviation below) the cutoff value may reflect high negative signals from true seronegative sera or may represent the initial stages of reactivity in sera from an individual undergoing incipient seroconversion. Because the immunoassay is not capable of differentiating these two possibilities, repeating the test on a fresh specimen, repeating the test with the same sera but using a different commercial assay, or a combination of these two approaches has been used as a means of attempting to resolve this diagnostic uncertainty. If borderline reactivity persists despite repetitive testing, a minimal recommendation would be to repeat the ELISA within a few weeks. Failure of the OD value to rise substantially over time suggests that the low level of reactivity does not represent true infection.

It was discovered that a strain of HIV-1 known as HIV-1 subtype O could be isolated from certain patients from Cameroon and other regions of West Africa.[94,95] Initial screening with several of the commercial ELISA kits commonly used in Europe and Africa failed to detect antibody reactivity in these patients. It appeared that the kits employing recombinant antigens were particularly prone to this defect. Assays using whole-virus lysate antigens may need to be used preferentially in this situation. Although endemic infection with this particular subtype of HIV-1 has yet to be documented in the United States, manufacturers in this country and abroad are revising their test kit antigens to enhance detection of antibodies against subtype O. Whether there may exist other, as yet uncharacterized, strains of HIV-1 that could also fail to show reactivity on current commercial assays is unknown.

The latest refinement in HIV-screening ELISA methodology in wide-scale use in this country and elsewhere has been the inclusion of test antigens for HIV-2 on the solid phase. Unlike the situation in parts of West Africa, documented cases of HIV-2 infection remain generally rare in the United States. Most cases identified have been imported into this country from elsewhere, such as in recent immigrants or expatriots with endemic exposure (eg, Peace Corps workers). Nonetheless, during the past 1 to 2 years, most major manufacturers of commercial ELISA kits have incorporated HIV-2 antigens in their preparations to enhance the sensitivity of these assays for both major types of HIV. It is standard practice in blood banks to screen donated blood samples with one of the new HIV-1/HIV-2 combination ELISA assays.

HIV-1 WESTERN BLOT

Because of the high degree of false positivity with commercial assays in screening low-risk populations, determination of a positive reaction on ELISA testing is not sufficient for the diagnosis of HIV infection. Essential to the diagnosis of a true serologic response to HIV is the requirement that a repeatedly positive result by ELISA or another rapid screening method be confirmed by a more specific assay such as a Western blot test. Because there are several explanations for why a positive ELISA result may occur, many of them having no relation to true HIV-1 infection, all ELISA readings having an OD falling within the positive range need to be verified by repeated testing before more detailed evaluation (Fig. 11-3). Although this algorithm should be followed on samples from all individuals, it is particularly true for individuals without risk factors for HIV-1 or HIV-2 exposure, for whom most positive ELISA test results are false positives. Only samples that are repeatedly reactive on two or more separate ELISA runs merit further diagnostic evaluation with a confirmatory assay.

In the United States and elsewhere, this confirmatory role most frequently involves the use of an HIV-1–specific (or HIV-2—specific) Western blot, of which numerous commercial preparations have been marketed.[30] A positive Western blot confirms the presence of antibodies reactive with HIV in the infected individual and permits identification of the specific viral components to which that individual has raised a detectable humoral response. By serial application, it can also be used to grade the intensity of the individual components of that response qualitatively and, in some cases, quantitatively during interval follow-up.

Commercial Western Blot Preparations

A conventional HIV Western blot is an immunoblot preparation consisting of a crude lysate of HIV-1 (or HIV-2) obtained from tissue culture, partially purified by differential centrifugation after cell lysis, separated by molecular weight into individual viral proteins through gel electrophoresis, and then electrophoretically transferred onto nitrocellulose paper (Fig. 11-4). The sensitivity of the newer generation of immunoblot preparations using recombinant antigens appears to be quite high.[45] The nitrocellulose paper is cut into narrow strips, which are then packaged in kit form along with an incubation tray and a set of developing reagents. Provision of seropositive and seronegative sera as controls is usually the responsibility of the individual laboratory performing the assay and should be included in each separate run as essential quality-control measures.

The standard assay is performed according to a modified method of Towbin and colleagues.[31] Test sera are allowed to react with the individual viral components on the nitrocellulose paper, which serves as the solid support for the detection of antibodies in a manner analogous to the antigen-coated microtiter well in a standard ELISA. After washing and removal of unbound antibodies, recognition of various viral proteins by antibodies within sera can be detected through addition of a second antibody directed against human immunoglobulin. The latter reagent is usually chemically tagged with a radioactive probe that can be detected by autoradiographic means or, as is common in commercial preparations, with an enzyme capable of generating a colorimetric reaction in the presence of substrate added during a subsequent development step. Performance of many com-

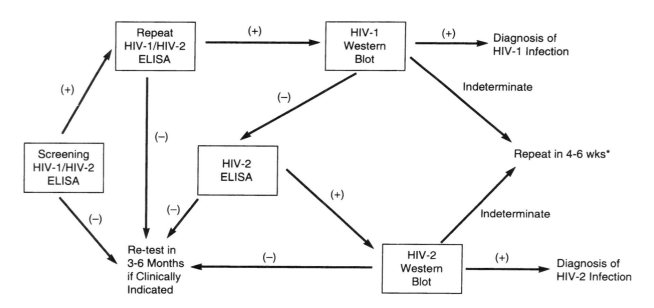

*Stable indeterminate Western blot over 4-6 weeks makes HIV infection unlikely. However, should be repeated at 3 month intervals x2 to rule-out HIV infection.

FIG. 11-3. Algorithm for the correct use and sequence of serologic testing in the diagnosis of HIV infection.

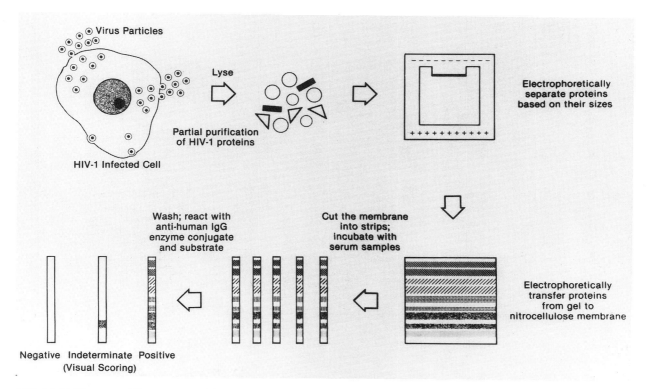

FIG. 11-4. Diagram of the commercial HIV-1 Western blot technique.

mercially available Western blot kits requires a minimal amount of sample handling and can be completed within a few hours. By comparison with control sera and with the internal reference standards usually provided in each kit, results can be scored visually in terms of the pattern and number of antibody bands. Alternatively, densitometry techniques allow antibody banding to be evaluated quantitatively as well; in the research setting, for example, this may have particular value for following serologic reactivity to specific HIV antigens over time. It has also been used to evaluate the humoral response to candidate AIDS vaccines in noninfected seronegative recipients after primary and booster immunizations.[22]

When used to confirm seroreactivity in a patient with presumed HIV infection, the Western blot generally reveals variable degrees of antibody reactivity with *env, gag,* and *pol* gene products of HIV-1 (Fig. 11-5). The specific pattern of banding may vary from individual to individual, and the intensity may fluctuate according to the relative amounts of specific anti–HIV-1 antibody circulating at any given time and the particular commercial preparation being used. Most commercial Western blot preparations are especially sensitive to the detection of anti-p24 antibody, and its appearance on immunoblotting may occur relatively early in the period after exposure, occasionally serving to herald the process of seroconversion. Appearance of detectable levels of antibody against *pol* and *env* gene products may be delayed until somewhat later, although this lag period is usually brief, and its impact on serodiagnosis is minor. Antibodies against other gene products of HIV-1, such as *nef* or other regulatory ele-

ments, are generally not detected by conventional immuno-blotting techniques.

Scoring of Western Blot Results

Official FDA licensure of the first commercial Western blot preparation (Biotech/Du Pont, Wilmington, DE) occurred in April of 1987. Since then, several different manufacturer's preparations have been introduced. Almost from the onset, however, the correct interpretation or scoring of a Western blot result has been an area of considerable controversy in the medical literature. All laboratories still have not agreed on a common algorithm for grading immunoblot banding patterns. Occasionally, this has led to some confusion in the reporting of test results, particularly when separate laboratories using different criteria have been asked to perform confirmatory assays on the same specimens.

Depending on the rigor of the definition applied, it is generally agreed that a negative Western blot result is one in which no bands are present at any location or one in which no bands corresponding to the molecular weights of known viral proteins can be detected. The presence of bands at locations not corresponding to known viral antigens is a fairly common finding and is presumed to reflect contaminants within the preparation to which some degree of antibody binding occurs. The molecular weights of these aberrant bands may vary from manufacturer to manufacturer or even from lot to lot in kits produced by the same manufacturer.

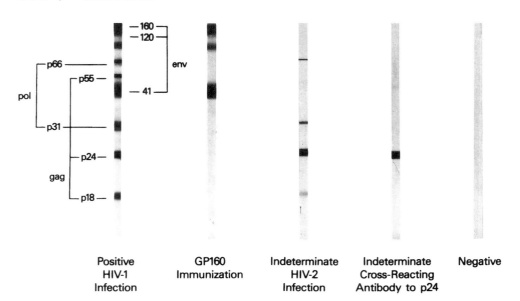

FIG. 11-5. Illustration of a positive HIV Western blot, showing antibody banding at the major viral proteins that can be identified using this technique. For comparision, both a negative Western blot, an example of an indeterminate Western blot, and the antibody profile of an HIV-2–infected patient are also shown.

The definition of what should constitute a positive Western blot result has been considerably more difficult to codify, particularly because there has been some disagreement among investigators about whether appropriate stringency of the definition should require the presence of antibody against two or all three of the major viral gene products. Antibody against a protein (or proteins) from all three groups has always been accepted as unequivocal evidence of a positive finding, and the Biotech/Du Pont kit was licensed with the manufacturer's recommendation that reactivity with all three gene products occur for a positive determination to be made.[32] This was also the position adopted by the American Red Cross at that time. Since that time, however, convincing evidence indicates that antibody against only two of the three major groups may be equally diagnostic of true seroreactivity to HIV-1.[21,30] In 1988, for example, the Consortium for Retrovirology Serology Standardization recommended that scoring of a positive Western blot could be made on the basis of the following pattern: anti-p24 or anti-p31 occurring in the presence of anti-gp41 or anti-gp160/gp120.[33] Other groups suggested that the presence or absence of antibody against *pol* gene products such as p31 should not be required within this definition.

Although this controversy still continues to some degree, the most widely accepted criteria are those adopted by the Centers for Disease Control in 1989.[30] These were based on the standards established by the Association of State and Territorial Public Health Laboratory Directors during the previous year.[34] According to these criteria, a Western blot can be considered reactive if it contains at least two of the three bands thought by the Association members to be of diagnostic significance: anti-p24, anti-gp41, and anti-gp160/gp120.

By definition, Western blot results that cannot be classified as negative or positive are categorized as indeterminate findings. Bands present may correspond to the molecular weights of known HIV-1 proteins[35] or to other proteins on the nitrocellulose paper of unknown (but presumably not viral) origin. Isolated or joint reactivity at the p24, p55, or both bands is particularly common in Western blots falling into the indeterminate category, regardless of whether the examiner is surveying patients whose histories might classify them as being at high risk[36] or low risk[37–43] for HIV-1 infection. However, most indeterminate Western blot results occur for patients with no other evidence of HIV-1 infection, and it is presumed that this limited antibody recognition represents reactivity by antibodies with various contaminants of the immunoblot preparation. For example, reactivity with class I and II HLA antigens present as cellular contaminants within the viral lysate appears to account for a significant percentage of false-positive banding. Newer immunoblot assays using recombinantly derived viral antigens rather than viral lysates may reduce the incidence of indeterminate reactivity, although this remains to be confirmed by large-scale testing.[44,45]

If clinically warranted (eg, possible recent HIV exposure), the finding of an indeterminate Western blot pattern in the presence of a positive HIV-1 ELISA result should prompt a repeat of the Western blot test using the same or, if available, a fresh serum specimen. If the repeated assay remains indeterminate, retesting the patient within a few weeks should be considered, because it is possible that the patient was first tested early in the process of seroconversion and that serial studies may reveal the full pattern of antibody reactivity. As several studies have confirmed, however, the likelihood that an indeterminate Western blot represents incipient seroconversion remains low for most patients. Serial testing after indeterminate findings usually produces repeated indeterminate findings (with identical or different patterns of banding), a reversion to full seronegativity, or a vacillation between the two categories. As with the ELISA, failure of the Western blot to evolve from an indeterminate to a positive test result within a few months strongly militates against the possibility that the patient is HIV-infected. Nonetheless, plagued by the anxiety generated during this period of diagnostic uncertainty, many physicians and patients understandably decide to consult other diagnostic procedures in an attempt to determine more conclusively the possibility of occult infection.

The Western blot is an inappropriate initial screening test for HIV infection. Among homosexual or bisexual men testing negative for HIV-1 by ELISA and polymerase chain reaction PCR), 20% to 30% may have one or more bands demonstrated on Western blot tests.[22,36] Moreover, during evaluations performed every 1 to 3 months over the course of 1 year or longer, 70% of an HIV-1 ELISA-negative, PCR-negative cohort of homosexual men with an initial indeterminate Western blot result continued to show one or more bands on serial immunoblots.[36] Other studies using low-risk populations have had similar findings.[37] Given this high frequency of indeterminate reactivity—the overwhelming preponderance of which represents nonspecific binding—the Western blot is not appropriate as a primary screening tool for the population at large. Its strength is as a confirmatory assay in the setting of a positive or indeterminate HIV-1 ELISA or other initial screening test.

Most commercial ELISA test kits in widespread use in the United States react with antibodies against HIV-1 or HIV-2. Given the preponderance of infection with HIV-1 in this country, a repeatedly reactive ELISA should prompt use of a specific HIV-1 Western blot as a confirmatory assay. If HIV-2 infection is suspected on epidemiologic grounds or the HIV-1 Western blot shows an atypical pattern of banding suggestive of HIV-2 cross-reactivity, the next level of evaluation should employ HIV-2 ELISA, and if it is positive or indeterminate, the evaluation should proceed to an HIV-2 immunoblot. No HIV-2 immunoblot kits are licensed by the FDA, but at least one company (Cambridge Biotech) manufacturers a kit commercially available for research purposes. The result for HIV-2 testing is positive when bands are seen (see Fig. 11-5) at env (gp120 plus gp34) and gag (p26) or pol (p31 or p68/58/55).

Although estimates for the sensitivity and specificity of the HIV-1 Western blot vary somewhat among manufacturers, comparative surveys have shown that most preparations afford a sensitivity of at least 96%.[21,33] Used properly as a confirmatory test in sequence with an initial positive screening assay, the combination of these two tests should have a positive predictive value greater than 99% for low-risk and high-risk populations.

INDIRECT IMMUNOFLUORESCENCE ASSAY

Although the performance time of commercially available Western blot kits is in the range of a few hours, some laboratories prefer to use the FDA-licensed indirect immunofluorescence assay (IFA) for screening or to substitute it for the conventional immunoblot as a confirmatory assay.[46–50]

Advantages of the IFA are that it is rapid, relatively simple to perform, and requires a minimum of technical skill. It does, however, require the use of a fluorescent microscope, elevating the equipment and training expenses. According to this technique, slides containing fixed monolayers of HIV-1–infected cell lines (ie, CEM lines) are coated with various dilutions of test sera for a defined period (Fig. 11-6). During this incubation step, anti–HIV-1 antibodies present in the sera bind to antigens contained within the monolayer. After washing, the slide preparation is allowed to react with anti-human IgG antibody tagged with an ultraviolet-activated dye such as fluorescein isothiocyanate (FITC). The slide is again washed, dried, and scored by microscopic examination using a fluorescent microscope. With the use of proper technique, background staining should be minimal. Fluorescent cells can be scored for number and intensity and for the character of the staining pattern. As a negative control, it is critical to measure immunofluorescence against a noninfected cell monolayer to reduce the possibility of nonspecific (false-positive) reactivity. As with any of the standard antibody detection methods, proper quality control requires that sera from a known seropositive individual also be included as a positive control.

The IFA is relatively easy to perform, and it usually turns positive earlier in the course of infection than a conventional ELISA or Western blot. Time to development of a positive IFA after an acute seroconversion to HIV-1 can be further reduced by substituting FITC-labeled anti-human IgM as the developing antiserum. Cooper and colleagues[12] studied eight individuals who presented with an acute mononucleosis-like illness consistent with primary infection with HIV-1. In their experience, the IFA using FITC-conjugated anti-IgM turned positive at a mean of 5 days after the onset of acute symptoms, compared with a mean of 11 days for a more conventional anti-IgG antiserum. Reactivity by what they regarded as their most sensitive HIV-1 ELISA did not develop until a mean of 31 days after the beginning of the illness. Most researchers agree that, in clinical use, the sensitivity and specificity of the IFA can match or exceed that of the Western blot, although there can be some variability in appropriate scoring of samples caused by inexperience with the technique. Its major limitation in the research setting is that, unlike the Western blot, it does not permit precise delineation of specific patterns of antibody reactivity, and it requires an experienced technician.

RADIOIMMUNOPRECIPITATION ASSAY

An alternative test that is sometimes used as a confirmatory assay over the conventional Western blot is the RIPA. However, its use is largely restricted to laboratories that have the facilities and expertise to propagate HIV-1 in continuous cell culture.[51] To perform this test, infected lymphocytic cells such as H9 cells are grown in the presence of amino acids radiolabeled with ^{35}S-methionine and ^{35}S-cysteine to permit incorporation of radiolabel into HIV-1

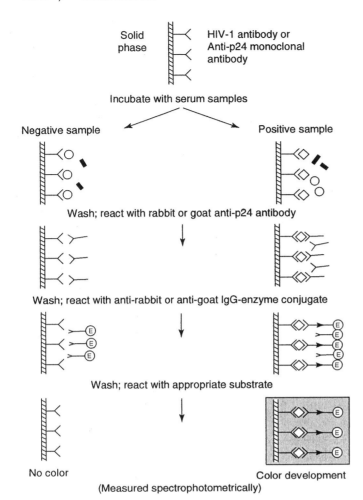

Solid phase — HIV-1 antibody or Anti-p24 monoclonal antibody

Incubate with serum samples

Negative sample   Positive sample

Wash; react with rabbit or goat anti-p24 antibody

Wash; react with anti-rabbit or anti-goat IgG-enzyme conjugate

Wash; react with appropriate substrate

No color   Color development
(Measured spectrophotometrically)

FIG. 11-6. Diagram of a conventional commercially-available p24 antigen capture assay.

proteins. Alternatively, surface labeling of HIV-1 with iodine 125 after purification of virus from a host cell line is used by some laboratories.[52] With metabolic radiolabeling, a cell lysate is then prepared by homogenization of cells in the presence of buffered detergent. Serum samples to be tested are reacted with the radiolabeled cell lysate, resulting in the generation of antigen-antibody complexes if anti–HIV-1 antibodies are present. The reaction mixture is next incubated with protein A–coated sepharose beads that bind to the heavy chain (Fc region) of IgG molecules in the immune complexes. Radiolabel-containing immune complexes become attached to a solid phase (ie, sepharose) by this protein A–binding mechanism. After binding, beads are isolated from the lysate by means of centrifugation. The antibody-antigen complexes are next eluted from the beads by heating and solubilization in detergent, and the resulting immunoprecipitates are separated electrophoretically according to molecular weight. Autoradiography of the separated proteins yields an immunoblot pattern similar to that produced by Western blotting, although resolution of the higher-molecular-weight envelope proteins is generally better.

Several aspects of the standard RIPA preclude its use by many clinical laboratories. The need to maintain viral stocks and active cell culture lines, the requirement for storing and handling of radioactive tracer materials, the time and technical expertise required in performing the assay properly, and the overall expense of this test have contributed to making the RIPA substantially less attractive than the Western blot for routine use. Most assays of this type are performed in research laboratories, where the skills and materials required are more readily accessible. Nonetheless, there are circumstances in which the clinician may find the RIPA helpful, such as detecting low levels of antibody positivity or evaluating individuals with indeterminate Western blot patterns. The sensitivity and specificity of the RIPA exceeds that of the Western blot under most circumstances, and it has provided insight into the nature of the antibody response to the higher-molecular-weight (eg, gp160, gp120) envelope proteins early in the process of seroconversion.[53] However, soon after infection, it may be relatively less sensitive than conventional immunoblotting as a means of monitoring the initial antibody response to other viral antigens, such as p24 or gp41. The availability of some of the newer direct viral detection methods have also limited the need for performing a RIPA under these circumstances.

RAPID LATEX AGGLUTINATION ASSAY

The technical complexity and expense associated with some of the more conventional anti–HIV-1 antibody detection methods fostered a search for simplified, less costly methods of serologic screening,[54-56] particularly those that could be more suitable for use under "field" conditions such as might be found in developing nations or other medically disadvantaged regions with a high incidence of HIV infection. These newer tests may also offer some practical advantages in developed nations.

One such test that has been developed is the rapid latex agglutination assay, a procedure that can be performed within a matter of a few minutes and that requires a minimum of reagents and technical skills.[57,58] This is a modification of a standard latex agglutination assay that is based on the use of recombinant proteins derived from a highly conserved region of the HIV-1 genome that are chemically linked to polystyrene beads. In this assay, the beads are incubated with various dilutions of test and control sera at room temperature and observed for the appearance of a characteristic agglutination reaction. HIV-1 envelope proteins commonly are used for this purpose, because anti-envelope antibodies generally arise early in the process of seroconversion and because they exhibit limited cross-reactivity with, for example, HIV-2 or other human retroviruses that may be endemic in a particular region. One nonglycosylated envelope preparation marketed by Cambridge BioScience Corporation, for example, consists of the carboxy-terminal third of gp120 linked with the amino-terminal half of gp41, minus 23 amino acids normally present at their junction.

The latex agglutination procedure is generally easy to perform but does require some skill and experience in the proper interpretation of results. As with all of the serologic assays, it should always be conducted with positive and negative controls. In using the latex agglutination assay to screen large panels of sera from several regions where HIV-1 infection is endemic, one group has reported estimates of sensitivity as high as 99.3% and specificity as high as 100% compared to Western blotting.[58] However, because such estimates were derived from populations in whom the incidence of infection was as high as 18%, the performance of this test as a screening tool in comparatively low-risk populations remains uncertain.

DOT-IMMUNOBINDING AND OTHER ASSAYS

Another rapid screening test that was developed as a cost-effective alternative to conventional ELISA and Western blot testing is the dot-blot immunoassay. In this assay, a lysate of viral antigens is prepared from HIV-1 harvested from cell culture and is dotted onto a grid of absorbent nitrocellulose paper.[59,60] Alternatively, recombinantly produced HIV-1 enve-lope or other proteins have also been used for this purpose.[54] Appropriate dilutions of test sera (with a panel of positive and negative controls) are spotted onto the areas containing bound viral antigens and allowed to react. After incubation, the nitrocellulose is washed to remove unbound antibody, and enzyme-linked goat anti-human IgG antibody is added to the paper. The dots are developed by the addition of an appropriate substrate for the bound enzyme, resulting in a colorimetric reaction whose intensity directly correlates with the amount of bound HIV-1–specific antibody. Using this method to screen sera from high-risk patients, one group reported a 93% concordance between results obtained by dot-blot and by ELISA.[60] Similarly, another group has reported a 98.2% concordance of the dot immunoassay with conventional Western blotting in evaluating sera from patients with and without risk factors for HIV exposure.[54]

Several other rapid and simple immunoassays have been proposed or developed for use in the detection of a serologic response to HIV-1, such as the passive hemagglutination assay.[61,62] One example is the autologous red cell agglutination assay developed by Kemp and colleagues.[63] According to this technique, a nonagglutinating mouse monoclonal antibody reactive with human red blood cells is chemically cross-linked to a synthetic peptide antigen derived from gp41 enveloped protein (other immunogenic proteins of HIV-1 could be adapted for this technique). Addition of this antigen-antibody complex to microliter quantities of whole blood obtained from a patient causes that patient's red cells to become coated with the complex. Anti–HIV-1 antibodies within the blood sample bind to the cell-bound antigen and cause agglutination of red cells into a visible mass. This assay can be completed within a few minutes and has the advantage of using the patient's own blood. It also offers the potential for quantitative assessment, because it may be possible to titer the amount of specific anti–HIV-1 antibody in a patient's blood by performing competitive inhibition of the agglutination reaction with added peptide antigen. A false-positive rate as low as 0.1% (compared with 0.2% using a commercial ELISA) has been described for seronegative blood donors using this assay, but the false-negative rate appears to be approximately 1%.

A test for detecting HIV-1 antibodies in oral fluid has been approved by the FDA.[110] A lollipop-style plastic stick with an absorbent pad containing a salt solution (Epitope,Inc., Beaverton, OR) draws serum transudate and gingival crevice fluid containing immunoglobulins into the oral cavity. The pad is tested with an ELISA. This new test is less sensitive and less specific than blood tests and must be administered by a trained technician. It has a relatively high false-positive rate, and positive results should be followed by confirmatory blood tests.

P24 ANTIGEN CAPTURE ASSAY

After the diagnosis of HIV-1 infection using the serologic methods previously outlined, several surrogate markers of

HIV-1 activity may be useful for guiding clinical decision making.[64–66] One serologic assay that has been useful in the staging and management of the infected individual is the serum p24 antigen capture assay.[67] This assay, also known as the HIV-1 antigen capture assay, is a solid-phase technique designed to provide a quantitative measure of the level of viral p24 antigen within serum or other body fluids. Viral p24 protein circulates in the bloodstream as free antigen or bound to anti-p24 antibody in the form of immune complexes. Earlier generations of the conventional p24 antigen capture assay detected only the unbound fraction. Later versions detect bound and free forms.

Although the levels of serum p24 antigen may vary from individual to individual, this antigen can be detected relatively early after HIV-1 exposure in many patients, and detection often precedes the process of seroconversion by several weeks (see Fig. 11-1B).[68] This rise in measurable p24 antigen presumably correlates with the burst in viral replication, detectable by other methods such as plasma viremia,[69,70] which occurs shortly after primary infection. However, because the timing of this p24 elevation and its rate of increase are not predictable, the p24 antigen capture assay typically is not useful as a primary screening tool in establishing independently an early diagnosis of HIV-1 infection. The p24 antigen level usually drops below the threshold of detection by conventional methods as anti-p24 antibody is formed during seroconversion and may remain in that state during the subsequent years of asymptomatic infection. Thereafter, depending on an individual's immune status as reflected in the dynamic equilibrium with levels of anti-p24 antibody, it may again become detectable as the infection proceeds to a more advanced stage.

Because only 20% to 30% of individuals with asymptomatic HIV-1 infection have detectable levels of serum p24 antigen by standard methods, this assay compares unfavorably to the conventional ELISA as a diagnostic tool for HIV-1 infection. Two large-scale studies of the utility of the serum p24 antigen capture assay in screening volunteer blood donors have shown that it provides little additional benefit over conventional screening for HIV-1 antibody in the detection of infected units of blood[71,72] although it has been recently licensed specifically for that purpose. The p24 assay is now included in the routine screening of blood donations at blood banks within the US, although estimates are that its use may only increase the detection of an additional 6–10 infected units per year. Other primary uses are in monitoring the levels of viral activity within the known infected host, such as in response to the initiation of antiretroviral chemotherapy, and in serving as an independent prognostic marker of disease activity over time. It is well established that conventional antiretroviral therapy with a nucleoside analog such as zidovudine can at least temporarily reduce the level of serum p24 antigen in antigenemic patients, presumably reflecting an overall inhibition of the level of viral activity within the treated patient.[73] Based

on these data, the p24 antigen test has been widely adopted for use as a surrogate marker of antiviral efficacy in several clinical drug trials of putative antiretroviral agents.[74,75] Whether there exists a strict correlation between a declining level of serum p24 antigen during therapy and an improved clinical status for an infected individual remains an area of considerable controversy.

The serum p24 antigen capture assay is used in prognostic stratification. Patients with detectable serum p24 antigen as a group may progress more rapidly to the development of AIDS-defining illnesses than a similar group of patients lacking this serum marker.[68,76–89] In a 1988 study of a cohort from San Francisco, it was found that over a 3-year period, serum antigenemic patients developed AIDS-defining conditions at a rate that was more than three times higher than within a similar cohort of p24 antigen-negative individuals.[90]

The serum p24 antigen capture assay is a solid-phase immunoassay that has been available since 1986; it is commercially marketed for research purposes in kit form by several different manufacturers, including Abbott, Coulter, and Du Pont Laboratories. Although specific reagents differ among manufacturers, the assay is generally performed in the same manner (see Fig. 11-6). Test sera and control sera are allowed to react with monoclonal or polyclonal anti–HIV-1 antibody (reactive to p24 antigen) bound to the bottom of a microtiter well or coated on polystyrene beads. After appropriate incubation and washing, the well or beads are incubated with goat or rabbit anti–HIV-1 antibody, which binds in proportionate amounts to any p24 antigen captured on the solid phase. After washing, an enzyme-tagged anti-goat (or anti-rabbit) immunoglobulin is added, which in the presence of an appropriate substrate, produces a colorimetric reaction whose intensity can be measured spectrophotometrically. Using dilutions of a serum with a known concentration of p24 antigen as a positive control, a standard curve of OD plotted against concentration can be generated for quantitative comparison of the absorbance values of test sera. Most commercially available kits define their lower limits of p24 antigen detection as being in the range of 50 pg/mL, although the actual linear portion of the standard curve often permits reliable measurements as low as 10 to 20 pg/mL. As a confirmation of the specificity of the assay, positive test sera can be retested in the presence of human sera containing a known high concentration of anti–HIV-1 antibody. With most kits, a reduction in the test sera's OD of 50% or greater by this "neutralization" procedure confirms the specificity of the p24 measurement.

A major limitation of the overall utility of the earlier forms of the p24 antigen capture assay was that they were only capable of detecting free p24 antigen and not antigen complexed with anti-p24 antibody. A significant improvement in the sensitivity of this test was achieved through incorporation of methods to disrupt immune complexes before the assay. It was found that alteration of the pH of samples through simple chemical pretreatment markedly increased the level of detectable p24 antigen in sera from asymptomatic and advanced-stage HIV-infected patients. One method involves the addition of dilute hydrochloric acid to samples and subsequent neutralization with alkali.[91] An alternative method involving acidification with a mild organic acid such as glycine (pH 2.2) offers the potential advantage of being less likely to denature epitopes on p24 antigen before measurement.[92,93]

DIRECT HIV DETECTION

The discussion to this point has focused on establishing a diagnosis of HIV infection by standard serologic means, usually by detection of circulating antibodies to viral proteins. Although some of the assays described are not routinely performed in all clinical laboratories, most of these techniques are readily available. To directly measure the presence of HIV or its components, however, more specialized techniques are required. Direct detection of HIV is useful in making or confirming the diagnosis of HIV infection and for studying the kinetics of viral load over time, identifying the particular quasispecies of virus with which an individual is infected, enabling genotypic mapping of viral isolates to address issues such as genetic drift and antiretroviral drug resistance, and numerous other purposes.

The HIV detection methods can be divided into three broad categories: those involving viral culture from cells or plasma; those that involve detection of discrete viral proteins, such as the p24 antigen capture assay; and those that involve direct detection of viral nucleic acids, such as the DNA PCR for measuring levels of proviral DNA, the reverse transcriptase PCR for measuring levels of viral RNA, and the branched-chain DNA (bDNA) assay for quantitating levels of particle-associated genomic RNA.

HIV Culture

Viral cultivation methods for HIV detection and isolation can be expensive and labor intensive, and they require sterile facilities and strict adherence to sterile technique. Isolation of HIV can be performed using plasma or peripheral blood mononuclear cells from the peripheral blood or lymphoid tissues of the infected patients (Fig. 11-7).[24–25,96–98,100] Viral isolation from mononuclear cells usually involves co-culturing the patient's cells with uninfected donor cells that have been stimulated with phytohemagglutinin (PHA) for 3 days. The stimulation leads to cellular activation, which enhances viral propagation from the infected to the uninfected cell population within the culture. These co-cultures are monitored approximately every 3 days for 28 days or longer to assess the formation of syncytia (ie, multinucleated giant cells that develop from cell-cell fusions) and the presence of HIV p24 antigen or reverse transcriptase (RT) in the culture supernatants. The presence of syncytia, p24 antigen, or RT is evidence of viral replication.

Viral isolation from plasma involves a variation of this approach. Plasma is derived from the peripheral blood of the infected host and then titered by a series of 3-fold to 5-fold dilutions. These dilutions are added to PHA-stimulated blasts that have been pelleted by centrifugation. Similar to cell co-cultivation, the plasma cultures are then monitored periodi-

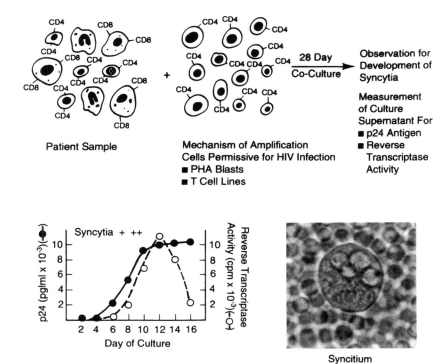

FIG. 11-7. Diagram of HIV isolation by co-cultivation methods.

cally for syncytia or p24 antigen or reverse transcriptase production during a minimum 28 days of cultivation. The viral titer of a culture is reported as the reciprocal of the lowest plasma dilution in which p24 antigen production is detectable during this period. A comparison of the changes in viral titer over time allows quantitation of the level of relative viral activity during an observation period, such as before and after the introduction of a new antiretroviral medication or therapy. A sustained reduction in plasma titer, for example, is likely to represent a favorable response to the new therapy.

Some investigators think that isolation of syncytia-inducing viral isolates from plasma culture is more likely to be associated with progressive immunologic deterioration in the host. As the name suggests, these isolates form large numbers of syncytia in viral co-cultivation. They also exhibit an enhanced tropism for T lymphocytes (as opposed to monocyte-macrophages), can be isolated with increasing frequency with advancing disease, and may negatively influence the overall response to certain antiretroviral medications. The predominance of non–syncytia-inducing strains in a culture has been associated with earlier stages of HIV infection, with a better antiretroviral response, and with a propensity for longer immunologic stability. There are numerous exceptions to these observations, and whether these findings are truly cause and effect situations has not been established. Nonetheless, some researchers choose to monitor the presence or absence of syncytia-inducing virus in cell culture as another surrogate marker of disease activity. Certain cell lines express large amounts of CD4 on their surface; the MT2 cell line can serve as a sensitive co-cultivation line in which to determine the syncytial phenotype of a patient's predominant viral strain.[99]

Measuring Viral Nucleic Acids

PCR methods enable the amplification of discrete fragments of the viral genome. This may be performed for diagnostic purposes (ie, as a confirmatory assay to supplement serologic diagnosis) or for research purposes to facilitate isolation and study of select portions of the viral genome.

The DNA PCR is a method for detecting and amplifying proviral DNA from the cells of an infected host.[26–29,100–102] Although HIV is an RNA virus, DNA copies of the RNA genome are rapidly produced by the enzyme RT after entry of HIV into a cell. These proviral DNA copies may remain in the cytoplasm of the cell or become integrated into the host cell genome. If integration into the host genome occurs, the proviral DNA serves as a template for the production of viral genomic RNA, which can then assemble at the cell surface with the relevant viral proteins to form new viral particles, or viral messenger RNA, which provides the genetic template encoding the production of viral proteins.

To perform DNA PCR (Fig. 11-8), the first step is to produce a lysate derived from mononuclear cells from the infected patient. Selected pairs of primers (ie, short oligonucleotide regions complementary to specific regions of the viral genome, such as segments of the *gag, ltr,* or *env* genes) that recognize and bind to specific sequences along the viral DNA strand are then added to the lysate. A separate primer pair such as the HLA-DQ-α genes, which recognize and bind to a specific sequence of host DNA, is often used as a positive internal control. Using the heat-stable Taq polymerase, an enzyme isolated from the thermophilic bacterium *Thermus aquaticus,* in the presence of appropriate nucleoside triphosphates and buffers, the mixture is subjected to an automated series of 20 to 30 cycles of repetitive heating and cooling that result in alternating periods of DNA polymerization followed by separation of the elongated strands. The separated strands, increasing in number geometrically as the cycling process proceeds, serve as the DNA templates for additional cycles of polymerization. By these means, an extremely high degree of selective amplification of the targeted DNA segments can be achieved. Specific DNA regions selectively amplified to a high copy number by this process can be further characterized by standard techniques of electrophoresis and nucleic acid hybridization.

DNA PCR is frequently employed for the early detection of HIV infection or to help resolve inconsistent findings obtained by the HIV ELISA and immunoblotting. Appropriate rigor must be applied in its use, however. At least two of the regions of the HIV genome plus the HLA-DQ-α region (or another internal standard serving as positive control) should be amplified unequivocally for a sample to be considered positive. By virtue of its extreme degree of sensitivity (ie, detection of one infected cell per 100,000 cells), the PCR technique is highly subject to false positivity by means of contamination or other common errors in laboratory processing of specimens. Suggested methods to minimize the problems associated with performance of the PCR are to use separate rooms for sample preparation and processing of the

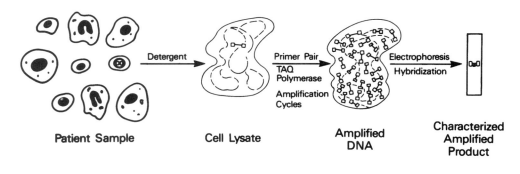

Patient Sample   Cell Lysate   Amplified DNA   Characterized Amplified Product

Detergent   Primer Pair TAQ Polymerase Amplification Cycles   Electrophoresis Hybridization

FIG. 11-8. Schematic of PCR methodology for the diagnosis of HIV infection.

specimens; to use special pipettors to minimize sample carryover; to use different primers and require that at least two primers are positive before concluding that the sample is reactive; to always use positive and negative controls in every run, including HLA-DQ-α to confirm the integrity of the lysate; and to consider repeating the PCR on a freshly obtained specimen from the same patient if the results do not agree with serologic data.

RT PCR provides a means for measuring viral RNA that allows quantitation of the viral load in plasma and differentiation of cells that contain replicating genomic RNA (and intact virions) from cells that are producing regulatory messages.[103-105] To use this technique to determine the viral burden in plasma, plasma from the infected host is centrifuged at high speed to pellet the viral particles. The pellet is extracted and treated with DNase to digest any DNA in the sample. Using standard techniques, cDNA copies are made of all RNA species within the treated sample. Assuming that HIV particles are contained within the sample, production of cDNA copies of the HIV RNA genome occurs in proportion to the amount of genomic RNA in the original sample. Using PCR amplification of the newly synthesized DNA, quantitation of the amount of RNA in the original sample can be accomplished. Although a highly sensitive means of viral quantitation, RT PCR has problems that are similar to those described for DNA PCR. This technique has a sensi-

tivity of detection down to 100 copies of HIV RNA per milliliter of plasma.

Quantitative competitive PCR (QC PCR) is a highly sensitive and reproducible method of HIV quantitation that measures the relative amounts of products produced from the target sequences of interest and a competitive template introduced into test specimens[104-107,111] to serve as an internal control. A plasmid or an infectious clone is created with a deletion or insertion such that it can be distinguished from the wild-type genome by gel separation. Titered quantities of known amounts of this competitive template are introduced into the clinical sample containing unknown amounts of the target sequence. The replicate samples are then processed for PCR or RT PCR. Increasing the amount of the known competitive template results in a progressive increase in the intensity of the product band for the competitive template and a corresponding progressive decrease in the intensity of band associated with the wild-type unknown. The interpolated point at which the intensity of the product band from the known amount of added competitive template is the same as the intensity obtained from the unknown corresponds to the relative amount of HIV-1 RNA or DNA contained in the unknown. This method can be used for quantitative analysis of mononuclear cell–associated HIV-1 DNA and plasma HIV-1 RNA (Fig. 11-9).

INTERNALLY CONTROLLED REVERSE TRANSCRIPTASE (RT) PCR FOR QUANTITATION OF HIV RNA

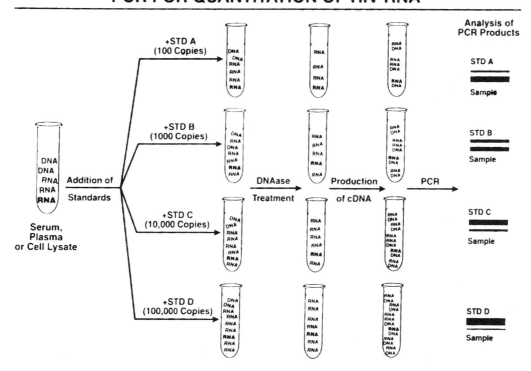

FIG. 11-9. Schematic of QCPCR methodology.

The bDNA is a method of quantitation of HIV-1 RNA in human plasma. It is a direct detection technique involving a series of nucleic acid hybridizations on the surface of microtiter wells.[108,109] This method differs fundamentally from PCR in that it relies on quantitation of HIV-1 RNA by signal amplification rather than the target amplification as used in PCR. The assay is done on solid phase similar to the ELISA but uses nucleic acid hybridization instead of antigen-antibody interactions (Fig. 11-10). To begin, virus in a plasma sample is concentrated by centrifuging the specimen at high speed. The pellet is solubilized and incubated with two types of target probes that are complementary to the multiple regions within the HIV *pol* gene. One half of these are also complementary to the capture protein bound to the bottom of the microtiter well. The other half are also complementary to the stem of the bDNA molecule. The sample-probe complex is spun down and added to microtiter wells that are coated with the capture probe. These capture probes are oligonucleotides complementary to the unbound regions of approximately one half of the target probes. During an overnight incubation, the RNA-probe complex is captured onto the surface of the microtiter well by way of hybridization of solid-phase capture probes with the subset of the target probe. After washing the wells to remove unbound material, the bDNA amplifier molecules

are hybridized to the immobilized target probe complex. These bDNA molecules have a comb-like structure (containing approximately 15 teeth/comb). The stem from the comb hybridizes with the half of the capture probes that are not complementary to the probes on the bottom of the well. Multiple bNDA molecules are captured in the well for each molecule of bound genomic RNA. The teeth of the comb contain repeating oligonucleotide sequences. Each tooth is capable of binding three oligonucleotide probes covalently linked to an alkaline phosphatase. Each bDNA molecule is capable of binding approximately 45 alkaline phosphatase molecules. After hybridization of the bDNA molecules to the microtiter well, the alkaline phosphatase-labeled probes are added and allowed to hybridize to the teeth of the bound bDNA molecules.

After the final hybridization step, the number of alkaline phosphatase molecules bound to the well are determined by incubation with a chemoluminescent substrate, dioxetane. The hydrolysis of the phosphate group on this molecule and subsequent breakdown of the unstable intermediate yields a chemoluminescent signal that can be measured with a luminometer. The light emission is directly proportional to the amount of HIV RNA in the plasma sample. The concentration of HIV RNA measured by the bDNA technique is expressed as HIV-1 RNA equivalents per milliliter of plasma.

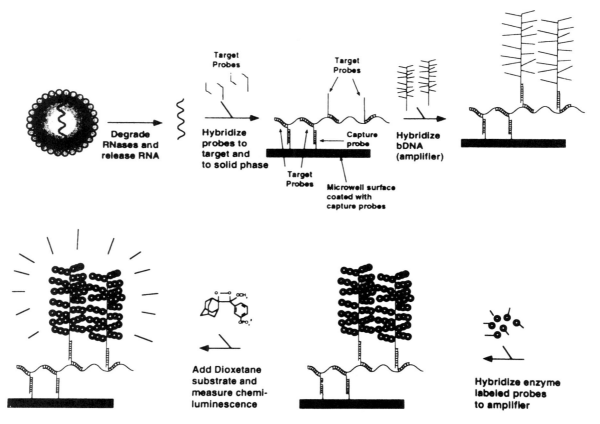

FIG. 11-10. Schematic of the bDNA assay for quantitation of HIV-1 viral load.

The bDNA assay exhibits good interassay reproducibility, is comparatively easy to perform, and has already been shown to be useful in monitoring changes in viral levels over time or monitoring responses to therapeutic interventions.[108] It compares favorably with more labor-intensive PCR methods in many of these parameters. However, the bDNA assay is less sensitive than the RT PCR. Its lower limitation of detection is 10,000 RNA molecules per milliliter. Patients at early stages of HIV infection may not have detectable signals using this assay. A second generation of bDNA assay being developed may increase the sensitivity of the technique at this lower end of the spectrum. An additional drawback is the comparatively high cost of the test kits in their current form.

SUMMARY

The procedure of choice for making the diagnosis of HIV infection is demonstration of antibodies to HIV using an ELISA combined with the confirmatory Western blot. Methods for detection of HIV and its components include assays such as viral culture, p24 antigen capture assay, PCR, and bDNA. Although these assays of viral load are generally confined to the research arena and are not part of the standard clinical laboratory, the clinical utility of some of the more rapid techniques is being explored.

ACKNOWLEDGMENT

We thank M.B. Vasudevachari for his invaluable help with this chapter.

REFERENCES

1. Gottlieb MS, Schroff R, Schanker HM, Weisman JD, Fan PT, Wolf RA, Saxon A. *Pneumocystis carinii* pneumonia and mucosal candidiasis in previously healthy homosexual men: evidence of a new acquired cellular immunodeficiency. N Engl J Med 1981;305:1425.
2. Masur H, Michelis MA, Greene JB, et al. An outbreak of community-acquired Pneumocystis carinii pneumonia: initial manifestation of cellular immune dysfunction. N Engl J Med 1981;305:1431.
3. Centers for Disease Control. Revision of the case definition of acquired immunodeficiency syndrome for national reporting—United States. MMWR 1985;34:373.
4. Centers for Disease Control. Revision of the CDC surveillance case definition for acquired immunodeficiency syndrome. Council of State and Territorial Epidemiologists; AIDS Program, Center for Infectious Diseases. MMWR 1987;36(Suppl 1):1S.
5. Barr`e-Sinoussi F, Cherman JC, Rey F, et al. Isolation of a T-lymphotropic retrovirus from a patient at risk for acquired immune deficiency syndrome (AIDS). Science 1983;220:868.
6. Popovic M, Sarngadharan MG, Read E, Gallo RC. Detection, isolation, and continuous production of cytopathic retroviruses (HTLV-III) from patients with AIDS and pre-AIDS. Science 1984;224:497.
7. Schleupner CJ. Diagnostic tests for HIV-1 infection. In: Mandell G, Douglas R, Bennett J, eds. Principles and practice of infectious diseases. New York: Churchill Livingstone, 1989:S3.
8. Sandler SG, Dodd RY, Fang CT. Diagnostic tests for HIV infection: serology. In: DeVita VT, Hellman S, Rosenberg SA, eds. AIDS: etiology, treatment, and prevention. 2nd ed. Philadelphia: JB Lippincott, 1988:121.
9. Levinson SS, Denys GA. Strengths and weaknesses in methods for identifying the causative agent(s) of acquired immunodeficiency syndrome (AIDS). CRC Crit Rev Clin Lab Sci 1988;26:277.
10. Houn HY, Pappas AA, Walker EM Jr. Status of current clinical tests for human immunodeficiency virus (HIV): applications and limitations. Ann Clin Lab Sci 1987;17:279.
11. Gaines H, Sydow MV, Sönnerborg A, et al. Antibody response in primary human immunodeficiency virus infection. Lancet. 1987;1:1249.
12. Cooper DA, Imrie AA, Penny R. Antibody response to human immunodeficiency virus after primary infection. J Infect Dis 1987;155;1113.
13. Ranki A, Valle SL, Krohn M, et al. Long latency precedes overt seroconversion in sexually transmitted human-immunodeficiency-virus infection. Lancet 1987;2:589.
14. Imagawa DT, Lee MH, Wolinsky SM, et al. Human immunodeficiency virus type 1 infection in homosexual men who remain seronegative for prolonged periods. N Engl J Med 1989;320:1458.
15. Horsburgh Jr CR, Ou CY, Jason J, et al. Duration of human immunodeficiency virus infection before detection of antibody. Lancet 1989;2:637.
16. Centers for Disease Control. Update: serologic testing for antibody to human immunodeficiency virus. MMWR 1988;36:833.
17. Centers for Disease Control. Problems created by heat-inactivation of serum specimens before HIV-1 antibody testing. MMWR 1989;38:407.
18. Evans RP, Shanson DC, Mortimer PP. Clinical evaluation of Abbott and Wellcome enzyme linked immunosorbent assays for detection of serum antibodies to human immunodeficiency virus (HIV). J Clin Pathol 1987;40:552.
19. Carlson JR, Bryant ML, Hinrichs SH, et al. AIDS serology testing in low and high risk groups. JAMA 1985;253:3405.
20. Ward JW, Holmberg SD, Allen JR, et al. Transmission of human immunodeficiency virus (HIV) by blood transfusions screened as negative for HIV antibody. N Engl J Med 1988;318:473.
21. Schwartz JS, Dans PE, Kinosian BP. Human immunodeficiency virus test evaluation, performance, and use. JAMA 1988;259:2574.
22. Kovacs JA, Megil ME, Deyton L, et al. Phase 1 trial of a recombinant gp160 candidate aids vaccine. Book II, meeting abstract. Fourth International Conference on AIDS, Stockholm, Sweden, June 12–16, 1988:289.
23. Redfield RR, Birx DL, Ketter N, et al. A phase I evaluation of the safety and immunogenicity of vaccination with recombinant gp160 in patients with early human immunodeficiency virus infection. N Engl J Med 1991;324:1677.
24. Coombs RW, Collier AC, Allain JP, et al. Plasma viremia in human immunodeficiency virus infection. N Engl J Med 1989;321:1626.
25. Ho DH, Moudgil T, Alam M. Quantitation of human immunodeficiency virus type 1 in the blood of infected persons. N Engl J Med 1989;321:1621.
26. Saiki RK, Gelfand DH, Stoffel S, et al. Primer-directed enzymatic amplification of DNA with a thermostable DNA polymerase. Science 1988;239:487.
27. Lifson AR, Stanley M, Pane J, et al. Detection of human immunodeficiency virus DNA using the polymerase chain reaction in a well-characterized group of homosexual and bisexual men. J Infect Dis 1990;161:436.
28. Phair JP, Wolinsky S. Diagnosis of infection with the Human Immunodeficiency Virus. J Infect Dis 1989;159:320.
29. Busch MP, Eble BE, Khayam-Bashi H, et al. Evaluation of screened blood donations for human immunodeficiency virus type 1 infection by culture and DNA amplification of pooled cells. N Engl J Med 1991;325:1.
30. Centers for Disease Control. Interpretation and use of the Western blot assay for serodiagnosis of human immunodeficiency virus type 1 infections. MMWR 1989;38:1.
31. Towbin H, Staehelin T, Gordon J. Electrophoretic transfer of proteins from polyacrylamide gels to nitrocellulose sheets: procedure and some applications. Proc Natl Acad Sci USA 1979;76:4350.
32. Du Pont Diagnostics. Human immunodeficiency virus (HIV): Biotech/Du Pont HIV Western blot kit for detection of antibodies to HIV. Wilmington, DE: Du Pont Diagnostics, 1987.
33. Consortium for Retrovirus Serology Standardization. Serologic diagnosis of human immunodeficiency virus infection by Western blot testing. JAMA 1988;260:674.
34. Hausler WJ Jr. Report of the Third Consensus Conference on HIV Testing sponsored by the Association of State and Territorial Public Health Laboratory Directors. Infect Control Hosp Epidemiol 1988;9:345.
35. Povolotsky J, Gold JWM, Chein N, Baron P, Armstrong D. Differences in human immunodeficiency virus type 1 (HIV-1) anti-p24 reactivities

in serum of HIV-1–infected and uninfected subjects: analysis of inde-terminate Western blot reactions. J Infect Dis 1991;163:247.

36. Davey R, Metcalf J, Easter M, et al. Western Blot and PCR reactivity pat-terns in individuals at high risk for HIV exposure. Abstract Th.B.P.179. The Fifth International Conference on AIDS, Montreal, June 1989.
37. Midthun K, Garrison L, Clements ML, et al. Frequency of indetermi-nate Western blot tests in healthy adults at low risk for human immun-odeficiency virus infection. J Infect Dis 1990;162:1379.
38. Dock NL, Lamberson HV, O'Brien TA, Tribe DE, Alexander SS, Poiesz BJ. Evaluation of atypical human immunodeficiency virus immunoblot reactivity in blood donors. Transfusion 1988;28:412.
39. Kleinman SH, Niland JC, Azen SP, et al. Prevalence of antibodies to human immunodeficiency virus type 1 among blood donors prior to screening. Transfusion 1989;29:572.
40. Leitman SF, Klein HG, Melpolder JJ, et al. Clinical implications of pos-itive tests for antibodies to human immunodeficiency virus type 1 in asymptomatic blood donors. N Engl J Med 1989;321:917.
41. Nusbacher J, Naiman R. Longitudinal follow-up of blood donors found to be reactive for antibody to human immunodeficiency virus (anti-HIV) by enzyme-linked immunoassay (EIA+) but negative by western blot (WB–). Transfusion 1989;29:365.
42. Jackson JB, MacDonald KL, Cadwell J, et al. Absence of HIV infection in blood donors with indeterminate Western blot tests for antibody to HIV-1. N Engl J Med 1990;322:217.
43. Genesca J, Shih JW, Jett B, Hewlett IK, Epstein JS, Alter HJ. What do Western blot indeterminate patterns for human immunodeficiency virus mean in EIA-negative blood donors? Lancet 1989;2:1023.
44. Hofbauer JM, Schulz TF, Hengster P, et al. Comparison of Western blot (immunoblot) based on recombinant-derived p41 with conventional tests for serodiagnosis of human immunodeficiency virus infections. J Clin Microbiol 1988;26:116.
45. Busch MP, el Amad Z, McHugh TM, Chien D, Polito AJ. Reliable confir-mation and quantitation of human immunodeficiency virus type 1 antibody using a recombinant-antigen immunoblot assay. Transfusion 1991;31:129.
46. Lennette ET, Karpatkin S, Levy JA. Indirect immunofluorescence assay for antibodies to human immunodeficiency virus. J Clin Microbiol 1987;25:199.
47. Hedenskog M, Dewhurst S, Ludvigsen C, et al. Testing for antibodies to AIDS-associated retrovirus (HLTV-III/LAV) by indirect fixed cell immunofluorescence: specificity, sensitivity, and applications. J Med Virol 1986;19:325.
48. Gallo D, Diggs JL, Shell GR, Dailey PJ, Hoffman MN, Riggs JL. Com-parison of detection of antibody to the acquired immune deficiency syn-drome virus by enzyme immunoassay, immunofluorescence, and West-ern blot methods. J Clin Microbiol 1986;23:1049.
49. Carlson JR, Yee J, Hinrichs SH, Bryant ML, Gardner MB, Pedersen NC. Comparison of indirect immunofluorescence and Western blot for detection of anti-human immunodeficiency virus antibodies. J Clin Mi-crobiol 1987;25:494.
50. McHugh TM, Stites DP, Casavant CH, et al. Evaluation of the indirect immunofluorescence as a confirmatory test for detecting antibodies to the human immunodeficiency virus. Diagn Immunol 1986;4:233.
51. Chiodi F, Bredberg-Raden U, Biberfeld G, et al. Radioimmunoprecipita-tion and Western blotting with sera of human immunodeficiency virus in-fected patients: a comparative study. AIDS Res Hum Retroviruses 1987;3:165.
52. Tersmette M, Lelie PN, van der Poel CL, et al. Confirmation of HIV seropositivity: comparison of a novel radioimmunoprecipitation assay to immunoblotting and virus culture. J Med Virol 1988;24:109.
53. Saah AJ, Farzadegan H, Fox R, et al. Detection of early antibodies in human immunodeficiency virus infection by enzyme-linked im-munosorbent assay, Western blot, and radioimmunoprecipitation. J Clin Microbiol 1987;25:1605.
54. Carlson JR, Yee JL, Watson-Williams EJ, et al. Rapid, easy, and eco-nomical screening tests for antibodies to human immunodeficiency virus. Lancet 1987;1:361.
55. Van de Perre P, Nzaramba D, Allen S, Riggin CH, Sprecher-Goldberger S, Butzler JP. Comparison of six serological assays for human immun-odeficiency virus antibody detection in developing countries. J Clin Mi-crobiol 1988;26:552.
56. Heyward WL, Curran JW. Rapid screening tests for HIV infection. JAMA 1988;260:542.
57. Riggin CH, Beltz GA, Hung CH, Thorn RM, Marciani DJ. Detection of antibodies to human immunodeficiency virus by latex agglutination with recombinant antigen. J Clin Microbiol 1987;25:1772.

58. Quinn TC, Riggin CH, Kline RL, et al. Rapid latex agglutination assay using recombinant envelope polypeptide for the detection of antibody to the HIV. JAMA 1988;260:510.
59. Heberling RL, Kalter SS. Rapid dot-immunobinding assay on nitrocel-lulose for viral antibodies. J Clin Microbiol 1986;23:109.
60. Heberling RL, Kalter SS, Marx PA, Lowry JK, Rodriquez AR. Dot im-munobinding assay compared with enzyme-linked immunosorbent assay for rapid and specific detection of retrovirus antibody induced by human or simian acquired immunodeficiency syndrome. J Clin Microbiol 1988;26:765.
61. Vasudevachari MB, Uffelman KU, Mast TC, Dewar RL, Natarajan V, Lane HC, Salzman NP. Passive hemagglutination test for detection of antibodies to human immunodeficiency virus type 1 and comparison of the test with enzyme-linked immunosorbent assay and Western blot (immunoblot) analysis. J Clin Microbiol 1989;27:179.
62. Scheffel JW, Wiesner D, Kapsalis A, Traylor D, Suarez A. Retrocell HIV-1 passive hemagglutination assay for HIV-1 antibody screening. J Acquir Immune Defic Syndr 1990;3:540.
63. Kemp BE, Rylatt DB, Bundesen PG, et al. Autologous red cell aggluti-nation assay for HIV-1 antibodies: simplified test with whole blood. Science 1988;241:1352.
64. Cooper EH, Lacey CJN. Laboratory indices of prognosis in HIV infec-tion. Biomed Pharmacother 1988;42:539.
65. Fahey JL, Taylor JMG, Detels R, et al. The prognostic value of cellular and serologic markers in infection with human immunodeficiency virus type 1. N Engl J Med 1990;322:166.
66. Muñoz A, Carey V, Saah AJ, et al. Predictors of decline in CD4 lym-phocytes in a cohort of homosexual men infected with human immun-odeficiency virus. J Acquir Immune Defic Syndr 1988;1:396.
67. Moss AR, Bacchetti P. Natural history of HIV infection. AIDS 1989;3:55.
68. Goudsmit J, Lange JM, Krone WJ, et al. Pathogenesis of HIV and its implications for serodiagnosis and monitoring of antiviral therapy. J Virol Methods 1987;17:19.
69. Clark SJ, Saag MS, Decker WD, et al. High titers of cytopathic virus in plasma of patients with symptomatic primary HIV-1 infection. N Engl J Med 1991;324:954.
70. Daar ES, Moudgil T, Meyer RD, Ho DD. Transient high levels of viremia in patients with primary human immunodeficiency virus type 1 infection. N Engl J Med 1991;324:961.
71. Busch MP, Taylor PE, Lenes BA, et al. Screening of selected male blood donors for p24 antigen of human immunodeficiency virus type 1. N Engl J Med 1990;323:1308.
72. Alter HJ, Epstein JS, Swensen SG, et al. Prevalence of human immun-odeficiency virus type 1 p24 antigen in U.S. blood donors—an assess-ment of the efficacy of testing in donor screening. N Engl J Med 1990;323:1312.
73. Jackson GG, Paul DA, Falk LA, et al. Human immunodeficiency virus (HIV) antigenemia (p24) in the acquired immunodeficiency syndrome (AIDS) and the effect of treatment with zidovudine (AZT). Ann Intern Med 1988;108:175.
74. Lane HC, Kovacs JA, Feinberg J, et al. Anti-retroviral effects of inter-feron-alpha in AIDS-associated Kaposi's sarcoma. Lancet 1988;2:1218.
75. Yarchoan R, Pluda JM, Thomas RV, et al. Long-term toxicity/activity profile of 2′,3′-dideoxyinosine in AIDS or AIDS-related complex. Lancet 1990;336:526.
76. Allain JP, Laurian Y, Paul DA, et al. Long-term evaluation of HIV anti-gen and antibodies to p24 and gp41 in patients with hemophilia. N Engl J Med 1987;317:1114.
77. Ras'ka K Jr, Kim HC, Ras'ka K 3rd, Martin E, Raskova J, Saidi P. Human immunodeficiency virus (HIV) infection in hemophiliacs: long-term prognostic significance of the HIV serologic pattern. Clin Exp Immunol 1989;77:1.
78. Eyster ME, Ballard JO, Gail MH, Drummond JE, Goedert JJ. Predictive markers for the acquired immunodeficiency syndrome (AIDS) in he-mophiliacs: persistence of p24 antigen and low T4 cell count. Ann In-tern Med 1989;110:963.
79. Hofmann B, Bygbjerg I, Dickmeiss E, et al. Prognostic value of im-munologic abnormalities and HIV antigenemia in asymptomatic HIV-infected individuals: proposal of immunologic staging. Scand J Infect Dis 1989;21:633.
80. Lindhardt BO, Ulrich K, Kusk P, Hofmann B. Serological response in patients with chronic asymptomatic human immunodeficiency virus in-fection. Eur J Clin Microbiol Infect Dis 1988;7:394.

81. Lindhardt BO, Gerstoft J, Hofmann B, et al. Antibodies against the major core protein p24 of human immunodeficiency virus: relation to immunological, clinical and prognostic findings. Eur J Clin Microbiol Infect Dis 1989;8:614.

82. Portera M, Vitale F, La Licata R, et al. Free and antibody-complexed antigen and antibody profile in apparently healthy HIV seropositive individuals and in AIDS patients. J Med Virol 1990;30:30.

83. Kamani N, Krilov LR, Wittek AE, Hendry RM. Characterization of the serologic profile of children with human immunodeficiency virus infection: correlation with clinical status. Clin Immunol Immunopathol 1989;53:233.

84. Sei Y, Tsang PH, Chu FN, et al. Inverse relationship between HIV-1 p24 antigenemia, anti-p24 antibody and neutralizing antibody responses in all stages of HIV-1 infection. Immunol Lett 1989;20:223.

85. Weber JN, Clapham PR, Weiss RA, et al. Human immunodeficiency virus infection in two cohorts of homosexual men: neutralising sera and association of anti-gag antibody with prognosis. Lancet 1987;1:119.

86. Forster SM, Osborne LM, Cheingsong-Popov R, et al. Decline of anti-p24 antibody precedes antigenaemia as correlate of prognosis in HIV-1 infection. AIDS 1987;1:235.

87. Andrieu JM, Eme D, Venet A, et al. Serum HIV antigen and anti-p24 antibodies in 200 HIV seropositive patients: correlation with CD4 and CD8 lymphocyte subsets. Clin Exp Immunol 1988;73:1.

88. Lange JM, Paul DA, Huisman HG, et al. Persistent HIV antigenaemia and decline of HIV core antibodies associated with transition to AIDS. Br Med J 1986;293:1459.

89. Murray HW, Godbold JH, Jurica KB, Roberts RB. Progression to AIDS in patients with lymphadenopathy or AIDS-related complex: reappraisal or risk and predictive factors. Am J Med 1989;86:533.

90. Moss AR, Bacchetti P, Osmond D, et al. Seropositivity for HIV and the development of AIDS or AIDS related condition: three year follow-up of the San Francisco General Hospital cohort. Br Med J 1988;296:745.

91. Nishanian P, Huskins KR, Stehn S, Detels R, Fahey JL. A simple method for improved assay demonstrates that HIV p24 antigen is present as immune complexes in most sera from HIV-infected individuals. J Infect Dis 1990;162:21.

92. Kestens L, Hoofd G, Gigase PL, Deleys R, van der Groen G. HIV antigen detection in circulating immune complexes. J Virol Methods 1991;31:67.

93. Vasudevachari MB, Salzman NP, Woll DR, et al. Clinical utility of an enhanced human immunodeficiency virus type-1 p24 antigen capture assay. J Clin Immunol 1993;13:185.

94. Loussert-Ajaka I, Ly TD, Chaix ML, et al. HIV-1/HIV-2 seronegativity in HIV-1 subtype O infected patients. Lancet 1994;343:1393.

95. Schable C, Zekeng L, Pau C-P, et al. Sensitivity of United States HIV antibody tests for detection of HIV-1 group O infections. Lancet 1994;344:1333.

96. Davey RT, Lane HC. Laboratory methods in the diagnosis and prognostic staging of infection with human immunodeficiency virus type 1. Rev Infect Dis 1990;12:912.

97. Davey RT, Dewar RL, Reed GF, et al. Plasma viremia as a sensitive indicator of the antiretroviral activity of L-697,661. Proc Natl Acad Sci USA 1993;90:5608.

98. Dewar RL, Sarmiento MD, Lawton ES, et al. Isolation of HIV-1 from plasma of infected individuals: an analysis of experimental conditions affecting successful virus propagation. J Acquir Immune Defic Syndr 1992;5:822.

99. Koot M, Keet IPM, Vos AHV, et al. Prognostic value of HIV-1 syncytium-inducing phenotype for rate of CD4+ cell depletion and progression to AIDS. Ann Intern Med 1993;118:681.

100. Dewar RL, Psallidopoulos MC, Salzman NP. Isolation and detection of human immunodeficiency virus. In: Rose NR deMarcario EC, Fahey J, et al., eds: Manual of clinical laboratory immunology. Washington, DC: American Society for Microbiology, 1992:371.

101. Montoya JG, Wood R, Katzenstein D, et al. Peripheral blood mononuclear cell human immunodeficiency virus type 1 proviral DNA quantification by polymerase chain reaction: relationship to immunodeficiency and drug effect. J Clin Microbiol 1993;31:2692.

102. Ou CY, Kwok S, Mitchell SW, et al. DNA amplification for direct detection of HIV-1 in DNA of peripheral blood mononuclear cells. Science 1988;239:295.

103. Bagnarelli P, Menzo S, Manzin A, et al. Detection of human immunodeficiency virus type 1 genomic RNA in plasma samples by reverse-transcription polymerase chain reaction. J Med Virol 1991; 34:89.

104. Menzo S, Bagnarelli P, Giacca M, et al. Alsolute quantitation of viremia in human immunodeficiency virus infection by competitive reverse transcription and polymerase chain reaction. J Clin Microbiol 1992;30:1752.

105. Scadden DT, Wang Z, Groopman JF. Quantitation of plasma human immunodeficiency virus type 1 by competitive polymerase chain reaction. J infect Dis 1992;165:1119.

106. Piatak M, Luk K-C, Williams B, Lifson JD. Quantitative competitive polymerase chain reaction for accurate quantitation of HIV DNA and RNA species. Biotechnology 1993;14:70.

107. Jurrians S, Dekker JT, de Ronde A. HIV-1 viral DNA load in peripheral blood mononuclear cells from seroconverters and long term infected individuals. AIDS 1992;6:635.

108. Dewar RL, Highbarger HC, Sarmiento MD, et al. Application of branched DNA signal amplification to monitor human immunodeficiency virus type 1 burden in human plasma. J Infect Dis 1994;170:1172.

109. Urdea M, Horn T, Fultz T, et al. Branched DNA amplification multimers for the sensitive, direct detection of human hepatitis viruses, Nucleic Acids Res Symp Ser 1991;24:197.

110. Wesley WE, Paparello SF, Decker CF, Sheffield JM, Lowe-Bey FH. A modified ELISA and western blot accurately determine anti-human immunodeficiency virus type 1 antibodies in oral fluids obtained with a special collecting device. J Infect Dis 1995;171: 1406.

111. Natarajan V, Plishka RJ, Scott EW, Lane HC, Salzman NP. An internally controlled virion PCR for the measurement of HIV-1 RNA in plasma. PCR Methods Appl 1994;3:346.

AIDS: Biology, Diagnosis, Treatment and
Prevention, fourth edition, edited by Vincent T.
DeVita, Jr., Samuel Hellman, and Steven A.
Rosenberg. Lippincott–Raven Publishers, © 1997

CHAPTER 12

Approach to the Individual Potentially Infected With the Human Immunodeficiency Virus

Jeffrey Moulton Benevedes and Donald I. Abrams

The approach to the potentially infected individual remains an infrequently discussed topic in the clinical literature, probably because of the lack of definition and delineation of this group. For the purpose of this discussion, the potentially infected individual may be a member of two subsets. The first includes the individual who presents to the clinical practice without knowledge of his or her human immunodeficiency virus (HIV) serostatus and who is at current or past risk for HIV infection by virtue of engaging in high-risk behaviors. The second group encompasses the individual who is HIV uninfected as determined by previous serology testing although remaining at continued risk for HIV acquisition by virtue of engaging in risk behavior. We are concerned with individuals who present with risk of HIV infection and require counseling to determine their current HIV status and individuals who require prevention counseling to help them maintain their current HIV seronegative status.

Any discussion of the role physicians and other health care providers can play in these prevention scenarios must be couched in an acknowledgement of the enormous burden health care professionals already bear. In this chapter, we ask physicians to don the hat of HIV prevention specialist, understanding that this is not a task they can or should pursue on their own. There are several obstacles to physicians engaging individuals in discussions about risk and prevention. Factors such as managed care and other changes in the health care delivery system have already presented physicians and other health care providers with increased paper work, larger case loads, and reduced decision-making autonomy.

Many physicians working in acquired immunodeficiency syndrome (AIDS) endemic areas with large HIV caseloads have seen their practices become more demanding because of the increasing proportion of patients with deteriorating health and social conditions. Such individuals present complex medical demands that stress the physician's time and expertise. To ask providers to become HIV prevention specialists in addition may seem preposterous, but we conceptualize the physician as being a partner on the front line of HIV information and prevention intervention provision. Ideally, physicians would then be able to refer at-risk patients to community-based prevention specialists who can provide HIV prevention education, individual counseling, and group interventions concerning risk reduction. However, the physician in clinical practice may be the only source of intervention, especially where few community supports exist or if the patient refuses ancillary interventions, and the added burden of the physician becoming a prevention specialist may make any but the most cursory interventions unrealistic.

WHO ARE THE POTENTIALLY INFECTED?

The populations most likely to be at greatest risk for HIV transmission in the United States demand the greatest focus of attention in terms of HIV education and prevention interventions: younger gay men, women, adolescents, and minorities. Those in need of HIV education and prevention interventions by physicians also include the gay men or injection drug users who have been targeted for many years with prevention messages and encouraged to seek HIV antibody testing but have not yet done so. HIV-seronegative gay men or injection drug users who have been reached by prevention messages and know every nuance of safe sex prac-

Jeffrey Moulton Benevedes, 1801 Bush Street, Suite 222, San Francisco, CA 94109.

Donald I. Abrams, Assistant Director, AIDS Program, San Francisco General Hospital and Professor of Clinical Medicine, University of California, San Francisco, Ward 84, 995 Potrero Avenue, San Francisco, CA 94110.

tice guidelines and safe needle use but who still choose to remain at risk for a variety of psychologic reasons constitute another group requiring intervention.

Several groups identified by the Centers for Disease Control and Prevention (CDC)[1,2] are at growing risk for HIV transmission. CDC surveillance data show that recent rates of increases in AIDS cases have been greatest among women, adolescents, persons infected through heterosexual contact, minorities and injection drug users. Gay and bisexual men no longer represent the majority of new cases of AIDS reported. In the United States, cases of heterosexually transmitted AIDS increased 114% among adult and adolescent males and 139% among adult and adolescent females from 1992 to 1993.

The number of cases among women of childbearing age has increased. AIDS has become one of the top five causes of death for women between 15 and 44 years of age. Women in urban areas have been especially hard hit by this epidemic. Although the prevalence of HIV infection among childbearing women fell in the Northeast, it rose in the South. The major risk factors for women were injection drug use (41%) or a male sex partner with HIV or HIV risk factors (38%).

There is an alarming increase in HIV infection among adolescents (10 to 18 years of age) as demonstrated by the growing number of 20 to 29 year olds with AIDS who have acquired HIV during adolescence.

Minorities constitute more than 50% of all AIDS cases. African-Americans made up more of a caseload in 1994 (39%) than in 1993 (36%), as did Hispanics (19% versus 18%), but the white proportion decreased (41% versus 45%).

AIDS is no longer an epidemic located solely in America's inner cities. AIDS in rural and suburban areas is beginning to grow.

The share of new AIDS cases with"no known risk factor reported" has increased from 6% to 12%. Although this may reflect poorer data collection, it may also reflect the possibility that HIV is spreading to persons who are less likely to recognize or acknowledge their risk.

WHO SHOULD BE ENCOURAGED TO UNDERGO HIV TESTING?

At-risk individuals are presenting to many clinical practices on a frequent basis. The decision to undergo HIV testing should be based on an assessment of risk for HIV infection that is mutually agreed on by the individual and physician. Only a collaborative assessment of risk can yield a valid assessment. Discussion of risk behaviors frequently represents a change in clinical practice, because detailed sex and drug histories are often not obtained as part of the routine clinical interview. Most physicians have not been trained to elicit such information from patients nor to manage the embarrassment and discomfort that may arise from initiating such discussions. Changes in clinical practice may be nec-

essary to incorporate frank and detailed discussions of risk behavior.

The clinician may be influenced by psychologic factors inhibiting his or her ability to initiate frank discussions with the patient. For example, a survey of senior medical students found that 50% felt poorly trained to take a sexual history, and 25% felt embarrassed to ask the necessary questions.[3] A nonsympathetic view of patient psychosocial problems was the variable most closely related to the belief that the sex history was of little importance in understanding a patient's problem. Students who believed this most were the same ones who were found to be most homophobic, authoritarian, and have the greatest fear of AIDS infection. It is not unlikely that physicians in practice would experience the same embarrassment and lack the acquired skill necessary in taking a detailed sex and drug history.

Thoroughly assessing sexual behavior and drug use begins with the need to encourage truth in self-reporting of these data. Developing rapport with the patient so that trust can be established is essential and leads to the elicitation of nuances of sexual behavior and drug use. The major purposes of taking a sex and drug history as part of an HIV risk evaluation are to accurately determine past risk and patterns of behavior, to evaluate current risk behaviors requiring intervention, and to provide the opportunity to plan with the individual what interventions may be needed. We strongly recommend that providers encountering potentially HIV-infected individuals use available resources to familiarize themselves with how to conduct a sex and drug history-taking session.

Beyond the logistics of taking a good sex and drug history, providers must encourage individuals to discuss transmission possibilities that lie more in the "gray zone." Some behaviors that are less straightforward and more complex may be difficult to discuss. Examples may include discussing the likelihood of infection in performing oral sex with one or multiple partners after an evening of drug use; specific lubricants to be used for anal or vaginal intercourse; or sexual encounters with persons who are known to be HIV seropositive.

WHY SHOULD AT-RISK INDIVIDUALS BE TESTED FOR HIV?

There are numerous compelling reasons for persons to be tested for HIV. For the individual testing HIV seronegative, a great relief would probably be experienced. Because all persons are potentially HIV seropositive before testing, several reasons supporting the usefulness of confirming an unconfirmed suspicion of seropositivity may be conveyed.

Establish baseline health indicators. Baseline health indicators can be established if the individual is found to be HIV seropositive. Tests results of viral burden and immunologic status dictate a treatment strategy.

Make decisions about long-term and short-term goals, including career, relationships, family life, finances, planning for services that may be needed. Because HIV disease radically alters the usual sequences of an individual's life, antibody testing sets into motion evaluation of many aspects of current and future plans.

Initiate treatment to slow the progress of HIV. Treat cofactors that may accelerate progression of HIV disease, and address treatment nihilism. Medical intervention for HIV disease based on a model of combination antiretroviral regimens and opportunistic infection prophylaxis may reduce symptoms, prolong life, and improve quality of life. Addressing the true limitations of treatment and potential side effects allows discussion of pessimism about the possibility of a relatively symptom-free life for many years.

Consider harm-reduction lifestyle changes. An individual testing HIV seropositive may want to consider addressing drug and alcohol problems, reducing unsafe sexual behavior, and accessing social service and community services developed for persons with HIV disease.

Initiate life changes that would improve overall health and quality of life.

Feeling an ability to influence the course of illness may be an important factor differentiating those persons who become psychosocially disabled from those who adapt to the challenge of their health condition. Changes made after a diagnosis thought to be salubrious (eg, changes in diet and exercise, adopting spiritual practices, stress reduction techniques) may be part of the coping process to restore psychologic and social equilibrium after a health crisis has occurred.

Fear of discrimination and breaches of confidentiality may inhibit those who suspect they are at risk from consenting to HIV antibody testing. Intravenous drug use is illegal in all 50 states, and one half the states still have laws against voluntary sodomy. Individuals who present at risk for HIV disease but have not been tested must be afforded access to strict confidentiality. This means that discussions must occur about how such information is to be handled in medical charts or wherever else it may appear. Individuals considering HIV antibody testing must consent before release of results to third parties.

Rejection of testing by some individuals may be valid. Many individuals feel that the possibility of an untoward emotional reaction to a positive result outweighs the benefits of knowing the status. Such a stance must be respected, but the practitioner may want to refer the individual to other prevention specialists for a more extensive discussion about the issue or continue discussions about the usefulness of testing during subsequent clinic visits.

WHY SOME MAY CONTINUE TO ENGAGE IN HIGH-RISK BEHAVIOR

As a way to understand why education efforts alone do not stem the tide of new HIV infections, even among individuals particularly well targeted for prevention messages, it is useful to describe the broader psychologic and social picture

of one subgroup still at risk for new infections: gay men. Important lessons may be learned from persistently at-risk individuals and applied to others who are increasingly at risk at this point in the trajectory of the epidemic.

Despite a decade of prevention efforts aimed at gay and bisexual men, a large number continue to become infected with HIV. Rates of seroconversion among gay men of color and gay youth are alarmingly high. Two studies projected that a majority of young, uninfected gay and bisexual men in the United States may eventually contract HIV.[4,5] Members of the slightly older at-risk cohort of gay men also continue to seroconvert despite being extensively reached by educational messages. What these data tell us is that factors beyond education lie at the heart of the continued rates of seroconversion. Large-scale prevention studies, clinical data, and anecdotal reports inform us that a social and cultural disaster has engulfed the gay community and has created a field in which deeper psychologic and social issues seem to determine who is likely to become infected with HIV.

From the proceedings of a 1994 national participatory summit conference organized in Dallas, Texas, by the Gay and Lesbian Medical Association (GLMA), several themes emerged concerning continued prevention efforts aimed at gay men.[6] These themes provide a broad social, psychologic, and behavioral context for physician understanding of the factors that are associated with continued seroconversion among young and older gay men of various race or ethnic groups. Many of the factors faced by these individuals after over a decade of the AIDS epidemic are beginning to be felt by other groups as well and have broader-scale applicability.

Gay men and persons of color in the United States are in an unacknowledged and unprecedented crisis, experiencing threats to their well-being on the political, social, and public health fronts. Many individuals seen by clinicians more than a decade into the epidemic are experiencing symptoms of posttraumatic stress disorder. The epidemic has psychologically transformed those directly infected and those at risk who have shared a community with many of the dead and dying. Any HIV prevention efforts must provide individuals with more than knowledge, although this is an important starting place for a prevention discussion. Prevention efforts must include discussions of loss, bereavement, posttraumatic stress disorder, dissociation, rage, love, and intimacy.

Many individuals at risk have witnessed the destruction of their communities by AIDS, lost their partners, lost entire sets of friends, and may believe that there is little opportunity for a future within their community. Some believe that the epidemic has made it too painful, too difficult, and too empty a life. Joining a community of those infected with HIV may be considered a way out, according to one San Francisco Bay Area psychologist counseling large numbers of at-risk gay men.[7] Individuals often present to the clinical practice with depression, numbness, and the belief that infection is inevitable. Alcohol and drug problems increase as a method of providing relief in the form of dissociation from the seeming impossible realities of living within the psychologic intensity of the epidemic. Another GLMA conference participant asked, "What impact does the failure to face the limits of education to swiftly and completely transform sexual activity have on our communities? . . . Workshops on eroticizing safer sex have limited impact when the landscapes of psyches are scorched wastelands. . . . Four-word slogans on the sides of buses are little use when souls suffer horrors parallel to the extreme historical events of this century."[6]

Gay men and communities of color have experienced a disruption of their social order because of AIDS and because of the insidious effects of increasing social marginalization and a high degree of drug availability and drug use among some of the most vulnerable subgroups. These factors have resulted in an accumulated sense of nihilism so deep that even the threat of the effects of HIV disease has little effect on the daily behaviors that put the individual at risk for infection.[8]

Prevention data demonstrate that one-shot interventions do not influence seroconversion rates.[9,10] It is unrealistic to expect that single visits to physicians' offices would have an impact on stemming the tide of new seroconversions. Although face-to-face interventions appear to be best for addressing the myriad of issues associated with risk for HIV infection, according to J.A. Kelly, Director of the Center for AIDS intervention Research of the Medical College of Wisconsin (written communication, 1995), it may take as much as 6 to 30 hours of one-on-one or group participation to achieve behavior changes in persons whose behavior puts them at risk. It also appears that most individuals who feel at risk turn to friends to discuss prevention matters rather than their physicians, ministers, or other authority figures in the community. One-shot interventions by physicians within the context of a clinical visit probably would yield little in the way of real effects on risk reduction.

WHAT CAN BE DONE?

Intervention with the potentially infected individual optimally demands nothing short of an intensive, multidisciplinary team approach to HIV education and prevention (Table 12-1). We think that physicians alone can constitute only one facet of what must be a team approach if the complexity and depth of the factors associated with HIV transmission in this latter stage of the epidemic are to be successfully addressed. The role of physicians is especially important in identifying patients at risk, providing education about the benefits of HIV antibody testing, and providing triage to other members of a diverse HIV prevention team. Such a team should also consist of clinically skilled mental health workers and persons from the at-risk individual's community to provide one-on-one counseling and group interventions. If such a care team is not available in the practice

TABLE 12-1. *Steps in a comprehensive evaluation and intervention with the potentially infected individual*

1. Take a thorough sex and drug history.
2. Assess the need for HIV antibody testing.
3. Educate about risky sex and drug use behaviors.
4. Educate about safer sex with an emphasis on effective condom use.
5. Assess psychologic factors associated with unsafe behaviors: posttraumatic stress disorder, depression, anxiety, dissociative disorders, grief, and bereavement.
6. Provide ongoing one-on-one or group interventions aimed at addressing psychologic factors and strengthening commitment to safer behavior.

setting, community resources should be used to address the many diverse challenges. The physician may be greatly challenged by being the only resource available to the potentially infected individual. In such a circumstance, extensive time must be allocated to develop the kind of clinical relationship which would elicit responses useful in an evaluation of HIV risk behavior. Such an investment of time is also required to facilitate frank discussions about the utility of HIV antibody testing and to evaluate how to approach persistent risk behaviors.

Interventions aimed at potentially HIV infected individuals will save lives. Providers and insurers should recognize that the investment made in counseling the potentially infected individual is well worth the time and effort in view of the enormous human and financial costs associated with each seroconversion.

REFERENCES

1. Centers for Disease Control and Prevention. Update: acquired immunodeficiency syndrome—United States, 1994. MMWR 1995;44:64.
2. Centers for Disease Control and Prevention. Update: AIDS among women—United States, 1994. MMWR 1995;44:81.
3. Merrill JM, Laux LF, Thornby JI. Why doctors have difficulty with sex histories. South Med J 1990;83:6.
4. Hoover DR, Muñoz A, Carey V, et al. Estimating the 1978–1990 and future spread of HIV virus type 1 in subgroups of homosexual men. (Abstract) Am J Epidemiol 1991;134:1190.
5. Osmond DH, Page J, Wiley J, et al. Human immunodeficiency virus infection in homosexual/bisexual men, ages 18–29: the San Francisco Young Men's Health Study. Am J Public Health 1994;84:1933.
6. Gerald G, Schatz B, Schechtel J, Novick A, Cortez J. The silent crisis: ongoing HIV infections among gay men, bisexuals and lesbians at risk. Report of the GLMA/AAPHR Summit on HIV prevention for gay men, bisexuals and lesbians at risk. San Francisco: Gay and Lesbian Medical Association, 1995.
7. Odets W. AIDS education: an American decision. AIDS Public Policy 1994;9:3.
8. West C. Race matters. New York: Vintage Books, 1994.
9. Choi KH, Coates TJ. Prevention of HIV infection. AIDS 1994;8:1371.
10. Stryker J, Coates TJ, DeCarlo P, Haynes-Sanstad K, Shriver M, Makadon H. Prevention of HIV infection: looking back, looking ahead. JAMA 1995;272:1143.

PART IV

Clinical Manifestations

AIDS: Biology, Diagnosis, Treatment and Prevention, fourth edition, edited by Vincent T. DeVita, Jr., Samuel Hellman, and Steven A. Rosenberg. Lippincott–Raven Publishers, © 1997

CHAPTER 13

Clinical Spectrum of Human Immunodeficiency Virus Diseases

Michael S. Saag

Infection with human immunodeficiency virus type 1 (HIV-1) induces an insidious, progressive loss of immune system function, which ultimately results in the opportunistic infections and malignancies of the acquired immunodeficiency syndrome (AIDS). The median time from initial infection to the development of AIDS is approximately 10 years, although the rate of disease progression varies substantially among patients. For any HIV-1–infected individual, the likelihood of disease progression is difficult to predict. However, CD4 count values, which can be easily measured, correlate with the relative risk of development of opportunistic diseases or death. Disease expression depends on host and viral factors and is altered significantly by treatment intervention and prophylaxis strategies. The natural history of HIV-1 infection is best described by disease stage, with special emphasis on viral pathogenesis and immune system function in each stage.

CLINICAL STAGING

In the early 1980s, the patients were staged primarily on the basis of whether they had an AIDS-defining opportunistic disease process.[1,2] By the mid-1980s, HIV-1 was discovered, and all patients with HIV-1 infection were categorized as having asymptomatic HIV-1 infection, AIDS-related complex (ARC), or AIDS.[3,4] ARC was defined as a compilation of symptoms and opportunistic processes that, although not

Michael S. Saag, The University of Alabama at Birmingham, 908 20th Street South, Birmingham, AL 35294-2050, phone 205-934-7349, fax 205-975-6120.

constituting an AIDS-defining condition, did result from immune dysfunction caused by HIV-1 infection. Common ARC-defining conditions included thrush, oral hairy leukoplakia, seborrheic dermatitis, weight loss, and lymphadenopathy. ARC symptoms and AIDS-defining conditions are listed in Table 13-1. Toward the end of the 1980s, as more information was accumulated about the natural history of HIV-1 disease, the terms ARC and AIDS became outdated from a clinical perspective. The term AIDS, which has little clinical meaning in terms of patient care, has been used since then to track the number of new cases, primarily for epidemiologic purposes.

Several clinical staging systems have been proposed to characterize HIV-1 disease. One of the first of these staging systems was the Walter Reed classification system, which was founded on clinical and immunologic features of HIV-1 infection.[5] The Walter Reed system never achieved widespread use, mainly because of its requirement of frequent skin testing to determine the cell-mediated immunity status of each patient, a procedure that most clinicians fail to obtain routinely. Other staging systems have been based on CD4 counts, a marker that is the best predictor of the relative risk for developing HIV-related opportunistic diseases.[6–14] In keeping with this concept, the Centers for Disease Control and Prevention (CDC) revised the case definition of AIDS to include all patients with CD4 counts of less than 200 cells/mm^3 or a CD4 percentage of less than 14%, whether the patients had developed a true AIDS-defining condition or not (see Table 13-1).[15] Part of the rationale behind this change was the impact of widespread use of *Pneumocystis* prophylaxis, which prevented the occurrence of the most common opportunistic infection in a large number of patients.[16–18] The revised CDC classification also added three new AIDS-defining conditions: pulmonary tuberculosis,

TABLE 13-1. *Centers for disease control 1993 classification system*

CD4 Count	Symptoms		
	A	B	C
>500	A1	B1	C1
200–520	A2	B2	C2
<200	A3	B3	C3

Symptom Category

A: Acute retroviral syndrome
    Generalized lymphadenopathy
    Asymptomatic disease

B: Symptoms of AIDS-related complex
    Candidiasis, mucosal
    Cervical dysplasia
    Constitutional symptoms
    Herpes zoster
    Idiopathic thrombocytopenic purpura
    Listeriosis
    Oral hairy leukoplakia
    Pelvic inflammatory disease
    Peripheral neuropathy

C: AIDS-defining conditions
    CD4 count < 200
    Candidiasis, pulmonary or esophageal
    Cervical cancer
    Coccidioidomycosis
    Crypotosporidiosis
    Cytomegalovirus infection
    Herpes esophagitis
    HIV encephalopathy
    Histoplasmosis
    Isosporiasis
    Kaposi's sarcoma
    Lymphoma
    Mycobacterial disease
    Pneumocystis carinii infection
    Pneumonia, bacterial
    Progressive multifocal leukoencephalopenia
    Salmonellosis

invasive cervical carcinoma, and recurrent bacterial pneumonia. Although the new CDC case definition staging system represents a substantial improvement over the previous version, it should be emphasized that the CDC staging system is intended primarily for use as an epidemiologic tool rather than as an instrument for use in clinical practice.

Although CD4 values are the best predictors of relative risk of disease progression, CD4 cell counts are imperfect surrogate markers of disease progression and are associated with some variability.[13,19–23] Diurnal changes of 50 to 150 cells/mm^3 have been described in normal adults, but the diurnal variability is diminished in patients with lower CD4 counts (Table 13-2).[19,21,22]

Laboratory variability is another source of difficulty in interpreting CD4 counts. Laboratories with little experience in performing CD4 enumeration tests may produce inaccurate results.[21] Ideally, clinicians should be familiar with the laboratory performing the tests they order and should use only one laboratory on a routine basis. Errors in specimen handling, especially refrigeration of the sample or long delays between specimen acquisition and testing, can lead to grossly inaccurate results. Refrigeration produces nonspecific binding of monoclonal antibodies, which may result in aberrantly high values. Prolonged delays between specimen acquisition and testing leads to reduced cell viability and inaccurate results.[20,21] Another source of variability is the reliance of CD4 count values on the total white cell count.[19] The circulating white blood cell count can vary substantially from day to day and is affected by medications, concomitant illnesses, and stress along with other factors. Although the use of CD4 percentage appears to represent a more stable value than the absolute CD4 count, most clinicians continue to use absolute CD4 counts as their primary means of following patients over time.[24,25]

Despite its limitations, the use of CD4 cell counts represents the best means of following the natural history of HIV disease.[26] Based on available data from several cohort studies, the average rate of CD4 cell count decline is 12% to 15% per year or approximately 80 to 90 cells/mm^3 per year.[6,7,23,27,28] A reasonable approach to categorizing HIV-1 disease is to divide the stages of illness into six categories based on a combination of clinical features and CD4 counts: initial infection (ie, acute seroconversion syndrome); early HIV-1 disease (CD4 count >500 cells/mm^3); intermediate HIV-1 disease (CD4 counts between 200 and 500 cells/mm^3); late HIV-1 disease (CD4 cell count between 50 and 200 cells/mm^3); advanced HIV-1 disease (CD4 counts <50 cells/mm^3); and terminal HIV-1 disease.

INITIAL INFECTION: ACUTE SEROCONVERSION SYNDROME

Although initial infection with HIV-1 may be asymptomatic, as many as 50% of individuals with acute infection report symptoms of a flu-like or mononucleosis-like illness.[29–32] Only 20% to 30% of these individuals seek medical attention while they are experiencing symptoms. Unfortunately, even when medical attention is sought, acute HIV-1 infection is usually not included in the differential diagnosis, and the patient diagnosed as having a "viral syndrome" or "Monospot-negative mononucleosis."

The symptoms of acute seroconversion syndrome usually occur within 2 to 6 weeks (median = 21 days) after exposure to the virus.[33–40] The most common symptom reported is fever, with lymphadenopathy, pharyngitis, aphthous ulcerations, esophagitis, myalgias, arthralgias, diarrhea, nausea, vomiting, and headache observed less frequently (Table 13-3).[31,33,34,41] One of the most distinguishing characteristics of acute seroconversion syndrome is the presence of a fleeting, morbilliform skin eruption.[42] Less commonly, neurologic manifestations occur, including asymptomatic meningitis, myopathy, peripheral neuropathy, brachial neuritis, isolated cranial nerve palsies (eg, Bell's palsy), and rarely, self-lim-

TABLE 13-2. *Diurnal variation of CD4 cell count and CD4 percentages*

Time	Asymptomatic HIV infection	Symptomatic HIV infection	Controls*
8:00 AM	426 (29%)	334 (26%)	81% (43%)
10:00 PM	495 (33%)	443 (28%)	1324 (48%)

*Controls are uninfected.

Adapted from Malone JL, Simms TE, Gray GC, Wagner KF, Burge JR, Burke DS. Sources of variability in repeated T-helper lymphocyte counts from human immunodeficiency virus type 1-infected patients: total lymphocyte count fluctuations and diurnal cycle are important. J Acquir Immune Defic Syndr 1990;3:144.

ited meningoencephalitis or Guillain-Barré syndrome.[34–35,41–48] Rarely, acute seroconversion is associated with significant immune deficiency, resulting in the development of *Pneumocystis carinii* pneumonia (PCP), esophageal candidiasis, or thrush.[49–51] Regardless of the type of symptoms, most symptoms resolve within 14 to 21 days. Individuals who have longer duration of symptoms have been reported to have more rapid progression to AIDS.[13,30,52]

The most striking laboratory feature of acute seroconversion syndrome is marked lymphopenia, with depletion of CD4 and CD8 T lymphocytes.[13,29,33,48] This initial lymphopenia is often followed by a period of relative lymphocytosis (predominantly CD8 cells), with a high degree of atypical lymphocytes. Around the time of resolution of symptoms, the CD4 lymphocyte count increases, but it usually does not return to baseline levels (Fig. 13-1).[13] In some individuals, number of CD4 cells remains profoundly suppressed, resulting in a more accelerated course of disease progression.[33,38,53,54]

To make an accurate diagnosis of the HIV-1 seroconversion syndrome, it is critical to understand the physiologic processes occurring at the time of seroconversion. Within 2 to 4 weeks after the initial infection, high levels of circulating virus can be detected by quantitative culture and quantitative polymerase chain reaction (PCR) techniques (see Fig. 13-1).[34,35,55] High levels of HIV-1 p24 antigen are also detected during this acute stage of disease, with values ranging from 100 to 5500 pg/mL.[34,35,39,40,44,49,53,54] During this period

TABLE 13-3. *Common symptoms of the acute retroviral syndrome*

Symptom	Percentage of Patients
Fever	57
Pharyngitis	73
Rash	70
Myalgias	58
Arthralgias	58
Diarrhea	33
Headache	30
Nausea/vomiting	20
Thrush	10
Altered mental status	3
Dysasthesias	8
Guillian Barré	1

Adapted from Clark SJ, Shaw GM. The acute retroviral syndrome and the pathogenesis of HIV-1 infection. Semin Immunol 1993; 5:149.

of high-level viremia, the immune system begins to recognize and respond to HIV-1 antigens. The immune system response is thought to be responsible for the development of clinical symptoms. Within 1 to 3 weeks after the onset of symptoms, HIV-1 antibodies become detectable.[34,35] IgM antibodies represent the initial immune response, reaching a peak between 2 and 5 weeks after the onset of clinical symptoms and becoming undetectable within 3 months.[56] Shortly after the appearance of IgM antibodies, IgG antibodies are produced. The initial antibody response is directed against gp160 and p24 antigens, followed shortly thereafter by antibodies to gp120 and gp41.[34,44,57] Antibodies against the envelope portion of the virus usually persist throughout the course of infection, but in some individuals, the p24 antibody response may be lost in the later stages of disease. Based on this conceptual understanding of HIV-1 replication and immune response during initial infection, a diagnosis of acute seroconversion can be easily established once the possibility of the diagnosis is considered. Before the development of antibody, p24 antigen, quantitative PCR, and branched-chain DNA (bDNA) values are easily detectable at high titer.[58] Serial determinations of anti–HIV-1 antibodies can also be used to document the seroconversion process.

Several studies have evaluated the effect of antiretroviral therapy during the acute seroconversion process.[59–61] The largest of these studies, conducted by Kinloch-deLoës and colleagues, demonstrated a significant reduction in opportunistic diseases and increasing CD4 counts with the use of zidovudine around the time of seroconversion.[61] However, the long-term sequela of any short-term antiretroviral effect is unknown, and as a result, routine use of antiretroviral treatment is not recommended during the acute seroconversion process. Nonetheless, based on knowledge about HIV-1 pathogenesis and the dynamic, ongoing replication of HIV-1 throughout the entire course of disease,[62,63] several investigators have suggested aggressive use of antiretroviral therapy during the time of seroconversion and beyond.[64] Additional studies are needed to address the validity of this recommendation.

EARLY HIV-1 DISEASE

Early-stage HIV-1 disease is defined by a CD4 cell count greater than 500 cells/mm[3]. Most HIV-1–Infected individuals with high CD4 counts are asymptomatic. Among those who have any symptoms of infection, lymphadenopathy is

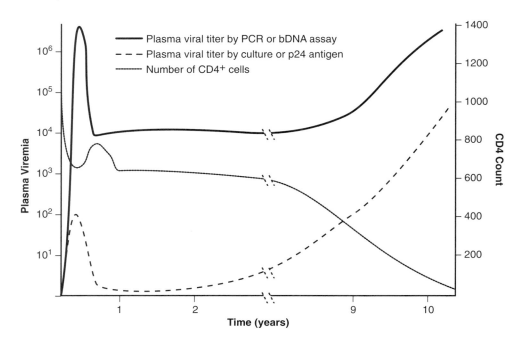

FIG. 13-1. Schematic representation of stylized course of HIV disease from the time of seroconversion until advanced disease. The CD$_4$ counts (*thin solid line*) decline slowly over time. The amount of plasma viremia, as measured by either quantitative viral copies/mL (PCR or bDNA, *thick solid line*) or culturable virus (*dotted line*) is very high during acute seroconverison; however, the culturable virus becomes undetectable soon after seroconversion while circulating viral particles remain detectable throughout all stages of disease.

the most common and usually persists from the time of acute seroconversion. In the mid-1980s, lymphadenopathy was considered evidence of more advanced disease or a precursor to the development of lymphoma.[65] As more data were collected, lymphadenopathy was shown to be associated with and improved outcome, and the loss of lymphadenopathy was understood to be a sign of impending disease progression. The anatomic pattern of enlarged lymph nodes are characteristic and usually involve the cervical, axillary, and inguinal chains, sparing the periaortic and mediastinal areas. Significant enlargement of thoracic or abdominal lymph nodes usually indicates an underlying secondary opportunistic process, such as pulmonary or disseminated tuberculosis, *Mycobacterium avium* complex (MAC) disease, histoplasmosis, or lymphoma.

Dermatologic abnormalities are the most common HIV-1–associated findings among patients with early HIV-1 disease.[66-68] Seborrheic dermatitis is a common manifestation, especially in the nasolabial fold or along the hairline.[67] New onset of psoriasis in a person older than 20 years of age is relatively uncommon and therefore suggests the possibility of occult HIV-1 infection. Patients with preexisting psoriasis may have more difficulty controlling their disease. Eosinophilic folliculitis, often characterized as "itchy, red bumps," may manifest on the thorax, back, and upper extremities. These lesions appear to be secondary to superficial bacterial or fungal disease and respond to specific topical or systemic antimicrobial therapy. Perifolliculitis also may be seen in early HIV-1 disease and usually is the result of insect bites. Disseminated scabies infection results in an intensely pruritic form of perifollicular dermatitis and should be considered as a possibility in all patients with itchy, red bump disorders.

Oral lesions, although more common in later stages, may occur in early HIV-1 disease. Aphthous ulcerations may be found in 2% to 5% of patients in the early stages of disease.[69] These idiopathic ulcers often respond to topical steroid applications. Although more common in the later stages of disease, herpes simplex labialis may occur in early HIV-1 disease.[70] These lesions usually erupt along the vermilion border of the lips and respond to oral acyclovir therapy. Oral hairy leukoplakia, a disorder caused by the Epstein-Barr virus, consists of white, plaque-like lesions along the lateral margins of the tongue bilaterally.[71,72] It is often confused with oral candidiasis, an entity that rarely occurs in patients with more than 500 CD4 cells/mm^3. More common in later stages of disease, oral hairy leukoplakia in early disease may be an indicator of impending disease progression; however, this is a relatively weak association. Oral hairy leukoplakia is usually asymptomatic and is virtually pathognomonic for underlying HIV-1 disease, making it a critical sign to observe during the physical examination. The common complications associated with the relative CD4 count at the time of onset are listed in Table 13-1.

Several studies have demonstrated an enormously high degree of viral production throughout all stages of infection.[62-63] Careful evaluation of viral changes in response to more potent antiretroviral therapy has demonstrated that 100 million to 1 billion new virions are produced in a 24-hour period within an infected individual. Such high levels of viral production and turnover, when viewed independently, strongly suggest that antiretroviral therapy should be used at every stage of HIV-1 disease. Nonetheless, conflicting clinical data exist to support the use of antiretroviral therapy when CD4 counts are greater than 500 cells/mm^3.[73,74] Even in the absence of antiretroviral therapy, the likelihood of a patient with early HIV-1 disease developing an AIDS-defining illness or death within 18 to 24 months is less than 5%.[75]

Ordinarily, an insidious, progressive decline in CD4 cells (40 to 80 cells/mm^3 per year) is expected in the absence of antiretroviral therapy (see Fig. 13-1).[13] Although some studies have shown this rate of decline can be blunted with the use of zidovudine therapy in patients with higher CD4 counts, no clinical data exist to indicate that this blunting of the CD4 decline correlates with a long-term improvement in survival. Several studies are underway to clarify this issue.

INTERMEDIATE STAGE OF HIV DISEASE

The intermediate stage of HIV disease is defined by a CD4 count between 200 and 500 cells/mm^3. Although the relative risk of developing new opportunistic infections is higher among patients with intermediate-stage disease than early disease, most patients with intermediate-stage disease remain asymptomatic or demonstrate only mild disease manifestations.

The frequency of skin and oral lesions becomes more common or worsens throughout this stage.[66,67] Among patients with symptoms, recurrent herpes simplex infection, varicella zoster virus infection (ie, shingles), recurrent diarrhea, intermittent fever, unexplained weight loss, and mild oropharyngeal or vaginal candidiasis represent the usual manifestations of illness at this stage. This symptom complex, previously referred to as ARC, usually indicates a higher likelihood of more rapid disease progression than in patients who do not develop these symptoms.[7,9,12,75] Other constitutional symptoms such as myalgias, arthralgias, headache, and fatigue are often present intermittently. HIV-1–associated nephropathy, a rare disorder characterized by progressive renal insufficiency and high-grade proteinuria, may manifest in some patients during this stage.[76] Bacterial sinusitis, bronchitis, and pneumonia become more frequent; however, these processes are generally caused by organisms usually present in the respiratory tract, such as *Streptococcus pneumoniae*, *Haemophilus influenzae*, *Moraxella catarrhalis*, and *Mycoplasma pneumoniae*, and not by the opportunistic pathogens associated with AIDS-defining illnesses.

Antiretroviral therapy is indicated for patients with CD4 counts less than 500/mm^3.[77] Historically, antiretroviral therapy was initiated with zidovudine monotherapy. Several pivotal studies have since indicated the advantage of starting with combination therapy (eg, zidovudine with zalcitabine, zidovudine with didanosine) or rapidly changing to didanosine monotherapy within 3 to 6 months over continuing long-term zidovudine monotherapy.[78,79] The AIDS Clinical Trials Group (ACTG) 175 study demonstrated comparable benefit of didanosine monotherapy to combination therapy among patients who were zidovudine experienced (ie, 6 to 12 months of prior zidovudine therapy).[79] Among antiretroviral-naive patients, the combination regimens appeared superior. Natural history studies indicate that patients who receive no antiretroviral therapy during intermediate stage HIV-1 disease have a 20% to 30% risk of progression to an

AIDS-defining condition or death over 18 to 24 months.[75] With the use of antiretroviral therapy, this risk is reduced twofold to threefold, especially when combination regimens are used.[77,80]

LATE-STAGE DISEASE

Late-stage HIV disease is defined by a CD4 cell count between 50 and 200 cells/mm^3. Based on the new CDC classification system, all patients with CD4 counts less than 200 cells/mm^3 are categorized as having AIDS.[15] This change in the classification system was based on natural history cohort data that indicated the risk of developing a new AIDS-defining condition rises dramatically when CD4 counts drop below 200 cells/mm^3. The most common opportunistic infection to affect this group of patients is PCP.[14,16] In 1988 and 1989, the value of primary and secondary prophylactic strategies markedly reduced the incidence of PCP from 80% to less than 15% among those taking prophylactic medication.[17–18] The risk of developing *Pneumocystis* infection while on PCP prophylaxis varies with the prophylactic agent used; trimethoprim-sulfamethoxazole is the most effective (0% to 2% risk of developing PCP), followed by dapsone (5% to 10% risk) and monthly aerosolized pentamidine treatments (15% to 20% risk).[18]

Patients with late-stage disease are also at substantial risk of developing other opportunistic infections, including *Toxoplasma gondii* infection, encephalitis, cryptosporidiosis, isoporoiasis, tuberculosis, B-cell lymphoma, Kaposi's sarcoma, and esophageal candidiasis.[9,11,15] Constitutional symptoms, such as myalgias, arthralgias, low-grade fever, and weight loss also become more common, along with other symptoms of ARC. Neurologic disorders, such as mononeuritis, cranial nerve palsies, vacuolar myelopathy, and peripheral neuropathy, occur with increased frequency. Although fundoscopic lesions of cytomegalovirus retinitis are uncommon among patients with CD4 counts greater than 50 cells/mm^3, well-circumscised cotton-wool spots of HIV retinopathy may occur in this population.[81] Cervical cancer in women, carcinoma of the rectum in men, and other disorders (eg, tracheal papillomas) associated with the human papillomavirus begin to appear more frequently when the CD4 count drops below 200 cells/mm^3. Hematologic abnormalities such as anemia, neutropenia, and idiopathic thrombocytopenia are commonly observed in this population. Abnormalities in luteinizing hormone and follicle-stimulating hormone may result in hypogonadism in men and menstrual irregularities in women.[82] Rarely, patients may develop occult hyperthyroidism or hypothyroidism, and they occasionally develop idiopathic adrenal insufficiency or adrenal insufficiency after invasion of the adrenal gland with an opportunistic pathogen.

Antiretroviral therapy should be continued throughout this disease stage, with special emphasis on continuation or initiation of combination chemotherapeutic approaches. Prophylactic therapy to prevent PCP is mandated in all patients with CD4 counts of less than 200 cells/mm³ and in some patients with higher CD4 counts (eg, CD4 count of 250 to 300 cells/mm³), especially if the patient has a history of oral candidiasis.[18] Unfortunately, many undiagnosed patients present with their initial symptoms at this stage, leading to their initial diagnosis. The diagnosis of HIV-1 at this stage of disease represents a failure of the health care delivery system through poor education of physicians to suspect HIV-1 disease, along with denial within the general population that individuals may be at risk for HIV-1 infection. Patients who receive no treatment at this stage have a 50% to 70% change of developing a new AIDS-defining condition or death within the next 18 to 24 months.[7,27,75,83]

ADVANCED HIV-1 DISEASE

Advanced HIV disease is defined as a CD4 count of less than 50 cells/mm³. The risk of developing certain opportunistic infections that are associated with more profound immunosuppression becomes significantly higher when the CD4 counts drop below 50 cells/mm³.[7,15,27] MAC disease, cryptococcal meningitis, cytomegalovirus retinitis, invasive aspergillosis, progressive multifocal leukoencephalopathy (PML), disseminated histoplasmosis, disseminated coccidioidomycosis, disseminated bartonellosis (ie, disseminated cat scratch disease), and disseminated *Penicillium marneffei* infection become much more common during this stage of HIV-1 infection. Unlike conditions for which a single entity is responsible for most symptoms, patients with advanced HIV-1 disease may develop coexisting opportunistic infections, with each infection contributing to the symptom complex. Another key feature of the advanced opportunistic diseases is their tendency to relapse after initially successful therapy. As a result, patients who receive treatment for the listed disorders usually require lifelong suppressive maintenance therapy to reduce the likelihood of relapse.

Disorders of the brain become especially common in advanced HIV-1 disease.[84] PML, caused by the JC polyomavirus, leads to a relentless decline in mental acuity and motor functioning over a periods of weeks to months. During the early stages, it can be difficult to differentiate the symptoms of PML from the symptoms of HIV-1–associated dementia, which is thought to result from direct infection of the central nervous system with HIV-1. In addition to several clinical and radiologic differences, the principal difference between these two disorders is the responsiveness to antiretroviral therapy that occasionally occurs in the treatment of HIV-1 dementia and the lack of treatment effect with virtually any agent for PML. The incidence of HIV-1–associated dementia has decreased substantially with the routine use of antiretroviral therapy in this patient population.[85,86]

A number of patients with advanced HIV-1 infection develop significant, involuntary weight loss. Often referred to as the HIV-1 wasting syndrome, patients who lose more than 10 lb of their usual body weight, with no obvious explanation, are diagnosed as having the syndrome.[87] Loss of appetite that results in decreased oral intake is a common cause of wasting in this population. Many patients have gastrointestinal malabsorption, which leads to weight loss and diarrhea. Wasting may result from metabolic changes and increased catabolism, which may be caused by the production of cytokines such as tumor necrosis factor-α and interleukin-6. Other factors that aggravate weight loss include the side effects of medications and endocrinopathies such as Addison's disease. Many approaches have been used to reverse the symptoms of weight loss in this population, including appetite stimulants such as megestrol acetate and marijuana derivatives (taken in pill form), hormone replacement, and steroid replacement in those with adrenal axis abnormalities.

Because of the substantially increased risk of opportunistic diseases when CD4 counts drop below 50 cells/mm³, several strategies for primary prophylaxis of common opportunistic diseases have been used by clinicians. In addition to standard prophylaxis for PCP, many clinicians initiate prophylaxis for disseminated MAC disease and invasive fungal infections.[88] Although some controversy persists, studies of primary MAC prophylaxis have demonstrated some degree of survival benefit.[89] In contrast, the use of primary fungal prophylaxis has not been associated with significant survival benefit, although there is a reduction of serious invasive fungal infections, such as cryptococcosis.[90] The use of antiviral therapy to prevent cytomegalovirus disease has led to mixed results in terms of preventing CMV retinitis, with no demonstrable survival benefit demonstrated. In general, patients with advanced-stage HIV-1 disease are living much longer than they did in the mid-1980s. The principal reasons for the increased survival in this population are improved awareness of potential opportunistic processes and newer approaches to control the expression of advanced opportunistic infections. Primary and secondary prophylaxis of many of these conditions plays a major role in prolonging survival. Antiretroviral therapy with suppression of viral replication through late-stage disease has also prolonged survival. As a result of all of these interventions, many clinicians have been following some patients with low CD4 counts (<10 cells/mm³) for as long as 5 to 7 years.

TERMINAL HIV-1 DISEASE

Although the rate of disease progression varies substantially among patients, it appears inevitable that all patients with HIV-1 infection will ultimately succumb to their disease. It is often difficult to define a precise moment when an individual makes the transition from advanced HIV-1 infection to the terminal stage of disease.[91] This determination is a clinical judgment based on a combination of medical status and, to a large degree, the patient's perspective and desires. From a medical standpoint, the diagnosis of terminal-stage HIV-1 disease is usually based on an inability to control the symptoms of disease, because no treatments are available for the particular disorder or, more commonly, because available treatments become ineffective. From a patient perspective, the transition to terminal stages of infection usually results from a decision by the patient to no longer take dozens of pills each day and a loss of desire to continue an aggressive fight against the disease. In such instances, it is appropriate for treating physicians to make the transition from one of providing primary treatment to the primary provision of comfort.[91] This includes psychological support, family support, and aggressive pain management.

PREDICTORS OF HIV-1 DISEASE PROGRESSION

The average time between initial infection and the development of an AIDS-defining illness is 10 to 12 years; however, the rate of disease progression is quite variable, with some individuals progressing to AIDS within months of the initial infection and others remaining free of AIDS-defining conditions for more than 15 to 20 years (ie, long-term nonprogressors).[7,27,92-94] Several studies have assessed the best predictive factors of potential disease progression for individual patients. The studies used clinical and laboratory evaluations of different patient populations based on risk factor assessments. The best cohort studies involve hemophiliacs, homosexual men, and transfusion recipients for whom the date of seroconversion is estimated or known.[6,7,9,10,12,16,95] A major limitation of these studies is the relative uncertainty of the precise time of seroconversion. Studies such as the multicenter AIDS cohort study (MACS) can determine the time of seroconversion within 6 months.[11,12] Other cohort studies involving individuals who received multiple transfusions, such as hemophiliacs, estimated the time of seroconversion based on patients' recollection of symptoms around the time of suspected seroconversion or based on the number of units of hemophilia factor transfused, the type of factor used, and the relative proportion of HIV-1 cases in the geographic regions from which the donated factor was collected.[9,96] Although some variability exists among cohorts, individuals who have received infected units of blood generally had more rapid progression to AIDS than hemophiliacs or homosexual men. No significant differences have been observed in the rate of disease progression between gay men and hemophiliacs.

Laboratory markers are generally better predictors of disease progression than clinical factors or modes of disease acquisition.[12,12,75,97-101] Oral candidiasis appears to be a good predictor of increased risk of PCP, and other clinical findings, such as oral hairy leukoplakia and dermatomal varicella zoster infection (ie, shingles) have been associated with some increased risk of progression, although usually not to the degree observed with oral candidiasis.[98,102] In a study of gay men followed at San Francisco General Hospital (SFGH), individuals with lymphadenopathy, shingles, thrush, hairy leukoplakia, and constitutional symptoms were 22%, 25%, 39%, 42%, and 100%, respectively, likely to develop AIDS over a period of 2 years compared with a 16% likelihood

among individuals who were asymptomatic.[7] This cohort was evaluated during a time when antiretroviral therapy and primary PCP prophylaxis were not used routinely.[86,103] The ability of data from studies such as this to predict outcome among contemporary patients remains unclear.

Among the laboratory markers, CD4 counts appear to be the best marker available in a series of cohort studies.[7-10,12,14,75,97-98,101] A single CD4 count can predict a relative likelihood of disease progression over a period of 1 to 2 years; however, the relative change in CD4 count over time appears to be the best predictor.[10,13,98,104] In one cohort, patients who had a decrease in CD4 percentage of greater than 7% during a 1-year period were 35 times more likely to develop AIDS than those who had stable CD4 percentages over the same period.[24] Based on this type of data, clinicians routinely obtain CD4 counts on their patients at 3- to 4-month intervals and more frequently around the times of critical therapeutic decisions, such as institution of PCP prophylaxis or changes in antiretroviral therapy.

Investigators have long sought reliable markers other than CD4 counts that could predict the likelihood of clinical disease progression. Several cohort studies, including the MACS cohort and SFGH cohort, evaluated the predictive value of serum β_2-microglobulin and neopterin when used in combination with CD4 counts and p24 antigen values.[7,8,11,12,75,99] In the SFGH study, β_2-microglobulin levels of 5 mg/dL or greater were associated with a 69% progression rate to AIDS over 3 years, compared with 12% among patients with levels 3 mg/dL or less.[7,27,101] When combined with the CD4 count in the presence of HIV-1 p24 antigenemia, this predictive value increased to 99% (Table 13-4). Despite these encouraging data, the applicability of β_2-microglobulin, neopterin, and p24 antigenemia has not gained favor among clinicians providing care for patients, in large part because of the lack of clinical utility of the tests. β_2-Microglobulin and neopterin have a relative small dynamic range, and p24 antigen is of limited benefit because of a substantial proportion of patients with advanced disease who continue to have with negative values.

Over the last several years, measurement of quantitative virion-associated RNA in plasma has been shown to be an accurate, direct measurement of circulating virions in plasma.[55,58,105-112] Plasma HIV RNA can be detected in virtually all patients at every stage of disease, and a strong correlation exists among the levels of viral RNA, stage of disease, and CD4 lymphocyte count (see Fig. 13-1).[58] Most importantly, plasma RNA levels change in a dynamic fashion with the initiation or modification of antiretroviral therapy.[58,113,114]

The most commonly used quantitative HIV RNA assays include quantitative competitive PCR and bDNA techniques, which have generated substantial enthusiasm in clinical and research settings.[55,110,111] Quantitative reverse transcriptase PCR and bDNA use different methods to measure the amount of HIV-1 RNA in plasma. The bDNA technique amplifies signal from captured viral RNA, and quantitative

TABLE 13-4. *Correlation of vitrologic markers*

	HIV p24 Ag	ICD p24 Ag	Plasma viremia[†]	Quant. PCR	bDNA
CD4	-0.26*	-0.12	-0.18	-0.62	-0.62
HIV p24 Ag		0.87	0.59	0.56	0.57
ICD p24 Ag			0.53	0.51	0.54
Plasma viremia[†]				0.72	0.67
Quant. PCR					0.89

*Spearman rank (R) values are given for all virologic markers.
[†]Culturable virus in plasma (TCID/mL).
Ag, antigen; bDNA, branched-chain DNA; ICD p24 Ag, immune complex (acid) disassociated p24 antigen; Quant. PCR, quantitative polymerase chain reaction.
Adapted from Cao Y, Ho DD, Todd J, et al. Clinical evaluation of branched DNA signal amplification for quantifying HIV type 1 in human plasma. AIDS Res Hum Retroviruses 1995; 11:353.

reverse transcriptase PCR amplifies target HIV-1 RNA into a measurable amount of nucleic acid product. Despite the differences in technique, plasma HIV-1 RNA, when measured with bDNA and quantitative PCR, correlates to a remarkable degree ($r = 0.89$; $P <0.001$; see Table 13-4).[58] Both assays have low intraassay sample variability, with an intrinsic intraassay variability of 0.14 to 0.2 log when single samples are tested multiple times.[105,110-111] When combined with the estimated biologic variability of 0.3 log, clinically significant changes in RNA values of more than 0.5 log (ie, threefold or greater change) is likely to reflect actual changes in the level of viral replication and viral burden. When compared with CD4 lymphocyte counts, which can vary by as much as 20% to 30% between sample time points, HIV-1 RNA assays show much promise as techniques to be used in clinical practice in the future.

Applications of these techniques in research settings have provided great insights into the pathogenesis of HIV.[62-63] Demonstration of a rapid drop in viral burden that was associated with novel protease inhibitor therapy led to the observation that the half-life of HIV-1 in plasma was less than 2 days (see Fig. 13-1). These data underscore the continuous nature of HIV replication in vivo and the dynamic, ongoing process of viral production and CD4 cell destruction. The data also highlight the ability of viral burden determinations to detect changes in response to antiretroviral therapy in a rapid and accurate fashion. Many clinicians believe that these markers will prove useful as a means of managing patients in the future.[115]

Although plasma viral RNA is established as a valuable tool in determining antiretroviral effects over a period of weeks to months, the ability of these changes to predict long-term clinical outcome remains unclear. Some natural history studies are beginning to demonstrate a correlation between higher viral load and more rapid decline in CD4 count and subsequent disease progression. In a subset of patients followed in the MACS cohort from the time of seroconversion, patients who maintained more than 100,000 HIV RNA copies/mL within 6 months of seroconversion were 10 times more likely to progress to AIDS over 5 years than those with less than 100,000 copies/mL.[116] Individuals who progressed to AIDS were more likely to have an increase in their HIV titers over time, and nonprogressors tended to have stable or decreasing viral load measurements. This study also demonstrated that CD4 counts and viral burden associates were *independent* predictors of response. Moreover, a single measurement of viral load provided information of at least equal prognostic value to a single CD4 lymphocyte count determination at any given time, especially among those with early-stage HIV disease.

Analysis of risk factors for clinical progression in trials of antiretroviral therapy have confirmed that plasma HIV-1 RNA levels and CD4 lymphocyte counts are independent predictors of disease progression. Among patients evaluated in a substudy of an ACTG 116B/117 trial, baseline plasma HIV-1 RNA levels greater than 100,000 copies/mL were associated with increased disease progression, regardless of treatment assignment.[117] Each twofold increase in the level of RNA measured at baseline was associated with a 26% increase in the risk of progression. Reduction in viral levels while on therapy was associated with a decreased risk of disease progression, with each twofold decrease in RNA level associated with a 27% reduction in the relative hazard of progression. Analysis of a subpopulation of patients who participated in the Department of Veterans Affairs trial of zidovudine, a fourfold decrease in mean plasma RNA levels determined during the first 6 months of treatment accounted for 60% of the treatment effect observed over 35 months.[118] In contrast, a 10% increase in the CD4 lymphocyte count accounted for approximately 30% of the effect. Among patients who experienced a fourfold decrease in plasma HIV-1 RNA levels and a 10% increase in CD4 count, these changes accounted for 80% of the treatment effect.

Plasma HIV-1 RNA determinations are not approved by the Food and Drug Administration for routine use in clinical practice. Nonetheless, many clinicians are using these tests "for research purposes." If these assays are used in clinical practice, it is probably best to use them in conjunction with CD4 cell counts with roughly the same intervals of testing. No single HIV-1 RNA determination should be relied on; the routine initial evaluation should consist of two measurements over a short period, because factors such as concurrent illness and immunization can cause dramatic spikes in HIV-1 RNA levels.[115,119]

Even with the paucity of available data regarding the use of the plasma HIV-1 RNA levels in patient management, the assays can be envisioned to play an important role in treatment decision making.[115] The assays may be particularly helpful in deciding when to stop drug therapy in patients who have developed dose-limiting toxicities or who have continued immunologic or a clinical deterioration with limited treatment options. Based on our understanding of HIV-1 pathogenesis, the most logical objective antiretroviral therapy is to lower the viral burden as much as possible for as long as possible. Viral burden assessments may add to the clinicians ability to tailor treatment regimens for optimal effects. Although the true benefit of maintaining a low viral burden over time is unknown, data from natural history studies suggest that a lower viral burden may prove to be a good predictor of long-term clinical outcome.

REFERENCES

1. Centers for Disease Control. Classification system for human T-lymphotropic virus type III/lymphadenopathy-associated virus infections. MMWR 1986;35:334.
2. Centers for Disease Control. Revision of the CDC surveillance case definition for acquired immunodeficiency syndrome. MMWR 1987;36(Suppl 1S):1S.
3. Popovic M, Sarngadharan MG, Read E, Gallo RC. Detection, isolation, and continuous production of cytopathic retroviruses (HTLV-III) from patients with AIDS and pre-AIDS. Science 1984;224:497.
4. Barré-Sinoussi F, Chermann JC, Rey F, et al. Isolation of a T-lymphotropic retrovirus from a patient at risk for acquired immune deficiency syndrome (AIDS). Science 1983;220:868.
5. Redfield RR, Wright DC, Tramont EC. The Walter Reed staging classification for HTLV-III/LAV infection. N Engl J Med 1986;314:131.
6. Lang W, Perkins H, Anderson RE, Royce R, Jewell N, Winkelstein W Jr. Patterns of T lymphocyte changes with human immunodeficiency virus infection: from seroconversion to the development of AIDS. J Acquir Immune Defic Syndr 1989;2:63.
7. Moss AR, Bacchetti P, Osmond D, et al. Seropositivity for HIV and the development of AIDS or AIDS-related condition: three year follow up of the San Francisco General Hospital Cohort. Br Med J 1988;296:745.
8. Kramer A, Biggar RJ, Fuchs D, et al. Levels of CD4+ lymphocytes, neopterin, and β_2-microglobulin are early predictors of acquired immunodeficiency syndrome. Monogr Virol 1990;18:61.
9. Goedert JJ, Kessler CM, Aledort LM, et al. A prospective study of human immunodeficiency virus type 1 infection and the development of AIDS in subjects with hemophilia. N Engl J Med 1989;321:1141.
10. Phillips AN, Lee CA, Elford J, et al. Serial CD4 lymphocyte counts and development of AIDS. Lancet 1991;337:389.
11. Kaslow RA, Phair JP, Friedman HB, et al. Infection with the human immunodeficiency virus: clinical manifestations and their relationship to immune deficiency. A report from the Multicenter AIDS Cohort Study. Ann Intern Med 1987;107:474.
12. Polk BF, Fox R, Brookmeyer R, et al. Predictors of the acquired immunodeficiency syndrome developing in a cohort of seropositive homosexual men. N Engl J Med 1987;316:61.
13. Stein DS, Korvick JA, Vermund SH. CD4+ lymphocyte cell enumeration for prediction of clinical course of human immunodeficiency virus disease: a review. J Infect Dis 1992;165:352.
14. Masur H, Ognibene FP, Yarchoan R, et al. CD4 counts as predictors of opportunistic pneumonias in human immunodeficiency virus (HIV) infection. Ann Intern Med 1989;111:223.
15. Centers for Disease Control. 1993 Revised classification system for HIV infection and expanded surveillance of definition for AIDS among adolescents and adults. MMWR 1992;41(RR-17):1.
16. Phair J, Munoz A, Detels R, et al. The risk of *Pneumocystis carinii* pneumonia among men infected with human immunodeficiency virus type 1. N Engl J Med 1990;322:161.
17. Leoung GS, Feigal DW Jr, Montgomery AB, et al. Aerosolized pentamidine for prophylaxis against *Pneumocystis carinii* pneumonia. The San Francisco community prophylaxis trial. N Engl J Med 1990;323:769.
18. Centers for Disease Control. Guidelines for prophylaxis against *Pneumocystis carinii* pneumonia for persons infected with human immunodeficiency virus. MMWR 1989;38(Suppl 5):1.
19. Malone JL, Simms TE, Gray GC, Wagner KF, Burge JR, Burke DS. Sources of variability in repeated T-helper lymphocyte counts from human immunodeficiency virus type 1-infected patients: total lymphocyte count fluctuations and diurnal cycle are important. J Acquir Immune Defic Syndr 1990;3:144.
20. Giorgi JV, Cheng HL, Margolick JB, et al. Quality control in the flow cytometric measurement of T-lymphocyte subsets: the Multicenter AIDS Cohort Study experience. Clin Immunol Immunopathol 1990;55:173.
21. Paxton H, Kidd P, Landay A, et al. Results of the flow cytometry ACTG quality control program: analysis and findings. Clin Immunol Immunopathol 1989;52:68.
22. Centers for Disease Control. Guidelines for the performance of CD4+ T-cell determinations in persons with human immunodeficiency virus infection. MMWR 1992;8(RR-8):1.
23. Hughes MD, Stein DS, Gundacker HM, Valentine FT, Phair JP, Volberding PA. Within-subject variation in CD4 lymphocyte count in asymptomatic human immunodeficiency virus infection: implications for patient monitoring. J Infect Dis 1994;169:28.
24. Burcham J, Marmor M, Dubin N, et al. CD4% is the best predictor of development of AIDS in a cohort of HIV-infected homosexual men. AIDS 1991;5:365.
25. Taylor JMG, Fahey JL, Detels R, Giorgi JV. CD4 percentage, CD4 number, and CD4:CD8 ratio in HIV infection: which to choose and how to use. J Acquir Immune Defic Syndr 1989;2:114.
26. Hoover DR, Graham NMH, Chen B, et al. Effect of CD4+ cell count measurement variability on staging HIV-1 infection. J Acquir Immune Defic Syndr 1992;5:794.
27. Moss AR, Bacchetti P. Natural history of HIV infection. AIDS 1989;3:55.
28. Margolick JB, Muñoz A, Vlahov D, et al. Changes in T-lymphocyte subsets in intravenous drug users with HIV-1 infection. JAMA 1992;267:1631.
29. Cooper DA, Gold JA, MacLean P, et al. Acute retrovirus infection. Definition of a clinical illness associated with seroconversion. Lancet 1985;1:137.
30. Pedersen C, Lindhardt BO, Jensen BL, et al. Clinical course of primary HIV infection: consequences for subsequent course of infection. Br Med J 1989;299:154.
31. Tindall B, Barker S, Donovan B, et al. Characterization of the acute clinical illness associated with human immunodeficiency virus infection. Arch Intern Med 1988;148:945.
32. Fox R, Eldred LJ, Fuchs EJ, et al. Clinical manifestations of acute infection with human immunodeficiency virus in a cohort of gay men. AIDS 1987;1:35.
33. Clark SJ, Shaw GM. The acute retroviral syndrome and the pathogenesis of HIV-1 infection. Semin Immunol 1993;5:149.
34. Clark SJ, Saag MS, Decker WD, et al. High titers of cytopathic virus in plasma of patients with symptomatic primary HIV-1 infection. N Engl J Med 1991;324:954.
35. Daar ES, Moudgio T, Meyer RD, Ho DD. Transient high levels of viremia in patients with primary human immunodeficiency virus type 1 infection. N Engl J Med 1991;324:961.
36. Goldman D, Lang W, Lyman D. Acute AIDS viral infection. Am J Med 1986;81:1122.
37. Oskenhendler E, Marzic M, Le Roux J-M, Rabian C, Clauvel JP. HIV infection with seroconversion after a superficial needlestick injury to the finger. (Letter) N Engl J Med 1986;315:582.
38. Valle SL. Febrile pharyngitis as the primary sign of HIV infection in a cluster of cases linked by sexual contact. Scand J Infect Dis 1987;19:13.
39. Isaksson B, Albert J, Chiodi F, Furucrona A, Krook A, Putkonen P. AIDS two months after primary human immunodeficiency virus infection. J Infect Dis 1988;158:866.
40. Bernard E, Dellamonica P, Michiels JF, et al. Heparin-like anticoagulant vasculitis associated with severe primary infection by HIV. AIDS 1990;4:932.

41. De Jong MD, Hulsebosch HJ, Lange JM. Clinical virological and immunological features of primary HIV-1 infection. Genitourin Med 1991;67:367.
42. McMillan A, Bishop PE, Aw D, Peutherer JF. Immunohistology of the skin rash associated with acute HIV infection. AIDS 1989;3:309.
43. Rabeneck L, Popovic M, Gartner S, et al. Acute HIV infection presenting with painful swallowing and esophageal ulcers. JAMA 1990;263:2318.
44. Kinloch-deLoës S, de Saussure P, Saurat JH, Stalder H, Hirschel B, Perrin LH. Symptomatic primary infection due to human immunodeficiency virus type 1: review of 31 cases. Clin Infect Dis 1993;17:59.
45. Biggar R, Johnson B, Musoke S, et al. Severe illness associated with appearance of antibody to human immunodeficiency virus in an African. Br Med J 1986;293:1210.
46. Elder G, Dalakas M, Pezeshkpour G, Sever J. Ataxic neuropathy due to ganglioneuronitis after probable acute human immunodeficiency virus infection. Lancet 1986;2:1275.
47. Hagberg L, Malmvall BE, Svennerholm L, Alestig K, Morkrans G. Guillain-Barré syndrome as an early manifestation of HIV central nervous system infection. Scand J Infect Dis 1986;18:591.
48. Calabrese LH, Proffitt MR, Levin KH, Yen-Lieberman B, Starkey C. Acute infection with human immunodeficiency virus (HIV) associated with acute brachial neuritis and an exanthematous rash. Ann Intern Med 1987;107:849.
49. Cila G, Perez TE, Furundarena JR, Cuadrado E, Iribarren JA, Neira F. Esophageal candidiasis and immunodeficiency associated with acute HIV infection. AIDS 1988;2:399.
50. Peña JM, Martínez-López MA, Arnalich F, Barbado FJ, Vásquez JJ. Esophageal candidiasis associated with acute infection due to human immunodeficiency virus. Rev Infect Dis 1991;13:872.
51. Ong EL, Mandal BK. Primary HIV-1 infection associated with pneumonitis. Postgrad Med J 1991;67:579.
52. Sinicco A, Fora R, Sciandra M, Lucchini A, Caramello P, Gioannini P. Risk of developing AIDS after primary acute HIV-1 infection. J Acquir Immune Defic Syndr 1993;6:575.
53. Kappes JC, Saag MS, Shaw GM, et al. Assessment of antiretroviral therapy by plasma viral load testing: standard and ICD HIV-1 p24 antigen and viral RNA (QC-PCR) assays compared. J Acquir Immune Defic Syndr 1995;10:139
54. Pedersen C, Nielsen JO, Dickmeis E, Jordal R. Early progression to AIDS following primary HIV infection. AIDS 1989;3:45.
55. Piatak M, Saag MS, Yang LC, et al. High levels of HIV-1 plasma during all stages of infection determined by competitive PCR. Science 1993;259:1749.
56. Lange JMA, Parry JV, De Wolf F, Mortimer PP, Goudsmit J. Diagnostic value of specific IgM antibodies in primary HIV infection. AIDS 1988;2:31.
57. Kessler HA, Blaauw B, Spear J, Paul DA, Falk LA, Landay A. Diagnosis of human immunodeficiency virus infection in seronegative homosexuals presenting with an acute viral syndrome. JAMA 1987;258:1196.
58. Cao Y, Ho DD, Todd J, et al. Clinical evaluation of branched DNA signal amplification for quantifying HIV type 1 in human plasma. AIDS Res Hum Retroviruses 1995;11:353.
59. Tindall B, Gaines H, Imrie A, et al. Zidovudine in the management of primary HIV-1 infection. AIDS 1991;5:477.
60. Tindall B, Carr A, Goldstein D, Penny R, Cooper DA. Administration of zidovudine during primary HIV-1 infection may be associated with a less vigorous immune response. AIDS 1993;7:127.
61. Kinloch-deLoës S, Hirschel BJ, Hoen B, et al. A controlled trial of zidovudine in primary human immunodeficiency virus infection. N Engl J Med 1995;333:408.
62. Wei X, Ghosh SK, Taylor M, et al. Viral dynamics in human immunodeficiency virus type 1 infection. Nature 1995;373:117.
63. Ho DD, Neumann AU, Perelson AS, Chen W, Leonard JM, Markowitz M. Rapid turnover of plasma virions and CD4 lymphocytes in HIV-1 infection. Nature 1995;373:123.
64. Ho DD. Time to hit HIV, early and hard. N Engl J Med 1995;333:450.
65. Osmond D, Chaisson RE, Moss AR, Bacchetti P, Krampf W. Lymphadenopathy in asymptomatic patients seropositive for HIV. N Engl J Med 1987;317:246.
66. Smith KJ, Skelton HG, Yeager J, et al. Clinical features of inflammatory dermatoses in human immunodeficiency virus type 1 disease and their correlation with Walter Reed stage. J Am Acad Dermatol 1993;28:167.
67. Soeprono FF, Schinella RA, Cockerell CJ, et al. Seborrheic-like dermatitis of acquired immunodeficiency syndrome. J Am Acad Dermatol 1986;14:242.
68. Valle S-L. Dermatologic findings related to human immunodeficiency virus infection in high-risk individuals. J Am Acad Dermatol 1987;17:951.
69. Feigal DW, Katz MH, Greenspan D, et al. The prevalence of oral lesions in HIV-infected homosexual and bisexual men: Three San Francisco epidemiology cohorts. AIDS 1991;5:519.
70. Quinnan GV, Masur H, Rook AH, et al. Herpes simplex infections in the acquired immune deficiency syndrome. JAMA 1984;252:72.
71. Greenspan D, Greenspan JS, Hearst NG, et al. Relation of oral hairy leukoplakia to infection with human immunodeficiency virus and the risk of developing AIDS. J Infect Dis 1987;155:475.
72. Greenspan JS, Greenspan D, Lennette ET, et al. Replication of Epstein-Barr virus within the epithelial cells of "hairy" leukoplakia, an AIDS-associated lesion. N Engl J Med 1985;313:1564.
73. Volberding PA, Lagakos SW, Grimes JM, et al. A comparison of immediate with deferred zidovudine therapy for asymptomatic HIV-infected adults with CD4 cell counts of 500 or more per cubic millimeter. N Engl J Med 1995;333:401.
74. Cooper DA, Gatell JM, Kroon S, et al. Zidovudine in persons with asymptomatic HIV infection and CD4+ cell counts greater than 400 per cubic millimeter. N Engl J Med 1993;329:297.
75. MacDonell KB, Chimiel JS, Poggensee L, Wu S, Phair JP. Predicting progression to AIDS: combined usefulness of CD4 lymphocyte counts and p24 antigenemia. Am J Med 1990;89:706.
76. Rao TKS, Friedman EA, Nicastri AD. The types of renal disease in the acquired immunodeficiency syndrome. N Engl J Med 1987;316:1062.
77. Volberding PA, Lagakos SW, Koch MA, et al. Zidovudine in asymptomatic human immunodeficiency virus infection. A controlled trial in persons with fewer than 500 CD4-positive cells per cubic millimeter. N Engl J Med 1990;322:941.
78. Kahn JO, Lagakos SW, Richman DD, et al. A controlled trial comparing continued zidovudine with didanosine in human immunodeficiency virus infection. N Engl J Med 1992;327:581.
79. Hammer S, Katzenstein D, Hughes M, et al. Preliminary results of ACTG 175. Abstract. The 35th Interscience Conference on Antimicrobial Agents and Chemotherapy, San Francisco, CA, 1995.
80. Volberding PA, Lagakos SW, Grimes JM, et al. The duration of zidovudine benefit in persons with asymptomatic HIV infection: prolonged evaluation of protocol 019 of the AIDS Clinical Trials Group. JAMA 1994;343:871.
81. Jabs DA, Green WR, Fox R, et al. Ocular manifestations of acquired immune deficiency syndrome. Ophthalmology 1989;96:1092.
82. Merenich JA, McDermott MT, Asp AA, et al. Evidence of endocrine involvement early in the course of human immunodeficiency virus infection. J Clin Endocrinol Metab 1990;70:566.
83. Hessol NA, Lifson AR, O'Malley PM, Doll LS, Jaffe HW, Rutherford GW. Prevalence, incidence and progression of human immunodeficiency virus infection in homosexual and bisexual men in hepatitis B vaccine trials, 1978–1988. Am J Epidemiol 1989;130:1167.
84. Levy RL, Bredesen DE, Rosenblum ML. Neurological manifestations of the acquired immunodeficiency syndrome (AIDS): experience at UCSF and review of the literature. J Neurosurg 1985;62:475.
85. Portegies P, de Gans J, Lange JMA, et al. Declining incidence of AIDS dementia complex after introduction of zidovudine treatment. Br Med J 1989;299:819.
86. Moore RD, Hidalgo J, Sugland BW, Chaisson RE. Zidovudine and the natural history of the acquired immunodeficiency syndrome. N Engl J Med 1991;324:1412.
87. Grunfeld C, Feingold KR. Seminars in medicine of the Beth Israel Hospital, Boston: metabolic disturbances and wasting in the acquired immunodeficiency syndrome. N Engl J Med 1992;327:329.
88. Kaplan JE, Masur H, Holmes KK, et al. USPHS/IDSA guidelines for the prevention of opportunistic infections in persons infected with human immunodeficiency virus: an overview. Clin Infect Dis 1995;21(Suppl 1):S12.
89. Pierce M. Early results of clarithromycin as maintenance therapy for Mycobacterium avium complex disease. Abstract. The 35th Interscience Conference on Antimicrobial Agents and Chemotherapy, San Francisco, CA, 1995.
90. Powderly WG, Finkelstein D, Feinberg J, et al. A randomized trial comparing fluconazole with clotrimazole troches for the prevention of fungal infections in patients with advanced human immunodeficiency virus infection. N Engl J Med 1995;332:700.
91. Stansell JD, Follansbee SE. Management of late-stage AIDS. In: Sande MA, Volberding PA, eds. The medical management of AIDS. 4th ed. Philadelphia: WB Saunders, 1995:665.

92. Pantaleo G, Menzo S, Vaccarezza M, et al. Studies in subjects with long-term nonprogressive human immunodeficiency virus infection. N Engl J Med 1995;332:209.
93. Baltimore D. Lessons from people with nonprogressive HIV infection. N Engl J Med 1995;332:259.
94. Cao Y, Qin L, Zhang L, Safrit J, Ho DD. Virologic and immunologic characterization of long-term survivors of human immunodeficiency virus type 1 infection. N Engl J Med 1995;332:201.
95. Selwyn PA, Alcabes P, Hartel D, et al. Clinical manifestations and predictors of disease progression in drug users with human immunodeficiency virus infection. N Engl J Med 1992;327:1697.
96. Biggar RJ and the International Registry of Seroconverters. AIDS incubation in 1891 HIV seroconverters from different exposure groups. AIDS 1990;4:1059.
97. Phillips A, Lee CA, Elford J, et al. Prediction of progression to AIDS by analysis of CD4 lymphocyte counts in a haemophilic cohort. AIDS 1989;3:737.
98. Saah AJ, Munoz A, Kuo V, et al. Predictors of the risk of development of acquired immunodeficiency syndrome within 24 months among gay men seropositive for human immunodeficiency virus type 1: a report from the multicenter AIDS cohort study. Am J Epidemiol 1992;135:1147.
99. De Wolf F, Lange JM, Houweling JT, et al. Numbers of CD4+ cells and the levels of core antigens of an antibodies to the human immunodeficiency virus as predictors of AIDS among seropositive homosexual men. J Infect Dis 1988;158:615.
100. Eyster ME, Ballard JO, Gail MH, Drummond JE, Goedert JJ. Predictive markers for the acquired immunodeficiency syndrome (AIDS) in hemophiliacs: persistence of p24 antigen and low T4 cell count. Ann Intern Med 1989;110:963.
101. Fahey JL, Taylor JMG, Detels R, et al. The prognostic value of cellular and serologic markers in infection with human immunodeficiency virus type 1. N Engl J Med 1990;322:166.
102. Melbye M, Goeddert JJ, Grossman RJ, Eyster ME, Biggar RE. Risk of AIDS after herpes zoster. Lancet 1987;1:728.
103. Jacobson MA, Bacchetti P, Kolokathis A, et al. Surrogate markers for survival in patients with AIDS and AIDS related complex treated with zidovudine. Br Med J 1991;302:73.
104. Lagakos SW. Surrogate markers in AIDS clinical trials: conceptual basis, validation, and uncertainties. Clin Infect Dis 1993;16(Suppl 1):S22.
105. Sninsky JJ, Kwok S. The application of quantitative polymerase chain reaction to therapeutic monitoring. AIDS 1993;7(Suppl 2):S29.
106. Winters MA, Tan LB, Katzenstein DA, Merigan TC. Biological variation and quality control of plasma human immunodeficiency virus type 1 RNA quantitation by reverse transcriptase polymerase chain reaction. J Clin Microbiol 1993;31:2960.
107. Lin HJ, Myers LE, Yen-Leiberman E, et al. Multicenter evaluation of quantification methods for plasma human immunodeficiency virus type 1 RNA. J Infect Dis 1994;170:553.
108. Holodniy M, Katzenstein DA, Sengupta S, et al. Detection and quantification of human immunodeficiency virus RNA in patient serum by use of the polymerase chain reaction. J Infect Dis 1991;163:862.
109. Holodniy M, Katzenstein DA, Israelski DM, Merigan TC. Reduction in plasma human immunodeficiency virus ribonucleic acid after dideoxynucleoside therapy as determined by the polymerase chain reaction. J Clin Invest 1991;88:1755.
110. Mulder J, McKinney N, Christopherson C, Sninsky J, Greenfield L, Kwok S. Rapid and simple PCR assay for quantitation of human immunodeficiency virus type 1 RNA in plasma: application to acute retroviral infection. J Clin Microbiol 1994;32:292.
111. Pachl C, Todd JA, Kern DG, et al. Rapid and precise quantification of HIV-1 RNA in plasma using a branched DNA (bDNA) signal amplification assay. J Acquir Immune Defic Syndr 1995;8:446.
112. Scadden DT, Wang Z, Groopman JE. Quantitation of plasma human immunodeficiency virus type 1 RNA by competitive polymerase chain reaction. J Infect Dis 1991;165:1119.
113. Holodniy M, Katzenstein DA, Winters M, et al. Measurement of Hiv virus load and genotypic resistance by gene amplification in asymptomatic subjects treated with combination therapy. J Acquir Immune Defic Syndr 1993;6:366.
114. Katzenstein DA, Winters M, Bubp J, Israelski D, Winger E, Merigan TC. Quantitation of human immunodeficiency virus by culture and polymerase chain reaction in response to didanosine after long-term therapy with zidovudine. J Infect Dis 1994;169:416.
115. Saag MS, Holodniy M, Kuritzkes DR, et al. Use of viral load markers in clinical practice: when, how , and why. Nature Medicine, 1996 (in press).
116. Mellors JW, Kinsley LA, Rinaldo Jr CR, et al. Quantitation of HIV-1 RNA in plasma predicts outcome after seroconversion. Ann Intern Med 1995;122:573.
117. Hooper C, Welles S, D'Aquila R, et al. HIV-1 RNA level in plasma and association with disease progression, zidovudine sensitivity phenotype and genotype, syncytium-inducing phenotype, CD4+ cell count and clinical diagnosis of AIDS. Abstract. Proceedings of Third International HIV Drug Resistance Workshop, Kauai, Hawaii, August 1994.
118. O'Brien W, Hartigan P, McCreedy B, Hamilton J. Plasma HIV RNA and β2-microglobulin as surrogate markers. Abstract. Proceedings of the Tenth International Conference on AIDS, Yokohama, Japan, August 7–12, 1994.
119. O'Brien WA, Grovit-Ferbas K, Namazi A, et al. Human immunodeficiency virus-type 1 replication can be increased in peripheral blood of seropositive patients after influenza vaccination. Blood 1995;86:001.

AIDS: Biology, Diagnosis, Treatment and Prevention, fourth edition, edited by Vincent T. DeVita, Jr., Samuel Hellman, and Steven A. Rosenberg. Lippincott–Raven Publishers, © 1997

CHAPTER 14 Infectious Complications

14.1 *Pneumocystis* and Other Protozoa

Catherine F. Decker and Henry Masur

PNEUMOCYSTIS CARINII

Although more than a decade has passed since the recognition of the acquired immunodeficiency syndrome (AIDS), *Pneumocystis carinii* pneumonia (PCP) continues to be acknowledged as the most common pulmonary infection in patients infected with the human immunodeficiency virus (HIV-1). Recent advances in early detection, primary and secondary prophylaxis, and aggressive treatment of PCP have resulted in a decline in the incidence of disease and significant reduction in associated morbidity and mortality.[1] As the AIDS epidemic grows, PCP remains a common problem, particularly in people who are unaware of their HIV infection until they develop PCP or who have poor access to health care, and in those who choose to be noncompliant. In addition, given that prophylaxis is not completely protective, breakthrough cases occur, especially in patients who are unable to tolerate optimal prophylaxis or who have far advanced HIV disease.[2]

Although hindered by the inability to cultivate *P carinii*, which interferes with the development of new drugs, investigators have learned much about the organism's microbiologic characteristics.[3] After its original identification by Chagas in 1906, *P carinii* was traditionally classified as a protozoan based on morphologic appearance and antibiotic susceptibilities. More recently, with the application of molecular biology techniques, it appears that the organism is phylogenetically more closely related to fungi.[3]

P carinii is a ubiquitous organism in the environment, although there may be geographic variation in its distribution.[4] Serologic data in the United States indicate that most humans become subclinically infected with *P carinii* during childhood and that this infection is usually well contained by an intact immune system.[5,6] The infection remains latent unless the host becomes immunosuppressed, usually from drugs or illness. If this occurs, latent infection may reactivate, depending on the duration and severity of immunosuppression, and clinically apparent PCP may develop. It has also been postulated that the ubiquitous nature of *P carinii* permits reinfection in immunosuppressed patients with a different strain of pneumocystis, but this has been confirmed only in murine models and a few humans.[7]

Infection with *P carinii* is transmitted by the respiratory route among rodents.[8] Direct person-to-person spread among humans has been suggested by intriguing clusters of cases, but it has never definitively been proven. Respiratory isolation of patients with acute PCP is not recommended by the Center for Disease Control and Prevention. Some authorities, however, feel it is prudent for susceptible patients not to be exposed to patients with acute PCP.

Based on the immunologic abnormalities found in patients with PCP, both humoral and cell-mediated immunity are important host defenses against infection.[9] The depletion of CD4-positive T-lymphocytes caused by HIV-1 infection strongly correlates with the likelihood of developing PCP.[10,11]

Epidemiologic studies and the correlation of levels of CD4+ T-lymphocyte (CD4 counts) with onset of infection have clarified when the period of vulnerability begins for patients with HIV infection. Retrospective and prospective studies have demonstrated that CD4 counts are excellent predictors of the risk of developing PCP in this patient population.[10,11] PCP has been seen primarily in patients with recent CD4 counts lower than 200 cells/mm^3. Some cases are seen in patients with higher CD4 counts. Prophylaxis should be initiated in HIV-infected patients whose absolute CD4 cell count falls below 200 cells/mm^3, in patients with oropharyngeal candidiasis or unexplained fever for longer than 2 weeks regardless of CD4 count, and in patients who have had a prior documented episode of PCP. The CD4 cell criterion for initiating prophylaxis is arbitrary, because the

Catherine F. Decker: Division of Infectious Disease, National Naval Medical Center, Bethesda, MD 20889. Henry Masur: Critical Care Medicine Department, Clinical Center, National Institutes of Health, Bethesda, MD 20892 frequency of PCP is inversely related to CD4 count. However, the criterion of 200 cells/mm^3 is reasonable in terms of the number of patients that need to be given prophylaxis in order to prevent cases of PCP.

CLINICAL MANIFESTATIONS

The most common presenting symptoms of PCP are fever and nonproductive cough, dyspnea, chest tightness, and shortness of breath. Fatigue and weight loss may also be seen, particularly if symptoms are prolonged. If patients are educated to seek medical attention early, many cases can be diagnosed when patients have only a slight cough, low fever, or substernal pressure. Health care providers must be aggressive in pursing diagnostic evaluations at this early stage. AIDS patients tend to have a more indolent course, with a longer duration of symptoms and less hypoxia on presentation, than do patients treated with cytotoxic chemotherapy or corticosteroids. The cough may be similar to that seen with a viral infection, and the shortness of breath may be noticed only with exertion.[12]

Extrapulmonary pneumocystosis has increasingly been recognized and has now been reported to occur at almost every anatomic site.[13] Extrapulmonary *P carinii* infection often produces no clinical symptoms and is present more often than is clinically appreciated. In some cases involving dysfunction of the brain, the retina, the liver, or the kidney, improvement of involved organ dysfunction has been noted after therapy for *P carinii*.[14,15]

The physical examination in patients with PCP is often nonspecific, although dry rales may be present on auscultation. Routine laboratory studies add little to diagnosis. The leukocyte count may be low or normal, and anemia is often seen. Elevations of serum lactate dehydrogenase (LDH) can occur, and it has been suggested that LDH levels could be used to aid in the diagnosis or determine prognosis.[16,17] However, given the nonspecific nature of LDH elevations, their use clinically is not helpful.

The radiologic findings are dictated by the stage of illness at the time the patient presents for evaluation.[18] Up to 20% of patients who present with minimal symptoms have normal chest radiographs.[19] The typical radiograph may vary from diffuse and symmetric increased interstitial markings to a diffuse alveolar pattern with infiltrations characterized by asymmetry, nodularity, or cavitation.[20] Bullae may be present, especially in patients receiving aerosolized pentamidine prophylaxis. Focal upper lobe disease often occurs with an aerosolized pentamidine breakthrough episode, although this can be seen in other patients as well.[21] Pleural effusions and intrathoracic adenopathy are very uncommon with PCP unless there is a concomitant process. The degree of hypoxemia is probably the most reliable prognostic marker. Other prognostic markers, including the percentage of neutrophils among bronchoalveolar lavage cells and the serum LDH, are less useful.[18,22] Quantitation of trophozoites is useful prognostically, but few laboratories are prepared to do careful quantitative studies.

Arterial blood gas abnormalities in patients with PCP characteristically include hypoxemia, hypocarbia, and an increase in the alveolar-arterial (A-a) oxygen gradient.[12,19,23] Normal arterial blood gases can be seen in up to 20% of patients who present with very mild disease, and this finding should not dissuade the clinician from initiating an evaluation in patients with compatible symptoms and a CD4 count lower than 200/mm^3.[24]

DIAGNOSIS

The definitive diagnosis of *P carinii* disease requires the demonstration of cysts or trophozoites within tissue or body fluids, given that the organism cannot be cultured from clinical material. Before the AIDS epidemic, the diagnosis of *P carinii* often required an open lung biopsy. With the increase in PCP associated with transplantation, cancer therapy, and then AIDS, bronchoscopy with bronchoalveolar lavage and transbronchial biopsy were used more frequently.[25,26] More recently, analysis of induced sputum has been shown to be a sensitive, simple, and noninvasive means to diagnose PCP, and it often precludes the need for bronchoscopy.[27-29] Examination of spontaneously expectorated sputum has not been a useful technique to recover *P carinii*; organisms can occasionally be seen, but the yield is low.[30] More than a dozen institutions report high yields for recovery of the organism through induced sputum, with the sensitivity of being 70% to 95%.[27,29,31] The yield in patients receiving prophylaxis, especially aerosolized pentamidine, appears to be lower in some but not all laboratories.[32] Some centers have not been as successful; this may result in part from inexperience by respiratory therapists in sputum induction and lack of expertise by the laboratory in processing and evaluating sputum specimens. Sputum induced by inhalation of a mist of 3% saline solution produced by a high-flow ultrasonic nebulizer is preferred. A nebulization lasting from 30 to 60 minutes may be required to induce patients to produce an adequate specimen. The use of mucolysis and centrifugation of the specimens seems to increase the sensitivity for detection of *P carinii*.[27] *P carinii* can be stained by a variety of tinctorial stains,[33,34] but more important than the stain used to detect the organism is the degree of expertise of the microbiologist who reviews the specimen.

The development of monoclonal antibodies has resulted in a rapid, sensitive, and easy to perform immunofluorescence assay, which is more sensitive in detecting *P carinii* in induced sputum specimens than conventional stains.[24,27,35,36] The use of polymerase chain reaction to diagnose *P carinii* in sputum, although sensitive, does not reliably differentiate acute clinical disease from other situations such as presumed latent infection.[37] It is therefore not clinically useful at the present time.

Bronchoscopy with bronchoalveolar lavage and transbronchial biopsy are very sensitive methods for diagnosis of PCP. If the procedures are performed together, sensitivity approaches 100%.[31,38] Bronchoalveolar lavage alone has been reported as having a sensitivity of up to 97% for the detection of *P carinii*.[28] In untreated patients or patients treated for only a few days, diagnoses of PCP should almost never be missed. The diagnostic yield of bronchoalveolar lavage has been reported to decrease to 60% in patients receiving aerosolized pentamidine, but this decrease in sensitivity has not been substantiated by several other experienced laboratories.[32,39]

The results of nuclear medicine scans and pulmonary function tests may be suggestive of the correct diagnosis, but the lack of specificity only delays definitive diagnosis and the initiation of appropriate therapy. Their cost also argues against their use.

The generally accepted approach to diagnosis of PCP in an HIV-infected patient begins with induced sputum. If *P carinii* is not identified in induced sputum, the next step should be bronchoscopy with bronchoalveolar lavage. If that procedure is not diagnostic, bronchoscopy is repeated with lavage and transbronchial biopsy, which, in addition to identifying *P carinii*, may lead to other diagnoses. Because processes other than *P carinii* can present with similar clinical and radiographic findings, some of which require alternative therapies, initiation of empiric therapy for *P carinii* in lieu of pursuit of a definitive diagnosis is not recommended.

TREATMENT

Currently, trimethoprim-sulfamethoxazole (TMP-SMX) is the first-line antimicrobial agent for the treatment of PCP. Intravenous pentamidine is highly effective but also highly toxic. There is increasing evidence that other regimens have clinical efficacy, including trimethoprim-dapsone,[40,41] primaquine-clindamycin,[42,43] and atovaquone[44] (Table 14.1-1).

TMP-SMX remains the agent of choice for initial therapy of acute PCP.[44,45] TMP-SMX acts sequentially to inhibit folate synthesis. Trimethoprim is an inhibitor of dihydrofolate reductase (DHFR), and sulfamethoxazole is an inhibitor of dihydropteroate synthetase (DHPS). TMP-SMX is well absorbed from the gastrointestinal tract and may be given orally or intravenously. Efficacy has been demonstrated with total doses of 15 to 20 mg/kg per day of trimethoprim and 75 to 100 mg/kg per day of sulfamethoxazole given in three or four divided doses. If a patient has mild disease (arterial partial pressure of oxygen [PaO_2] higher than 70 mm Hg) and is able to tolerate oral medications, TMP-SMX may be given in the dosage of two double-strength tablets (160 mg TMP and 800 mg SMX) every 8 hours. There is no evidence that doses of higher than 5 mg/kg trimethoprim and 25 mg/kg sulfamethoxazole every 8 hours are necessary. Total duration of therapy is 21 days, but there is no hard evidence that 3 weeks of therapy is more effective than 2 weeks.[46]

Symptoms of toxicity associated with TMP-SMX include fever, rash, headache, nausea, vomiting, bone marrow suppression, and elevation of liver transaminases.[46–49] Nephrotoxicity, hypokalemia, aseptic meningitis, and a sepsis-like syndrome can also occur. Additional myelosuppression may occur with simultaneous use of zidovudine. Toxicity occurs more frequently in HIV-infected patients than in patients without HIV infection. Treatment-limiting toxicities usually occur between day 6 and day 10 of therapy. Recent trials suggest that approximately 25% of patients are unable to tolerate a full course of TMP-SMX.[50,51] Most adverse reactions appear to be caused by the sulfamethoxazole component of therapy. The toxicity has been hypothesized to be related to the hydroxylamine metabolite of sulfamethoxazole, but evidence for this is scant.[52] Some patients may be able to continue taking TMP-SMX despite mild toxicity. Clinicians should be aware that life-threatening reactions can occur and that a few cases of fatal Stevens-Johnson–type exfoliative skin reactions have been reported. Some advocate desensitization to TMP-SMX as a way to reduce the likelihood of adverse outcomes in patients with a history of hypersensitivity reactions, but the usefulness of this approach remains unproven and controversial.[53] There have been reports of severe systemic reactions that resemble anaphylaxis or septic shock occurring in HIV-infected patients who are rechallenged with TMP-SMX after experiencing toxicity within the previous 6 to 8 weeks. Although its mechanism remains unclear, the reaction has features of cytokine-mediated effects.[54,55]

TABLE 14.1-1. *Drug regimens for treatment of Pneumocystis carinii pneumonia*

Agent	Total Daily Adult Dose	Route	Interval	Days of Therapy
Trimethoprim plus sulfamethoxazole	15–20 mg/kg 75–100 mg/kg	IV or PO	6–8 h	21
Pentamidine isethionate	4 mg/kg	IV	24 h	21
Trimethoprim plus dapsone	15–20 mg/kg 100 mg	PO PO	8 h 24 h	21 21
Clindamycin plus primaquine	1.35–1.8 g 15–30 mg	PO PO	8 h 24 h	21 21
Atovaquone	2250 mg	PO	8 h	21
Trimetrexate	45 mg/m^2	IV	24 h	21
ADJUNCTIVE AGENTS				
Prednisone	40 mg	PO	12 h	5
	40 mg	PO	24 h	5
	20 mg	PO	24 h	11

For many years, pentamidine was the only available agent for the treatment of PCP. It is now one of several alternative agents to TMP-SMX as initial therapy. Pentamidine is not absorbed from the gastrointestinal tract, and therefore parenteral administration is necessary. The standard dose of pentamidine is 4 mg/kg per day, given intravenously over a period of at least 1 hour for a minimum of 14 to 21 days. Some small studies suggest that a lower dose of 3 mg/kg per day may also be effective,[56,57] but whether the lower dose is equally effective is unknown. The dosing interval of 24 hours should probably be increased in patients with impaired renal function, although there are no precise guidelines.

Between 50% and 60% of both AIDS and non-AIDS patients experience adverse reactions with the use of pentamidine.[12,30] Nephrotoxicity, hypoglycemia, hyperglycemia, hypotension, neutropenia, and pancreatitis are the major toxicities seen.[12,58] In addition, hyponatremia, abnormal liver function, and azotemia can occur. Torsades de pointes has been reported. Hypoglycemia, which may lead to seizures and death, is seen more frequently in patients who also have nephrotoxicity and in those who receive a longer duration of therapy and greater total dose.[59,60] Pentamidine can cause an acute release of insulin, followed by inhibition of insulin release and damage to pancreatic islet cells. Dysglycemias can occur weeks after pentamidine use. Hyperglycemia may be irreversible and may result in insulin dependence. In one prospective study, pentamidine was discontinued in 55% of 20 patients because of adverse events. However, in another study, pentamidine could be continued in all patients despite toxicity by reducing the dose by 30% to 50% in patients who had a rise in serum creatinine of greater than 1 mg/dL rise during therapy.[61] Most reactions occurred between day 7 and 14 of therapy. There is an impression among some clinicians that intravenous pentamidine is associated with increased risk of pancreatitis among patients who have received didanosine or zalcitabine, but this remains to be substantiated. There have been scattered reports of the use of aerosolized pentamidine in the treatment of PCP.[62-64] There is usually a lower success rate with its use and it cannot be recommended as a therapeutic option.

Dapsone is a sulfone and, like sulfonamides, inhibits the enzyme DHPS. As a single agent, dapsone appears to be less than optimal for the treatment of PCP, with failure rates of approximately 40%.[65,66] In combination with trimethoprim (20 mg/kg per day), its efficacy has been demonstrated to be higher.[67] In a small randomized study and a subsequent three-arm controlled study, TMP-dapsone was shown to be as effective as and better tolerated than TMP-SMX.[41] TMP-dapsone is now a commonly used alternative oral regimen in mild to moderate disease for patients who are intolerant of TMP-SMX. Adverse reactions to dapsone include fever, rash, liver function abnormalities, nausea, and methemoglobinemia. This regimen can be given only orally and is therefore not suitable for patients with severe disease or gastrointestinal dysfunction.

The combination of clindamycin and primaquine has emerged as another reasonable alternative in the treatment of PCP.[42,43] Investigators report success rates of 80% in open, noncomparative trials with patients who were intolerant to or had failed standard treatment and 75% with patients who had not been treated previously.[42,43] A recently completed randomized trial found the combination to be comparable in efficacy to TMP-SMX or TMP-dapsone. The most commonly experienced adverse reactions are skin rash (which occurred in 50% of patients), diarrhea, and hepatitis. Clindamycin is given either orally (300 mg to 450 mg every 6 to 8 hours) or intravenously (600 mg to 900 mg every 6 to 8 hours) and primaquine (30 mg/day).

Atovaquone (formerly BW 566C80), a hydroxynaphthoquinone, is another oral agent effective in the treatment of *P cariini* infection. After the demonstration of efficacy in open trials,[68] a randomized, blinded study was undertaken of atovaquone (750 mg orally three times per day; 160 patients) versus TMP-SMX (162 patients) in mild to moderate disease (A-a gradient <45 mm Hg and PaO_2 >60 mm Hg). There was a significantly higher proportion of treatment failures in the atovaquone arm (20% versus 7%), whereas the TMP-SMX arm had a higher incidence of treatment-limiting toxicities (20% versus 7%). Death was also significantly more frequent with atovaquone treatment than with TMP-SMX.[44] Rash and elevation of liver-associated enzymes were the most common adverse reactions to atovaquone. Recently, oral atovaquone and intravenous pentamidine were found to have similar success rates in mild and moderate PCP in patients who were intolerant to TMP-SMX, and atovaquone was better tolerated. Patients receiving atovaquone more frequently failed to respond to therapy, and patients receiving pentamidine had more treatment-limiting adverse drug toxicities.[69] Low plasma atovaquone levels are associated with a poor response.[44] Low plasma levels are in part caused by the poor bioavailability of the drug. The drug should be taken with a fatty meal to facilitate absorption. Although the drug half-life is long (2 to 3 days), bioavailability of the drug is erratic. Recently, a new formulation of atovaquone in suspension has become available that is more bioavailable than the tablet formulation. Whether this improved bioavailability will translate into improved efficacy remains to be determined.

Trimetrexate, a potent inhibitor of DHFR, is an effective agent that has very few adverse effects despite concerns about its potential for bone marrow toxicity.[70] When compared with TMP-SMX in patients with moderate to severe disease, trimetrexate was found to be less effective and to be associated with more relapses. Its role is as an alternative agent for patients who are intolerant of TMP-SMX and who cannot tolerate or do not respond to intravenous pentamidine.[71]

Other agents that have been evaluated include piritrexim, an orally bioavailable DHFR inhibitor,[68] and difluoromethylornithine.[72] Neither is currently available for therapy of PCP. Other agents under current investigation include analogs of primaquine, analogs of pentamidine, albendazole, and echinocandins or pneumocandins.[73]

As the host response to *Pneumocystis* infection becomes better defined, there has been an increased interest in immunotherapy or immunoprophylaxis for *P carinii*, especially with agents such as interferon-γ,[74] monoclonal or polyclonal antibodies against pneumocystis,[5,75] and CD4+ lymphocytes.[76,77] Agents that interfere with attachment of the organism to the host cells[78] and those that affect the inflammatory response to *P carinii*, such as various cytokines and surfactants, are also being studied.[77,79–82] These agents are all experimental and as yet have no defined role in treating human disease.

The use of corticosteroids in conjunction with antimicrobial agents has become the standard of care in the treatment of moderate to severe PCP. After anecdotal reports suggested that corticosteroids used as adjunctive therapy in combination with specific antimicrobial agents were beneficial in ameliorating the hypoxemia associated with initial treatment for PCP, three randomized, controlled studies were conducted to further define their role in the treatment of *P carinii* disease.[79–82] In the largest study, 123 patients were randomly assigned to standard therapy plus corticosteroids and 128 to standard therapy alone. The corticosteroid group had a significantly decreased frequency of early deterioration in oxygenation and, in addition, had significantly greater survival benefit than the control group. The survival benefit could be shown only for patients who had an initial PaO_2 on room air of less than 70 mm Hg.[79] The study was not large enough to show benefit for patients with higher PaO_2s given that death is uncommon in this setting, but patients who are less hypoxic may derive some symptomatic and functional benefit. Two other randomized trials supported this finding. The corticosteroid regimen used is presented in Table 14.1-2. The use of corticosteroids was not associated with life-threatening complications, although oral candidiasis and perirectal herpes simplex did occur more frequently with corticosteroid treatment; an increased number of other opportunistic infections was not noted. As a result of these and other trials, a consensus panel recommended the use of adjunctive corticosteroids in patients with PCP who exhibit hypoxia (PaO_2 <70 mm Hg) at any time during the first 72 hours of therapy. Corticosteroid therapy is not recommended unless the diagnosis of *P carinii* is confirmed promptly.[82]

If a patient has mild to moderately severe PCP, outpatient therapy with an oral agent, preferably TMP-SMX, is a reasonable treatment strategy. Patients who are more severely ill with moderate to severe disease or who cannot tolerate oral agents should be given intravenous TMP-SMX. In sulfa-intolerant patients, intravenous pentamidine or perhaps intravenous trimetrexate should be administered.

The median time to respond to therapy is usually 4 to 6 days; many patients get worse before clinical improvement is observed. This decline has been attributed to treatment-induced deterioration, probably occurring because dying organisms elicit intense inflammatory response during the first week of therapy. A reported decline of 10 to 30 mm Hg in the PaO_2 has been associated with the initiation of therapy.[81]

There are no factors that differentiate slow responders from treatment failures, and the initial regimen should probably be continued for 5 to 10 days or longer (a minimum of 4 days) before being considered a failure. Fluid status should be monitored carefully, because PCP may cause increased permeability of alveolar capillary membranes, which can lead to accumulation of interstitial and alveolar fluid and respiratory failure. Concomitant congestive heart failure also may occur.

Survival from an episode of PCP correlates with several factors other than the choice of drug, the most important being pretreatment oxygenation.[19,69] Other factors that influence outcome include number of tachyzoites in the bronchoalveolar lavage, degree of chest radiograph abnormality, severity of hypoxia, magnitude of A-a oxygen difference, level of LDH elevation, and degree of lymphopenia.[12,19,83] For a patient with an initial PaO_2 higher than 70 mm Hg on room air, expected response rates are at least 60% to 80% in non-AIDS patients and 80% to 95% in patients with AIDS.[19]

Evaluation of response to therapy should be based on clinical and radiographic examination. The use of bronchoscopy to assess response to drug therapy is not helpful, because *P carinii* is present in bronchoalveolar lavage specimens for many weeks after initiation of therapy, even in patients who rapidly improve.[84]

The management of respiratory failure in patients with PCP should follow the same general guidelines as for any patients with diffuse lung injury. Although studies undertaken early in the AIDS epidemic suggested that survival in patients requiring ventilatory support was dismal, with mortality rates ranging from 86% to 100%,[19,49,85,86] more recently prognosis has improved substantially.[87–89] Some large institutions have observed a decrease in mortality rate in ventilated patients from 87% to 60%,[88] perhaps secondary to the use of corticosteroids and more aggressive attempts to diagnose concurrent infections.

TABLE 14.1-2. *Recommendations for the use of corticosteroids in the treatment of acute* Pneumocystis carinii Pneumonia

Population	Patients with acute *P. carinii* pneumonia and PaO_2 < 70 mm Hg on room air or alveolar-arterial gradient >35 mm Hg at presentation
Dosage	Prednisone 40 mg twice daily for 5 days, 20 mg twice daily for 5 days, then 20 mg/day until the end of antimicrobial therapy
Timing	Initiate during first 72 hours of antipneumocystis therapy

PROPHYLAXIS

Prophylaxis for PCP is well defined and has been shown to decrease morbidity and mortality (Table 14.1-3). It has been recommended based on large databases that prophylactic agents should be initiated if an HIV-infected patient's absolute CD4 cell count falls below 200 cells/mm^3. This threshold is based largely on the results of the prospective Multicenter AIDS Cohort Study (MACS), a natural history study that began monitoring 1665 HIV-infected men at 6-month intervals in 1984.[11] The MACS study also suggests that the presence of unexplained persistent daily fever higher than 37.7°C for more than 2 weeks or oropharyngeal candidiasis (unrelated to antibiotic or steroid use) is indicative of enhanced susceptibility to P cariini independent of CD4 count. Any patient who develops an opportunistic infection, regardless of measured CD4 cell count, should also receive prophylaxis.[11]

Long-term preventive therapy (secondary prophylaxis) is indicated for patients with a history of PCP. Although zidovudine has been shown to decrease the frequency of second episodes of PCP, there continues to be a substantial rate of subsequent episodes without the use of prophylaxis.[90] Historically, TMP-SMX has been used successfully as a primary prophylactic agent in the prevention of P cariini disease in pediatric oncology patients,[91] and, subsequently, it has been found to be effective in HIV-infected patients.[92]

TMP-SMX has become the preferred agent in patients who can tolerate it, because it is more effective than any other regimen for preventing PCP. The relative efficacy and toxicity of TMP-SMX as a primary or secondary prophylactic agent has been assessed in randomized prospective trials. In a European trial evaluating primary prophylaxis,[50,51] either high-dose (1 DS per day TMP 160 mg, SMX 800 mg) or low-dose (1 SS per day TMP 80 mg, SMX 400 mg) TMP-SMX was found to be significantly more effective in preventing PCP than aerosolized pentamidine. The rate of discontinuation of study drug because of toxicity was higher in the TMP-SMX groups than in the placebo group. The incidence and types of adverse reactions were similar in both TMP-SMX groups, but the toxic effects occurred significantly sooner in the group receiving the higher dose. These adverse events may represent a dose-related cumulative toxicity.[51] In a large trial that was recently completed (ACTG 081),[93] 843 patients were randomly assigned to receive TMP-SMX (1 DS tablet twice per day TMP 160 mg, SMX 800 mg), dapsone (50 mg twice per day), or aerosolized pentamidine (300 mg once monthly). Fewer episodes of PCP occurred among patients receiving TMP-SMX than in the other two arms when patients with CD4 counts less than 100 cells/mm^3 were considered but not when patients with higher CD4 counts were assessed. In this trial, the efficacy of dapsone appeared to be better than that of aerosolized pentamidine. Dapsone given at doses of 50 mg/day or less was not as effective as twice-daily doses of 50 mg.[93]

In a secondary prophylaxis study in the United States, 310 patients were randomly assigned either to administration of aerosolized pentamidine (300 mg/month) by a Respirgard II nebulizer (Marquest, Englewood, Colorado) or to ingestion of one double-strength tablet of TMP-SMX daily (HTMP 160 mg, SMX 800 mg).[50] As analyzed by intent-to-treat method, the recurrence rate of P carinii was significantly higher among the patients assigned to aerosolized pentamidine (18%) than among those who received TMP-SMX (4%). As expected, more patients who received TMP-SMX (27%) experienced sufficient toxicity to result in discontinuation of the agent.

Although it is associated with the potential toxicities previously described, TMP-SMX has advantages not provided by aerosolized pentamidine, including low cost, oral preparation, and probable protective effect against disseminated pneumocystis. In addition, because of its broad spectrum of antimicrobial activity, it offers protection against toxoplasmosis. It is also apparent that TMP-SMX confers protection against *Haemophilus influenzae* and *Streptococcus pneumoniae*.[50,94]

Aerosolized pentamidine delivered by the Fisons (Rochester, New York) hand-held ultrasonic nebulizer at a dose of 60 mg every 2 weeks (after five loading doses) has also been shown to be highly effective for prophylaxis in a prospective, randomized trial.[95,96] Other delivery systems have not been as extensively evaluated and cannot be recommended. Aerosolized pentamidine (300 mg/month) is usually well tolerated if delivered by the Respirgard II nebulizer in the indicated dosing regimens. Coughing or wheezing occurs in 30% to 40% of patients, but this reaction may be dimin-

TABLE 14.1-3. *Drug regimens for prophylaxis for* Pneumocystis carinii Pneumonia

Agent	Total Daily Adult Dose (mg)	Route	Frequency
Trimethoprim plus Sulfamethoxazole	160/800	Oral	Daily
	160/800	Oral	Twice daily
	80/400	Oral	Daily
Pentamidine	300	Aerosol (Respigard)	Monthly
	60	Aerosol (Fisoneb)	Every other week
Pyrimethamine plus Sulfadoxine	50/100	Oral	Every other week
Dapsone	100	Oral	Daily in 1 or 2 divided doses
Pyrimethamine plus dapsone	75/200	Oral	Weekly

ished or prevented by the administration of β-adrenergic agonists such as albuterol.[40,56,95,96] If aerosolized pentamidine is delivered by the Fisons nebulizer at the doses indicated, it is similarly well tolerated. Bronchospasm rarely necessitates discontinuation of prophylaxis with aerosolized pentamidine treatment. Effective delivery to the lungs depends on numerous factors, including the size of the particle generated by the nebulizer, the efficacy of the nebulizer, and the patient's breathing pattern.[97,98] Patients with reactive airway disease or bullous lung disease may not distribute aerosolized pentamidine effectively and therefore may not obtain maximum protection. Systemic toxicities such as nephrotoxicity, hypoglycemia, and pancreatitis rarely occur in patients receiving aerosolized pentamidine. There have been reports of disseminated pneumocystosis in patients receiving aerosolized pentamidine for prophylaxis.[99,100]

There is increasing concern about outbreaks of *Mycobacterium tuberculosis* among health care workers and HIV-infected patients associated with the coughing induced by aerosolized pentamidine. All patients should be screened for tuberculosis before aerosolized pentamidine is administered, and health care workers should follow guidelines provided by the Centers for Disease Control and Prevention to minimize the risk of spread of tuberculosis to other patients and health care workers.[101] Ideally, aerosolized pentamidine should be administered in individual booths or rooms with negative-pressure ventilation and direct exhaust to the outside. After the administration of aerosolized pentamidine, patients should not return to common waiting areas until coughing has subsided.

Dapsone has received the most attention as a prophylactic agent because it can be administered orally and is convenient. In addition to the data dapsone alone, weekly doses of dapsone (200 mg) and pyrimethamine (75 mg) have been shown to be well tolerated but less effective than TMP-SMX.[102] Dapsone-pyrimethamine has efficacy as a prophylactic regimen against PCP that is similar to that of aerosol pentamidine but less effective than TMP-SMX. This has been assessed as a daily regimen (dapsone, 50 mg orally every day, plus pyrimethamine, 75 mg weekly) or as a weekly regimen (dapsone, 200 mg, plus pyrimethamine, 75 mg). It is not clear whether pyrimethamine truly adds potency, given the results of the ACTG 981 study mentioned previously.

Other potential prophylactic agents that have been used empirically or evaluated in clinical trials include pyrimethamine-sulfadoxine (Fansidar), trimethoprim-dapsone, primaquine-clindamycin, and atovaquone. Although the other agents probably have some efficacy, data dealing with these forms of prophylaxis are limited and not yet sufficient to warrant their recommendation, except in patients who require an alternative to TMP-SMX or aerosolized pentamidine.

TOXOPLASMA GONDII

Toxoplasmic encephalitis was one of the sentinel opportunistic infections observed early in the AIDS epidemic.[103]

Currently, it is recognized as one of the most frequent and most treatable opportunistic infections of the central nervous system (CNS) and the most common cause of a focal intracerebral lesion in patients with AIDS.[104]

Toxoplasma gondii, an obligate intracellular protozoan whose definitive host is the cat, exists in three forms—tachyzoite, tissue cyst, and oocyst—all of which are potentially infectious for humans. The infection is usually acquired by ingestion of cysts present in inadequately cooked meat or of oocysts excreted in cat feces.[103] After acute infection in normal hosts, cysts persist in the CNS in a dormant state. If an individual becomes immunocompromised, particularly with defective cellular immunity as is present in AIDS patients, he or she is at risk for reactivation and dissemination of toxoplasmic infection.[105] In AIDS patients, reactivation of latent infection usually manifests as toxoplasmic encephalitis,[106] although chorioretinitis,[105] pneumonia,[107] and disseminated disease have also been reported. Some cases of toxoplasmosis in AIDS patients may conceivably represent primary infection, either in a previously uninfected individual or in an individual previously infected.

Investigators have reported that between 20% and 40% of AIDS patients who are seropositive for *T gondii* ultimately reactivate and develop toxoplasmic encephalitis if their CD4 count declines below cells 100/mm³.[103] Seroprevalence studies vary according to geographic location. In the United States, 10% to 40% of adults with AIDS are seropositive for *Toxoplasma*.[108] In Europe, Latin America, and Africa, where the incidence of latent infection is between 75% to 90%, the number of AIDS patients who develop toxoplasmic encephalitis may be three to four times greater than in the United States.

Clinical Presentation

Toxoplasmosis almost always occurs in HIV-infected patients with preexisting antibody to *Toxoplasma* and a CD4 count below 100 cells/mm³. Clinical presentation of toxoplasmic encephalitis can vary from motor weakness to neuropsychiatric manifestations, depending on the size, location, and number of lesions, but it usually consists of focal neurologic abnormalities. Altered mental status may be present in 60% of patients; it is characterized by confusion, psychosis or other neuropsychiatric disturbance, cognitive impairment, or coma. Seizures are also a frequent finding.[109–114] Pulmonary disease caused by *T gondii* has been reported, especially in Europe; patients experience a febrile illness with cough. Ocular disease is an infrequent occurrence in AIDS patients[107] and is usually characterized by necrotizing retinochoroiditis.[105] Concurrent toxoplasmic encephalitis has also been reported with these conditions.[105,115]

Routine laboratory studies add little in the diagnosis of toxoplasmic encephalitis. The cerebrospinal fluid may be normal or may reveal mild pleocytosis (predominately mononuclear) with elevated protein and a normal glucose.[112,116]

Neuroradiologic studies play an extremely important role in the diagnosis and management of toxoplasmic encephalitis. Results of magnetic resonance imaging (MRI) or computed tomography (CT) are highly suggestive of toxoplasmosis.[117] CNS lesions are characteristically multiple, bilateral, hypodense, enhancing masses with a predilection for the basal ganglia and corticomedullary junction,[112,118–121] but any pattern may be seen. It is less common for lesions to fail to enhance or to be solitary. In such cases, alternative diagnoses should be entertained, including lymphoma.[122] MRI is more sensitive in the detection of masses than CT.[123,124]

AIDS patients who have immunoglobulin G (IgG) *Toxoplasma* antibody should be regarded as being at high risk for the development of toxoplasmosis. Rarely are AIDS patients with toxoplasmic encephalitis seronegative.[103,125] If the serologic status is unknown in an AIDS patient with a CNS lesion, an IgG antibody evaluation should be obtained.

Diagnosis

Definitive diagnosis of toxoplasmic encephalitis is made by demonstration of organisms histopathologically in brain tissue. The presence of tachyzoites in cysts surrounded by an inflammatory reaction is diagnostic. The inflammatory reaction can vary from a granulation reaction with gliosis to necrotizing encephalitis.[112,118,121,126] Cysts or organisms not identified on routine examination can be demonstrated using the peroxidase-antiperoxidase method to stain *Toxoplasma* antigens and organisms in brain tissue.[113,117,127] Because CT-directed needle biopsy specimens are typically small, organisms may be missed because of sample error. Abnormal lymphocytes recovered by needle biopsy or aspiration may led to a mistaken diagnosis of lymphoma.[117] Wright-Giemsa stain is useful to demonstrate tachyzoites in cerebrospinal fluid and bronchoalveolar lavage fluid.[127,128] Isolation of *Toxoplasma* in culture requires tissue culture techniques or animal inoculation, which are not readily available.[129] Polymerase chain reaction has enabled detection of *T gondii* in cerebrospinal fluid,[130,131] brain,[132] bronchoalveolar lavage fluid,[133] and blood,[134] but it is currently a research tool only.

For patients who have characteristic findings on neuroradiographic imaging, especially those with CD4 counts lower than 100 cells/mm³ who have not been taking TMP-SMX prophylaxis, it is reasonable to initiate empiric therapy for toxoplasmosis. Brain biopsy should be pursued in the patient who fails to respond clinically or radiographically, usually within 14 days. Time to response varies according to location and the degree of necrosis (signal intensity); with peripheral lesions with less necrosis take 3 to 5 weeks to resolve completely. Clinical response is much faster, with up to 90% of patients experiencing partial or complete response within 2 weeks.[135] Negative serology for *T gondii*, a single lesion on MRI, a CD4 count higher than 100 cells/mm³, and adherence to TMP-SMX prophylaxis are clues suggesting another cause (eg, lymphoma); early biopsy should be considered.[136]

Treatment

First-line therapy for the treatment of toxoplasmosis includes pyrimethamine in combination with sulfadiazine.

Pyrimethamine plus clindamycin appears to be efficacious for the treatment of toxoplasmic encephalitis as well[110] (Table 14.1-4). The combination of pyrimethamine and sulfadiazine (sequentially) blocks folic acid metabolism of the proliferative form of the organism.[137] Loading doses of pyrimethamine are used to ensure adequate serum levels during early therapy.[109,138,139] If sulfadiazine is unavailable, sulfamethoxazole can be used. TMP-SMX is a convenient and available source for the sulfamethoxazole, but it must be used in conjunction with pyrimethamine, because trimethoprim has little anti-*Toxoplasma* activity.

Hematologic toxicity is commonly seen in patients who are treated with pyrimethamine. Gastrointestinal disturbances are observed in patients treated with clindamycin.[111] Skin rash may be seen with either sulfadiazine or clindamycin. Folinic acid reduces the likelihood of bone marrow toxicity and may aid in the treatment of marrow suppression.[139] Studies have revealed that as many as 40% of AIDS patients who receive sulfadiazine and pyrimethamine for toxoplasmic encephalitis experience adverse reactions that necessitate discontinuation of drug.[111,113]

Although not studied in large prospective trials, other regimens have been used successfully, including pyrimethamine and dapsone. The new macrolide agents, including clarithromycin,[140] azithromycin,[141] and roxithromycin,[140] are also promising agents and demonstrate in vivo and in vitro activity against *T gondii*. One small clinical study with clarithromycin plus pyrimethamine demonstrated some efficacy in the treatment of toxoplasmic encephalitis.[142] Atovaquone, a hydroxynaphthoquinone with excellent activity against *T gondii*,[143] has been used in small salvage studies and was found to be safe and effective, but there was a high relapse rate.[144,145] It is currently being assessed in combination with pyrimethamine. Other intriguing investigational agents in the treatment of toxoplasmosis include biologic response modifiers such as interferon-γ, which is a known important mediator of host resistance to *T gondii* and may be a helpful adjunct to standard therapy.[146,147]

Corticosteroids may be required in the acute management of toxoplasmic encephalitis in patients who demonstrate increased intracranial pressure secondary to mass effect from their lesions. However, it has been suggested that there is no significant difference in response rate or time in patients who receive corticosteroids compared with those who do not.[148] Corticosteroids are not contraindicated and should be used if necessary. Patients who present with seizures should also receive anticonvulsant agents during primary therapy, but their use as a prophylactic measure is not recommended.

Lifelong maintenance therapy is essential in the treatment of toxoplasmosis in AIDS patients. The relapse rate approaches 100% on withdrawal of therapy, which is attributed to the cyst form of the organism.[149] Pyrimethamine and sulfadiazine are active against the proliferative form but are not effective against the cysts. Approximately 10% of patients on maintenance therapy relapse, but this may reflect noncompliance.[150] A variety of dosing regimens are used.

TABLE 14.1-4. *Drug regimens for treatment of toxoplasmic encephalitis*

Agent	Total Daily Adult Dose	Route	Interval
FIRST CHOICES			
Pyrimethamine plus	200 mg load, followed by 50–75 mg	PO	24 h
Folinicacid plus	10–20 mg	PO	24 h
Sulfadiazine or	4–6 g	PO	6 h
Clindamycin	1.35–1.8 g	PO	8 h
ALTERNATIVE AGENTS			
Dapsone	100 mg	PO	24 h
Clarithromycin	2 g	PO	12 h
Atovaquone	3 g	PO	6 h
Azithromycin	1.2–1.5 g	PO	24 h

Continuation of the initial regimens is probably the most reasonable approach. The regimen of pyrimethamine and sulfadiazine appears to have a low rate of relapse and is recommended.[150-152] Patients on this regimen do not require PCP prophylaxis.[153] Fansidar (pyrimethamine-sulfadoxine) administered twice a week has also been effective for maintenance therapy but is rarely used because of concern about hypersensitivity reactions.[154]

The use of primary prophylaxis for toxoplasmic encephalitis is particularly attractive because the patient population at risk can be targeted to include patients with CD4 counts lower than 100 cells/mm^3 who are seropositive for *T gondii*. HIV-infected adults who are seronegative for *T gondii* are at risk of acquiring acute toxoplasmosis, but this risk appears to be low, at least in North America.[6] Patients should be educated about the prevention of toxoplasmosis, including avoidance of reservoirs for *T gondii* (eg, cat litter boxes) and to avoidance of ingestion of undercooked meats.[103]

The most convincing evidence for the use of prophylaxis for toxoplasmic encephalitis has originated from trials of prophylaxis for PCP,[50,51,94] and few trials have been designed to specifically evaluate prophylaxis for toxoplasmic encephalitis.[155-158] In a retrospective study of 155 patients who received TMP-SMX or pentamidine for secondary PCP prophylaxis over a 3-year period, TMP-SMX was significantly more effective in preventing toxoplasmic encephalitis. None of the 22 patients seropositive for *T gondii* who received TMP-SMX developed disease, whereas 12 of 36 patients seropositive for *T gondii* who received pentamidine developed toxoplasmic encephalitis. No patient seronegative for *T gondii* developed disease.[94] The AIDS Clinical Trial Group study of secondary prophylaxis for PCP, ACTG 021, also suggests a protective effect for TMP-SMX.[50] This analysis was also a retrospective data review.

Pyrimethamine has been assessed as a prophylactic agent. A three-arm study by The National Institute of Allergy and Infectious Diseases Community Programs for Clinical Research on AIDS compared clindamycin (300 mg twice daily), pyrimethamine (25 mg three times a week) without folinic acid, and placebo. Entry criteria were seropositivity

for *T gondii* and a CD4 count lower than 200 cells/mm^3. Early into the study, the clindamycin arm was terminated prematurely because of excessive toxicity (diarrhea and rash). During the study, possibly because of the protective effects of TMP-SMX, there was a low event rate. The study was terminated because it was unlikely that a protective effect could be demonstrated. Analysis of the data on an intent-to-treat basis indicated a higher death rate among the pyrimethamine recipients (28.9% versus 15.7%). However, for those actually receiving study drug, there was no difference. The possibility that pyrimethamine may increase mortality has not been supported by two other studies, although each used folinic acid in conjunction with pyrimethamine.[156] In ACTG 154, a placebo-controlled study of more than 500 participants evaluating pyrimethamine (50 mg three times a week) plus folinic acid (15 mg three times a week) versus placebo for primary prophylaxis, pyrimethamine was protective against toxoplasmic encephalitis if the results were analyzed on the basis of those actually receiving drug (38 cases of toxoplasmic encephalitis in the placebo group versus 15 cases in pyrimethamine group) as opposed to the intent-to-treat analysis (42 in the placebo group versus 43 in the pyrimethamine group). There were four deaths in the placebo group and none in the pyrimethamine group. A third trial, sponsored by the American Federation for Clinical Research, has been stopped, suggesting that pyrimethamine has not been shown to be associated with excess mortality.

Dapsone plus pyrimethamine has also been assessed for prophylaxis. In a randomized prospective study, 349 patients with CD4 counts lower than 200 cells/mm^3 were randomly assigned to receive dapsone (50 mg per day) and pyrimethamine (50 mg per day) with folinic acid (25 mg per week) or aerosolized pentamidine (300 mg/month) for primary prevention of both PCP and toxoplasmic encephalitis.[157] The study was discontinued early because dapsone-pyrimethamine demonstrated a significant protective effect against toxoplasmic encephalitis, although no difference in the occurrence of PCP was observed. Another European trial assessing weekly therapy with dapsone (200 mg) and pyrimethamine (75 mg) showed similar results.[158]

Atovaquone and the macrolides (azithromycin and clarithromycin) warrant further evaluation for prophylaxis and treatment.

CRYPTOSPORIDIOSIS

With the advent of the AIDS epidemic, *Cryptosporidium* has been more widely appreciated as a cause of diarrheal disease.[159,160] It has been estimated that 10% to 15% of patients with AIDS in the United States and as many as 30% to 50% in the developing world have developed chronic cryptosporidiosis.[161,162]

Although outbreaks of cryptosporidiosis are common among immunocompetent hosts (eg, travelers, health care workers, persons in day care centers), these episodes are predominantly self-limited. The clinical course in HIV-infected patients can be varied. Patients who develop cryptosporidial infections at a time when their CD4 counts are high resolve spontaneously, in most cases.[163–165] Patients with low CD4 counts, especially counts lower than 100 cells/mm^3, experience severe, unremitting diarrhea. The diarrhea caused by cryptosporidiosis is usually characterized as profuse, watery, and nonbloody, with no evidence of leukocytes on stool examination, but mucus may be seen. Although it may be cholera-like in character, less fulminant diarrhea is also seen. Diarrhea is often associated with crampy abdominal pain, fatigue, anorexia, nausea, and vomiting, and it may lead to malnutrition and dehydration. Fever may be present, but it may be attributed to other coinfections.[164–167]

After it is ingested, the oocyst excysts in the small intestine, and sporozoites invade the small intestine. Although infection in the small bowel predominates, other sites of the gastrointestinal tract have been involved, and invasion of extrahepatic bile ducts may result in acalculous biliary disease.[168,169] The clinical significance of the isolation of *Cryptosporidium* from extraintestinal sites (eg, lung) remains unclear because patients usually have coinfection with other opportunistic pathogens.[170]

Diagnosis of cryptosporidiosis is usually made by examination of stool (either fresh stool or samples fixed with formalin) with modified acid-fast staining.[167,168] If few oocysts are present, concentration techniques employing sucrose flotation method may be useful.[164] A monoclonal antibody directed against oocyst wall and an enzyme-linked immunoabsorbent assay have become commercially available.

Until recently, no treatment had been proven to be consistently effective in the treatment of diarrhea,[159,164] even though there were sporadic reports of response to spiramycin,[164] diclazuril,[171] hyperimmune bovine colostrum or globulin,[172] and azithromycin.[173] Paromomycin, an oral nonabsorbable aminoglycoside, has been shown to have some clinical activity for limited time periods in uncontrolled, prospective trials.[174] In small studies, paromomycin was effective in the abatement of diarrhea, patients gained weight, and the drug was well tolerated.[174–176] Octreotide, a synthetic cyclic octapeptide analog of somatostatin, was not shown to be useful in the control of cryptosporidiosis in AIDS patients in a prospective multicenter trial.[174] Symptom-directed therapy with loperamide or Lomotil and diet modification may be helpful.

MICROSPORIDIOSIS

Microsporidiosis has become increasingly recognized as a cause of refractory unexplained diarrhea in 15% to 20% of AIDS patients.[177,178] Microsporidia, like cryptosporidia, can cause mild, self-limited diarrheal disease in normal hosts, although usually it has been observed in immunocompromised patients. Colonization with microsporidia has been identified in asymptomatic HIV-infected patients with higher CD4 cell counts, and patients may only become symptomatic with enteric disease as their immune function wanes.[179]

Microsporidia are primitive obligate intracellular spore-producing protozoa. Although several species have been recognized as causing disease in humans, only two species have been found to infect the gut: *Enterocytozoon bieneusi* and *Septata intestinalis*.[177,180] Microsporidia appear to invade the enterocyte of the intestine, which may serve as the portal of entry preceding dissemination.[181] Although infection with *E bieneusi* is limited to the intestine, the organism has also been found in the biliary system and has been implicated in acalculous cholecystitis and, most recently, identified in bronchoalveolar lavage fluid in AIDS patients.[182–184] *S intestinalis* can cause more disseminated disease because of its propensity to invade macrophages in addition to enterocytes and to cause disease in the lungs, liver, and kidneys.[185,186]

Infection with microsporidia is characterized by nonbloody diarrhea with cramping abdominal pain and gradual weight loss, but it can be severe enough to necessitate electrolyte replacement. Patients usually lack fever and anorexia. Malabsorption may be present.[187,188] Diagnosis may be delayed because of the intermittent nature of the illness. Repeatedly negative results of stool studies, including fecal leukocytes, bacteria, mycobacteria, and other protozoa or parasites, suggests infection with microsporidia. Usually, patients have prolonged and severe immunosuppression, with CD4 counts lower than 50 cells/mm^3. Elevated alkaline phosphatase levels may be suggestive of biliary involvement.[182,183,186] The mechanism by which microsporidia produce diarrhea and wasting is unknown. Malabsorption may play a part; some have suggested that the parasite has the ability to induce a secretory process within the small intestine.[187]

The diagnosis of microsporidial infection may be difficult to establish, especially in inexperienced laboratories, and its prevalence is probably underestimated among AIDS patients with diarrhea. Usually, electron microscopic examination of enteric biopsies is required.[188,189] Recently, light microscopy and concentrated Giemsa staining of stool specimens or a modified trichrome or chromotrope stain have been used to detect organisms.[190,191]

No therapeutic agent has consistently been effective against microsporidia, although recently albendazole appears to be a promising agent, particularly in patients infected with *S intestinalis*.[187] Response to therapy is often dramatic in patients with *S intestinalis* infection, with rapid improvement of symptoms within days and eradication of organisms from the stool.[187] Albendazole is less effective in patients with *E bieneusi*.[187] No well controlled trial has been done to assess albendazole therapy, and optimal dose and length of therapy are unknown. In addition, albendazole does not currently have approval of the US Food and Drug Administration and must be obtained on a compassionate-use basis. There are anecdotal reports of variable responses to metronidazole.[177,178,192] Patients frequently experience improvement in symptoms with the use of antisecretory drugs such as loperamide or Lomotil. Nutritional therapy directed at minimizing the symptoms of malabsorption through change in diet from fat to simple carbohydrates and nutritional supplements may also be of some benefit.[187]

ISOSPORIASIS

Infection of AIDS patients with *Isospora belli*, another coccidian, can cause severe and protracted diarrhea that clinically resembles cryptosporidiosis. Crampy abdominal pain, weight loss, malaise, and fever are part of this syndrome. Steatorrhea may result. Eosinophilia may be present.[168] Although a relatively uncommon cause of diarrhea in AIDS patients in the United States, it can be implicated in enteric infection in 15% to 20% of Haitian and African patients with AIDS.[168,193,194] Although the organism is predominately found in the small intestine, *I belli* has been identified throughout the gastrointestinal tract and, rarely, in other organs.[193]

The diagnosis of isosporiasis is made by the detection of large oval oocysts (20 to 30 μm by 10 to 20 μm) in the stool by the modified acid-fast method or by wet mount.[195] *I belli* oocysts can be differentiated from *Cryptosporidium* cysts by size, shape, and number of oocysts. Biopsy of the small intestine may show organisms within the lumen or within cytoplasmic vacuoles in enterocytes, localized mucosal inflammation, and atrophy.[196]

A 10-day course of therapy with TMP-SMX is highly effective in the treatment of *I belli*; symptoms resolve rapidly, and oocysts are eradicated from the stool.[194,197] Maintenance therapy with TMP-SMX three times weekly for continual suppression is recommended because of reports of relapses occurring in half of treated patients after the completion of therapy. In patients who are intolerant of sulfa, pyrimethamine, metronidazole, or quinacrine may be used.[168,198]

CYCLOSPORIASIS

Cyclospora has been isolated from the stools of AIDS patients with diarrhea.[199–203] The organism is classified in this genus based on in vitro sporulation and excystation studies and by appearance on electron microscopy.[204] This organism has been reported to cause prolonged but ultimately self-limited diarrheal illness in travelers. It was initially recovered from Haitian patients with AIDS who had diarrhea.[200–204]

Examination of the stools revealed acid-fast cryptosporidium-like organisms that uncharacteristically responded to TMP-SMX. The organism was called "Big crypto" and was characterized by its size (8 to 9 μm), which was between those of *Cryptosporidium* and *I belli*. Limited epidemiologic and environmental data support the hypothesis that this organism is waterborne.[205]

The response to therapy with TMP-SMX is similar to that observed in isosporiasis; symptoms resolve within 2 to 3 days. Secondary prophylaxis is also successful and is recommended, given the high rate of recurrence.[206]

Several theories may explain the low incidence of cyclosporiasis as an opportunistic infection in patients with AIDS in the United States, including the lack of routine screening of stool samples for acid-fast organisms, confusion with *Cryptosporidium* given the size of oocysts, the frequent use of TMP-SMX for therapy and prophylaxis for *T gondii* and *P carinii*.[206]

REFERENCES

1. Kovacs JA, Masur H. Prophylaxis for *Pneumocystis carinii* pneumonia in patients infected with human immunodeficiency virus. Clin Infect Dis 1992;14:1005.
2. US Public Health Service Task Force on Antipneumocystis Prophylaxis in Patients with Human Immunodeficiency Virus Infection. Recommendations for prophylaxis against *Pneumocystis carinii* pneumonia for persons infected with human immunodeficiency virus. J Acquir Immune Defic Syndr 1993;6:46.
3. Masur H, Lane HC, Kovacs JA, et al. Advances in *Pneumocystis* pneumonia: from bench to clinic. Ann Intern Med 1989;111:813.
4. Hughes WT. Geographic distribution. In: Hughes WT, ed. *Pneumocystis carinii* pneumonitis, vol 1. Boca Raton, FL: CRC Press, 1987:33.
5. Kovacs JA, Halpern JL, Swan JC, eet al. Identification of antigens and antibodies specific for *Pneumocystis carinii*. J Immunol 1988;140:2023.
6. Peglow SL, Smulian AG, Linke MJ, et al. Serologic responses to *Pneumocystis carinii* antigens in health and disease. J Infect Dis 1990;161:296.
7. Peters SE, Wakeneld AE, Sinclair K, et al. A search for *Pneumocystis carinii* in post-mortem lungs by DNA amplification. J Pathol 1992;166:195.
8. Hughes WT. Natural mode of acquisition for de novo infection with *Pneumocystis carinii*. J Infect Dis 1982;145:842.
9. Roths JB, Sidman CL. Single and combined humoral and cell mediated immunotherapy of *Pneumocystis carinii* pneumonia in immunodeficient SCID mice. Infect Immun 1993;61:1641.
10. Masur H, Ognibene FP, Yarchoan R, et al. CD4 counts as predictors of opportunistic pneumonias in human immunodeficiency virus (HIV) infection. Ann Intern Med 1989;111:223.
11. Phair J, Munoz A, Detels R, et al. The risk of *Pneumocystis carinii* pneumonia among men infected with HIV-1. N Engl J Med 1990;322:1607.
12. Kovacs JA, Hiemenz JW, Macher AM, et al. *Pneumocystis carinii* pneumonia: a comparison between patients with the acquired immunodeficiency syndrome and patients with other immunodeficiencies. Ann Intern Med 1984;100:663.
13. Raviglione MC. Extrapulmonary pneumocystosis: the first 50 cases. Rev Infect Dis 1990;12:1127.
14. Coulman CU, Greene I, Archibald RW. Cutaneous pneumocystosis. Ann Intern Med 1987;106:396.
15. Gherman CR, Ward RR, Bassis ML. *Pneumocystis carinii* otitis media and mastoiditis as the initial manifestation of the acquired immunodeficiency syndrome. Am J Med 1988;85:250.
16. Smith RL, Ripps CS, Lewis ML. Elevated lactate dehydrogenase values in patients with *Pneumocystis carinii* pneumonia. Chest 1988;93:987.

17. Zaman MK, White DA. Serum lactate dehydrogenase levels and *Pneumocystis carinii* pneumonia: diagnostic and prognostic significance. Am Rev Respir Dis 1988;37:796.
18. Goodman PC. *Pneumocystis carinii* pneumonia. J Thorac Imaging 1991;6:16.
19. Brenner M, Ognibene FP, Lack EE, et al. Prognostic factors and life expectancy of patients with acquired immunodeficiency syndrome and *Pneumocystis carinii* pneumonia. Am Rev Respir Dis 1987;136:1199.
20. DeLorenzo LJ, Huang CT, Maguire GP, et al. Roentgenographic patterns of *Pneumocystis carinii* pneumonia in 104 patients with AIDS. Chest 1987;91:323.
21. Metersky ML, Catanzaro A. Diagnostic approach to *Pneumocystis carinii* pneumonia in the setting of prophylactic aerosolized pentamidine. Chest 1991;100:1345.
22. Garay S, Greene J. Prognostic indicators in the initial presentation of *Pneumocystis* pneumonia. Chest 1989;95:769.
23. Murray JF, Felton CP, Garay SM, et al. Pulmonary complications of the acquired immunodeficiency syndrome: report of a National Heart, Lung, and Blood Institute workshop. N Engl J Med 1984;310:1682.
24. Elvin KM, Lunbwo CM, Luo NP, et al. *Pneumocystis carinii* is not a major cause of pneumonia in HIV-infected patients in Lusada, Zambia. Trans R Soc Trop Med Hyg 1989;83:553.
25. Hartman B, Koss M, Hui A, et al. *Pneumocystis carinii* pneumonia in the acquired immunodeficiency syndrome (AIDS): diagnosis with bronchial brushings, biopsy, and bronchoalveolar lavage. Chest 1985;87:603.
26. Ognibene FP, Shelhamer J, Gill V, et al. The diagnosis of *Pneumocystis carinii* pneumonia in patients with the acquired immunodeficiency syndrome using subsegmental bronchoalveolar lavage. Am Rev Respir Dis 1984;129:929.
27. Kovacs JA, Ng VL, Masur, et al. Diagnosis of *Pneumocystis carinii* pneumonia: improved detection in sputum with the use of monoclonal antibodies. N Engl J Med 1988;318:589.
28. Ng, Virani NA, Chaisson RE, et al. Rapid detection of *Pneumocystis carinii* using a direct fluorescent monoclonal antibody stain. J Clin Microbiol 1990;128:2228.
29. Bigby TD, Margolskii D, Curtis JL, et al. The usefulness of induced sputum in the diagnosis of *Pneumocystis carinii* pneumonia in patients with the acquired immunodeficiency syndrome. Am Rev Respir Dis 1986;133:515.
30. Walzer PD, Perl DP, Krogstad DJ, Rawson PG, Schultz MG. *Pneumocystis carinii* pneumonia in the United States: epidemiologic, diagnostic, and clinical features. Ann Intern Med 1974;80:83.
31. Pitchenik AE, Ganjei P, Torres A, et al. Sputum examination for the diagnosis of *Pneumocystis carinii* pneumonia in the acquired immunodeficiency syndrome. Am Rev Respir Dis 1986;33:226.
32. Levine SJ, Masur H, Gill VJ, et al. Effect of aerosolized pentamidine prophylaxis on the diagnosis of *Pneumocystis carinii* pneumonia by induced sputum examination in patients infected with the human immunodeficiency virus. Am Rev Respir Dis 1991;144:760.
33. Hughes WT. Current status of laboratory diagnosis of *Pneumocystis carinii* pneumonitis. Crit Rev Clin Lab Sci 1975;6:145.
34. Smith JW, Bartlett MS. Laboratory diagnosis of *Pneumocystis carinii* infection. Clin Lab Med 1982;2:393.
35. Gill VJ, Evans G, Stock F, et al. Detection of *Pneumocystis carinii* by fluorescent-antibody stain using a combination of three monoclonal antibodies. J Clin Microbiol 1987;25:1837.
36. Kovacs JA, Halpern JL, Lundgren B, et al. Monoclonal antibodies to *Pneumocystis carinii*: identification of specific antigens and characterization of antigenic differences between rat and human isolates. J Infect Dis 1989;159:60.
37. Lipschik GY, Gill VJ, Lundgren JD, et al. Improved diagnosis of *Pneumocystis carinii* infection by polymerase chain reaction on induced sputum and blood. Lancet 1992;340:203.
38. Broaddus VC, Dake MD, Stulbarg MS, et al. Bronchoalveolar lavage and transbronchial biopsy for the diagnosis of pulmonary infections in patients with the acquired immunodeficiency syndrome. Ann Intern Med 1985;102:747.
39. McKenna RJ Jr, Campbell A, McMurtrey MJ, et al. Diagnosis for interstitial lung disease in patients with acquired immunodeficiency syndrome (AIDS): a prospective comparison of bronchial washing, alveolar lavage, transbronchial lung biopsy, and open-lung biopsy. Ann Thorac Surg 1986;41:318.
40. Leoung GS, Feigel DW Jr, Montgomery AB, et al. Aerosolized pentamidine for prophylaxis against *Pneumocystis carinii* pneumonia: the San Francisco community prophylaxis trial. N Engl J Med 1990;323:769.
41. Medina I, Mills J, Leoung G, et al. Oral therapy for *Pneumocystis carinii* pneumonia in the acquired immunodeficiency syndrome: a controlled trial of trimethoprim-sulfamethoxazole versus trimethoprim-dapsone. N Engl J Med 1990;323:776.
42. Ruf B, Rohde I, Pohle HD. Efficacy of clindamycin-primaquine vs. trimethoprim-sulfamethoxazole in primary treatment of *Pneumocystis carinii* pneumonia. Eur J Clin Microbiol Infect Dis 1991;10:207.
43. Toma E. Clindamycin-primaquine for treatment of *Pneumocystis carinii* pneumonia in AIDS. Eur J Clin Microbiol Infect Dis 1991;10:210.
44. Hughes WT, Leoung G, Kramer R, et al. Comparison of atovaquone (566C80) with trimethoprim-sulfamethoxazole to treat *Pneumocystis carinii* pneumonia in patients with AIDS. N Engl J Med 1993;328:1521.
45. Masur H. Drug therapy: prevention and treatment of pneumocystis pneumonia. N Engl J Med 1992;327:1853.
46. Catterall JR, Potasman I, Remington JS. *Pneumocystis carinii* pneumonia in the patient with AIDS. Chest 1985;88:758.
47. Castellano AR, Nettlemen MD. Cost and benefit of secondary prophylaxis for *Pneumocystis carinii* pneumonia. JAMA 1991;266:820.
48. Gordin FM, Simon GL, Wofsy CD, Mills J. Adverse reactions to trimethoprim-sulfamethoxazole in patients with acquired immunodeficiency syndrome. Ann Intern Med 1984;100:495.
49. Wachter RM, Luce JM, Turner J, et al. Intensive care of patients with the acquired immunodeficiency syndrome: outcome and changing patterns of utilization. Am Rev Respir Dis 1986;134:891.
50. Hardy WD, Reinberg J, Finkelstein DM, et al. A controlled trial of trimethoprim-sulfamethoxazole or aerosolized pentamidine for secondary prophylaxis of *Pneumocystis carinii* pneumonia in patients with the acquired immunodeficiency syndrome: AIDS Clinical Trials Group 021. N Engl J Med 1992;327:1842.
51. Schneider MME, Hoepelman AI, Eeftinck Schattenkerk JK, et al. A controlled trial of aerosolized pentamidine or trimethoprim-sulfamethoxazole as primary prophylaxis against *Pneumocystis carinii* pneumonias in patients with human immunodeficiency virus infection. N Engl J Med 1992;327:1836.
52. Van der Ven AJAM, Koopmans PP, Vree TB, Van der Meer JWM. Adverse reactions to co-trimoxazole in HIV infection. Lancet 1991;338:431.
53. Rubin RH, Iwamoto GK, Richerson HB, Flaherty JP. Trimethoprim-sulfamethoxazole desensitization in the acquired immunodeficiency syndrome. (Letter) Ann Intern Med 1987;106:355.
54. Kelly JW, Dolley DP, Lattuada CP, Smith CE. A severe unusual reaction to trimethoprim-sulfamethoxazole in patients infected with human immunodeficiency virus. Clin Infect Dis 1992;14:1034.
55. Martin GJ, Paparello SF, Decker CF. A severe systemic reaction to trimethoprim-sulfamethoxazole in a patient infected with the human immunodeficiency virus. Clin Infect Dis 1992;16:175.
56. Conte JE Jr, Hollander H, Golden JA. Inhaled pentamidine or reduced dose intravenous pentamidine for *Pneumocystis carinii* pneumonia: a pilot study. Ann Intern Med 1987;107:495.
57. Conte JE Jr, Chernoff D, Feigel DW Jr, et al. Intravenous or inhaled pentamidine for treating *Pneumocystis carinii* pneumonia in AIDS. Ann Intern Med 1990;113:203.
58. Mallory DL, Parrillo JE, Bailey DR, et al. Cardiovascular effects and safety of intravenous and intramuscular pentamidine isethionae. Crit Care Med 1987;15:503.
59. Stahl Bayliss CM, Kalman CM, Laskin OL. Pentamidine-induced hypoglycemia in patients with the acquired immune deficiency syndrome. Clin Pharmacol Ther 1986;39:271.
60. Waskin H, Stehr Green JK, Helmick CG, et al. Risk factors for hypoglycemia associated with pentamidine therapy for *Pneumocystis* pneumonia. JAMA 1988;260:345.
61. Wharton JM, Coleman DL, Wofsy CB, et al. Trimethoprim-sulfamethoxazole or pentamidine for *Pneumocystis carinii* pneumonia in the acquired immunodeficiency syndrome: a prospective randomized trial. Ann Intern Med 1986;105:37.
62. Conte JE Jr, Upton RA, Phelps RT, Wofsy CB, Zurlinden E, Lin ET. Use of a specific and sensitive assay to determine pentamidine pharmacokinetics in patients with AIDS. J Infect Dis 1986;154:923.
63. Montgomery AB, Debs RJ, Luce JM, et al. Aerosolized pentamidine as a second-line therapy in patients with the acquired immunodefi-

ciency syndrome and *Pneumocystis carinii* pneumonia. Chest 1989;95:747.

64. Montgomery AB, Eidson RE, Sattler F, et al. Aerosolized pentamidine vs. trimethoprim-sulfamethoxazole for acute *Pneumocystis carinii* pneumonia: a randomized double-blind trial. Abstract ThB395. Sixth International Conference on AIDS, San Francisco, 1990.

65. Mills J, Leoung G, Medina I, et al. Dapsone treatment of *Pneumocystis carinii* pneumonia in the acquired immunodeficiency syndrome. Antimicrob Agents Chemother 1988;32:1057.

66. Safrin S, Sattler FR, Lee BL, et al. Dapsone as a single agent as suboptimal therapy for *Pneumocystis carinii* pneumonia. J Acquir Immune Defic Syndr 1991;4:244.

67. Leoung GS, Mills J, Hopewell PC, et al. Dapsone-trimethoprim for *Pneumocystis carinii* pneumonia in the acquired immunodeficiency syndrome. Ann Intern Med 1986;105:45.

68. Falloon J, Kovacs J, Hughes W, et al. A preliminary evaluation of 566C80 for the treatment of *Pneumocystis carinii* pneumonia in patients with the acquired immunodeficiency syndrome. N Engl J Med 1991;325:1534.

69. Dohn MN, Weinberg WG, Torres RA, et al. Oral atovaquone compared with intravenous pentamidine for *Pneumocystis carinii* pneumonia in patients with AIDS. Ann Intern Med 1994;121:174.

70. Allegra CJ, Chabner BA, Tuazon CU, et al. Trimetrexate for the treatment of *Pneumocystis carinii* pneumonia in patients with the acquired immunodeficiency syndrome. N Engl J Med 1987;317:978.

71. Sattler FR, Frame P, Davis R, et al. Comparison of trimetrexate with leucovorin versus trimethoprim-sulfamethoxazole for moderate to severe episodes of *Pneumocystis carinii* pneumonia in patients with AIDS. J Infect Dis 1994;170:165.

72. Golden JA, Sjoerdsma A, Santi DV. *Pneumocystis carinii* pneumonia treated with alpha-difluoromethylornithine. West J Med 1984;141:613.

73. Kovacs JA, Allegra CJ, Beaver J, et al. Characterization of de novo folate synthesis in *Pneumocystis carinii* and *Toxoplasma gondii*: Potential utilization for screening therapeutic agents. J Infect Dis 1989;160:312.

74. Shear HL, Valladares G, Naachi MA. Enhanced treatment of *Pneumocystis carinii* pneumonia in rats with interferon-gamma and reduced doses of trimethoprim-sulfamethoxazole. J Acquir Immune Defic Syndr 1990;3:943.

75. Gigliotti F, Hughes WT. Passive immunoprophylaxis with specific monoclonal antibody confers partial protection against *Pneumocystis carinii* pneumonitis in animal models. J Clin Invest 1988;81:1666.

76. Harmsen AG, Stankiewicz M. Requirement for CD4+ cells in resistance to *Pneumocystis carinii* pneumonia in mice. J Exp Med 1990;172:937.

77. Pesanti EL. Interaction of cytokines and alveolar cells with *Pneumocystis carinii* in vitro. J Infect Dis 1991;163:661.

78. Pottratz ST, Martin WJ II. Role of fibronectin in *Pneumocystis carinii* attachment to cultured lung cells.

79. Bozzette SA, Sattler FR, Chiu J, et al. A controlled trial of early adjunctive treatment with corticosteroids for *Pneumocystis carinii* pneumonia in acquired immunodeficiency syndrome. N Engl J Med 1990;323:1451.

80. Gagnon S, Botta AM, Fischl MA, Daier H, Kirksey OW, LaVoie L. Corticosteroids as adjunctive therapy for severe *Pneumocystis carinii* pneumonia in the acquired immunodeficiency syndrome: a double-blind, placebo-controlled trial. N Engl J Med 1990;323:1444.

81. Montaner JSG, Lawson LM, Levitt N, Belzberg A, Schechter MT, Ruedy J. Corticosteroids prevent early deterioration in patients with moderately severe *Pneumocystis carinii* pneumonia and the acquired immunodeficiency syndrome (AIDS). Ann Intern Med 1990;113:14.

82. The National Institutes of Health University of California Expert Panel for Corticosteroids as Adjunctive Therapy for *Pneumocystis* Pneumonia. Consensus statement on the use of corticosteroids as adjunctive therapy for *Pneumocystis* pneumonia in the acquired immunodeficiency syndrome. N Engl J Med 1990;323:1500.

83. Kales CP, Murren JR, Torres RA, et al. Early predictors of in hospital mortality for *Pneumocystis carinii* pneumonia in the acquired immunodeficiency syndrome. Arch Intern Med 1987;147:1413.

84. Shelhamer JH, Ognibene FP, Macher AM, et al. Persistence of *Pneumocystis carinii* in lung tissue of acquired immunodeficiency syndrome patients treated for *Pneumocystis* pneumonia. Am Rev Respir Dis 1984;130:1161.

85. el Dasr WM, Simberkoff MS. Survival and prognostic factors in severe *Pneumocystis carinii* pneumonia requiring mechanical ventilation. Am Rev Respir Dis 1988;137:1264.

86. Schein RM, Fischl MA, Pitchenik AE, Sprung CL. ICU survival of patients with the acquired immunodeficiency syndrome. Crit Care Med 1986;14:1026.

87. Kovacs JA, Masur H. *Pneumocystis carinii* pneumonia: therapy and prophylaxis. J Infect Dis 1988;158:254.

88. Wachter RM, Russi MB, Block DA, et al. *Pneumocystis carinii* pneumonia and respiratory failure in AIDS: improved outcomes and increased use of intensive care units. Am Rev Respir Dis 1991;143:251.

89. Wachter RM, Luce JM, Hopewell PC. Critical care of patients with AIDS. JAMA 1992;267:541.

90. Fischl MA, Richman DD, Grieco MH, et al. The efficacy of azidothymidine (AZT) in the treatment of patients with AIDS and AIDS related complex. N Engl J Med 1987;317:185.

91. Hughes WT, Kuhn S, Chaudhary S, et al. Successful chemoprophylaxis for *Pneumocystis carinii* pneumonitis. N Engl J Med 1877;297:1419.

92. Fischl M, Dickinson GM, LaVoie. Safety and efficacy of sulfamethoxazole and trimethoprim chemoprophylaxis for *Pneumocystis carinii* pneumonia in AIDS. JAMA 1988;259:1185.

93. Bozzette SA, Finkelstein DM, Spector SA, et al. A randomized trial of three antipneumocystis agents in patients with advanced human immunodeficiency virus infection. N Engl J Med 1995;332:693.

94. Carr A, Tindall D, Brew BJ, et al. Low-dose trimethoprim-sulfamethoxazole prophylaxis for toxoplasmic encephalitis in patients with AIDS. Ann Intern Med 1992;117:106.

95. Montaner JSG, Lawson LM, Gervais A, et al. Aerosol pentamidine for secondary prophylaxis of AIDS-related *Pneumocystis carinii* pneumonia: a randomized placebo-controlled study. Ann Intern Med 1991;114;948.

96. Murphy RL, Lavelle JF, Allan JD, et al. Aerosol pentamidine prophylaxis following *Pneumocystis carinii* pneumonia in AIDS patients: results of blinded dose-comparison study using ultrasonic nebulizer. Am J Med 1991;90:418.

97. Baskin MI, ABD AG, Howitz JS. Regional deposition of aerosolized pentamidine: effects of body position and breathing pattern. Ann Intern Med 1990;113:677.

98. O'Doherty MJ, Thomas S, Page C, Bradeer C, Nunan TO, Bateman NT. Does inhalation of pentamidine in the supine position increase deposition in the upper part of the lung? Chest 1990;97:1343.

99. Hardy WD, Northfelt DW, Drake TA. Fatal disseminated pneumocystosis in patient with acquired immunodeficiency syndrome receiving prophylactic aerosolized pentamidine. Am J Med 1989;87:329.

100. Telzak EE, Cote RJ, Gold JWM, Campbell SW, Armstrong D. Extrapulmonary *Pneumocystis carinii* infection. Rev Infect Dis 1990;12:380.

101. Centers for Disease Control. Guidelines for preventing the transmission of mycobacterium tuberculosis in health-care settings with special focus on HIV-related issues. MMWR 1990;39(RR17);1.

102. Lavelle J, Falloon J, Morgan A, et al. Weekly dapsone and dapsone/pyrimethamine for *Pneumocystis* pneumonia prophylaxis. Abstract 233. Seventh International Conference on AIDS, Florence, 1991.

103. Hauser WE, Luft BJ, Conley BK, et al. Central nervous system toxoplasmosis in homosexual and heterosexual adults. N Engl J Med 1982;307:498.

104. Luft BJ, Remington JS. Toxoplasmic encephalitis in AIDS. Clin Infect Dis 1992;15:211.

105. Cochereau-Massin I, LeHoang P, Lautier-Frau. Ocular toxoplasmosis in human immunodeficiency virus-infected patients. Am J Ophthalmol 1992;114:130.

106. Frenkel JK, Nelson BM, Arias-Stella J. Immunosuppression and toxoplasmic encephalitis. Hum Pathol 1975;6:97.

107. Oskenhendler E, Cadranel J, Sarfati C, et al. *Toxoplasma gondii* pneumonia in patients with the acquired immunodeficiency syndrome. Am J Med 1990;88:18N.

108. Partisani M, Candolfi H, DeMautort E, Bethencourt S, Lang JM. Seroprevalence of latent *Toxoplasma gondii* infection in HIV-infected individuals and long-term follow-up of *Toxoplasma* seronegative subjects. Abstract WP2294. Seventh International Conference on AIDS, Florence, June 1991.

109. Cohn JA, McMeeking A, Cohen W, et al. Evaluation of the policy of empiric treatment of suspected *Toxoplasma* encephalitis in patients with acquired immunodeficiency syndrome. Am J Med 1989;86:521.

110. Dannemann BR, McCutchan JA, Israelski DM, et al. Treatment of toxoplasmic encephalitis patients with AIDS: a randomized trial com-

paring pyrimethamine plus clindamycin to pyrimethamine plus sulfonamides. Ann Intern Med 1992;116:33.

111. Haverkos HW: Assessment of therapy for *Toxoplasma* encephalitis. Am J Med 1987;82:907.

112. Navia BA, Petito CK, Gold JWM, et al: Cerebral toxoplasmosis complicating AIDS: clinical and neuropathological findings in 27 patients. Ann Neurol 1986;19:224.

113. Leport C, Raffi F, Katlama C, et al. Treatment of central nervous system toxoplasmosis with pyrimethamine/sulfadiazine combination in 35 patients with acquired immunodeficiency syndrome. Am J Med 1988;84:94.

114. Levy RM, Bredesen DE. Central nervous system dysfunction in acquired immunodeficiency syndrome. J Acquir Immune Defic Syndr 1988;1:41.

115. Holland GN, Engstrom RE Jr, Glasgow BJ, et al. Ocular toxoplasmosis in patients with the acquired immunodeficiency syndrome. Am J Ophthalmol 1988;106:653.

116. Wanke C, Tuazon CU, Kovacs A, et al. *Toxoplasma* encephalitis in patients with acquired immune deficiency syndrome. Am J Trop Med Hyg 1987;36:509.

117. Levy RM, Breit R, Russell R, DalCanto MC. MRI-guided stereotaxic brain biopsy in neurologically symptomatic AIDS patients. J Acquire Immune Defic Syndr 1991;4:254.

118. Farkash AE, MacCabbee PJ, Sher JH. Central nervous system toxoplasmosis in AIDS: a clinical-pathological-radiological review of 12 cases. J Neurol Neurosurg Psychiatry 1986;49:744.

119. Elkin CM, Leon E, Grenell SL, et al. Intracranial lesions in the acquired immunodeficiency syndrome: radiological (CT) features. JAMA 1985;253:393.

120. Post MJD, Kursunoglu SJ, Hensley GT, et al. Cranial CT in AIDS: spectrum of disease and optimal contrast enhancement technique. AJNR Am J Neuroradiol 1984;6:743.

121. Post MJD, Chan JC, Hensley GT, et al. *Toxoplasma* encephalitis in Haitian adults with AIDS: a clinical-pathologic-CT correlation AJNR Am J Neuroradiol 1983;140:861.

122. Goldstein J, Dickson D, Moser F, et al. Primary central nervous system lymphoma in acquired immunodeficiency. Cancer 1991;67:2765.

123. Kupfer M, Zee CS, Colletti PM, et al. MRI evaluation of AIDS-related encephalopathy: toxoplasmosis vs. lymphoma. Magn Reson Imaging 1990;8:51.

124. Levy RM, Mills CM, Posin JP, et al. The efficacy and clinical impact of brain imaging in neurological symptomatic AIDS patients: a prospective CT/MRI study. J Acquir Immune Defic Syndr 1990;3:461.

125. Suzuki Y, Israelski DM, Dannemann BR, et al: Diagnosis of toxoplasmic encephalitis in patients with AIDS by using a new serologic method. J Clin Microbiol 1988;26:2541.

126. Luft BG, Remington JS. Toxoplasmosis of the central nervous system. In: Remington JS, Swartz MN, eds. Current topics in infectious diseases, vol 6. New York: McGraw-Hill, 1985:315.

127. Dement SH, Cox MC, Grupta PK. Diagnosis of central nervous system *Toxoplasma gondii* from the cerebrospinal fluid in a patient with AIDS. Diagn Cytopathol 1987;3:148.

128. Bottone EJ. Diagnosis of acute pulmonary toxoplasmosis by visualization of invasive and intracellular tachyzoites in Giemsa-stained smears of bronchoalveolar lavage fluid. J Clin Microbiol 1991;29:2626.

129. Derouin R, Mazeron MC, Garin YJF. Comparative study of tissue culture and mouse inoculation methods for demonstration of *Toxoplasma gondii*. J Clin Microbiol 1987;25:1597.

130. Parmley S, Goebel F, Remington JS. Detection of *Toxoplasma gondii* in cerebrospinal fluid from AIDS patients by polymerase chain reaction. J Clin Microbiol 1992;30:3000.

131. Ostergaard L, Nielsen AK, Black FT. DNA amplification on cerebrospinal fluid for diagnosis of cerebral toxoplasmosis among HIV-positive patients with signs or symptoms of neurological disease. Scand J Infect Dis 1993;25:227.

132. Holliman RE, Johnson JD, Savva D. Diagnosis of cerebral toxoplasmosis in association with AIDS using polymerase chain reaction. Scand J Infect Dis 1990;22:243.

133. Bretagne S, Costa J, Vidaud M, et al. Detection of *Toxoplasma gondii* by competitive DNA amplification of bronchoalveolar lavage samples. J Infect Dis 1993;168:1585.

134. Filice G, Hitt J, Mitchell C, et al. Diagnosis of *Toxoplasma* parasitemia in patients with AIDS by gene detection after amplification with polymerase chain reaction. J Clin Microbiol 1993;31:2327.

135. DeLaPaz R, Enzman D. Neuroradiology of acquired immunodeficiency syndrome. In: Rosenblum ML, ed. AIDS and the nervous system. New York: Raven Press, 1988:200.

136. Ciricillo SR, Rosenblum ML. Imaging of solitary lesions in AIDS. J Neurosurg 1991;74:1029.

137. Weiss LM, Harris C, Berger M, et al. Pyrimethamine concentrations in serum and cerebrospinal fluid during treatment of acute *Toxoplasma* encephalitis in patients with AIDS. J Infect Dis 1988;157:580.

138. Luft BJ, Remington JS. Toxoplasmic encephalitis. J Infect Dis 1988;157:1.

139. Kaufman HE, Geisler PH. The hematologic toxicity of pyrimethamine (daraprim) in man. Arch Ophthalmol 1960;64:140.

140. Chang HR, Perchere JC. In vitro effects of four macrolides roxithromycin, spiramycin, azithromycin (CP-62,93) and A-56268 on *Toxoplasma gondii*. Antimicrob Agents Chemother 1988;32:524.

141. Araujo FG, Shepard RM, Remington JS. In vivo activity of the macrolide antibiotics azithromycin, roxithromycin and spiramycin against *Toxoplasma gondii*. Eur J Clin Microbiol Infect Dis 1991;10:519.

142. Fernandez-Martin J, Leport C, Morlat P, et al. Pyrimethamine-clarithromycin combination for therapy of acute *Toxoplasma* encephalitis in patients with AIDS. Antimicrob Agents Chemother 1991;35:2049.

143. Araujo FG, Huskinson J, Remington JS. Remarkable in vitro and in vivo activities of the hydroxynaphthoquinone 566C80 against tachyzoites and tissue cysts of *Toxoplasma gondii*. Antimicrob Agents Chemother 1991;35:293.

144. Kovacs JA. Efficacy of atovaquone in treatment of toxoplasmosis in patients with AIDS. Lancet 1992;340:637.

145. Clumeck N, Katlama C, Ferrero T, et al. Atovaquone (14 hydroxynaphthoquinone 566C80) in the treatment of acute cerebral toxoplasmosis in AIDS patients. Abstract 1217. Eighth International Conference on AIDS, Amsterdam, 1992.

146. Suzuki Y, Orellana MA, Schreiber RD, et al. Interferon-gamma: the major mediator of resistance against *Toxoplasma gondii*. Science 1988;240:516.

147. McCabe RE, Luft BJ, Remington JS. Effect of murine interferon gamma on murine toxoplasmosis. J Infect Dis 1084;150:961.

148. Luft BJ, Hafner R, Korzun AH, et al. Toxoplasmic encephalitis in patients with the acquired immunodeficiency syndrome. N Engl J Med 1993;329:995.

149. Walckenaer G, Leport C, Longuet P, et al. Relapses of brain toxoplasmosis in 15 AIDS patients. Abstract 251. Thirty-first Interscience Conference on Antimicrobial Agents Chemotherapy, Chicago, 1991.

150. Renold C, Sugar, Chave J-P, et al. Toxoplasmic encephalitis in patients with the acquired immunodeficiency syndrome. Medicine (Baltimore) 1992;71:224.

151. Leport C, Tournerie C, Raguin G, et al. Long-term follow-up of patients with AIDS on maintenance therapy for toxoplasmosis. Eur J Clin Microbiol 1989;160:312.

152. Leport C, Tournerie C, Raguin G, et al. Long-term follow-up of patients with AIDS on maintenance therapy for toxoplasmosis. Eur J Clin Microbiol Infect Dis 1991;10:191.

153. Heald A, Flepp M, Chave J-P, et al: Treatment of cerebral toxoplasmosis protects against *Pneumocystis cariini* pneumonia in patients with AIDS. Ann Intern Med 1991;115:760.

154. Ruf B, Schurmann D, Bergmann F, et al. Efficacy of pyrimethamine/sulfadoxine in the prevention of toxoplasmic encephalitis relapses and *Pneumocystis cariini* pneumonia in HIV-infected patients. Eur J Clin Microbiol Infect Dis 1993;12:325.

155. Jacobson MA, Beach CL, Child C, et al. Toxicity of clindamycin as prophylaxis for AIDS-associated toxoplasmic encephalitis. Lancet 1992;339:333.

156. Girard PM, Landman R, Gaudebout C, et al. Dapsone-pyrimethamine vs. aerosol pentamidine for primary prophylaxis of pneumocystosis and neurotoxoplasmosis. Abstract WeB1017. Seventh International Conference on AIDS/Third STD World Congress, Amsterdam, 1992.

157. Opravil M, Heald A, Lazzarin A, Hirschel B, Luthy R. Combined prophylaxis of *Pneumocystis cariini* pneumonia and toxoplasmosis: prospective, randomized trial of dapsone and pyrimethamine vs. aerosolized pentamidine. Abstract PoB3315. Eighth International Conference on AIDS/Third STD World Congress, Amsterdam, 1992.

158. Jacobson MA, Besch CL, Child C, et al. Primary prophylaxis with pyrimethamine for toxoplasmic encephalitis in patients with advanced human immunodeficiency virus disease: results of a randomized trial. J Infect Dis 1994;169:384.

159. Peterson C. Cryptosporidiosis in patients infected with the human immunodeficiency virus. Clin Infect Dis 1992;15:903.

160. Godwin TA. Cryptosporidiosis in the acquired immunodeficiency syndrome: a study of 15 autopsy cases. Hum Pathol 1991;22:1215.

161. Laughon BE, Druckman DA, Vernon A, et al. Prevalence of enteric pathogens in homosexual men with and without acquired immunodeficiency syndrome. Gastroenterology 1988;29:593.

162. Colbunders R, Francis H, Mann JM, et al. Persistent diarrhea strongly associated with HIV infection in Kinshasa, Zaire. Am J Gastroenterol 1987;82:859.

163. Saltzberg DM, Kotloff KL, Newman JL, Fastiggi R. *Cryptosporidium* infection in acquired immunodeficiency syndrome: not always a poor prognosis. J Clin Gastroenterol 1991;13:94.

164. Connolly GM, Dryden MS, Shanson DC, Gazzard BG. Cryptosporidial diarrhoea in AIDS and its treatment. Gut 1988;29:593.

165. Greenberg RE, Mir R, Bank S, Siegal FP. Resolution of intestinal cryptosporidiosis after treatment of AIDS with AZT. Gastroenterology 1989;97:1327.

166. Flanigan T, Whalen C, Turner J, et al. *Cryptosporidium* infection and CD4 counts. Ann Intern Med 1992;116:840.

167. Soave R, Armstrong D: *Cryptosporidium* and cryptosporidiosis. Rev Infect Dis 1986;8:1012.

168. Soave R, Johnson WD Jr. *Cryptosporidium* and *Isospora belli* infections. J Infect Dis 1988;157:225.

169. Schneiderman DJ, Cello Jp, Laing FC. Papillary stenosis and sclerosing cholangitis in the acquired immunodeficiency syndrome. Ann Intern Med 1987;106:546.

170. Brady E, Margolis ML, Korzeniowski OM. Pulmonary cryptosporidiosis in acquired immune deficiency syndrome. JAMA 1984;252:89.

171. Connolly GM, Youle M, Gazzard BG. Diclazuril in the treatment of severe cryptosporidial diarrhoea in AIDS patients. AIDS 1990;4:700.

172. Nord J, Ma P, DiJohn D, Tzipori S, Tacket CO. Treatment with bovine hyperimmune colostrum of cryptosporidial diarrhoea in patients. AIDS 1990;4:581.

173. Blanshard C, Shanson DS, Gazzard BG. Azithromycin, paromomycin and letrazuril in the treatment of cryptosporidiosis. Abstract. Third European Conference on Clinical Aspects and Treatment of HIV Infection, Paris, 1992:P28.

174. Cello JP, Grendell JH, Basul P, et al. Effect of octreotide on refractory AIDS-associated diarrhea: a prospective, multicenter clinical trial. Ann Intern Med 1991;115:705.

175. Fichtenbaum CJ, Ritchie DJ, Powderly WG. Use of paromomycin for treatment of cryptosporidiosis in patients with AIDS. Clin Infect Dis 1993;16:298.

176. Bissuel R, Cotte I, Rabodonirina M, Rougier P, Piens M-A, Trepo C. Paromomycin: an effective treatment for cryptosporidial diarrhea in patients with AIDS. Clin Infect Dis 1994;18:447.

177. Eeftinck-Schattenkerk JK, van Gool T, van Ketel RJ, et al. Clinical significance of small-intestinal microsporidiosis in HIV-2–infected individuals. Lancet 1991;337:895.

178. Molina JM, Sarfati C, Beauvais B, et al. Intestinal microsporidiosis in human immunodeficiency virus-infected patients with chronic unexplained diarrhea: prevalence and clinical and biologic features. J Infect Dis 1993;167:217.

179. Rabeneck L, Gyorky F, Gerta RM, et al. The role of microsporidia in the pathogenesis of HIV-related chronic diarrhea. Ann Intern Med 1993;119:895.

180. Cali A, Kotler DP, Orenstein JM. *Septata intestinalis* N.G., N. Sp., an intestinal microsporidian associated with chronic diarrhea and dissemination in AIDS patients. J Eur Microbiol 1993;40:101.

181. Orenstein JM, Tenner M, Kotler DP. Localization of infection by the microsporidian *Enterocytozoon bieneusi* in the gastrointestinal tract of AIDS patients with diarrhea. AIDS 1992;6:195.

182. Beaugerie L, Teilhac M-F, Deluol A-M, et al. Cholangiopathy associated with *Microsporidia* infection of the common bile duct mucosa in a patient with HIV infection. Ann Intern Med 1992;117:401.

183. Pol S, Romana CA, Richard S, et al. Microsporidia infection in patients with the human immunodeficiency virus and unexplained cholangitis. N Engl J Med 1993;328:95.

184. Weber R, Kuster H, Keller R, et al. Pulmonary and intestinal microsporidiosis in a patient with the acquired immunodeficiency syndrome. Am Rev Respir Dis 1992;146:1603.

185. Orenstein JM, Tenner M, Cali A, Kotler DP. A microsporidian previously undescribed in humans, infecting enterocytes and macrophages, and associated with diarrhea in an acquired immunodeficiency syndrome patient. Hum Pathol 1992;23:722.

186. Orenstein JM, Dieterich DT, Kotler DP. Systemic dissemination by a newly recognized intestinal microsporidia species in AIDS. AIDS 1992;6:1143.

187. Asmuth DM, DeGirolami PC, Federman M, et al. Clinical features of microsporidiosis in patients with AIDS. Clin Infect Dis 1994;18:819.

188. Modigliani R, Bories C, Le Charpentier Y, et al. Diarrhoea and malabsorption in acquired immune deficiency syndrome: a study of four cases with special emphasis on opportunistic protozoan infestations. Gut 1985;26:179.

189. Dobbins WO III, Weinstein WM. Electron microscopy of the intestine and rectum in acquired immunodeficiency syndrome. Gastroenterology 1985;88:738.

190. van Gool T, Hollister WS, Eeftinck-Schattenkerk J, et al. Diagnosis of *Enterocytozoon bieneusi* microsporidiosis in AIDS patients by recovery of spores from faeces. Lancet 1990;336:697.

191. Rijpstra AC, Canning EU, van Ketel RJ, Edftinck-Schattenkerk JK, Laarman JJ. Use of light microscopy to diagnose small-intestinal microsporidiosis in patients with AIDS. J Infect Dis 1988;157:827.

192. Hing M, Field A, Harkness J, Marriott D. Enteric microsporidiosis: incidence and response to albendazole or metronidazole therapy. Abstract PoB3344. In: Poster abstracts of the Eighth International Conference on AIDS, Amsterdam, 1992;2:B144.

193. Restrepo C, Macher AM, Radany EH. Disseminated extraintestinal isosporiasis in a patient with acquired immunodeficiency syndrome. Am J Clin Pathol 1987;87:536.

194. DeHovitz JA, Pape JW, Boncy M, Johnson WD Jr. Clinical manifestations and therapy of *Isospora belli* infections in patients with the acquired immunodeficiency syndrome. N Engl J Med 1986;315:87.

195. Ng E, Markell EK, Fleming RL, Fried M. Demonstration of *Isospora belli* by acid-fast stain in a patient with acquired immune deficiency syndrome. J Clin Microbiol 1984;20:384.

196. Quinn TJ. Protozoan infections. In: Smith PD, moderator. Gastrointestinal infections in AIDS. Ann Intern Med 1992;116:66.

197. Pape JW, Verdier R-I, Johnson WD Jr. Treatment and prophylaxis of *Isospora belli* infection in patients with the acquired immunodeficiency syndrome. N Engl J Med 1989;320:1044.

198. Weiss LM, Perlman DC, Sherman J, et al. *Isospora belli* infection: treatment with pyrimethamine. Ann Intern Med 1988;109:474.

199. Hart AS, Ridinger MT, Soundarafan R, Peters CS, Swiatio AL, Kocka FE. Novel organisms associated with chronic diarrhoea in AIDS. Lancet 1990;335:169.

200. Long EG, Ebrahimzadeh A, White EH, Swisher B, Callaway CS. Alga associated with diarrhea in patients with acquired immunodeficiency syndrome and in travelers. J Clin Microbiol 1990;28:1101.

201. Bendall RP, Lucas S, Moody A, Tovey G, Chiodini PL. Diarrhoea associated with cyanobacterium-like bodies: a new coccidian enteritis of man. Lancet 1993;341:590.

202. Wurtz RM, Kocka FE, Peters CS, Weldon-Linne CM, Kuritza A, Yungbluth P. Clinical characteristics of seven cases of diarrhea associated with a novel acid-fast organism in the stool. Clin Infect Dis 1993;16:136.

203. Hoge CW, Shlim DR, Rajah R, et al. Epidemiology of diarrheal illness associated with coccidian-like organism among travelers and foreign residents in Nepal. Lancet 1993;341:1175.

204. Ortega YR, Sterling CR, Gilman RH, Cama VA, Diaz F. *Cyclospora* species: a new protozoan pathogen of humans. N Engl J Med 1993;328:1308.

205. Shlim DR, Cohen MT, Eaton M, Rajah R, Long EG, Ungar BL. An alga-like organism associated with an outbreak of prolonged diarrhea among foreigners in Nepal. Am J Trop Med Hyg 1991;45:383.

206. Pape JW, Verdier R-I, Boncy M, Boncy J, Johnson WD Jr. *Cyclospora* infection in adults infected with HIV. Ann Intern Med 1994;121:654.

AIDS: Biology, Diagnosis, Treatment and Prevention, fourth edition, edited by Vincent T. DeVita, Jr., Samuel Hellman, and Steven A. Rosenberg. Lippincott–Raven Publishers, © 1997

14.2

Fungal Infections in Patients with the Acquired Immunodeficiency Syndrome

Michael A. Polis and Joseph A. Kovacs

Fungal infections are common complications of infection with the human immunodeficiency virus (HIV). Such infections can result in life-threatening meningitis or in discomforting but not debilitating oral thrush. This chapter reviews the clinical presentation and management of fungal infections in AIDS patients.

CRYPTOCOCCUS NEOFORMANS

C neoformans is the major cause of meningitis in AIDS patients, and it can also cause local organ dysfunction and disseminated disease. *C neoformans* is a yeast-like fungus that reproduces by budding.[1] It produces no known toxins, but it does have a large polysaccharide capsule that appears to play a role in protecting the organism from host defense mechanisms. There are four serotypes of *C neoformans*; based on several characteristics, including mating abilities, serotypes A and D are classified as *C neoformans* var *neoformans*, and B and C are classified as *C neoformans* var *gattii*.[1] Although B and C serotypes occasionally cause disease in non-AIDS patients, cryptococcosis in AIDS patients, both in the United States and in Africa, is caused almost exclusively by serotypes A and D.[2–4] Organisms isolated from AIDS patients have been reported to differ from those isolated from non-AIDS patients.[5] On primary culture in one study, isolates from AIDS patients grew as nonmucoid, pasty colonies, in contrast to the mucoid colonies of non-AIDS isolates. Further, the capsule of AIDS isolates has been reported to be significantly smaller than that of non-AIDS isolates.[5]

Epidemiology and Pathogenesis

C neoformans var *neoformans* is a ubiquitous fungus that can be isolated from a variety of environmental sites, including soil, and is found in especially high concentrations in pigeon feces[1]; *C neoformans* var *gattii* is found environmentally only in association with certain species of eucalyptus trees.[6] Initial infection occurs by the respiratory route, through inhalation of aerosolized organisms after exposure to environmental sources. There is no evidence that *C neoformans* can be contracted directly from humans or animals, and isolation of patients with active infection therefore is not necessary. In patients with intact immune systems, the infection is controlled in the lung, usually without causing serious complications. In immunocompromised patients, however, especially in patients with AIDS, the organism is inadequately controlled and can cause life-threatening extrapulmonary disease, primarily meningitis. Because there are no reliable serologic markers for prior exposure, it cannot at present be determined whether disease in immunosuppressed hosts results from primary infection or, as with many other opportunistic infections (eg, toxoplasmosis), from reactivation of latent, previously controlled infection.

The incidence of cryptococcosis in AIDS patients in the United States has been reported in larger studies to range from approximately 6% to 12%.[7–10] Among 160,000 AIDS patients reported to the Centers for Disease Control, cryptococcosis was identified, usually as the AIDS-defining diagnosis, in 1.5%. The annual prevalence among HIV-infected patients in New York City with clinical AIDS or CD4-positive T-lymphocyte counts lower than 200 cells/mm³ has been estimated at 6.1% to 8.5%.[11] Among 1115 homosexual men with AIDS in San Francisco who were observed until death occurred, 8.6% were diagnosed with cryptococcal disease at some point.[12] Longitudinal studies have suggested that cryptococcal disease is increasing in frequency, but this trend is

Michael A. Polis: Laboratory of Immunoregulation, National Institute of Allergy and Infectious Diseases.

Joseph A. Kovacs, CCMD, National Institutes of Health, Building 10, Room 7D43, 10 Center Drive MSC 1662, Bethesda, MD 20892-1662.

lost after correction for CD4 count.[13] Cryptococcosis has been reported to occur in 3.7% of AIDS patients in Great Britain, and it is a very common opportunistic infection in Africa, occurring in 13% to 17% of patients in one report.[14,15]

Cryptococcosis can present in HIV-infected patients either as the initial, AIDS-defining opportunistic process (42% to 75% of cases) or as a later process. If cryptococcosis is the initial manifestation, other opportunistic processes, such as *Pneumocystis carinii* pneumonia, are often identified simultaneously.[7–9,16] HIV-infected patients with low CD4 counts are at greatest risk for the development of cryptococcosis. A prospective prophylaxis study found a median CD4 count of well under 50 cells/mm³ immediately before the diagnosis of cryptococcosis.[17] In another report, 30 of 31 patients had CD4 counts lower than 100 cells/mm³ at the time of diagnosis.[18]

Clinical Manifestations

The most common site of infection with *C neoformans* in both AIDS and non-AIDS patients is the central nervous system (CNS).[7–9,16] *C neoformans* usually infects both the brain and the meninges diffusely, producing both meningitis and encephalitis. Occasionally, cryptococcomas, which are large focal lesions, develop. In four published series, meningitis, alone or together with extrameningeal disease, has been reported to occur in 67% to 85% of AIDS patients with cryptococcosis.[7–9,16] Cryptococcal meningitis in AIDS patients frequently presents in a subtle manner. Headache and fever are the most common manifestations, occurring in 60% to 100% of patients, and they may be the only presenting symptoms (Table 14.2-1).[7–9,16] Nausea or vomiting have been reported in about 40%. Meningeal signs and an altered mental status are seen in only about one fourth of patients, and seizures or focal neurologic abnormalities are seen infrequently. Symptoms are usually present for 2 to 4 weeks before diagnosis, although occasionally they may be present for up to 4 months.[16]

Abnormal computed tomography or magnetic resonance scans of the head have been reported in 20% to 30% of patients with meningitis, although the abnormalities were not always related to cryptococcosis. Abnormalities attributable to cryptococcosis have included multiple ring-enhancing lesions in patients with cryptococcomas, nonenhancing focal lesions, and meningeal enhancement.[8,9,16,19]

Examination of cerebrospinal fluid (CSF) in AIDS patients with cryptococcal meningitis usually reveals a large organism burden but often a minimal inflammatory response. Ten percent to 35% of patients have a CSF leukocyte count higher than 20 cells/mm³; 35% to 70% have an elevated CSF protein, and 17% to 64% have a low glucose concentration.[7–9,16] In one study, all three parameters were normal in 15% of patients[7]; in another, only 41% had at least one abnormality.[8] Despite the minimal CSF abnormalities, India ink preparations are positive in 64% to 88% of patients, and often many organisms are seen. CSF crypto-

TABLE 14.2-1. *Incidence of symptoms, signs, and laboratory values in patients with cryptococcal meningitis*

Characteristic	Incidence (%)
Headache	67–100
Fever	62–95
Altered mental status	18–28
Meningeal signs	25–30
Seizures	4–9
Focal neurologic abnormality	6–17
Positive serum cryptococcal antigen	94–100
Positive CSF cryptococcal antigen	91–100
Positive CSF India ink	64–88
Positive CSF culture	95–100
Abnormal CSF glucose	17–64
Abnormal CSF protein	35–69
Abnormal CSF leukocyte count	13–35

CSF, cerebrospinal fluid.
Data from references 7, 8, 9, and 16.

coccal antigen is present in more than 90% of patients with meningitis, and titers are often very elevated; titers were greater than 1:1024 in 39% to 48% of patients in two reports.[8,9] Patients with cryptococcomas may have a negative CSF cryptococcal antigen test.[16] Serum cryptococcal antigen is present in an even higher proportion of patients with meningitis (94% to 100%).[7–9,16] CSF culture for *C neoformans* is positive in almost 100% of patients with meningitis. Patients with cryptococcomas may have negative CSF cultures but positive biopsy cultures.[16]

Disease exclusively outside the CNS has been reported in 10% to 33% of AIDS patients with cryptococcosis. Pneumonia and fungemia are the most common extraneural presentations. Four percent to 10% of patients with cryptococcosis have presented with pneumonia without meningitis; up to 40% of all patients with cryptococcosis have evidence of pulmonary infection. Patients with pneumonia may present with fever, productive cough, dyspnea, and, occasionally, hemoptysis. On chest radiograph, a variety of abnormalities have been seen, including lobar consolidation, nodules that may cavitate, diffuse interstitial infiltrates, bilateral miliary infiltrates, pleural effusions, and hilar adenopathy. Chest radiographs may also be normal. Histopathologically, cryptococci are most often located in the interstitium of the alveoli but occasionally within capillaries and lymphatics[20] (Fig. 14.2-1). There is often little or no inflammatory response despite the presence of large numbers of organisms.

Fungemia as the sole manifestation of *C neoformans* infection has been noted in 4% to 8% of patients.[7,9] Positive blood cultures have also been reported in 33% to 68% of patients with meningitis.[7,8,16] Fungemia may be associated with minimal complaints; fever, malaise, and fatigue are often the only symptoms suggesting a systemic infection. Disseminated disease can also be documented by bone marrow biopsy.[21] In rare patients, all cultures are negative but serum cryptococcal antigen assays are positive.[7,9]

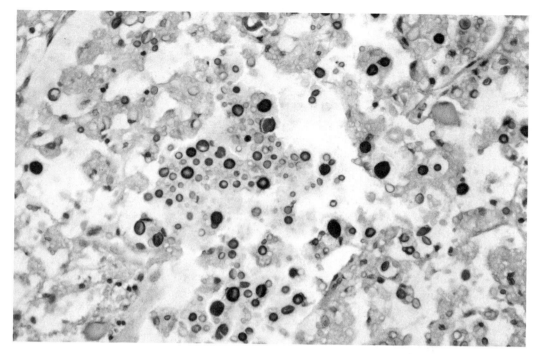

FIG. 14.2-1. Mucicarmine stain of cryptococcus in the lung showing massive disruption of the pulmonary architecture in a patient with AIDS and cryptococcal pneumonia.

Other sites of infection are occasionally seen. Eye involvement, including retinitis, papilledema, and abducens nerve palsy, may be seen in patients with meningitis.[22] Oral manifestations have included palatal and tongue ulcers, which are indurated and tender to palpation.[23,24] Skin lesions can present in a variety of forms: papules, plaques, nodules, and ulcerated lesions have all been reported.[24–29] Frequently, the lesions have characteristics resembling other processes commonly seen in AIDS patients, such as Kaposi's sarcoma, herpes simplex or herpes zoster, and molluscum contagiosum. Cryptococcal arthritis is a rare complication of infection.[30] Gastrointestinal involvements, including infection of the stomach, duodenum, colon, pancreas, and liver, have also been reported.[31] Omental involvement presented as an incarcerated hernia in one case, and massive abdominal adenopathy was initially thought to be caused by a lymphoma in another.[7,32] Cryptococcal myocarditis, presenting with or without heart failure, has also been seen.[33] Rarely, asymptomatic patients have positive urine, blood, or bone marrow cultures for *C neoformans* without evidence of clinically significant disease attributable to cryptococcal infection.[16] The prostate may also be a site of asymptomatic infection, especially in patients who have completed a course of antifungal therapy.[34]

Diagnosis

Diagnosis of cryptococcosis in AIDS patients relies on culture of the organism or detection of cryptococcal antigen in a clinical specimen. Histopathologic diagnosis without culture confirmation is also used; however, other fungal pathogens with similar morphology should then be considered, and the diagnosis of cryptococcosis should be confirmed by staining with mucicarmine. Although the diagnosis can usually be established quickly and easily when it is considered, a high index of suspicion is necessary to ensure that appropriate specimens are obtained and cultured. Given the subtle manifestations of *C neoformans* infection in AIDS patients, it is easy for both physicians and patients to dismiss seemingly minor complaints such as headache or fever, because such symptoms are common and most often are not caused by cryptococcosis. Patients at highest risk for developing cryptococcosis, especially those with a history of other life-threatening opportunistic infections or with CD4 counts lower than 100 cells/mm³, should be diligently evaluated.

The simplest and most rapid method for diagnosing cryptococcosis at any site is the serum cryptococcal antigen test. This test can be performed in a few hours; it is positive in more than 90% of patients with meningitis and also in most infected patients without meningitis.[7–9,16] Although occasional false-positive results are seen, the use of appropriate controls minimizes these. The serum cryptococcal antigen test is a useful screening test in patients with or without a headache, especially those with fever, in whom fungal blood culture should also be obtained. The utility of routine screening in asymptomatic patients is limited and depends in part on the incidence of cryptococcosis in a given population.[35,36] Urine antigen tests also may be positive in patients with meningitis, although the titers tends to be lower than in serum.[37]

All patients suspected of having cryptococcal meningitis should undergo a lumbar puncture. The diagnosis is confirmed by detection of cryptococcal antigen in CSF, by visualization of organisms in CSF with the use of India ink, and by culture of the organism from CSF. Because CSF protein, glucose, and cell counts are often normal in AIDS patients, all CSF samples should be cultured and assayed for antigen regardless of the characteristics of the fluid. Patients with detectable antigen should be started on therapy immediately, while cultures are pending. Although the India ink test is positive in most patients with meningitis, it is less sensitive than antigen detection and requires greater experience for correct interpretation. Some laboratories perform only the antigen test.[7–9,16]

Diagnosis of extraneural cryptococcosis depends on culturing the organism or detecting it histopathologically in biopsy or other clinical specimens. For patients with pneumonitis, bronchoscopy appears to be very useful in making the diagnosis. Transbronchial biopsy was positive in 6 (75%) of 8 patients in one series.[20] Cryptococci were also identified in 5 (63%) of 8 bronchial brush specimens, 5 (83%) of 6 bronchoalveolar lavage specimens, and 7 (100%) of 7 cell blocks prepared from bronchoalveolar lavage fluid.[20] Bronchoscopy specimens may also be positive without radiographic or histopathologic evidence of pneumonitis.[38]

Isolation of C neoformans from any site should be considered significant and an indication for further evaluation and therapy. Although the organism may be detected in the urine or bronchoalveolar lavage fluid of patients with no evidence of disease, such patients should probably receive antifungal therapy because of the risk of life-threatening dissemination or meningitis. As previously noted, some patients have fungemia without localized infection, and the diagnosis relies on positive blood cultures exclusively. Lysis-centrifugation techniques and radiometric techniques appear to increase the sensitivity of cultures, although occasionally cultures are falsely negative by the radiometric techniques alone.[39] In rare patients, positive serum cryptococcal antigen is the exclusive evidence for cryptococcal infection.[9,16] Although the site of infection in such patients may not be identified, again it is prudent to begin treatment in order to prevent life-threatening complications.

Differential Diagnosis

In AIDS patients, meningitis is caused predominantly by C neoformans. Other organisms (eg, Listeria, other fungi, mycobacteria) can occasionally cause meningitis. Headaches can be caused by cryptococcal meningitis or by focal mass lesions, including those caused by toxoplasmosis, lymphoma, and tuberculosis. Sinusitis also is commonly seen in HIV-infected patients, although it may coexist with another, more life-threatening process.

Therapy

Before AIDS, C neoformans infections were routinely treated with amphotericin B (0.3 to 0.6 mg/kg per day) alone or combined with flucytosine (150 mg/kg per day) for 6 to 10 weeks.[40] For patients with AIDS and cryptococcal infection, it became clear early in the epidemic that treatment with similar regimens, although successful in many patients, was associated with a high relapse rate after therapy was discontinued. In two series, a combined response rate of 54% (28 of 52 patients) was seen, but the relapse rate in the absence of suppressive therapy was 56% (10 of 18 patients) among those who had initially responded to therapy.[7,16] Although amphotericin B remains a mainstay of therapy, the benefit of flucytosine in the AIDS setting remains unclear, because it has not been adequately evaluated in a controlled study. In a retrospective study of 89 patients with cryptococcal meningitis, no difference in survival rate was found between patients receiving amphotericin B alone and those receiving amphotericin B plus flucytosine.[9]

Important new advances in the management of cryptococcal infection have been made based on the availability of fluconazole and its evaluation in well designed randomized studies. Fluconazole is a triazole with good activity against C neoformans; it crosses the blood-brain barrier efficiently, achieving levels in the CSF that are 25% to 88% of serum levels.[41] Preliminary uncontrolled studies suggested that fluconazole is effective in treating cryptococcal meningitis in AIDS patients.[41,42] However, in a small, randomized study, failure rates and death rates were higher in patients receiving fluconazole than in those receiving amphotericin B plus flucytosine.[43] More recently, a randomized study of 194 patients conducted by the National Institute of Allergy and Infectious Diseases Mycoses Study Group compared fluconazole (200 to 400 mg/day) with amphotericin B (mean 0.4 mg/kg per day, with or without flucytosine) and found no significant difference in outcome between the two groups. However, the time to sterilization of CSF in successfully treated patients was shorter in the amphotericin B group (2 weeks versus 4 weeks), and a higher proportion of the patients receiving fluconazole died during the first 2 weeks of therapy.[44]

Other regimens for acute therapy, including high-dose fluconazole, fluconazole combined with flucytosine, itraconazole, and liposomal amphotericin B have been evaluated in the treatment of cryptococcosis, but they cannot be recommended as primary therapy until well controlled studies have defined their relative efficacy.[45–49] Although intrathecal amphotericin B has been advocated for treatment of cryptococcal meningitis, there is currently no evidence that such therapy is beneficial or necessary in AIDS patients.[50]

In AIDS patients, there is a high rate of recurrence of cryptococcosis after discontinuation of antifungal therapy, presumably from inadequately treated sites of infection. The prostate appears to be one such nidus. In one report, cultures of prostatic secretions were positive in 22% of patients who had no evidence of active disease elsewhere.[34] Molecular studies also suggest relapse rather than reinfection as the mechanism behind recurrences.[51] Although the use of fluconazole as initial therapy is controversial, the role of fluconazole as a suppressive agent has been validated in two randomized trials. In the first, fluconazole was shown to be significantly more effective than placebo in preventing relapse at any site in patients with cryptococcal meningitis who had previously responded to standard therapy.[52] Ten (37%) of 27 placebo patients but only 1 (3%) of 34 patients receiving fluconazole (100 or 200 mg/day) had recurrence during a median follow-up period of 4 to 5 months. Another study compared the efficacies of amphotericin B (1 mg/kg per week) and fluconazole (200 mg/day) as suppressive regimens after successful treatment with amphotericin B. A significantly higher proportion of patients receiving amphotericin B (14 of 78, or 18%) relapsed during a median follow-up period of 9 months, compared with patients receiving fluconazole (3 of 111, or 3%).[53] Relapses that occur during suppressive therapy do not appear to be caused by the development of resistance.[54]

Based on these data, treatment of cryptococcal meningitis should begin with amphotericin B (0.3 to 0.7 mg/kg per day), either alone or together with flucytosine (100 mg/kg per day, a lower dose that has been recommended to decrease the incidence of toxicity[55-57]). One recommended approach is to continue this regimen for at least 2 to 3 weeks, until CSF cultures have become negative or clinical symptoms have resolved, at which time fluconazole, at therapeutic rather than suppressive doses (400 mg/day), should be administered to complete at least 10 weeks of therapy.[55,56] Suppressive therapy with fluconazole (200 mg/day) should then be continued for the life of the patient. An alternative approach is to administer amphotericin B plus flucytosine for 6 to 10 weeks, after which fluconazole at suppressive doses is administered for life. Although therapy for extrameningeal disease has not been as thoroughly evaluated, the described regimen should be used for such patients also. However, patients with isolated positive serum cryptococcal antigen may respond well to initial therapy with fluconazole.

Prognostic Factors

In non-AIDS patients, a number of factors, such as low CSF glucose or leukocyte count and positive India ink smear, have been associated with a poor prognosis.[58] Among AIDS patients, however, such factors appear less important in prognosis. In a large retrospective study, only a low sodium level at presentation and positive cultures obtained from extrameningeal sites were associated with shorter survival.[9] In a prospective trial, however, altered mental status at presentation, low CSF leukocyte count, and high CSF cryptococcal antigen titer (>1:1024) were associated with a poor prognosis.[44]

Changes in serum antigen titers do not appear to be helpful in predicting responses to therapy or relapse during chronic suppression.[59] Changes in CSF antigen titers are more helpful, although the utility of follow-up lumbar punctures in asymptomatic patients receiving chronic suppression appears to be limited because most relapses are clinically apparent.[59]

Prophylaxis

A number of retrospective studies have suggested that fluconazole is effective in decreasing the incidence of cryptococcal infection in HIV-infected patients with low CD4 counts, and the use of antifungal prophylaxis has become increasingly common.[60,61] A recent prospective, randomized study[17] comparing fluconazole (200 mg/day) to clotrimazole troches (10 mg five times daily) in patients with CD4 counts lower than 200 cells/mm^3 demonstrated that during a median follow-up period of 35 months, fluconazole decreased the incidence of deep-seated fungal infections from 11% (23 of 211 patients) to 4% (9 of 217 patients).[17] The benefit derived exclusively from a decrease in cryptococcal infections (15 cases versus 2 cases), and it was most pronounced for patients with CD4 counts lower than 50 cells/mm^3. Although fluconazole was also superior in preventing esophageal and oropharyngeal candidiasis, recent experience has suggested that the broader use of fluconazole results in the development of resistant mucosal *Candida* infections, which may require therapy with amphotericin B.[62] Thus, the optimal implementation of antifungal prophylaxis must take into account the relatively low incidence of invasive fungal infections, the risk of inducing resistance, and the costs, inconveniences, and potential drug interactions associated with prophylactic therapies.

CANDIDA SPECIES

Candida are yeasts that exist predominantly in unicellular forms. They are 2.5- to 6-μm ovoid cells that reproduce by budding. More than 150 species exist, and at least 10 are pathogenic in humans. *Candida* organisms are ubiquitous; they have been recovered from soil, hospital environments, and food.

Clinical Manifestations

Candida species are the most common causative agents of fungal infection in HIV-infected persons. Fortunately, these infections are seldom invasive, can usually be easily treated, and, with appropriate management, can often be prevented. It was established early in the course of the HIV epidemic that oral candidiasis is a marker of an impaired immune system and a prognostic marker for the subsequent development of opportunistic infections.[63] Candidal infections of the esophagus, trachea, bronchi, or lungs are recognized as indicator diseases for AIDS.[64] Whereas oropharyngeal candidal infections (and candidal vaginosis in women) regularly occur in HIV-infected persons with CD4 counts higher than 200 cells/mm^3, esophageal candidiasis is indicative of more advanced immunodeficiency and seldom occurs with CD4 counts higher than 100 cells/mm[3].[65] Oropharyngeal and vaginal candidiasis may recur frequently.[65,66] *Candida* species seldom cause disseminated infections in patients with AIDS unless there are associated factors such as the presence of chronic indwelling catheters or neutropenia.

Diagnosis

Oropharyngeal candidiasis (thrush) is usually diagnosed by the characteristic appearance of white plaques on the tongue, buccal mucosa, or palate. Microscopic examination of a scraping of the plaque, using Gram's stain or potassium hydroxide, reveals sheets of hyphae, pseudohyphae, and yeast forms.

Candida esophagitis is frequently diagnosed on the basis of the characteristic clinical presentations of odynophagia, dysphagia, a feeling of obstruction, substernal chest pain, or a combination of these symptoms, often accompanied by oropharyngeal candidiasis.[67] Radiographically, an esophageal contrast study may reveal discrete, widely separated plaques on a normal background mucosa, diffuse plaque formation without ulcers, or a grossly irregular esophagus caused by multiple plaques and ulcers[68] (Fig. 14.2-2). In one study, with radiologists experienced in the diagnosis of esophageal disease in persons with AIDS, *Candida* esophagitis was distinguished from esophagitis caused by herpes virus or cytomegalovirus without the need for endoscopy.[68] Blind brushings of the esophagus through a nasogastric tube have a high sensitivity and specificity in the diagnosis of *Candida* esophagitis.[69] Most often, however, the diagnosis of *Candida* esophagitis is made on its characteristic clinical presentation without the need for endoscopy or radiologic intervention.[70,71] Esophagoscopy or radiographic contrast procedures may be reserved for persons not responding to empiric therapy.

Differential Diagnosis

Oropharyngeal candidiasis may often be mistaken for oral hairy leukoplakia. Although *Candida* is the most common cause of esophagitis in patients with HIV infection, cytomegalovirus and herpes simplex virus may produce a similar constellation of radiographic and clinical findings.[68,72] Other causes of esophageal lesions in these patients include Kaposi's sarcoma, *Mycobacteria*, and lymphoma.

Therapy

Oropharyngeal candidiasis usually responds readily to topical agents such as nystatin or clotrimazole troches, and these agents should be the initial treatment of choice because of their ease of administration and relatively low cost. Before the introduction of the azoles, there were no oral antifungal agents available that could effectively treat esophageal candidiasis. Ketoconazole, an imidazole, is well tolerated when administered orally at 200 mg/day and can successfully treat esophageal and oropharyngeal candidiasis. Ketoconazole

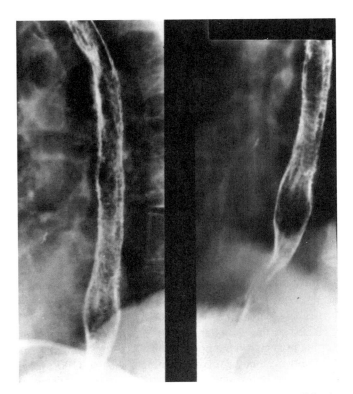

FIG. 14.2-2. Esophagogram of esophageal candidiasis showing a markedly irregular esophagus due to multiple plaques in a patient with AIDS and severe odynophagia.

requires an acidic pH for dissolution, however, and may not be well absorbed in patients with hypochlorhydria or in those taking H_2-blocking agents or antacids.[73] Some patients have had persistent *Candida* esophagitis despite prolonged therapy with ketoconazole.[74] Fluconazole, a triazole, is given at a dose of 50 to 100 mg daily and may be better tolerated and more effective than ketoconazole for oropharyngeal candidiasis.[71,75] In spite of its higher cost, fluconazole (100 to 200 mg daily for 14 days) has become the standard of care for the treatment of *Candida* esophagitis. Fluconazole may be successful in treating some cases of refractory oral candidiasis.[76] For severe cases of esophageal candidiasis not responding to the azoles, amphotericin B (0.6 mg/kg intravenously for 7 to 10 days) may still be necessary.[62]

Prophylaxis

Oropharyngeal candidiasis frequently recurs after treatment is stopped. The data for routine prophylaxis against candidal infections is controversial. Although data from a recent randomized trial demonstrated *Candida* esophagitis in 17 (8.1%) of 211 persons receiving clotrimazole troches, compared with 3 (1.4%) of 217 persons receiving fluconazole,[17] the cost of fluconazole is considerable and *Candida* esophagitis is easy to diagnose and may be treated on a case-by-case basis. There was no increased survival among persons receiving the prophylactic fluconazole in this study.[17] Further, there appears to be an increased development of resistance to fluconazole among *Candida* species, including *C albicans, C krusei, C stellatoidea,* and *C glabrata,* after prolonged prophylactic therapy.[62,77-81] Lifelong therapy with the least expensive effective agent may be recommended for patients with frequent recurrences.

An additional caution should be addressed with the use of the azole agents. Drugs that are commonly used in the treatment of advanced HIV infection and induce hepatic drug-metabolizing enzymes, such as rifampin, rifabutin, and phenytoin, may accelerate the metabolism of fluconazole, ketoconazole, and itraconazole. Conversely, these antifungal agents may increase drug levels of phenytoin or rifabutin, leading to adverse drug effects.[82-85]

HISTOPLASMA CAPSULATUM

Histoplasma capsulatum exists in the soil in the mycelial phase but converts to the yeast form at the body temperature of mammals. The mycelial form has septate, branching hyphae (1 to 2.5 μm across) with lateral and terminal spores. The yeast form is ovoid, 1.5 to 2.0 μm by 3.0 to 3.5 μm, and reproduces by budding.

Epidemiology and Pathogenesis

The major endemic focus of histoplasmosis is in the central United States. Examination of soil specimens has shown that the organism is present in large numbers in areas frequented by birds or bats. An estimated 500,000 new cases occur in the United States per year, but most are either asymptomatic or acute, self-limited illnesses. Because histoplasmosis is endemic in the central United States and the initial presentation and propagation of the HIV epidemic occurred on the coasts, histoplasmosis has been reported in fewer than 0.5% of patients with AIDS.[86] As the AIDS epidemic spreads through the central United States, the numbers of cases of histoplasmosis will correspondingly increase. Although *H capsulatum* rarely disseminates in immunocompetent patients,[87] disseminated disease is the primary presentation in patients with AIDS.[88-91] Disseminated histoplasmosis (at a site other than the lungs or cervical or hilar lymph nodes), diagnosed definitively, with laboratory evidence of HIV infection, is included in the Centers for Disease Control surveillance case definition for AIDS.[64]

Clinical Manifestations

The most common presentation of disseminated histoplasmosis is that of fever and weight loss. Respiratory complaints are common, but chest radiographs may be normal in more than 40% of patients. Hepatomegaly, splenomegaly, and lymphadenopathy each occur in about one quarter of patients.[88,89,91,92] CNS involvement is common, presenting as a meningitis or a space-occupying lesion, and occurs in about 15% of patients.[88,90,93] Hematologic abnormalities, including thrombocytopenia, neutropenia, and anemia, are found in more than 20% of patients at presentation.[91,93] A syndrome resembling bacterial septicemia has been reported in about 10% of cases.[88,92,94] Disseminated histoplasmosis may not uncommonly present with various types of cutaneous lesions, including maculopapular rashes,[95] tender pustules,[96,97] papules, skin or oral ulcers,[96,98] and ulcerated palatal nodules.[99] Gastrointestinal masses,[100,101] chorioretinitis,[102] and pleural effusion[103] have also been reported in association with disseminated histoplasmosis. CD4 counts obtained within 60 days of diagnosis of disseminated histoplasmosis in one series of patients showed a median count of 33 cells/mm³; only 2 of 17 patients had counts higher than 250 cells/mm³.[104]

Diagnosis

The definitive diagnosis of disseminated histoplasmosis rests on biopsy and culture of the organism from tissue. Positive cultures are often obtained from bone marrow, blood, lung biopsy or lavage, sputum, lymph node, skin, or CSF.[88,89,91,104] Diff-Quik, Wright-Giemsa, or methenamine silver stains, among others, can lead to a rapid diagnosis from tissue, sputum, or lavage specimens (Fig. 14.2-3). Immunodiffusion or complement fixation anti–*H capsulatum* antibody tests are frequently negative but may be helpful if positive.[88] Detection of *H capsulatum* polysaccharide antigen by radioimmunoassay from blood and urine has been reported to correlate well with response to therapy and relapse. The test may prove useful in diagnosis and management of patients with disseminated histoplasmosis and AIDS.[105]*

Differential Diagnosis

The presentation of histoplasmosis in the patient with AIDS is similar to that of tuberculosis or *P carinii* pneumonia. Less commonly, pulmonary cryptococcosis, coccidioidomycosis, nocardiosis, cytomegalovirus, or Kaposi's sarcoma may be seen. Because the infection may endogenously reactivate, patients may not have a recent history of travel to endemic areas.

Therapy

Treatment with amphotericin B (0.6 mg/kg per day intravenously) is the standard treatment and is highly effective.[105] Almost all patients, however, relapse within 1 year, even after receiving more than 35 mg/kg, an observation that supports the use of maintenance therapy to prevent recurrence. Weekly or biweekly doses of 1 mg/kg of amphotericin B appear to be better in preventing relapses than ketoconazole.[88,106] In a prospective, multicenter, open trial of 42 patients who had completed induction therapy of at least 15

---

*The assay is available only at the Histoplasmosis Reference Laboratory of Dr. L. Joseph Wheat by calling 1-800-HISTO-DG.

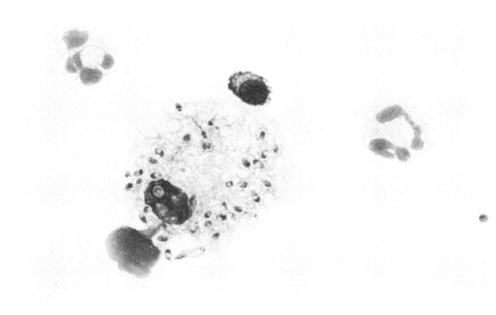

FIG. 14.2-3. Diff-Quik stain of a cytopathologic specimen from a bronchoalveolar lavage showing multiple *Histoplasma capsulatum* organisms within a macrophage in a patient with AIDS and pulmonary histoplasmosis.

mg/kg of amphotericin B, follow-up therapy with itraconazole (200 mg given orally twice daily) resulted in only 2 relapses[107]; this should be the standard of care for patients with moderate or severe disseminated histoplasmosis. In a study of persons without CNS involvement or severe clinical manifestations of disseminated histoplasmosis, 50 (85%) of 59 patients responded to therapy with oral itraconazole (300 mg twice daily for 3 days, then 200 mg twice daily for 12 weeks).[108] This oral regimen may be considered for persons with mild histoplasmosis. For persons unable to tolerate itraconazole, fluconazole (200 mg or more per day) may be an alternative regimen for maintenance.[109]

Prophylaxis

The efficacy of prophylaxis for a disease of low incidence is difficult to ascertain. Only in areas highly endemic for histoplasmosis would it be reasonable to consider prophylaxis.

COCCIDIOIDES IMMITIS

Coccidioides immitis is a fungus that lives in the soil as a mold. Arthroconidia, produced from the hyphae of the mycelial phase, infect the host after they are released into the air and inhaled. In tissues, the fungus grows as spherules, large structures containing hundreds of endospores.[110]

Epidemiology and Pathogenesis

Coccidioidomycosis is endemic in certain areas in North, Central, and South America, including the deserts of the southwestern United States. Most cases are concentrated in these regions, and in susceptible persons without AIDS the annual rate of infection has been estimated to be about 3%.[110] Early in the course of the AIDS epidemic, coccidioidomycosis was only rarely seen as a complication of AIDS.[111–113] Although disseminated disease occurs in 1.2% of immunocompetent patients with coccidioidomycosis who require hospitalization, dissemination is more common in patients with AIDS.[114] Disseminated coccidioidomycosis (other than to lungs or cervical or hilar lymph nodes), diagnosed definitively and with laboratory evidence of HIV infection, is included in the Centers for Disease Control surveillance definition of AIDS.[64]

It has not been established whether coccidioidomycosis in patients with AIDS represents reactivation of latent infection or primary infection. In the largest reported series, positive serology results were reported for complement-fixing antibodies, indicative of an immunoglobulin G (IgG) response, and were generally negative for tube precipitin serologies, which would indicate an IgM response.[115] This suggests that much of the disease incidence results from reactivation rather than primary infection. A smaller study calculated an annual rate of coccidioidal infection in some AIDS patients in Tucson, Arizona, to be 27%, much larger than the annual rate of less than 4% among non-AIDS patients in the same city. This suggests that either the disease reactivates or susceptibility to infection is enhanced in patients with AIDS.[114]

Clinical Manifestations

Because the route of infection of *C immitis* is by inhalation of arthroconidia, coccidioidomycosis most frequently involves the lungs. The most common presentation is that of fever, weight loss, and cough. Diffuse reticulonodular infiltrates on chest radiography are characteristic of its presentation in patients with AIDS[114–116] (Fig. 14.2-4). In contrast to the presentation in patients with AIDS, a review of 300 non-AIDS patients hospitalized with coccidioidomycosis identified only 13 patients with the same extent of disease.[114]

In the largest reported series of AIDS patients with coccidioidomycosis, 77 patients were grouped in six clinical categories: focal pulmonary disease, diffuse pulmonary disease, cutaneous disease, meningitis, lymph node or liver involvement, and positive serology only.[115] Twenty patients (26%) presented with focal pulmonary disease, most commonly as a focal alveolar infiltrate, but also as discrete nodules, pulmonary cavities, hilar adenopathy, and bilateral pleural effusions. Thirty-one patients (40%) presented with diffuse reticulonodular infiltrates. Four patients (5%) presented with cutaneous disease; 3 of them also had pulmonary involvement. Nine patients (12%) presented with coccidioidal meningitis. The CSF usually had an elevated leukocyte count (range, 2 to 772 cells/mm³), decreased glucose, increased protein, and a positive complement-fixing antibody titer to *C immitis*. *C immitis* was cultured from the CSF in 5 of 9 patients. Seven patients (9%) presented with localized extrathoracic lymph node or liver involvement. An additional 6 patients (8%) were positive only by coccidioidal serology.[115] Of the patients who had CD4 counts obtained at the time of diagnosis, 84% had counts lower than 250 cells/mm³. Those patients with diffuse pulmonary disease had a lower median CD4 count, only 44 cells/mm³. Isolated cases of peritonitis[117] and fungemia[118] caused by *C immitis* have also been reported.

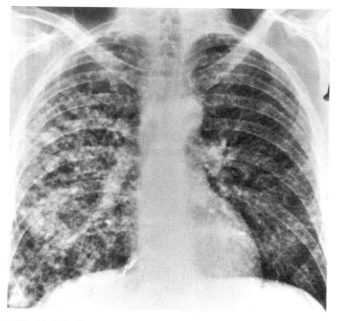

FIG. 14.2-4. Chest radiograph of a patient with AIDS and pulmonary coccidioidomycosis showing a characteristic difuse, reticulonodular pattern.

Diagnosis

The diagnosis of coccidioidomycosis is easily made because the fungus can readily be cultured with most media. Visualization of the distinctive spherule in tissues is also diagnostic of invasive disease (Fig. 14.2-5). Coccidioidal serologies may be helpful in the diagnosis of the disease, but both complement-fixing antibodies and tube precipitin serologies may be negative in as many as 25% of patients.[115,119] A high index of suspicion must be maintained for the diagnosis of coccidioidomycosis in the patient with AIDS and negative coccidioidal serologies who has traveled through an endemic area.

Differential Diagnosis

The pulmonary manifestations of coccidioidomycosis may mimic the more common presentations of pulmonary disease in patients with AIDS, particularly *P carinii* pneumonia, tuberculosis, and histoplasmosis. The reticulonodular pattern may be similar to that seen with pulmonary Kaposi's sarcoma. The presentation of meningitis may be similar to that of cryptococcal meningitis.

Therapy

Standard treatment for disseminated or diffuse pulmonary coccidioidomycosis remains amphotericin B, 1 to 1.5 mg/kg per day intravenously, up to a total of at least 1 to 2.5 g before maintenance therapy with oral agents is considered.[120] The optimal treatment of patients with AIDS and limited disease caused by coccidioidomycosis is unknown. Ketoconazole has been used in doses of 400 mg/day orally. However, three patients on ketoconazole for other reasons developed active coccidioidomycosis.[115] The experience with the triazole itraconazole (200 mg twice daily by mouth) and fluconazole (400 mg/day by mouth) has been limited but encouraging.[115,120] Itraconazole for coccidioidal meningitis has shown some anecdotal success in non–HIV-infected patients,[121] and fluconazole induced prolonged suppression of disease in 37 of 47 patients in another study.[122]

Prognostic Factors

Patients with diffuse pulmonary disease appear to have a worse prognosis than do patients with more limited disease; median survival time was only 1 month from the date of diagnosis in the former group, though it ranged up to 17 months. Correspondingly, a high mortality rate was seen in patients with low CD4 counts.[115]

ASPERGILLUS SPECIES

Aspergillus is a common mold found in the soil that frequently causes invasive pulmonary and obstructing bronchial disease in immunocompromised patients. Pul-

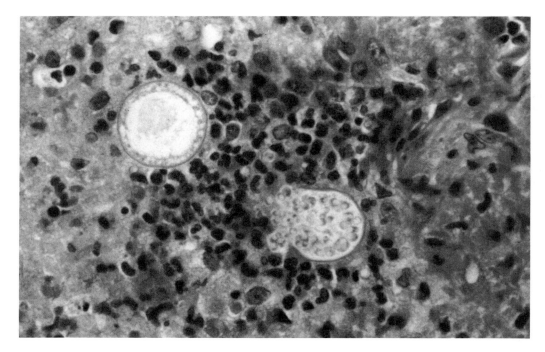

FIG. 14.2-5. Hematoxylin-eosin stain of a lung biopsy from the patient in Figure 14.2-4 showing a rupturing endosporulating spherule and an empty spherule.

monary aspergillosis, however, is a relatively uncommon complication of AIDS and predominantly occurs as a late manifestation of the disease.[123–126] Spores (conidia) of *Aspergillus* are approximately 3 μm in size, and their hyphae, which are 2 to 5 μm wide, are often septate and exhibit Y-shaped branching. The hyphae cannot easily be differentiated from those of other pathogenic molds. *A fumigatus* and *A flavus* are the most common causes of aspergillosis.

Clinical Manifestations

Both invasive pulmonary and obstructing bronchial aspergillosis have been described in patients with AIDS.[123] In one report, the most common clinical presentation was the insidious development of cough and fever in a profoundly immunocompromised patient with neutropenia.[123] Four of 13 patients were reported to have received corticosteroids previously, and 4 patients were users of marijuana. Radiographically, cavitary lung disease and diffuse infiltrates were the most common findings. Ten of the 13 patients died a median of 3 months after diagnosis.

Other organs, including the heart,[127,128] the pancreas,[129] and the brain and spinal cord,[130] may rarely be infected by *Aspergillus* in patients with AIDS.

Diagnosis

Isolation of *Aspergillus* from biopsy cultures together with microscopic identification in tissue assures the diagnosis of aspergillosis. Isolation of *Aspergillus* from sputum or the appearance of hyphae in a smear or biopsy sample can be suggestive of the diagnosis and, in the appropriate clinical setting, should prompt further investigation.

Differential Diagnosis

Because pulmonary aspergillosis is seen only infrequently in patients with AIDS, the diagnosis of invasive pulmonary aspergillosis in an AIDS patient must be made with caution. More common causes of pulmonary disease, such as *P carinii*, nonspecific interstitial pneumonitis, tuberculosis, histoplasmosis, cytomegalovirus, and Kaposi's sarcoma, must be ruled out.

Therapy

Response to treatment has been poor. Intravenous amphotericin B and oral itraconazole have been used with limited success.[123] Because of the paucity of data, treatment of invasive pulmonary aspergillosis in the patient with AIDS should be the same as in other immunocompromised patients: intravenous amphotericin B, 0.5 to 1.0 mg/kg per day. Early treatment may be beneficial.[131] Itraconazole, 200 to 400 mg daily for extended periods, has shown promise in the treatment of aspergillosis in other immunocompromised patients.[132–134] Its utility in the treatment of aspergillosis in patients with AIDS is still unknown.[123,126]

BLASTOMYCES DERMATITIDIS

Blastomyces dermatitidis is an 8- to 15-μm yeast cell with daughter cells forming a bud with a broad base. Pulmonary or miliary blastomycosis has only rarely been reported in persons with AIDS.[135–138] Persons with advanced disease traveling through the endemic areas of the Ohio and Mississippi River basins may be at risk for development of disease with *Blastomyces*. Early therapy with amphotericin B, followed by lifetime therapy with ketoconazole or itraconazole, may be of benefit.[137,138]

PENICILLIUM MARNEFFEI

Penicillium marneffei is a dimorphic fungus that grows in tissue as a 3- by 8-µm yeast. It is endemic in Southeast Asia and China and has been reported to be the third most common opportunistic infection associated with HIV infection in northern Thailand.[139] The disease most frequently presents with a generalized papular skin rash associated with fever, weight loss, lymphadenopathy, and anemia. Chest radiographs were abnormal in 30 (38%) of 80 persons with disseminated *P marneffei* infection in one study.[139] Diagnosis can be made by bone marrow or lymph node biopsy or, less commonly, by blood culture. Approximately 75% of persons with disseminated *P marneffei* infection responded clinically and microbiologically to therapy with amphotericin B or itraconazole.[140]

REFERENCES

1. Diamond RD. *Cryptococcus neoformans*. In: Mandell GL, Douglas RG Jr, Bennett JE, Dolin R, eds. Principles and practice of infectious diseases, 4th ed. New York: Churchill Livingstone, 1995:2331.
2. Bottone EJ, Salkin IF, Hurd NJ, Wormser GP. Serogroup distribution of *Cryptococcus neoformans* in patients with AIDS. J Infect Dis 1987;156:242.
3. Swinne D, Nkurikiyinfura JB, Muyembe TL. Clinical isolates of *Cryptococcus neoformans* from Zaire. Eur J Clin Microbiol Infect Dis 1986;5:50.
4. Rinaldi MG, Drutz DJ, Howell A, Sande MA, Wofsy CB, Hadley WK. Serotypes of *Cryptococcus neoformans* in patients with AIDS. (Letter) J Infect Dis 1986;153:642.
5. Bottone EJ, Toma M, Johansson BE, Wormser GP. Poorly encapsulated *Cryptococcus neoformans* from patients with AIDS: I. Preliminary observations. AIDS Res 1986;2:211.
6. Levitz SM. The ecology of *Cryptococcus neoformans* and the epidemiology of cryptococcosis. Rev Infect Dis 1991;13:1163.
7. Kovacs JA, Kovacs AA, Polis M, et al. Cryptococcosis in the acquired immunodeficiency syndrome. Ann Intern Med 1985;103:533.
8. Clark RA, Greer D, Atkinson W, Valainis GT, Hyslop N. Spectrum of *Cryptococcus neoformans* infection in 68 patients infected with human immunodeficiency virus. Rev Infect Dis 1990;12:768.
9. Chuck SL, Sande MA. Infections with *Cryptococcus neoformans* in the acquired immunodeficiency syndrome. N Engl J Med 1989;321:794.
10. Dismukes WE. Cryptococcal meningitis in patients with AIDS. J Infect Dis 1988;157:624.
11. Currie BP, Casadevall A. Estimation of the prevalence of cryptococcal infection among patients infected with the human immunodeficiency virus in New York City. Clin Infect Dis 1994;19:1029.
12. Katz MH, Hessol NA, Buchbinder SP, Hirozawa A, O'Malley P, Holmberg SD. Temporal trends of opportunistic infections and malignancies in homosexual men with AIDS. J Infect Dis 1994;170:198.
13. Bacellar H, Munoz A, Miller EN, et al. Temporal trends in the incidence of HIV-1 related neurologic diseases: multicenter AIDS cohort study, 1985–1992. Neurology 1995;44:1892.
14. Mackenzie DW. Cryptococcosis in the AIDS era. Epidemiol Infect 1989;102:361.
15. Clumeck N, Carael N, Van de Perre P. The African AIDS experience in contrast with the rest of the world. In: Leoung G, Mills J, eds. Opportunistic infections in patients with the acquired immunodeficiency syndrome. New York: Marcel Dekker, 1989:43.
16. Zuger A, Louie E, Holzman RS, Simberkoff MS, Rahal JJ. Cryptococcal disease in patients with the acquired immunodeficiency syndrome: diagnostic features and outcome of treatment. Ann Intern Med 1986;104:234.
17. Powderly WG, Finkelstein DM, Feinberg J, et al. A randomized trial comparing fluconazole with clotrimazole troches for the prevention of fungal infections in patients with advanced human immunodeficiency virus infection. N Engl J Med 1995;332:700.
18. Lecomte I, Meyohas MC, De Sa M. Relation between decreasing serial CD4 lymphocytes count and outcome of cryptococcosis in AIDS patients: a basis for new diagnosis strategy. International Conference on AIDS 1990;6:235 .
19. Andreula CF, Burdi N, Carella A. CNS cryptococcosis in AIDS: spectrum of MR findings. J Comput Assist Tomogr 1993;17:438.
20. Gal AA, Koss MN, Hawkins J, Evans S, Einstein H. The pathology of pulmonary cryptococcal infections in the acquired immunodeficiency syndrome. Arch Pathol Lab Med 1986;110:502.
21. Witt D, McKay D, Schwam L, Goldstein D, Gold J. Acquired immune deficiency syndrome presenting as bone marrow and mediastinal cryptococcosis. Am J Med 1987;82:149.
22. Kestelyn P, Taelman H, Bogaerts J, et al. Ophthalmic manifestations of infections with *Cryptococcus neoformans* in patients with the acquired immunodeficiency syndrome. Am J Ophthalmol 1993;116:721.
23. Glick M, Cohen SG, Cheney RT, Crooks GW, Greenberg MS. Oral manifestations of disseminated *Cryptococcus neoformans* in a patient with acquired immunodeficiency syndrome. Oral Surg Oral Med Oral Pathol 1987;64:454.
24. Lynch DP, Naftolin LZ. Oral *Cryptococcus neoformans* infection in AIDS. Oral Surg Oral Med Oral Pathol 1987;64:449.
25. Hernandez AD. Cutaneous cryptococcosis. Dermatol Clin 1989;7:269.
26. Jones C, Orengo I, Rosen T, Ellner K. Cutaneous cryptococcosis simulating Kaposi's sarcoma in the acquired immunodeficiency syndrome. Cutis 1990;45:163.
27. Borton LK, Wintroub BU. Disseminated cryptococcosis presenting as herpetiform lesions in a homosexual man with acquired immunodeficiency syndrome. J Am Acad Dermatol 1984;10:387.
28. Rico MJ, Penneys NS. Cutaneous cryptococcosis resembling molluscum contagiosum in a patient with AIDS. Arch Dermatol 1985;121:901.
29. Concus AP, Helfand RF, Imber MJ, Lerner EA, Sharpe RJ. Cutaneous cryptococcosis mimicking molluscum contagiosum in a patient with AIDS. J Infect Dis 1988;158:897.
30. Ricciardi DD, Sepkowitz DV, Berkowitz LB, Bienenstock H, Maslow M. Cryptococcal arthritis in a patient with acquired immune deficiency syndrome: case report and review of the literature. J Rheumatol 1986;13:455.
31. Bonacini M, Nussbaum J, Ahluwalia C. Gastrointestinal, hepatic, and pancreatic involvement with *Cryptococcus neoformans* in AIDS. J Clin Gastroenterol 1990;12:295.
32. Scalfano FP, Prichard JG, Lamki N, Athey PA, Graves RC. Abdominal cryptococcoma in AIDS: a case report. J Comput Tomogr 1988;12:237.
33. Lewis W, Lipsick J, Cammarosano C. Cryptococcal myocarditis in acquired immune deficiency syndrome. Am J Cardiol 1985;55:1240.
34. Larsen RA, Bozzette S, McCutchan JA, Chiu J, Leal MA, Richman DD. Persistent *Cryptococcus neoformans* infection of the prostate after successful treatment of meningitis: California Collaborative Treatment Group. Ann Intern Med 1989;111:125.
35. Desmet P, Kayembe KD, De Vroey C. The value of cryptococcal serum antigen screening among HIV-positive/AIDS patients in Kinshasa, Zaire. AIDS 1989;3:77.
36. Hoffmann S, Stenderup J, Mathiesen LR. Low yield of screening for cryptococcal antigen by latex agglutination assay on serum and cerebrospinal fluid from Danish patients with AIDS or ARC. Scand J Infect Dis 1991;23:697.
37. Chapin-Robertson K, Bechtel C, Waycott S, Kontnick C, Edberg SC. Cryptococcal antigen detection from the urine of AIDS patients. Diagn Microbiol Infect Dis 1993;17:197.
38. Masur H, Ognibene FP, Yarchoan R, et al. CD4 counts as predictors of opportunistic pneumonias in human immunodeficiency virus (HIV) infection. Ann Intern Med 1989;111:223.
39. Robinson PG, Sulita MJ, Matthews EK, Warren JR. Failure of the Bactec 460 radiometer to detect *Cryptococcus neoformans* fungemia in an AIDS patient. Am J Clin Pathol 1987;87:783.

40. Bennett JE, Dismukes WE, Duma RJ, et al. A comparison of amphotericin B alone and combined with flucytosine in the treatment of cryptococcal meningitis. N Engl J Med 1979;301:126.

41. Stern JJ, Hartman BJ, Sharkey P, et al. Oral fluconazole therapy for patients with acquired immunodeficiency syndrome and cryptococcosis: experience with 22 patients. Am J Med 1988;85:477.

42. Sugar AM, Saunders C. Oral fluconazole as suppressive therapy of disseminated cryptococcosis in patients with acquired immunodeficiency syndrome. Am J Med 1988;85:481.

43. Larsen RA, Leal MA, Chan LS. Fluconazole compared with amphotericin B plus flucytosine for cryptococcal meningitis in AIDS: a randomized trial. Ann Intern Med 1990;113:183.

44. Saag MS, Powderly WG, Cloud GA, et al. Comparison of amphotericin B with fluconazole in the treatment of acute AIDS-associated cryptococcal meningitis. N Engl J Med 1992;326:83.

45. Haubrich RH, Haghighat D, Bozzette SA, Tilles J, McCutchan JA, The California Collaborative Treatment Group: High-dose fluconazole for treatment of cryptococcal disease in patients with human immunodeficiency virus infection. J Infect Dis 1994;170:238.

46. Larsen RA, Bozzette SA, Jones BE, et al. Fluconazole combined with flucytosine for treatment of cryptococcal meningitis in patients with AIDS. Clin Infect Dis 1994;19:741.

47. de Gans J, Portegies P, Tiessens G, et al. Itraconazole compared with amphotericin B plus flucytosine in AIDS patients with cryptococcal meningitis. AIDS 1992;6:185.

48. Coker RJ, Viviani M, Gazzard BG, et al. Treatment of cryptococcosis with liposomal amphotericin B (AmBisome) in 23 patients with AIDS. AIDS 1993;7:829.

49. Nightingale SD. Initial therapy for acquired immunodeficiency syndrome-associated cryptococcosis with fluconazole. Arch Intern Med 1995;155:538.

50. Polsky B, Depman MR, Gold JWM, Galicich JH, Armstrong D. Intraventricular therapy of cryptococcal meningitis via a subcutaneous reservoir. Am J Med 1986;81:24.

51. Spitzer ED, Spitzer SG, Freundlich LF, Casadevall A. Persistence of initial infection in recurrent Cryptococcus neoformans meningitis. Lancet 1993;341:595.

52. Bozzette SA, Larsen RA, Chiu J, et al. A placebo-controlled trial of maintenance therapy with fluconazole after treatment of cryptococcal meningitis in the acquired immunodeficiency syndrome. N Engl J Med 1991;324:580.

53. Powderly WG, Saag MS, Cloud GA, et al. A controlled trial of fluconazole or amphotericin B to prevent relapse of cryptococcal meningitis in patients with the acquired immunodeficiency syndrome. N Engl J Med 1992;326:793.

54. Casadevall A, Spitzer ED, Webb D, Rinaldi MG. Susceptibilities of serial Cryptococcus neoformans isolates from patients with recurrent cryptococcal meningitis to amphotericin B and fluconazole. Antimicrob Agents Chemother 1993;37:1383.

55. Powderly WG. Cryptococcal meningitis and AIDS. Clin Infect Dis 1993;17:837.

56. Bozzette SA. The management of cryptococcal disease in patients with AIDS. Curr Clin Top Infect Dis 1993;13:250.

57. White MH, Armstrong D. Management of infection in HIV disease: cryptococcosis. Infect Dis Clin North Am 1994;8:383.

58. Diamond RD, Bennett JE. Prognostic factors in cryptococcal meningitis: a study in 111 cases. Ann Intern Med 1974;80:176.

59. Powderly WG, Cloud GA, Dismukes WE, Saag MS. Measurement of cryptococcal antigen in serum and cerebrospinal fluid: value in the management of AIDS-associated cryptococcal meningitis. Clin Infect Dis 1994;18:789.

60. Nightingale SD, Cal SX, Peterson DM, et al. Primary prophylaxis with fluconazole against systemic fungal infections in HIV-positive patients. AIDS 1992;6:191.

61. Quagliarello VJ, Viscoli C, Horwitz RI. Primary prevention of cryptococcal meningitis by fluconazole in HIV-infected patients. Lancet 1995;345:548.

62. Sanguineti A, Carmichael JK, Campbell K. Fluconazole resistant Candida albicans after long term suppressive therapy. Arch Intern Med 1993;153:1122.

63. Klein RS, Harris CA, Small CB, Moll B, Lesser M, Friedland GH. Oral candidiasis in high-risk patients as the initial manifestation of the acquired immunodeficiency syndrome. N Engl J Med 1984;311:354.

64. Centers for Disease Control. Revision of the CDC surveillance case definition for acquired immunodeficiency syndrome. MMWR 1987;36:1S.

65. Imam N, Carpenter CCJ, Mayer KH, Fisher A, Stein M, Danforth SB. Hierarchical pattern of mucosal candida infections in HIV-seropositive women. Am J Med 1990;89:142.

66. Carpenter CCJ, Mayer KH, Fisher A, Desai MB, Durand L. Natural history of acquired immunodeficiency syndrome in women in Rhode Island. Am J Med 1989;86:771.

67. Tavitian A, Raufman JP, Rosenthal LE. Oral candidiasis as a marker for esophageal candidiasis in the acquired immunodeficiency syndrome. Ann Intern Med 1986;104:54.

68. Levine MS, Woldenberg R, Herlinger H, Laufer I. Opportunistic esophagitis in AIDS: radiographic diagnosis. Radiology 1987;165:815.

69. Bonacini M, Laine L, Gal AA, Lee MH, Martin SE, Strigle S. Prospective evaluation of blind brushing of the esophagus for Candida esophagitis in patients with human immunodeficiency virus infection. Am J Gastroenterol 1990;85:385.

70. Porro GB, Parente F, Cernushi M. The diagnosis of esophageal candidiasis in patients with acquired immune deficiency syndrome: is endoscopy always necessary? Am J Gastroenterol 1989;84:143.

71. Rabeneck L, Laine L. Esophageal candidiasis in patients infected with the human immunodeficiency virus: a decision analysis to assess cost-effectiveness of alternative management strategies. Arch Intern Med 1994;154:2705.

72. Gould E, Kory WP, Raskin JB, Ibe MJ, Redlhammer DE. Esophageal biopsy findings in the acquired immunodeficiency syndrome (AIDS): clinicopathologic correlation in 20 patients. South Med J 1988;81:1392.

73. Lake-Bakaar G, Tom W, Lake-Bakaar D, et al. Gastropathy and ketoconazole malabsorption in the acquired immunodeficiency syndrome (AIDS). Ann Intern Med 1988;109:471.

74. Tavitian A, Raufman JP, Rosenthal LE, Weber J, Webber CA, Dincsoy HP. Ketoconazole-resistant Candida esophagitis in patients with acquired immunodeficiency syndrome. Gastroenterol 1991;90:443.

75. DeWit S, Weerts D, Goossens H, Clumeck N. Comparison of fluconazole and ketoconazole for oropharyngeal candidiasis in AIDS. Lancet 1989;1:746.

76. Lucatorto FM, Franker C, Hardy WD, Chafey S. Treatment of refractory oral candidiasis with fluconazole: a case report. Oral Surg Oral Med Oral Pathol 1991;71:42.

77. Cameron ML, Schell WA, Bruch S, Bartlett JA, Waskin HA, Perfect JR. Correlation of in vitro fluconazole resistance of Candida isolates in relation to therapy and symptoms of individuals seropositive for human immunodeficiency virus type I. Antimicrob Agents Chemother 1993;37:2449.

78. Newman SL, Flanigan TP, Fisher A, Rinaldi MG, Stein M, Vigilante K. Clinically significant mucosal candidiasis resistant to fluconazole treatment in patients with AIDS. Clin Infect Dis 1994;19:684.

79. Redding S, Smith J, Farinacci G, et al. Resistance of Candida albicans to fluconazole during treatment of oropharyngeal candidiasis in a patient with AIDS: documentation by in vitro susceptibility testing and DNA subtype analysis. Clin Infect Dis 1994;18:240.

80. Sangeorzan JA, Bradley SF, He X, et al. Epidemiology of oral candidiasis in HIV-infected patients: colonization, infection, treatment, and emergence of fluconazole resistance. Am J Med 1994;97:339.

81. Horn CA, Washburn RG, Givner LB, Peacock JE Jr, Pegram PS. Azole-resistant oropharyngeal and esophageal candidiasis in patients with AIDS. AIDS 1995;9:533535.

82. Narang PK, Trapnell CB, Schoenfelder JR, Lavelle JP, Bianchine JR. Fluconazole and enhanced effect of rifabutin prophylaxis. (Letter) N Engl J Med 1994;330:1316.

83. Cadle RM, Zenon GJ III, Rodriguez-Barradas MC, Hamill FJ. Fluconazole-induced symptomatic phenytoin toxicity. Ann Pharmacother 1994;28:191.

84. Drayton J, Dickinson G, Rinaldi MG. Coadministration of rifampin and itraconazole leads to undetectable levels of serum itraconazole. Clin Infect Dis 1994;18:266.

85. Havlir D, Torriani F, Dube M. Uveitis associated with rifabutin prophylaxis. Ann Intern Med 1994;121:510.

86. Graybill JR. AIDS commentary: histoplasmosis and AIDS. J Infect Dis 1988;158:623.

87. Sathapatayavongs B, Batteiger BE, Wheat J, Slama TG, Wass JL. Clinical and laboratory features of disseminated histoplasmosis

during two large urban outbreaks. Medicine (Baltimore) 1983;62:263.

88. Wheat LJ, Connolly-Stringfield PA, Baker RL, et al. Disseminated histoplasmosis in the acquired immune deficiency syndrome: clinical findings, diagnosis and treatment, and review of the literature. Medicine (Baltimore) 1990;69:361.

89. Johnson PC, Hamill RJ, Sarosi GA. Clinical review: progressive disseminated histoplasmosis in the AIDS patient. Semin Respir Infect 1989;4:139.

90. Anaissie E, Fainstein V, Samo T, Bodey GP, Sarosi GA. Central nervous system histoplasmosis: an unappreciated complication of the acquired immunodeficiency syndrome. Am J Med 1988;84:215.

91. Johnson PC, Khardori N, Najjar AF, Butt F, Mansell PWA, Sarosi GA. Progressive disseminated histoplasmosis in patients with acquired immunodeficiency syndrome. Am J Med 1988;85:152.

92. Ankobiah WA, Vaidya K, Powell S, et al. Disseminated histoplasmosis in AIDS: clinicopathologic features in seven patients from a non-endemic area. N Y State J Med 1990;90:234.

93. Wheat LJ, Batteiger BE, Sathapatayavongs B. *Histoplasma capsulatum* infections of the central nervous system. Medicine (Baltimore) 1990;69:244.

94. Huang CT, McGarry T, Cooper S, Saunders R, Andavolu R. Disseminated histoplasmosis in the acquired immunodeficiency syndrome: report of five cases from a nonendemic area. Arch Intern Med 1987;147:1181.

95. Barton EN, Roberts L, Ince WE, et al. Cutaneous histoplasmosis in the acquired immune deficiency syndrome: a report of three cases from Trinidad. Trop Geogr Med 1988;40:153.

96. Cohen PR, Bank DE, Silvers DN, Grossman ME. Cutaneous lesions of disseminated histoplasmosis in human immunodeficiency virus-infected patients. J Am Acad Dermatol 1990;23:422.

97. Ibanez HE, Ibanez MA. Case report: a new presentation of disseminated histoplasmosis in a homosexual man with AIDS. Am J Med Sci 1989;298:407.

98. Eisig S, Boguslaw B, Cooperband B, Phelan J. Oral manifestations of disseminated histoplasmosis in acquired immunodeficiency syndrome: report of two cases and review of the literature. J Oral Maxillofac Surg 1991;49:310.

99. Oda D, McDougal L, Fritsche T, Worthington P. Oral histoplasmosis as a presenting disease in acquired immunodeficiency syndrome. Oral Surg Oral Med Oral Pathol 1990;70:631.

100. Graham BD, McKinsey DS, Driks MR, Smith DL. Colonic histoplasmosis in acquired immunodeficiency syndrome: report of two cases. Dis Colon Rectum 1991;34:185.

101. Haggerty CM, Britton MC, Dorman JM, Marzoni JFA. Gastrointestinal histoplasmosis in suspected acquired immunodeficiency syndrome. West J Med 1985;143:244.

102. Macher A, Rodrigues MM, Kaplan W, et al. Disseminated bilateral chorioretinitis due to *Histoplasma capsulatum* in a patient with the acquired immunodeficiency syndrome. Ophthalmology 1985;92:1159.

103. Marshall BC, Cox JK, Carroll KC, Morrison RE. Case report: histoplasmosis as a cause of pleural effusion in the acquired immunodeficiency syndrome. Am J Med Sci 1990;300:98.

104. Nightingale SD, Parks JM, Pounders SM, Burns DK, Reynolds J, Hernandez JA. Disseminated histoplasmosis in patients with AIDS. South Med J 1990;83:624.

105. Wheat LJ, Connolly-Stringfield P, Kohler RB, Frame PT, Gupta MR. *Histoplasma capsulatum* polysaccharide antigen detection in diagnosis and management of disseminated histoplasmosis in patients with acquired immunodeficiency syndrome. Am J Med 1989;87:396.

106. McKinsey DS, Gupta MR, Riddler SA, Driks MR, Smith DL, Kurtin PJ. Long-term amphotericin B therapy for disseminated histoplasmosis in patients with the acquired immunodeficiency syndrome (AIDS). Ann Intern Med 1989;111:655.

107. Wheat J, Hafner R, Wulfsohn M, et al. Prevention of relapse of histoplasmosis with itraconazole in patients with the acquired immunodeficiency syndrome. Ann Intern Med 1993;118:610.

108. Wheat J, Hafner R, Korzun AH, et al. Itraconazole treatment of disseminated histoplasmosis in patients with the acquired immunodeficiency syndrome. Am J Med 1995;98:336.

109. Norris S, Wheat J, McKinsey D, et al. Prevention of relapse of histoplasmosis with fluconazole in patients with the acquired immunodeficiency syndrome. Am J Med 1994;96:504.

110. Knoper SR, Galgiani JN. Coccidioidomycosis. Infect Dis Clin North Am 1988;2:861.

111. Abrams DI, Robia M, Blumenfeld W, Simonson J, Cohen MB, Hadley WK. Disseminated coccidioidomycosis in AIDS. (Letter) N Engl J Med 1984;310:986.

112. Roberts CJ. Coccidioidomycosis in acquired immune deficiency syndrome: depressed humoral as well as cellular immunity. Am J Med 1984;76:734.

113. Kovacs JA, Forthal DN, Kovacs JA, Overturf GD. Disseminated coccidioidomycosis in a patient with acquired immune deficiency syndrome. West J Med 1984;140:447.

114. Bronnimann DA, Adam RD, Galgiani JN, et al. Coccidioidomycosis in the acquired immunodeficiency syndrome. Ann Intern Med 1987;106:372.

115. Fish DG, Ampel NM, Galgiani JN, et al. Coccidioidomycosis during human immunodeficiency virus infection: a review of 77 patients. Medicine (Baltimore) 1990;69:384.

116. Galgiani JN, Ampel NM. *Coccidioides immitis* in patients with human immunodeficiency virus infections. Semin Respir Infect 1990;5:151.

117. Byrne WR, Dietrich RA. Disseminated coccidioidomycosis with peritonitis in a patient with acquired immunodeficiency syndrome: prolonged survival associated with positive skin test reactivity to coccidioidin. Arch Intern Med 1989;149:947.

118. Ampel NM, Ryan KR, Carry PJ, Wieden MA, Schifman RB. Fungemia due to *Coccidioides immitis*: an analysis of 16 episodes in 15 patients and a review of the literature. Medicine (Baltimore) 1986;65:312.

119. Antoniskis D, Larsen RA, Akil B, Rarick MU, Leedom JM. Seronegative disseminated coccidioidomycosis in patients with HIV infection. AIDS 1990;4:691.

120. Galgiani JN, Ampel NM. AIDS commentary: coccidioidomycosis in human immunodeficiency virus-infected patients. J Infect Dis 1990;162:1165.

121. Tucker RM, Denning DW, Dupont B, Stevens DA. Itraconazole therapy for chronic coccidioidal meningitis. Ann Intern Med 1990;112:108.

122. Galgiani JN, Catanzaro A, Cloud GA, et al. Fluconazole therapy for coccidioidal meningitis: The NIAID-Mycoses Study Group. Ann Intern Med 1993;119:28.

123. Denning DW, Follansbee SE, Scolaro M, Norris S, Edelstein H, Stevens DA. Pulmonary aspergillosis in the acquired immunodeficiency syndrome. N Engl J Med 1991;324:654.

124. Lortholary O, Meyohas MC, Dupont B, et al. Invasive aspergillosis in patients with acquired immunodeficiency syndrome: report of 33 cases. Am J Med 1993;95:177.

125. Minamoto GY, Barlam TF, Vander Els NJ. Invasive aspergillosis in patients with AIDS. Clin Infect Dis 1992;14:66.

126. Keating JJ, Rogers T, Petrou M, et al. Management of pulmonary aspergillosis in AIDS: an emerging clinical problem. J Clin Pathol 1994;47:805.

127. Cox JN, diDio F, Pizzolato GP, Lerch R, Pochon N. Aspergillus endocarditis and myocarditis in a patient with the acquired immunodeficiency syndrome (AIDS): a review of the literature. Virchows Archiv A Pathol Anat Histopathol 1991;417:255.

128. Henochowicz S, Mustafa M, Lawrinson WE, Pistole M, Lindsay J. Cardiac aspergillosis in acquired immune deficiency syndrome. Am J Cardiol 1985;55:1239.

129. Bhatt B, Cappell MS. A perihepatic abscess containing *Aspergillus* in a patient with the acquired immune deficiency syndrome. Am J Gastroenterol 1990;85:1200.

130. Woods GL, Goldsmith JC. *Aspergillus* infection of the central nervous system in patients with acquired immunodeficiency syndrome. Arch Neurol 1990;47:181.

131. Aisner J, Schimpff SC, Wiernik PH. Treatment of invasive aspergillosis: relation of early diagnosis and treatment to response. Ann Intern Med 1977;86:539.

132. Denning DW, Tucker RM, Hanson LH, Stevens DA. Itraconazole in opportunistic mycoses: cryptococcosis and aspergillosis. J Am Acad Dermatol 1990;23:602.

133. Dupont B. Itraconazole therapy in aspergillosis: study in 49 patients. J Am Acad Dermatol 1990;23:607.

134. Viviani MA, Tortorano AM, Langer M, et al. Experience with itraconazole in cryptococcosis and aspergillosis. J Infect 1989;18:151.

135. Kitchen LW, Clark RA, Hoadley DJ, Wisniewski TL, Janney FA, Greer DL. Concurrent pulmonary *Blastomyces dermatitidis* and *Mycobacterium tuberculosis* infection in an HIV-1 seropositive man. J Infect Dis 1991;160:911.

136. Herd AM, Greenfield SB, Thompson WS, Brunham RC. Miliary blastomycosis and HIV infection. Can Med Assoc J 1990; 143:1329.

137. Pappas PG, Pottage JC, Powderly WG, et al. Blastomycosis in patients with acquired immunodeficiency syndrome. Ann Intern Med 1992;116:847.

138. Witzig RS, Hoadley DJ, Greer DL, Abriola KP, Hernandez RL. Blastomycosis and human immunodeficiency virus: three new cases and review. South Med J 1994;87:715.

139. Supparatpinyo K, Khamwam C, Baosoung V, Nelson KE, Sirisanthana T. Disseminated *Penicillium marneffei* infection in Southeast Asia. Lancet 1994;344:110.

140. Supparatpinyo K, Nelson KE, Merz WG, et al. Response to antifungal therapy by human immunodeficiency virus infected patients with disseminated *Penicillium marneffei* infections and in vitro susceptibilities of isolates from clinical specimens. Antimicrob Agents Chemother 1993;37:2407.

AIDS: Biology, Diagnosis, Treatment and Prevention, fourth edition, edited by Vincent T. DeVita, Jr., Samuel Hellman, and Steven A. Rosenberg. Lippincott–Raven Publishers, © 1997

14.3

Tuberculosis and Human Immunodeficiency Virus Infection

Michael O. Rigsby and Gerald Friedland

After years of decline in many parts of the world, tuberculosis (TB) has returned as a major public health problem in the United States and other developed countries, while remaining highly prevalent in many developing countries. In addition, the emergence of multidrug-resistant strains has increased the morbidity and mortality associated with TB, significantly diminishing the remarkable advances in treatment that followed the discovery of streptomycin in 1944. The resurgence of TB in the past decade is closely linked to the acquired immunodeficiency syndrome (AIDS) pandemic. The high susceptibility of patients infected with the human immunodeficiency virus (HIV) to TB and other mycobacterial infections is unique, creating for the clinician many diagnostic and therapeutic challenges. The epidemiology, pathophysiology, clinical manifestations, treatment, and prevention of TB in persons and populations infected with HIV are the subject of this chapter.

EPIDEMIOLOGY

The worldwide epidemic of HIV infection has resulted in a major secondary epidemic of TB. In the United States, this has reversed a 20-year decline in the annual incidence of TB cases, which reached its lowest point in 1985. Since then, the annual incidence rates first leveled off and then rose to a high of 26,673 cases in 1992.[1] In 1993, the number of new cases

Michael O. Rigsby: Assistant Professor of Medicine, Yale University School of Medicine, Director, HIV Program, West Haven VA Medical Center, 950 Campbell Avenue, 111-I, West Haven, CT 06516, phone 203-937-3446, fax 203-937-3476. Gerald Friedland: Professor of Medicine and Epidemiology and Public Health, Director, AIDS Program, Yale University School of Medicine, 135 College Street, Suite 323, New Haven, CT 06520, phone 203-737-2450, fax 203-737-4051.

decreased to 25,313.[2] But despite such indications that the resurgence may be abating, an excess of approximately 64,000 reported cases, compared with the number that would have been predicted had the declining trend from 1980 through 1984 continued, has been observed since 1985.[3]

Several lines of evidence suggest that these excess TB cases can be attributed in large part to the AIDS epidemic. The largest increases in TB rates have been observed in the 25- to 44-year-old age group, which is also the group in which most HIV infections occur.[4] In addition, the increase in TB cases has been greatest in geographic areas with high prevalence of HIV infection.[5-10] The overlap in demographic and geographic characteristics of the two diseases has been particularly pronounced in areas such as Dade County, Florida, and New York City; striking increases in TB rates have been observed in these cities among nonwhites in the 25- to 44-year-old age group, population groups which also account for 80% of HIV infections.

More direct evidence of association between HIV infection and TB has been provided by matching case registries of AIDS and TB. Such studies have been conducted in many areas of the United States and reveal incidence rates of TB among AIDS patients as high as 10%. These rates, even when adjusted for age, race, and sex, are many times higher than those of the general population.[4-6] Even more striking has been the association in some smaller population groups. In one state prison system, 56% of inmates with TB were listed in the HIV and AIDS registry.[11]

These epidemiologic associations could be explained, at least in part, by the fact that in many areas HIV infection is prevalent among groups already known to be at high risk for TB: drug users, the homeless, and foreign-born individuals. However, evidence also suggests that there is a more direct association between HIV infection and the development of TB. The high risk of reactivation of latent *Mycobacterium tuberculosis* infection was documented in a study of injection drug users in a New York City methadone maintenance program. Over a 2-year period, 8 cases of active TB occurred among 215 HIV-seropositive persons and none among 298 HIV-seronegative individuals. Of the 8 cases, 7 occurred among the 49 patients who were known to have had a previously reactive skin test with purified protein derivative (PPD). No cases of active TB occurred among 62 persons who were PPD-positive but HIV-seronegative.[12] These data indicated a rate of reactivation of 7.9% per year among persons coinfected with HIV and *M tuberculosis*, in contrast to an estimated lifelong risk of 5% to 10% among those infected with *M tuberculosis* alone. Further observations in this cohort demonstrated that the increased risk of developing active TB extended to those HIV-seropositive subjects who were anergic by skin testing as well.[13]

Although many cases of TB in HIV-infected individuals are caused by this increased risk of reactivation of latent infection, recent data suggest that new infection may be an even more important factor in the co-epidemic. There have been many reports of outbreaks of TB characterized by temporal and geographic clustering, similarity in drug susceptibility patterns, and, in some cases, similarity in DNA fingerprints of isolates.[14–16] Such outbreaks have occurred among HIV-infected groups in correctional facilities, AIDS clinics, and hospital wards. The risk of exposure to *M tuberculosis* in these settings is probably related to nonbiologic factors such as patient cohorting and environmental factors and is not known to be any higher because of HIV infection. However, the risk of developing active TB in a short period of time after exposure does appear to be greatly enhanced by HIV-related immune dysfunction. In one study of nosocomial transmission in a hospital ward, the case rate of active TB in HIV-infected patients after exposure to an infectious patient was 35.7 per 100 person-years.[14]

More recent documentation of community spread of TB, in part in association with HIV, has been provided by two recent studies that used restriction fragment length polymorphism (RFLP) patterns to type large numbers of isolates from persons with TB in New York and San Francisco.[17,18] This DNA fingerprinting technique makes it possible to identify patterns of strain identity within populations and to make estimates of the relative contributions of recent infection and reactivation disease to the overall TB case rate. In both the cities studied, the RFLP pattern analyses suggested that recent transmission accounted for higher numbers of cases than was previously believed: one third of the cases in San Francisco and 40% of the New York cases. Although the contribution of HIV infection to this apparent increase in new TB cases can only be inferred, it is plausible that such an association may exist, based on the higher risk of developing active TB after exposure.

For all these reasons—overlap in at-risk groups, increased risk of reactivation of latent *M tuberculosis* infection, high rates of infection after exposure, and rapid progression to disease—the connection between the HIV epidemic and TB is important at both individual clinical and societal public health levels. The Centers for Disease Control (CDC) has recommended, therefore, that HIV testing and counseling should be offered to everyone diagnosed with TB.[19] Because recommendations for prophylactic therapy may differ based on HIV serostatus, this recommendation can reasonably be extended to anyone with a positive PPD skin test as well.

In contrast to the United States, which has for several decades experienced relatively low rates of TB, the magnitude of the TB problem worldwide has never been diminished. Among adults, TB is the leading infectious cause of death worldwide, and approximately 90 million new cases are expected to occur during the current decade.[20] It is estimated that in 1990 more than 1.7 billion people worldwide were infected with *M tuberculosis*.[21] The majority of these infections occurred in the developing countries of Africa and Asia, where dramatically high rates of HIV infection and AIDS have been observed. Estimates of the prevalence of HIV infection and TB have produced predictions that more than 5.6 million people worldwide were dually infected by 1994, of whom 3.8 million lived in sub-Saharan Africa.[21,22] The high rate of coinfection has resulted in TB becoming the most common opportunistic infection associated with HIV disease in many parts of the world. In some reports, more than 50% of AIDS patients in Africa, India, and Thailand developed clinical TB.[23–27] Further evidence of the significant overlap in epidemiology is provided by a study from Kinshasa, Zaire, which reported that 33% to 47% of residents of a TB sanatorium were HIV-seropositive. Seropositivity was highest among patients between 20 to 40 years old, especially women in that age group, and patients with extrapulmonary TB.[28]

PATHOPHYSIOLOGY

HIV-infected individuals have an increased risk of developing TB by either of two mechanisms: failure to contain a primary infection (leading to rapid progression) or reactivation of latent infection. In both cases, the development of active disease results from the loss of cell-mediated immune responses as a result of HIV infection.

Most people are exposed to *M tuberculosis* through the inhalation of droplet nuclei containing the bacteria. If a person with pulmonary TB coughs, respiratory secretions and mycobacteria are aerosolized in droplet nuclei, which can remain suspended in the air for hours. The chance of being infected with *M tuberculosis* is a function of the density of these droplets in the air and the time spent in the local environment in which they are present. Prolonged contact in an enclosed space with a person who has cavitary pulmonary TB carries a high risk of infection, whereas brief exposure in open spaces to a person with a lower burden of organisms represents a much smaller risk.

After the infected droplet nuclei are inhaled, the mycobacteria multiply within macrophages in the bronchioles or alveoli and then spread to the regional lymph nodes in the hilum of the lung. Dissemination of organisms at this stage occurs when mycobacteria pass into the bloodstream through lymphatic channels. In most infected people, this primary infection is contained after several weeks by a robust cell-mediated immune response that contains the multiplication of mycobacteria. However, organisms can remain within granulomas for decades. The immune response in the infected host is manifested by proliferation of CD4-positive T-lymphocytes after exposure to mycobacterial antigens as well as a delayed-type hypersensitivity (DTH) response, which is responsible for the skin test reaction to PPD. Reactivation of disease occurs when organisms escape the immune-mediated containment mechanisms, leading to liquefaction of caseous material, cavity formation, and fibrosis.

The exact mechanism of the immune response to *M tuberculosis* is complex and not completely understood. It appears that a number of cell types are involved, including CD4+ T cells, γδ T cells, CD8-positive T cells, and mononuclear phagocytes.[29] Although overly simplistic, the traditional notion that the CD4+ T lymphocytes stimulates killing by macrophages through the production of cytokines is certainly a central feature of mycobacterial immunity. The lymphocyte clones responsible for this response produce large amounts of interferon-γ and little or no interleukin-4 or interleukin-5. This pattern has been ascribed to the so-called T_{H1} functional phenotype of CD4 cells; however, some studies suggest a more complex picture, with predominant production of interferon-γ early in the immunologic response and interleukin-4 later.[30]

Like the normal immunologic responses to mycobacteria, the immunologic defects that result from HIV infection are multiple and complex. The most obvious is a steady decline in the number of circulating CD4+ lymphocytes. In addition to this quantitative defect, there is a qualitative change in CD4-lymphocyte effector function, which may decline significantly before the fall in CD4 cells approaches a level associated with most opportunistic infections. This dysfunction is characterized by loss of the ability to recognize various antigens, and it can be detected in vitro by a decline in lymphocyte proliferation and in vivo as loss of DTH responses (ie, anergy).[31] A characteristic pattern of anergy has consistently been noted in association with HIV: response to HIV-associated antigens is lost first, followed by response to recall antigens, and, finally, response to mitogens.[32] In addition, and perhaps linked to the development of anergy, is a functional shift in favor of T_{H2} responses, which decreases production of interferon-γ and interleukin-2.[33] Because of these qualitative changes in lymphocyte function (even if the absolute number of CD4 cells remains relatively high) and because of the inherent pathogenicity of the organism, the HIV-infected patient is at risk for development of TB much sooner than for other opportunistic infections such as *Pneumocystis carinii* pneumonia.

CLINICAL MANIFESTATIONS OF TUBERCULOSIS IN HIV DISEASE

Several reports have suggested that TB usually occurs before AIDS is clinically diagnosed (on the basis of criteria other than TB) and therefore is one of the earliest infectious complications of HIV. In one series from Florida,[5] TB was diagnosed at least 1 month before AIDS diagnosis in 57% of patients. In a report from San Francisco,[10] among HIV-positive patients with TB the median CD4 count was 326 cells/mm³ (range, 23 to 742 cells/mm³), significantly higher than the levels associated with development of other opportunistic infections. Because it appears that new infections, as opposed to reactivation, are becoming an important mechanism of TB disease, it is possible that a shift toward higher incidence of TB will be seen among people with more advanced HIV disease, who appear to be at particularly high risk after nosocomial exposures.

General Characteristics

In general, the traits that characterize TB in HIV-seropositive patients include the potential for rapid progression from primary infection to disseminated disease, atypical radiographic features of pulmonary disease, increased frequency of extrapulmonary disease, and involvement of unusual sites of infection. All of these atypical features seem to occur more commonly with more advanced stages of immunosuppression, and the paradigm that emerges is one of typical TB early in the course of HIV infection and atypical manifestations with advanced HIV disease.

The spectrum of clinical features described here has been compiled from a number of case series and individual case reports. These may tend to overreport unusual or atypical features because, in most cases, the cohorts described were defined by the presence of known HIV infection. Because it is more likely that HIV infection will be recognized if it is more advanced, and because clinical manifestations of TB may be less typical in advanced HIV disease, such reports contain a potential bias. This possibility has been avoided in two studies, in which all patients with TB in a given area were evaluated systematically for HIV infection. In one report from Florida,[34] 31% of patients with TB evaluated during a 6-month period were HIV positive. These patients had significantly more extrapulmonary manifestations of TB, more adenopathy on chest radiographs, and fewer cavitary lesions than HIV-seronegative patients. The majority of the HIV-positive patients (64%) had no clinical evidence of AIDS or AIDS-related complex. In contrast to these findings, a similar study from San Francisco[10] reported no significant differences in clinical or radiographic features among 17 HIV-positive TB patients (median CD4 cell count, 326 cells/mm³), compared with 43 HIV-seronegative TB patients. It can be concluded that there do appear to be real differences in TB associated with HIV, but the extent of those differences is variable.

Primary Infection

Reports of the manifestations of primary TB disease have resulted from investigations of outbreaks associated with nosocomial or institutional exposure and therefore may not be entirely representative of larger populations. In addition, many of these reports have involved infection with antibiotic-resistant strains of *M tuberculosis*, which may have a more aggressive course because of the lack of effective therapy. Nonetheless, it seems apparent that HIV infection increases the risk of rapid progression from initial infection to serious disease.[15] This has been demonstrated in several reports of outbreaks in which very high numbers of HIV-positive patients exposed to an index case of TB developed active disease shortly thereafter. In one such report from New York, 12 residents of a housing facility for people living with HIV developed TB during a 4-month period. The strains were all identical by RFLP analysis, indicating a common source of exposure, probably the first patient with active TB. This group represented 37% of the HIV-positive subjects potentially exposed. The median CD4 count in the group that developed TB was 68 cells/mm^3, but the range was broad (5 to 623 cells/mm^3) and included several patients who had CD4 counts higher than 200 cells/mm^3. Therefore, the attack rate among exposed individuals was very high and was not limited to those with the most advanced stages of HIV infection. The time between exposure and development of active disease was also very short, as little as 4 weeks in one subject.

Latent Infection and Reactivation

In people with HIV infection who were previously infected with *M tuberculosis* or who recover from primary infection, the ensuing period of latent infection is characterized by an increased likelihood of skin test anergy and increased risk of progression to active disease. Skin test anergy, defined as lack of reaction to trichophytin, mumps, and *Candida* antigens, has been reported to be present in up to 72% of HIV-positive patients with CD4 counts lower than 200 cells/mm^3 and in 25% of patients with counts higher than 600 cells/mm^3.[35]

If reactivation of latent TB infection occurs, the signs and symptoms in HIV-positive patients are similar to those in other groups and frequently overlap with signs and symptoms of other complications of HIV. In a series of more than 100 patients from Florida, fever and night sweats were the most common complaints. Dyspnea and productive cough affected the majority of the patients, and weight loss was reported in 36%.[16] Pulmonary involvement occurs in most patients, either alone or with extrapulmonary sites of involvement. The clinical and radiographic features of pulmonary disease may be atypical and appear to depend both on the stage of HIV-related immunosuppression and the mode of infection (ie, primary or reactivation). However, the distinction between new and reactivated infection is more difficult in this population because of the presence of atypical features. In the previously cited series from Florida, radiographic features were described for patients with multidrug-resistant isolates, all or most of which were presumed to represent recent infection, as well as for control patients who had drug-susceptible isolates. In the former group (40 chest radiographs), alveolar infiltrates occurred in 76%, interstitial infiltrates in 23%, cavitation in 18%, pleural effusions in 40%, and mediastinal adenopathy in 45%. Among the controls, who presumably represented a mixture of new and reactivated infections, interstitial infiltrates were significantly more likely (49%), but cavitation was rare (3%), and the frequencies of mediastinal adenopathy (42%) and pleural effusions (42%) were similar frequency to those seen in the cases with drug resistance.

Another study examined the radiographic features of pulmonary TB as a function of CD4 cell count.[37] Radiographs from subjects with HIV infection and proven pulmonary TB were characterized as either typical of reactivation TB or atypical. Among patients with CD4 counts higher than 200 cells/mm^3, only 1 of 9 had atypical features. However, atypical features were present in radiographs from 21 of 26 patients with CD4 counts lower than 200/mm^3 ($P<.001$). The atypical features included lower lobe alveolar opacities, multifocal alveolar opacities, interstitial infiltrates, mediastinal adenopathy, and pleural effusions. There were insufficient data to determine how many of these cases were the result of recent infection. In general, classic upper lobe infiltrates and cavitary lesions seem to be less frequently seen in HIV-positive subjects with TB compared with those without HIV infection.[34] This may be a result of the absence of destructive changes associated with intact DTH responses. This diminished inflammatory response presumably also accounts for the consistent observations that a small percentage of HIV-infected patients have sputum cultures positive for *M tuberculosis* with normal chest radiographs.

Extrapulmonary involvement is one of the most frequently reported features of TB in HIV infection, and it occurs in 40% to 75% of patients with both diagnoses. The proportion of extrapulmonary cases increases as HIV disease progresses. In San Francisco, 60% of patients with AIDS and TB had at least one extrapulmonary site of disease, compared with 28% of non-AIDS patients with TB ($P<.001$).[38] An increase in extrapulmonary sites of TB infection has been observed in nationwide surveys coincident with the previously described increase in TB incidence rates during the period of 1986 to 1993, and this increase has been substantially more common among AIDS patients who were black or whose risks for acquisition of HIV included injection drug use or heterosexual sexual contact.[39] Many extrapulmonary sites have been reported, including the central nervous system, bone, viscera, skin, pericardium, eye, and pharynx. In one large series from Spain,[40] tuberculous meningitis occurred in 10% of HIV-infected patients with TB, compared with only 2% of HIV-seronegative patients during the same time period ($P<.001$). The clinical characteristics, spinal fluid profile, and response to treatment did not differ significantly in relation to HIV status. In 14 of the 18 patients for whom results were available, CD4 counts were below 200 cells/mm^3.

Diffuse lymph node involvement and mycobacteremia also appear to be more common in HIV-infected persons[41,42]; these may represent easily accessible sites for diagnostic examination. Mycobacteremia occurs in up to 26% of HIV-infected patients with TB and has been associated with poor outcomes.[43] Most of these patients have clinical evidence of widespread disease with abnormal chest radiographs, although not necessarily a miliary pattern, and abnormal liver function tests.[43,44] Marked elevations of serum lactate dehydrogenase (mean, 585 U/L) were seen in all patients in one series[44]; this finding, along with radiographic abnormalities, may erroneously suggest a diagnosis of *P carinii* pneumonia.

The prognosis of HIV-infected patients with TB depends on many variables, but, in general, response to appropriate therapy is good. However, there is some suggestion that active TB may have additional impact on the course of HIV disease. In a retrospective cohort study, Whalen and colleagues[45] compared HIV-positive patients who had active TB with HIV-positive control subjects without TB who were matched for CD4+ T-lymphocyte counts. Patients with TB tended to develop AIDS-defining opportunistic infections at a greater rate and had significantly shorter survival times than controls. The odds ratio for death associated with TB in a multivariate analysis was 2.17 (1.06 to 2.73). This is similar to the results of a retrospective study of HIV-infected women from Zaire, in whom the relative risk of death associated with TB was estimated to be 2.7.[46] In neither of these studies were the poor outcomes clearly the result of poor response to TB treatment. The possibility that TB may augment or accelerate the immunosuppression of HIV is plausible based on observations that TB can trigger immune activation and stimulate production of cytokines such as tumor necrosis factor (TNF).[47] However, the true impact of and mechanisms for TB-induced HIV disease progression await further study.

DIAGNOSIS

As in other patients, the diagnosis of TB in HIV-infected patients is based on assessment of risk of infection, clinical presentation, direct examination of appropriately collected patient specimens, and isolation and identification of mycobacteria from cultures. Although recent advances in methodology have opened the door to more rapid diagnosis, there remains no reliable rapid method for identification of *M tuberculosis* directly from patient materials. Given the slow growth rate of these organisms in vitro, diagnosis is often a long and frustrating process. In this situation, a knowledge of the clinical features of TB and a high index of suspicion are of great importance.

The risk of *M tuberculosis* infection varies with both demography and geography. The excess cases of TB and of AIDS observed during the past few years are concentrated in the 25- to 44-year-old age group, in minority and foreign-born populations, in homeless populations, and in substance abusers.[48,49] However, HIV-associated TB is not confined to these populations and occurs in all risk and demographic groups. The approach must therefore be individualized and should take into account the potential for exposure in nosocomial settings, homeless shelters, and correctional facilities; contact with a known or suspected case of TB; and any history, including remote history, of PPD skin test reactivity. Because skin test anergy may occur early in the course of HIV infection, information about PPD testing at earlier times (eg, at entry into military service, during drug treatment programs, when starting school or a new job) should be sought.

The clinical features associated with TB and the possibility of atypical features in HIV-infected patients have been previously discussed. TB should be suspected not only in patients with pulmonary disease but also in those with unexplained fevers, systemic symptoms, lymphadenopathy (particularly mediastinal), or symptoms localized to any of the extrapulmonary sites that *M tuberculosis* may infect.

PPD skin testing is less useful as a diagnostic tool in HIV-infected patients than in other groups, and the sensitivity of the test decreases with advancing HIV disease. At the time of presentation with active TB, more than 60% of HIV-infected patients have PPD skin reactions smaller than 10 mm.[49] In a large study of skin test reactivity in Haiti,[50] subjects with HIV infection were significantly less likely than HIV-negative subjects to have a PPD reaction of at least 10 mm. However, the percentage of HIV-seropositive subjects with reactions of 5 mm or greater was similar to that of HIV-seronegative persons with reactions of 10 mm or greater. Therefore, even small PPD reactions are likely to be significant indicators of TB infection in HIV-positive patients.

Direct examination of patient specimens with the use of stains for mycobacteria remains the most useful rapid diagnostic method for TB. This is especially true for pulmonary TB, in which the number of organisms seen in expectorated sputum correlates well with infectivity and with response to therapy. Acid-fast microscopy of a single specimen, however, is a relatively insensitive test because of the small amount of material that is examined. Examination of multiple sputum specimens significantly enhances the sensitivity for detection of pulmonary TB.[51] Fluorescent staining allows for faster scanning of slides and may therefore increase sensitivity by increasing the amount of sample examined.

There has been concern that the utility of sputum acid-fast smears may be reduced in HIV-infected populations. The sensitivity of smear examination may be reduced if the blunted inflammatory response and relative absence of cavitary lesions results in fewer organisms expectorated in sputum. Two studies have specifically addressed this possibility. A retrospective study from New York[52] found that significantly fewer HIV-seropositive patients with con-firmed pulmonary TB had positive smears (45%), compared with control patients without HIV (81%). The number of sputum specimens examined in the two groups was similar (mean, 3.82). A larger study from Haiti[53] of 289 patients with pulmonary TB also found that the sensitivity of sputum smear examination was decreased in subjects who were HIV seropositive (79% versus 66%). However, two other studies have shown no difference in the sensitivity of acid-fast smears between HIV-seropositive and -seronegative patients.[10,54]

Another potential limitation in HIV-infected patients is the inability to differentiate *M tuberculosis* from other mycobacterial species, which frequently colonize immuno-compromised patients. Several studies have reported that acid-fast organisms visualized in expectorated sputum sam-ples are more likely to be *M tuberculosis* than *Mycobac-terium avium* complex (MAC) organisms. In a large study from a hospital where MAC was the predominant mycobac-terial isolate, sputum smears and culture results were com-pared over a 3-year period.[54] Subjects included patients with and without known HIV infection. Of 2139 specimens that yielded positive mycobacterial cultures during the study period, MAC was identified from 51% and *M tuberculosis* from 43%. However, *M tuberculosis* was cultured from 92% of smear-positive expectorated sputum specimens. The pos-itive predictive value for *M tuberculosis* of an acid-fast smear was 92% for expectorated sputum, 71% for induced sputum samples, and 71% for bronchoalveolar lavage spec-imens. Similarly, in the previously described study from Haiti,[53] the positive predictive value of sputum acid-fast smear for TB remained high (80%) in HIV-seropositive sub-jects, although somewhat lower than in controls (90%). Given the imperfect sensitivity of examinations of expecto-rated sputum, more invasive tests may be pursued if the clin-ical suspicion for TB is high but multiple sputum smears are negative. In one study of 31 such patients with or at risk for HIV infection, the role of fiberoptic bronchoscopy was eval-uated. In this study, transbronchial biopsy provided the highest yield for an immediate diagnosis of TB.[55]

Definitive identification and testing for drug susceptibil-ity depend on the ability to grow mycobacteria in culture media. Conventional and more recently developed tech-niques are outlined in Table 14.3-1. Traditional culture mate-rials include egg-based solid media, such as Löwenstein-Jensen medium, and synthetic solid media, such as Middle-brook 7H10 and 7H11 agars. With either, identification depends on the visualization of mycobacterial colonies and is limited by the slow growth rate of these organisms. A major advance in laboratory diagnosis of TB has been the development of systems based on detecting growth in liquid media with the use of radiometric methods (Bactec system, Becton-Dickenson Diagnostic Instrument Systems, Sparks, MD). In these systems, the medium contains palmitic acid labeled with carbon-14. The metabolism of this fatty acid by the growing mycobacteria liberates radioactive carbon diox-

TABLE 14.3-1. *Laboratory diagnosis of mycobacteria*

Test or Procedure	Conventional (C) or Rapid (R)	Time From Initiation of Work-up
SPECIMEN COLLECTION		
Decontamination (if nonsterile site), concentration, and acid-fast staining	R	24–48 h
Growth in Bactec*	R	1–4 wk
Growth on solid media	C	2–6 wk
Species identification by genetic probe or high-performance liquid chromatography	R	2–6 wk
Species identification with biochemical tests	C	4–8 wk
SUSCEPTIBILITY TESTING†		
Broth-based radiometric method (Bactec)*	R	3–8 wk
Agar-based proportional method	C	4–10 wk

*Bactec is an automated radiometric system for detection of growth in liquid media.

†Drug susceptibility testing can be performed simul-taneously with culture and speciation (direct susceptibility testing) if the suspicion for tuberculosis is high and drug resistance is likely.

ide; periodic sampling of the gasses in the culture-containing flask permits rapid detection of mycobacterial growth. Species identification was accomplished in the past with biochemical tests that often involved additional diagnostic delays. Genetic probes are now available for the identifica-tion of *M tuberculosis* and several other common mycobac-terial species. These probes recognize species-specific sequences of ribosomal RNA. The combination of radio-metric growth detection methods and specific genetic probes has significantly shortened the time needed for defin-itive laboratory diagnosis of TB.

Other techniques currently being evaluated in a number of clinical settings include identification based on high-performance liquid chromatography or polymerase chain reaction (PCR) technology. PCR-based methods have the potential advantage of identification and speciation of very small numbers of mycobacteria. Theoretically, these meth-ods may permit diagnosis directly from patient specimens, eliminating the need for culture of organisms. In practice, the utility of PCR has been limited by problems with the sensitivity and, particularly, the specificity of results. In some laboratories, sensitivity and specificity have been reported to exceed 85%.[56] However, in a European study that provided prepared specimens to seven laboratories for PCR testing, considerable variability was observed. In several laboratories, false-positive rates ranged from 3% to 20%, and in one, 77% of positive results were false.[57] Sensitivity also varied widely among the different sites. Although these problems currently limit the practical utility of PCR diagno-sis, it is likely this or similar methods will continue to make possible the more rapid identification of smaller numbers of organisms, thus speeding the diagnosis of TB.

Diagnosis of TB in extrapulmonary sites presents special challenges, including difficulty in sampling and low concentrations of organisms in some sites. Careful thought should be given to sampling the site most likely to yield useful diagnostic information and to assuring that specimens are cultured appropriately; in many instances, samples should also be examined histologically for evidence of mycobacterial disease. One report has suggested that in HIV-positive patients with fever of undetermined cause, liver biopsy is of greater utility in diagnosing mycobacterial infection than blood culture or bone marrow examination.[58] Fine-needle aspiration of enlarged lymph nodes may also be a relatively sensitive test for detection of mycobacterial infection in patients with suspected disseminated infection.

Drug susceptibility testing should be performed on all *M tuberculosis* isolates and can be accomplished by any of several methods based on inhibition of growth on agar or in liquid media in the presence of specified concentrations of antibiotics. In most cases, drug susceptibility testing is performed only after definitive isolation and identification of *M tuberculosis.* However, if there is a high suspicion of drug resistance, it is sometimes possible to perform drug susceptibility tests simultaneously with isolation and identification (direct susceptibility testing). If information about drug susceptibility is needed rapidly, the clinician should communicate directly with the diagnostic laboratory to see whether such arrangements are possible. In the near future, rapid tests based on increasing knowledge of the mechanisms and biology of drug resistance may become available.

TREATMENT

Chemoprophylaxis

In patients with HIV infection, as in others, chemoprophylaxis with isoniazid appears to be highly effective in preventing the progression from TB infection to tuberculous disease.[59,60] The increased risk of developing active disease associated with HIV infection has provoked a number of questions, however, regarding who should receive prophylactic therapy, how long it should be continued, and whether isoniazid alone is the most effective agent. Although some uncertainty remains in these areas and clinical trials are ongoing, some data are available.

The risk of developing active TB in HIV-infected persons with positive PPD skin test reactions may be as high as 7.9% per year. This figure comes from the previously cited study by Selwyn and colleagues in a methadone maintenance program in New York. All of these cases occurred in patients who did not take prophylactic isoniazid. In a subsequent report from the same cohort in which the overall prevalence of PPD reactivity was 20%, the risk of developing TB among anergic, HIV-positive drug injectors was found to be similar to that in PPD reactors. Similar results were obtained

in a study of HIV-infected patients from Spain, most of whom were also injecting drug users.[59] These observations have led to recommendations that all HIV-infected patients undergoing PPD skin testing be tested for anergy and to speculation that anergic patients may benefit from preventive therapy with isoniazid. However, a recent study among injecting drug users in Baltimore, Maryland,[61] found that there was considerable change in DTH status over time, particularly among persons infected with HIV. During a median follow-up period of 17.5 months, 24% of HIV-seropositive persons who were initially DTH positive became anergic, and 15% who were initially anergic became DTH positive. Stable anergy and change from DTH-positive status to anergy were both associated with lower CD4 cell counts.

Others have suggested that establishing the likelihood of *M tuberculosis* infection on grounds other than skin testing is a more useful means for determining who should receive prophylactic therapy.[62] Factors such as community rates of infection and active disease, demographic information, history of exposure, and abnormalities on chest radiographs can all be used to identify those HIV-infected patients at highest risk. These individuals may be considered for prophylactic therapy regardless of skin test results. The CDC has recommended that preventive therapy for anergic HIV-infected persons be considered if the patient has had known contact with an active TB case or belongs to a group in which the prevalence of TB infection is at least 10%.[63]

The American Thoracic Society has recommended that isoniazid prophylactic therapy be continued for 12 months in persons with HIV infection, although there are no studies comparing the efficacy of this approach with that of either shorter of longer courses.[64] Because of the difficulty of such long courses, considerable attention has been given to development of shorter regimens using multiple drugs. This approach is currently being evaluated in a large trial conducted by the AIDS Clinical Trials Group and the Community Program for Clinical Research on AIDS; 12 months of isoniazid therapy is being compared with 2 months of rifampin plus pyrazinamide. Preliminary results are available from a similar study of HIV-positive patients in Haiti.[65] In this trial, subjects received either isoniazid twice weekly for 6 months or rifampin plus pyrazinamide twice weekly for 2 months. The rate of development of active TB was similar in the two groups after 3 years, but patients who received rifampin and pyrazinamide had significantly more cases of active TB during the first 10 months.

Treatment of Active Disease

Despite the impaired cell-mediated immune response to *M tuberculosis* in persons with HIV infection, the response to therapy, if it is appropriately selected and instituted in a timely manner, is usually excellent. Mortality from TB in HIV-infected patients appears to result in most cases from failure to make the diagnosis, poor compliance with therapy, or the presence of drug resistance.

In a large, retrospective series of 132 coinfected patients from San Francisco,[66] standard regimens of isoniazid and rifampin plus ethambutol for the first 2 months (42%), isoniazid and rifampin plus pyrazinamide and ethambutol for the first 2 months (31%), isoniazid and rifampin (10%), isoniazid and rifampin plus pyrazinamide for the first 2 months (3%), and other combinations (14%) were employed. The intended treatment duration was 6 months for regimens containing pyrazinamide and 9 months for the others. Sixty-six patients completed a full course of therapy and were monitored for a median period of 9.6 months. Among treated patients, 8 (6.4%) died of what were thought to TB-related causes, most within the first month of therapy. One patient's therapy failed because of multidrug-resistant organisms and poor compliance. Three additional relapses after completion of therapy were seen in patients who were believed to be poorly compliant. Therefore, it was concluded that the response among compliant patients who survived the first month of treatment was excellent.

The optimal duration of therapy in HIV-infected patients has been at least partially addressed in a report from Zaire.[67] In a prospective, open-label study, more than 400 patients with TB received isoniazid, rifampin, ethambutol, and pyrazinamide daily for 2 months, followed by twice-weekly isoniazid and rifampin for 4 months. One hundred eighty-six HIV-infected patients were then randomly assigned to receive either an additional 6 months of twice-weekly isoniazid and rifampin, or placebo. Patients were assessed for treatment efficacy after completion of 6 months of therapy and for relapse through 24 months after diagnosis. Patients who received the additional 6 months of treatment had a relapse rate of 1.9%, compared with 9% among those who received only 6 months of treatment ($P<.01$). However, there was no difference in survival rate between the two groups.

The American Thoracic Society and the CDC have formulated recommendations for initial treatment regimens for TB.[64] The initial phase of treatment should consist of isoniazid, rifampin, and pyrazinamide, with the addition of ethambutol or streptomycin until drug susceptibility information is available. The addition of a fourth drug is not necessary if the possibility of drug resistance is remote. Given that recent increases in drug resistance have been observed predominantly in HIV-infected populations and that the margin of error in treatment of immunosuppressed patients may be small, it would seem prudent to treat all HIV-infected patients with four drugs initially. After the initial 2-month phase, patients who are responding adequately and who have susceptible isolates can be continued on isoniazid and rifampin alone for at least 4 months. Many authorities recommend extending therapy in HIV-infected patients to a minimum total duration of 9 months. This question is being addressed in a large, ongoing study by the AIDS Clinical Trials Group in which HIV-infected subjects with sensitive TB isolates are randomly assigned to total treatment courses of 6 or 9 months.

Intermittent dosing of anti-TB drugs has been shown to be effective and may improve compliance. Recommended regimens are described in Table 14.3-2.

If resistance or intolerance to isoniazid or rifampin is present, longer treatment regimens are required. Rifampin and ethambutol given together for 18 months, or for 12 months after cultures become negative, are effective if isoniazid cannot be used. Alternatively, if an initial four-drug regimen was used, isoniazid can be discontinued and rifampin, ethambutol, and pyrazinamide continued for 6 months. If an isolate is resistant to multiple drugs, a regimen based on known susceptibility should be devised. Ideally, at least three agents to which the isolate is susceptible should be given, and response to treatment should be carefully assessed. Treatment should continue for 12 months after results of bacteriologic culture are negative.

The problem of toxicities from anti-TB medication is complicated by the frequent use of multiple other drugs and the presence of other complications of HIV disease that can mimic adverse drug effects. This is particularly true in monitoring and assessing abnormalities in liver function. In addition, it appears likely that such reactions, particularly with rifampin, actually do occur more commonly in HIV-infected patients.[68] In a series from San Francisco, 18% of patients required a change in therapy because of drug reactions, primarily rashes and hepatitis. Two thirds of these reactions were attributed to rifampin.[69] There are also a number of drug interactions that are potentially important in these patients. Rifampin induces hepatic enzymes, which rapidly metabolize methadone. Therefore, rifampin frequently induces symptoms of opiate withdrawal in patients on methadone maintenance. Besides the unpleasant effects that result, the symptoms of opiate withdrawal may be misinterpreted as toxicity to rifampin, leading to poor patient compliance or to unnecessary changes in treatment. Some methadone programs routinely increase dosage by 25% to 50% if treatment with rifampin is begun. The commonly used antifungal agents ketoconazole and fluconazole interact with isoniazid and rifampin, with resultant reduced serum levels and ineffective antifungal therapy in some patients.[70] Finally, rifampin absorption may be inhibited by ketoconazole, with resultant failure of treatment for TB.[71] Overlapping toxicities as well as true drug interactions may also occur. For example, peripheral neuropathy may develop as a complication of the antiretroviral agents didanosine, zalcitabine, and stavudine as well as from isoniazid.

Drug-Resistant Tuberculosis

One of the most alarming features of the resurgence of TB in the past decade has been the increased prevalence of strains that are resistant to one or more of the first-line anti-TB drugs. In the past, most cases of drug-resistant TB involved secondary, or acquired, resistance—that is, resistance developed after exposure to antimycobacterial drugs through selection for drug-resistant mutants. This type of

TABLE 14.3-2. *Recommended initial drug regimens for tuberculosis in adults*

Agent	Daily Dose	Maximum Daily Dose	Twice-weekly Dose	Adverse Effects
Isoniazid	5 mg/kg PO or IM	600 mg	10 mg/kg (maximum 900 mg)	Hepatitis, peripheral neuropathy, hypersensitivity
Rifampin	10 mg/kg PO	600 mg	10 mg/kg (maximum 600 mg)	Nausea, vomiting, fever, rash, hepatitis; drug interactions; methodaone, ketoconazole, fluconazole
Pyrazinamide	15–25 mg/kg PO	2 g	50–70 mg/kg	Hepatitis, hyperuricemia
Ethambutol	15–25 mg/kg PO	2.5 g	50 mg/kg	Optic neuritis* (decreased red-green discrimination, decreased visual acuity), rash
Streptomycin	15 mg/kg	1 g	25–30 mg/kg	Ototoxic, nephrotoxic effects*

*Potential for toxicity is increased by renal insufficiency.

resistance is associated with the use of inappropriate treatment regimens, poor compliance with appropriate regimens, and inadequate duration of therapy. Among the therapeutic mistakes that lead to acquired drug resistance, selection of an inappropriate initial regimen, failure to recognize drug resistance, and addition of a single drug to a failing regimen are the most common.[72] Acquired resistance, as well as treatment failure, can also result from inadequate levels of antimycobacterial drugs. This can be a particular problem in HIV-infected patients because of impaired absorption of oral medications. In one study of AIDS patients with disseminated MAC infection, serum levels of oral antimycobacterial drugs were consistently lower than expected.[73] In ongoing pharmacokinetic studies at the National Jewish Center for Immunology and Respiratory Medicine, this situation appears to be true for patients with HIV infection and TB as well, particularly with rifampin and ethambutol.[74] If these findings are confirmed in additional subjects, it may become necessary to monitor therapeutic drug levels in HIV-positive patients being treated for TB.

Primary resistance is the term used to describe drug resistance in a person never previously treated with anti-TB therapy. It results from the spread of drug-resistant strains, from an index patient with acquired resistance to additional susceptible hosts. Under usual circumstances, most of these hosts would not develop active TB and there would be little indication of an overall increase in drug resistance. However, in patients infected with HIV, the increased risk of progression to disease after exposure, the frequent difficulty in assuring adequate therapy for TB, and the concentration of highly susceptible hosts in situations such as hospital wards, prisons, and homeless shelters has produced increases in drug resistance that have alarmed public health professionals and the general public. The enormous impact of HIV on drug-resistant TB was illustrated in a study from New York City, in which 75% of isolates resistant to isoniazid and rifampin from previously untreated TB patients came from patients known to be infected with HIV.[75] A number of outbreaks of multidrug-resistant TB among hospitalized

patients with HIV have been reported, pointing out the importance of nosocomial transmission.

The implications of increased resistance are profound. The effect of resistance to a single agent may not be great if appropriate multidrug regimens are employed and if drug susceptibility testing is available so that regimens can be tailored appropriately. Resistance to multiple drugs raises the stakes considerably. For *M tuberculosis*, resistance to rifampin and isoniazid (ie, the definition of multidrug resistance in this context) is associated with poor response to treatment, prolonged shedding of infectious organisms, increased cost of providing care, need for prolonged treatment, and poor clinical outcomes.[76] This is particularly true for patients with HIV infection, in whom mortality resulting from infection with multidrug-resistant *M tuberculosis* strains has approached 80%.[75,77] In an outbreak involving 62 HIV-seropositive patients with multidrug-resistant TB in Florida, median survival time was 2.1 months, compared with 14.6 months for patients with TB strains that were resistant to no more than one drug, although patients with earlier stages of HIV disease and multidrug-resistant TB had significantly longer survival than those with AIDS.[16] More recently, better results have been reported from a group of 10 patients with multidrug-resistant TB in New York.[78] Despite relatively advanced HIV infection (median CD4 count, 114 cells/mm^3), 9 of 10 patients survived with sterilized cultures after median follow-up of 10.2 months. Earlier recognition of drug resistance and the use of directly observed therapy were believed to be significant factors in the success with these patients.

The prompt recognition of drug resistance and the use of appropriate regimens are essential for successful treatment. Acquired drug resistance should be suspected in patients with a history of TB within 2 years before presentation who received at least 8 weeks of anti-TB therapy or who were treated with inadequate courses of anti-TB therapy. Primary drug resistance should be suspected if there is known or potential exposure to resistant TB or if infection may have been acquired in a medical facility, prison, or shelter in which other cases of drug-resistant TB are known to have occurred. Clinical or radiographic progression of TB despite more than 4 weeks of supervised therapy with an appropriate regimen of three or more drugs should also suggest drug resistance.

Treatment regimens for multidrug-resistant TB must be based on drug susceptibility results, but if drug resistance is considered very likely, empiric regimens (pending results of drug susceptibility testing) can be designed based on knowledge of the patient's prior treatment history (at least two drugs not previously used should be incorporated) or on known susceptibility of other isolates in an outbreak or cluster. After susceptibility test results are available, treatment regimens can be adjusted appropriately. Ideal regimens for multidrug-resistant TB should include at least three (preferably four) drugs to which the isolate is fully susceptible in vitro and which the patient has not previously received. This therapy always involves use of some agents considered second line in terms of their efficacy or safety (Table 14.3-3). Because many of these drugs are unfamiliar to clinicians, expert guidance should be sought in the management of multidrug-resistant TB. Long courses of treatment are required, and surgical treatment of localized disease, if possible, is often necessary for eventual cure.

Adherence to Therapy

Effective pharmacologic regimens for the prevention and treatment of TB entail long courses of therapy—in the case of treatment for active disease, with multiple medications. Although these drugs are usually well tolerated, many patients perceive or actually experience one or more untoward effects from the treatment. Adherence to treatment recommendations is no better than 50% in some studies, and it can be as low as 10% among certain populations.[79,80] About 8% of patients with TB develop multiple relapses, leading to long periods of potential infectivity.[81] Besides producing more cases of primary infection, nonadherence is the largest factor in the development of drug resistance. Because of the increased risk of transmitting infection and the increased cost of treating drug-resistant TB, failure to ensure adherence to prescribed treatment has profound public health and financial consequences.

Many individual patient characteristics have been associated with poor adherence to TB therapy, including homelessness, alcohol abuse, lower educational level, poor understanding of the disease, and inability to understand treatment instructions. However, some authors have pointed out that it is perhaps even more important to recognize the environmental, structural, and operational factors that are beyond the patient's control.[82] Effective interventions to improve adherence are likely to be those that include attention to overcoming obstacles to effective therapy as well as patient education and close supervision of therapy. Programs that have been shown to work have incorporated use of patient incentives (eg, food, clothing), enablers (eg, transportation, bus tokens) and directly observed therapy.[83]

Directly observed therapy is an especially effective tool. In a study from New York that compared TB patients treated with directly observed therapy to a historical cohort that had received traditional, unsupervised treatment,[84] direct observation was associated with significant decreases in the frequencies of primary drug resistance, acquired drug resistance, and disease relapse. The CDC and the American Thoracic Society currently recommend that consideration be given to treating all patients with directly observed therapy.[85]

PREVENTION

Prevention of TB is a multidimensional effort that includes case finding, contact tracing, effective preventive and curative therapy, environmental controls to prevent spread of disease, and the use of personal protective devices. A full discussion of these topics is beyond the scope of this chapter; the reader is directed to several excellent reviews of these subjects and to the CDC Guidelines for Preventing the Transmission of *M tuberculosis* in Health-Care Facilities.[86] However, several aspects of TB prevention are of particular significance to HIV-infected and at-risk groups and warrant further discussion.

The high risk for development of active disease after infection with *M tuberculosis* in HIV-positive patients makes it important to identify these patients and to provide preventive therapy with isoniazid if there is no active disease. For this reason, most recommendations for primary

TABLE 14.3-3. *Second-line agents for treatment of tuberculosis in adults*

Agent	Daily dose	Major adverse effects
Ciprofloxacin	750–1500 mg PO	Gastrointestinal upset, headache, variable absorption (do not administer with antacids)
Ofloxacin	600–800 mg PO	Similar to ciprofloxacin
Kanamycin, amikacin, capreomycin	15 mg/kg IM or IV 1000	Auditory and renal toxicity
Ethionamide	500–1000 mg PO	Gastrointestinal upset, hepatitis
Cycloserine	750–1000 mg PO	Psychosis, depression, seizures, rash (administer with pyridoxine)
Para-aminosalicylic acid (PAS)	8–12 gm PO	Gastrointestinal upset, sodium load, hypersensitivity

medical care of HIV-positive patients include periodic screening with PPD skin testing. Our practice has been to test all patients in our HIV clinic yearly with PPD and two control antigens. Issues concerning the utility of anergy testing and the appropriate indications for treatment of anergic patients have been discussed previously. Our approach is to individualize decisions about prophylaxis in anergic patients based on assessment of potential exposures and evaluation of chest radiographs for evidence of old TB infection.

Early identification and treatment of patients with active TB decreases the time of infectivity and minimizes exposure to others. In HIV-infected patients, this requires a heightened awareness of atypical clinical and radiographic presentations and access to excellent diagnostic laboratory facilities. In response to the increased incidence of TB and the emergence of multidrug-resistant strains, many laboratories have been able to reduce the time between specimen acquisition and reporting of culture and drug susceptibility results.

Institutional spread of TB is of particular concern to people living with HIV because of the clustering of persons at high risk for acquisition of new infection in such settings as HIV clinics, hospital wards, correctional facilities, and homeless shelters. Decreasing the possibility of TB spread in these settings requires maintenance of a high index of suspicion for TB in patients with undiagnosed pulmonary disease, avoidance of cough-inducing procedures, and proper use of environmental controls such as respiratory isolation rooms. Rooms for housing of patients with known or suspected pulmonary TB should have ventilatory systems that prevent movement of air from the room to other patient areas. This usually involves creation of a pressure gradient, with the isolation room at negative pressure to surrounding corridors or rooms, and a method of frequent air exchanges that are vented to the outside. The CDC guidelines contain detailed information regarding systems that comply with these principles.

The allocation and proper use of respiratory isolation rooms can create strains for institutions, medical care providers, and patients. To avoid inconsistencies and to ensure proper use of resources, clear guidelines explaining when respiratory isolation is required and when it can be discontinued are helpful. In our institution, all patients in whom a diagnosis of pulmonary TB is being considered or has been established are admitted to respiratory isolation rooms. Respiratory isolation is continued until the patient is determined to be noninfectious based on three negative sputum smears, or, if the diagnosis if confirmed, until the patient is on effective therapy, has exhibited clinical improvement, and has had negative results for acid-fast bacilli on sputum smears collected on three consecutive days.

Health care workers with and without HIV infection are at risk for occupational exposure to TB. The most important tool for prevention of infection in health care workers is the ability to recognize and appropriately isolate patients who potentially have active TB. This requires proper education and training of clinical manifestations and modes of transmission of TB. Other strategies to protect health care workers include screening for latent TB with periodic PPD skin testing and use of personal respiratory protection devices (masks). Detailed information regarding these and other recommendations to prevent transmission of TB in health care facilities is contained in the CDC guidelines previously mentioned.

Correctional facilities are another setting in which spread of TB is a special concern. In a study from the New York state correctional system, incidence of TB among inmates rose from 15.4 cases per 100,000 in 1976 through 1978 to 105.5 cases per 100,000 in 1986.[11] More than half of the cases in 1985 and 1986 occurred among inmates who were known to be HIV positive. This increased incidence probably represents a confluence of several factors: high prevalence of latent TB among inmate populations, rising prevalence of HIV infection with consequent increased incidence of reactivation, and acquisition of new infection because of crowding and the potential for delayed recognition of infectious inmates. Most of the cases in the New York report were believed to be reactivation cases, although genetic analysis of isolates revealed at least one cluster of three patients, suggesting inmate-to-inmate transmission. The recognition of increased risk of TB to both inmates and workers in correctional facilities has led to new recommendations from the Advisory Council for the Elimination of Tuberculosis. These recommendations emphasize the inadequacy of relying exclusively on PPD skin testing to identify inmates with TB. Prompt identification and isolation of inmates with symptoms indicative of pulmonary TB, along with medical evaluation, PPD skin testing, and chest radiography, is recommended as a more reliable screening method. Indications for preventive therapy and regimens for treatment of active disease do not differ from those for other populations, although special problems may arise in providing adequate treatment if the period of incarceration is short or if inmates are transferred from one correctional facility to another. The use of designated TB treatment coordinators who work closely with other correctional facilities and with public health departments may help to overcome some of these difficulties.

CONCLUSION

Tuberculosis is a highly contagious disease, spread through the air, for which there are effective drugs and for which cure can reasonably be anticipated in most cases. On the other hand, HIV infection is spread only by sexual or blood-to-blood contact, is so far invariably fatal, and can be treated only with therapeutic agents of limited efficacy. The approach to controlling and ultimately eliminating each of these diseases, therefore, is quite different, but the need to confront the two diseases together is compelling.

In order to advance the battle against TB, new tools are needed. More rapid diagnostic tests, including rapid tests of drug susceptibility, are especially important for HIV-positive patients because of the atypical clinical presentations and increased drug resistance. New drugs active against drug-resistant strains and with favorable toxicity profiles are once again a priority. Better understanding of the complexities of the immunologic response to TB may make possible additional therapeutic options, such as cytokine therapy, or may lead to the development of a more effective vaccine. However, the lessons of the past suggest that technology alone is insufficient. Ultimately, the most powerful tool may be the creation of more effective public health structures to ensure the availability, distribution, and proper utilization of existing effective diagnostic and treatment technologies. The fact that TB is still with us despite the availability of very effective antimicrobial therapies should also be a sobering warning to those who believe that better drugs alone can win the war against AIDS.

REFERENCES

1. Centers for Disease Control. Summary of notifiable diseases, United States, 1992. MMWR 1993;41:1.
2. Centers for Disease Control. Summary of notifiable diseases, United States, 1993. MMWR 1994;42:1.
3. Centers for Disease Control. Expanded tuberculosis surveillance and tuberculosis morbidity, United States, 1993. MMWR 1994;43:361.
4. Reider HL, Cauthen GM, Kelly GD, Block AB, Snider DE. Tuberculosis in the United States. JAMA 1989;262:385.
5. Centers for Disease Control. Tuberculosis in acquired immunodeficiency syndrome, Florida. MMWR 1986;35:587.
6. Centers for Disease Control. Tuberculosis and AIDS, New York City. MMWR 1987;36:785.
7. Centers for Disease Control. Tuberculosis and AIDS, Connecticut. MMWR 1987;36:133.
8. Pitchenik AE, Cole C, Russell BW, Fischl MA, Spira TJ, Snider DE. Tuberculosis, atypical mycobacteriosis, and the acquired immunodeficiency syndrome among Haitian and non-Haitian patients in South Florida. Ann Intern Med 1984;101:641.
9. Sunderm A, McDonald RJ, Maniatis T, et al. Tuberculosis as a manifestation of the acquired immunodeficiency syndrome (AIDS). JAMA 1986;256:363.
10. Theuer CP, Hopewell PC, Elias DK, Schecter GF, Rutherford GW, Chaisson RE. Human immunodeficiency virus infection in tuberculosis patients. J Infect Dis 1990;162:8.
11. Braun MM, Truman BL, Maguire B et al. Increasing incidence of tuberculosis in a prison inmate population: association with HIV infection. JAMA 1989;261:393.
12. Selwyn PA, Hartel D, Lewis VA, et al. A prospective study of the risk of tuberculosis among intravenous drug users with human immunodeficiency virus infection. N Engl J Med 1989;320:545.
13. Selwyn PA, Sckell B, Alcabes P, Friedland GH, Klein RS, Schoenbaum EE. High risk of active tuberculosis in HIV-infected drug users with cutaneous anergy. JAMA 1992;268:504.
14. Dooley SW, Villarino ME, Lawrence M, et al. Nosocomial transmission of tuberculosis in a hospital unit for HIV-infected patients. JAMA 1992;267:2632.
15. Daley CL, Small PM, Schecter GF, et al. An outbreak of tuberculosis with accelerated progression among persons infected with the human immunodeficiency virus: an analysis using restriction-fragment-length-polymorphisms. N Engl J Med 1992;26:231.
16. Fischl MA, Uttamchandani RB, Daikos GL, et al. An outbreak of tuberculosis caused by multiple-drug-resistant tubercle bacilli among patients with HIV infection. Ann Intern Med 1992;117:177.
17. Small PM, Hopewell PC, Singh SP, et al. The epidemiology of tuberculosis in San Francisco: a population based study using conventional and molecular methods. N Engl J Med 1994;330:1703.
18. Alland D, Kalbut GE, Moss AR, et al. Transmission of tuberculosis in New York City: an analysis of DNA fingerprinting and conventional epidemiologic methods. N Engl J Med 1994;330:1710.
19. Centers for Disease Control. Tuberculosis and human immunodeficiency virus infection: recommendations of the advisory committee for the elimination of tuberculosis. MMWR 1989;38:236.
20. Dolin PJ, Raviglione MC, Kochi A. Global tuberculosis incidence and mortality during 1990–2000. Bull World Health Organ 1994;72:213.
21. Sudre P, ten Dam G, Kochi A. Tuberculosis: a global overview of the situation today. Bull World Health Organ 1992;70:149.
22. Narain JP, Raviglione MC, Kochi A. HIV-associated tuberculosis ind eveloping countries: epidemiology and strategies for precention. Tuber Lung Dis 1992;73:311.
23. Mbaga JM, Pallangyo KJ, Bakari M, Aris EA. Survival time of patients with acquired immunodeficiency syndrome: experience with 274 patients in Dar-Es-Salaam. East Afr Med J 1990;67:95.
24. Lucas SB, Nounnou A, Peacock C, et al. The mortality and pathology of HIV infection in a West African city. AIDS 1993;7:1569.
25. McLeod DT, Neill P, Robertson W, et al. Pulmonary disease in patients infected with the human immunodeficiency virus in Zimbabwe, Central Africa. Trans R Soc Trop Med Hyg 1989;83:691.
26. Kaur A, Babu PG, Jocob M, et al. Clinical and laboratory profile of AIDS in India. J Acquir Immune Defic Syndr 1992;5:883.
27. Raviglione MC, Snider DE, Kochi A. Global epidemiology of tuberculosis. JAMA 1995;273:220.
28. Colebunders RL, Ryder RW, Nzilambi N, et al. HIV infection in patients with tuberculosis in Kinshasa, Zaire. Am Rev Respir Dis 1989;139:1082.
29. Orme IM, Anderson P, Boom WH. T cell response to *Mycobacterium tuberculosis*. J Infect Dis 1993;167:1481.
30. Orme IA, Roberts AD, Griffin JP, Abrams JS. Cytokine secretion by CD4 T lymphocytes acquired in response to *Mycobacterium tuberculosis* infection. J Immunol 1993;151:518.
31. Wahren B, Morfeldt-Mansson L, Biberfeld G, et al. Characteristics of the specific cell-mediated immune response in human immunodeficiency virus infection. J Virol 1987;61:2017.
32. Schrier RD, Gnann JW, Landes R, et al. T cell recognition of HIV synthetic peptides in a natural infection. J Immunol 1989;142:1166.
33. Clerici M, Hakim FT, Venzon DJ, et al. Changes in interleukin-2 and interleukin-4 production in asymptomatic human immunodeficiency virus-seropositive individuals. J Clin Invest 1993;91:759.
34. Pitchenik AE, Burr J, Suarez M, et al. Human T-cell lymphotropic virus-III (HTLV-III) seropositivity and related disease among 71 consecutive patients in whom tuberculosis was diagnosed. Am Rev Respir Dis 1987;135:875.
35. Markowitz N, Hansen NI, Wilcosky TC, et al. Tuberculin and anergy testing in HIV-seropositive and HIV-seronegative persons. Ann Intern Med 1993;119:185.
36. Fischl MA, Daikos GL, Uttamchandani RB, et al. Clinical presentation and outcome of patients with HIV infection and tuberculosis caused by multiple-drug-resistant bacilli. Ann Intern Med 1992;117:184.
37. Keiper MD, Beumont M, Elshami A, Lunglotz CP, Miller WT. CD4 T lymphocyte count and the radiographic presentation of pulmonary tuberculosis. Chest 1995;107:74.
38. Chaisson RE, Schecter GF, Theuer CP, et al. Tuberculosis in patients with the acquired immunodeficiency syndrome. Am Rev Respir Dis 1987;136:570.
39. Braun MM, Byers RH, Heyward WL, Rutherford GW, Echenberg DF, Hopewell PC. Acquired immunodeficiency syndrome and extrapulmonary tuberculosis in the United States. Arch Intern Med 1990;150:1913.
40. Berenguer J, Moreno S, Laguna F, et al. Tuberculous meningitis in patients infected with the human immunodeficiency virus. N Engl J Med 1992;326:668.
41. Barnes PF, Bloch AB, Davidson DT, Snider DE. Tuberculosis in patients with human immunodeficiency virus infection. N Engl J Med 1991;324:1644.
42. Saltzman BR, Motyl MR, Friedland GH, et al. *Mycobacterium tuberculosis* bacteremia in the acquired immunodeficiency syndrome. JAMA 1986;256:390.

43. Shafer RW, Goldberg R, Sierra M, Glatt AE. Frequency of *Mycobacterium tuberculosis* bacteremia in patients with tuberculosis in an area endemic for AIDS. Am Rev Respir Dis 1989;140:1611.

44. Barber TW, Craven DE, McCabe WR. Bacteremia due to *Mycobacterium tuberculosis* in patients with human immunodeficiency virus infection. Medicine (Baltimore) 1990;69:375.

45. Whalen C, Horsburgh CR, Hom C, et al. Accelerated course of human immunodeficiency virus infection after tuberculosis. Am J Respir Crit Care Med 1995;151:129.

46. Braun MM, Badi N, Ryder RW, et al. A retrospective cohort study of the risk of tuberculosis among women of childbearing age with HIV infection in Zaire. Am Rev Respir Dis 1991;143:501.

47. Wallis RS, Vjecha M, Amir-Tahmassab M, et al. Influence of tuberculosis on human immunodeficiency virus (HIV-1): enhanced cytokine expression and elevated beta-2-microglobulin in HIV-1 associated tuberculosis. J Infect Dis 1993;176:43.

48. Torres RA, Mani S, Altholz J, Brickner PW. Human immunodeficiency virus infection among homeless men in a New York City shelter: association with *Mycobacterium tuberculosis* infection. Arch Intern Med 1990;150:2030.

49. Pitchenis AE, Fertel D. Tuberculosis and nontuberculous mycobacterial disease. Med Clin North Am 1992;76:121.

50. Johnson MP, Coberly JS, Clarmont HC, et al. Tuberculin skin test reactivity among adults infected with human immunodeficiency virus. J Infect Dis 1992;166:194.

51. Lipsky BA, Gates J, Tenover FC, Plorde JJ. Factors affecting the clinical value of microscopy for acid-fast bacilli. Rev Infect Dis 1984;6:214.

52. Klein NC, Duncanson FP, Lenox TH, Pitta A, Cohen S, Wormser GP. Use of mycobacterial smears in the diagnosis of pulmonary tuberculosis in AIDS/ARC patients. Chest 1989;95:1190.

53. Long R, Scalcini M, Manfreda J, Jean-Baptiste M, Hershfield E. The impact of HIV on the usefulness of sputum smears for the diagnosis of tuberculosis. Am J Public Health 1991;81:1326.

54. Yajko DM, Nassos DM, Sanders CA, Madej JJ, Hadley WK. High predictive value of the acid-fast smear for *Mycobacterium tuberculosis* despite the high prevalence of *Mycobacterium avium* complex in respiratory specimens. Clin Infect Dis 1994;19:334.

55. Salzman SH, Schindel ML, Aranda CP, Smith RL, Lewis ML. The role of bronchoscopy in the diagnosis of pulmonary tuberculosis in patients at risk for HIV infection. Chest 1992;102:143.

56. Forbes SA, Hicks KE. Direct detection of *Mycobacterium tuberculosis* in respiratory specimens in a clinical laboratory by polymerase chain reaction. J Clin Microbiol 1993;31:1688.

57. Noordhoek GT, Kolk AH, Bjune G, et al. Sensitivity and specificity of PCR for detection of *Mycobacterium tuberculosis*: a blind comparison study among seven laboratories. J Clin Microbiol 1994;32:277.

58. Prego V, Glatt AE, Roy V, Thelmo W, Dincsoy H, Raufman JP. Comparative yield of blood culture for fungi and mycobacteria, liver biopsy, and bone marrow biopsys in the diagnosis of fever of undetermined origin in human immunodeficiency virus–infected patients. Arch Intern Med 1990;150:333.

59. Moreno S, Baraaaia-Etxaburu J, Bouza E, et al. Risk for developing tuberculosis among anergic patients infected with HIV. Ann Intern Med 1993;119:194.

60. Pape JW, Jean SS, Ho JL, et al. Effect of isoniazid prophylaxis on incidence of active tuberculosis and progression of HIV infection. Lancet 1993;342:268.

61. Caiaffa WT, Graham NM, Galai N, Rizzo RT, Nelson KE, Vlahov D. Instability of delayed-type hypersensitivity skin test anergy in human immunodeficiency virus infection. Arch Intern Med 1995;155:2111.

62. Jordan TJ, Lewit E, Montgomery RL, Reichman LB. Isoniazid as preventive therapy in HIV-infected intravenous drug abusers: a decision analysis. JAMA 1991;265:2987.

63. Centers for Disease Control. Purified protein derivative (PPD)-tuberculin anery and HIV infection. MMWR 1991;40(RR-5):27.

64. American Thoracic Society. Treatment of tuberculosis and tuberculosis infection in adults and children. Am J Respir Crit Care Med 1994;149:1359.

65. Halsey N, Coberly J, Losikoff P, et al. Twice weekly INH vs RIF and PZA for TB prophylaxis in HIV infected adults. Second National Conference on Human Retroviruses and Related Infections. Washington, DC, January 1995.

66. Small PM, Schecter GF, Goodman PC, et al. Treatment of tuberculosis in patients with advanced human immunodeficiency virus infection. N Engl J Med 1991;324:289.

67. Perriens JH, St Louis ME, Mukadi YB, et al. Pulmonary tuberculosis in HIV-infected patients in Zaire. N Engl J Med 1995;332:779.

68. Chaisson RE, Slutkin G. Tuberculosis and human immunodeficiency syndrome. J Infect Dis 1989;159:96.

69. Small PM, Schecter GF, Goodman PC, et al. Treatment of tuberculosis in patients with advanced human immunodeficiency virus infection. N Engl J Med 1991;324:289.

70. Barnes PF, Bloch AB, Davidson PT, Snider DE. Tuberculosis in patients with HIV infection. N Engl J Med 1991;324:1644.

71. Enselhard D, Stutman HR, Marks MI. Interaction of ketoconazole with rifamin and isoniazid. N Engl J Med 1984;311:1681.

72. Mahmoudi A, Iseman MD. Pitfalls in the care of patients with tuberculosis. JAMA 1993;270:65.

73. Gordon SM, Horsburgh CR, Peloquin CA, et al. Low serum levels of oral antimycobacterial agents in patients with disseminated *Mycobacterium* avium complex disease. J Infect Dis 1993;168:1559.

74. Peloquin C, MacPhee AA, Berning SE. Malabsorption of antimycobacterial medications. (Letter) N Engl J Med 1993;329:1122.

75. Frieden TR, Sterling T, Pablos-Mendez A, Kilburn JO, Cauthen GM, Dooley SW. The emergence of drug-resistant tuberculosis in New York City. N Engl J Med 1993;328:521.

76. Goble M, Iseman MD, Madsen LA, Waite D, Ackerman L, Horsburgh CR. Treatment of 171 patients with pulmonary tuberculosis resistant to isoniazid and rifampin. N Engl J Med 1993;328:527.

77. Busillo C, Lassnau K, Sanjana V, et al. Multidrug resistant *Mycobacterium tuberculosis* in patients with human immunodeficiency virus infection. Chest 1992;102:745.

78. Salomon N, Perlman DC. Improved outcomes in a cohort of HIV-infected patients with multidrug-resistant tuberculosis enrolled in a directly observed therapy tuberculosis program. Abstract 4. Programs and Abstracts: Second National Conference on Human Retroviruses and Related Infections, Washington, DC, January 1995.

79. Brudney K, Dobkin J. Resurgent tuberculosis in New York City: human immunodeficiency virus, homelessness, and the decline of tuberculosis control programs. Am Rev Respir Dis 1992;144:1459.

80. Werhane MJ, Snukst-Torbeck G, Schraufnagel D. The tuberculosis clinic. Chest 1989;96:815.

81. Kopanoff DE, Snider D, Johnson M. Recurrent tuberculosis: why do patients develop disease again? A United States Public Health Service cooperative survey. Am J Public Health 1988;78:30.

82. Sumartojo E. When tuberculosis treatment fails: a social behavioral account of patient adherence. Am Rev Respir Dis 1993;147:1311.

83. Centers for Disease Control. Approaches to improving adherence to antituberculosis therapy, South Carolina and New York, 1986–1991. MMWR 1993;42:74.

84. Weiss SP, Slocum F, Blais B, et al. The effect of directly observed therapy on the rates of drug resistance and relapse in tuberculosis. N Engl J Med 1994;330:1179.

85. American Thoracic Society. Control of tuberculosis in the United States. Am Rev Respir Dis 1992;146:1624.

86. Centers for Disease Control. Guidelines for preventing the transmission of *Mycobacterium tuberculosis* in health-care facilities, 1994. MMWR 1994;43:1.

AIDS: Biology, Diagnosis, Treatment and Prevention, fourth edition, edited by Vincent T. DeVita, Jr., Samuel Hellman, and Steven A. Rosenberg. Lippincott–Raven Publishers, © 1997

14.4

Other Bacterial Infections

John J. Zurlo and H. Clifford Lane

Although such agents as *Pneumocystis carinii*, *Cryptococcus neoformans*, and cytomegalovirus have been long recognized as principal pathogens causing disease in patients infected with the human immunodeficiency virus (HIV), common bacterial pathogens such as *Streptococcus pneumoniae* and *Haemophilus influenzae* were not formally recognized for their role in causing morbidity related to the acquired immunodeficiency syndrome (AIDS) until recently. The Centers for Disease Control and Prevention first included recurrent bacterial pneumonias in their case definition of AIDS only in 1993.[1] Although the true incidence of bacterial infections is difficult to discern and varies with the population surveyed, such diseases as pneumonia occur at a rate many times higher than in the general population.[2,3] The incidence is highest in patients whose CD4-positive T-lymphocyte counts are lower than 200 cells/mm^3.[1] This chapter describes the clinical features of the major nonmycobacterial, bacterial infections seen in HIV-infected patients, including pneumonia, sinusitis, bacteremia, and bacillary angiomatosis (BA). Host defense abnormalities that may predispose to the development of these infections are also discussed, as are preventative strategies. Bacterial infections of the gastrointestinal tract are discussed in Chapter 10.

HOST DEFENSE DEFECTS THAT MAY PREDISPOSE TO BACTERIAL INFECTIONS

Given the protean nature of the immune system defects that have been described in HIV-infected patients, it is little wonder that bacterial infections are part of the spectrum of clinical disease seen in these patients. Table 14.4-1 lists

some of the host defense defects that may predispose patients with HIV infection to bacterial infections.

Humoral immune defects have been recognized since the earliest part of the HIV epidemic. In comparison with healthy controls, B cells from HIV-infected individuals proliferate poorly in response to mitogens. Cells from patients with more advanced disease tend to have a worse response than those from patients with early-stage disease.[4] Similarly, B cells that spontaneously secrete immunoglobulin have been found to be present in much higher numbers than they are in control subjects.[5] Both defects point to polyclonal B-cell activation, the clinical manifestation of which, hypergammaglobulinemia, is present in most HIV-infected patients, even in the earliest stages of infection. Although immunoglobulin A (IgA) and IgM are variably elevated, IgG is elevated persistently throughout the course of infection.[6] Circulating levels of certain IgG subclasses, particularly IgG2, have been reported to be decreased in HIV-infected patients.[7,8] IgG2 deficiency may be of particular importance, because antibodies directed against bacterial polysaccharide antigens commonly belong to this subclass. Concentrations of secretory IgA also have been reported to be decreased in HIV-infected patients as a result of decreased numbers of IgA-secreting plasma cells.[9,10]

Despite the high circulating levels of immunoglobulin, antibody responses to specific antigens have been shown to be markedly diminished if either protein or polysaccharide antigens are employed.[6,11] For a variety of potentially useful vaccines, including *H influenzae* conjugate vaccine, polyvalent pneumococcal vaccine, and inactivated influenza vaccine, antibody responses have been shown to vary inversely with stage of disease.[6,11,12] This diminished response to neoantigen challenge has significant implications for the development of immunization strategies.

Quantitative and qualitative defects in phagocytic cells may also predispose some HIV-infected patients to recurrent bacterial infections. Mild to moderate leukopenia is seen commonly in patients with low CD4 counts. Against this background, patients can experience even further drops in the

John J. Zurlo, Associate Professor of Medicine, Pennsylvania State University, Milton S. Hershey Medical Center, Division of Infectious Diseases, P.O. Box 850, Hershey, PA 17033.

H. Clifford Lane, Clinical Director, National Institute of Allergy and Infectious Diseases, National Institutes of Health, Building 10, Room 11B13, 10 Center Drive, Bethesda, MD 20892.

TABLE 14.4-1. *Host defense defects that may predispose HIV-infected patients to bacterial infections*

Diminished antibody response to protein and
  polysaccharide antigens
Diminished B-cell mitogenic response
Immunoglobulin G subclass deficiencies
Decreased production of secretory Immunoglobulin A
Quantitative and qualitative abnormalities of neutrophils
Macrophage dysfunction
Long-term urinary and intravenous catheterization
Encephalopathy
Malnutrition

neutrophil count as a result of exposure to certain drugs such as ganciclovir or zidovudine or as a result of the infiltration of the bone marrow by tumor cells or infection. Yet, the incidence of infectious complications associated with neutropenia may not be as great for HIV-infected patients as for patients with hematologic malignancies, who typically experience more profound and prolonged neutropenic episodes.[13] Sustained neutropenia at levels between 500 and 1000 cells/mm^3 as a result of zidovudine treatment is not associated with a major increase in the incidence of bacterial infections.[14]

In addition to quantitative neutrophil defects, abnormalities in neutrophil function, including chemotaxis, bacteriocidal activity, and binding for phagocytosis, also have been described and may be important determinants of susceptibility to bacterial infection.[15,16] Among other phagocytic cells, macrophages are targets for HIV infection.[17] Such cells are part of the reticuloendothelial system and have been shown to be defective in the clearance of complement and IgG opsonized particles in both the liver and spleen.[18,19]

Along with defects intrinsic to immune and phagocytic defense mechanisms, other host defense defects develop, particularly in patients with late-stage disease. HIV dementia complex can result in bladder dysfunction and ineffective clearance of respiratory secretions, leading to bacterially-induced urosepsis and pneumonia, respectively. The use of long-term indwelling intravenous and bladder catheters also predisposes to invasive bacterial infections. Finally, the weight loss and malnutrition that occur with HIV wasting syndrome frequently lead to cachexia, immobility, and resultant decubiti, which can become bacterially infected.

BACTERIAL INFECTIONS OF THE RESPIRATORY TRACT

Pneumonia

The lower respiratory tract is one of the most common sites of bacterial infection observed in HIV-infected patients. Pneumonia may be community-acquired or nosocomial. In most series, *S pneumoniae* and *H influenzae* are the two most common pathogens causing community-acquired pneumonia. Other pathogens that have been described include *Staphylococcus aureus*, *Moraxella catarrhalis*, and other *Haemophilus* and *Streptococcus* species.[20] More recently,

reports of pneumonia and other invasive infections caused by *Pseudomonas aeruginosa* have appeared.

Streptococcus pneumoniae

The importance of the pneumococcus was recognized early in the AIDS epidemic.[21] Polsky and colleagues estimated the yearly attack rate for pneumococcal pneumonia in New York to be 17.9 per 1000 patients with AIDS, which was 6.9 times higher than in the general population.[2] Witt and colleagues in Boston noted a yearly incidence of pneumococcal pneumonia to be 45.5 per 1000, 17.5 times higher than in the general population.[22]

One characteristic that makes pneumococcal pneumonia different in HIV-infected patients is the high rate of associated bacteremia. The incidence of pneumococcal bacteremia in one cohort of HIV-infected patients in San Francisco between the ages of 20 and 55 years was approximately 100-fold greater than in the general age-matched population.[23]

With the exception of a higher incidence of bacteremia, the clinical presentation of pneumococcal pneumonia is very similar to that in patients without HIV infection. Presenting symptoms include the typically abrupt onset of high fever, productive cough, dyspnea, and pleuritic chest pain.[3] Leukocytosis may be modest or absent, particularly in patients with low CD4 counts and patients receiving myelosuppressive agents. The leukocyte differential often reveals large numbers of band neutrophils. The chest radiograph most commonly reveals lobar or multilobar consolidation; diffuse or patchy infiltrates are less commonly seen.[2] Pleural effusions are occasionally seen, but frank empyema is unusual.[3]

A presumptive diagnosis can be made if a high-quality sputum specimen is obtained and reviewed after Gram's staining. The finding of numerous neutrophils along with a predominance of gram-positive diplococci is suggestive of pneumococcal pneumonia. However, culture confirmation is required to establish the diagnosis, because Gram's stain readings can sometimes be misleading. The organism also is isolated commonly from blood cultures. Prevention, treatment, and prognosis of pneumococcal disease are discussed later in this chapter.

Haemophilus influenzae

Along with the pneumococcus, *H influenzae* is one of the well recognized causes of bacterial pneumonia in this patient group. In San Francisco, the overall incidence of invasive *H influenzae* disease in HIV-infected men between the ages of 20 and 49 years was reported by Steinhart and colleagues to be 79.2 and 14.6 per 100,000 for patients with and without AIDS, respectively.[24] This compares with an overall rate of invasive *H influenzae* disease in this age group of 0.65 to 2.8 per 100,000 adults.[24] Yet, the incidence rate reported in Steinhart's series may underestimate the true incidence of significant *H influenzae* disease in this population, because the study included only patients from whom the organism was grown from normally sterile sites. Most *H influenzae* isolates reported from HIV-infected patients and in the general adult population have been nontypeable.[24,25] In the Steinhart series, isolates from approximately one third of the patients were type B.[24]

Presenting symptoms of *H influenzae* pneumonia almost invariably include fever and cough.[26] Most patients also present with pleuritic chest pain and dyspnea. Laboratory abnormalities include leukocytosis and a left-shifted leukocyte differential. Accompanying bacteremia occurs less frequently that it does with pneumococcal pneumonia. In a group of 34 patients with *H influenzae* pneumonia reported by Schlamm and colleagues, only 4 were bacteremic.[26] The chest radiograph reveals unilateral or bilateral lobar infiltrates. In a significant number of patients, diffuse infiltrates are seen, which can resemble the radiographic findings commonly observed in patients with *P carinii* pneumonia. Pleural effusions are uncommon, as is frank empyema.[26] Gram's staining of sputum specimens reveals a predominance of gram-negative coccobacilli, which can easily be overlooked if the background is thick with proteinaceous material and inflammatory cells. The diagnosis is established by finding heavy growth of the organism in culture from sputum or from blood culture isolation. Prevention, treatment, and prognosis of *H influenzae* disease are described later in this chapter.

Pseudomonas aeruginosa

Invasive pseudomonal infections were not recognized until relatively recently as a problem for HIV-infected patients. In an early study by Eng and colleagues, the incidence of pseudomonal bacteremia was significantly lower in AIDS patients than in a non-AIDS control population.[27] In a report on a series of community-acquired pneumonias in HIV-infected patients by Burack and colleagues, *P aeruginosa* was the etiologic agent in 2.3% of cases.[20] Along with pneumonia, the organism has been found to cause bacteremia, empyema, endocarditis, urosepsis, osteomyelitis, sinusitis, and otitis externa.[28,29] Treatment and prognosis of pseudomonal pneumonia are discussed later in this chapter.

Other Community-Acquired Pathogens

Variable numbers of cases of pneumonia secondary to other bacterial pathogens have been reported. *S aureus* is frequently reported in case series of pneumonia in HIV-infected patients.[20,30,31] In the series by Burack, 10 (4.6%) of 216 cases of pneumonia were caused by *S aureus*.[20] The more common clinical syndrome associated with this organism, however, is bacteremia, which is often associated with soft tissue infections and infected intravascular catheters.[32] Streptococci other than pneumococcus also have been reported to cause pneumonia. Species have included α-hemolytic streptococci such as *Streptococcus milleri*[20,31] and group B streptococci (*Streptococcus agalactiae*).[2,22,30] In the series by Burack, nonpneumococcal streptococci were the identified pathogens

in 6.9% of HIV-infected patients with community-acquired pneumonia.[20] A host of other bacterial species have been reported to cause community-acquired pneumonia, including *M catarrhalis*, noninfluenzal *Haemophilus* species, *Klebsiella pneumoniae*, and other gram-negative enteric organisms.[20] *Rhodococcus equi* has been reported to cause cavitary lung disease in a small number of HIV-infected patients.[33] *Nocardia* has also been reported to cause lobar consolidation and cavitary lung disease along with focal infection at extrapulmonary locations, including brain and bone.[34,35] Finally, pertussis has been reported in an HIV-infected patient who had paroxysmal cough and dyspnea for several months.[36]

Nosocomial Pneumonia

Hospital-acquired pneumonias occur in HIV-infected patients, often in those with late-stage disease who have been hospitalized for treatment of other opportunistic infections.[22] The risk factors for nosocomial pneumonia may not be much different from those of equally debilitated, hospitalized patients without HIV infection, including aspiration, cachexia, and endotracheal intubation. The organisms involved are also similar and include gram-negative enteric bacilli such as *Enterobacter* spp. and *K pneumoniae*, along with *P aeruginosa* and *S aureus*.[22,37]

Treatment and Prognosis of Bacterial Pneumonia

Trimethoprim-sulfamethoxazole (TMP-SMX) is an appropriate empiric choice for treatment of community-acquired bacterial pneumonia in an HIV-infected patient. With the exception of *P aeruginosa*, TMP-SMX covers the common bacterial pathogens. In addition, it also treats *P carinii*, which may be present concurrently. For patients allergic to TMP-SMX, second-generation cephalosporins such as cefuroxime have been used, especially in areas in which there is a high incidence of ampicillin-resistant *H influenzae*.[20] Macrolides such as erythromycin are often added to treat *Legionella* spp. and *Mycoplasma* spp., although the true incidence of infection caused by these organisms is unknown. After the correct pathogens have been identified by sputum culture or by more invasive procedures such as bronchoscopy, antimicrobial therapy should be adjusted. The prognosis for most community-acquired pneumonias is excellent; most patients recover without serious sequelae.[3,22,26] Relapse rates may be higher for some pathogens, particularly *H influenzae*. Treatment continuing beyond the standard 7 to 10 days for uncomplicated *H influenzae* pneumonia should be contemplated. Patients with pseudomonal or nosocomial pneumonia sustain not only a high relapse rate but also a higher rate of morbidity and mortality, even with optimal antimicrobial therapy.[28,29]

Sinusitis

Sinusitis is perhaps the most common but least well defined bacterial infection seen among HIV-infected patients. Both the incidence and severity of sinusitis are greater in patients with low CD4 counts.[38,39] In addition, chronicity of disease tends to ensue, particularly among patients with late-stage HIV disease. Along with the possible predisposing factors for bacterial infections listed in Table 14.4-1, increased IgE levels have been associated with a greater degree of sinusitis severity in this patient group. It has been postulated that sinusitis may be one manifestation of acquired atopy, which occurs with HIV disease progression.[40]

Although they have not been evaluated systematically, there appear to be some differences in the microbiology of HIV-associated sinusitis compared with sinusitis in the non-HIV–infected population. The principal isolates are *S pneumoniae* and *H influenzae*, as in immunocompetent hosts. In contrast, however, *P aeruginosa* and *S aureus* have also been reported with some frequency.[41,42] *M catarrhalis* and gram-negative enteric bacilli are also likely to be important, and anaerobes probably play a prominent role in chronic sinusitis in patients with HIV infection.

The clinical presentation of sinusitis is often nonspecific. Patients commonly complain of symptoms such as nasal congestion, facial pain, postnasal drip, and fever. Radiographs can be misleading. Although plain sinus radiographs visualize the maxillary and frontal sinuses reasonably well, the ethmoid and sphenoid sinuses are poorly seen.[43] Computed tomography and magnetic resonance imaging of the sinuses provide more detailed views, including the osteomeatal complex.[43] However, these scans are costly and may have low specificity.[38] The maxillary and ethmoid sinuses are involved in 75% and 55% of sinusitis cases in this patient group, respectively[38] (Fig. 14.4-1). A significant proportion of patients suffer from isolated sphenoid disease.[39]

Treatment of sinusitis in this patient group has been poorly defined. The initial treatment should include an oral antimicrobial agent such as TMP-SMX, cefuroxime axetil, or amoxicillin-clavulanate to treat the most likely pathogens, along with a combination decongestant and expectorant. Guaifenesin has been reported to reduce the quantity and viscosity of nasal discharge and may promote faster resolution of sinus disease.[44] Antibiotics should be continued for 14 to 21 days. For patients with maxillary sinusitis who fail initial treatment, maxillary antral puncture should be considered as a means of obtaining a proper specimen for microbiologic culture and to drain the sinus. For patients with either refractory disease or frequent relapses, endoscopic or traditional sinus surgery may be of benefit in reestablishing proper sinus drainage. Long-term antibacterial prophylaxis also may be useful to reduce the relapse rate.[45]

BACTEREMIA AND CATHETER-ASSOCIATED INFECTIONS

Bacteremia as a distinct clinical entity in HIV-infected patients has been the focus of several clinical reports.[22,27,30] In the early 1980s, Whimbey and colleagues described 38 episodes of bacteremia among 336 patients with AIDS.[30] Eng and colleagues described 35 episodes of bacteremia among 125 febrile AIDS patients from whom blood was drawn for culture.[27] Witt and colleagues described 34 episodes of bacteremia among 59 patients admitted to Boston City Hospital between 1983 and 1985; all patients were diagnosed with AIDS or AIDS-related complex.[22]

In most cases, a primary focus of infection is identified as a source of bacteremia, although some cases of primary bacteremia have been described. The best recognized associations include *S pneumoniae* bacteremia secondary to pneumonia (described previously), *Salmonella* spp. bacteremia secondary to gastrointestinal disease, and *S aureus* bacteremia secondary to catheter infections. Nosocomial

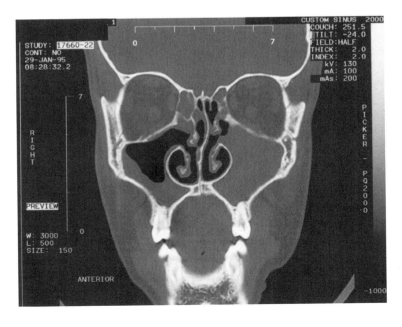

FIG. 14.4-1. Computed tomogram (CT) image, coronal projection, of the paranasal sinuses of a 20-year-old patient with late stage HIV infection and recurrent sinusitis caused by *P aeruginosa*. Extensive bilateral maxillary and ethmoid sinusitis are evident.

bacteremias in which enteric gram-negative bacilli and staphylococci are isolated also occur and typically result from intravascular catheter infections, pneumonia, or infections of the urinary tract.

Staphylococcal bacteremia is a common complication in patients with long-term intravenous catheters, including implanted catheters such as Hickman or Broviac devices and peripherally inserted central catheters. Raviglione and colleagues calculated the rate of Hickman catheter infection among a cohort of patients with AIDS to be 0.47 per 100 catheter-days, compared with a rate of 0.09 per 100 catheter-days among a non-HIV–infected control group.[46] S aureus was responsible for 87% of the cases, whereas coagulase-negative staphylococcus, alone or in combination with S aureus, was present in 25%. Two (12.5%) of 16 patients died as the result of the infection, a case-fatality rate that is much higher than what has been reported in non-HIV–infected populations.[46,47] Jacobson and colleagues described 22 episodes of S aureus bacteremia occurring between 1984 and 1987, most of which (73%) occurred secondary to an infected intravascular catheter.[32] They described a high rate of late metastatic complications (43%) despite courses of antimicrobial therapy averaging 18 days.[32]

Treatment of catheter-associated infections should first be preemptive. For both short- and long-term intravascular catheterization, careful attention to aseptic technique is crucial in preventing infection. After an infection has been diagnosed, early and aggressive antimicrobial therapy should be directed at the causative organisms. Short-term catheters should be removed. The decision to remove long-term, implanted catheters is more difficult, because replacement is expensive and sometimes there is a paucity of other potential access sites. Tunnel infections probably require catheter removal in all cases, whereas exit site infections and bacteremias presumed to be catheter related can probably be treated with appropriate antimicrobial agents through the catheter.

BACILLARY ANGIOMATOSIS (BARTONELLOSIS)

BA was described near the beginning of the AIDS epidemic in a patient who presented with numerous subcutaneous nodules.[48] Organisms were identified in a biopsy specimen of one of the lesions by Warthin-Starry stain. Since that initial report, the causative organisms of BA have been identified, and the clinical characteristics of the disease have been defined. Two organisms in the genus Bartonella, B henselae and B quintana, were identified by first extracting 16S ribosomal gene fragments from infected tissue samples. The DNA sequences of the amplified fragments were compared with the sequences of other bacteria and found to be unique but closely related to Bartonella bacilliformis, the causative agent of Carrión's disease (bartonellosis).[49]

BA typically occurs in patients with late-stage HIV infection who have CD4 counts lower than 100 cells/mm^3.[50] Most disease manifestations are accompanied by constitutional symptoms, which include fever, chills, night sweats, and weight loss. Cutaneous disease is the most common manifestation, and it can take different forms. Raised, erythematous or violaceous nodules are the classic cutaneous manifestation. The lesions can be clinically indistinguishable from those associated with Kaposi's sarcoma. In such cases, biopsy and appropriate staining are required to distinguish between the two diseases (Fig. 14.4-2). Cellulitis and subcutaneous abscess formation also are seen, the latter commonly associated with underlying osteomyelitis. Bony lesions appear lytic and most commonly involve the long bones of the extremities.[50] Hepatic and splenic involvement, termed peliosis, also occurs. The syndrome was first described in a group of patients who presented with fever and abdominal pain of 1 week to 2 months duration.[51] Organisms were identified by Warthin-Starry staining of liver biopsy specimens. Two patients had concurrent cutaneous involvement.[51] Other organs of involvement include lymph nodes, typically those that drain affected organs and soft tissues, the gastrointestinal and respiratory tracts, and the brain.[52,53] Bacteremia without obvious organ involvement also occurs.[54]

The diagnosis of BA first requires the appropriate clinical suspicion. A common mistake is to misdiagnose BA cutaneous lesions as Kaposi's lesions without obtaining a biopsy. Furthermore, if the possibility of BA is not considered, the diagnosis may be missed if the biopsy specimen is not properly stained. The Warthin-Starry staining method remains the most reliable way to visualize the causative bacilli. Usually, organisms are numerous and clearly identified in tissue. The organism also can be identified in blood culture by the lysis-centrifugation technique. Culture of the organism is difficult, however, and requires special media.

The optimal treatment of BA has not been systematically established. Erythromycin should be considered the agent of choice. It is given by mouth unless the patient is severely ill or cannot reliably take oral agents.[48,55] The tetracyclines, particularly doxycycline, are also active and have been used successfully in a number of patient reports.[50] Overall, BA is a responsive disease, and most patients can be successfully treated with oral therapy. Duration of treatment has not been well established but should vary with the clinical manifestations. Isolated cutaneous disease should be treated for at least 1 month, whereas bony or hepatosplenic involvement may require many months of treatment in order to eradicate the organism and prevent relapses.[50]

PREVENTION OF BACTERIAL INFECTIONS

Prevention of bacterial infections centers on the use of vaccinations and antibacterial prophylaxis. Vaccinations are available for two HIV-related bacterial pathogens, S pneumoniae and H influenzae. Polyvalent pneumococcal vaccine contains antigens to 23 pneumococcal types, which are responsible for 85% to 90% of cases of invasive pneumococcal infection. In comparison with non-HIV–infected patients, the antibody titer after vaccination among HIV-infected patients is lower.[6,56]

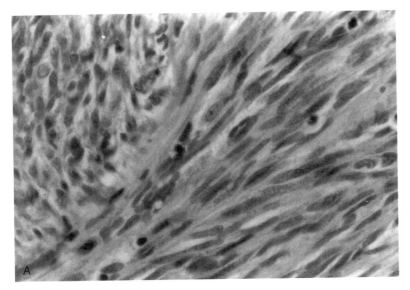

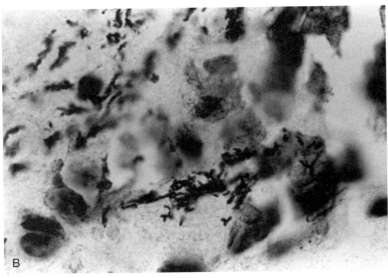

FIG. 14.4-2. Microscopic comparision of Kaposi Sarcoma (KS) and Bacillary Angiomatosis (BA). **(A)** Photomicrograph of a biopsy from a cutaneous KS lesion stained with hematoxylin and eosin showing the typical spindle cell appearance of (KS) ×400 magnification). **(B)** Photomicrograph of a biopsy from a cutaneous BA lesion stained by the Warthin-Starry staining method showing numerous small bacilli ×1000.

In addition, patients with AIDS develop a lower titer than patients who have earlier-stage disease.[6] Vaccine failures have been reported.[21] *H influenzae* conjugate vaccines have been shown to be immunogenic and offer significant protection against invasive *H influenzae* type b infection in children. As with the pneumococcal vaccine, the quantitative antibody response after vaccination with *H influenzae* type b polysaccharide-mutant diphtheria toxoid conjugate vaccine (PRP-CRM) has been shown to vary directly with the CD4 count.[12] Also, the majority of invasive *H influenzae* infections in HIV-infected patients are nontypeable. Efficacy in reducing the incidence or severity of infection in this population has not been demonstrated with either pneumococcal or *H influenzae* vaccine. Nevertheless, because the vaccines are relatively inexpensive and have few serious side effects, all patients should be vaccinated, preferably as early as possible during their course of HIV infection.

Antimicrobial prophylaxis against bacterial infections has not been advocated on a routine basis in HIV-infected patients, although for individual patients with a history of frequent recurrence, long-term prophylaxis may be considered. It appears that the incidence of bacterial infections may be reduced for patients who receive TMP-SMX for *P carinii* pneumonia prophylaxis.[45,57] Because TMP-SMX has the added benefits of providing more effective and less expensive *P carinii* pneumonia prophylaxis than other agents and because it may also provide prophylaxis against toxoplasmosis, it is the best possible choice in this setting.

REFERENCES

1. Centers for Disease Control. 1993 Revised classification system for HIV infection and expanded surveillance case definition for AIDS among adolescents and adults. MMWR Morb Mortal Wkly Rep 1992;41(RR-17):1.

2. Polsky B, Gold JWM, Whimbey E, et al. Bacterial pneumonia in patients with the acquired immunodeficiency syndrome. Ann Intern Med 1986;104:38.

3. Janoff EN, Breiman RF, Daley CL, Hopewell PC. Pneumococcal disease during HIV infection: epidemiologic, clinical and immunologic perspectives. Ann Intern Med 1992;117:314.

4. Pahwa SG, Quilop MTJ, Lange M, Pahwa RN, Grieco MH. Defective B-lymphocyte function in homosexual men in relation to the acquired immunodeficiency syndrome. Ann Intern Med 1984;101:757.

5. Lane HC, Masur H, Edgar LC, Whalen G, Rook AH, Fauci AS. Abnormalities of B-cell activation and immunoregulation in patients with the acquired immunodeficiency syndrome. N Engl J Med 1983;309:453.

6. Janoff EN, Douglas JM, Gabriel M, et al. Class-specific antibody response to pneumococcal capsular polysaccharides in men infected with human immunodeficiency virus type 1. J Infect Dis 1988;158:983.

7. Aucouturier P, Couderc LJ, Gouet D, et al. Serum immunoglobulin G subclass dysbalances in the lymphadenopathy syndrome and acquired immune deficiency syndrome. Clin Exp Immunol 1986;63:234.

8. Parkin JM, Helbert M, Hughes CL, Pinching AJ. Immunoglobulin G subclass deficiency and susceptibility to pyogenic infections in patients with AIDS-related complex and AIDS. AIDS 1989;3:37.

9. Kotler DP, Scholes JV, Tierney AR. Intestinal plasma cell alterations in acquired immunodeficiency syndrome. Dig Dis Sci 1987;32:129.

10. Muller F, Froland SS, Hvatum M, Radl J, Brandtzaeg P. Both IgA subclasses are reduced in parotid saliva from patients with AIDS. Clin Exp Immunol 1991;83:203.

11. Miotti PG, Nelson KE, Dallabetta GA, Farzadegan H, Margolick J, Clements ML. The influence of HIV infection on antibody responses to a two-dose regimen of influenza vaccine. JAMA 1989;262:779.

12. Steinhoff MC, Auerbach BS, Nelson KE, et al. Antibody responses to Haemophilus influenzae type B vaccines in men with human immunodeficiency virus infection. N Engl J Med 1991;325:1837.

13. Farber BF, Lesser M, Kaplan MH, Woltmann J, Napolitano B, Armellino D. Clinical significance of neutropenia in patients with human immunodeficiency virus infection. Infect Control Hosp Epidemiol 1991;12:429.

14. Shaunak S, Bartlett JA. Zidovudine-induced neutropenia: are we too cautious? Lancet 1989;2:91.

15. Ellis M, Gupta S, Galant S, et al. Impaired neutrophil function in patients with AIDS or AIDS-related complex: a comprehensive evaluation. J Infect Dis 1988;158:1268.

16. Murphy PM, Lane HC, Fauci AS, Gallin JI. Impairment of neutrophil bactericidal capacity in patients with AIDS. J Infect Dis 1988;158:627.

17. Embretson J, Zupancic M, Ribas JL, et al. Massive covert infection of helper T lymphocytes and macrophages by HIV during the incubation period of AIDS. Nature 1993;362:359.

18. Bender BS, Bohnsack JF, Sourlis SH, Frank MM, Quinn TC. Demonstration of defective C3-receptor–mediated clearance by the reticuloendothelial system in patients with acquired immunodeficiency syndrome. J Clin Invest 1987;79:715.

19. Bender BS, Frank MM, Lawley TJ, Smith WJ, Brickman CM, Quinn TC. Defective reticuloendothelial system Fc-receptor function in patients with acquired immunodeficiency syndrome. J Infect Dis 1985;152:409.

20. Burack JH, Hahn JA, Saint-Maurice D, Jacobson MA. Microbiology of community-acquired bacterial pneumonia in persons with and at risk for human immunodeficiency virus type 1 infection. Arch Intern Med 1994;154:2589.

21. Simberkoff MS, El Sadr W, Schiffman G, Rahal JJ. Streptococcus pneumoniae infections and bacteremia in patients with acquired immune deficiency syndrome, with report of a pneumococcal vaccine failure. Am Rev Respir Dis 1984;130:1174.

22. Witt DJ, Craven DE, McCabe WR. Bacterial infections in adult patients with the acquired immune deficiency syndrome (AIDS) and AIDS-related complex. Am J Med 1987;82:900.

23. Redd SC, Rutherford GW III, Sande MA, et al. The role of human immunodeficiency virus infection in pneumococcal bacteremia in San Francisco residents. J Infect Dis 1990;162:1012.

24. Steinhart R, Reingold AL, Taylor R, Anderson G, Wenger JD. Invasive Haemophilus influenzae infections in men with HIV infection. JAMA 1992;268:3350.

25. Farley MM, Stephens DS, Brachman PS, et al. Invasive Haemophilus influenzae disease in adults: a prospective, population-based surveillance. Ann Intern Med 1992;116:806.

26. Schlamm HT, Yancovitz SR. Haemophilus influenzae pneumonia in young adults with AIDS, ARC, or risk of AIDS. Am J Med 1989;86:11.

27. Eng RHK, Bishburg E, Smith SM, Geller H, Kapila R. Bacteremia and fungemia in patients with acquired immune deficiency syndrome. Am J Clin Pathol 1986;86:105.

28. Kielhofner M, Atmar RL, Hamill RJ, Musher DM. Life-threatening Pseudomonas aeruginosa infections in patients with human immunodeficiency virus infection. Clin Infect Dis 1992;14:403.

29. Lozano F, Corzo JE, Nogales C, Garcia-Bragado F. Life-threatening Pseudomonas aeruginosa infections in patients with infection due to human immunodeficiency virus. Clin Infect Dis 1992;15:751.

30. Whimbey E, Gold JWM, Polsky B, et al. Bacteremia and fungemia in patients with the acquired immunodeficiency syndrome. Ann Intern Med 1986;104:511.

31. Magnenat J-L, Nicod LP, Auckenthaler R, Junod AF. Mode of presentation and diagnosis of bacterial pneumonia in human immunodeficiency virus-infected patients. Am Rev Respir Dis 1991;144:917.

32. Jacobson MA, Gellermann H, Chambers H. Staphylococcus aureus bacteremia and recurrent staphylococcal infection in patients with acquired immunodeficiency syndrome and AIDS-related complex. Am J Med 1988;85:172.

33. Scannel KA, Portoni EJ, Finkle HI, Rice M. Pulmonary malacoplakia and Rhodococcus equi infection in a patient with AIDS. Chest 1990;97:1000.

34. Rodriquez JL, Barrio JL, Pitchenik AE. Pulmonary nocardiosis in the acquired immunodeficiency syndrome: diagnosis with bronchoalveolar lavage and treatment with non–sulphur containing drugs. Chest 1986;90:912.

35. Holtz HA, Lavery DP, Kapila R. Actinomycetales infection in the acquired immunodeficiency syndrome. Ann Intern Med 1985;102:203.

36. Doebbeling BN, Feilmeier ML, Herwaldt LA. Pertussis in an adult man infected with the human immunodeficiency virus. J Infect Dis 1990;161:1296.

37. Nichols L, Balogh K, Silverman M. Bacterial infections in the acquired immune deficiency syndrome: clinicopathologic correlations in a series of autopsy cases. Am J Clin Pathol 1989;92:787.

38. Zurlo JJ, Feuerstein IM, Lebovics R, Lane HC. Sinusitis in HIV-1 infection. Am J Med 1992;93:157.

39. Godofsky EW, Zinreich J, Armstrong M, Leslie JM, Weikel CS. Sinusitis in HIV-infected patients: a clinical and radiographic review. Am J Med 1992;93:163.

40. Small CB, Kaufman A, Armenaka M, Rosenstreich DL. Sinusitis and atopy in human immunodeficiency virus infection. J Infect Dis 1993;167:283.

41. O'Donnell JG, Sorbello AF, Condoluci DV, Barnish MJ. Sinusitis due to Pseudomonas aeruginosa in patients with human immunodeficiency virus infection. Clin Infect Dis 1993;16:404.

42. Hadderingh RJ. Recurrent maxillary sinusitis in AIDS patients. Abstract MBP 203. Proceedings of the Fifth International Conference on AIDS, Montreal, 1989:255.

43. Davidson TM, Brahme FJ, Gallagher ME. Radiographic evaluation for nasal dysfunction: computed tomography versus plain films. Head Neck 1989;11:405.

44. Wawrose SF, Tami TA, Amoils CP. The role of guaifenesin in the treatment of sinonasal disease in patients infected with the human immunodeficiency virus (HIV). Laryngoscope 1992;102:1225.

45. Mayer HB, Rose DN, Cohen S, Gurtman AC, Cheung TW, Szabo S. The effect of Pneumocystis carinii pneumonia prophylaxis regimens on the incidence of bacterial infections in HIV-infected patients. AIDS 1993;7:1687.

46. Raviglione MC, Battan R, Pablos-Mendez A, Aceves-Casillas P, Mullen MP, Taranta A. Infections associated with Hickman catheters in patients with acquired immunodeficiency syndrome. Am J Med 1989;86:780.

47. Press OW, Ramsey PG, Larson EB, Fefer A, Hickman RO. Hickman catheter infections in patients with malignancies. Medicine (Baltimore) 1984;63:189.

48. Stoler MH, Bonfiglio TA, Steigbigel RT, Pereira M. An atypical subcutaneous infection associated with acquired immune deficiency syndrome. Am J Clin Pathol 1983;80:714.

49. Relman DA, Loutit JS, Schmidt TM, Falkow S, Tompkins LS. The agent of bacillary angiomatosis: an approach to the identification of uncultured pathogens. N Engl J Med 1990;323:1573.

50. Koehler JE, Tappero JW. Bacillary angiomatosis and bacillary peliosis in patients infected with human immunodeficiency virus. Clin Infect Dis 1993;17:612.

51. Perkocha LA, Geaghan SM, Yen TSB, et al. Clinical and pathological features of bacillary peliosis hepatitis in association with human immunodeficiency virus infection. N Engl J Med 1990;323:1581.
52. Cockerell CJ, Whitlow MA, Webster GF, Friedman-Kien AE. Epithelioid angiomatosis: a distinct vascular disorder in patients with the acquired immunodeficiency syndrome or AIDS-related complex. Lancet 1987;2:654.
53. Spach DH, Panther LA, Thorning DR, Dunn JE, Plorde JJ, Miller RA. Intracerebral bacillary angiomatosis in a patient with human immunodeficiency virus. Ann Intern Med 1992;116:740.
54. Slater LN, Welch DF, Hensel D, Coody DW. A newly recognized fastidious gram-negative pathogen as a cause of fever and bacteremia. N Engl J Med 1990;323:1587.
55. Koehler JE, LeBoit PE, Egbert BM, Berger TG. Cutaneous vascular lesions and disseminated cat-scratch disease in patients with the acquired immunodeficiency syndrome (AIDS) and AIDS-related complex. Ann Intern Med 1988;109:449.
56. Klein RS, Selwyn PA, Maude D, Pollard C, Freeman K, Schiffman G. Response to pneumococcal vaccine among asymptomatic heterosexual partners of persons with AIDS and intravenous drug users infected with human immunodeficiency virus. J Infect Dis 1989;160:826.
57. Hardy WD, Feinberg J, Finkelstein DM, et al. A controlled trial of trimethoprim-sulfamethoxazole or aerosolized pentamidine for secondary prophylaxis of *Pneumocystis carinii* pneumonia in patients with the acquired immunodeficiency syndrome. N Engl J Med 1992;327:1842.

AIDS: Biology, Diagnosis, Treatment and Prevention, fourth edition, edited by Vincent T. DeVita, Jr., Samuel Hellman, and Steven A. Rosenberg. Lippincott–Raven Publishers, © 1997

14.5

Herpesvirus Infections In Human Immunodeficiency Virus–Infected Persons

Timothy Schacker and Lawrence Corey

Herpesvirus infections are among the most common opportunistic infections in persons infected with the human immunodeficiency virus (HIV). Herpes simplex virus (HSV), varicella zoster virus (VZV), and cytomegalovirus (CMV) were some of the earliest recognized viral infections complicating HIV infection. Human herpesvirus 6 (HHV6), which apears to be the cause of roseola in infants, and Kaposi's sarcoma–associated herpesvirus (HHV8) also have been detected in HIV-infected persons. Seroepidemiologic studies have shown that infection with one or more of these viruses is almost universal among those at highest risk for HIV, and the family of herpesviruses are therefore important pathogens to consider in the management of any HIV-infected person.

A cardinal feature of all herpesviruses is their ability to establish latency after primary infection and then reactivate at some later time,[1] each with a unique clinical syndrome or set of syndromes. Herpes simplex virus type 1 (HSV1) and type 2 (HSV2) cause recurrent oral, genital, and rectal ulcerations and occasionally disseminate to cause visceral and central nervous system (CNS) disease. CMV reactivation can lead to pneumonia, encephalitis, retinitis, gastroenteritis, adrenalitis; VZV reactivation can cause shingles and occasionally disseminate; and Epstein-Barr virus (EBV) is the cause of oral hairy leukoplakia (OHL) and has been associated with lymphoproliferative disorders in immunocompromised persons. Primary EBV infections in HIV-infected persons may lead to a malignancy of muscle tissue. No specific clinical syndrome has been attributed to HHV6 or HHV7 reactivation in HIV-infected persons. The

Kaposi's sarcoma–associated herpesvirus (ie, HHV8) has been identified in acquired immunodeficiency syndrome (AIDS)-related Kaposi's sarcoma lesions and the Kaposi's sarcoma found in immunocompetent persons of Mediterranean descent, but because no serologic assay has been established, its epidemiologic pattern has not been characterized. Table 14.5-1 lists the known human herpesviruses and their most common manifestations as initial infections and as reactivation infections.

HERPES SIMPLEX 1 AND 2

HSV1 and HSV2 are highly prevalent infections in HIV-seropositive persons. In the United States and Europe, 95% of homosexual men are seropositive for HSV1, HSV2, or both,[2-6] and 40% to 60% of injection drug users are HSV2 seropositive. In Africa and Asia, HSV2 is also found more frequently in persons who are HIV seropositive than in the general population.

Clinical Manifestations

The acquisition of HSV usually occurs before the acquisition of HIV, and the HSV infection is usually subclinical. In many persons, the first recognized reactivation may occur years after the initial acquisition of HSV infection.[7] In 30% to 50% of persons, the acquisition of HSV is clinically symptomatic. Classically, the clinical manifestations of primary HSV infection include fever, adenopathy, malaise, and painful ulcerative lesions involving mucosal and cutaneous sites.[8] The initial signs and symptoms of primary oral or labial HSV infection are sore throat with mild to moderate pharyngeal edema and erythema. Small, painful vesicles develop on oral mucosa, rapidly ulcerate, and increase in number. The lesions may extend onto the lips and cheeks

Timothy Schacker, Acting Assistant Professor, Department of Medicine, University of Washington, 1001 Madison, Suite 320, Seattle, WA 98122.

Lawrence Corey, Professor, Laboratory Medicine, Microbiology and Medicine, University of Washington, 1200 12th Avenue South, Room 9301, Seattle, WA 98144.

TABLE 14.5-1. *Clinical manifestations of herpes virus infections*

Virus	Primary Infection	Reactivation from latent stage
HSV1	Primary HSV gingivostomatis HSV encephalitis (rare) Neonatal HSV Genital HSV	Recurrent oral/labial HSV Recurrent anogenital HSV HSV encephalitis HSV esophagitis HSV hepatitis
HSV2	Genital/rectal herpes Neonatal HSV Meningoencephalitis Sacral radiculitus	Genital HSV Mollaret's meningitis HSV encephalitis (rare) Chronic mucocutaneous lesions
CMV	Subclinical infection Heterophile-negative mononucleosis	CMV retinitis CMV colitus/cholangitis CMV pneumonia (rare) CMV adrenal insufficiency (rare) Marrow failure
HHV6	Roseola subitum	Possible hepatitis Possible interstitial pneumonia in the immunocompromised host
HHV7	Possible childhood exanthem	None identified
EBV	Mononucleosis Sarcoma of muscle Encephalitis (young adult)	Oral hairy leukoplakia EBV-associated lymphoproliferative syndrome EBV-related CNS lymphoma Lymphoid interstitial pneumonia of children
KSHV (HHV8)	Unknown	Associated with Kaposi's sarcoma Body cavity lymphoma Casselman's disease

CMV, cytomegalovirus; EBV, Epstein-Barr virus; HHV, human herpesvirus; HSV, herpes simplex virus; KSHV, Kaposi's sarcoma–associated herpesvirus; VZV, varicella zoster virus.

and usually resolve within 10 to 21 days. Primary genital or rectal infection is usually associated with fever, malaise, anorexia, and tender, bilateral inguinal adenopathy. Vesicular lesions develop on the glans or penile shaft, vulva, perineum, rectum, cervix, or vagina. Primary HSV proctitis may be associated with severe rectal bleeding, friability, and rectal discharge.[9] Sacral radiculomyelitis can occur with primary anogenital HSV, and it is usually caused by HSV2. It may lead to sacral distribution sensory loss or parasthesias, urinary retention, neuralgia, constipation, and impotence.

After primary infection, HSV becomes latent in sacral and trigeminal ganglia. Reactivation is often heralded by a prodromal illness or constellation of symptoms that the patient associates with a herpes outbreak: aching, pain, tingling, and a feeling of heaviness. Within hours, one or more vesicular lesions appears. However, reactivation can be subclinical (ie, no lesions)[10–12] and can occur at any time, and most HSV transmissions occur during periods of subclinical reactivation.[13–15] The frequency of anogenital recurrence varies; some persons have frequent outbreaks after primary infection, and others have no recognized clinical reactivations.[16] However, almost all HSV2- and HIV-seropositive persons eventually have a reactivation in the anogenital region.

Herpes Simplex Infection in HIV-Infected Persons

Persistent perirectal ulceration from HSV2 infection was one of the original descriptions of an opportunistic infection associated with AIDS.[17] Among persons with AIDS, HSV2 infections can be persistent, erosive, and associated with fever, pain, friability, and subcutaneous necrosis, but dissemination to visceral organs is rare. The natural history of mucocutaneous HSV infection in HIV-infected persons has only recently been systematically studied. When compared with HIV-negative persons matched for sexual lifestyle, HSV2 reactivates three to five times more often in HIV-infected persons than in noninfected persons.[18,19] Most reactivations are perirectal and occur on days the patient is not aware of having lesions (Table 14.5-2).

The degree of immunosuppression appears to influence the reactivation rate and severity of disease,[19,20] and persons with lower CD4 cell counts appear to have larger and more persistent ulcerating lesions. As for HIV-negative persons, there is great variability among HIV-infected persons in the frequency and severity of HSV reactivation. Lesions typically start as small, localized ulcerations and can spread contiguously to cover large areas of the perineum and buttocks (Fig. 14.5-1). This "zosteriform" appearance of HSV can occur in persons with high CD4 cell counts. The zosteriform appearance of HSV may make it more difficult to differentiate from VZV and underscores the need for a specific diagnosis, because treatment options for the two viral infections differ. The frequency of reactivation of HSV1 is less than HSV2 in HIV-positive persons, and in our experience, extensive zosteriform lesions are more often HSV2 reactivations. Other complications, such as bleeding and sec-

TABLE 14.5-2. *Therapy of herpes simplex virus infections in persons with HIV or AIDS*

Indication	Drug	Dose	Frequency	Cost[#]
Primary HSV	Acyclovir*	200 mg PO	5×/d for 10d	$36.60
	Acyclovir	400 mg PO	3×/d for 10d	$64.35
Recurrent HSV	Acyclovir	200 mg PO	5×/d for 5d	$20.00
	Acyclovir	400 mg PO	3×/d for 5d	$34.05
	Famciclovir	250 mg PO	2×/d for 5d	$57.10
	Valaciclovir	500 mg PO	2×/d for 5d	$26.90
Suppressive therapy[†]	Acyclovir	400 mg PO	TID	$185/mo
	Famciclovir	500 mg PO	BID	$323.95/mo
Severe mucocutaneous involvement[‡]	Acyclovir IV	5.0 mg/kg IV (infuse over 1 hr)	q 8 h × 7	Approximately $2100 for 7d
Neurologic involvement (including encephalitis)	Acyclovir IV	10 mg/kg IV (infuse over 1 h)	q 8 h × 10–21d	Approximately $6200 for 10d
Acyclovir-resistant HSV[§]	Foscarnet	40 mg/kg IV	q 8 h until healed (10–24 days)	$7138 for 24d

*Acyclovir side effects include occasional diarrhea, nausea, vertigo and rash. Bone marrow suppression is not a typical side effect of acyclovir. In our experience, standard doses of acyclovir will adequately treat most primary or recurrent episodes of HSV. For those with lower CD4 cell counts, higher doses (800 mg PO TID or 400 mg PO QID) may be useful.

†Suppressive therapy may be indicated if the patient experiences > 6 recurrence/year. Higher doses may be needed in some persons.

‡Immunosuppressed patients with severe mucocutaneous involvement (including esophagitis), or patients who fail conventional oral therapy should be treated with intravenous acyclovir.

§Lesions that do not heal with high-dose oral or intravenous therapy may be acyclovir resistant. To verify resistantce, obtain a viral culture and ask for acyclovir sensitivity testing. The cost for this is $300 to $400. Foscarnet can cause acute renal failure. Electrolytes (especially calcium, potassium, and magnesium) and serum creatinine should be monitored. Adequate hydration should be given to reduce the chances of developing renal failure. Famvir (at doses similar to those used for varicella zoster virus) may be useful when thymidine kinase–altered variants are detected in the lesion. Topical triflouridine (Viroptic) mixed with interferon-α and applied topically effectively cures about 50% of lesions.

#Cost to a patient at our hospital-based outpatient pharmacy.

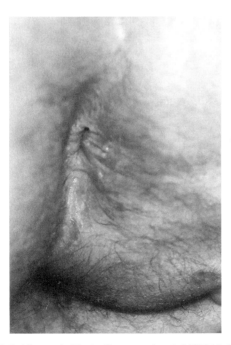

FIG. 14.5-1. Photo 1: Zosteriform perirectal HSV infection in an HIV-infected male. See also Color Figure 14.5-1.

ondary bacterial infections, may arise, especially in lesions that spread throughout the perineum.

Although mucocutaneous infections are the most common problem with HSV- and HIV-positive persons, extensions of infection to visceral organs has been reported, including esophagitis,[21] encephalitis,[22–24] retinitis,[25] thoracic myelitis,[26] and thrombocytopenia.[27] HSV esophagitis is seen in persons with long-standing HIV disease and manifests with dysphagia, retrosternal pain, and odynophagia.[21] The physical examination results may be normal, and concomitant oral candidiasis is common. HSV encephalitis is relatively rare in AIDS patients, but there are case reports of HSV2 meningoencephalitis in these patients, including encephalitis from acyclovir-resistant HSV2.[22] Signs and symptoms of encephalitis include headache, fever, behavioral disorders, speech difficulties, and seizures. In immunocompetent persons, the mortality rate for untreated, biopsy-proven cases is 60% to 80%, with more than 90% of survivors having significant neurologic sequelae.

Resistance to acyclovir is an important complication of herpes in HIV-infected persons.[28–30] The natural history of acyclovir resistance has not been well defined, but risk factors appear to include a CD4 cell count of less than 50 cells/mm³ and prolonged duration of the herpes lesion.[31] The mechanism leading to the emergence of resistant virus is unknown. During reactivation, there are very high titers of replicating virus in epithelial cells, and therapy with acyclovir may select for replication of variants with altered thymidine kinase (TK) proteins. Such variants do not phosphorylate acyclovir well, and adequate levels of acyclovir triphosphate, which inhibits HSV DNA polymerase, are not achieved in virally infected cells. Because the original population of ganglionic isolates are primarily TK positive, subsequent HSV reactivations (after healing from a resistant lesion) may be acyclovir sensitive.[32]

Acyclovir-resistant HSV lesions have been described in the mouth, on the lips and face, on fingers (whitlow), on the genitals, and in the perirectal area (Fig. 14.5-2).[21,22,30,33,34] These lesions are persistent and almost never resolve without targeted therapy. Acyclovir-resistant HSV should be suspected when HSV culture–positive lesions persist despite adequate serum concentrations of acyclovir (documented by demonstrating serum concentrations of acyclovir >2 µg/mL). Initially, it is useful to determine if higher therapeutic levels of acyclovir or penciclovir can achieve healing. This can be accomplished by higher oral dosing of acyclovir (up to 800 mg every 5 hours) or substituting one of the newer prodrugs, such as valaciclovir (1000 mg, taken orally three times daily) or using famciclovir (500 mg, taken orally three times daily). These oral regimens are less toxic and expensive than the only alternative, intravenous foscarnet. Foscarnet inhibits HSV-specific DNA polymerase and does not require viral TK for phosphorylation.[35-38] It is effective against TK-altered and TK-deficient variants. The major toxicities of foscarnet are

renal effects, with azotemia and profound electrolyte abnormalities being common. Because of the increased risk of acute renal failure, profound hypocalcemia, hypomagnesemia, and hypophosphatemia, it is useful to hospitalize the patient for the first few days of therapy. After a stable dosing regimen is achieved (including an assessment for the hydration and electrolyte replacement requirements), the patient can be managed on an outpatient basis.

Reports of a topical preparation containing Viroptic (ie, trifluridine) are encouraging, and studies are underway to evaluate its efficacy as a single agent and in combination with interferon-α.[39] The antiviral drug called HPMPC (Cidofovir, Gilead Sciences Inc., Foster City, CA) has in vitro activity against TK-deficient strains of HSV2. A clinical trial of 3% topical HPMPC applied once daily demonstrated a modest effect in speeding cutaneous healing.[40] Anecdotal reports suggest systemic HPMPC may also be useful.

Acyclovir-resistant herpes lesions often take weeks to completely heal, and supportive care is an important aspect of the management of these lesions. Daily dressing changes and peroxide debridement are helpful.

Herpes Simplex Virus as a Risk Factor for Acquisition and Transmission of HIV

Several studies have established HSV2 as a significant risk factor for acquisition and transmission of HIV. In a study of 123 men at risk for HIV, 32 (68%) of 47 with preexisting HSV2 antibody seroconverted to HIV positive, but only 24 (46%) of 52 without HSV2 antibody seroconverted.[41] HSV2 seropositivity is an independent risk factor for acquisition of HIV.[42] Among heterosexual men and women, genital ulcers appear to facilitate the transmission and ability to acquire HIV.[43] These epidemiologic studies demonstrate the need for an understanding of the precise mechanism by which HSV facilitates transmission and acquisition of HIV, because an effective therapy for HSV exists.

Herpes Simplex Virus as a Cofactor in HIV Pathogenesis

In vitro studies suggest that coinfection of certain cell lines with HSV and HIV can change the rate of HIV replication.[44-46] Addition of HSV1 or HSV2 to T-cell lines such as MT-2, MT-4, and ACH-2 has markedly upregulated expression of HIV.[47,48] ICP0 and ICP4, the early regulatory proteins of HSV1, transactivate the long terminal repeat (LTR) of HIV-1, and ICP0 and ICP27 can upregulate HIV expression in CEM cells.[49,50] The transactivating protein of HSV, Vp16, acts synergistically with the HIV-1 Tat protein to increase HIV transcription from the HIV-1 LTR.[51] However, this phenomenon has not been observed in vivo, and studies are underway to determine if this does occur in vivo. We reported that HIV RNA levels in plasma significantly increase in some patients with active herpes lesions (Fig. 14.5-3).[52] Studies are underway to determine how frequently

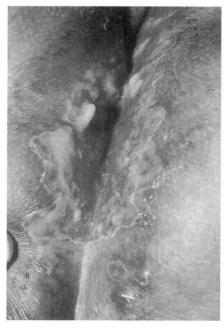

FIG. 14.5-2. Acyclovir-resistant perirectal HSV2 infection in an HIV-infected male. See also Color Figure 14.5-2.

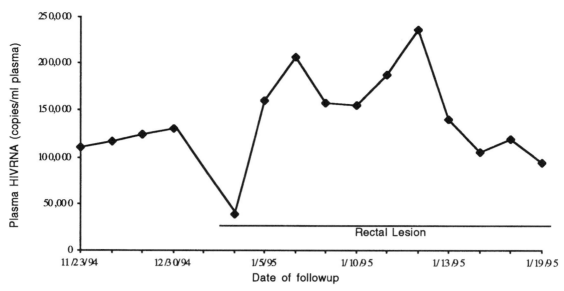

FIG. 14.5-3. Elevated plasma HIV RNA during an outbreak of rectal HSV in one patient during follow-up.

that phenomenon occurs, but some studies already have shown a survival benefit for persons taking acyclovir,[53,54] suggesting that suppression of HSV2 may lead to less frequent expression of HIV. However, not all studies have shown this survival benefit.[55,56] Until controlled studies are completed that define the precise role of HSV in the pathogenesis of HIV, there is no indication for the routine use of antiviral therapy in HIV-infected persons, unless they have frequent clinical reactivations of HSV2.

Diagnosis

The most common methods used to detect HSV are serology, microscopic evaluation of lesional exudates, culture, and demonstration of HSV antigen by immunofluorescence or enzyme immunoassay. The ability of each method to provide relevant clinical information varies. During the last decade, excellent serologic assays that clearly define HSV1 and HSV2 antibodies in humans have been developed. Unfortunately, commercially available enzyme immunoassays are not accurate.[57,58] Paired serologies can be used to establish primary infection with an initial negative result and a positive convalescent result. HSV serology is probably not important to obtain for HIV-infected persons, except for defining HSV seroconversion in HIV-infected children or adolescents. The physician should always attempt to confirm a diagnosis of mucocutaneous HSV by culture, immunofluorescence, enzyme immunoassay, or polymerase chain reaction (PCR) methods.

Microscopic evaluation with a Tzanck smear is done by scraping the margin of the lesion and staining with Wright or Giemsa stain, which reveals multinucleated giant cells characteristic of HSV or VZV infection. The sensitivity and specificity of this technique is poor and depends on the experience of the person reading the slide. Moreover, because zosteriform HSV can occur in these patients, the

Tzanck smear cannot help to differentiate HSV from VZV, and because therapy differs for these two infections, we usually recommend a more complete workup that includes culture or an antigen detection assay.

Because HSV is easily isolated from lesions, culture remains the gold standard. Typing of the virus (ie, HSV1 or HSV2) is helpful in defining subsequent reactivation rates, because HSV1 reactivates subclinically and clinically less frequently. Moreover, a culture is needed to define antiviral sensitivity. Rectal HSV cultures are often negative because of bacterial or fungal overgrowth, and if HSV proctitis is suspected, biopsy material should be sent for pathologic evaluation and viral culture.

The diagnosis of HSV infection of the CNS has changed, because HSV-specific PCR has become clinically available. Several studies have shown that HSV DNA is present in cerebrospinal fluid (CSF) during HSV encephalitis and meningoencephalitis.[59,60] PCR is the method of choice for determining CNS and unusual HSV infections.

Treatment

Acyclovir is the first-line therapy for mucocutaneous HSV infection. It is available in topical, oral, and intravenous forms.[61] Oral acyclovir (400 mg, taken orally three times daily) and its congener valaciclovir (500 mg, taken orally twice daily) can limit the duration of viral shedding and decrease the time to healing of mucocutaneous HSV infection in persons with HIV. Famciclovir (125 mg, taken orally twice daily), can speed the healing of mucocutaneous HSV infections in immunocompetent persons with genital HSV, but data are not yet available to evaluate its efficacy in HIV-infected persons. For persons with frequent reactivations (>6 recurrences/year), reactivation may be suppressed with chronic, daily doses of acylcovir, starting with 400 mg taken orally two to three times daily, but other regimens, such as

800 mg taken orally twice daily, have also been used.[62,63] Famciclovir (500 mg, taken orally twice daily) has been effective in reducing the signs and symptoms of HSV reactivation in HIV-seropositive persons. Table 14.5-2 lists the indication, route, frequency, and cost options for the treatment of HSV in HIV-infected persons.

CYTOMEGALOVIRUS

Epidemiology

As with other herpesviruses, the age-specific prevalence of CMV in HIV-positive persons is higher than in the general population. More than 95% of men who have sex with men and 80% of injection drug users have antibodies to CMV.[2,64–66] However, as the transmission patterns of HIV change, with more women and teenagers becoming infected, it is likely that the CMV seroprevalence associated with HIV may change, resulting in an overall lower seroprevalence rate among HIV-infected persons. Reactivation of CMV during the course of HIV is common; CMV retinitis and CMV-associated gastrointestinal disease are among the most formidable challenges in the diagnosis and management of HIV-infected persons.

Clinical Manifestations

Clinically important CMV infections in the setting of HIV infection occur in those with advanced AIDS (usually with a CD4 cell count <100 cells/mm^3). Infections of the eye, gastrointestinal tract, and CNS are the most common. As many as 40% of patients with AIDS are estimated to have some form of CMV-related problem during the course of their disease. In a study of 1002 HIV-infected persons with CD4 cell counts of 250 cells/mm^3 or less, 110 (11%) developed end-organ CMV disease; 94 (85%) of 110 had CMV retinitis, 10 (7%) of 110 had colitis, and 4 (3%) of 110 had gastritis, hepatitis, or encephalitis.[67] The ability to diagnose CMV disease clinically appears to underestimate the true prevalence of end-organ disease, because autopsy studies have shown that most persons dying of complications of AIDS have evidence of CMV reactivation at death. Despite the nearly universal seroprevalence, some have retinitis, some have gastroenteritis, some have encephalitis, and some may have infections of multiple organ systems, illustrating that the pathogenesis of CMV disease in HIV-infected persons is not well understood.

Ocular Infection

CMV infection of the retina is the most common intraocular infection and cause of blindness in patients with AIDS.[68] Symptoms include complaints of "floaters" in the affected eye, decreased visual acuity or field loss, and unilateral vision loss. Ophthalmologic examination reveals large, creamy to yellow-white granular areas with perivascular exudates and hemorrhages. The differential diagnosis includes cotton-wool spots, toxoplasmosis, syphilis, HSV infection, VZV infection, and tuberculosis. CMV retinitis usually occurs in patients with CD4 counts less than 50 cells/mm^3, and left untreated, it can result in total blindness of the affected eye. Any patient with advanced HIV disease complaining of these symptoms should be referred for evaluation by an ophthalmologist experienced in HIV retinal pathology. Some clinicians send patients with low CD4 cell counts for routine ophthalmologic screening every 3 to 6 months, but others think that careful patient education and referral for symptoms is sufficient.

Central Nervous System Infection

The importance of CMV infection of the central nervous system has only recently been appreciated. CMV encephalitis, polyradiculopathy, and myelitis are the most common manifestations. Patients with CMV encephalitis commonly present with dementia accompanied by a decreased level of consciousness, cranial nerve abnormalities, and seizures.[69] The CSF may be normal or show a nonspecific mononuclear pleocytosis and mildly elevated protein level. Cultures of CSF are usually negative, and neuroimaging may be normal or show only atrophy. CMV PCR of the CSF is sensitive and specific for CNS infection.[70] Higher DNA copy numbers correlate with more extensive and clinically significant disease. Radiculomyelitis typically manifests with a triad of lower extremity weakness, sacral sensory loss, and urinary incontinence.[71,72] The CSF has a characteristic polymorphonuclear pleocytosis with hypoglycorrhachia. This condition can rapidly (over hours) progress to flaccid paraplegia or quadriplegia, and prompt evaluation and treatment is essential.

Gastrointestinal Infection

Common symptoms of CMV esophagitis include odynophagia, retrosternal chest pain, and dysphagia.[73–75] Patients usually have lost a significant amount of weight at the time of initial evaluation. Endoscopically, the esophagus may contain a large, shallow ulcer with candidal overgrowth. Cultures of biopsy specimens are not helpful because they are often negative, or if positive, they may reflect CMV blood contamination from the biopsy procedure. The diagnosis is made by histopathologic examination of biopsy material, revealing multinucleated giant cells or CMV inclusion bodies. The differential diagnosis includes *Candida albicans* infection, HSV infection, syphilis, and invasive fungal infections.

Patients with CMV-related colitis usually experience watery diarrhea (≤20 liquid stools/day), fever (>38.5°C), significant weight loss, crampy abdominal pain, and hematochezia.[76–78] Seventy percent of patients report persistent, unremitting diarrhea, but some have only intermittent episodes. The differential diagnosis includes common enteric pathogens (eg, *Escherichia coli*, *Shigella*, *Salmonella*), as well as infections with *Mycobacterium avian* complex, *Microsporidium, Cryptosporidium,* or *Isospora* and HIV enteropathy. The clinician should be alert for several pathogens contributing to the cause of diarrhea, because 25% to 40% of cases have more than one cause. Definitive diagnosis is best made by histopathologic examination of biopsy material. As many as 25% of patients have normal-appearing colonic mucosa, 40% have patchy colitis (primarily limited to the left colon and cecum), and 15% have diffuse colitis.[77] Because of the patchy involvement of mucosa, flexible sigmoidoscopic examination and biopsy may miss the involved area.

Other Manifestations of Cytomegalovirus Infection in the HIV-infected Person

CMV is an uncommon cause of pneumonia in persons with HIV or AIDS. No effect on mortality has ever been demonstrated by the presence of CMV in the respiratory tract of persons with AIDS,[79,80] despite the fact that it is often isolated in cases of *Pneumocystis carinii* pneumonia.

The isolated finding of CMV reactivation in the blood or urine of an HIV-infected person is difficult to interpret, because 36% of urine and semen cultures done for CMV-seropositive homosexual men without HIV infection are positive.[65] In a retrospective study, the presence of viremia or viruria did not correlate with the development of CMV end-organ disease.[81] CMV viremia did not correlate with weight loss or the presence of fever, but in one study, treatment of persons with CMV reactivations detected by the presence of antigen in the blood reduced the frequency of CMV end-organ disease. Studies are underway to further characterize the relation of antigen or HSV DNA in blood and the development of end-organ disease.[82–84]

Treatment

Primary therapy for CMV end-organ disease is limited to foscarnet and ganciclovir. HPMPC (Cidofovir) appears to be useful in the treatment of CMV infection in HIV-infected persons.[85] All three drugs inhibit CMV DNA polymerase, each at a different site of the polymerase molecule. Each of the compounds has a different toxicity profile. The main toxic effect of ganciclovir is bone marrow depression, usually neutropenia, with 16% of patients developing neutropenia (absolute neutrophil count <500 cells/mm^3).[68] This toxicity is usually reversible, but there are case reports of persistent granulocytopenia after ganciclovir administration. Other toxicities are uncommon, but 15% of patients report gastrointestinal disturbances (primarily nausea), and 17% report CNS disturbances (primarily confusion). After 3 months of therapy with ganciclovir, 10% of patients begin to excrete ganciclovir-resistant CMV, but not much is known about the frequency of CMV isolates that are resistant to foscarnet or HPMPC.

In addition to its anti-CMV activity, foscarnet has reverse transcriptase activity and may act synergistically with other antiretroviral agents against HIV.[86,87] The main toxic effect of foscarnet is renal, causing electrolyte abnormalities, azotemia, anemia, hypocalcemia, and hypophosphatemia. HPMPC also has renal toxicity, which can be reduced with probenecid therapy. Treatment options for CMV are outlined in Table 14.5-3, and with the exception of ocular infection, they are limited to intravenous ganciclovir or foscarnet.

The choice of therapy for CMV retinitis is controversial. Results of the Studies of Ocular Complications of AIDS (SOCA) trial comparing foscarnet to ganciclovir showed a clear survival benefit with foscarnet (8 versus 12 months), but time to progression of CMV retinitis was the same for both drugs (56 days).[88] The difference in mortality probably is explained by more persons in the ganciclovir group discontinuing zidovudine (AZT) therapy because of AZT-induced neutropenia (granulocyte colony-stimulating factor was not available at the time) and the fact that foscarnet has antiretroviral activity, providing combination therapy for patients randomized to foscarnet. At standard maintenance doses (see Table 14.5-3), most patients progress within 2 to 4 months, regardless of the initial choice of antiviral agent, but results of one small study suggested that higher maintenance doses of

TABLE 14.5-3. *Therapy for cytomegalovirus infection in HIV-positive persons*

Agent		Dose	Frequency	Cost*	Indication	Comment
Monotherapy						
Ganciclovir		5 mg/kg IV	q12 h × 14 d	$2000 for 14 d	Induction	Neutrapenia
	or	6 mg/kg IV	q d × 5 d/wk	$1510/mo	Maintenance	Neutrapenia
		1 g PO	TID	$1350/mo	Maintenance	
Foscarnet		40 mg/kg IV	q 8 h × 10–21 d	$2974 for 10 d	Induction	Adjust for renal function
		90 mg/kg IV	qd	$2719/mo	Maintenance	Adjust for renal function
Combination ganciclovir + foscarnet						
Ganciclovir		5 mg/kg IV	q12h × 14–21 d	$2000 for 14 d	Failed	Neutrapenia
Foscarnet		60 mg/kg IV	q 8 h × 14–21 d	$4079 for 14 d	Monotherapy	Adjust for renal function
Ganciclovir		3.75 mg/kg IV	qd	$1510/mo	Maintenance	Neutrapenia
Foscarnet	or	60 mg/kg IV	qd	$2719/mo		Adjust for renal function
Ganciclovir		6 mg/kg IV	qod (alternating)	$755/mo	Maintenance	Neutrapenia
Foscarnet		120 mg/kg IV	qod (alternating)	$1359/mo		Adjust for renal function

*Cost to a patient at our hospital-based outpatient pharmacy.

TABLE 14.5-4. *Frequency of HSV2 reactivation in HIV-infected homosexual men compared with HIV-negative homosexual men**

HIV status	Number of days HSV isolated/total days cultured	Overall HSV shed rate (%)
HIV positive		
Oral	7/4112	0.2
Genital	44/2313	1.9
Perirectal	335/4109	8.6
HIV negative		
Oral	1/762	0.1
Genital	2/235	0.9
Perirectal	12/763	1.6

*HSV reactivation rates are obtained from a group of 50 HIV-infected men completing at least 60 days of daily home HSV cultures of the mouth, genitals, and rectum and a group of 13 HIV-negative men (with a sexual lifestyle similar to the HIV-infected persons) who completed the same protocol.
†Total consecutive days cultured.

foscarnet significantly increased survival time and delayed progression to retinitis,[89] suggesting that more potent antiviral activity is critical for relapsing disease. Results of a second SOCA trial suggest that the combination of ganciclovir and foscarnet may be superior to single-drug therapy for recurrent CMV retinitis. When progression occurs, switching to the other intravenous agent may be of some benefit.

Intravitreal therapy with a surgical implant containing a sustained-release ganciclovir pellet has been successfully used for the treatment of CMV infection. In one trial, patients randomized to the surgical implant had a significantly longer period until clinical progression than those in the deferred-treatment group (226 days versus 15 days).[90] The local therapy was well tolerated, with few toxic or other side effects. The ganciclovir implants, if approved by the Food and Drug Administration, will offer patients a much easier approach to the management of their disease, avoiding the systemic toxicity of ganciclovir and foscarnet and the need for multiple intravenous infusions each day. However, the surgical placement of the pellet is associated with a somewhat increased incidence of retinal detachment and endophthalmitis. Moreover, local therapy has the disadvantage of not protecting the other eye from infection. Whether intermittent systemic therapy can be used in addition to local therapy is unclear.

HPMPC, an intravenous or intravitreal agent with broad anti-CMV activity, has also been evaluated in the treatment of CMV retinitis.[85] HPMPC has been used locally and systemically. It has a long half-life, and studies suggest it has activity in preventing the progression of CMV retinitis at a dose of 5 mg/kg given weekly combined with 1g of probenecid taken orally each day.

Oral ganciclovir has been licensed for maintenance therapy after induction with parenteral ganciclovir.[91] Clinical studies have shown that the time to retinitis progression is relatively similar to the time for intravenous therapy used for maintenance. In 117 patients randomized to oral ganciclovir or to intravenous ganciclovir for maintenance therapy for CMV retinitis, the mean time to retinitis progression was 62 days for the intravenous ganciclovir group and 57 days for the oral ganciclovir group ($P = 0.63$). Survival and adverse gastrointestinal symptoms events were similar in the two groups, but there was a higher incidence of neutropenia, anemia, intravenous catheter–related events, and sepsis in the intravenous group. Oral ganciclovir is being used for chronic maintenance therapy.

There is some controversy about the use of these antivirals for prevention of CMV disease in AIDS patients. Oral ganciclovir and high-dose valaciclovir have been evaluated in this setting, but because the incidence of CMV disease among enrollees in the oral ganciclovir study was low (<25%), the economics of prophylactic use for all patients has been questioned. Data on the valaciclovir prophylaxis study are under analysis.

VARICELLA ZOSTER VIRUS

Epidemiology

Approximately 90% of HIV-infected persons are seropositive for VZV, the causative agent of chickenpox. This rate is similar to that for the general population, because only 10% of persons 15 years of age or older are susceptible. However, reactivation of latent VZV from nerve root ganglia is more common in HIV-positive persons, and they are 17 times more likely to have shingles than HIV-negative persons.[92]

Clinical Manifestations

Primary VZV infection usually results in chickenpox. In immunocompetent children, this is typically an illness with a benign outcome. Primary VZV in immunocompromised persons may be associated with more numerous lesions, prolonged healing time, bacterial superinfection, and dissemination. Primary VZV in persons with HIV or AIDS may have a fatal outcome,[93] and varicella in adults with HIV should be treated with antiviral therapy. CNS manifestations of varicella dissemination include encephalitis and cerebellar ataxia. Pneumonitis, hepatitis, and hemorrhagic skin lesions are seen with visceral dissemination.[93] Pneumonitis is common in persons with primary VZV infections, and it may be fatal in immunocompromised persons. Because as many as 10% of HIV-infected persons are VZV seronegative and a primary infection could be fatal, all patients with HIV or AIDS should be questioned about a history of chickenpox. If they have no clinical history of chickenpox or are unsure, a VZV serologic profile should be obtained. This allows the clinician to advise the patient about avoiding possible exposures and to promptly institute antiviral therapy at the time of exposure. Whether such persons should be vaccinated for VZV with the live attenuated vaccine is unclear.

The most common clinical manifestations of VZV reactivation is herpes zoster. As many as 20% of HIV-infected persons may have recurrent episodes of shingles,[92] often in the form of multidermatomal zoster. Zoster is seen in persons with high and low CD4 cell counts, and prolonged shingles is often the first manifestation of HIV infection.[94] Diagnosis of zoster in an HIV-infected person does not appear to be a prognostic sign for rapid progression of HIV.[92,95,96]

Symptoms of zoster in HIV-infected persons are similar to those in immunocompetent persons. The patient typically experiences a radicular pain, followed by a vesicular rash over the involved dermatomes. VZV can be differentiated from disseminated HSV or zosteriform HSV by documenting lesions in different stages of development. Crusted lesions can be adjacent to vesicular or healed lesions. Zoster

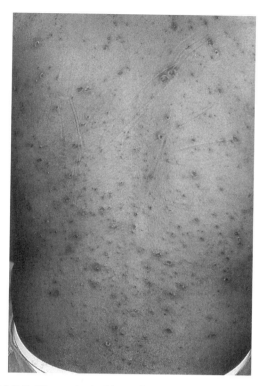

FIG. 14.5-5. Disseminated hyperkeratotic zoster in an HIV-infected person (photo courtesy of Dr. David Spach). See also Color Figure 14.5.5.

ophthalmicus occurs when the ophthalmic branch of the trigeminal nerve (V_1) is involved and is suggested by lesions appearing on the tip of nose. Such patients should be referred for an ophthalmologic examination, because anterior uveitis, corneal scarring, and permanent vision loss may occur. Hematogenous dissemination to other cutaneous sites (>20 vesicles outside of a single dermatome) is unusual in immunocompetent persons but more common in those with AIDS.[97] Visceral dissemination of VZV in the HIV-infected person is uncommon, but CNS involvement may occur. CNS symptoms, including polyneuritis, myelitis, and encephalitis, become apparent 9 to 12 days after the onset of skin symptoms.[98,99]

Although dissemination of VZV in HIV-infected persons is atypical, persistent cutaneous infection is common, especially with indistinguishable lesions. The lesions may mimic ecthymatous lesions, consisting of erythema with central necrosis (Fig. 14.5-4).[100,101] Persistent cutaneous VZV may also manifest as hyperkeratotic, verrucous lesions that are prolonged and widely distributed throughout the body, often with more than 20 lesions outside of a single dermatome (Fig. 14.5-5). These are often resistant to acyclovir and are usually seen in patients on suppressive acyclovir therapy.[102–105] Susceptibility testing confirms that the isolates are resistant by the absence of TK activity.

Recurrences of zoster are more common in the HIV-positive person. Between 20% and 30% have two to three recur-

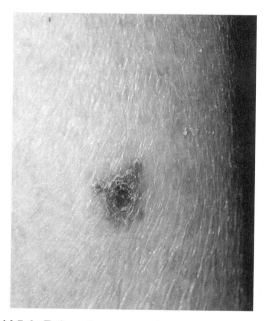

FIG. 14.5-4. Ecthymatous zoster lesion in an HIV-infected person (photo courtesy of Dr. David Spach, University of Washington, Seattle, WA). See also Color Figure 14.5-4.

rences of VZV infection. The viruses isolated during these recurrences are usually still sensitive to TK-dependent antivirals.

Another complication of VZV infection in HIV-infected persons is acute retinal necrosis. This infection is uncommon, but it can rapidly cause blindness, and both eyes commonly are involved. Therapy with high-dose ganciclovir, foscarnet, or a combination of the two drugs is advised.

The diagnosis of zoster is usually clinical, with characteristic lesions appearing over a single dermatome. Because of the confusion with zosteriform HSV, we recommend obtaining a culture or using an antigen-based test to determine if the lesion is caused by VZV or HSV. Atypical presentations may complicate the diagnosis, and if a laboratory diagnosis is warranted, immunofluorescent assays that detect virally infected cells from the base of a lesion can verify the presence of the virus. If acyclovir resistance is suspected, culture is necessary to obtain an isolate for sensitivity testing.

Treatment

Three agents are licensed for oral therapy of shingles: acyclovir (Zovirax), valaciclovir (Valtrex), and famciclovir (Famvir). Most of the therapeutic studies on VZV have been conducted with immunocompetent persons. In a trial comparing valaciclovir to acyclovir, valaciclovir was associated with faster relief of pain and better healing. Famciclovir was studied in a placebo-controlled trial and shown to be effective in speeding healing and reducing post-herpetic neuralgia in elderly patients.[106] No results of a trial comparing valaciclovir with famciclovir are available.

Sorivudine, a new antiviral agent, has been compared with acyclovir. In this trial, Sorivudine (40 mg once daily)

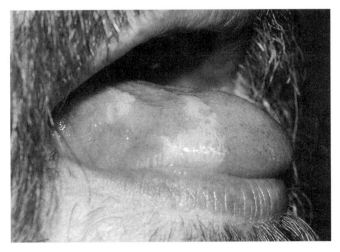

FIG. 14.5-6. Oral hairy leukoplakia on the sides of the tongue in an HIV-infected person (photo courtesy of Dr. David Spach). See also Color Figure 14.5-6.

was slightly better than acyclovir in reducing the time to healing of herpes zoster in HIV-positive persons. The major complication of Sorivudine is a drug interaction with 5-fluorouracil, a chemotherapeutic agent used in the therapy of many solid tumors. Sorivudine blocks the enzyme that metabolizes 5-fluorouracil, allowing accumulation of 5-fluorouracil and its metabolites. Fatal marrow toxicity has occurred in this setting.

We recommend famciclovir (500 mg, taken orally twice daily) or valaciclovir (1000 mg, taken twice daily for 7 days) for the therapy of zoster in HIV seropositive persons. For disseminated zoster in HIV-infected persons, intravenous acyclovir at a dose of 10 mg/kg three times daily for 3 to 5 days, followed by oral therapy, is appropriate. For persons with neurologic sequelae, the relapse rate is often high and long-term suppressive therapy is often recommended. Foscarnet is used at a dose of 40 mg/kg (administered intravenously three times daily for 14 to 28 days) when acyclovir-resistant VZV is suspected.

EPSTEIN-BARR VIRUS

Primary EBV in HIV-infected adults is uncommon, because the seroprevalence is so high in the adult population (>90% by early adolescence). The most common clinical manifestation of primary EBV is infectious mononucleosis. A recent report of children with HIV or AIDS has described the development of aggressive muscle tumors[107] during primary EBV infection. These tumors are the result of a clonal expansion of smooth muscle cells that were presumably transformed by EBV. Reactivation of EBV after primary infection is typically restricted to immunosuppressed persons and is associated with hematopoietic malignancies such as endemic (African) Burkitt's lymphoma, CNS lymphoma, and nasopharyngeal carcinoma.[108–111]

In persons with asymptomatic HIV infection, the primary clinical manifestation is OHL (Fig. 14.5–6). OHL has been documented in other immunocompromised populations and rarely in immunocompetent persons. This is a benign, self-limited condition of the tongue that is caused by replication of EBV in epithelial cells, and it is associated with frequent viral recombination events.[112] It may occur at any stage of HIV disease, and it has not been shown to be a sign of advancing HIV disease. Despite the very high seroprevalence of EBV among persons with HIV or AIDS, OHL occurs in only 25% of patients. Acyclovir, given in very high doses, can reduce the size of the lesion or cause it to disappear. However, because of the high cost of therapy and benign nature of the condition, the drug is usually not indicated.

HUMAN HERPESVIRUSES 6 AND 7

HHV6 and HHV7 have only recently been discovered as herpesviruses whose homology is closest to CMV. These viruses appear to be T-cell tropic, but specific sites of latency have not been identified. These viruses are ubiquitous; most persons become seropositive during infancy and early childhood.[113]

HHV6 seroconversion has been documented during the acute phase of roseola, suggesting it is the etiologic agent of that disease.[114] Two other illnesses occasionally associated with HHV6 seroconversion are heterophile-negative mononucleosis[115,116] and hepatitis.[117,118] Other complications of primary HHV6 infection mentioned in the literature include anemia, granulocytopenia, and Kawasaki's disease.[119–121] Reactivation of HHV6 (documented by elevated levels of IgM antibody) appears to be associated with interstitial pneumonitis in patients undergoing bone marrow transplantation[122–124] and spontaneous abortions.[125] HHV6 reactivation has also been associated with febrile seizures in children.[126]

There has been no demonstration of HHV6 as an opportunistic infection in HIV-infected persons. Using immunocytochemistry methods, HHV6-infected cells have been identified in the lymphoid organs of patients with AIDS and may have been associated with a case of pneumonitis.[127] We have demonstrated that HHV6 is found in higher copy numbers in HIV-infected men with high CD4 cell counts,[128] supporting the hypothesis that HHV6 is latent in CD4 cells. However, despite numerous studies demonstrating significant in vitro interactions between HHV6 and HIV, no clinical disease has been documented to be caused by HHV6 or HHV7. A prospective, longitudinal study of HHV6 reactivation in peripheral blood mononuclear cells (PBMCs) of HIV-infected persons at all stages of infection have shown a very low incidence of HHV6 reactivation in this cohort, as measured by PCR (T. Schacker, unpublished data).

HUMAN HERPESVIRUS 8

HHV8 is a member of the herpesvirus family and was discovered through identification of unique DNA sequences associated with Kaposi's sarcoma lesions in patients with AIDS.[129] The epidemiology of AIDS-related Kaposi's sarcoma suggests it is a sexually transmitted agent, and HHV8 may follow the epidemiologic patterns seen in other HIV-associated sexually transmitted diseases.

HHV8 sequences have been detected by PCR in in Kaposi's sarcoma lesions from patients with AIDS and those with Mediterranean Kaposi's sarcoma.[130–133] HHV8 sequences have been detected in a subset of body cavity B-cell lymphomas characterized by pleural, pericardial, and peritoneal lymphomatous effusions. Although most of these tumors have had HHV8 and EBV genomic sequences detected in the same tissue,[134] Reene and colleagues identified a tumor using just HHV8 sequences. These genomic sequences have also been found in PBMCs of patients with asymptomatic HIV infection. The sensitivity of detection of HHV8 in the PBMCs of asymptomatic HIV-infected persons for predicting risk of Kaposi's sarcoma is unknown. One study showed that of HIV-infected persons in whom HHV8 genomic sequences

were identified in PBMCs went on to develop Kaposi's sarcoma. Larger studies will be needed to settle this issue and to determine if treatment of HHV8 infection can alter the progression of Kaposi's sarcoma.

REFERENCES

1. Banks T, Rouse B. Herpesviruses—immune escape artists? Clin Infect Dis 1992;14:933.
2. Enzensberger R, et al. Prevalence of antibodies to human herpesviruses and hepatitis B virus in patients at different stages of human immunodeficiency virus (HIV) infection. Infection 1991;19:140.
3. Johnson RE, et al. A seroepidemiologic survey of the prevalence of herpes simplex virus type 2 infection in the United States. N Engl J Med 1989;321:7.
4. Mann SL, et al. Prevalence and incidence of herpesvirus infections among homosexually active men. J Infect Dis 1984;149:1026.
5. Siegel D, et al. Prevalence and correlates of herpes simplex infections. The population-based AIDS in multiethnic neighborhoods study. JAMA 1992;268:1702.
6. Quinn TC, et al. Serologic and immunologic studies in patients with AIDS in North America and Africa. The potential role of infectious agents as cofactors in human immunodeficiency virus infection. JAMA 1987;257:2617.
7. Frenkel LM, et al. Clinical reactivation of herpes simplex virus type 2 infection in seropositive pregnant women with no history of genital herpes. Ann Intern Med 1993;118:414.
8. Corey L, Spear P. Infections with herpes simplex viruses. N Engl J Med 1986;314:749.
9. Rompalo AM, et al. Oral acyclovir for treatment of first-episode herpes simplex virus proctitis. JAMA 1988;259:2879.
10. Wald A, et al. Virologic characteristics of subclinical and symptomatic genital herpes infections. N Engl J Med 1995;333:770.
11. Koelle DM, et al. Asymptomatic reactivation of herpes simplex virus in women after the first episode of genital herpes. Ann Intern Med 1992;116:433.
12. Brock B, et al. Frequency of asymptomatic shedding of herpes simplex virus in women with genital herpes. JAMA 1990;263:418.
13. Rooney JF, et al. Acquisition of genital herpes from an asymptomatic sexual partner. N Engl J Med 1986;314:1561.
14. Mertz GJ, et al. Transmission of genital herpes in couples with one symptomatic and one asymptomatic partner: a prospective study. J Infect Dis 1988;157:1169.
15. Mertz GJ, et al. Risk factors for the sexual transmission of genital herpes. Ann Intern Med 1992;116:197.
16. Benedetti J, Corey L, Ashley R. Recurrence rates in genital herpes after symptomatic first-episode infection. Ann Intern Med 1994;121:847.
17. Siegal FP, et al. Severe acquired immunodeficiency in male homosexuals, manifested by chronic perianal ulcerative herpes simplex lesions. N Engl J Med 1981;305:1439.
18. Schacker T, et al. Efficacy of famciclovir for suppressing HSV2 infections among HIV+ persons. Third National Conference on Retroviruses and Opportunistic Infections, Washington DC, 1966.
19. Augenbraun M, et al. Increased genital shedding of herpes simplex virus type 2 in HIV-seropositive women. Ann Intern Med 1995;123:845.
20. Bagdades EK, et al. Relationship between herpes simplex virus ulceration and CD4+ cell counts in patients with HIV infection. AIDS 1992;6:1317.
21. Sacks S, et al. Progressive esophagitis from acyclovir-resistant herpes simplex. Ann Intern Med 1989;111:893.
22. Gateley A, et al. Herpes simplex virus type 2 meningoencephalitis resistant to acyclovir in a patient with AIDS. J Infect Dis 1990;161:711.
23. Laskin OL, Stahl BCM, Morgello S. Concomitant herpes simplex virus type 1 and cytomegalovirus ventriculoencephalitis in acquired immunodeficiency syndrome. Arch Neurol 1987;44:843.
24. Nicoll JA, Kinrade E, Love S. PCR-mediated search for herpes simplex virus DNA in sections of brain from patients with multiple sclerosis and other neurological disorders. J Neurol Sci 1992;113:144.

25. Rummelt V, et al. Triple retinal infection with human immunodeficiency virus type 1, cytomegalovirus, and herpes simplex virus type 1. Light and electron microscopy, immunohistochemistry, and in situ hybridization. Ophthalmology 1994;101:270.

26. Britton CB, et al. A new complication of AIDS: thoracic myelitis caused by herpes simplex virus. Neurology 1985;35:1071.

27. Koike K, et al. Herpes simplex virus type 1 and human immunodeficiency virus type 1 antigens in platelets from a hemophilia B patient with human immunodeficiency virus type 1-related thrombocytopenia. Int J Hematol 1992;55:205.

28. Erlich KS, et al. Acyclovir-resistant herpes simplex virus infections in patients with the acquired immunodeficiency syndrome. N Engl J Med 1989;320:293.

29. Englund JA, et al. Herpes simplex virus resistant to acyclovir. A study in a tertiary care center. Ann Intern Med 1990;112:416.

30. Marks G, et al. Mucocutaneous dissemination of acyclovir-resistant herpes simplex virus in a patient with AIDS. Rev Infect Dis 1989;2:474.

31. Safrin S, Elbaggari A, Elbeik T. Risk factors for the development of acyclovir-resistant herpes simplex virus (HSV) infection. Presented at the VIII International Conference on AIDS/III STD World Conference, Amsterdam, 1992.

32. Bevilacqua F, et al. Acyclovir resistance/susceptibility in herpes simplex virus type 2 sequential isolates from an AIDS patient. J Acquir Immune Defic Syndr 1991;4:967.

33. Norris S, Kessler H, Fife K. Severe, progressive herpetic whitlow caused by an acyclovir-resistant virus in a patient with AIDS. J Infect Dis 1987;157:209.

34. Erlich KS, et al. Acyclovir-resistant herpes simplex virus infections in patients with the acquired immunodeficiency syndrome. N Engl J Med 1989;320:293.

35. Erlich KS, et al. Foscarnet therapy for severe acyclovir-resistant herpes simplex virus type-2 infections in patients with the acquired immunodeficiency syndrome (AIDS). An uncontrolled trial. Ann Intern Med 1989;110:710.

36. Crumpacker CS. Mechanism of action of foscarnet against viral polymerases. Am J Med 1992;92:2A.

37. Safrin S, et al. Foscarnet therapy for acyclovir-resistant mucocutaneous herpes simplex virus infection in 26 AIDS patients: preliminary data. J Infect Dis 1990;161:1078.

38. Safrin S, et al. A controlled trial comparing foscarnet with vidarabine for acyclovir-resistant mucocutaneous herpes simplex in the acquired immunodeficiency syndrome. The AIDS Clinical Trials Group. N Engl J Med 1991;325:551.

39. Birch CJ, et al. Clinical effects and in vitro studies of trifluorothymidine combined with interferon-alpha for treatment of drug-resistant and -sensitive herpes simplex virus infections. J Infect Dis 1992;166:108.

40. Polis MA, et al. Anticytomegaloviral activity and safety of cidofovir in patients with human immunodeficiency virus infection and cytomegalovirus viruria. Antimicrob Agents Chemother 1995;39:882.

41. Holmberg SD, et al. Prior herpes simplex virus type 2 infection as a risk factor for HIV infection. JAMA 1988;259:1048.

42. Hook EWD, et al. Herpes simplex virus infection as a risk factor for human immunodeficiency virus infection in heterosexuals. J Infect Dis 1992;165:251.

43. Cameron DW, et al. Female to male transmission of human immunodeficiency virus type 1: risk factors for seroconversion in men [see comments]. Lancet 1989;2:403.

44. Mosca JD, et al. Herpes simplex virus type 1 can reactivate transcription of latent human immunodeficiency virus. Nature 1987;325:67.

45. Mosca JD, et al. Activation of human immunodeficiency virus by herpesvirus infection: identification of a region within the long terminal repeat that responds to a trans-acting factor encoded by herpes simplex virus 1. Proc Natl Acad Sci U S A 1987;84:7408.

46. Heng MC, Heng SY, Allen SG. Co-infection and synergy of human immunodeficiency virus-1 and herpes simplex virus-1. Lancet 1994;343:255.

47. Kroner BL, et al. HIV-1 infection incidence among persons with hemophilia in the United States and western Europe, 1978–1990; Multicenter Hemophilia Cohort Study. J Acquir Immune Defic Syndr 1994;7:279.

48. Golden MP, et al. Activation of human immunodeficiency virus by herpes simplex virus. J Infect Dis 1992;166:494.

49. Albrecht MA, et al. The herpes simplex virus immediate-early protein, ICP4, is required to potentiate replication of human immunodeficiency virus in CD4+ lymphocytes. J Virol 1989;63:1861.

50. Margolis DM, et al. Transactivation of the HIV-1 LTR by HSV1 immediate-early genes. Virology 1992;186:788.

51. Ghosh S, Selby MJ, Peterlin BM. Synergism between Tat and VP16 in trans-activation of HIV-1 LTR. J Mol Biol 1993;234:610.

52. Schacker T, et al. Changes in HIV viral load during clinical episodes of HSV. Presented at the 33rd International Conference on Antimicrobial Agents and Chemotherapy, San Francisco, 1995.

53. Stein D, et al. The effect of the interaction of acyclovir with zidovudine on progression to AIDS and survival. Ann Intern Med 1994;121:100.

54. Youle MS, et al. Effects of high-dose oral acyclovir on herpesvirus disease and survival in patients with advanced HIV disease: a double-blind, placebo-controlled study. European-Australian Acyclovir Study Group. AIDS 1994;8:641. [Published erratum appears in AIDS 1994;8:following 859.]

55. Pederson C, et al. The effect of treatment with zidovudine with or without acyclovir on HIV p24 antigenemia in patients with AIDS and AIDS-related complex. AIDS 1992;6:821.

56. Cooper DA, et al. Zidovudine in persons with asymptomatic HIV infection and CD4+ cell counts greater than 400 per cubic millimeter. The European-Australian Collaborative Group [see comments]. N Engl J Med 1993;329:297.

57. Ashley RL, et al. Comparison of western blot (immunoblot) and glycoprotein G-specific immunodot enzyme assay for detecting antibodies to herpes simplex virus types 1 and 2 in human sera. J Clin Microbiol 1988;26:662.

58. Ashley R, et al. Inability of enzyme immunoassays to discriminate between infections with herpes simplex virus types 1 and 2. Ann Intern Med 1991;115:520.

59. Aurelius E, et al. Rapid diagnosis of herpes simplex encephalitis by nested polymerase chain reaction assay of cerebrospinal fluid. Lancet 1991;337:189.

60. Rowley AH, et al. Rapid detection of herpes-simplex-virus DNA in cerebrospinal fluid of patients with herpes simplex encephalitis [see comments]. Lancet 1990;335:440.

61. Reichman R, et al. Treatment of recurrent genital herpes simplex infections with oral acyclovir. JAMA 1984;251:2103.

62. Straus S, et al. Suppression of frequently recurring genital herpes. N Engl J Med 1984;310:1545.

63. Douglas J, et al. A double-blind study of oral acyclovir for suppression of recurrences of genital herpes simplex virus infection. N Engl J Med 1984;310:1551.

64. Drew L, et al. Prevalence of cytomegalovirus infection in homosexual men. J Infect Dis 1981;143:188.

65. Collier A, et al. Cytomegalovirus infection in homosexual men. Am J Med 1987;82:593.

66. Berry NJ, et al. Seroepidemiologic studies on the acquisition of antibodies to cytomegalovirus, herpes simplex virus, and human immunodeficiency virus among general hospital patients and those attending a clinic for sexually transmitted diseases. J Med Virol 1988;24:385.

67. Gallant JE, et al. Incidence and natural history of cytomegalovirus disease in patients with advanced human immunodeficiency virus disease treated with zidovudine. The Zidovudine Epidemiology Study Group [see comments]. J Infect Dis 1992;166:1223.

68. Henderly DE, Jampol LM. Diagnosis and treatment of cytomegalovirus retinitis. J Acquir Immune Defic Syndr 1991;1:S6.

69. Berman SM, Kim RC. The development of cytomegalovirus encephalitis in AIDS patients receiving ganciclovir. Am J Med 1994;96:415.

70. Achim CL, et al. Detection of cytomegalovirus in cerebrospinal fluid autopsy specimens from AIDS patients. J Infect Dis 1994;169:623.

71. Cohen BA, et al. Neurologic prognosis of cytomegalovirus polyradiculomyelopathy in AIDS [see comments]. Neurology 1993;43(Pt 1):493.

72. Tokumoto JI, Hollander H. Cytomegalovirus polyradiculopathy caused by a ganciclovir-resistant strain [see comments]. Clin Infect Dis 1993;17:854.

73. Rusconi S, Meroni L, Galli M. Tracheoesophageal fistula in an HIV-1–positive man due to dual infection of Candida albicans and cytomegalovirus. Chest 1994;106:284.

74. Goodgame RW, et al. Esophageal stricture after cytomegalovirus ulcer treated with ganciclovir. J Clin Gastroenterol 1991;13:678.

75. Wilcox CM, Straub RF, Schwartz DA. Cytomegalovirus esophagitis in AIDS: a prospective evaluation of clinical response to ganciclovir therapy, relapse rate, and long-term outcome. Am J Med 1995;98:169.

76. Mentec H, et al. Cytomegalovirus colitis in HIV-1–infected patients: a prospective research in 55 patients. AIDS 1994;8:461.

77. Dieterich DT, Rahmin M. Cytomegalovirus colitis in AIDS: presentation in 44 patients and a review of the literature. J Acquir Immune Defic Syndr 1991;1:S29.

78. Beaugerie L, et al. Etiology and management of toxic megacolon in patients with human immunodeficiency virus infection. Gastroenterology 1994;107:858.

79. Millar AB, et al. Cytomegalovirus in the lungs of patients with AIDS. Respiratory pathogen or passenger? Am Rev Respir Dis 1990;141:1474.

80. Miles PR, Baughman RP, Linnemann CC Jr. Cytomegalovirus in the bronchoalveolar lavage fluid of patients with AIDS. Chest 1990;97:1072.

81. Zurlo JJ, et al. Lack of clinical utility of cytomegalovirus blood and urine cultures in patients with HIV infection [see comments]. Ann Intern Med 1993;118:12.

82. Mazzuli T, et al. Cytomegalovirus antigenemia: clinical correlations in transplant recipients and in persons with aids. J Clin Microbiol 1993;31:3824.

83. Landry ML, Ferguson D. Comparison of quantitative cytomegalovirus antigenemia assay with culture methods and correlation with clinical disease. J Clin Microbiol 1993;31:2851.

84. Erice A, et al. Cytomegalovirus (CMV) antigenemia assay is more sensitive than shell vial cultures for rapid detection of CMV in polymorphonuclear blood leukocytes [see comments]. J Clin Microbiol 1992;30:2822.

85. Flores-Aguilar M, et al. Long-acting therapy of viral retinitis with (S)-1-(3-hydroxy-2-phosphonylmethoxypropl)cytosine. J Infect Dis 1994;169:642.

86. Kong X-B, Zhu Q-Y, Ruprecht R-M, et al. Synergistic inhibition of human immunodeficiency virus type 1 replication in vitro by two-drug and three-drug combination of 3′-azido-3′-deoxythymidine, phosphonoformate, and 2′,3′-dideoxythymidine. Antimicrob Agents Chemother 1991;35:2003.

87. Eriksson BF, Schinazi RF. Combinations of 3′-azido-3′-deoxythymidine (zidovudine) and phosphonoformate (foscarnet) against human immunodeficiency virus type 1 and cytomegalovirus replication in vitro. Antimicrob Agents Chemother 1989;33:663.

88. Ocular Complications of AIDS Research Group with the AIDS Clinical Trials Group. Mortality in patients with the acquired immunodeficiency syndrome treated with either foscarnet or ganciclovir for cytomegalovirus retinitis [see comments]. N Engl J Med 1992;326:213. [Published erratum appears in N Engl J Med 199223;326:1172.]

89. Jacobson MA, et al. A dose-ranging study of daily maintenance intravenous foscarnet therapy for cytomegalovirus retinitis in AIDS. J Infect Dis 1993;168:444.

90. Martin DF, et al. Treatment of cytomegalovirus retinitis with an intraocular sustained-release ganciclovir implant. A randomized controlled clinical trial. Arch Ophthalmol 1994;112:1531.

91. Drew W, et al. Oral ganciclovir as maintenance treatment for cytomegalovirus retinitis in patients with AIDS. N Engl J Med 1995;333:615.

92. Buchbinder SP, et al. Herpes zoster and human immunodeficiency virus infection [see comments]. J Infect Dis 1992;166:1153.

93. Perronne C, et al. Varicella in patients infected with the human immunodeficiency virus [see comments]. Arch Dermatol 1990;126:1033.

94. Veenstra J, et al. Herpes zoster, immunological deterioration and disease progression in HIV-1 infection. AIDS 1995;9:1153.

95. Rogues AM, et al. Herpes zoster and human immunodeficiency virus infection: a cohort study of 101 coinfected patients. Groupe d'Epid'emiologie clinique du SIDA en aquitaine [see comment]. (Letter) J Infect Dis 1993;168:245.

96. Moss AR and K. Vranizan, Charting the epidemic: the case study of HIV screening of injecting drug users in San Francisco, 1985–1990. Br J Addict 1992;87:467.

97. Cohen PR, Beltrani VP, Grossman ME. Disseminated herpes zoster in patients with human immunodeficiency virus infection. Am J Med 1988;84:1076.

98. Ryder JW, et al. Progressive encephalitis three months after resolution of cutaneous zoster in a patient with AIDS. Ann Neurol 1986;19:182.

99. Grant AD, et al. Detection of varicella-zoster virus DNA using the polymerase chain reaction in an immunocompromised patient with transverse myelitis secondary to herpes zoster. Genitourin Med 1993;69:273.

100. Gilson I, et al. Disseminated ecthymatous herpes varicella-zoster virus infection in patients with acquired immunodeficiency syndrome. J Am Acad Dermatol 1989;20:637.

101. Hoppenjans WB, et al. Prolonged cutaneous herpes zoster in acquired immunodeficiency syndrome [see comments]. Arch Dermatol 1990;126:1048.

102. Pahwa S, et al. Continuous varicella-zoster infection associated with acyclovir resistance in a child with AIDS. JAMA 1988;260:2879.

103. Jacobson MA, et al. Acyclovir-resistant varicella zoster virus infection after chronic oral acyclovir therapy in patients with the acquired immunodeficiency syndrome (AIDS). Ann Intern Med 1990;112:187.

104. Linnemann CCJ, et al. Emergence of acyclovir-resistant varicella zoster virus in an AIDS patient on prolonged acyclovir therapy. AIDS 1990;4:577.

105. Safrin S, et al. Foscarnet therapy in five patients with AIDS and acyclovir-resistant varicella-zoster virus infection. Ann Intern Med 1991;115:19.

106. Tyring S, et al. Famciclovir for the treatment of acute herpes zoster: effects on acute disease and postherpetic neuralgia. A randomized, double-blind, placebo-controlled trial. Collaborative Famciclovir Herpes Zoster Study Group [see comments]. Ann Intern Med 1995;123:89.

107. Pathmanathan R, et al. Clonal proliferations of cells infected with Epstein-Barr virus in preinvasive lesions related to nasopharyngeal carcinoma [see comments]. N Engl J Med 1995;333:693.

108. Samoszuk M, Ravel J. Frequent detection of Epstein-Barr viral deoxyribonucleic acid and absence of cytomegalovirus deoxyribonucleic acid in Hodgkin's disease and acquired immunodeficiency syndrome-related Hodgkin's disease. Lab Invest 1991;65:631.

109. Samoszuk M, et al. Incidence of Epstein-Barr virus in AIDS-related lymphoma specimens. J Acquir Immune Defic Syndr 1993;6:913.

110. Cohen JI. Epstein-Barr virus lymphoproliferative disease associated with acquired immunodeficiency. Medicine (Baltimore) 1991;70:137.

111. Cinque P, et al. Epstein-Barr virus DNA in cerebrospinal fluid from patients with AIDS-related primary lymphoma of the central nervous system. Lancet 1993;342:398.

112. Walling DM, et al. Epstein-Barr virus coinfection and recombination in non-human immunodeficiency virus-associated oral hairy leukoplakia [see comments]. J Infect Dis 1995;171:1122.

113. Clark DA, et al. Prevalence of antibody to human herpesvirus 7 by age. (Letter) J Infect Dis 1993;168:251.

114. Yamanishi K, et al. Identification of human herpesvirus-6 as a causal agent for exanthem subitum [see comments]. Lancet 1988;1:1065.

115. Steeper TA, et al. The spectrum of clinical and laboratory findings resulting from human herpesvirus-6 (HHV-6) in patients with mononucleosis-like illnesses not resulting from Epstein-Barr virus or cytomegalovirus. Am J Clin Pathol 1990;93:776.

116. Irving WL, Cunningham AL. Serological diagnosis of infection with human herpesvirus type 6. BMJ 1990;300:156.

117. Asano Y, et al. Fatal fulminant hepatitis in an infant with human herpesvirus-6 infection. (Letter) Lancet 1990;335:862.

118. Sobue R, et al. Fulminant hepatitis in primary human herpesvirus-6 infection. (Letter) N Engl J Med 1991;324:1290.

119. Takikawa T, et al. Liver dysfunction, anaemia, and granulocytopenia after exanthema subitum. (Letter) Lancet 1992;340:1288.

120. Huang LM, et al. Human herpesvirus-6 associated with fatal haemophagocytic syndrome [see comments]. (Letter) Lancet 1990;336:60.

121. Hagiwara K, et al. Isolation of human herpesvirus-6 from an infant with Kawasaki disease. (Letter) Eur J Pediatr 1992;151:867.

122. Carrigan DR, et al. Interstitial pneumonitis associated with human herpesvirus-6 infection after marrow transplantation. Lancet 1991;338:147.

123. Cone R, et al. Human herpesvirus 6 in lung tissue from bone marrow transplant patients with pneumonia. N Engl J Med 1993;329(3):156.

124. Cone RW, Huang ML, Hackman RC. Human herpesvirus 6 and pneumonia. Leuk Lymphoma 1994;15:235.

125. Ando Y, et al. HHV-6 infection during pregnancy and spontaneous abortion. (Letter) Lancet 1992;340:1289.

126. Breese C, et al. Human herpesvirus-6 infection in children. N Engl J Med 1994;331:432.

127. Knox KK, Carrigan DR. Disseminated active HHV-6 infections in patients with AIDS [see comments]. Lancet 1994;343:577.

128. Fairfax MR, et al. Human herpesvirus 6 DNA in blood cells of human immunodeficiency virus-infected men: correlation of high levels with high CD4 cell counts. J Infect Dis 1994;169:1342.

129. Chang Y, et al. Identification of herpesvirus-like DNA sequences in AIDS-associated Kaposi's sarcoma [see comments]. Science 1994;266:1865.

130. Huang YQ, et al. Human herpesvirus-like nucleic acid in various forms of Kaposi's sarcoma [see comments]. Lancet 1995;345:759.

131. Moore PS, Chang Y. Detection of herpesvirus-like DNA sequences in Kaposi's sarcoma in patients with and without HIV infection [see comments]. N Engl J Med 1995;332:1181.

132. Dupin N, et al. Herpesvirus-like DNA sequences in patients with Mediterranean Kaposi's sarcoma [see comments]. Lancet 1995;345:761.

133. Rady PL, et al. Herpesvirus-like DNA sequences in non-Kaposi's sarcoma skin lesions of transplant patients. Lancet 1995;345:1339.

134. Cesarman E, et al. Kaposi's sarcoma-associated herpesvirus-like DNA sequences in AIDS-related body-cavity-based lymphomas [see comments]. N Engl J Med 1995;332:1186.

AIDS: Biology, Diagnosis, Treatment and Prevention, fourth edition, edited by Vincent T. DeVita, Jr., Samuel Hellman, and Steven A. Rosenberg. Lippincott–Raven Publishers, © 1997

14.6

Human Papillomavirus and Hepatitis Viral Infections In Human Immunodeficiency Virus–Infected Persons

Nancy B. Kiviat

Even before the human immunodeficiency virus (HIV) epidemic, it was clear that the courses of human papillomavirus (HPV), hepatitis B (HBV), and hepatitis C virus (HCV) were altered in immunosuppressed patients. During the last decade, numerous studies have examined the associations among HPV, HCV, HBV, and HIV. Most individuals infected with HIV are also infected with at least one of the other viruses. Understanding how these infections interact is of practical importance for those caring for HIV-infected persons.

INTERACTIONS BETWEEN HIV AND HUMAN PAPILLOMAVIRUSES

Epidemiology of HPV Infection

More than 85 types of HPV have been identified. These viruses demonstrate considerable site-specific tissue trophism, and the clinical manifestations of HPV infection vary with the type of virus, the site infected, and the age and immune status of the host.[1] Traditional techniques used for culturing most viruses cannot be employed for HPV, because viral replication and capsid production are tightly linked to terminal squamous epithelial cell differentiation. The diagnosis is made by clinical, colposcopic, or microscopic evaluation or by the use of hybridization technology. The inability to grow the virus has made it difficult to develop a reliable serologic assay for acute or past infection.

"Genital types" of HPV preferentially infect the epithelium of the male and female genital tract, where infection produces visible genital warts or, more frequently, estab-

lishes subclinical disease, which can be detected only with the aid of magnification (eg, colposcopy, microscopy) or DNA probes. Because most genital tract infections are asymptomatic and because sensitive type-specific serologic assays have not been available, relatively little is known about the natural history of genital tract HPV infection. On the basis of hybridization assay results, it appears that sexually transmitted HPVs are probably the most common of all sexually transmitted diseases (STDs). Although most genital HPV infections are self-limited, infection with specific types of genital HPVs, most commonly HPV type 16 or 18, is associated with an increased risk of developing genital tract squamous cancers (ie, cervical, vaginal, vulvar, penile, and anal cancers) and intraepithelial cancer precursor lesions. Endocervical adenocarcinomas have also been associated with HPV infection.

HPV Infection and Immunosuppression Before the HIV Epidemic

Before the acquired immunodeficiency syndrome (AIDS) epidemic, it was already well documented that immunosuppressed patients were at increased risk for the benign and malignant manifestations of HPV infection.[2] Patients with epidermodysplasia verruciformis, a rare genetic defect of cell-mediated immunity, were known to be at increased risk for large numbers of warts, many containing HPV types only rarely found in persons with normal immune systems. Unlike warts in individuals with normal immunity, the warts in persons with epidermodysplasia verruciformis frequently developed into squamous cell cancers.[3] Iatrogenic immunosuppression, such as that of transplantation patients, confers an increased risk for genital warts and for HPV-associated neoplasms. The risks of carcinoma in

Nancy B. Kiviat, HPV Research Group, 6 Nickerson Street, Suite 310, Seattle, WA 98109.

situ of the cervix, vulva, and anus are estimated to be from 14-fold to 100-fold higher in renal transplantation patients than in normal women.[3-8]

The HPV types detected in immunosuppressed patients have been found to be similar to those associated with warts in immunocompetent persons, rather than types seen in epidermodysplasia verruciformis. Although at least one investigator found a selective increase of high-risk HPV types among transplantation patients,[9] another investigator reported "nononcogenic" HPV viruses, such as HPV types 6 and 11, associated with cancers in immunosuppressed patients.[8] A few studies suggested that intraepithelial neoplasia develops into cancer at an accelerated rate[10,11] and that the natural history of cancers is altered by immunosuppression.[10] Given such data, it was expected that similar changes would be seen in the natural history of HPV infection among those with HIV-induced immunosuppression.

Viral Acquisition and Transmission

It is unknown whether persons with existing HPV or HIV infection are at increased risk for acquisition of the other virus. Without a well-characterized, type-specific HPV serologic assay, it is impossible to differentiate reactivation of latent HPV virus from the acquisition of new HPV infection. Moreover, HPV infection is exceedingly common, even among low-risk individuals with fewer than five sexual partners in a lifetime. It is likely that most HIV-seropositive adults acquired HPV before acquiring HIV.

It is unknown whether persons who are coinfected with HIV and HPV may be more efficient at transmitting HPV to susceptible sexual partners than are HPV-positive, HIV-seronegative persons. However, compared with HIV-seronegative, HPV-positive persons, those infected with HPV and HIV have higher levels of HPV DNA.[12,13]

HIV-1 Infection and Genital Warts

The incidence of genital warts, which are common among all homosexual men, has significantly increased among HIV-1–infected men.[14-16] Holmberg[17] followed 1073 homosexual and bisexual men and found that the incidence of anal warts among HIV-1 seroconverters was elevated compared with men who remained HIV-1 seronegative (incidence of 5.8 cases per 100 person-years; incident risk ratio [IRR]=2.7). HIV-1–infected women also have increased rates of prevalent[18] and incidental genital warts. Chirgwin[19] reported that the incidence of venereal warts was 8.2 compared with 0.8 per 100 person-years of follow-up for HIV-1–seropositive and HIV-1–seronegative women, respectively.

HIV-1 Infection, HPV DNA, and Immunosuppression

Numerous cross-sectional studies of HIV-seropositive and HIV-seronegative women and homosexual men have corre-lated HIV seropositivity with detection of cervical or anal HPV DNA, as demonstrated by hybridization methods with or without prior amplification of HPV DNA (Tables 14.6-1 and 14.6-2). Studies examining HIV-infected women in the United States,[20-26] Europe,[27,28] East Africa,[29,30] and West Africa[31-33] found genital HPV DNA in 8% to more than 50% of HIV-seronegative women and 37% to 78% HIV-seropositive women; the crude odds ratios (OR) for the association between HIV and detection of HPV DNA ranges from 1.9 to 16.9. My colleagues and I also have seen an association between HIV-2 and detection of cervical HPV DNA in our studies of commercial sex workers, STD patients, and women presenting to the University of Dakar Infectious Disease Services.[32,40]

One of the largest studies of the associations among anal HPV infection, HIV infection, and immunosuppression examined homosexual men presenting to a community-based clinic for HIV testing and counseling (ie, patients were not selected on the basis of signs or symptoms of anal pathology). Anal HPV DNA was detected in 78% of HIV-seronegative men and 92% of HIV-seropositive men. After adjusting for factors known to be associated with the detection of HPV DNA, such as age and sexual activity, HIV-1 seropositivity was associated with genital tract HPV DNA detected by Southern transfer hybridization (STH) or by more sensitive polymerase chain reaction (PCR)–based assays (STH: OR=3.1, 95% confidence interval [CI]=1.6, 5.8; PCR: OR=4.0, 95% CI=2.7, 6.2).[12] In this study, but not all such studies,[34] HIV-seropositive men had higher levels of HPV DNA than HIV-seronegative men. Smaller studies[13,21,26,35–37] have reported that 26% to 60% of HIV-seropositive men and 15% to 29% of HIV-seronegative men have anal HPV DNA.

All types of HPV DNA appear to be found more frequently among HIV-seropositive persons than HIV-seronegative persons.[12,21,27,29,32,38] Detection of multiple types within a single patient has been found to be more common among men and women with HIV infection than among those without HIV infection.[12,21,39] Coll Seck and colleagues[32] reported that, among women in whom cervical HPV DNA was detected, HIV-seropositive women were more likely to harbor high-risk HPV types 16 and 18 than were HIV-seronegative women (OR=9.23, 95% CI=0.97, 433.3).

Increasing HIV-induced immunosuppression, as measured by CD4 counts, correlates with increased likelihood of detecting of HPV DNA in men and women.[12,21,23,32,39–41] Among all men presenting for HIV testing and counseling, HIV-1–infected men, even those with CD4 counts above 800/μL, were at increased risk for having HPV DNA compared with HIV-1–seronegative men. Among HIV-1–infected men, the likelihood of detection of HPV DNA by STH methods increased with increasing immunosuppression (compared with those with CD4 counts of >800 × 10/μL, chi square for test of trend=7.24, P=0.007). Palefsky[21] also found low CD4 counts (200/mμL) to be a risk factor for detection of anal HPV DNA. A similar association

TABLE 14.6-1. *Detection of cervical HPV DNA in women with HIV-1 or HIV-2 infection*

Investigation and HIV type	Study population	HIV+ subjects HPV+/total %	HIV– HPV+/total (%)	HPV assays*	Odds ratio	95% Confidence interval
ter Meulen, 1992 HIV-1	Gyn service, Tanzania	22/32 (69%)	131/269 (49%)	PCR	2.3	1.0, 5.5
N. Kiviat (unpublished data) HIV-1 and/or HIV-2	Prostitutes, Senegal	75/133 (56%)	237/603 (39%)	PCR	2.0	1.3, 3.0
Coll-Seck, 1993 HIV-1 and/or HIV-2	ID service, Senegal	23/31 (74%)	11/53 (21%)	PCR	11.0	3.5, 36
Johnson, 1992 HIV-1	HIV outpatients, USA	13/32 (41%)	ND[†]	DBH/PCR	NA[†]	NA
Laga, 1992 HIV-1	Prostitutes, Zaire	18/47 (38%)	4/48 (8%)	DBH/STH	6.8	1.9, 30.0
Kreiss, 1992 HIV-1	Prostitutes, Kenya	54/147 (37%)	12/51 (24%)	DBH/STH	1.9	0.9, 4.3
Vermund, 1991 HIV-1	IVDU[‡] & partners, USA	27/51 (53%)	10/45 (22%)	STH	3.9	1.5, 10.8
Feingold, 1990 HIV-1	IVDU & partners, USA	17/35 (49%)	8/32 (25%)	STH	2.8	0.9, 9.3
St. Louis, 1993 HIV-1	General population, Zaire	20/52 (38%)	1/28 (4%)	DBH/STH	15.9	3.2, 88
Spinillo, 1992 HIV-1	ID clinic, Italy	13/25 (52%)	ND[†]	ISH	NA[†]	NA[‡]
Sun, 1995 HIV-1	HIV clinics, USA	206/344 (60%)	117/325 (36%)	PCR		
Van Doornum, 1993 HIV-1	IVDU/prostitutes, USA	8/25 (32%)	3/44 (7%)	PCR	7.8	1.8, 34.6
Williams, 1994 HIV-1	IVDU, USA	37/53 (70%)	7/55 (13%)	PCR	8.9	32-27

*STH, Southern transfer hybridization; ISII, in situ hybridization; DBH, dot blot hybridization; PCR, polymerase chain reaction.
[†]ND, not done; NA, not applicable.
[‡]IVDU, intravenous drug user.

between detection of anal HPV DNA and immunosuppression was observed by Breese[35] and by Melbye and associates[37] among homosexual men. However, Williams and coworkers[26] found no association between detection of cervical or anal HPV DNA and CD4 counts in 55 HIV-1–seropositive and 59 HIV-1–seronegative women. Smith[41] examined 50 HIV-seropositive and 43-HIV seronegative women and failed to find associations among HIV, detection of HPV, and CD4 counts. This study also failed to find an association between HPV and cervical intraepithelial neoplasia (CIN), which has been universally found by other investigators.

HIV-1 Infection and HPV-Related Neoplasia

Cross-sectional and cohort studies have shown that HIV-infected persons are at increased risk for HPV-related neoplasia. Melbye[36] found that the relative risk (RR) of invasive anal cancer among homosexual men, compared with the general population, was 13.9 (95% CI=6.6, 29.2) for up to 5 years before a diagnosis of AIDS. This relative risk increased to more than 84 (95% CI=46.4, 152) after a diagnosis of AIDS.[36] Support for an association between HIV

and invasive cervical cancer is limited to case reports and small case series.[40,42–45] A comparison of the actual number of cases of cervical cancer in those with HIV with the expected number of cases of cervical cancer in the United States in the general population failed to show a significant increase in invasive cervical cancer among HIV-seropositive women.[46] Neither has an increase in invasive cervical cancer been documented among women in developing countries where HIV has been present for longer periods.[29] Despite these findings, cervical cancer is considered an AIDS-defining illness in women.

It is not surprising that an association between HIV and cervical cancer has not been detected in industrialized countries. HIV infection has been introduced into the population relatively recently. Most women in such countries have access to routine screening and treatment. In developing countries, where large numbers of women have been infected with HIV since the onset of the epidemic, neither routine screening or treatment for cervical cancer precursor lesions nor tumor registries are widely available. In such settings, it is possible that women are dying of HIV-associated disease before the development of cancer or without the detection of cervical cancer.

TABLE 14.6-2. *Prevalence of anal HPV DNA among homosexual men with or without HIV infection*

Investigation	Study population	HIV+ subjects HPV+/total (%)	HIV− subjects HPV+/total (%)	HPV assays*	Odds ratio	95% Confidence interval
Kiviat, 1993	HIV screening clinic	221/241 (92)%	119/152 (78%)	PCR	3.1	1.6, 5.8
		156/285 (55%)	47/204 (23%)	STH	4.0	2.7, 6.2
Caussy, 1990	Patients of 1 of 3 primary care providers, USA	23/43 (54%)	18/62 (29%)	DBH/PCR	2.8	1.2, 6.9
Critchlow, 1992	HIV serology screening clinic	8/26 (31%)	10/119 (8%)	DBH/STH	4.4	1.4, 13
Kiviat, 1990	STD clinic, GI‡ symptoms, USA	13/49 (26%)	3/47 (6%)	DBH/STH	5.3	1.3, 31
Melbye, 1990	Danish cohort	11/18 (61%)	22/102 (22%)	DBH	5.7	1.8, 19
Palefsky, 1990 [147]	Group IV HIV disease, San Francisco	52/97 (54%)	ND†	DBH	NA†	NA†
Breese	Denver, USA	57/93 (61%)	20/116 (17%)	DBH	7.6	3.85, 15.18
Palefsky, 1994	San Francisco General Hospital Cohort Study	10/28 (36%)	19/37 (51%)	DBH	1.9	0.62, 5.91

*STH, Southern transfer hybridization; DBH, dot blot hybridization; PCR, polymerase chain reaction.
†ND, not done; NA, not applicable.
‡GI, gastrointestinal.

Studies in the United States, Europe, and West and East Africa (Table 14.6-3) have shown HIV-1–infected women to be at increased risk for cytologically proven squamous intraepithelial lesions (SIL), a cancer precursor lesion. Between 2% and 19% of women without HIV and 5% to 63% of women with HIV infection have changes consistent with SIL (OR=1.0 to 10). Similar findings have been reported for patients with HIV-1 and biopsy-confirmed CIN.[39,47] Associations among HIV-2 infection, HPV infection, and SIL have been observed for Senegalese prostitutes and women presenting to the Infectious Disease Out Patient Clinic (Coll Seck A, Kiviat NB: unpublished data). Although early studies suggested that the sensitivity of cytologic analysis was low for HIV-infected women for the detection of cancer,[48] other studies found the sensitivity of cytology for the detection of CIN to be similar for those with and without HIV.[49]

Anal intraepithelial lesions (AIN) are increased among those with HIV infection. In one of the larger studies addressing this issue, men who were not selected or referred on the basis of anal rectal signs or symptoms were found to have high rates of anal dysplasia. Twenty-six percent of HIV-1–seropositive men and 8% of HIV-1–seronegative men had anal SIL (ASIL) detected by cytologic smears,[12] and high-grade lesions were associated with HIV-seropositive status. High rates of dysplasia among homosexual men have also been reported.[37,50,51] Palefsky and associates[21] found cytologic abnormalities in 39% of ASIL cases and in 15% of 97 men with group IV HIV infection.

High-grade lesions are associated with high-risk types of HPV.[12,13] Wright and colleagues[39] found a high rate of HPV type 18 infection, an HPV type usually associated with high-grade lesions in HIV-seronegative women, to be present in 47% of low-grade CIN (CIN 1) lesions in HIV-infected women. A cohort study by Critchlow and colleagues[13] examining the associations among HIV infection, specific types of HPV, and the development of high-grade ASIL found HPV types 16 and 18 were associated with the risk of developing AIN 2 or 3 in HIV-seropositive and HIV-seronegative men but that HPV types other than 16 and 18 were associated with development of high-grade ASIL only in HIV-seropositive men.

Among HIV-infected persons, cytologically documented SIL and histologically proven intraepithelial neoplasia have been associated with various degrees of immunosuppression. Among HIV-infected women, CIN has been associated with decreased CD4 counts or advanced clinical disease.[20,24,52] Schafer[40] found a significant correlation between blastogenic responses of peripheral blood leukocytes to various mitogens (eg, pokeweed, phytohemagglutinin, tetanus toxin) and the presence of CIN. Kiviat and colleagues[12] reported that the prevalence of ASIL among HIV-seropositive men increased from 8% to 36% with decreasing CD4 counts (chi test for trend=13.5, $P<0.001$).

Few longitudinal studies have addressed the natural history of SIL or HPV infection or the risk conferred by HIV infection for development of CIN or AIN 2 or 3. Heard and coworkers[53] monitored HIV-infected women for SIL by cytologic examination every 6 months for 18 months and found a 95% (18 of 19) rate of persistent disease in those who presented with SIL and who were not treated and a 61% (8 of 13) rate of recurrent disease among those treated. Petry and colleagues[11] examined the natural history of low-grade lesions in persons with immunosuppression (ie, 48 HIV-infected women and 52 female renal allograft recipients) along with matched immunocompetent controls. Low-grade lesions in those with abnormal immune systems progressed

TABLE 14.6-3. *Prevalence of cervical intraepithelial neoplasia or squamous intraepithelial neoplasia in women with or without HIV-1 or HIV-2*

Investigation	Study population	HIV infected CIN/total (%)	HIV uninfected CIN/total (%)	Odds ratio	95% Confidence interval
Feingold, 1990	IVDU, USA	11/35 (31%)	1/23 (4%)	10.1	1.2, 453
Vermund, 1991	IVDU, USA	14/35 (40%)	3/32 (9%)	6.4	1.5, 38.3
Rellihan, 1990		46/111 (41%)	7/76 (9%)	7.0	2.8, 19.5
Lags, 1992	Prostitutes, Zaire	2/10 (20%)	2/10 (20%)	1.0	0.06, 17.1
Smith, 1993	Hospital/outpatients, London	11/42 (26%)	5/21 (24%)	1.1	0.3, 4.9
Kreiss, 1992	Prostitutes, Kenya	11/41 (27%)	1/41 (3%)	14.7	1.8, 647
Williams, 1994*	IVDU, USA	18/88*	2/98*	12.3	2.78, 111.83
Langley, 1995	Prostitutes, Senegal	15/43 (35%)	15/43 (19%)	2.3	0.8, 7.1
Wright	Outpatients, New York, New Jersey	80/398 (20%)	15/357 (4%)	5.7	3.19, 10.93
Coll-Seck, 1993 HIV-1	Infectious disease service, Senegal	6/14 (43%)	3/50 (6%)	23.3	2.9, 209
HIV-2		4/15 (33%)	3/50 (6%)	9.3	1.1, 79

*CIN plus atypical squamous cells of undetermined significance (ASCUS).

more often than lesions in controls, and an increased rate of recurrent lesions after destructive treatment was associated with immune system dysfunction. All patients with CD4 counts less than 400/μL or immunosuppression for more than 3 years had progressive lesions.

In our studies of homosexual men with and without HIV infection, my colleagues and I found that HIV-seronegative men were more likely to regress to a negative status (defined as two consecutive negative cytologic smear results during follow-up) from a low-grade ASIL status (defined as two consecutive low-grade anal cytologic smear results) than were HIV-seropositive men. The disease of 6 (40%) of 15 HIV-seronegative men resolved, compared with resolution for 4 (11%) of 37 HIV-seropositive men (RR=2.0, 95%=1.1, 3.4; Hawes SE, Kiviat NB: unpublished data). Vernon and colleagues[54] tested 124 HIV-seronegative and 126 HIV-seropositive women over 8 months for HPV DNA by vaginal wash methods. She and her group found that 26.9% of HIV-seropositive and 2% of HIV-seronegative women were positive for HPV DNA on entry into the study. Cumulative detection of HPV DNA differed by HIV serostatus: 42.8% of those with and 13.4% of those HIV infection (*P*<0.001).[54]

Published longitudinal studies of SIL and HIV infection include that by Palefsky and coworkers[21], who examined development of high-grade ASIL among 37 HIV-seropositive men with Centers for Disease Control (CDC) group IV disease followed for 17 months. Ten of the men had abnormal cytologic results at study entry; the disease of five regressed, four progressed, and one persisted. Virtually all men who were cytologically negative but in whom anal HPV DNA was detected developed AIN. Although development of anal neoplasia was not associated with immunosuppression, addressing this issue within this population was difficult because of the narrow range of CD4 counts among the men studied; only four men had entry CD4 counts above 500/μL at study entry.

A prospective cohort study by Critchlow and coworkers[13] defined the risk of developing high-grade ASIL in relation to HIV infection after controlling for the effects of HPV infection. High-grade ASIL developed in 8 of 147 HIV-seronegative men and 24 of 158 HIV-seropositive men, all of whom initially had negative anal cytologic and colposcopic findings. Among HIV-seronegative men, the risk of high-grade ASIL was associated with the detection of anal HPV types 16 or 18 by the STH method (RR=16.5, 95% CI=1.4, 190) and with detection of HPV types 16 or 18 at lower levels by PCR methods (RR=7.1, 95% CI=0.6, 80). Among HIV-seropositive men, the risk of high-grade ASIL was associated with finding HPV types 16 or 18 only at the higher levels detectable by STH (RR=3.0, 95% CI=1.0, 9.1) and with finding HPV types other than 16 or 18 (RR=2.2, 95% CI=0.9, 58). After adjusting for detection of HPV, HIV-seropositive men with CD4 counts below 500/μL were 7.5 times (95% CI=2.2, 25.2) more likely and HIV-seropositive men with CD4 counts greater than 500/μL were 1.4 times (95% CI=0.4, 5.1) more likely to develop high-grade ASIL than HIV-seronegative men. HIV infection remained an independent predictor of high-grade ASIL after taking into account the number of tests positive for HPV DNA. The association of high-grade ASIL with HIV independent of HPV type, level of HPV detection, and number of tests positive for HPV suggested that HIV might be acting directly on HPV to effect an increase in the risk of ASIL.

HIV-Induced Alterations in Response to Treatment

The responses of HIV-infected women to traditional treatments for cervical neoplasia are not well characterized, and little is known about the response of HIV-infected individuals to treatment of anal neoplasia. Spinillo and collaborators[27] examined 18 HIV-infected women, including 10 with CIN 1 treated with electrocautery and 8 with CIN 2 or 3 treated with electrocautery or cold knife cone. Only one of the women treated for CIN 2 or 3 developed recurrent disease.[27] In contrast, high recurrence rates after using cryosurgery have been reported by McGuiness and LaGuardia,[55] who found a 78% recurrence rate among 18 HIV-infected women, and by Adachi and colleagues,[56] who found a 50% recurrence rate among five HIV-infected women treated with cryosurgery.

Maiman and colleagues[48] described treatment by cryotherapy, laser, or cone biopsy of 44 HIV-infected women and 125 HIV-seronegative women with CIN. Thirty-nine percent of the HIV-infected women, compared with 9% of the HIV-seronegative women, developed biopsy-proven recurrent CIN ($P<0.01$). Recurrence was associated with mean CD4 counts of 239 cells/μL for those with HIV and 367 cells/μL for those without HIV.[48] Wright[20] found that 56% of HIV-seropositive and 13% of HIV-seronegative women treated for CIN by loop electrosurgical excision had recurrent disease. The outcome was associated with the level of immune system function (as measured by CD4 counts), with 61% of those with CD4 counts less than 500 cells/μL and 20% of those with CD4 counts greater than 500 cells/μL developing recurrent disease.[20]

Mechanisms of Interactions Between HIV and HPV

Alterations in the natural history of HPV infection and of HPV-related neoplasia among HIV-seropositive individuals are probably the result of general or local HIV-induced immune system dysfunction. It is possible, for example, that control of HPV is impaired when large numbers of lymphocytes or Langerhans' cells in the area are infected with HIV. Some small studies found that, among HIV-seronegative women, those with SIL had fewer Langerhans' cells than those without SIL[57–59] and that HIV-seropositive women with cervical SIL had even fewer Langerhans' cells than HIV-seronegative women with SIL. It is also possible that HIV acts directly on HPV. In vitro studies have shown that intracellular HIV-1 Tat mRNA can transactivate HPV type 16 E6 and E7, an action that is important in the development of squamous cell cancers. In vitro studies have also shown that extracellular HIV-1 Tat protein can enter HPV-infected cells and upregulate HPV type 16 E6 and E7.[60,61] The HIV-1 Tat protein enhances E2-dependent HPV type 16 transcription. It is possible that extracellular Tat migrates from Langerhans' cells or other HIV-infected mononuclear cells that abut HPV-infected epithelial cells and upregulates HPV. However, although several in vitro studies suggested that HIV could enter and establish infection in epithelial cells, this remains controversial.[58,60,61]

INTERACTIONS BETWEEN HIV AND THE HEPATITIS VIRUSES

Virus Transmission and At-Risk Populations

HIV replicates in CD4 cells, macrophages, microglial cells of the central nervous system, and gut epithelial cells. Replication of HBV and HCV occurs primarily in hepatocytes and, to a small extent, in lymphocytes.[62–64] However, all three viruses are present and available for transmission in blood and in genital tract secretions. All can be parenterally or sexually transmitted, although sexual transmission is markedly inefficient for HCV.[37,65] HBV and HIV are also spread to offspring by exposure of infants to infected maternal fluids (ie, blood, vaginal secretions, and in the case of HIV, breast milk) or by in utero passage of virus across the placenta to the fetus. Because these viruses are transmitted in similar fashions,[66] it is not surprising that most HIV-seropositive persons are also infected with HBV or HCV.

Several other aspects of the epidemiology of HIV, HCV, and HBV increase the likelihood of coinfection. In the Eastern hemisphere and in many parts of Africa, exposure to HBV at or near birth is virtually universal, and the prevalence of HBV serum markers is high in the general adult population. In the Western hemisphere, HBV is primarily sexually or parenterally transmitted and is relatively uncommon among the general population. The highest prevalence of HBV occurs among those engaging in high-risk sexual behavior (eg, frequent partner change, anal intercourse) or intravenous drug abuse or among those requiring frequent exposure to blood or blood products. Before the HIV epidemic, 50% to 70% of homosexual men, most hemophiliacs,[67–69] and many intravenous drug users (IDUs) in the United States and Europe already had evidence of HBV infection[70–72] by the late 1970s.[73] HCV infection also affected most hemophiliacs who received clotting factor concentrates before 1984, at which time viral inactivation standards were put in place.[74–78] Seventy-nine percent of HIV-seronegative hemophiliacs seen at nine U.S. regional treatment centers between 1987 and 1988 were HCV seropositive.[79] Similar trends were noticed among intravenous drug abusers; 40% to 75% were HCV seropositive, compared with a prevalence of 1% to 2% in the general population.[80,81,82] Because HCV does not seem to be efficiently sexually transmitted, it is much less prevalent among homosexual men who are not intravenous drug abusers; HCV infects fewer than 10% of such populations.[37,65]

The same populations that had already become widely infected with HBV and HCV before the appearance of HIV were those at highest risk for the acquisition of HIV infection. Strong associations between infection with HIV and infection with HBV, HCV, or both were reported early in the HIV epidemic. Rustgi[83] and others[79] reported that almost 90% of HIV-seropositive men had evidence of HBV infection. Flo and colleagues[84] observed that 42% of HIV-seropositive men from western Norway were HBV seropositive, compared with 3% of the general populations of Oslo and Sweden. Troisi and colleagues[79] reported that 53% of 382 hemophilia A and B patients tested between 1987 and 1988 were HIV seropositive, with 75% of 382 HIV-seropositive hemophiliacs having serologic evidence of HBV infection. A similarly high rate of HBV infection has been found among HIV-seropositive patients in countries where HBV is primarily acquired early in life. Because of the high prevalence of serum markers for HBV in the general population in such areas, it is not surprising that a statistical association between infection with HBV and HIV was not always detected.

Kashala and colleagues[85] undertook a study of several different groups in Zaire, including 500 healthy pregnant women, 145 persons recruited from a major medical care clinic in Lubumbashi, and 100 patients with hepatocellular carcinoma and controls. Between 77.7% and 97.9% of patients had serum markers for HBV. Overall, there was no significant difference between HIV-positive and HIV-negative serostatus, which was in part a reflection of the high prevalence of HBV in all persons in this study.[75,76,85]

Detection of HCV is frequently associated with detection of antibody to HIV and to HBV. Makris and associates[75] reported that HCV was detected in 75% or those with and 46% of those without antibodies to HIV and in 88% of those with and 39% of those without antibodies to HBV. Worldwide coinfection with HIV is exceedingly common among persons with hepatitis virus infection.

Acquisition and Course of HIV in HBV-Infected Persons

Acquisition of HIV and Preexisting HBV Infection

A number of studies have addressed the question of whether preexisting HBV infection increases the risk of subsequent acquisition of HIV. Solomon[86] analyzed the relation between the risk of HIV-1 seroconversion and the baseline HBV serostatus of 2421 men enrolled in the Multicenter AIDS Cohort Study (MACS) who were unvaccinated for HBV and HIV-1 seronegative at study entry. The presence of hepatitis antibodies (ie, HBsAb or HBcAb) at entry was only weakly associated with HIV-1 acquisition during the 6 and 24 months of follow-up (for HBsAg with or without HBcAb at 6 months, OR=2.2, 95% CI=0.8, 6.5; at 24 months, OR=1.3, 95% CI=0.7, 2.7).

Because differences in sexual behavior could have resulted in biased conclusions, Twu and colleagues[87] reexamined the issue after adjusting for changes in sexual behavior and reported STDs (but not HBV status) at each visit. Logistic regression analysis, adjusting for possible confounders of sexual behavior such as incident syphilis and gonorrhea, changes in the number of partners, and frequency of anogenital intercourse over time, demonstrated a positive association between HBV and incident HIV infection, although it is difficult to know if this association resulted from residual confounding by sexual behavior. Another possible explanation of such findings is that chronic HBV infection is characterized by high numbers of activated lymphocytes, which are thought to be particularly susceptible to HIV infection. This remains only a theoretical possibility. However, van Ameijden and associates[88] examined the prevalence and transmission of HIV and HBV in IDUs in Amsterdam but did not find HIV seroconversion to be significantly related to HBV serostatus.

Progression of HIV and Coinfection With HBV

Solomon and coworkers[86] examined the question of whether HBV infection altered the rate of development of AIDS and specifically the decline of CD4 and CD8 counts. Prospective data from unvaccinated HIV-infected men with and without HBsAg or HBcAb were assessed for CD4 counts at 6 months (n=1348), 18 months (n=1131), and 30 months (n=929). After controlling for CD4 counts at study entry, those who were seropositive for HBV on enrollment were not found to be at increased risk for more rapid development of AIDS or a more rapid decline in CD4 counts than were those who were HBV seronegative on entry. Scharschmidt and colleagues[90] reported similar findings for 35 HIV-seropositive, HBsAg-positive persons and 70 HIV-matched controls who were followed for a mean of 18 months (relative hazard attributable to HBsAg stratified for a diagnosis of AIDS=1.2, 95% CI=0.7, 2.0).

Eskild and associates[91] analyzed data on 80 HIV-seropositive men who were followed for a mean of 62 months. When evaluating the risk for progression of HIV in relation to HBV infection, the investigators controlled for age, year of first positive HIV test, and other behavior variables, but they did not control for CD4 counts on entry. Compared with the men without HBV, those coinfected with HIV and HBV appeared to be at increased risk of progression to AIDS (RR=3.6, 95% CI=1.3, 10.1).[91] Such data are difficult to interpret because of the failure to adjust for entry-level CD4 counts.

HBV infection was also identified as a risk factor for progression to AIDS by Greenspan and colleagues[92] in a case-control study examining risk factors for progression to AIDS among homosexual men presenting with hairy leukoplakia. Twenty-seven men who did not progress to AIDS within 1000 days of the diagnosis of hairy leukoplakia were compared with 28 who did progress within this time. Those with a history of HBV were at a fourfold higher risk (95% CI=1.4, 14.3) for progression than those without such a history.[92] Although a few studies (some with significant problems in study design) have reported an association between HBV infection and the risk of HIV-1 seroconversion or progression to AIDS, solid support for this hypothesis has not yet appeared.

Acquisition and Course of HBV Infection in HIV-Infected Persons

Acquisition of HBV and Preexisting HIV Infection

Results of a few studies have suggested that HIV-infected individuals are at increased risk for acquisition of HBV compared with those without HIV infection. In one of the largest studies, Kingsley and colleagues[93] examined sexual transmission of HBV and HIV among a subset of 1062 homosexual men enrolled in MACS and found prior infection with HIV-1 to be an independent risk factor for subsequent acquisition of HBV infection (OR=3.4). Although these findings could be the result of increased host susceptibility to HBV infection because of

HIV-induced immune system dysfunction, it is also possible that such findings reflect confounding by sexual behavior. HIV-infected individuals may be more likely to engage in high-risk behavior, such as sex with high-risk partners who have a high likelihood of being HBV and perhaps HIV seropositive. If it is true that HIV-seropositive individuals are more likely to have partners who are HIV and HBV seropositive, the increased risk for acquisition of HBV may result from exposure to extremely high levels of HBV, which are characteristic of HIV-seropositive individuals infected with HBV. In contrast, van Ameijden and colleagues[88] studied IDUs in Amsterdam and reported that the presence of HIV infection was not correlated with an increased risk for acquisition of HBV.

Progression of HBV and Coinfection With HIV

Most investigators have reported that the manifestations and course of acute HBV infection, the development and course of chronic HBV infection, and the frequency of reactivation of HBV are altered by coinfection with HIV. The frequency and type of changes seen in the course of HBV infection among HIV-seropositive persons appear to vary with the order and age at which HBV and HIV are acquired. For this reason, prospective cohort studies in well-characterized populations are of particular importance in understanding HBV infection in HIV-seropositive persons.

Acute HBV Infection With Coexisting HIV Infection

Hadler and coworkers[94] studied the effect of HIV-1 infection on subsequently acquired HBV infection among homosexual or bisexual men enrolled in a large CDC multicenter study of HBV vaccine. Peak alanine aminotransferase (ALT) levels during acute HBV infection did not differ between HIV-seropositive and HIV-seronegative groups. However, HIV-infected men who acquired HBV had elevated ALT levels (>200 IU) for a mean of 22.1 days, compared with 15.8 days for HIV-negative men. Compared with HIV-seronegative men, HIV-infected men tended to develop more severe clinical illness but without jaundice, although this factor was not statistically significant. Overall, approximately 20% of HIV-seropositive and HIV-seronegative men became jaundiced. Similar findings regarding enzyme levels were reported in a prospective study by Taylor[95] and a study by Bodsworth.[96] However, acute HBV infection in HIV-infected men is generally anicteric, similar to what has been described in HIV-seronegative individuals with immunologic dysfunction.[71,97,98]

Chronic HBV Infection With Coexisting HIV Infection

Several studies have shown that HIV-infected persons who acquire HBV are at increased risk for chronic HBV infection.[94–96,99] Hadler[94] found that 21.4% of HIV-seropositive men who acquired HBV became carriers, compared with 7% of HIV-seronegative men (P=0.097). Similar findings were reported by Taylor and colleagues[95] for unvaccinated men. Bodsworth[96] reported that 7 (23%) of 31 of HIV-seropositive, compared with 2 (4%) of 46 of HIV-seronegative men, with a documented seroconversion to anti-hepatitis B core antibody developed chronic HBV infection. Still higher rates of chronic HBV occurred among those who had acquired HBV and HIV during the same interval. Several investigators reported that the development of chronic HBV infection was also influenced by the degree of immunosuppression in HIV-infected men.[85,94,96]

The course of chronic HBV infection appears to be altered by coexisting HIV infection. Liver function profiles of chronic carriers of HBV are less abnormal when they are coinfected with HIV, perhaps reflecting less severe hepatitic inflammation.[94,100,101] Increased serum levels of HBV DNA, increased HBV DNA polymerase levels, and lower HBV DNA clearance rates are characteristic of chronic HBV carriage among those with HIV infection.[100,102–105] Bodsworth[99] examined 82 HIV-seropositive and 68 HIV-seronegative men with chronic HBV infection from a group known to be free of hepatitis D and A viruses and not on zidovudine or corticosteroid therapy. Compared with those without HIV, HIV-seropositive men were more likely to have HBeAg and HBV DNA (P<0.001 and P<0.0005, respectively). Overall, the presence of HBeAg was not related to levels of CD4 or CD8 cells or to CDC class, and associations remained after IDUs and those with possible recent acute hepatitis were removed from the analyses. Among the subset of HIV-seropositive, HBeAg-positive persons, lower CD4 counts were correlated with lower ALT levels. These observations provide some support for the hypothesis that HIV-induced immunosuppression leads to increased HBV replication and decreased hepatic inflammation.

However, not all investigators have found that chronic HBV infection among HIV-seropositive men is characterized by increased HBV replication[106] and decreased levels of liver enzymes.[105,107] Monno and colleagues[108] studied 48 HIV-seropositive and 22 HIV-seronegative HBsAg chronic carriers who were IDUs and found that HBV DNA was detected more frequently in HIV-seronegative than HIV-seropositive men (50% versus 35%). There was no difference between HIV-seropositive and HIV-seronegative men with regard to severity of liver damage, as assessed by biopsy or HBV seroconversion from ongoing to inactive infection. Viral replication was not related to CD4 cell counts. Similar results were reported by Govindarajan and colleagues[109] for patients who acquired HIV parenterally.

Not all studies have reported positive associations for immunosuppression, hepatic inflammation, and HBV replication among those coinfected with HIV and HBV. Rector and colleagues[101] examined the relation between cellular immune function (as measured by skin test reactivity; lymphocyte transformation responses to mitogens, *Candida*, and tetanus antigens; and CD4 counts) and hepatic inflammation (as measured by serum aspartate transaminase [AST] concentration) or HBV replication (as measured by serum HBV DNA concentration) among 20 HIV-seropositive chronic HBV carriers. No associations were found among cellular immune function, serum AST concentration, and HBV replication. Such results could reflect different behavioral characteristics of the study populations, fashion of acquisition of HIV, or the order of acquisition of HIV and HBV. In Monno's[108] study, HIV was acquired after HBV. It is also possible that many of these manifestations of HBV change over time, a factor that could not be accurately taken into account in comparing study results.

The histopathology of HBV in HIV-seropositive and HIV-seronegative persons has been described by McDonald[110] and Goldin.[111] Using immunofluorescent staining of liver biopsies with monoclonal antibodies to HbeAg and HBcAg, McDonald[110] showed that, compared with HIV-seronegative chronic HBV carriers, HIV-seropositive chronic HBV carriers had significantly more hepatocyte nuclear staining ($P<0.0003$ for HBeAg and $P=0.02$ for HBcAg). Goldin[111] reported that HIV-seronegative men had more scarring and active liver disease than HIV-infected men.

Most studies suggest that HIV-seropositive men with chronic HBV infection, especially those with marked immunosuppression, are more likely to have HBV replication, serum HBV DNA, and DNA polymerase than HIV-seronegative HBV carriers. Positive HIV serostatus among HBV carriers is associated with decreased hepatic inflammation, as reflected by decreased ALT levels and less severe disease seen on biopsy. Whether or how all these findings may be influenced by time since acute HBV infection and by the presence of other hepatitis viruses is unclear.

Reactivation of HBV in HIV-Infected Persons

Although few large studies have focused on the reactivation of HBV in HIV-infected persons, some small reports suggest that HIV-seropositive men may be more likely to lose HBsAb than those without HIV infection.[112] Asymptomatic reactivation or reinfection with HBV appears to be relatively common among HIV-infected persons, especially if they have marked immunosuppression. Symptomatic reactivation of HBV infection in HIV-seropositive men is a relatively rare occurrence. Homann and colleagues[113]followed 138 HIV-seropositive men with AIDS, AIDS-related complex, or CD4 counts less than 200/µL who were initially positive for HBsAb at study entry for a median of 18 months; 10 became HBsAb negative or had elevations in transaminase levels without symptoms.

Response of HIV-Seropositive Persons to HBV Vaccine

There is general agreement that the response of HIV-infected persons to vaccination against HBV is impaired. Collier and associates[114] found vaccination with three doses of 20 µg of plasma-derived HBV vaccine (repeated after 1 and 6 moths) to result in low or no responses in 7 of 16 HIV-seropositive men, compared with 6 of 68 HIV-seronegative

men ($P=0.002$). Loke and colleagues[115] reported that, among 27 HIV-seropositive and 77 HIV-seronegative patients given three doses of recombinant DNA vaccine, 9 (33%) of the HIV-seropositive and 69 (89.6%) of the HIV-seronegative patients had a detectable antibody response 2 months after the last dose ($P<0.001$). A lack of response appeared to be associated with immunosuppression.

Rutstein[116] examined antibody response to hepatitis B immunization according to the CDC control and prevention recommended schedule in HIV-infected and uninfected infants. After the three recommended doses, 22 (92%) of 24 HIV-exposed but uninfected infants demonstrated an antibody response, compared with 6 (35%) of 17 HIV-infected infants ($P<0.0005$). No significant difference was observed between the HIV-seropositive responders and nonresponders, although CD4 counts were different for HIV-seropositive and HIV-seronegative infants. Similar data were reported by Choudhury and Peters,[117] who followed 24 HIV-infected children; 25% developed protective antibody titers, but 18 (75%) had undetectable antibodies 2 to 4 months after the third dose of HBV vaccine.[118] Sixteen of the 18 children who failed to respond to the standard CDC protocol for immunization against HBV received one or two booster doses at twice the standard dose at a mean of 5 months after the third vaccine dose. Follow-up serologic testing was performed within 14 months of the third vaccination dose and within 11 months of the initial postimmunization. Only 2 (14%) of the children developed protective antibody levels. HBsAg was not detected in any of the children.[117]

Mechanisms of Interactions Between HIV And HBV

HBV Influence on HIV Replication

In vitro studies[119] have shown that the HBV-encoded "protein X" interacts with NF-κB or κB-like cellular transcriptional factors produced in B lymphocytes to form complexes that are capable of binding at the long terminal repeats of HIV-1 and HIV-2, the regions associated with upregulation of HIV replication.[120,121] The implications of such in vitro observations are unclear, although the findings may be important, because HBV and HIV can infect lymphocytes.[62,63] If the two viruses were routinely found within the same lymphocytes, HBV might indirectly increase HIV replication through the action of an HBV pol-encoded protein that is able to decrease production of interferon and interfere with the cellular response to interferon, allowing increased replication of HIV.[122]

Compared with those without chronic HBV, patients with chronic hepatitis B have elevated levels of tumor necrosis factor-α.[123] Tumor necrosis factor-α is able to upregulate HIV in cell culture[124] and to induce NF-κB. HBV infection may also indirectly upregulate HIV through the cytokine pathway, although there are no in vivo or in vitro data supporting this theory.[125]

HIV Influence on HBV Replication

Active HIV gene expression can alter the natural history of HBV in several ways. The outcome of HBV infection is tightly linked to cell-mediated immunity through direct destruction of HBV-infected hepatocytes. Cytotoxic T-cell activity directed against the e and core antigens of HBV-infected hepatocytes plays a central role in the resolution of HBV infection[66,126] and in the development of hepatic HBV-related pathology. It appears that HIV-seropositive persons are more likely to be chronic carriers of HBV, just as organ transplantation or cancer patients who receive immunosuppressive therapy are less able to resolve HBV infection. One of the most important effects of HIV infection is a decrease in the competence of cell-mediated immunity, and it is likely that the immunosuppression is the basis of the observed inability to resolve HBV infection.

Mechanisms of Interactions Between HIV and HCV

HIV Influence on HCV Acquisition and Transmission

Studies done during the last 5 years suggest that HIV infection may alter several important aspects of HCV infection. Sexual transmission of HCV to susceptible individuals appears to be altered by the coexistence of HIV in the index case. Among those who have acquired HCV parenterally, the risk of developing severe liver disease appears to be increased if they are coinfected with HIV.

Even after controlling for intravenous drug abuse, HCV is more common in those with than those without HIV infection.[127] On the basis of such findings, several studies have asked whether persons coinfected with HIV and HCV might more effectively sexually transmit HCV to susceptible sexual partners.[128–130] Soto and associates[128] examined sexual transmission of HCV from 423 HCV-seropositive IDUs to their stable (not intravenous drug abusing) sexual partners and found transmission of HCV to stable sexual partners was three times more frequent among 120 IDUs who were HIV seropositive than it was among 22 IDUs (matched for age and mean time of sexual activity) who were HIV seronegative (24.2% versus 9.2%). Results, however, were not significant for this relatively small sample. Eyster[130] reported similar results. Examining 234 female partners of 231 hemophiliac men, she found that men who were dually infected with HIV and HCV were more likely to transmit HCV to susceptible partners than were the index cases who were infected with HCV alone; 5 (3%) of 164 women whose male partners were HIV and HCV seropositive became seropositive, compared with none of 30 women whose male partner was HIV-negative but HCV positive. Because HIV appears to increase the level of HCV RNA, HIV infection may also increase the likelihood of parental transmission of HCV to susceptible persons.

HIV Influence on the Natural History of HCV

Several studies have examined the associations among HCV RNA levels, HIV infection, immunosuppression, and severe liver disease. Most studies suggest that HIV-infected persons have an impaired response to HCV and that HCV RNA levels are higher in those coinfected with HIV. The data are conflicting regarding the relation of such changes to hepatic pathology, CD4 counts, and abnormalities of hepatic enzymes. These differences may reflect longer periods of exposure, different sequences of exposure, and different modes of acquisition of HCV and HIV.

Several groups have shown that, compared with hemophiliacs infected with HIV or HCV alone, those who are infected with both viruses are at increased risk for developing severe hepatic pathology. Eyster[130,131] examined a cohort of 223 HCV-seropositive hemophiliacs (determined by a second-generation four-antigen recombinant immunoblot assay, RIBA-2) and found that 8 (9%) of 91 HCV-seropositive, HIV-seropositive (non-AIDS) patients and none of 58 HCV-seronegative, HIV-seropositive patients developed liver failure. This low rate of liver pathology among those who are HIV positive but HCV negative was also observed in several other studies.[132] Liver failure occurs more frequently in those infected with HCV for 10 years or longer and in those with low CD4 counts.[131]

Other investigators have documented that persons dually infected with HCV and HIV appear to be at high risk for developing serious liver pathology. Martin and colleagues[133] reported that, of 97 persons referred with non-A, non-B hepatitis, three were HIV seropositive, and all developed symptomatic cirrhosis within 3 years of the onset of hepatitis. Only 8 of the 94 HIV-seronegative men had clinically apparent cirrhosis. Telfer and associates[134] reported a similar association between dual HIV and HCV infection and the risk of liver decompensation among 255 hemophiliacs.

Quan[135] analyzed samples from 226 consecutive HIV-seropositive outpatients for HCV by enzyme immunoassay (EIA; 145 by a first-generation EIA and 81 by a second-generation EIA for HCV) and by PCR. The prevalence of anti-HCV antibody was 8%; 52.4% of those admitting to intravenous drug abuse were positive, and 16% of those who were HCV positive had AIDS. Slightly elevated liver function test results were more common for those with than those without HCV. The mild disease found with dual HIV and HCV infection contrasts with that reported for hemophiliacs and may reflect a shorter exposure to HCV and less-advanced HIV disease. Similar results were described by Guido and colleagues,[136] who concluded that the study supports the role of the host immune system in the development of hepatic pathology.

The influence of HIV on the level of HCV RNA and the correlation of the HCV RNA level with development of hepatic pathology have been explored by several groups. Eyster[131] used stored samples to prospectively examine the associations among HIV infection, levels of HCV, CD4 counts, and hepatic dysfunction. Serial samples accrued over 5 to 12 years or longer from 17 HCV-seropositive, HIV-seropositive hemophiliacs and 17 HCV-seropositive, HIV-seronegative hemophiliacs who had similar mean baseline HCV levels were available for analysis. Among those who remained HIV seronegative, HCV RNA levels increased approximately threefold, and among those who became HIV seropositive, HCV RNA levels increased 58-fold. Overall, this is an eightfold faster rate of increase among those who seroconverted to become HIV seropositive than among those who remained HIV seronegative (P=0.009). The HCV load increased as immunodeficiency became more profound. HCV RNA levels and levels of AST correlated with CD4 levels and HCV RNA levels. The rate of increase of HCV RNA was higher among those who developed liver failure than those who did not, although this difference was not significant among the 17 patients considered in this analysis.[137] Telfer and colleagues[134] and Sherman and coworkers[138] also reported HCV RNA levels to be higher in those with HIV infection than those without HIV.

Telfer[134] analyzed the HCV RNA levels of HIV-seropositive and matched HIV-seronegative, HCV-positive hemophiliacs. HIV infection was associated with increased HCV RNA levels but not (within the HIV-seropositive group) with CD4 counts. HCV RNA levels were not associated with ALT levels. Sherman and coworkers[138] examined 13 HIV-seropositive and 30 HIV-seronegative persons and found a positive association between HIV and HCV RNA levels but no association between mean HCV RNA levels and CD4 counts, perhaps because the median CD4 counts were too high compared with studies in which such an association was found.[138] By examining paired serum and biopsy specimens from persons with chronic HBV, Lau and colleagues[139] found that high levels of HCV RNA were associated with lobular inflammation, lymphoid aggregates, and bile duct lesions.

CONCLUSIONS

Studies conducted during the last decade have convincingly shown that the natural courses of infection with HPV, HBV, and HCV are altered by HIV infection. The efficiency of transmission of HCV and perhaps of HBV also appears to be increased in those who are infected with HIV. Data do not support the hypothesis that acquisition, transmission, or the natural history of HIV is altered by concomitant HBV, HCV, or HPV infection. Many of the important pathologic consequences of infection with HBV, HCV, and HPV, such as malignancy, occur only after many years of chronic infection, and it is likely that studies done were unable to accurately describe the risk for such disease that might be conferred by HIV infection.

REFERENCES

1. Kiviat NB, Koutsky LA. Human papillomavirus infection. In: Murray PR, et al, eds. Manual of clinical microbiology. 6th ed. Washington, DC: American Society for Microbiology Press, 1995:1082.

2. Krone MR, Kiviat NB, Koutsky LA. The epidemiology of cervical neoplasms. In: Luesly D, Jordan J, Richart RM, eds. Intraepithelial neoplasia of the lower genital tract. Singapore: Pearson Professional Limited, 1995:49.
3. Orth G. Epidermodysplasia verruciformis: a model for understanding the oncogenicity of human papillomaviruses. Ciba Found Symp 1986;120:157.
4. Sillman FH, Sedlis A. Anogenital papillomavirus infection and neoplasia in immunodeficient women. Obstet Gynecol Clin North Am 1987;15:537.
5. Schneider V, Kay S, Lee HM. Immunosuppression as a high risk factor in the development of condyloma acuminatum and squamous neoplasia of the cervix. Acta Cytologica 1983;27:220.
6. Halpert R, Fruchter RG, Sedlis A, Butt K, Boyce J, Sillman FH. Human papillomavirus and lower genital neoplasia in renal transplant patients. Obstet Gynecol 1986;68:251.
7. Dyall-Smith D, Trowell H, Dyall-Smith ML. Benign human papillomavirus infection in renal transplant recipients. Int J Dermatol 1991;30:785.
8. Rovere GQ, Oliver RTD, McCance DJ, Castro JE. Development of bladder tumour containing HPV type 11 DNA after renal transplantation. Br J Urol 1988;62:36.
9. Alloub MI, Barr BBB, McLaren KM, Smith IW, Bunney MH, Smart GE. Human papillomavirus infection and cervical intraepithelial neoplasia in women with renal allografts. BMJ 1989;298:153.
10. Sillman FH, Boyce JG, Macaset MA, Nicastri AD. 5-Fluorouracil/chemosurgery for intraepithelial neoplasia of the lower genital tract. Obstet Gynecol 1981;58:356.
11. Petry KU, Scheffel D, Bode U, et al. Cellular immunodeficiency enhances the progression of human papillomavirus-associated cervical lesions. Int J Cancer 1994;57:836.
12. Kiviat NB, Critchlow CW, Holmes KK, et al. Association of anal dysplasia and human papillomavirus with immunosuppression and HIV infection among homosexual men. AIDS 1993;7:43.
13. Critchlow CW, Surawickz CM, Holmes KK, et al. Prospective study of high grade anal squamous intraepithelial neoplasia in a cohort of homosexual men: influence of HIV infection, immunosuppression and human papillomavirus infection. AIDS 1995;9:1255.
14. Van Doornum GJ, Van den Hoek JA, Van Ameijden EJ, et al. Cervical HPV infection among HIV-infected prostitutes addicted to hard drugs. J Med Virol 1993;41:185.
15. Healy E, Meenan J, Maulcahy F, Barnes L. The spectrum of HIV related skin disease in an Irish population. Ir Med J 1993;86:188.
16. Law CL, Qassim M, Thompson CH, et al. Factors associated with clinical and sub-clinical anal human papillomavirus infection in homosexual men. Genitourin Med 1991;67:92.
17. Holmberg SD, Buchbinder SP, Conley LJ, et al. The spectrum of medical conditions and symptoms before acquired immunodeficiency syndrome in homosexual and bisexual men infected with the human immunodeficiency virus. Am J Epidemiol 1995;141:395.
18. Temmerman M, Chomba EN, Ndinya AJ, Plummer FA, Coppens M, Piot P. Maternal human immunodeficiency virus-1 infection and pregnancy outcome. Obstet Gynecol 1994;83:495.
19. Chirgwin KD, Feldman J, Augenbraun M, Landesman S, Minkoff H. Incidence of venereal warts in human immunodeficiency virus infected and uninfected women. J Infect Dis 1995;172:235.
20. Wright TC. CIN in HIV-infected women. In: Luesly D, Jordan J, Richart R, eds. Intraepithelial neoplasia of the lower genital tract. Singapore: Pearson Professional Limited, 1995:263.
21. Palefsky JM, Shiboski S, Moss A. Risk factors for anal human papillomavirus infection and cytologic abnormalities in HIV-positive and HIV-negative homosexual men. J Acquir Immune Defic Syndr 1994;7:599.
22. Sun X-W, Ellerbrock TV, Lungu O, Chiasson MA, Bush TJ, Wright TC. Human papillomavirus infection in human immunodeficiency virus–seropositive women. Obstet Gynecol 1995;85:680.
23. Johnson JC, Burnett AF, Wilet GD, Young MA, Dongier J. High frequency of latent and clinical human papillomavirus cervical infections in immunocompromised human immunodeficiency virus infected women. Obstet Gynecol 1992;79:321.
24. Vermund SH, Kelley KF, Klein RS, et al. High risk of human papillomavirus infection and cervical squamous intraepithelial lesions among women with symptomatic human immunodeficiency virus infection. Am J Obstet Gynecol 1991;165:392.

25. Feingold AR, Vermund SH, Burk RD, et al. Cervical cytologic abnormalities and papillomavirus in women infected with human immunodeficiency virus. J Acquir Immune Defic Syndr 1990;3:896.

26. Williams AB, Darragh TM, Vranizan K, Ochia C, Moss A, Palefsky JM. Anal and cervical human papillomavirus infection and risk of anal and cervical epithelial abnormalities in human immunodeficiency virus-infected women. Obstet Gynecol 1994;82:205.

27. Spinillo A, Tenti P, Zappatore R, et al. Prevalence, diagnosis and treatment of lower genital neoplasia in women with human immunodeficiency virus infection. Eur J Obstet Gynecol Reprod Biol 1992; 43(3):235.

28. Johnstone FD, McGoogan E, Smart GE, Brettle RP, Prescott RJ. A population based, controlled study of the relation between HIV infection and cervical neoplasia. Br J Obstet Gynecol 1994;101:986.

29. ter Meulen, Eberhardt HC, Luande J, et al. Human papillomavirus (HPV) infection, HIV infection and cervical cancer in Tanzania, East Africa. Int J Cancer 1992;51:515.

30. Kreiss JK, Kiviat NB, Plummer FA, et al. Human immunodeficiency virus, human papillomavirus, and cervical intraepithelial neoplasia in Nairobi prostitutes. Sex Trans Dis 1992;19:54.

31. Laga M, Icenogle JP, Marsella R, et al. Genital papillomavirus infection and cervical dysplasia—opportunistic complications of HIV infection. Int J Cancer 1992;50:45.

32. Coll Seck A, Awa Faye M, Critchlow, CW, et al. Cervical intraepithelial neoplasia and human papillomavirus infection among Senegalese women seropositive for HIV-1 or HIV-2 or seronegative for HIV. Int J STD AIDS 1994;5:189.

33. St Louis ME, Icenogle JP, Manzila T, et al. Genital types of papillomavirus in children of women with HIV-1 infection in Kinshasa, Zaire. Int J Cancer 1993;54:181.

34. Brown DR, Bryan JT, Cramer H, Katz BP, Handy V, Fife KH. Detection of multiple human papillomavirus types in condylomata acuminata from immunosuppressed patients. J Infect Dis 1994;170:759.

35. Breese PL, Judson FN, Penley KA, Douglas JM Jr. Anal human papillomavirus infection among homosexual and bisexual men: prevalence of type-specific infection and association with human immunodeficiency virus. Sex Transm Dis 1995;226:7.

36. Melbye M, Cote TR, Kessler L, Gail M, Bigger RJ, and the AIDS/Cancer Working Group. High incidence of anal cancer among AIDS patients. Lancet 1994;343:636.

37. Melbye M, Biggar RJ, Wantzin P, Krogsgraard K, Ebbesen P, Becker NG. Sexual transmission of hepatitis C virus: cohort study (1981–9) among European homosexual men. 1990;301:210.

38. Van Landuyt H, Mougin C, Drobacheff C, et al. HIV infection: comparison of colposcopic, histopathological and virological results. Ann Dermatol Venerol 1993;120:281.

39. Wright TC, Ellerbrock TV, Chiasson MA, Devanter NV, Sun X-W, and The New York Cervical Disease Study. Cervical intraepithelial neoplasia in women infected with human immunodeficiency virus: prevalence, risk factors, and validity of Papanicolaou smears. Obstet Gynecol 1994; 84:591.

40. Schafer A, Friedmann W, Mielke M, Schwartlander B, Koch MA. The increased frequency of cervical dysplasia-neoplasia in women infected with the human immunodeficiency virus is related to the degree of immunosuppression. Am J Obstet Gynecol 1991;164:593.

41. Smith JK, Kitchen VS, Botcherby M, et al. Is HIV infection associated with an increase in cervical neoplasia? Br J Obstet Gynecol 1993;100:149.

42. Tirelli U, Vaccher E, Zagonel V, et al. Malignant tumors other than lymphoma and Kaposi's sarcoma in association with HIV infection. Cancer Detect Prev 1988;12:267.

43. Maiman M, Frutcher R, Serur E, Remy JC, Feuer G, Boyce J. Human immunodeficiency virus infection and cervical neoplasia. Gynecol Oncol 1990;38:377.

44. Rellihan MA, Dooley DP, Burke TW, Berkland ME, Longfield RN. Rapidly progressing cervical cancer in a patient with human immunodeficiency virus infection. Gynecol Oncol 1990;36:435.

45. Schwartz LB, Carcangiu ML, Bradham L, Schwartz PE. Rapidly progressive squamous cell carcinoma of the cervix coexisting with human immunodeficiency virus infection: clinical opinion. Gynecol Oncol 1991;41:255.

46. Rabkin CS, Biggar RJ, Baptiste MS, Abe T, Kohler BA, Nasca PC. Cancer incidence trends in women at high risk of human immunodeficiency virus (HIV) infection. Int J Cancer 1993;55:208.

47. Conti M, Agarossi A, Parazzini F, et al. HIV infection, and risk of cervical intraepithelial neoplasia in former intravenous drug abusers. Gynecol Oncol 1993;49:344.

48. Fink MJ, Fruchter RG, Maiman M, et al. The adequacy of cytology and colposcopy in diagnosing cervical neoplasia in HIV-seropositive women. Gynecol Oncol 1994;554:133.

49. Del Priore G, Maag T, Bhattacharya M, Garcia PM, Till M, Lurain JR. The value of cervical cytology in HIV-infected women. Gynecol Oncol 1995;56:395.

50. Caussy D, Goedert JJ, Palefsky J. Interaction of human immunodeficiency and papillomaviruses: association with anal epithelial abnormality in homosexual men. Int J Cancer 1990;46:214.

51. Frazer IH, Medley G, Crapper RM, Brown TC, Mackay IR. Association between anorectal dysplasia, human papillomavirus, and human immunodeficiency virus infection in homosexual men. Lancet 1986;2:657.

52. Marte C, Kelly P, Cohen M, et al. Papanicolaou smear abnormalities in ambulatory care sites for women infected with human immunodeficiency virus. Am J Obstet Gynecol 1991;166:1232.

53. Heard I, Bergeron C, Jeannel D, Henrion R, Kazatchkine MD. Papanicolaou smears in human immunodeficiency virus seropositive women during follow-up. Obstet Gynecol 1995;86:749.

54. Vernon SD, Reeves WC, Clancy KA, et al. A longitudinal study of human papillomavirus DNA detection in human immunodeficiency virus type 1-seropositive and seronegative women. J Infect Dis 1994;169:1108.

55. McGuiness K, La Guardia K. Cryotherapy in the management of cervical dysplasia (CIN) in HIV infected women. Presented at the Ninth International Conference on AIDS, Berlin, Germany,1994.

56. Adachi A, Fleming I, Burk RD, Ho GY, Klein RS. Women with HIV infection and abnormal PAP smears: a prospective study of colposcopy and clinical outcome. Obstet Gynecol 1993;81(3):372.

57. Lehtinen M, Rantala I, Toivonen A, et al. Depletion of Langerhans' cells in cervical HPV infection is associated with replication of the virus. APMIS 1993;101:833.

58. Tay SK, Jenkins D, Maddox P, Campion M, Singer A. Subpopulations of Langerhans' cells in cervical neoplasia. Br J Obstet Gynecol 1987;94:10.

59. Hughes RG, Norval M, Howie SE. Expression of major histocompatibility class II antigens by Langerhans' cells in cervical intraepithelial neoplasia. J Clin Pathol 1989;41:2.

60. Vernon SD, Hart CE, Reeves WC, Icenogle JP. The HIV-1 tat protein enhances E2-dependent human papillomavirus 16 transcription. Virus Res 1993;27:133.

61. Tornesselo ML, Buonguro FM, Giraldo BE, Giraldo G. Human immunodeficiency virus type 1 tat gene enhances human papillomavirus early gene expression. Intervirology 1993;36(2):57.

62. Chemin I, Vermot-Desroches C, Baginski I, et al. Selective detection of human hepatitis B virus surface and core antigens in some peripheral blood mononuclear cell subsets by flow cytometry. J Clin Lab Immunol 1992;38:63.

63. Roisman FR, Castello A, Fainboim H, Morelli A, Fainboim L. Hepatitis B virus antigens in peripheral blood mononuclear cells during the course of viral infection. Clin Immunol Immunopathol 1994;70:99.

64. Moldvay J, Deny P, Pol S, Brechot C, Lamas E. Detection of hepatitis C virus RNA in peripheral blood mononuclear cells of infected patients by in situ hybridization. Blood 1994;83:269.

65. Lissen E, Alter HJ, Abad MA, et al. Hepatitis C virus infection among sexually promiscuous groups and the heterosexual partners of hepatitis C virus infected index cases. Eur J Clin Microbiol Infect Dis 1993;12:827.

66. Hilleman M. Comparative biology and pathogenesis of AIDS and hepatitis B viruses: related but different. AIDS Re Hum Retroviruses 1994;10:1409.

67. Islam M, Banatvalaj. The prevalence of hepatitis B antigen (Hbs Ag) and its antibody (anti-HBs) among London hemophiliacs and blood donors from London and two tropical areas. Transfusion 1976; 16:237.

68. Hansson B. Antibodies to hepatitis B surface and core antigens in haemophiliacs and their contacts among hospital personnel. Scan J Infect Dis 1977;9:167.

69. Burrell C, Black S, Ramsay D. Antibody to hepatitis B surface antigen in hemophiliacs on long-term therapy with Scottish factor VIII. J Clin Pathol 1978;31:309.

70. Schreeder MT, Thompson SE, Hadler SC, et al. Hepatitis B in homosexual men: prevalence of infection and factors related to transmission. J Infect Dis 1982;146:7.

71. Szumess W, Much MI, Prince AM, et al. On the role of sexual behavior in the spread of hepatitis B infection. Ann Intern Med 1975; 83:489.

72. Rogers MF, Morens DM, Stewart JA, et al. National case control study of Kaposi's sarcoma and *Pneumocystis carinii* pneumonia in homosexual men: part 2, laboratory results. Ann Intern Med 1983;99:151.

73. van Griensven G, Hessol NA, Koblin BA, et al. Epidemiology of human immunodeficiency virus type 1 infection among homosexual men participating in hepatitis B vaccine trials in Amsterdam, New York City, and San Francisco, 1978–1990. Am J Epidemiol 1993;137:909.

74. Schramm W, Roggendorf M, Rommel F, et al. Prevalence of antibodies to hepatitis VC virus (HCV) in haemophiliacs. Blut 1989;59:390.

75. Makris M, Preston FE, Triger DR, et al. Hepatitis C antibody and chronic liver disease in haemophilia. Lancet 1990;335:1117.

76. Brettler DB, Alter HJ, Dienstag JL, Forsberg AD, Levine PH. Prevalence of hepatitis C virus antibody in a cohort of hemophilia patients. Blood 1990;76:254.

77. Blanchette VS, Vorstman E, Shore A, et al. Hepatitis C infection in children with hemophilia A and B. Blood 1991;78:285.

78. Rumi GM, Colombo M, Gringeri A, Mannucci PM. High prevalence of antibody to hepatitis C virus in multitransfused hemophiliacs with normal transaminase levels. Ann Intern Med 1990;112:379.

79. Troisi CL, Hollinger FB, Hoots WK, et al. A multicenter study of viral hepatitis in a United States hemophilic population. Blood 1993;81:412.

80. Brettler DB, Alter HJ, Dienstag JL, Forsberg AD, Levine PH. Prevalence of hepatitis C virus antibody in a cohort of hemophilia patients. Blood 1990;76(1):254.

81. Bell J, Batey RG, Farrell GC, Crewe EB, Cunningham AL, Byth K. Hepatitis C virus in intravenous drug users. Med J Aust 1990;153:274.

82. Van Den Hoek JAR, Van Haastrecht HJA, Goudsmit J, de Wolf F, Coutinho RA. Prevalence, incidence, and risk factors of hepatitis C virus infection among drug users in Amsterdam. J Infect Dis 1990;162(4):823.

83. Rustgi VK, Hoffnagle JH, Gerin JL, et al. Hepatitis B virus infection in the acquired immunodeficiency syndrome. Ann Intern Med 1984;101:795.

84. Flo RW, Nilsen A, Voltersvik P, Haukenes G. Serum antibodies to viral pathogens and Toxoplasma gondii in HIV-infected individuals. APMIS 1993;101:946.

85. Kashala O, Mubikayi L, Kayembe K, Mukeba P, Essex M. Hepatitis B virus activation among Central Africans infected with human immunodeficiency virus (HIV) type 1: pre s2 antigen is predominantly expressed in HIV infection. J Infect Dis 1994;169:628.

86. Solomon RE, VanRaden M, Kaslow RA, et al. Association of hepatitis B surface antigen and core antibody with acquisition and manifestations of human immunodeficiency virus type 1 (HIV-1) infection. Am J Pub Health 1990;80:12.

87. Twu JS, Schloemer RH. Transcriptional transactivating function of hepatitis B virus. J Virol 1987;61:3448.

88. van Ameijden, van den Hoek, Mientjes GHC, Couthino RA. A longitudinal study on the incidence and transmission patterns of HIV, HBV, and HCV infection among drug users in Amsterdam. Eur J Epidemiol 1993;9:3.

89. Solomon et al, 1994.

90. Scharshmidt BF, Held MJ, Hollander H, et al. Hepatitis B in patients with HIV infection: relationship to AIDS and patient survival. Ann Intern Med 1992;117:10.

91. Eskild A, Magnus P, Petersen G, et al. Hepatitis B antibodies in HIV-infected homosexual men are associated with more rapid progression to AIDS. AIDS 1992;6:6.

92. Greenspan D, Greenspan JS, Overby G, et al. Risk factors for rapid progression from hairy leukoplakia to AIDS: a nested case-control study. J Acquir Immune Defic Syndr 1991;4:652.

93. Kingsley LA, Rinaldo CR, Lyter DW, Valdiserri RO, Belle SH, Monto H. Sexual transmission efficiency of hepatitis B virus and human immunodeficiency virus among homosexual men JAMA 1990;264:2.

94. Hadler SC, Judson FN, O'Malley PM, et al. Outcome of hepatitis B virus infection in homosexual men and its relation to prior human immunodeficiency virus infection. J Infect Dis 1991;163:454.

95. Taylor PE, Stevens CELL, de Cordoba SR, Rubinstein P. Hepatitis B virus and human immunodeficiency virus: possible interactions. In: Zuckerman AJ, ed. Viral hepatitis and liver disease. New York: Alan R Liss. 1988:198.

96. Bodsworth, NJ, Cooper DA, Donovan B. The influence of human immunodeficiency virus type 1 infection on the development of the hepatitis B virus carrier state. J Infect Dis 1991;163:1138.

97. Beasley RP, Hwang LY, Lin CC, et al. Incidence of hepatitis B virus infections in preschool children in Taiwan. J Infect Dis 1982; 146:198.

98. Sutnick AI, London WT, Gerstley BJS, Cronlund MM, Blumberg BS. Anicteric hepatitis associated with Australia antigen: occurrence in patients with Down's syndrome. JAMA 1068;205:670.

99. Bodsworth N, Donovan B, Nightingale B. The effect of concurrent human immunodeficiency virus infection on chronic hepatitis B: a study of 150 homosexual men. J Infect Dis 1989;160:577.

100. Krogsgaard K, Lindhardt BO, Nielsen JO, et al. The influence of HTLV-III infection on the natural history of hepatitis B virus infection in male homosexual HBsAg carriers. Hepatology 1987;7:37.

101. Rector WG, Govindarajan S, Horsburgh CR, Penley KA, Cohn DL, Judson FN. Hepatic inflammation, hepatitis B replication, and cellular immune function in homosexual males with chronic hepatitis B and antibody to human immunodeficiency virus. Am J Gastroenterol 1988;83:3.

102. Mills CT, Lee E, Perrillo R. Relationship between histology, aminotransferase levels, and viral replication in chronic hepatitis B. Gastroenterology 1990;99:519.

103. Pastore G, Santantonio T, Monno L, Milella M, Luchena N, Angarano G. Effects of HIV superinfection on HBV replication in a chronic HBsAg carrier with liver disease. J Hepatol 1988;7:164.

104. Perillo RP, Regenstein FG, Roodman ST. Chronic hepatitis B in asymptomatic homosexual men with antibodies to human immunodeficiency virus. Ann Intern Med 1986;105:382.

105. Housset C, Pol S, Carnot F, et al. Interactions between human immunodeficiency virus-1, hepatitis delta virus and hepatitis B virus infections in 260 chronic carriers of hepatitis B virus. Hepatology 1992;15:578.

106. Bonacini M, Govindarajan S, Redeker AG. Human immunodeficiency virus infection does not alter serum transaminases and hepatitis B virus (HBV) DNA in homosexual patients with chronic infection. Am J Gastroenterol 1991;86:570.

107. Favre O, Heyraud JP, Chossegros P, et al. Influence de l'infection a VIH sur l'infection par le virus de l'hepatite B chez les patients homosexuels. Gastroenterol Clin Biol 1989;13:696.

108. Monno L, Angarano G, Santanonio T, et al. Lack of HBV and HDV replicative activity in HBsAg-positive intravenous drug addicts with immune deficiency due to HIV. J Med Virol 1991;34:199.

109. Govindarajan S, Edwards VM, Stuart ML, Operskalki EA, Mosley JW, Transfusion Safety Study Group. Influence of human immunodeficiency virus infection on expression of chronic hepatitis B and D virus infection. In: Zuckerman AJ, ed. Viral hepatitis and liver disease. New York: Alan R Liss, 1988:201.

110. McDonald JA, Caruso L, Karayiannis P, et al. Diminished responsiveness of male homosexual chronic hepatitis B virus carriers with HTLV III antibodies to recombinant interferon. Hepatology 1987;7:719.

111. Goldin RD, Fish DE, Hay A, et al. Histological and immunohistochemical study of hepatitis B virus in human immunodeficiency virus infection. J Clin Pathol 1990;43:203.

112. Biggar RJ, Goedert JJ, Hoofnagle J. Accelerated loss of antibody to hepatitis B surface antigen among immunodeficient homosexual men infected with HIV. N Engl J Med 1987;316:630.

113. Homann C, Krogsgaard K, Pedersen C, Andersson P, Nielsen JO. High incidence of hepatitis B infection and evolution of chronic hepatitis B infection in patients with advanced HIV infection. J Acquir Immune Defic Syndr 1991;4:416.

114. Collier AC, Corey L, Murphy VL, et al. Antibody to human immunodeficiency virus (HIV) and suboptimal response to hepatitis B vaccination. Ann Intern Med 1988;15:101.

115. Loke RHT, Murray-Lyon LM, Coleman JC, et al. Diminished response to recombinant hepatitis B vaccine in homosexual with HIV antibody: an indicator of poor prognosis. J Med Virol 1991;31:109.

116. Centers for Disease Control. Hepatitis B virus: a comprehensive strategy for eliminating transmission in the United States through universal childhood vaccination. Recommendations of the Immunization Practices Advisory Committee (ACIP). MMWR 1991;40(RR-13):1.

117. Choudhury SA, Peters VB. Responses to hepatitis B vaccine boosters in human immunodeficiency virus-infected children. Pediatr Infect Dis J 1995;14:65.
118. Diamant EP, Schecter C, Hodes DS, Peters VB. Immunogenicity of hepatitis B vaccine in human immunodeficiency virus infected children. Pediatr Infect Dis J 1993;12:877.
119. Levero M, Balsano C, Natoli G, et al. Hepatitis B virus X protein transactivates the long terminal repeats of human immunodeficiency virus types 1 and 2. Am Soc Microbiol 1990;64:3082.
120. Twu JS, Robinson WS. Hepatitis B virus X gene can transactivate heterologous viral sequences. Proc Natl Acad Sci USA 1989;86:2046.
121. Seto E, Yen TSB, Peterlin BM, Ou JH. Transactivation of the human immunodeficiency virus long terminal repeat by the hepatitis B virus X protein. Proc Natl Acad Sci USA 1988;85:8286.
122. Foster GR, Ackrill AM, Goldin RD, et al. Expression of the terminal protein region of hepatitis B virus inhibits cellular responses to interferons alpha and gamma and double-stranded RNA. Proc Natl Acad Sci USA 1991;88:2888.
123. Sheron N, Lau J, Daniels H, et al. Increased production of tumour necrosis factor alpha in chronic hepatitis B virus infection. J Hepatol 1991;12:241.
124. Israel N, Hazan U, Alcami J, et al. Tumor necrosis factor-alpha stimulates transcription of HIV-1 in human T-lymphocytes independently and synergistically with mitogens. J Immunol 1989;143:3956.
125. Clouse KA, Robbins PB, Fernie B, Ostrove JM, Fauci AS. Viral antigen stimulation of the production of human monokines capable of regulating HIV 1 expression. J Immunol 1989;143:470.
126. Carman W, Thomas H, Domingo E. Viral genetic variation: hepatitis B as a clinical example. Lancet 1993;341:349.
127. Sonnerborg A, Abebe A, Strannegard O. Hepatitis C virus infection in individuals with or without human immunodeficiency virus type 1 infection. Infection 1990;18:347.
128. Soto B, Rodrigo L, Garcia Bengoechea M, et al. Heterosexual transmission of hepatitis C virus and the possible role of coexistent human immunodeficiency virus infection in the index case: a multicentre study of 423 pairings. J Intern Med 1994;236:515.
129. Gabrielli C, Zannini A, Corradini R, Gafa S. Spread of hepatitis C virus among sexual partners of HCVAb positive intravenous drug users. J Infect 1994;29:17.
130. Eyster ME. Transfusion and coagulation factor-acquired human immunodeficiency virus infection. Pediatr Infect Dis J 1991;10:50.
131. Eyster ME, Diamondstone LS, Lien J-M, Ehmann WC, Quan S, Goedert JJ for the Multicenter Hemophilia Cohort Study. Natural history of hepatitis C virus infection with human immunodeficiency virus. J Acquir Immune Defic Syndr 1993;6:602.
132. Schneiderman DJ, Arenson DM, Cello JP, Margaretten W, Weber TE. Hepatic disease in patients with the acquired immune deficiency syndrome (AIDS). Hepatology 1987;7:925.
133. Martin P, Bisceglie AMD, Kassianides C, Lisker-Melman M, Hoffnagle J. Rapidly progressive non-A, non-B hepatitis in patients with human immunodeficiency virus infection. Gastroenterology 1989;97:1559.
134. Telfer PT, Devereuex HL, Dusheiko F, Lee CA. The progression of HCV-related liver disease in a cohort of haemophilic patients. Br J Haematol 1994;87:557.
135. Quan CM, Krajden M, Grigoriew GA, Salit IE. Hepatitis C virus infection in patients infected with the human immunodeficiency virus. Clin Infect Dis 1993;17:117.
136. Guido M, Rugge M, Fattovich G, et al. Human immunodeficiency virus infection and hepatitis C pathology. Liver 1994;14:314.
137. Eyster ME, Fried MW, Bisceglie D, Goedert JJ, for the Multicenter Hemophilia Cohort Study. Increasing hepatitis C Virus RNA levels in hemophiliacs: relationship to human immunodeficiency virus infection and liver disease. Blood 1994;84:1020.
138. Sherman KE, O'Brien J, Gutierrez AG, et al. Quantitative evaluation of hepatitis C virus RNA in patients with concurrent human immunodeficiency virus infections. J Clin Microbiol 1993;31:2679.
139. Lau JY, Davis GL, Kniffen J, et al. Significance of serum hepatitis C virus RNA levels in chronic hepatitis C. Lancet 1993;342:1501.
140. Langley Cl, Benga-De E, Critchlow CW, et al. HIV-1, HIV-2, Human papillomavirus infection and cervical neoplasia in high-risk African women. AIDS 1996;10:413.

AIDS: Biology, Diagnosis, Treatment and Prevention, fourth edition, edited by Vincent T. DeVita, Jr., Samuel Hellman, and Steven A. Rosenberg. Lippincott–Raven Publishers, © 1997

CHAPTER 15 Tumors in HIV Infection

15.1 Kaposi's Sarcoma and Acquired Immunodeficiency Syndrome

Bijan Safai

In early 1981, acquired immunodeficiency syndrome (AIDS) was initially recognized by the outbreak of Kaposi's sarcoma (KS) and *Pneumocystis carinii*[1,2] KS was among the first of AIDS-defining conditions and has remained one of the major diseases associated with human immunodeficiency virus type 1 (HIV-1) infection. The sudden increase in the incidence of KS provided challenging opportunities for clinicians and scientists and resulted in investigations focused on what was once considered a rare and indolent tumor. Considerable information on KS has accumulated, and some of the previously held views have been challenged. This chapter summarizes the developments in KS research and proposes a coherent model of its pathogenesis.

HISTORICAL INFORMATION

In 1872, the Hungarian physician Moriz Kaposi first described this disease as "multiple idiopathic pigmented hemangiosarcoma."[3] He described the condition as localized, nodular, brown-red to blue-red tumors that appeared first on the soles and then on the hands. He recognized the disease as a rare, chronic, cutaneous disorder affecting men older than 40 years of age. He was also aware of the multifocal nature of the disease, the occurrence of visceral involvement, and the vascular nature of the tumor. This form of KS, known as classic KS, occurs most commonly in eastern Europe and North America among men of Italian or Jewish ancestry.[4]

In the 1950s and 1960s, endemic KS, a more aggressive form of the disease that occurred in younger individuals, was described in central Africa, accounting for 9% of all cancers

in Uganda.[5-7] During the 1970s, KS was reported among a new group of patients receiving immunosuppressive therapy for renal transplants and other medical conditions.[8-11]

In early 1980, clusters of KS cases were reported from New York and San Francisco among young homosexual and bisexual men who engaged in promiscuous sexual activities and who had signs of cellular immune defects.[1,2,12-16] HIV-infected homosexual and bisexual men now are the group with the highest incidence of an aggressive form of KS known as epidemic or AIDS-associated KS.

EPIDEMIOLOGY

Before the AIDS epidemic, KS was considered to be a rare disease, appearing in patients originating from eastern Europe, Italy, and Russia.[4] The annual incidence of classic KS in the United States was estimated to be 0.021 to 0.061 per 100,000 persons.[4,17,18] Although this form of KS is mostly seen in persons of European descent, it has been seen in other groups, including three persons of pure Eskimo inheritance.[19] In the late 1960s, large series of classic KS cases were observed in Northern European countries of Sweden and Norway, where only small Jewish populations reside.[20-22] A twofold increase in the incidence of classic KS occurred in Sweden in the late 1960s, which was reported in the late 1980s.[20] Other clusters of classic KS have been reported from the Mediterranean Island of Sardinia and the Peloponnisos Peninsula.[23]

The older literature indicates a male to female ratio of 15 : 1 for classic KS, but in later reports, this ratio is 2 : 1 to 3 : 1.[4,23,24] A distinct male predominance is reported in Africa, ranging from 3 : 1 among children to 10 : 1 among adults.[24-26] The ratio of male to female iatrogenic KS has been reported as 3 : 1 to 7 : 1.[8,27-29] The age of onset of KS varies considerably, with most cases appearing after the age of 50, with means reported

Bijan Safai, Department of Dermatology, New York Medical College, Valhalla, NY 10595.

between 64 and 66 years of age.[4] In African endemic cases, onset usually occurs is in the third and fourth decades of life, with a mean age of 48 years for men and 36 years for women.[26] The lymphadenopathic form occurs in children and young adults. For AIDS-associated KS, the typical age of onset is between 34 and 36 years.[6]

Endemic KS is most common in black Africans.[6,17,18,25–27] It accounts for 1.3% of all cancers in Durham and South Africa, 4% of cancer cases in Tanzania, and 9% to 10% in equatorial African countries, such as Uganda and the Congo.[25–27]

Iatrogenic KS has been reported with increasing frequency in children and adults because of the increased number of organ transplantation cases and more frequent use of immuno-suppressive therapy for autoimmune disorders and in cytostatic chemotherapy for cancer patients.[8–11,29–39] The drugs most often associated with the development of KS include corticosteroids, azathioprine, cyclophosphamide, and cylcosporin A.[30,31,40] KS occurs two to four times more frequently in patients receiving cyclosporin A than other agents. The time to the onset of the disease is also shorter with cyclosporin A (20 versus 60 months).[30] The highest incidence of KS (2.5%) among renal transplant recipients has been reported from Israel, providing further support for the hypothesis of a genetic predisposition for KS.[11] In organ transplant recipients, the overall prevalence for KS is reported to be 0.52%. The prevalence is 1:24% for liver, 0.45% for kidney, and 0.41% for heart transplantations.[41] Cyclosporine is reported to increase the severity of the disease.

The discovery of HIV and availability of the serologic testing made it possible to determine with more accuracy the actual frequency of KS among HIV-infected individuals.[42,43] KS occurs mostly in homosexual and bisexual men and to a much lesser degree in female partners of the bisexual men and in women from certain regions of the Caribbean Island and Africa, who had heterosexually acquired HIV infections.[44,45] KS is reported in other AIDS risk groups, although to a lesser degree. Approximately 95% of all reported cases of AIDS-associated KS in the United States have been in homosexual and bisexual men, representing 26% of all homosexual men with AIDS. AIDS-associated KS is reported in 9% of Haitians, 3% of heterosexual intravenous drug abusers, 3% of transfusion recipients, 3% of women with AIDS, 3% of children with AIDS, and 1% of hemophiliacs. AIDS-associated KS has not been seen in women with AIDS who acquired their HIV infections through heterosexual contacts, in those with transfusion-acquired AIDS, or in iatrogenically infected hemophiliacs.[44–46]

The incidence of AIDS-associated KS is very high among homosexual and bisexual men who meet their partners in places where anonymous casual sex was common, such as bath houses. Specifically sexual practices involving rimming (ie, oral-anal contacts) and fisting (ie, insertion of the hand and foot into the partner's rectum) were more commonly practiced among the homosexual and bisexual men who developed AIDS-associated KS.

The incidence of AIDS-associated KS has declined steadily since the mid-1980s (Tables 15.1-1 and 15.1-2). In 1992, only 9% of all reported cases of AIDS had KS. The overall incidence of AIDS-associated KS since the beginning of the epidemic is 13%.[47,48] Changes in the definition of AIDS-defining conditions will help reduce the ratio of AIDS-associated KS in future reports.

This trend has been the subject of several reviews and discussions.[44,49,50] One explanation may be the decreased use of unlabeled amyl nitrate, an inhalant recreational drug and a possible mitogen.[48,49,51,52] Other epidemiologic studies suggest that changes in certain sexual practices may account for the decreasing incidence of KS.[53,54] AIDS-associated KS tends to appear among the homosexual men who engaged in promiscuous sexual activities, reported histories of sexually transmitted diseases, and were more likely to have had partners from areas with a high frequency of AIDS-associated KS, such as New York City and San Francisco.[44,45,51–62]

The steady decline in the incidence of AIDS-associated KS has been paralleled by a decrease in the incidence of seroconversion in homosexual men. It is thought that changes in the sexual behavior of homosexual and bisexual men and avoidance of high-risk behaviors for contracting HIV have attributed to this decline.[63–66]

AIDS-associated KS has been reported in pediatric population, mostly in the form of lymphadenopathic KS detected generally at postmortem.[67–69] Mucocutaneous KS has also been reported in children who developed HIV infections through blood transfusions.[70,71]

In Africa, AIDS-associated Kaposi's sarcoma appears to be transmitted by heterosexual contact and has an approximately equal incidence among men and women.[72] This is in contrast to the male predominance observed in all other populations, and a male to female ratio of approximately 8 : 1 for AIDS-associated KS in the United States.[73]

TABLE 15.1-1. *AIDS cases with presumptive or definitive Kaposi's sarcoma by risk exposure category reported to the CDC through December 1992*

Risk	Total AIDS Cases	Patients With KS (%)
Homo/bisexual men ± IDU*	158,742	30,513 (19.2)
IDU, heterosexual	57,483	1,510 (2.6)
Heterosexual contact		
Pattern 2 country†	2,957	154 (5.2)
Not pattern 2	13,377	266 (2.0)
Adult transfusion recipients	6,989	177 (2.5)
Adults, unidentified risk	9,513	530 (5.6)
All pediatric cases	4,261	20 (0.5)
Total	253,322	33,170 (13.1)

CDC, Centers for Disease Control and Prevention; IDU, injecting drug users.

*Odds ratio, homo/bisexual men vs. other = 8.23 (7.90, 8.57 Cornfield 95% confidence limits).

†The CDC defines 37 countries in Africa and the Caribbean as pattern 2.

Data provided by Dr. H. Haverkos.

TABLE 15.1-2. *AIDS cases with presumptive or definitive Kaposi's sarcoma by year of report to CDC through December 1992*

Year of Report	Total AIDS Patients	Patients With KS (%)
1981–1983	2,931	957 (32.7)
1984	4,510	1,252 (27.8)
1985	8,308	1,859 (22.4)
1986	13,262	2,560 (19.3)
1987	21,276	3,306 (15.5)
1988	31,964	4,051 (12.7)
1989	35,085	4,251 (12.1)
1990	43,336	5,212 (12.0)
1991	45,456	5,063 (11.1)
1992	47,194	4,659 (9.9)
Total	253,322	33,170 (13.1)

Data provided by Dr. H. Haverkos.

CLINICAL FEATURES

Four categories of KS are recognized: classic, endemic African, iatrogenic, and AIDS-associated. Classic KS usually manifests with blue to reddish purple macules, plaques, or nodules (Color Figs. 15.1-1 through 15.1-4). Untreated lesions may coalesce to form large plaques and tumors that may produce fungating masses with ulceration. In classic KS, Lesions are frequently located on the extremities, most often on the feet and lower leg, but they may appear anywhere on the skin or mucous membranes. Older lesions become brown and may develop a verrucous and hyperkeratotic surface. The lesions may erode and ulcerate, and the

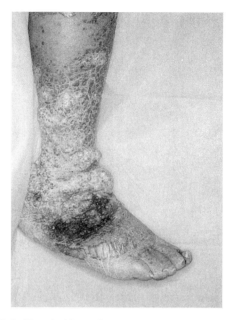

FIG. 15.1-2. Classic Kaposi's sarcoma, showing extensive infiltration, tumor, and secondary lymphedema. Also see Color Figure 15.1-2.

patients may present with large, infected, ulcerated wounds. The lesions are initially soft and spongy, but they later become hard and solid. In addition to cutaneous lesions, KS may appear on oral or other mucosal surfaces. Gastrointestinal lesions are often asymptomatic in classic KS and are usually detected at autopsy.

Edema of the lower extremities, often nonpitting and painful, may precede or follow tumor invasion into the superficial and deep lymphatics. Lymph nodes and internal organs are rarely involved (Color Figs. 15.1-5 and 15.1-6).[25] Classic KS usually runs a benign, protracted course. Rarely, rapid courses with involvement of the internal organs (eg,

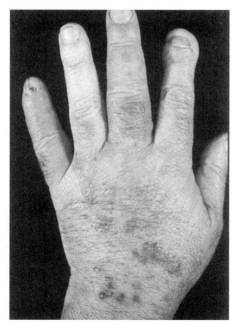

FIG. 15.1-1. Classic Kaposi's sarcoma plaque and nodular lesion. Also see Color Figure 15.1-1.

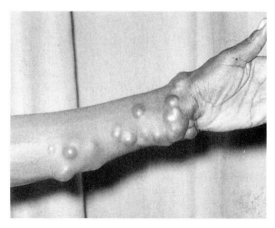

FIG. 15.1-3. Endemic Kaposi's sarcoma, nodular form. Also see Color Figure 15.1-3.

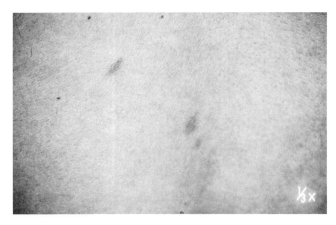

FIG. 15.1-4. Early patch lesion of Kaposi's sarcoma in an AIDS patient. Also see Color Figure 15.1-4.

lungs, gastrointestinal tract, liver, spleen, heart) are reported.

In Africa, clinical forms of KS have been described[26] as nodular, florid, infiltrative, and lymphadenopathic (Table 15.1-3 and Color Fig. 15.1-7). This classification is based on the clinicopathologic presentation of the disease. The lymphadenopathic form is usually seen in African children and young adults. It manifests mainly with involvement of the lymph nodes, and the disease is often rapidly fatal.[27,74]

In transplant recipients, KS is the second most common tumor, after lymphoma, to arise. It occurs more often (10% versus 3% of all transplant-associated neoplasms) in patients

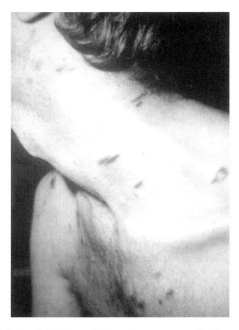

FIG. 15.1-6. Patch lesions of Kaposi's sarcoma distributed symmetrically along Langer's (skin cleavage) lines. Also see Color Figure 15.1-6.

who receive cyclosporin A as part of their immunosuppressive regimen.[28] The mean duration of therapy before the development of KS is 23 months.[28,29] In iatrogenic KS, cutaneous involvement is typical, but lymphatic and visceral dissemination also occur. The disease runs a clinical course similar to classic KS, but in some cases, the course may be more aggressive. Resolution of the disease has been reported after withdrawal or reduction of immunosuppressive therapy.[35,36]

The clinical features of AIDS-associated KS are markedly different from those seen in the other forms (Color Figs. 15.1-8 through 15.1-15). The disease is characterized by a multifocal, widespread distribution that may involve any location on the skin or mucous membranes, as well as the lymph nodes,

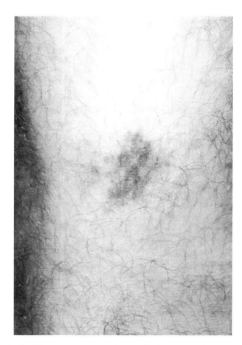

FIG. 15.1-5. More advanced patch lesion of Kaposi's sarcoma in an AIDS patient. Also see Color Figure 15.1-5.

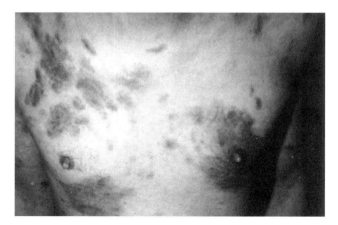

FIG. 15.1-7. Hemorrhagic presentation of Kaposi's sarcoma in an AIDS patient. Also see Color Figure 15.1-7.

TABLE 15.1-3. *Taylor classification of Kaposi's sarcoma*

Clinical Type	Behavior	Age	Bone Involvement	Lymph Node Involvement	Predominant Skin Tumor
Nodular plaques	Indolent	>25	Rare	Rare	Nodules
Florid (exophytic)	Locally aggressive	>25	Often	Rare	Fungating
Infiltrative	Locally aggressive	>25	Always	Rare	Diffuse
Lymphadenopathic	Disseminated aggressive	<25	Rare	Always	Nodules

Taylor JF, Templeton AC, Vogel CL, Ziegler JC, Kyalwazi SK. Kaposi's sarcoma in Uganda: a clinicopathological study. Int J Cancer 1971;8:122.

gastrointestinal tract, and other visceral organs.[75–77] There is considerable variability in the timing of the initial development of KS in HIV-infected individuals. We have seen patients with AIDS-associated KS who lacked evidence of immune impairment.[75–78] KS may be the first sign of HIV infection, especially in populations where HIV testing is not routinely performed. It can also arise in the later stages of HIV infection, when patients are suffering from various degrees of immunodeficiency and opportunistic infections,[78] or it may occur during their last months or weeks of life.

Early lesions of AIDS-associated KS appear as pink to red macules or tense, purple papules. The lesions mostly appear on the face, especially on the nose, eyelids, ears, and trunk. The lower extremities may be involved as well with early lesions and edema. The lesions may progress to form plaques, nodules, and tumors, which may erode and ulcerate. The oral mucosa may be involved, with KS lesions appearing on the palate, gingiva, epipharynx, and larynx. Between 10% and 15% of AIDS-associated KS is initially observed in the oral cavities of patients. Considerable discomfort and difficulty in eating and swallowing may be caused by oral KS lesions.

Extracutaneous KS is observed almost in every internal organ, including the gastrointestinal tract, lymph nodes, and lungs. The lymph nodes and gastrointestinal tract may be the initial or exclusive site of KS lesions.[79–82] In the gastrointestinal tract, KS lesions are most commonly found in the stomach and duodenum. The lesions are frequently symptomatic, and patients have nausea, ulcers, bleeding, and ileus. Because the lesions are localized mostly to submucosa, they are readily visible by gastroscopy, but they are underdiagnosed by superficial biopsies.[79]

Pulmonary KS often manifests with intractable cough, bronchospasm, and respiratory insufficiency.[83–85] These symptoms are very much similar to that of *Pneumocystis carinii* pneumonia (PCP), and accurate diagnosis is achieved by bronchoscopy, bronchoalveolar lavage, and bronchial biopsy. The prognosis of pulmonary KS is poor, even with aggressive systemic chemotherapy and radiation therapy.[83–85] Involvement of bone, subcutaneous tissues and skeletal muscle, bone marrow, the peritoneal cavity and omentum, and the heart occurs but is rare.[87–92]

The natural course of the disease and the rate of the progression of KS vary greatly with the clinical form of the disease. In classic KS, most cases follow a slow and indolent course. Endemic KS follows a more aggressive course,

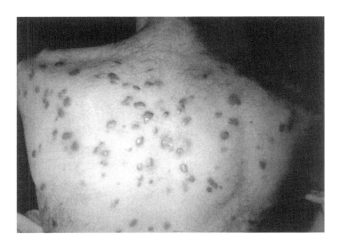

FIG. 15.1-8. Extensive symmetric distribution of plaque and tumor lesions of Kaposi's sarcoma in an AIDS patient. Also see Color Figure 15.1-8.

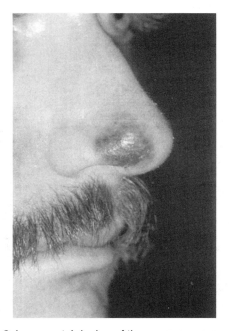

FIG. 15.1-9. Large patch lesion of the nose, a common site for AIDS-related Kaposi's sarcoma. Also see Color Figure 15.1-9.

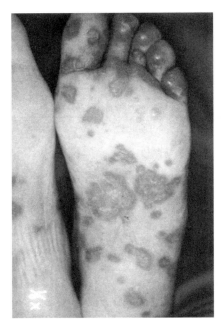

FIG. 15.1-10. Kaposi's sarcoma patches, plaques, and nodules on the sole of an AIDS patient. Also see Color Figure 15.1-10.

especially in children with the lymphadenopathic form. Most AIDS-associated KS cases have a rapidly progressive course. Skin lesions appear most often on the lower extremity, followed by upper extremity, trunk, and less commonly, the face, oral mucosa, and genitalia.[77] The initial few localized lesions frequently progress to widespread skin and mucosal involvement and, in some cases, to involvement of lymph nodes, solid visceral organs, and most commonly the gastrointestinal tract.

Although AIDS-associated KS is more aggressive than other forms of the disease, patients usually succumb to opportunistic infections rather than to the KS itself. In a report on 112 patients followed for a minimum of 15

months, 65 died within that period. All but 10 of the deaths were attributed to opportunistic infections. Two of the 10 patients died of non-Hodgkin's lymphoma, and the other 8 apparently died of AIDS-associated KS.[93,94] Many of the fatal cases of KS result from pulmonary involvement, and although infrequent, pulmonary involvement carries a poor prognosis (Color Figs. 15.1-12 through 15.1-16, *insert*).[95,96] At the other extreme are a few cases of indolent disease that show minimal progression over several years.[75,78,97]

Patients with AIDS-associated KS who do not develop opportunistic infections are estimated to have an 80% survival at 28 months from diagnosis, compared with a less than 20% survival rate for those with opportunistic infections.[98] We have observed a small group of patients with AIDS-associated KS who lived at least 36 months from the time of biopsy diagnosis of KS without developing opportunistic infections. These patients survived 36 to 124 months (average, 69 months; Safai B: unpublished observations).[75,78] These long-term survivors of AIDS-associated KS have normal immune reactivity, indicating that immunodeficiency is not a prerequisite for the development of KS.

Spontaneous regression has been reported for cases of classic and AIDS-associated KS. The regression normally occurs early in the disease and affects only some of the lesions. In cases of iatrogenic KS, discontinuation of immunosuppressive therapies has resulted in complete regression of the disease.[35,36,99]

STAGING

A successful staging classification system should yield prognostic information, be a useful guide to therapeutic interventions, and simplify analysis of different clinical trials. Because it is a multicentric neoplasm, KS does not lend itself to a TNM classification, as do other solid tumors. There are, however, certain clinical features that can identify different presentations of KS and, in general, the overall clinical course.

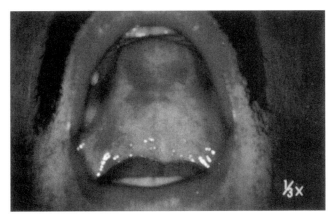

FIG. 15.1-11. Involvement of the hard and soft palate by Kaposi's sarcoma. Also see Color Figure 15.1-11.

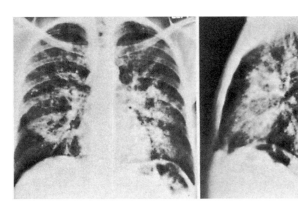

FIG. 15.1-12. Chest x-ray films show extensive central infiltration by Kaposi's sarcoma. Also see Color Figure 15.1-12.

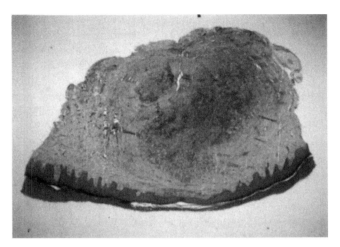

FIG. 15.1-13. Gross microscopic view shows the hemorrhagic and cellular nature of Kaposi's sarcoma. Also see Color Figure 15.1-13.

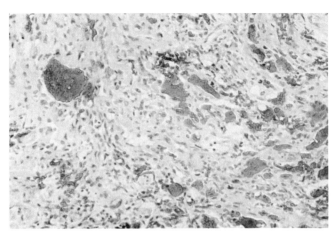

FIG. 15.1-15. High-power view shows irregularly shaped vascular channels, extravasated erythrocytes, and spindle cells of AIDS-associated Kaposi's sarcoma. Also see Color Figure 15.1-15.

The most widely used staging system for KS before the AIDS epidemic was based on the experience from equatorial Africa (see Table 15.1-3).[26] With the emergence of epidemic KS and its aggressive features, it became apparent that a new staging system was needed to identify the distinctive features of this new group of patients. The initial classification[93] took into account the clinical presentation of KS and subtypes A (without) and B (with) systemic B symptoms (Table 15.1-4).[100]

A later classification system, specifically for AIDS-associated KS, takes into account clinical and laboratory factors and recognizes the importance of the helper T count, as did the earlier Walter Reed staging system for HIV disease.[101,102] A multivariate analysis of nine variables employed in the study of 212 patients showed three variables to be significant: a T4 cell count below 300 cells/mm^3, B symptoms, and a prior or coexisting opportunistic infection. A staging system based on these three variables, which identifies four distinct prognostic groups, has been proposed (Table 15.1-5). The variables found not to be significant on multivariate analysis were age, the T4 : T8 ratio, β_2-macroglobulin, acid-labile interferon-α (INF-α), skin or lymph node disease only, and gastrointestinal or palate lesions. Only on univariant analysis was the factors of extent of disease (defined as limited skin or extensive skin involvement) and skin or lymph node involvement versus gastrointestinal tract or palate involvement found to be significant.

Another proposed staging classification uses three parameters (ie, extent of tumor, immune status, and severity of systemic illness) divided into good- and poor-risk groups (Table 15.1-6).[103] Only with use in prospective trials can the value in predicting treatment outcome and survival of these much needed staging systems be realized.

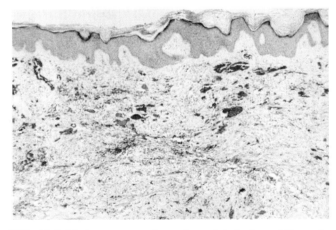

FIG. 15.1-14. Low-power view of a patch lesion of Kaposi's sarcoma shows slit-like vascular spaces and inflammatory cell infiltrate of the dermis. Also see Color Figure 15.1-14.

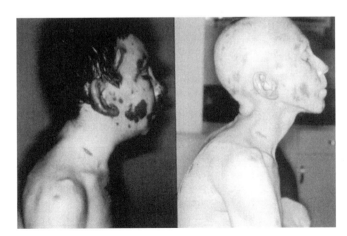

FIG. 15.1-16. Extensive facial tumors of Kaposi's sarcoma before and after radiation therapy. Also see Color Figure 15.1-16.

TABLE 15.1-4. *Staging classification for Kaposi's sarcoma*

Stage	Clinical Manifestation
I	Cutaneous, locally indolent
II	Cutaneous, locally aggressive with or without lymph nodes
III	Generalized mucocutaneous and/or lymph node involvement
IV	Visceral
A	No systemic signs or symptoms
B	Systemic signs: weight loss (10%) or fever
	(>100°F orally, unrelated to an identifiable source of infection lasting >2 weeks)

Redfield RR, Wright DC, Tramont EC. The Walter Reed staging classification for HTLV-III/LAV infection. N Engl J Med 1986;314:131.

HISTOPATHOLOGIC FEATURES

The histopathologic process is thought to start in the middle dermis and extend upward toward the epidermis. A fully developed lesion has a characteristic histopathologic picture consisting of interweaving bands of spindle cells and vascular structures embedded in a network of reticular and collagen fibers. Spindle cells may demonstrate a wide range of nuclear pleomorphism. The vascular component may appear as slit-like spaces between the spindle cells or as very early, delicate capillaries. Extravasated erythrocytes and hemosiderin-laden macrophages are also present. Mononuclear cell infiltrates are seen, especially in younger lesions.

Based on the quantity of the vascular component, the presence of nuclear pleomorphism, the number of spindle cells, and the amount of fibrosis in the tumor, three histopathologic patterns have been identified: a mixed cellular pattern, containing equal proportions of vascular slits, well-formed vascular channels, and spindle cells; a mononuclear pattern, consisting of proliferation of one cell type, usually spindle cells; and an anaplastic pattern, characterized by cellular pleomorphism and frequent mitoses. The mixed cellular pattern is seen in all clinical forms of KS, but the anaplastic pattern has only been reported in the florid type, associated with African endemic and some AIDS-associated KS.[26,104]

TABLE 15.1-5. *Staging classification of AIDS-associated Kaposi's sarcoma based on multivariate analysis of nine clinical and laboratory variables in 212 patients*

Stage	Characteristics
I	No OI, no B symptoms, T4 cells >300
II	No OI, no B symptoms, T4 cells <300
III	No OI, B symptoms
IV	OI

OI, opportunistic infection.
Chachoua A, Krigel R, Lafleur F, et al. Prognostic factors and staging classification of patients with epidemic Kaposi's sarcoma. J Clin Oncol 1989;7:774.

The histopathologic features of AIDS-associated KS has been the subject of many reports describing the pathologic changes that take place in various clinical presentations, such as patch, plaque, and nodular forms of KS.[104]

In early patch stages (ie, macular lesions), a distinct proliferation of spindle-shaped cells in proximity to the superficial vascular plexus within the interstitium of the upper dermis is observed.[105,106] These oval cells form small, irregularly shaped slits and clefts, sometimes giving the appearance of lymphangioma. Sparse mononuclear cells infiltrate composed of lymphocytes and plasma cells in perivascular areas is observed.[107,108] The papular and plaque stage of KS is characterized by proliferation of the dilated and angulated vascular spaces outlined by thin endothelial cells. These structures are interspaced between collagen bundles of the dermis and give a spongy network appearance. The characteristic histologic finding of this stage is the presence of solid condensed fascicles of spindle cells arranged between jagged shaped vascular slits. This produces the special KS morphology, which exhibits solid tumor and angiomatous features. The mononuclear cell infiltration is increased and quite pronounced.

The histology of the nodular tumor consists of a few thin endothelium-lined vascular channels in a matrix of dense, interweaving and bundles of spindle-shaped cells. The mononuclear infiltration is absent or sparse, but extravasated erythrocytes and hemosiderin-laden macrophages are present. Nuclear and cytologic atypia and a few mitotic cells are seen.

The histopathology of KS in lymph nodes and viscera is similar to that seen in skin. Foci of KS tumor located in the sinusoid and capsular areas of the lymph node and a generalized lymphoid hyperplasia are characteristic of KS at this site[107] (see Color Figs. 15.1-13 through 15.1-15).

PATHOGENESIS

The increased incidence of KS among HIV-infected individuals and advances in biotechnology have made it possible to investigate the cellular and molecular events leading to the development and progression of KS. The resulting wealth of knowledge about the pathogenesis of KS is summarized here.

Cell of Origin

The nature of the cells lining the irregular, vascular-like structures and the cells composing the solid tumor fascicles has been the subject of extensive investigations; however, histochemical staining, cell culture, and ultrastructural studies have resulted in controversial information (Table 15.1-7).[109–122] Endothelial cells, pericytes, smooth muscle cells, fibroblasts, Schwann cells, and undifferentiated mesenchymal cells have been suspected as KS cells of origin.[123–127]

In situ immunohistochemical studies have provided insights about the cells involved in KS tumors. KS cells are shown to be reactive with antibodies EN-4, E-92,

TABLE 15.1-6. *Staging classification for Kaposi's sarcoma*

Component	Good Risk (0)	Poor Risk (1)
Tumor (T)	Confined to skin and/or lymph nodes and/or minimal oral disease*	Tumor associated edema or ulceration Extensive oral KS Gastrointestinal KS KS in other nonnodal viscera
Immune system (I) Systemic illness (S)	CD4 cells > 200/μL No history of OI or thrush No B symptoms† Karnofky performance status >70	CD4 cells < 200/μL History of IO and/or thrush B symptoms present Performance status <70 Other HIV-related illnesses (eg, lymphoma, neurologic disease)

KS, Kaposi's sarcoma; OI, opportunistic infections.
*Minimal oral disease is nonnodular KS confined to the palate.
†B symptoms are unexplained fever, night sweats, > 10% involuntary weight loss, or diarrhea persisting more than 2 weeks.
Krown SE, Metroka C, Wernz JC, et al. Kaposi's sarcoma in the acquired immune deficiency syndrome: a proposal for a uniform evaluation, response, and staging criteria. J Clin Oncol 1989;7:1201.

JC70/CD31, Q-bend/CD34, OKM5/CD36, and BMA-120.[116,128–137] The extracellular matrix contains the basal lamina protein, type IV collagen, and laminin.[138–140] KS cells similar to normal vascular endothelium demonstrate 5'-nucleotidase and ATPase activity.[115,141] KS cells do not react with the blood vessel–specific antibody PAL-E, but they react with monoclonal antibodies directed against determinants on lymphatic and vascular endothelial cells.[130–133,142–144] Ultrastructural studies indicate that KS cells are derived from lymphatic endothelium rather than vascular endothelium.[107,144–151] One study indicated that KS tumors express endothelial and macrophage markers.[152] The endothelial markers include von Willebrand factor, vascular endothelial cadherin, endothelium-specific adhesion molecules, and PECAM/CD31. The macrophage markers seen on KS tumors are PAM-1, CD68, and CD14. KS tumors also stain for vitronectin receptors and α_1, α_5, α_6, and β_1 integrin. Staining for intercellular adhesion molecule-1 (ICAM-1) (ICAM-1) is reported to be weak, and staining for VCAM-1 and E-selectin is negative.[152]

A major breakthrough in the study of the nature of KS cells has been the establishment of a long-term culture of AIDS-associated KS derived spindle cells. The growth of these cells is supported by conditioned media obtained from CD4+ T cells infected with human T-cell lymphotropic virus (HTLV)-II.[122,153] Conditioned media from HTLV-I– and HIV-1–infected CD4+ T cells similarly maintained the growth of KS cells, although to a lesser degree. These long-term cultured cells have been characterized by phenotypic markers and cytochemical studies, and it has been shown that the KS spindle cells have features of vascular channel and endothelial cell lineage.[118,154,155] The same cells have some features of vascular smooth muscle when grown on a three-dimensional matrix.[120] One study showed that KS spindle cells share morphology with vascular smooth muscle cells and stain for and express the gene for smooth muscle α-actin.[121] The conclusion drawn from these studies suggests that the spindle cells originate from a mesenchymal precursor cell. Some reports suggest involvement of dermal dendrocytes.[156–158] AIDS-associated KS cell lines express several antigens linking

TABLE 15.1-7. *Cell of origin of Kaposi's sarcoma*

Reference	Year	Putative Cell of Origin	Method of Analysis
Pepler WJ[109]	1959	Neural origin	Histochemistry
Pepler WJ, Theron JJ[110]	1962	Schwann cell	Electron microscopy
Hashimoto K, et al[111]	1964	Endothelial, perithelial	Histochemistry, electron microscopy
Dayan AD, Lewis PD[112]	1967	Reticuloendothelial	Silver staining
Harrison AC, Kahn LB[113]	1978	Pluripotential mesenchymal cell	Electron microscopy
Nadji M, et al[114]	1981	Endothelial cell	Immunohistochemistry
Beckstead JH, et al[115]	1985	Lymphatic endothelium	Enzyme-, immuno-, lectin-histochemistry
Rutgers JL, et al[116]	1986	Vascular endothelium	Immunohistochemistry
Jones RR, et al[117]	1986	Lymphatic endothelium	Immuno-, lectin-histochemistry
Salahuddin SZ, et al[118]	1988	Lymphatic endothelium	Cytochemical, immuno-, enzyme-histochemistry
Nickoloff BJ, Christopher EM[119]	1989	Dermal dendrocyte (reticuloendothelial)	Immunohistochemistry
Thompson EW, et al[120]	1991	Smooth muscle	Cell culture, matrigel culture
Weich HA, et al[121]	1991	Vasc. smooth muscle precursor	Northern blot, immunohistochemistry

them to dermal dendrocytes such as factor XIII A, CD4, and CD14.[156-159] Despite the abundance of new information and the available technology, the identity of the cells in KS tumor remains contested.

Preliminary data indicate that KS represents a monoclonal expansion of the KS cells (Bigger R: personal communication), but what is not yet clear is whether this monoclonality is the same in different KS lesions of a given patient. Each of the KS tumors may be a separate monoclonal expansion, or they may all be the same.

Another area of research is the possible malignant nature and metastasis of KS. Although mitotic figures are observed in KS tissues, cytogenetic abnormalities have not been reported, and there is no well-documented evidence showing that KS tumors metastasize. However, some later reports described cultivation of an immortal neoplastic cell line grown from an AIDS-associated KS tissue which had abnormal cytogenetic features. This cell line was capable of causing angiogenesis, tumor formation, and metastasis in immunodeficient mice.[160,161] Inoculation of this cell line produces tumor at the site of injection, as well as metastatic tumors in the lungs, spleen, pancreas, gastrointestinal tract, and skin. All of these tumors have shown tetraploid karyotypes of human origin.[160,162] These findings suggest that KS cells may develop features of malignant neoplastic cells and become capable of metastasizing. Cytometric DNA analysis demonstrated that the cells were diploid if the clinical course was benign and the cells were aneuploid if the course was aggressive.

Cytokine Cascade

In 1988, a new milestone in the history of KS was reached by the reports that demonstrated successful culture and propagation of spindle cells derived from the pleural effusions of patients with AIDS-associated KS.[118,122] These cells exhibited some features of the endothelial cell, such as *Ulex europaeus* agglutinin and tissue plasminogen activator inhibitors, but they lacked von Willebrand factor, PAL-E, and EN-4. They were positive for vimentin, indicating their mesenchymal origin. Other investigators cultured KS-like spindle cells from KS tumors obtained from skin or internal organs. They showed that cultured KS cells react with endothelium-specific antibodies, anti–von Willebrand factor, PAL-E, EN-4, and BMA 120.[137,163,164] Similar to KS tissues, cultured KS cells demonstrate considerable heterogeneity in phenotypic markers and growth requirements.

An initial report by Nakamara an coworkers[122] demonstrated that conditioned media obtained from HTLV-II–infected CD4+ T cells was necessary for the growth of KS cells. Further studies indicated that the major growth-promoting components in these conditioned media were basic fibroblast growth factor (bFGF), interluekin-1 (IL-1), and a new 30-kd molecule. This new cytokine was later identified to be a 28- to 36-kd polypeptide produced by activated T cells and monocytic cells.[165] The new cytokine was shown to be the same polypeptide previously described as oncostatin M, a cytokine originally defined by its ability to inhibit the growth of a certain melanoma cell line.[165,166] Oncostatin M is produced by macrophages and activated T lymphocytes and has a mitogenic effect on KS cells; it is an autocrine growth factor for KS.[166-168] Oncostatin M acts as mitogen for cells obtained from KS lesions[167,169] but does not induce or maintain the proliferation of normal human endothelial cells.[169] The selective effect of oncostatin M on KS cells, but not on the endothelial cells, indicates that KS cells are different from their normal counterparts.[167,170,171] These differences could reflect an indigenous property of the KS stem cells or result from the transformation of normal endothelial cells.

Interleukin-6 (IL-6) also functions as an autocrine growth factor for AIDS-associated KS.[171,172] The alpha chain of the IL-6 receptors is expressed in AIDS-associated KS, and an IL-6–dependent autocrine growth loop exists in KS tumors.[173] After exposure to oncostatin M, KS cells acquire the ability to secrete increased amounts of IL-6.[167,173] IL-6 is a multifunctional cytokine and has been shown to be highly inducible at the mRNA and protein levels in KS cell cultures by a variety of agents, such as IL-1β and tumor necrosis factor-α (TNF-α).[172] IL-1β induces high levels of IL-6 mRNA and protein expression, but lipopolysaccharide and TNF-α cause modest increases in IL-6 protein and mRNA. Exogenous IL-6 induces the proliferation of KS cells, but there has been a dramatic inhibition of proliferation in response to poly(I:C), despite the high levels of IL-6 produced.[172]

Detailed studies[118,153] of long-term KS cell lines demonstrate that these cells produce a variety of potent biologic agents. KS cell cultures and their products demonstrate growth-promoting activities for KS spindle cells, normal capillary endothelial cells, fibroblasts, and some other mesenchymal cells. They show angiogenic activities in cellular adhesion molecule (CAM) assays and in nude mice. They induce a murine tumor that is histologically similar to KS when the cells are inoculated subcutaneously into nude mice. They have chemotactic and chemoinvasive activities for KS spindle cells, normal endothelial cells, and fibroblasts.[120] They manifest IL-1 and granulocyte-macrophage colony-stimulating factor (GM-CSF)-like activities.[153] The mRNA extracted from the long-term KS cell cultures and probed for a number of cytokines showed the cells expressed high levels of mRNA for GM-CSF and TGF-β.[153] GM-CSF is reported to increase the growth of KS tumors and KS cells in cultures.[174] Messenger RNA for platelet-derived growth factor-α (PDGF-α) and IL-6 has also been shown in significant quantities.[171] The expression of platelet-activating factor, adhesion molecules, and chemokines by KS cells has also been reported.[175]

These results have been confirmed by determining the rate of production and release of these cytokines in conditioned media obtained from the KS cell cultures using ELISA and radioimmunoprecipitation assays. The sequence analysis of several cDNA clones, Southern blot analysis, and quantitative slot-blot analysis further confirm high levels of expression of bFGF and IL-1β by KS cells.[176]

Both bFGF and IL-1β, which are found in high levels along with other cytokines expressed by KS cell cultures, exert significant effects on KS cells, mesenchymal cells, and immune cells.[176,177] The KS cells proliferate in response to the mitogenic effects of recombinant IL-1α, IL-1β, PDGF, TNF-α, and TNF-β, but smooth muscle cells respond to acidic and basic FGF, IL-1, and PDGF.[177] Some of the KS cell cultures express PDGF-β receptors, and these cells are highly responsive to PDGF.[178–181] These observations indicate that KS cells produce cytokines that support their own growth (ie, autocrine) and the growth of other cells (ie, paracrine) and that these cytokines may play a major role in the pathogenesis of AIDS-associated KS.[176,177]

Of special interest is the isolation of a vascular permeability factor from the conditioned media that is thought to be responsible for the development of the tissue edema that sometimes precedes development of KS tumor. This new factor has been shown to synergies the effects of FGF (Insoli B: unpublished data).

The expression of CAM is necessary for the immune cells to accumulate in the pre-KS sites. CAM expression is induced by several agents, such as IL-1β, TNF-α, and lipopolysaccharide.[182] The levels of serum-soluble intercellular adhesion molecule-1 (SICAM-1) is increased in AIDS-associated KS, and these levels correlates directly with the decline of CD4+ T cell count. SICAM-1 therefore may play a pathogenic role in the development of immunodeficiency in AIDS-associated KS.[183] In another study, immunohistochemical staining and in situ hybridization methods were used to demonstrate that KS tumors express endothelial leukocyte adhesion molecule-1, thrombomodulin, and tissue factor antigens.[184] Tissue staining for ICAM-1 is reported to be weak, and staining for VCAM-1 and E-selectin is negative.[152]

HIV-1 Transactivating Gene

Investigations have demonstrated that the HIV-1 transactivating (*tat*) gene and its product, the Tat protein, are important in the pathogenesis of KS.[170] An experimental model has been developed by inserting the *tat* gene into the genome of nude mice. These transgenic mice were found to express *tat*-encoded mRNA only in skin, and most went on to develop skin lesions histologically suggesting early KS.[185] KS-like lesions developed only in male mice, which suggested a possible hormonal influence in the development of this tumor. The *tat*-encoded mRNA was not found in tumor cells. This implies that the *tat* gene product (ie, Tat protein), released by nearby or perhaps distant cells, is able to exert influence on the growth of the KS cells.[187] The Tat protein induces the expression of inflammatory cytokines.[186,188] Further investigations showed that supernatant containing Tat protein stimulated the growth of KS cells in culture, but it did not stimulate normal mesenchymal cells. This growth-promoting effect was inhibited by anti-Tat antibodies and

antisense for Tat.[170] Studies have demonstrated the uptake of Tat protein in tissue culture and localization of Tat protein to the nucleus.[189] This is the first example of a human retrovirus regulatory gene product that is released, that has biologic activity, and that acts as a growth factor for tumor cells.[170,187] bFGF and Tat protein have synergistic effects on KS cells.[190] Tat may produce the primary growth stimulus for the development of KS cells in HIV-1 infected individuals. HIV-1 Tat protein has been shown to transactivates TNF-β gene expression through a transacting-response element–like structure.[191]

Tat protein adheres to AIDS-associated KS cells and normal vascular cells through its RGD (Arg-Gly-Asp) amino acid sequence. This attachment is achieved through a specific interaction with integrin receptors $\alpha_5\beta_1$ and $\alpha_v\beta_3$. It has been demonstrated that inflammatory cytokines increase the expression of both of these integrin receptors. The growth-promoting effects of Tat on vascular endothelial cells and KS cells appears to be mediated through the RGD-recognizing integrin sites.[192]

Immune Activation

Previously reported data suggested that activation of the immune system might play a role in the pathogenesis of AIDS-associated KS.[57,193–196] This appears to be true in the cases of classic, endemic, and iatrogenic KS. Patients with classic KS cases have high levels of anti-cytomegalovirus (CMV) antibodies,[197,198] which suggests that persistent infection with this virus could provide the necessary stimulus for immune activation. In the African endemic KS, parasitic infestation and a variety of different infections could be the source of continuous antigenic stimulation. In the case of iatrogenic KS, infections with CMV, Epstein-Barr virus, and herpes simplex virus may serve as immune activators. Immune stimulation may result from transplanted tissue alloantigens. Moreover, corticosteroids have a direct stimulatory growth effect on AIDS-associated KS cells, and drugs such as cyclosporine can reduce suppressor T-cell activity.[199] Removal of these suppressor cells may result in disregulation and activation of the immune system.

Homosexual and bisexual men are exposed to chronic antigenic stimuli in the form of multiple viral, bacterial, fungal, and parasitic infections and sperm alloantigens.[57,200] Homosexual men with AIDS-associated KS, compared with a group of healthy homosexual controls, had a much higher rate of passive (receptive) anal-genital intercourse associated with rectal deposition of the sexual partner's semen and traumatic sexual practices such as fisting, which would allow entry of infections and exposure to sperm alloantigens.[54] Further support for this hypothesis of pathogenesis comes from the observation that patients with early AIDS-associated KS often show no evidence of immunosuppression and instead show signs of immune activation.[57,75,195,196] Patients with AIDS who develop KS as their initial AIDS manifestation live much longer than those presenting with opportunistic infections.[98] Later reports describe KS in individuals doubly infected with HTLV-II and HIV-1, in whom HTLV-II may act as the source of antigenic stimulation.[201] It is unclear why doubly infected intravenous drug abusers are not developing KS at a greater rate. These observations support the view that immune stimulation plays a major role in the initiation of KS tumors.

Some laboratory studies have strongly supported the role of immune activation in the pathogenesis of KS. Conditioned media, which is necessary for the long-term culture of AIDS-associated KS cells, contains several cytokines normally produced by activated immune cells. Conditioned media from phytohemagglutinin-stimulated peripheral blood mononuclear cells, enriched T cells, and HTLV-I–infected CD4+ cells contain cytokines (eg, IL-1α, IL-1β, IL-2, IL-6, TNF-α, TNF-β, GM-CSF) with additive or synergistic mitogenic effects on the AIDS-associated KS cells, human umbilical vein endothelial cells (hUVE), and adult aortic smooth muscle cells (aa-SMC).[202] The hUVE cells and aa-SMC cells could become responsive to the mitogenic effects of Tat (similar to AIDS-associated KS-derived cells) after exposure to these conditioned media. Several studies indicate that increased levels of intracellular and extracellular cytokines may interrupt HIV-1 latency and increase *tat* gene expression.[203–205] TNF-α has enhanced the progression of KS lesions and augmented HIV-1 replication in AIDS-associated KS.[206–209]

Other investigations have demonstrated that the products of activated immune cells affect the development of AIDS-associated KS. These products induce vascular endothelial cells and KS progenitor cells to acquire features of KS cells, such as spindle cell morphology and growth responsiveness to the mitogenic effects of extracellular Tat protein.[210] They induce AIDS-associated KS cells to produce and release bFGF and enhance KS-like lesions in nude mice.[211] They promote HIV-1 gene expression, rescue defective HIV-1 proviruses, interrupt HIV-1 latency, and increase Tat production. These cellular and viral effects of inflammatory cytokines are synergistically increased with picomolar concentrations of extracellular Tat.[200,212] bFGF and HIV-1 Tat protein have synergistic effects on the induction of angiogenic KS-like lesions in mice.[190] This synergy is attributed to Tat, which enhances endothelial cell growth, and type IV collagenase expression in response to bFGF mimicking extracellular matrix protein. The bFGF, extracellular Tat, and Tat receptors are present in KS cells.[190] The cells proliferate in response to extracellular HIV-1 Tat protein. Normal endothelial cells must be incubated with inflammatory cytokines to demonstrate Tat responsiveness and spindle cell morphology. These cytokines are increased in HIV-1–infected individuals, suggesting that immune stimulation rather than immunodeficiency is a component of AIDS-associated KS pathogenesis.[192] These observations suggest that, under appropriate conditions, some cells of mesenchymal origin could be made responsive to Tat protein by the conditioned media from activated lymphocytes.[192]

One proposed model for the pathogenesis of AIDS-associated KS (Fig. 15.1-17) brings together much of the current knowledge of this disease.[176,177] In this model, excessive T-cell activation in an HIV-1–infected individual leads to the release of cytokines at levels sufficient to stimulate proliferation of the AIDS-associated KS cells and normal mesenchymal cells, induce Tat responsiveness in SMC and endothelial cells, and activate HIV-1 replication and *tat* gene expression. The extracellular Tat protein, which is released transiently, also may stimulate proliferation of AIDS-associated KS cells and preactivated mesenchymal cells. It may induce transactivation of the HIV-1 long terminal repeat and amplify HIV-1 gene expression and replication. Tat protein increases the effects of T-cell activation products on cell growth and HIV-1 transactivation. The proliferation of KS cells leads to the release of cytokines by means of autocrine and paracrine activities; the cytokines induce neoangiogenesis and proliferation of mesenchymal cell types.[176,177]

HIV-1 infection and immunostimulation, through the effects of their extracellular products, may act together to initiate pathologic cellular and molecular events leading to the proliferation of spindle and mesenchymal cells observed in KS lesions.[176,177] Experimental observations delineate some of the mechanisms that explain the increased appearance of KS among HIV-1–infected homosexual and bisexual men. Nevertheless, other factors, such as hormonal influences,[185] sexual practices,[44,54] genetics,[214] environmental factors,[56] and other infectious agents,[44] also may play roles in the initiation and development of KS.

Immunodeficiency

It has been assumed that immunodeficiency is one of the prerequisites for the development of KS. This notion stemmed from the observation that some renal transplant recipients, who were taking immunosuppressive drugs to prevent organ rejection, developed KS, and after the immunosuppressive drugs were discontinued, the KS lesions regressed.[101] The appearance of KS as one of the first manifestations of the AIDS epidemic gave further support to the possible role of immunodeficiency in the development of this disease. However, only a few years into the AIDS epidemic, a small population of HIV-1–infected patients were identified who developed KS without any clinical or laboratory evidence of impaired immunity (Safai B: unpublished observations). It became apparent that HIV-1 could cause KS without immunodeficiency and that the mechanism by which HIV-1 causes KS is different from the mechanism causing immunodeficiency. Studies of classic and endemic KS did not show any evidence of immunodeficiency in these patients.[214] Based on this information and the studies implicating immune activation in the development of KS, immunodeficiency is no longer considered necessary for the development of KS. It is more likely that chronic antigenic stimulation and

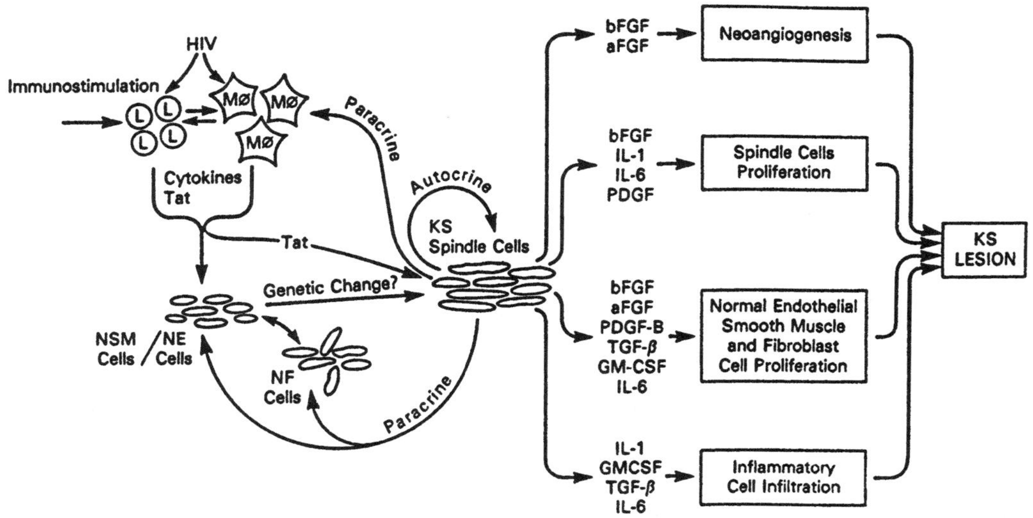

FIG. 15.1-17. Model for the pathogenesis of the Kaposi's sarcona (KS) lesion in AIDS patients, showing normal endothelial cells (NE), normal smooth muscle cells (NSM), normal fibroblasts (NF), lymphocytes (L), and monocyte-macrophages (M). HIV-infected and activated cells (L and M) release Tat or other viral and cellular factors capable of stimulating activation and proliferation of particular cell type of mesenchymal origin. These cells (eg, smooth muscle cells, endothelial cells?) then acquire the peculiar spindle-shaped morphology characteristic of KS cells. The KS cells begin to produce and release several cytokines that maintain and amplify the cellular response through autocrine and paracrine pathways. Paracrine activation of normal cells (NE, NSM, NF, L, and M) leads to endothelial, smooth muscle cell, and fibroblast proliferation; neoangiogenesis; neoangiogenesis; and inflammatory cell infiltrates. These phenomena, together with the spindle cell proliferation, could underlie the typical histologic changes observed in early KS lesions. Later, interactions between cells of the immune system and mesenchymal cells could amplify cell activation and cytokine produciton. If the initial stimulus persists, a vicious cycle could be established that under circumstances such as specific genetic changes, would lead to tumor transformation. Ensoli B, Salahuddin SZ, Gallo RC. Pathogenesis of AIDS-associated Kaposi's sarcoma, Hematol. Oncolo Clin North Am 1991;5:281.

disregulation of the immune system are important in the development of AIDS-associated KS and other forms of this disease.

Host Genetics

The appearance of KS in elderly Italian and Jewish men, the endemic form of KS seen in localized areas of Africa, and the occurrence of AIDS-associated KS among a subpopulation of HIV-infected individuals all demonstrate cluster distribution of this disease and point to a possible genetic susceptibility for KS. However, the number of reported cases of KS among members of the same family is very small and argues against involvement of a mendelian recessive or dominant inheritance pattern.[4] An increased frequency of human leukocyte antigen (HLA)-DR5 in Italian and Jewish patients with KS and of HLA-DR2 in patients of other European descent with the disease had been reported and confirmed for classic and AIDS-associated KS.[215-222] However, HLA typing in a larger population with AIDS-associated KS did not show an increased frequency of any HLA antigen (Safai B: unpublished data). Several other studies have yielded variable or even contradictory results. One possible reason may be that in the group of HIV-1–infected persons, KS developed first

among those most susceptible, perhaps those with HLA-DR5. This would result in the currently observed smaller percentage of HIV-1–infected persons with KS who do not show increased frequency of genetic markers. The absence of familial cases and the lack of increased frequency of one or more HLA subtype do not rule out the possibility of a genetic susceptibility factor in KS.

Etiologic Model

The latest model proposed for the pathogenic mechanism involved in AIDS-associated KS fails to answer many of the perplexing questions that exist about this disease. Although the actual cause of KS remains unknown, there are series of data hat suggest that development of KS cannot be explained by immunosuppression. These data support the hypothesis that a transmissible agent other than HIV may be involved in the development of KS:

1. HIV-1 gene products are not found in KS lesions but are found in their vicinity.
2. Available clinical and laboratory data indicate that immunodeficiency is not a prerequisite for development of KS (Safai B: unpublished data).[75,78]

3. The propensity for developing KS among HIV-infected individuals does not correlate with the extent of immunosuppression in these cases.[59–61,75]

4. The observed decline in the number of AIDS-associated KS cases in the United States and Europe is thought to result from changes in the sexual behavior of HIV-infected homosexual and bisexual men.[45,57,61–65,223,224]

5. KS is 300 times more common in AIDS patients than in iatrogenically immunosuppressed individuals, but the incidence (3%) of non-Hodgkin's lymphomas in both groups is the same.[44]

6. More than 90% of AIDS-associated KS is seen among homosexual or bisexual men.[44,45,60,224] The incidence of KS among HIV-positive homosexual men is higher than for other HIV-infected groups.[225,226]

7. There is a higher incidence of AIDS-associated KS among homosexual and bisexual men who were more promiscuous and engaged in high-risk sexual activities, such as rimming, fisting, and being the receptive sexual partner.[45,54,224]

8. Homosexual men who live in New York and San Francisco have a greater risk of developing KS than men from the central United States.

9. AIDS-associated KS is four times more common among women who had sex with bisexual men than with other HIV-1–seropositive men.[44]

10. Women from Great Britain who developed AIDS-associated KS were more likely to have contracted HIV-1 infection through sexual contact with bisexual men from the United States.[44]

11. The increase incidence of KS in Sweden observed in late 1960s was reported in the mid-1980s.[20–22]

12. Clusters of KS cases are found in Sardinia and the Peloponnesus Peninsula.[23]

Although the cited data support the hypothesis that a sexually transmitted agent other than HIV is involved in KS, this appears unlikely for a number of reasons.[1] No single causative agent has been consistently isolated in KS tissue, and the theory of another agent does not explain the male predominance in African AIDS-associated KS, where HIV-1 is transmitted through heterosexual contact. It also does not explain the development of classic or transplantation-associated KS, in which there is no evidence of sexual transmission.

The search for a putative agent of KS was started long before the outbreak of the AIDS epidemic. Geraldo and coworkers described herpesvirus-like particles in tissue cultures derived from classic and endemic KS. They described a close serologic association between CMV and classic KS in North American and European populations.[197,198,226–229] Later, CMV RNA and CMV early antigens were demonstrated in KS tumors and tissue cultures from classic endemic and iatrogenic KS.[230–232] These observations do not substantiate a casual relation between KS and CMV, but they indicate a close association between the two. CMV may play a part in the development of KS, may act as facilitator or promotor, and may provide the initial cytokines needed for the development of initial KS lesion. At least one study further supports the association of CMV and KS.[233]

Hepatitis B virus DNA and human papillomavirus DNA and proteins have been observed in AIDS-associated KS.[234–236] However, neither of these viruses appears to be truly associated with KS or its pathogenesis.[237]

Retroviruses have been suspected agents in the pathogenesis of KS. In animals, KS-like lesions are caused by retroviruses. Moloney murine sarcoma virus 349 causes KS-like lesions in Balb/c mice,[238] and the lymphoid leukosis group causes avian hemangiomatosis.[239] In humans, attempts to isolate a retrovirus from KS tumors have not been successful. Several reports, however, demonstrated retrovirus-like particles in KS tumors.[240–244] Other studies further support the true retroviral origin of the reported particles.[245–251] Antibodies to GP41 and Nef have been reported in a patient with KS who was seronegative for HIV infection and had normal immune function.[252] The reactivity to HIV-1 antigens observed in this patient may represent involvement of a retrovirus in the development of KS in the form of a defective virus or a close subtype of HIV-1.

Chang and coworkers[253] identified herpes-like DNA sequences in AIDS-associated KS. These investigators employed "representational difference analysis" and were able to isolate unique sequences in more than 90% of KS tumors obtained from AIDS-associated KS. These sequences were found in 15% of non-KS tissue DNA samples from AIDS cases but were absent in tissue DNA from non-AIDS cases. The investigators have reported that these sequences are homologous to, but distinct from, capsid and tegument protein genes of the γ-Herpesvirinae, herpesvirus saimiri, and Epstein-Barr virus. These KS-associated herpesvirus-like sequences are thought to define a new human herpesvirus. This initial report was rapidly followed by reports from the same authors and other investigators indicating the presence of the herpes-like DNA sequences in the classic, endemic, and iatrogenic forms of KS.[253–258] These sequences were found in only 1 of 21 control samples and in 3 of 14 uninvolved skin samples from the patients with KS.

These DNA sequences were also found in AIDS-related body-cavity-based lymphomas.[259] Body-cavity-based lymphomas are characterized by pleural, pericardial, or peritoneal lymphomatous effusions. Later reports, however, indicated an absence of these fragments in KS cell cultures and their presence in tumors such as squamous cell carcinoma, seborrheic keratosis, and others. The initial data, although appearing to be very convincing, still are not sufficient to prove a correlation. The data are available only for the sequence analyses, and the actual virus has yet to be isolated. The wide distribution of these viral sequences further argues against their role as an etiologic agent.

TREATMENT

The choice of therapy for KS depends on the type and location of the lesions, the course and extent of the disease, and the status of the patient's HIV infection.

Local Treatment

The local treatment of KS is important for the control of pain, edema, improvement of function, and cosmetic appearance. There are numerous relatively safe therapeutic modalities for the control of local lesions. Small, isolated lesions can be treated by excision, by electrodesiccation and curettage, or by intralesional injections of chemotherapeutic agents such as bleomycin or vinblastine.[260]

Cryotherapy is another common treatment, although it is often leaves residual brown pigmentation and cosmetically unacceptable hypopigmentation or hyperpigmentation. Cryotherapy is mostly useful for macular lesions.

Radiotherapy, which has been frequently employed in the treatment of classic KS, has become the most important therapeutic modality in the local treatment of AIDS-associated KS.[261–263] Different dosages and kinds of radiation and a variety of techniques have been used. Large-field irradiation has been achieved using high-energy electron beams. Cobalt therapy has been used for large tumors and infiltrative lesions. Radiotherapy is especially useful for the treatment of lesions in difficult anatomic sites, such as the oral mucosa, conjunctiva, face, and soles (see Color Figs. 15.1-14 and 15.1-15). In a review article of 226 lesions in 129 patients that were treated with radiation therapy, there was complete regression of 68% of the lesions. Only 9% of the lesions regrew locally within the radiation field.[264] This mode of therapy is, however, expensive and requires specialized treatment facilities and repeated visits because of fractionation of the radiation dose over 2 to 3 weeks.

Infrared coagulation is reported to be useful in palliative therapy of small KS lesions.[265] Sclerosing agents such as sodium tetradecyl sulfate has been used for the treatment of local lesions with good results.[266]

Local treatment employing intralesional vinblastine in 190 lesions resulted in a complete response in 13% and a partial response in 78%.[267] The side effects were mainly local pain (100%) and skin irritation (90%). Intralesional

interferon has resulted in mixed responses.[268] Future trials of intralesional biologic response modifiers may result in safer and more effective treatment for mucocutaneous KS.

Systemic Chemotherapy

The systemic treatment of KS has been a challenge since the onset of the AIDS epidemic. There was relatively little experience with systemic chemotherapy for KS, because the classic form of the disease is usually indolent and responds well to local therapy.

The aggressive nature of AIDS-associated KS, often manifesting with widespread disease, lymph node, and visceral involvement, dictates the use of intensive chemotherapy. However, the anemia, multiple infections with opportunistic organisms, and immunodeficiency often associated with AIDS-associated KS are serious obstacles to aggressive chemotherapeutic regimens. Nevertheless, several trials using chemotherapy for KS were undertaken, and some reported successful results. The initial trials for AIDS-associated KS followed the recommendations of the National Cancer Institute,[269] which recommended single-drug therapy used for minimal disease and combination chemotherapy for advanced disease. Partial response rates have ranged from 26% to 76%, with tolerable side effects in the later regimens using low-dose therapy (Table 15.1-8).[269–281]

The most successful regimen, with an overall response rate of 88%, has been low-dose ABV (Adriamycin, bleomycin, and vincristine).[278] The frequency of opportunistic infections in this group was 25%, compared with 61% in patients treated with the same regimen with a standard dose.[278] Another promising treatment is the use of oral etoposide (VP-16), which may be more effective than parenteral vinblastine monotherapy and has the additional advantage of ease of administration.[270]

There are considerable difficulties in comparing different chemotherapeutic trials for patients with AIDS-associated KS. A uniform staging system has not been used to group patients in most of the clinical trials. The high partial remission rates seen in some trials employing a single drug may reflect patients who are in a better prognostic group or have limited disease. Some of the more aggressive regimens with multiple drugs have been employed only after single-drug treatment failure or in patients with aggressive, widespread disease.

Variables that have been found to predict a poor therapeutic response have been low T4 counts, anemia, an increased erythrocyte sedimentation rate, and systemic B symptoms. Some of these variables correlate with those used in the proposed prognostic staging classification.[102] Later treatment regimens have fewer immunosuppressive effects, but it is still difficult to determine whether they lead to a decreased survival, owing to death from opportunistic infections, and lack of matched control patients. The mean duration of remission, even among those reported with favorable response, is less than 8 months. Durable response

TABLE 15.1-8. *AIDS-related Kaposi's sarcoma chemotherapy trials*

Regimen	N	CR	PR	OR (%)	Reference
VP-16	41	12	19	31 (76)	270
ABV	31	7	19	26 (84)	270
Vb	38	1	9	10 (26)	275
ABV/AdVcD	27	8	12	20 (74)	276
Vc	18	0	11	11 (61)	277
VcVb	21	1	8	9 (42)	278
BVel	31	0	24	24 (62)	279
B	9	0	7	7 (78)	279
Vel/MTX	9	3	4	7 (77)	280
BVc	18	2	11	13 (72)	281
ABV	24	9	12	21 (88)	282
A	29	1	13	14 (48)	281

N, number of patients; CR, complete response; PR, partial response; OR, overall response; A, adriamycin; B, bleomycin; Vc, vincristine; Vb, vinblastine; Vel, velbane; MTX, methotrexate; Ad, actinomycin D; D, dacarbazine.

TABLE 15.1-9. *Interferon trials for AIDS-related Kaposi's sarcoma*

Regimen	N	CR	PR	TR (%)	Reference
Interferon α-2a					
3 mu daily IM	36	0	1	1 (3)	283
3–36 mu daily IM	30	3	2	5 (17)	283
36 mu daily IM	34	8	5	13 (38)	283
36 mu daily IM + VBL	20	1	5	6 (30)	284
Interferon-α-2b					
1 mu/mm² 5 d/wk QOW SC	10	1	1	2 (20)	285
1–50 mu/mm² 5 d/wk QOW SC-IV	4	1	1	2 (50)	285
50 mu/mm² 5 d/wk QOW IV	10	0	4	4 (40)	285
1 mu/mm² 5 d/wk QOW SC	9	2	1	3 (33)	286
30 mu/mm² 3 d/wk SC	65	5	13	18 (28)	286
50 mu/mm² 5 d/wk QOW IV	33	4	11	15 (45)	286
Interferon-α-N1 (lymphoblastoid)					
6–15 mu/mm² daily × 28 d IM	27	3	1	4 (15)	287
20 mu/mm² daily × 2 mo IM	12	4	4	8 (67)	288
20 mu/mm² daily × 8 wk IV	20	3	9	12 (60)	289
20 mu/mm² daily × 8 wk + VBL	12	1	7	8 (67)	289
Interferon + zidovudine					
4.5, 9, 18 mu daily IM + zidovudine 100–200 mg q 4 h	37	1	16	17 (46)	290
9, 18, 27 mu daily IM + zidovudine 100–200 mg q 4 h	43	16	4	20 (47)	291
9–18 mu daily SC + zidovudine 300 mg bid	20	0	1	1 (5)	291

N, number of patients; CR, complete response; mu, million units; PR, partial response; TR, response; VBL, vinblastine.

rates are not usually seen. Much work needs to be done to find the optimal regimen for the treatment of KS patients.

Immune Response Modifiers

IFN-α has emerged as the only immunomodulating agent effective in the treatment of AIDS-associated KS, and it has been approved for this use by the U.S. Food and Drug Administration. Besides its antiproliferative effects, IFN-α has antiviral and immune stimulatory properties, which make it theoretically advantageous over cytotoxic and immunosuppressive regimens. Although the exact mechanism of action of IFN-α in KS is unknown, its action probably results from its antiproliferative properties, because no improvement in immunologic parameters has been reported in patients who received this biologic agent.[282–288]

Clinical trails using high-dose (≥20 MU) IFN-α have shown response rates in the range of 20% to 50% (Table 15.1-9).[283–289] The rate of response and the time to response have been found to be dose related, although a complete remission has been reported with low-dose therapy (1 MU/day).[285] In one large study, the median disease-free interval and the duration of the median response were 13 and 18 months, respectively, which were improvements over the results achieved with chemotherapy.[288] IFN-α can be used safely as a long-term therapy for KS. In one study, five patients were treated for 24 to 30 months with medium-dose therapy, and there was one sustained remission; regression and stabilization occurred in two other patients.[290] None of

the patients developed opportunistic infections requiring interruption of the protocol side effects. This demonstrates that early and sustained treatment with IFN-α may lead to prolonged disease control and increased survival.

The clinical trials with biologic response modifiers have led to recognition of certain features that are predictive of a positive or negative response to IFN-α. Clinical features associated with a poor response include opportunistic infections, systemic B symptoms, and anemia. The most important laboratory factor is the number of CD4+ lymphocytes. Patients with CD4 counts above than 600 cells/mm³ have response rates greater than 80%. Patients with CD4+ counts below 200 cells/mm³ are unlikely to respond to the therapy.[286–291]

The subjective toxic effects associated with IFN-α are common and can be severe. Frequent symptomatic complaints include flu-like symptoms, which occur in almost all patients receiving high-dose IFN-α. Other adverse effects include somnolence, headache, dizziness, and gastrointestinal disturbances. Fortunately, tolerance increases as treatment progresses. Hematologic and hepatic toxicities occur infrequently, are usually mild, and rarely necessitate a dose reduction.

The combination of IFN-α and zidovudine has resulted in synergistic suppression of HIV replication in vitro. Studies have been conducted to evaluate the combined effects of these drugs in AIDS-associated KS. In two reports,[291–293] the maximum tolerated dose combinations were 18 MU of IFN-α daily and 100 mg of zidovudine every 4 hours. The dose-limiting toxic effects were anemia and neutropenia for zidovudine and hepatotoxicity for IFN-α. Tumor response rates were higher than expected given the relatively low dose of IFN-α used, suggesting antitumor synergy. However, one study showed no treatment advantage with the addition of zidovudine.[293] As in studies of IFN-α alone, tumor response was associated with CD4+ T-cell counts of greater than 200 cells/mm[3].

Studies have also used IFN-α in combination with vinblastine and etoposide.[280,289] There was no positive synergistic effect found in either study, and the hematologic and subjective toxic effects were more severe. Although the antitumor mechanisms for cytotoxic chemotherapy and IFN-α are unknown, tumor response and survival benefits can only be expected in earlier stages of immunodeficiency, as measured by CD4+ T-cell counts higher than 200 to 300 cells/mm[3].

New and Experimental Treatments

During the past few years many new treatment approaches have been reported for KS, and although some of these modalities are still experimental, it is promising to see so many different approaches being tried. Most of these treatment approaches are based on recently acquired information about the pathogenesis of KS and the availability of KS cell cultures.

Perhaps the most promising experimental therapeutic approach for KS is the use of human chorionic gonadotropin (hCG). One report indicated that KS cells in culture were inhibited or killed by the addition of hCG.[161] Another report indicated the successful use of hCG in the treatment of KS patients.[294]

Retinoids are a group of natural and synthetic vitamin A analogs. All-*trans* retinoic acid and 13-*cis*-retinoic acid have been shown to inhibit proliferation of AIDS-associated KS cells, suggesting their possible therapeutic use for KS patients. The growth of KS cells inhibited by retinoic acid was potentiated by forskolin, an intracellular cyclic AMP-inducing agent.[295,296] In a clinical trial, all-*trans* retinoic acid was reported to be effective therapy in AIDS-associated KS patients.[297]

A liposomal delivery system has been shown to be useful in achieving high-efficiency therapy while reducing toxicity. Liposomal doxorubicin has been reported to be effective in the treatment of AIDS-associated KS, demonstrating impressive results.[298,299] This report indicated that a higher dose of drug can be used with fewer toxic effects.

Metalloproteinase inhibitors are potential therapeutic agents for AIDS-associated KS. Their use is based on the observation that collagenase inhibitors such as tissue inhibitor of metalloproteinase (ie, TIMP-2) has been demonstrated to inhibit the angiogenic effects of AIDS-associated KS cells, their products, bFGF, and recombinant Tat protein when injected into laboratory animals.[300,301]

Pentosan polysulfate inhibits bFGF, and FGF-like-dependent tumor growth in vivo and in vitro. It has also been shown to inhibit the growth of AIDS-associated KS cells. However, KS patients, although the agent is tolerated well, no objective tumor response is seen.[302]

Intravenous immunoglobulin used for the treatment of polymyositis has caused regression of iatrogenically induced KS.[303] Enediynes, a unique class of antitumor agents, have been shown to have potent inhibitory effects on the growth of AIDS-associated KS cells and may be effective in the treatment of KS patients.[304]

Systemic hyperthermia has been useful in the treatment of AIDS-associated KS. A low-flow extracorporeal perfusion hyperthermia was effective in the treatment of HIV-1 infection and AIDS-associated KS tumors.[305,306]

A chimeric protein (DAB389-IL-6), engineered by fusion of a truncated diphtheria toxin structural gene plus the gene encoding for IL-6, is reported to be effective on the protein synthesis and cell viability of AIDS-associated KS cell cultures.[307] One study indicated that a naturally occurring bacterial wall component, a polysaccharide peptidoglycan product known as SP-PG, was effective in tissue culture in controlling growth of KS cells and inhibiting angiogenesis in a KS animal model of this disease. This compound will most likely be in clinical trials within the next year.[308]

Antisense oligonucleotide targeting bFGF has been shown to block AIDS-associated KS growth and angiogenesis and block lesion formation in nude mice, providing a novel therapeutic approach for AIDS-associated KS.[309]

FUTURE PROSPECTS

The interest generated in KS after the AIDS epidemic has resulted in considerable new information about this disease. The cause, epidemiology, pathogenesis, and treatment of KS have been the focus of major investigative work. Undoubtedly, as the investigations continue, many of the intriguing questions, especially those concerning concomitant etiologic agents, the role of host genetics, and the contribution by hormones, will be answered. A more effective treatment remains the ultimate goal.

ACKNOWLEDGEMENT

The author wishes to acknowledge the invaluable assistance of Dr. Jun Ling Huang in the preparation of the manuscript.

REFERENCES

1. Centers for Disease Control. *Pneumocystis* pneumonia—Los Angeles. MMWR 1981;30:250.
2. Centers for Disease Control, Friedman-Kien A, et al. Kaposi's sarcoma and *Pneumocystis* pneumonia among homosexual men–New York and California. MMWR 1981;30:305.
3. Kaposi M. Classics in oncology: idiopathic multiple pigmented sarcoma of the skin. Cancer 1982;31:3.
4. Digiovanna JJ, Safai B. Kaposi's sarcoma: retrospective study of 90 cases with particular emphasis on the familial occurrence, ethnic background and prevalence of other diseases. Am J Med 1981;71:779.
5. Loethe R. Kaposi's sarcoma in Ugandan Africans. Acta Pathol Microbiol Scand 1963;161:1.
6. Dutz W, Stout AP. Kaposi's sarcoma in infants and children. Cancer 1960;13:684.

7. Davies JNP, Loethe R. Kaposi's sarcoma in African children. Acta Union Int Contra Cancrum 1962;18:394.
8. Myers BD, Kessler E, Levi J, et al. Kaposi's sarcoma in kidney transplant recipients. Arch Intern Med 1974;133:307.
9. Gange RW, Wilson JE. Kaposi's sarcoma and immunosuppressive therapy: an appraisal. Clin Exp Dermatol 1978;3:135.
10. Penn I. Kaposi's sarcoma in organ transplant recipients. Transplantation 1979;27:8.
11. Shmueli D, Shapira Z, Yussim A, Nakache R, Ram Z, Shaharabani E. The incidence of Kaposi's sarcoma in renal transplant patients and its relation to immunosuppression. Transplant Proc 1989; 21:3209.
12. Haverkos HW, Curran JW. The current outbreak of Kaposi's sarcoma and opportunistic infections. CA Cancer J Clin 1982;32:330.
13. Gottlieb MS, et al. *Pneumocystis carinii* pneumonia and mucosal candidiasis in previously healthy men. Evidence of a new acquired cellular immunodeficiency. N Engl J Med 1981;305:1425.
14. Masur HV, et al. An outbreak of community acquired *Pneumocystis carinii* pneumonia. Initial manifestation of cellular immune dysfunction. N Engl J Med 1981;304:1431.
15. Siegal FR, et al. Severe acquired immunodeficiency in male homosexuals, manifested by chronic perianal ulcerative herpes simplex lesions. N Engl J Med 1981;305:1439.
16. Center for Disease Control. Task Force on Kaposi's sarcoma and opportunistic infections. Special report: epidemiologic aspects of the current outbreak of Kaposi's sarcoma and opportunistic infections. N Engl J Med 1982;306:258.
17. Oettle AG. Geographical and racial differences in the frequencies of Kaposi's sarcoma as evidence of environmental or genetic causes. Acta Union Int Contra Cancrum 1962;18:330.
18. Rothman S. Remarks on sex, age, and racial distribution of Kaposi's sarcoma and on possible pathogenetic factors. Acta Union Int Contra Cancrum 1962;18:326.
19. Mikkelsen F, Nielsen N, Hansen JP. Kaposi's sarcoma in polar Eskimos. Acta Derm Venereol (Stockh) 1977;57:539.
20. Dictor M, Attewell R. Epidemiology of Kaposi's sarcoma in Sweden prior to the acquired immunodeficiency syndrome. Int J Cancer 1988;42:346.
21. Bendsoe N. Increased incidence of Kaposi's sarcoma in Sweden before the AIDS epidemic. Eur J Cancer 1990;26:699.
22. Klepp O, et al. Association of Kaposi's sarcoma and prior immunosuppressive therapy. A 5 year study of Kaposi's sarcoma in Norway. Cancer 1978;42:2626.
23. Cottoni F, et al. Kaposi's sarcoma in Northeast Sardinia: an epidemiologic, geographic and statistical study. In: Cerimele D, ed. Kaposi's sarcoma. New York: SP Medical & Scientific Books, 1985:19.
24. Safai B, Good RA. Kaposi's sarcoma: a review and recent development. CA Cancer J Clin 1981;31:2.
25. Rothman S. Some clinical aspects of Kaposi's sarcoma in the European and North American populations. Acta Union Int Contra Cancrum 1962;18:364.
26. Taylor JF, Templeton AC, Vogel CL, Ziegler JC, Kyalwazi SK. Kaposi's sarcoma in Uganda: a clinicopathological study. Int J Cancer 1971;8:122.
27. Slavin G, Cameron HM, Forbes C, et al. Kaposi's sarcoma in East African children: a report of 51 cases. Lab Pathol 1970;100:187.
28. Civati G, Busnach G, Brando B, et al. Occurrence of Kaposi's sarcoma in renal transplant recipients treated with cyclosporine. Transplant Proc 1988;20(Suppl 3):924.
29. Harwood AR, Osoba SD, Hofstadler SL, et al. Kaposi's sarcoma in recipients of renal transplants. Am J Med 1979;67:759.
30. Penn I. Cancer following cyclosporine therapy. Transplantation 1987;43:32.
31. Penn I. The changing pattern of posttransplant malignancies. Transplant Proc 1991;23:1101.
32. Akhtar M, et al. Kaposi's sarcoma in renal transplant recipients. Ultrastructural and immunoperoxidase study of four cases. Cancer 1984;53:258.
33. Klein MB, et al. Kaposi's sarcoma complicating systemic lupus erythematosus treated with immunosuppression. Arch Dermatol 1974;110:602.
34. Fenoglio CM, et al. Kaposi's sarcoma following chemotherapy for testicular cancer in a homosexual man: demonstration of CMV-RNA in sarcoma cells. Hum Pathol 1982;13:955.
35. Zisbrod Z, et al. Kaposi's sarcoma after kidney transplantation. Report of complete remission of cutaneous and visceral involvement. Transplantation 1980;30:383.
36. Wijnveen AC, Persson H, Bjorck S, et al. Disseminated Kaposi's sarcoma-full regression after withdrawal of immunosuppressive therapy of a case. Transplant Proc 1987;19:3735.
37. al Sulaiman MH, Mousa DH, Rassoul Z, Abdalla AH, Abdur Rehman M, al Khader AA. Transplant-related Kaposi sarcoma in children. Nephrol Dial Transplant 1994;9:443.
38. al Sulaiman MH, al Khader AA. Kaposi's sarcoma in renal transplant recipients. Transplant Sci 1994;4:45.
39. Drut R, Drug RM. EBV-associated Kaposi's sarcoma in a pediatric renal transplant recipient. Pediatr Pathol 1994;14:863.
40. Casoli P, Tumiati B. Rheumatoid arthritis, corticosteroid therapy and Kaposi's sarcoma: a coincidence? A case and review of literature. Clin Rheumatol 1992;11:432.
41. Farge D. Kaposi's sarcoma in organ transplant recipients. The Collaborative Transplantation Research Group of Ille de France. Eur J Med 1993;2:339.
42. Jaffe HW, et al. Acquired immune deficiency syndrome in the United States. The first one thousand cases. J Infect Dis 1983;148:339.
43. Biggar R, et al. AIDS related Kaposi's sarcoma in New York City in 1977. (Letter) N Engl J Med 1988;318:252.
44. Beral V, Peterman TA, Berkelman RL, et al. Kaposi's sarcoma among persons with AIDS: a sexually transmitted infection? Lancet 1990;335:123.
45. Beral V. Epidemiology of Kaposi's sarcoma. In: Franks LM, ed. Cancer surveys, vol X. Cold Spring Harbor, NY: Cold Spring Harbor Laboratory Press, 1991:5.
46. Velez-Garcia E, et al. Kaposi's sarcoma in transfusion associated AIDS. (Letter) N Engl J Med 1985;312:648.
47. Haverkos HW. The epidemiology of AIDS-related Kaposi's sarcoma. Oncology (in press).
48. Haverkos HW, Friedman-Kien AE, Drotman P, et al. The changing incidence of Kaposi's sarcoma among patients with AIDS. J Am Acad Dermatol 1990;22:1250.
49. Selik RM, Starcher ET, Curran JW. Opportunistic diseases reported in AIDS patients: frequencies, associations, and trends. AIDS 1987;1:175.
50. Elford J, McDonald A, Kaldor J. Kaposi's sarcoma as a sexually transmissible infection: an analysis of Australian AIDS surveillance data. The National HIV Surveillance Committee. AIDS 1993;7:1667.
51. Dunkel VC, Rogers-Back AM, Lawlor TE, Harbell JW, Cameron TP. Mutagenicity of some alkyl nitrites used as recreational drugs. Environ Mol Mutagen 1989;14:115.
52. Archibald CP, Schechter MT, Le TN, Craib KJ, Montaner JS, O'Shaughnessy MV. Evidence for a sexually transmitted cofactor for AIDS-related Kaposi's sarcoma in a cohort of homosexual men [see comments]. Epidemiology 1992;3:203.
53. Jaffe HW, Choi K, Thomas PA, et al. National case-control study of Kaposi's sarcoma and *Pneumocystis carinii* pneumonia in homosexual men: Part I. Epidemiologic results. Ann Intern Med 1983;99:145.
54. Darrow WW, Jaffe HW, Curran JW. Passive anal intercourse as a risk factor for AIDS in homosexual men. Lancet 1983;2:160.
55. Lifson AR, Darrow WW, Hessol NA, et al. Kaposi's sarcoma in a cohort of homosexual and bisexual men. Am J Epidemiol 1990;131:221.
56. Haverkos HW, Pinsky PF, Dortman DP, Bergman DJ. Disease manifestation among homosexual with acquired immunodeficiency syndrome: a possible role of nitrites in Kaposi's sarcoma. Sex Transm Dis 1985;12:203.
57. Jacobson LP, Munos A, Fox R, et al. Incidence of Kaposi's sarcoma in a cohort of homosexual men with human immunodeficiency virus type 1. J Acquir Immune Defic Syndr 1990;3(Suppl 1):S24.
58. Rutherford GW, et al. The epidemiology of AIDS-related Kaposi's sarcoma in San Francisco. J Acquir Immune Defic Syndr 1990;3(Suppl l):S4.
59. Goedert JJ, et al. Effect of T4 count and cofactors on the incidence of AIDS in homosexual men infected with human immunodeficiency virus. JAMA 1987;257:331.
60. Archibald CP, et al. Risk factors for Kaposi's sarcoma in the Vancouver lymphadenopathy–AIDS study. J Acquir Immune Defic Syndr 1990;3(Suppl 1):18.
61. Beral V, et al. Risk of Kaposi's sarcoma in AIDS patients in the British Isles: is it increased if sexual partners come from the USA or Africa? Br Med J 1991;325:624.

62. Piot P, et al. Acquired immunodeficiency syndrome in a heterosexual population in Zaire. Lancet 1984;2:65.

63. Drew WL, et al. Declining prevalence of Kaposi's sarcoma in homosexual AIDS patients paralleled by fall in cytomegalovirus transmission. (Letter) Lancet 1988;327:66.

64. Moss AR, et al. Risk factors for AIDS and HIV seropositivity in homosexual men. Am J Epidemiol 1987;125:1035.

65. Detels R, et al. Seroconversion, sexual activity and condom use among 2915 HIV-seronegative men followed for up to 2 years. J Acquir Immune Defic Syndr 1989;2:77.

66. Peters BS, et al. Changing disease patterns in patients with AIDS in a referral centre in the United Kingdom. The changing face of AIDS. Br Med J 1991;302:203.

67. Scott GB, et al. Acquired immunodeficiency syndrome in infants. N Engl J Med 1986;310:76.

68. Rogers M, et al. Acquired immunodeficiency syndrome in children: report of the Centers for Disease Control. National Surveillance, 1982–1985. Pediatrics 1987;79:1008.

69. Buch BE, et al. Kaposi's sarcoma in two infants with acquired immune deficiency syndrome. J Pediatr 1983;103:911.

70. Connor E, et al. Cutaneous acquired immunodeficiency syndrome-associated Kaposi's sarcoma in pediatric patients. Arch Dermatol 1990;126:791.

71. Gutierrex-Ortega P, et al. Kaposi's sarcoma in a 6-day old infant with human immunodeficiency virus. Arch Dermatol 1989; 125:432.

72. Bayley AC, Downing RG, Cheingsong-Popov R, et al. HTLV-III serology distinguishes atypical and endemic Kaposi's sarcoma in Africa. Lancet 1985;1:359.

73. Haverkos HW, Friedman-kien Ae, Drotman P, et al. The changing incidence of Kaposi's sarcoma among patients with AIDS. J Am Acad Dermatol 1990;22:1250.

74. Dutz W, Stout AP. Kaposi's sarcoma in infants and children. Cancer 1959;12:289.

75. Safai B, Johnson KG, Myskowski PL, et al. The natural history of Kaposi's sarcoma in the acquired immunodeficiency syndrome. Ann Intern Med 1985;103:744.

76. Niedt GW, Schinella RA. Acquired immunodeficiency syndrome: a clinicopathologic study of 56 autopsies. Arch Pathol Lab Med 1985;109:727.

77. Myskowski PL, Niedzwiecki D, Shurgot BA, et al. AIDS-associated Kaposi's sarcoma: variables associated with survival. J Am Acad Dermatol 1988;18:1299.

78. Safai B, Sarngadharan MG, Koziner B, et al. Spectrum of Kaposi's sarcoma in the epidemic of AIDS. Cancer Res 1985;45:4646s.

79. Friedman SL, et al. Gastrointestinal Kaposi's sarcoma in patients with the acquired immunodeficiency syndrome. Gastroenterology 1985;89:102.

80. Rose HS, et al. Alimentary track involvement in Kaposi's sarcoma: radiographic and endoscopic findings in 25 homosexual men. Am J Radiol 1982;139:661.

81. Frager DH, et al. Gastrointestinal complications of AIDS: radiologic features. Radiology 1986;158:597.

82. Galtz RK. Kaposi's sarcoma. Gastrointestinal involvement correlation with skin findings an immunologic functions. Dig Dis Sci 1984;29:817.

83. Kaplan LD, et al. Kaposi's sarcoma involving the lung in patients with the acquired immunodeficiency syndrome. J Acquir Immune Defic Syndr 1988;1:23.

84. Ognibene FP, et al. Kaposi's sarcoma causing pulmonary infiltrates and respiratory failure in the acquired immunodeficiency syndrome. Ann Intern Med 1985;102:471.

85. Pitchenik AF, et al. Kaposi's sarcoma of the tracheobronchial tree. Clinical, bronchoscopic and pathologic features. Chest 1985;87:122.

86. Chin R Jr, Jones DF, Pegram PS, Haponik EF. Complete endobronchial occlusion by Kaposi's sarcoma in the absence of cutaneous involvement. Chest 1994;105:1581.

87. Nicholas CM, Flaitz CM, Hicks MJ. Primary intraosseous Kaposi's sarcoma of the maxilla in human immunodeficiency virus infection: review of literature and report of case. J Oral Maxillofac Surg 1995;53:325.

88. Leal R, Lewin M, Ahman I, Korul AJ. Peritoneal Kaposi's sarcoma: a cause of ascites in acquired immunodeficiency syndrome. Dig Dis Sci 1994;39:206.

89. Levin M. Hertzbrg L. Kaposi's sarcoma of the bone marrow presenting with fever of unknown origin. Med Pediatr Oncol 1994;22:410.

90. Lopez Rubio F, Anguita M, Arizon JM, et al. Visceral Kaposi's sarcoma mucocutaneous involvement in a heart transplant recipient. J Heart Lung Transplant 1994;13:913.

91. Lin O, Scholes JV, Lustbader IJ. Chylous ascites resulting from Kaposi's sarcoma in an AIDS patient. Am J Gastroenterol 1994;89:2252.

92. Martinez Sapina MJ, Mosquera J, Castro JM, Comesana ML, Rodriguez E, Menendez MD. Kaposi sarcoma involving bone in an HIV negative patient. Eur J Radiol 1992;15:200.

93. Krigel RL. The treatment and nature history of Kaposi's sarcoma. Ann N Y Acad Sci 1984; 437:447.

94. Krigel R. Prognostic factors in Kaposi's sarcoma. In: Friedman-Kien AE, Laubenstein LJ, eds. Epidemic Kaposi's sarcoma and opportunistic infections in homosexual men. New York: Masson, 1984.

95. Meduri GU, Stover DE, Lee M, et al. Pulmonary Kaposi's sarcoma in the acquired immunodeficiency syndrome. Am J Med 1986;81:11.

96. Hamm PG, Judson MA, Aranda CP. Diagnosis of pulmonary Kaposi's sarcoma with fiberoptic bronchoscopy and endobronchial biopsy. Cancer 1987;59:807.

97. Hardy AM. Characterization of long term survivors of acquired immunodeficiency syndrome. J Acquir Immune Defic Syndr 1991;4:386.

98. Rothenberg R, Woelfel M, Stoneburner R, et al. Survival with the acquired immunodeficiency syndrome. Experience with 5,833 cases in New York City. N Engl J Med 1987;317:1297.

99. Pilgrim M. Spontaneous manifestation of regression of a Kaposi's sarcoma under cyclosporin A. Hautarzt 1988;39:368.

100. Krigel RL, Laubenstein LJ, Muggia FM. Kaposi's sarcoma: a new staging classification. Cancer Treat Rep 1983;67:531.

101. Redfield RR, Wright DC, Tramont EC. The Walter Reed staging classification for HTLV-III/LAV infection. N Engl J Med 1986;314:131.

102. Chachoua A, Krigel R, Lafleur F, et al. Prognostic factors and staging classification of patients with epidemic Kaposi's sarcoma. J Clin Oncol 1989;7:774.

103. Krown SE, Metroka C, Wernz JC, et al. Kaposi's sarcoma in the acquired immune deficiency syndrome: a proposal for a uniform evaluation, response, and staging criteria. J Clin Oncol 1989;7:1201.

104. Gottlieb GJ, Ackerman AB, eds. Kaposi's sarcoma: a text and atlas. Baltimore: Lea & Febiger, 1988.

105. Ackerman AB. Subtle clues to diagnosis by conventional microscopy: the patch stage of Kaposi's sarcoma. Am J Dermatopathol 1979;1:165.

106. Gange WR, Wilson Jones E. Lymphangioma-like Kaposi's sarcoma. A report of three cases. Br J Dermatol 1979;100:327.

107. McNutt NS, Fletcher V, Conant MA. Early lesions of Kaposi's sarcoma in homosexual men. An ultrastructural comparison with other vascular proliferations in skin. Am J Pathol 1983;11:62.

108. Gottlieb GJ, Ackerman AB. Kaposi's sarcoma: an extensive disseminated form in young homosexual men. Hum Pathol 1982;13:882.

109. Pepler WJ. The origin of Kaposi's haemangiosarcoma: a histochemical study. J Pathol Bacteriol 1959;78:553.

110. Pepler WJ, Theron JJ. An electron microscopic study of Kaposi's haemangiosarcoma. J Pathol Bacteriol 1962;83:521.

111. Hashimoto K, Lever WF. Kaposi's sarcoma: histochemical and electron microscopic studies. J Invest Dermatol 1964;43:539.

112. Dayan AD, Lewis PD. Origin of Kaposi's sarcoma from the reticuloendothelial system. Nature 1967;2:889.

113. Harrison AC, Kahn LB. Myogenic cells in Kaposi's sarcoma: an ultrastructural study. J Pathol 1978;124:157.

114. Nadji M, Morales AR, Ziegles-Weissman J, Penneys NS. Kaposi's sarcoma: immunohistologic evidence for an endothelial origin. Arch Pathol Lab Med 1981;105:274.

115. Beckstead JH, Wood GS, Fletcher V. Evidence for the origin of Kaposi's sarcoma from lymphatic endothelium. Am J Pathol 1985;119:294.

116. Rutgers JL, Wieczorek R, Bonetti F, et al. The expression of endothelial cell surface antigens by AIDS-associated Kaposi's sarcoma: evidence for a vascular endothelial cell origin. Am J Pathol 1986;122:493.

117. Jones RR, Spaull J, Spry C, et al. Histogenesis of Kaposi's sarcoma in patients with and without acquired immunodeficiency syndrome (AIDS). J Clin Pathol 1986;39:742.

118. Salahuddin SZ, Nakamura S, Biberfeld, et al. Angiogenic properties of Kaposi's sarcoma-derived cells after long-term culture in vitro. Science 1988;242:430.

119. Nickoloff BJ, Griffiths CEM. The spindle-shaped cells in cutaneous Kaposi's sarcoma. Am J Pathol 1989;135:793.

120. Thompson EW, Nakamura S, Shima TB, et al. Supernatants of acquired immunodeficiency syndrome-related Kaposi's sarcoma cells induce endothelial cell chemotaxis and invasiveness. Cancer Res 1991;51:2670.

121. Weich HA, Salahuddin SZ, Nakamura S, et al. AIDS-Kaposi's derived cells in long-term culture express and synthesize smooth muscle α-actin. (in press).

122. Nakamura S, Salahuddin SZ, Biberfeld P, et al. Kaposi's sarcoma cells: long-term culture with growth factor from retrovirus-infected CD4+ T cells. Science 1988;242:426.

123. Harrison AC, et al. Myogenic cells in Kaposi's sarcoma: an ultrastructural study. J Pathol 1978;124:256.

124. Sterry W, Steigleer G. Kaposi's sarcoma: venous capillary hemangioblastoma: a histochemical and ultrastructural study. Arch Dermatol Res 1979;266:253.

125. Witte MH, Witte CL. AIDS-Kaposi's sarcoma complex: evolution of a full blown lymphologic syndrome. Lymphology 1988;21:4.

126. Dorfman RF. Kaposi's sarcoma: evidence supporting its origin from the lymphatic system. Lymphology 1988;21:45.

127. Dictor M. Vascular remodeling in Kaposi's sarcoma and avian hemangiomatosis: relation to the vertebrate lymphatic system. Lymphology 1988;21:53.

128. Burgdorf W, et al. Immunohistochemical identification of factor VIII-related antigen in endothelial cells of cutaneous lesions of alleged vascular nature. Am J Clin Pathol 1981;75:167.

129. Guarda LG, et al. Factor VIII in Kaposi's sarcoma. Am J Clin Pathol 1981;76:197.

130. Russell-Jones R, et al. Histogenesis of Kaposi's sarcoma in patients with and without acquired immune deficiency syndrome (AIDS). J Clin Pathol 1986;39:742.

131. Schlingemann RO, et al. Monoclonal antibody PLA-E specific for endothelium. Lab Invest 1985;52:71.

132. Cui YC, et al. A vascular endothelial cell antigen with restricted distribution in human fetal, adult and malignant tissue. Immunology 1983;49:183.

133. Nadimi H, et al. Expression of endothelial cell markers PLA-E and EN-4 and Ia antigen in Kaposi's sarcoma. J Oral Pathol 1988;17:416.

134. Parums DV, et al. JC70: a new monoclonal antibody that detects vascular endothelium-associated antigen on routinely processed tissue sections. J Clin Pathol 1990;43:752.

135. Nickoloff BJ. The human progenitor cell antigen (CD34) is localized on endothelial cells, dermal dendritic cells, and perifollicular cells in formalin-fixed normal skin, and on proliferating endothelial cells and stromal spindle shaped cells in Kaposi's sarcoma. Arch Dermatol 1991;127:523.

136. Knowles DM, et al. Monoclonal antihuman monocyte antibodies OKM1 and OKM5 possess distinctive tissue distribution including differential reactivity with vascular endothelium. J Immunol 1984;132:2170.

137. Roth WK, et al. Culture, AIDS-related Kaposi sarcoma cells express endothelial cell markers and are weakly malignant in vitro. Int J Cancer 1988;42:767.

138. Kramer RH, et al. Basement membrane and connective tissue proteins in early lesions of Kaposi's sarcoma associated with AIDS. J Invest Dermatol 1985;84:516.

139. Green TL, et al. Kaposi's sarcoma in AIDS. Basement membrane and endothelial cell markers in late stage lesion. J Oral Pathol 1988;17:266.

140. Barsky SH, et al. Use of antibasement membrane antibodies to distinguish blood vessel capillaries from lymphatic capillaries. Am J Surg Pathol 1983;7:667.

141. Roth WK, et al. Cellular and molecular features of HIV-associated Kaposi's sarcoma. AIDS 1992;6:895.

142. Rappersberger K, et al. Endemic Kaposi's sarcoma in human immunodeficiency virus type 1-seronegative persons. Demonstration of retrovirus-like particles in cutaneous lesions. J Invest Dermatol 1990;95:371.

143. Holden CA. The detection of endothelial cell antigens in cutaneous tissue using methacarn and periodate lysin paraformaldehyde fixation. J Immunol Methods 1986;4:45.

144. Scully PA, et al. AIDS-related Kaposi's sarcoma displays differential expression of endothelial surface antigen. Am J Pathol 1988;130:244.

145. Leak LV. Studies on the permeability of lymphatic capillaries. J Cell Biol 1971;50:300.

146. Leak LV, Kato F. Electron microscopic studies of lymphatic capillaries during early inflammation. Lab Invest 1972;26:572.

147. Leak LV. The structure of lymphatic capillaries in lymph formation. Fed Proc 1976;35:1863.

148. Dictor M. Kaposi sarcoma. Origin and significance of lymphaticovenous connections. Virchows Arch A Pathol Anat Histopathol 1966;409:23.

149. Kuntz AA, et al. Ultrastructural findings in oral Kaposi's sarcoma (AIDS). J Oral Pathol 1987;16:372.

150. Daroczy J. The dermal lymphatic capillaries. Berlin: Springer-Verlag, 1988.

151. Dictor M, Anerson C. Ultrastructural development of Kaposi's sarcoma in relation to the dermal microvasculature. Virchows Arch A Pathol Anat Histopathol 1991;419:35.

152. Uccini S, Ruco LP, Monardo F, et al. Co-expression of endothelial cell and macrophage antigens in Kaposi's sarcoma cells. J Pathol 1994;173:23.

153. Ensoli B, Nakamura S, Salahuddin SZ, et al. AIDS-Kaposi's sarcoma-derived cells express cytokines with autocrine and paracrine growth effects. Science 1989;243:223.

154. Benelli R, Repetto L, Carlone S, Parravicini C, Albini A. Establishment and characterization of two new Kaposi's sarcoma cell cultures from an AIDS and a non-AIDS patient. Res Virol 1994;145:252.

155. Herndier BG, Werner A, Arnstein P, et al. Characterization of a human Kaposi's sarcoma cell line that induces angiogenic tumors in animals. AIDS 1994;8:575.

156. Huang YQ, Friedman Kien AE, Li JJ, Nickoloff BJ. Cultured Kaposi's sarcoma cell lines express factor X111a, CD14, and VCAM-1, but not factor VIII or ELAM-1. [Published erratum appears in Arch Dermatol 1993;12:1622.] Arch Dermatol 1993;.129:1291.

157. Kanitakis J, Roca Miralles M. Factor-X111a-expressing dermal dendrocytes in Kaposi's sarcoma. A comparison between classical and immunosuppression-associated types. Virchows Arch A Pathol Anat Histopathol 1992;420:227.

158. Kumar D, Sanchez RL, KUMAR S. Dendrocyte population in cutaneous and extracutaneous Kaposi's sarcoma. Am J Dermatopathol 1992;14:298.

159. Regezi JA, MacPhail LA, Daniels TE, DeSouza YG, Greenspan JS, Greenspan D. Human immunodeficiency virus-associated oral Kaposi's sarcoma. A heterogeneous cell population dominated by spindle-shaped endothelial cells. Am J Pathol 1993;143:240.

160. Lunardi-Iskander Y, Gill P, Lam VH, et al. Isolation and characterization of an immortal neoplastic cell line (KSY-1) from AIDS-associated Kaposi's sarcoma. J Natl Cancer Inst 1995;87:974.

161. Lunardi-Iskander Y, Bryant JL, Zeman RA, et al. Tumor-genesis and metastasis of neoplastic Kaposi's sarcoma cell line in immunodeficient mice blocked by a human pregnancy hormone. Nature 1995;375:64.

162. Eto H, Toriyama K, Tsuda N, Tagawa Y, Itakura H. Flow cytometric DNA analysis of vascular soft tissue tumors, including African endemic-type Kaposi's sarcoma. Hum Pathol 1992;23:1055.

163. Werner S, et al. Cells derived from sporadic and AIDS-related Kaposi's sarcoma reveal identical cytochemical and molecular properties in vitro. Int J Cancer 1989;43:1137.

164. Corbeli J, et al. Culture and properties of cells derived from Kaposi's sarcoma. J Immunol 1991;146:2972.

165. Nair BC, et al. Identification of a major growth factor for AIDS-Kaposi's sarcoma cells as oncostatin M. Science 1992;255:1430.

166. Zarling JM, et al. Onco M: a growth regulator produced by differentiated histiocytic lymphoma cells. Proc Natl Acad Sci USA 1986;83:9739.

167. Miles SA, et al. Oncostatin M as a potent mitogen for AIDS-Kaposi's sarcoma-derived cells. Science 1992;255:1432.

168. Cai J, Gill PS, Masood R, et al. Oncostatin-M is an autocrine growth factor in Kaposi's sarcoma. Am J Pathol 1994;145:74.

169. Brown TJ, et al. Regulation of IL-6 expression by oncostatin M. J Immunol 1991;147:2175.

170. Ensoli B, et al. Tat protein of HIV-1 stimulates growth of cells derived from Kaposi's sarcoma lesions of AIDS patients. Nature 1990;345:84.

171. Miles SA, et al. AIDS Kaposi's sarcoma-derived cells produce and respond to interleukin 6. Proc Natl Acad Sci USA 1990;87:4068.

172. Yang J, Hagan MK, Offermann MK. Induction of IL-6 gene expression in Kaposi's sarcoma cells. J Immunol 1994;152:943.

173. Miles SA. Pathogenesis of human immunodeficiency virus-related Kaposi's sarcoma. Curr Opin Oncol 1992;4:875.

174. Hermans P, Gori A, Lemone M, Franchioly P, Clumeck N. Possible role of granulocyte-macrophage colony stimulating factor (GM-CSF) on the rapid progression of AIDS-related Kaposi's sarcoma lesions in vivo. Br J Haematol 1994;87:413.

175. Sciacca FL, Sturzl M, Bussolino F, et al. Expression of adhesion molecules, platelet-activating factor and chemokines by Kaposi's sarcoma cells. J Immunol 1994;153:4816.

176. Ensoli B, Salahuddin SZ, Gallo RC. AIDS-associated Kaposi's sarcoma: a molecular model for its pathogenesis. Cancer Cells 1989;1:93.

177. Ensoli B, Barillari G, Gallo RC. Pathogenesis of AIDS-associated Kaposi's sarcoma. Hematol Oncol Clin North Am 1991;5:281.

178. Roth WK, et al. Depletion of PDGF from serum inhibits growth of AIDS-related and sporadic Kaposi's sarcoma cells in culture. Oncogene 1989;4:483.

179. Sturzl M, et al. Expression of platelet-derived growth factor and its receptor in AIDS-related Kaposi's sarcoma in vivo suggests paracrine and autocrine mechanisms of tumor maintenance. Proc Natl Acad Sci USA 1992;89:7046.

180. Sturzl M, Roth WK, Brockmeyer NH, Zietz C, Speiser B, Hofschneider PH. Expression of platelet-derived growth factor and its receptor in AIDS-related Kaposi sarcoma in vivo suggests paracrine and autocrine mechanisms of tumor maintenance. Proc Natl Acad Sci USA 1992;89:7046.

181. Pistritto G, Ventura L, Mores N, Lacal PM, D'Onofrio C. Regulation of PDGF-B and PDGF receptor expression in the pathogenesis of Kaposi's sarcoma in AIDS. Antibiot Chemother 1994;46:73.

182. Yang J, Xu Y, Zhu C, Hagan MK, Lawley T, Offermann MK. Regulation of adhesion molecule expression in Kaposi's sarcoma cells. J Immunol 1994;152:361.

183. De Paoli P, Caffau C, D'Andrea M, Tavio M, Tirelli U, Santini G. Serum levels of intercellular adhesion molecule 1 in patients with HIV-related Kaposi's sarcoma. J Acquir Immune Defic Syndr 1994;7:695.

184. Zhang YM, Bachmann S, Hmmer C, et al. Vascular origin of Kaposi's sarcoma. Expression of leukocyte adhesion molecule-1, thrombomodulin, and tissue factor. Am J Pathol 1994;144:51.

185. Vogel J, Hinrichs SH, Reynolds RK, et al. The HIV *tat* gene induces dermal lesions resembling Kaposi's sarcoma in transgenic mice. Nature 1988;335:606.

186. Buonaguro L, Barillari G, Chang HL, et al. Effects of the human immunodeficiency virus type 1 Tat protein on the expression of inflammatory cytokines. J Virol 1992;66:7159.

187. Fiorelli V, Barillari G, Gallo RC, Ensoli B. Biological properties of human immunodeficiency virus type-1 Tat protein: angiogenic effects and adhesive interactions of extracellular Tat. In: Preissner KT, Rosenblatt S, Kost C, Wegerhoff J, Mosher DF, eds. Biology of vitronectins and their receptors. Amsterdam: Excerpta Medica, 1993:351.

188. Ensoli B, Buonaguro L, Barillari G, et al. Release, uptake, and effects of extracellular HIV-1 Tat protein on cell growth and viral transactivation. J Virol 1993;67:277.

189. Frankel AD, Paba CO. Cellular uptake of the Tat protein from human immunodeficiency virus. Cell 1988;55:1189.

190. Ensoli B, Gendelman R, Markham P, et al. Synergy between basic fibroblast growth factor and HIV-1 Tat protein in induction of Kaposi's sarcoma. Nature 1994;371:674.

191. Buonaguro, L, Buonaguro FM, Giraldo G, Ensoli B. The human immunodeficiency virus type 1 Tat protein transactivates tumor necrosis factor beta gene expression through a TAR-like structure. J Virol 1994;68:2677.

192. Barillari G, Gendelman R, Gallo RC, Ensoli B. The Tat protein of human immunodeficiency virus type 1, a growth factor for AIDS Kaposi sarcoma and cytokine-activated vascular cells, induces adhesion of the same cell types by using integrin receptors recognizing the RGD amino acid sequence. Proc Natl Acad Sci USA 1993;90:7941.

193. Rabkin CS, Goedert JJ, Biggar RJ, et al. Kaposi's sarcoma in three HIV-1–infected cohorts. J Acquir Immune Defic Syndr 1990;3(Suppl 1):S38.

194. Mitsuyasu RT, Taylor JMG, Glaspy J, et al. Heterogeneity of epidemic Kaposi's sarcoma. Cancer 1986;57:1657.

195. Ballard HS. Dissemination of Kaposi's sarcoma without lymphocyte abnormalities. Arch Intern Med 1985;145:547.

196. Lane HC, Masur H, Gelman EP, et al. Correlation between immunologic function and clinical subpopulations of patients with the acquired immunodeficiency syndrome. Am J Med 1985;78:417.

197. Giraldo G, et al. Antibody patterns to herpesvirus in Kaposi's sarcoma: I. Serological association of European Kaposi's sarcoma with cytomegalovirus. Int J Cancer 1975;15:839.

198. Giraldo G, et al. Antibody patterns to herpes virus in Kaposi's sarcoma: II. Serological association of American Kaposi's sarcoma with cytomegalovirus. Int J Cancer 1978;22:126.

199. Cohen DJ, Loertscher R, Rubin MF, et al. Cyclosporine: a new immunosuppressive agent for organ transplantation. Ann Intern Med 1984;101:667.

200. Mavligit GM, Talpaz M, Hsia FT, et al. Chronic immune stimulation by sperm alloantigens. JAMA 1984;251:237.

201. Gorter RW, Osmond D, Gallo D, et al. Coinfection of HIV-I and HTLV-I/II in intravenous drug users in treatment programs in San Francisco. Seventh International Conference on AIDS. Florence, Italy, June 1991.

202. Barillari G, Buonaguro K. Fiorelli V, et al. Effects of cytokines from activated immune cells on vascular cell growth and HIV-1 gene expression. Implications for AIDS-Kaposi's sarcoma pathogenesis. J Immunol 1992;149:3727.

203. Folks T, Justement J, Kinter A, et al. Cytokine-induced expression of HIV-1 in a chronically infected promonocyte cell line. Science 1988;238:800.

204. Koyanagi Y, O'Brien WA, Zhao JQ. Cytokines alter production of HIV-1 from primary mononuclear phagocytes. Science 1988;241:1673.

205. Latham PS, Lewis AM, Varesio L, et al. Expression of human immunodeficiency virus long terminal repeat in the human promonocyte cell line U937: effect of endotoxin and cytokines. Cell Immunol 1990;129:513.

206. Aboulafia D, Miles SA, Saks SR, Mitsuyasu RT. Intravenous recombinant tumor necrosis factor in the treatment of AIDS-related Kaposi's sarcoma. J Acquir Immune Defic Syndr 1989;2:54.

207. Duh EJ, Maury WJ, Folks TM, et al. Tumor necrosis factor α activates human immunodeficiency virus type 1 through induction of nuclear factor binding to the NF-kB sites in the long terminal repeat. Microbiology 1989;86:5974.

208. Poli G, Kinter A, Justement JS, et al. Tumor necrosis factor α functions in an autocrine manner in the induction of human immunodeficiency virus expression. Immunology 1990;87:782.

209. Osborn L, Kunkel S, Nabel GJ. Tumor necrosis factor α and interleukin 1 stimulate the human immunodeficiency virus enhancer by activation of the nuclear factor kB. Proc Natl Acad Sci USA 1989;86:2336.

210. Fiorelli V, Genelman R, Samaniego F, Markham PD, Ensoli B. Cytokines from activated T cells induce normal endothelial cells to acquire the phenotypic and functional features of AIDS-Kaposi's sarcoma spindle cells. J Clin Invest 1995;95:1723.

211. Samaniego R, Markah P, Gallo RC, Ensoli B. Inflammatory cytokines induce AIDS-Kaposi's sarcoma-derived spindle cells to produce and release basic fibroblast growth factor and enhance Kaposi's sarcoma-like lesion formation in nude mice. J Immunol 1995;154:3582.

212. Ensoli B, Barillari G, Gallo RC. Cytokines and growth factors in the pathogenesis of AIDS-associated Kaposi's sarcoma. Immunol Rev 1992;127:147,1992.

213. Pollack MS, Safai B, DuPont B. HLA-DR5 and DR2 are susceptibility factors for acquired immunodeficiency syndrome with Kaposi's sarcoma in different ethnic subpopulations. Dis Markers 1983;1:135.

214. Safai B, Mike V, Giraldo G, et al. Association of Kaposi's sarcoma with second primary malignancies. Cancer 1980;45:1472.

215. Pollack MS, et al. Frequencies of HLA and Gm immunogenetic markers in Kaposi's sarcoma. Tissue Antigens 1983;21:1.

216. Pollack MS, Mastrota F, Robinson H, et al. Lymphocytotoxic antibodies to non-HLA antigens with sera of patients with acquired immune deficiency syndrome (AIDS). In: Liss AR, ed. Proceedings of the meeting on non-HLA antigens in health, aging, and malignancy. Roswell Park Memorial Institute, Buffalo, NY, March 28 and 29, 1983.

217. Prince HE, et al. HLA studies in acquired immune deficiency syndrome patients with Kaposi's sarcoma. J Clin Immunol 1984;4:242.

218. Papasteriades C, et al. Histocompatibility antigens HLA-A, B, DR in Greek patients with Kaposi's sarcoma. Tissue Antigens 1984;24:313.

219. Marinig C, et al. Immunologic and immunogenetic features of primary Kaposi's sarcoma. Cancer 1985;55:1899.

220. Friedman-Kien AE, at al. Disseminated Kaposi's sarcoma in homosexual men. Ann Intern Med 1982;96:693.

221. Mann DL, et al. HLA antigen frequencies in HIV-1 related Kaposi's sarcoma. J Acquir Immune Defic Syndr 1990;3(Suppl 1):S551.

222. Brunson ME, et al. HLA and Kaposi's sarcoma in solid organ transplantation. Hum Immunol 1990;29:56.

223. Lifson AR, et al. Kaposi's sarcoma among homosexual and bisexual men enrolled in the San Francisco City Clinic Cohort Study. J Acquir Immune Defic Syndr 1990;3(Suppl 1):S32.

224. Beral V, et al. Risk of Kaposi's sarcoma and sexual practices associated with faecal contact in homosexual or bisexual men with AIDS. Lancet 1992;339:632.

225. Safai B, Peralta H, Menzies K, et al. Kaposi's sarcoma among HIV-seronegative high risk population. Seventh International Conference on AIDS. Florence, Italy, June 1991.

226. Friedman-Kien AE, Saltzman BR, Cao Y, et al. Kaposi's sarcoma in HIV-negative homosexual men. Lancet 1990;335:168.

227. Giraldo G, et al. Kaposi's sarcoma: a new model in the search for viruses associated with human malignancies. J Natl Cancer Inst 1972;49:1495.

228. Giraldo G, et al. Herpes-type virus particles in tissue culture of Kaposi's sarcoma from different geographic regions. J Natl Cancer Inst 1972;49:1509.

229. Giraldo G, et al. Kaposi's sarcoma and its relationship to cytomegalovirus (CMV) III. CMV-DNA and CMV early antigen in Kaposi's sarcoma. Int J Cancer 1980;26:23.

230. Boldogh L, et al. Kaposi's sarcoma. IV: Detection of CMV DNA, CMV RNA and CMNA in tumor biopsies. Int J Cancer 1981;28:469.

231. McDougal JK, et al. HSV, CMV and HPV in human neoplasia. J Invest Dermatol 1984;83:72s.

232. Siegal B, et al. Kaposi's sarcoma in immunosuppression. Possibly the result of a dual viral infection. Cancer 1990;65:492.

233. Ioachim HL, Dorsett B, Melamed J, Adsay V, Santagada EA. Cytomegalovirus, angiomatosis, and Kaposi's sarcoma: new observations of a debated relationship [see comments]. Mod Pathol 1992;5:169.

234. Siddiqui A. Hepatitis B virus DNA in Kaposi's sarcoma. Proc Natl Acad Sci USA 1983;80:4861.

235. Nickoloff BJ, et al. Immunohistochemical detection of papillomavirus antigens in Kaposi's sarcoma. Lancet 1992;339:548.

236. Huang YQ, Li JJ, Rush MG. HPV-16–related DNA sequences in Kaposi's sarcoma. Lancet 1992;339:515.

237. Biggar RJ, Dunsmore N, Kurman RJ, et al. Failure to detect human papillomavirus in Kaposi's sarcoma. (Letter; comment) Lancet 1992;339:1604.

238. Stoica G, et al. Moloney murine sarcoma virus 349 induces Kaposi's sarcoma-like lesions in Babl/c mice. Am J Pathol 1990;136:933.

239. Dictor M. Jarplid B. The case of Kaposi's sarcoma. J Am Acad Dermatol 1988;18:398.

240. Rappersberger K, et al. Demonstration of (im)mature Oncovirinae in tumour cells from patients with Mediterranean and classic Kaposi's sarcoma. Arch Dermatol Res 1991;283:58.

241. Gyorkey F, et al. retroviruses in Kaposi's sarcoma cells in AIDS. N Engl J Med 1984;311:1183.

242. Schenk P, Konrad K. Ultrastructure of Kaposi's sarcoma in acquired immune deficiency syndrome (AIDS). Arch Otorhinolaryngol 1985;242:305.

243. Schenk P. Retroviruses in Kaposi's sarcoma in acquired immune deficiency syndrome (AIDS). Acta Otolaryngol (Stockh) 1986;202:295.

244. Crovari PC, et al. Kaposi's sarcoma and HTLV-III infection virus-like particles in skin lesions: experimental observations. Virologica 1985;64:352.

245. Gyorkey F, et al. Tubuloreticular structures in Kaposi's sarcoma. Lancet 1982;2:984.

246. Sidhu GS, et al. Ultrastructural markers of AIDS. Lancet 1983;2:990.

247. Kostianovsky M, Grimley PM. Ultrastructural findings in the acquired immunodeficiency syndrome (AIDS). Ultrastruct Pathol 1985;8:123.

248. Orenstein JM, et al. Ultrastructural markers in circulating lymphocytes of subjects at risk for AIDS. Am J Clin Pathol 1985;84:603.

249. Yoffee B, et al. In vivo and in vitro ultrastructural alterations induced by human immunodeficiency virus in human lymphoid cells. Lab Invest 1989;61:303.

250. Luu J, et al. Tubuloreticular structures and cylindrical confronting cisternae: a review. Hum Pathol 1989;20:617.

251. Marquart KH, Philip M. Tubuloreticular structures in classic Kaposi's sarcoma. Ultrastruct Pathol 1988;12:255.

252. Bowden FJ, et al. Antibodies to gp41 and nef in otherwise HIV-negative homosexual men with Kaposi's sarcoma. Lancet 1991;337:1313.

253. Chang Y, Cesarman E, Pessin MS, Lee F, Culpepper J, Knowles D, Moore PS. Identification of herpesvirus-like DNA sequence in AIDS-associated Kaposi's sarcoma. Science 1994;266:1865.

254. Huang YQ, Li JJ, Kaplan MH, et al. Human herpesvirus-like nucleic acid in various forms of Kaposi's sarcoma. Lancet 1995;345:759.

255. Jones JL, Hanson DL, Chu SY, Wand J, Jaffe HW. AIDS-associated Kaposi's sarcoma. (Letter) Lancet 1995;345:759.

256. Ambrogiak JA, Blackbourne DJ, Herndier BQ, et al. Herpes-like sequences in HIV-infected and uninfected Kaposi's sarcoma patients. Science 1995;268:582.

257. Moore PS, Chang Y. Detection of herpesvirus-like NA sequences in Kaposi's sarcoma in patients with and those without HIV infection. N Engl J Med 1995;332:1181.

258. Su I-J, Hsu Y-S, Chang Y-C, Wang I-W. Herpesvirus-like DNA sequence in Kaposi's sarcoma from AIDS and non-AIDS patients, in Taiwan. Lancet 1995;345:722.

259. Cesarman E, Chang Y, Moore PS, Said JW, Knowles DE. Kaposi's sarcoma-associated herpesvirus-like DNA sequences in AIDS-related body-cavity-based lymphomas. N Engl J Med 1995;332:1186.

260. Boudreaux AA, Smith LL, Cosby CD, Bason MM, Tappero JW, Berger TG. Intralesional vinblastine for cutaneous Kaposi's sarcoma associated with acquired immunodeficiency syndrome. A clinical trial to evaluate efficacy and discomfort associated with infection. J Am Acad Dermatol 1993;28:61.

261. Nisce L, Safai B. Radiation therapy of Kaposi's sarcoma in AIDS. Front Radiat Ther Oncol 1985;19:126.

262. Le Bourgeois JP, Frikha H, Piedbois P, Le Pechoux C, Martin L, Haddad E. Radiotherapy in the management of epidemic Kaposi's sarcoma of the oral cavity, the eyelid and the genitals. Radiother Oncol 1994;30:263.

263. Stelzer KJ, Griffin TW. A randomized prospective trial of radiation therapy for AIDS-associated Kaposi's sarcoma. Int J Radiat Oncol Biol Phys 1993;27:1057.

264. Cooper JS, Steinfeld AD, Lerch I. Intentions and outcomes in the radiotherapeutic management of epidemic Kaposi's sarcoma. Int J Radiat Oncol Biol Phys 1991;20:422.

265. Langtry JA, Bottomley DM, Phillips RH, Staughton RC. The infra-red coagulator in the treatment of AIDS-related Kaposi's sarcoma and a comparison with radiotherapy. Clin Exp Dermatol 1994;19:23.

266. Lucatorto FM, Sapp JP. Treatment of oral Kaposi's sarcoma with a sclerosing agent in AIDS patients. A preliminary study. Oral Surg Oral Med Oral Pathol 1993;75:192.

267. Newman SB. Treatment of epidemic Kaposi's sarcoma (KS) with intralesional vinblastine injection (IL-VBL). Proc Annu Meet Am Soc Clin Oncol 1988;7:A19.

268. Trattner A, Reizis Z, David M, Ingber A, Hagler J, Sandbank M. The therapeutic effect of intralesional interferon in classical Kaposi's sarcoma. Br J Dermatol 1993;129:590.

269. DeWys WD, Curran J, Henle W, Johnson G. Workshop on Kaposi's sarcoma: meeting report. Cancer Treat Rep 1982;66:1387.

270. Laubenstein LJ, Krigel RL, Odajnyk CM, et al. Treatment of epidemic Kaposi's sarcoma with etoposide of a combination of doxorubicin, bleomycin, and vincristine. J Clin Oncol 1984;2:1115.

271. Volberding PA, Abrams DI, Conant M, et al. Vinblastine therapy for Kaposi's sarcoma in the acquired immunodeficiency syndrome. Ann Intern Med 1985;103:335.

272. Gelmann E, Longo D, Lane H, et al. Combination chemotherapy of disseminated Kaposi's sarcoma in patients with the acquired immune deficiency syndrome. Am J Med 1987;82:456.

273. Minzter D, Real F, Jovino F, et al. Treatment of Kaposi's sarcoma and thrombocytopenia with vincristine in patients with the acquired immunodeficiency syndrome. Ann Intern Med 1985;102:200, 1985

274. Kaplan L, Abrams D, Volberding P. Treatment of Kaposi's sarcoma in acquired immunodeficiency syndrome with an alternating vincristine-vinblastine regimen. Cancer Treat Rep 1986;70:1121.

275. Wernz J, Laubenstein L, Hymes K, et al. Chemotherapy and assessment of response in epidemic Kaposi's sarcoma (EKS) with bleomycin and velbane. (Abstract) Proc Am Soc Clin Oncol 1986;5:4.

276. Minor R, Brayes T. Velban and methotrexate combination chemotherapy for epidemic Kaposi's sarcoma. (Abstract) Proc Am Soc Clin Oncol 1986;5:1.

277. Gill PS, Rarick M, Bernstein-Singer M. Treatment of advanced Kaposi's sarcoma using a combination of bleomycin and vincristine. Am J Oncol 1990;13:315.

278. Gill PS, Rarick M, McCutchan LA, et al. Systemic treatment of AIDS-related Kaposi's sarcoma: results of a randomized trail. Am J Med 1991;90:427.

279. Glaspy J, Miles S, McCarthy S, et al. Treatment of advanced stage Kaposi's sarcoma with vincristine and bleomycin. (Abstract) Proc Am Soc Clin Oncol 1986;5:3.

280. Krigel RL, Slywotzky VW, Lonberg M, et al. Treatment of epidemic Kaposi's sarcoma with a combination of interferon-alpha 2b and etoposide. J Biol Response Mod 1988;7:359.

281. Brambilla L, Fossati S, Boneschi V, Clerici M. Oral etoposide verses parenteral vinblastine in chemotherapy for Kaposi's sarcoma. (Abstract) Fourth European Conference on Clinical Oncology and Cancer Nursing, Nov 1–4, 1987.

282. Krown SE, Real FX, Cunningham-Rundles S, et al. Preliminary observations on the effect of recombinant leukocyte A interferon in homosexual men with Kaposi's sarcoma. N Engl J Med 1983; 308:1071.

283. Real FX, Oettgen HF, Krown SE. Kaposi's sarcoma and the acquired immunodeficiency syndrome: treatment with high and low doses of recombinant leukocyte A interferon. J Clin Oncol 1986;4:544.

284. Krown SE, Gold JWM, Real FX, et al. Interferon alpha-2a ± vinblastine (VLB) in AIDS-associated Kaposi's sarcoma (KS/AIDS): therapeutic activity, toxicity and effects on HTLV-III/LAV viremia. (Abstract) J Interferon Res 1986;6:3.

285. Groopman JE, Gottlieb MS, Goodman J, et al. Recombinant alpha-2 interferon therapy for Kaposi's sarcoma associated with acquired immunodeficiency syndrome. Ann Intern Med 1984;100:671.

286. Volberding PA, Mitsuyasu RT, Golando JP, Spiegel RJ. Treatment of Kaposi's sarcoma with interferon alpha-2b (intron A). Cancer 1987;59:620.

287. Gelmann EP, Preble OT, Steis R, et al. Human lymphoblastoid interferon treatment of Kaposi's sarcoma in the acquired immune deficiency syndrome. Clinical response and prognostic parameters. Am J Med 1985;78:737.

288. Rios A, Mansell PWA, Newell GA, et al. Treatment of acquired immunodeficiency syndrome-related Kaposi's sarcoma with lymphoblastoid interferon. J Clin Oncol 1985;3:506.

289. Fischl M, Lucas S, Gorowski E, et al. Interferon alfa-N1 Welferon (WFN) in Kaposi's sarcoma: single agent of combination with vinblastine (VBL). (Abstract) J Interferon Res 1986;6(Suppl 1):4.

290. Schaart FM, Bratzke B, Ruszczak Z, et al. Long-term therapy of HIV-associated Kaposi's sarcoma with recombinant interferon α-2a. Br J Dermatol 1991;124:62.

291. Krown SE, Gold JWM, Niedzwiecki D, et al. Interferon-α with zidovudine: safety, tolerance, and clinical and virologic effects in patients with Kaposi's sarcoma associated with the acquired immunodeficiency syndrome (AIDS). Ann Intern Med 1990;112:812.

292. De Wit R, Danner SA, Bakker JM, et al. Combined zidovudine and interferon-alpha treatment in patients with AIDS-associated Kaposi's sarcoma. J Intern Med 1991;229:35.

293. Fischl MA, Uttamchandani, RB, Resnick L, et al. A phase I study of recombinant human interferon-α_{2a} or human lymphoblastoid interferon-α_{n1} and concomitant zidovudine in patients with AIDS-related Kaposi's sarcoma. J Acquir Immune Defic Syndr 1991;4:1.

294. Gill PS, Harrington W Jr, Kaplan MH, et al. Treatment of adult cell leukemia-lymphoma with a combination of interferon alpha and zidovudine. N Engl J Med 1995;332:1744.

295. Guo WX, Gill PS, Antakly T. Inhibition of AIDS-Kaposi's sarcoma cell proliferation following retinoic acid receptor activation. Cancer Res 1995;55:823.

296. Corbeil J, Rapaport E, Rihmann DD, Looney DJ. Antiproliferative effect of retinoid compounds on Kaposi's sarcoma cells. J Clin Invest 1994;93:1981.

297. Gill PS, Espina BM, Moudgil T, et al. All-*trans* retinoic acid for the treatment of AIDS-related Kaposi's sarcoma; results of a pilot phase II study. Leukemia 1994;8(Suppl 3):S26.

298. Bogner JR, Kronawitter U, Rolinski B, Truebenbach K, Goebel FD. Liposomal doxorubicin in the treatment of advanced AIDS-related Kaposi sarcoma. J Acquir Immune Defic Syndr 1994;7:463.

299. James ND, Coker RJ, Tomlinson D, et al. Liposomal doxorubicin (Doxil); an effective new treatment for Kaposi's sarcoma in AIDS. Clin Oncol R Coll Radiol 1994;6:294.

300. Albini A, Fontanini G, Masiello L, et al. Angiogenic potential in vivo by Kaposi's sarcoma cell-free supernatants and HIV-1 tat product: inhibition of KS-like lesions by tissue inhibitor of metalloproteinase-2. AIDS 1994;8:1237.

301. Benelli R, Datia R, Ensoli B, Stetler-Stevenson WG, Santi L, Albini A. Inhibition of AIDS-associated Kaposi's sarcoma cell induced vascular cell invasion by TIMP-2 an synthetic peptide from the metalloproteinase pre-propeptide: implication for an anti-angiogenic therapy. Oncol Res 1994;6:251.

302. Pluda JM, Shay LE, Foli A, et al. Administration of pentosan polysulfate to patients with human immunodeficiency virus-associated Kaposi's sarcoma. J Natl Cancer Inst 1993;85:1585.

303. Carmeli Y, Mevorach D, Kaminski N, Raz E. Regression of Kaposi's sarcoma after intravenous immunoglobulin treatment for polymyositis. Cancer 1994;73:2859.

304. Corbeil J, Richman DD, Wrasidlo W, Nicolaou KC, Looney DJ. Antiproliferative effects of enediynes on AIDS-derived Kaposi's sarcoma. Cancer Res 1994;54:4270.

305. Alonso K, Pontiggia P, Sabato A, et al. Systemic hyperthermia in the treatment of HIV-related disseminated Kaposi's sarcoma. Long-term follow-up of patients treated with low-flow extracorporeal perfusion hyperthermia. Am J Clin Oncol 1994;17:353.

306. Alonso K, Pontiggia P, Nardi C, Sabato A, Cuppone Curto F. Systemic hyperthermia in the treatment of HIV-related Kaposi's sarcoma. A phase 1 study. Biomed Pharmacother 1992;46:21.

307. Masood R, Lunardi Iskandar Y, Jean LF, et al. Inhibition of AIDS-associated Kaposi's sarcoma cell growth by DAB389-interleukin 6. AIDS Res Hum Retroviruses 1994;10:969.

308. Nakamura S, Sakurada S, Salahuddin SZ, et al. Inhibition of development of Kaposi's sarcoma-related lesions by a bacterial cell wall complex [see comments]. Science 1992;255:1437.

309. Ensoli B, Markham P, Kao V, et al. Block of AIDS-Kaposi's sarcoma (KS) cell growth, angiogenesis and lesion formation in nude mice by antisense oligonucleotide targeting basic fibroblast growth factor: a novel strategy for the therapy of KS. J Clin Invest 1994;94:1736.

AIDS: Biology, Diagnosis, Treatment and Prevention, fourth edition, edited by Vincent T. DeVita, Jr., Samuel Hellman, and Steven A. Rosenberg. Lippincott–Raven Publishers, © 1997

15.2

Lymphomas and Other Cancers Associated With Acquired Immunodeficiency Syndrome

David M. Aboulafia and Ronald T. Mitsuyasu

In 1981, Gottlieb and colleagues detailed the development of *Pneumocystis carinii* pneumonia (PCP) and mucosal candidiasis in young homosexual men with profound defects in humoral and cell-mediated immunity.[1] Subsequently, the high frequency of lymphoma among patients with acquired immunodeficiency syndrome (AIDS) was identified in the publication of a large number of cases, and the importance of this phenomenon was ultimately acknowledged by the inclusion of specific types of high-grade non-Hodgkin's lymphoma (NHL) in the 1985 U.S. Center for Disease Control and Prevention (CDC) revised definition of AIDS.[2] Although other tumors, most notably Hodgkin's disease, have been suggested to be human immunodeficiency virus (HIV) related, only Kaposi's sarcoma and carcinoma of the uterine cervix are included in the surveillance definition of AIDS.

HIV-associated malignancies are similar to cancers seen in other acquired or congenital immunodeficiencies, although some information suggests a unique but indirect role for HIV in the pathogenesis of these malignancies. Studies of HIV-associated cancer provide an opportunity to define mechanisms for the development of neoplasia in acquired immunodeficiency states. Because AIDS is not yet a curable condition, therapeutic efforts are implemented to lengthen survival and improve functional status. As opportunistic infections yield to newer strategies in prophylaxis and treatment, further improvements in the therapy of AIDS malignancies will depend on knowledge derived from clinical trials that integrate antiretroviral therapy with antineoplastic drugs, hematopoietic growth factors, and novel agents that offer the promise of reconstituting a compromised immune system.

Accurate tools to measure financial costs, toxicity, and quality of life are assuming increasing importance in this era of shrinking medical resources and data-based decision making. Treatment must therefore also take into account other non–tumor-related factors, such as degree of immunologic impairment, the stage of HIV infection, and the usual criteria of histology and tumor stage.

This chapter explores the epidemiology, pathogenesis, and therapy of HIV-associated peripheral NHL. We also discuss briefly other cancers seen in AIDS, including primary central nervous system (CNS) lymphoma, Hodgkin's disease, cervical cancer, and anorectal carcinoma.

IMMUNODEFICIENCY AND MALIGNANCY

The emergence of NHL and Kaposi's sarcoma as the two most common and characteristic malignancies of AIDS was not surprising, because the association of with various other states of congenital and acquired immune deficiency had been documented for several decades.[3] For example, organ transplant recipients on long-term immunosuppression therapy to prevent graft rejection have more than 100 times the incidence of NHL than those in an age-matched population.[4] Kaposi's sarcoma is most common in patients with iatrogenic immunosuppression; it is 150 to 500 times more common in kidney transplant recipients than in the general population. Reports of Kaposi's sarcoma lesions and lymphomas spontaneously regressing when immunosuppression is reduced or eliminated underscores the importance of immune surveillance in inhibiting carcinogenesis.[5,6]

Studies have shown impaired cell-mediated immunity to be a risk factor for anogenital cancer. Immunosuppressed

David M. Aboulafia, Section of Hematology and Oncology, Virginia Mason Clinic, P.O. Box 900 (C2-S), Seattle, WA 98111.

Ronald T. Mitsuyasu, UCLA Care Center, BH-412 Le Conte Avenue, Los Angeles, CA 190024-1793.

organ transplant recipients have a 100-fold increase in the incidence of vulvar and anal carcinomas and a 144-fold increase in the incidence of cervical carcinoma compared with controls. The prevalence of human papillomavirus (HPV) infection is 5 to 17 times greater in these patients than in the general population.[7,8] An increased incidence of malignancy also is observed in patients with autoimmune diseases, as documented in patients with Sjögren's syndrome, Hashimoto's thyroiditis, rheumatoid arthritis, and sarcoidosis.[9–11]

Why immunosuppressed individuals are particularly prone to specific neoplasms remains a vexing question. Among patients with the X-linked lymphoproliferative syndrome, a congenital disorder characterized by uncontrolled B-cell proliferation after an initial exposure to Epstein-Barr virus (EBV) infection, male infants have roughly a 50% risk of developing fulminant NHL before the age of 3 years, presumably because of a defect in T-cell regulation of EBV-stimulated B-cell clones.[12] If the predilection to NHL and Kaposi's sarcoma were attributable only to compromised immunologic surveillance, a variety of neoplasms would be expected to appear. In the setting of HIV infection, in particular, there are multiple factors favoring the emergence of cancers, including chronic and protracted defects in cellular and humoral immunity.

EPIDEMIOLOGY

The incidence of NHL in the United States is growing, perhaps because of an increased exposure to a variety of agents, including benzene and herbicides.[13–15] Superimposed on this underlying trend, it was expected that increased numbers of AIDS-related NHLs would be diagnosed as patients with AIDS live longer because of better supportive strategies. This supposition has proven true and is best reflected in the San Francisco linkage study, which assessed cancer risk among AIDS patients during the period 1980 to 1987.[16] Relative to pre-epidemic levels of NHL (1973–1977), the observed number of cases of NHL among the homosexual AIDS cohort was 97-fold greater than expected. In San Francisco and New York City, the risk has been estimated to be 100 times greater than that seen in the general population.[17,18] This devastating complication of immunodeficiency is an important factor limiting survival in approximately 8% to 10% of all HIV-infected individuals who develop NHL. Unlike Kaposi's sarcoma, however, this risk if not confined primarily to homosexuals. NHL affects the various HIV transmission categories approximately equally, and the clinical and pathologic spectrum of disease appears similar among drug users, homosexuals, hemophiliacs, heterosexuals, and transfusion recipients.[19,20] This finding suggests that environmental cofactors are probably less important in the cause of NHL than Kaposi's sarcoma and makes identification of preventive strategies more difficult.

Similar examples of secular trends in NHL rates were reported in an updated study of a relatively small cohort of patients with severe HIV infection who received prolonged antiretroviral therapy and in a cohort of hemophilia patients. In the former, the frequency of NHL among long-term survivors who participated in zidovudine (AZT) or dideoxyinosine clinical trials at the National Institutes of Health (NIH) was 8% 2 years after starting therapy and 29% at 3 years, with no significant differences seen between the two antiretrovirals.[21] An earlier report from the NIH suggesting that the incidence and clinical manifestations of NHL were different in this group compared with HIV cohorts who were antiretroviral naive has not been confirmed with additional follow-up.[22] Among hemophilia patients, 14 cases of NHL were reported in a group of 1295, for an overall incidence of 0.16 per hundred person-years, more than a 36-fold increase.[23] In an overlapping cohort of HIV-infected hemophiliacs, the incidence of NHL increased exponentially as the duration of HIV infection was extended, with the risk doubling every 2.4 years.[24] This finding is consistent with a previous report showing that the risk of peripheral NHL appears more intimately related to duration of HIV infection rather than to CD4+ level.[25]

Based on data collected from the National Cancer Institute, it is estimated that between 8% and 27% of the approximately 40,000 cases of NHL diagnosed yearly in the United States are HIV related.[26] This contrasts with the findings of the CDC, which described a 3% incidence of NHL among the first 100,000 patients reported with AIDS, a figure that probably underestimated the incidence of NHL because lymphoma was not an AIDS-defining illness until 1985 and because CDC reporting requires only the first AIDS diagnosis, potentially missing 25% of NHL occurring as a second or later AIDS diagnosis.[27,28]

PATHOGENESIS

Although several models have been proposed, the pathogenesis and reason for the high incidence of NHL in AIDS remains incompletely understood. It was initially presumed that HIV was a transforming retrovirus whose presence was requisite for the development of NHL. However, results of subsequent molecular studies indicate HIV is rarely involved directly in B-cell oncogenesis. More apparent is the great molecular heterogeneity that exists among AIDS-related NHLs. Specific characteristics that distinguish the various subtypes include monoclonal or polyclonal origin of the lymphoma, presence or absence in lymphoma cells of EBV genome or *MYC* rearrangements, and type of immunoglobulin gene rearrangements. The role of cytokines and tumor suppressor genes in promoting and maintaining uncontrolled B-cell growth and differentiation are additional areas of active research.

The foundation for molecular studies of AIDS-related NHL stems from information garnered during tumor analyses of samples from patients with non–HIV-associated Burkitt's lymphoma. Elegant genetic probe studies have demonstrated activation of the *MYC* (c-*myc*) oncogene on chromosome 8 by chromosomal translocation to immuno-globulin encoding regions in these B-cell neoplasms on chromosomes 14, 2 or 22, with subtle differences in site of translocation distinguishing the endemic African variant from the sporadic pleomorphic variant typically seen in the United States. This suggests different mechanisms of patho-genesis.[29]

In roughly 50% to 80% of AIDS-associated Burkitt's lymphomas, similar chromosomal changes of the sporadic type are found.[30,31] The high frequency of rearranged MYC genes appears primarily confined to the Burkitt's (small, non-cleaved cell) histology. In one study, MYC rearrange-ments were seen in 100% of Burkitt's cases but in only 33% or fewer of large cell or immunoblastic cases.[32] In another study, only 15% of large cell lymphomas collected from AIDS patients showed evidence of MYC rearrangements, but roughly 50% of the Burkitt's-like lymphomas possessed MYC rearrangements.[33]

Pelicci and colleagues provided the clearest evidence for a multistep progression to lymphoma involving MYC rearrangement.[34] They described oligoclonal B-cell expan-sions in hyperplastic lymph nodes from patients with HIV disease and MYC rearrangements only after lymphoma developed. In this model, EBV mitogenically stimulates oligoclonal B-cell proliferation, and only after MYC activa-tion does a tumor develop. Therefore, translocation leading to MYC rearrangement may play a critical role in the patho-genesis of HIV-associated NHL, predominantly those of the Burkitt's lymphoma subset.

Immune suppression, EBV infection, polyclonal B-cell activation, and aberrant B-cell regulation are of central importance in the development of epidemic Burkitt's lym-phoma and in NHL occurring in individuals with congenital or iatrogenically induced immune suppression.[35-37] HIV-infected persons are prone to EBV infections, have a pro-found defect in T-cell immunity to EBV, and possess abnormally high numbers of circulating EBV-infected B cells.[38] The role of EBV in EBV-associated lymphomagene-sis therefore has been the subject of much investigation. The principal hypothesis advanced by various groups is that, in the setting of HIV-induced immunodeficiency, EBV infec-tion results in polyclonal stimulation and immortalization of B-cell clones.[34,39,40] Such clones are presumably predisposed to MYC gene rearrangements, resulting in the development of a fully transformed EBV-containing monoclonal B-cell NHL. Findings cited to bolster this hypothesis include the presence of monoclonal or oligoclonal B-cell populations infected with EBV in the lymph nodes of patients with per-sistent, generalized lymphadenopathy and the concomitant occurrence or subsequent development of EBV-containing NHL.[34,41] This hypothesis is further supported by studies demonstrating that the introduction of an activated MYC gene into EBV-infected lymphoblasts obtained from HIV-infected persons leads to their malignant conversion.[42]

Possibly conflicting with this model is the finding that a substantial number of the AIDS-related NHLs do not show evidence of EBV genome detection. EBV-positive tumors are more likely to be immunoblastic phenotype. Only 30% to 50% of Burkitt's lymphomas have EBV genome sequence present.[31,32,43] When no etiologic evidence of EBV is present, it is possible that bacterial, fungal, or viral agents cause chronic antigenic stimulation and, in a comparable fashion to EBV, make the risk of chromosomal translocations, immunoglobulin gene rearrangements, and ultimately growth of NHL more likely.[44]

McGrath and colleagues have emphasized that a wide histologic and molecular spectrum of HIV-associated lym-phoma exists. They identified six distinct molecular subsets of aggressive B-cell lymphomas among 40 AIDS-associ-ated NHL tumor specimens, based on studies of tumor clonality, EBV genome presence, and MYC arrangements (Table 15.2-1).[45] In 43% of these tumors, no clonal rearrangements were identified, signifying that polyclonal lymphoproliferations are occurring in a significant propor-tion. The precise frequency of polyclonal lymphoprolifera-tive processes will require additional study, because not all investigators have been able to document significant num-bers among HIV-tumor specimens.[44,46-48] Like the polyclonal lymphoproliferations occurring in the setting of iatrogenic immunosuppression, HIV polyclonal lymphomas may have an aggressive clinical course. Unlike their transplant coun-terparts, EBV infection and MYC gene rearrangements are notably absent.

Heightened cytokine production in response to HIV infection (and perhaps to other viruses) may also contribute to the development of lymphomas in AIDS. Of the many lymphohematopoietic growth factors released under normal and virus-perturbed conditions, interleukin-6 (IL-6) is a potent stimulator of B-cell proliferation.[48] Monocytes obtained from HIV-infected patients express high levels of IL-6, and Emile and associates reported that IL-6 was local-ized to the lymphoma-associated macrophages.[49,50] In analo-gous fashion to how IL-6 may drive through paracrine and autocrine loops B-cell proliferation in multiple myeloma and Castleman's disease, IL-6 interaction with lymphoma-

TABLE 15.2-1. *Molecular classification of HIV non-Hodgkin's lymphoma*

Molecular Class	Number of Cases (%)	Clonality	Presence EBV Genome	MYC Rearrangement
1	14 (35)	Polyclonal	–	–
2	3 (8)	Polyclonal	+	–
3	4 (10)	Monoclonal	–	–
4	10 (25)	Monoclonal	+	–
5	7 (18)	Monoclonal	–	+
6	2 (5)	Monoclonal	+	+

EBV, Ebstein-Barr virus; +, yes; –, no.
Adapted from Shiramizu B, Herndier B, Meeker T, et al. Molecular and immunophenotypic characterization of AIDS-associated Epstein-Barr virus negative, polyclonal lymphoma. J Clin Oncol 1992;10:383.

associated IL-6 receptors may drive subsets of HIV-associated lymphoma. Data linking IL-6 to the pathogenesis of AIDS-related NHL may also be seen in the study conducted by Pluda and coworkers, who found elevated IL-6 levels in patients with symptomatic HIV infection.[21]

In addition to mechanisms that directly stimulate B-cell expansion, suppression of helper T-cell antiviral or cytotoxic surveillance activities can permit the establishment of malignant clones.[51] Interleukin-10 (IL-10), also known as cytokine synthesis inhibiting factor, is a suppressor of T-cell function and has been implicated in the development of AIDS-related NHL.[52,53] Excess IL-10 may permit viral replication (particularly EBV and possibly HIV) to go unchecked, promoting the cascade of events culminating in the establishment of a clonal B-cell malignancy. Although the actual steps and factors responsible for malignant transformation are not well understood, it appears to be a multistep process that necessitates activation of protooncogenes such as *MYC* in almost one half of patients with AIDS-related NHLs. The production of various cytokines may also favor the manufacture of growth factors, stimulating B-cell proliferation and differentiation.

Occasionally, oncogenic alterations and retroviral proteins may contribute to AIDS-related NHL lymphomagenesis. *P53* and *BCL6* rearrangement mutations have been observed in a relatively high frequency in HIV-associated NHLs.[32,54,56] Alterations in their tumor suppressor function could result in increased genomic instability and changes in cell cycle interactions. Shiramizu and colleagues described four cases of large cell lymphomas in which cells expressed large amounts of HIV antigen p24, and HIV integration was found in the same region of the cellular genome upstream to the oncogene *FES/FPS*.[57] Several mechanisms by which the insertions could be causing cell transformation have been proposed: the provirus could cause an insertional mutation which is upregulating the oncogene; the retrovirus could have acquired an oncogene before insertion and introduced it into the cell's genome; the insertion could have produced a mutation in a regulatory gene, causing cellular transformation; or the HIV virus, possibly a particular variant of the virus, may have properties that cause cell transformation by itself.

PATHOLOGIC AND CLINICAL MANIFESTATIONS

Approximately 90% of NHLs in patients with HIV are of B-cell origin. Large cell immunoblastic lymphoma is the most common histologic subtype, representing more than 60% of AIDS-defining NHL diagnoses, and small, non-cleaved cell (Burkitt's-like) lymphoma represents approximately 20%.[58,59] The predominance of Burkitt's and immunoblastic lymphoma is especially noteworthy in HIV patients, because these lymphomas make up only 10% of all NHLs seen in the general population. The remaining tumors are mainly large cell and diffuse lymphomas of intermediate grades. Low-grade B-cell NHL and T-cell phenotypes are

rarely encountered in patients with HIV and are not considered to be AIDS-defining illnesses.[60–62] Their natural history appears to be largely unaffected by the patient's underlying immune status.

Most systemic AIDS-related NHLs express monotypic surface immunoglobulin or B-cell–associated antigens (eg, CD19, CD20, CD22) and generally lack T-cell–associated antigens.[39,58] Such immunophenotypes resemble morphologically similar lymphomas seen in the non–HIV-infected population. A minority of AIDS-related NHLs that preferentially involve body cavities exhibit an indeterminate immunophenotype, characterized by lack of surface immunoglobulin and B-cell–associated antigens, but they express leukocyte common antigen and various antigens associated with activation and late stages of B-cell differentiation.[39,63,64]

Extranodal sites of disease at time of diagnosis are typical of AIDS-related NHL; they are reported in 60% to 95% of patients and are the only site of disease in as many as one third of patients.[58,59,65] This contrasts with non–HIV-associated lymphomas, because approximately 40% of these patients present with extranodal involvement. The CNS is a frequent extranodal site of involvement at presentation and may involve the brain parenchyma as the only site of disease (ie, primary CNS lymphoma) or the leptomeninges. Primary CNS lymphomas are principally immunoblastic or large cell malignancies, unlike the Burkitt's subtype, and are associated with EBV in almost 100% of tested cases.[66,67] Other common extranodal sites include the bone marrow (33%), the gastrointestinal tract (27%), and the liver (9%).[58–60,65,68] Numerous reviews and case reports detail the occurrence of NHL in unusual extranodal sites, including the heart and pericardium, conjunctiva, and popliteal fossa. The disease, therefore, should be considered in a variety of clinical circumstances.

PROGNOSTIC FACTORS AND CLINICAL EVALUATION

Several factors have been shown to imply an ominous prognosis in the patient with AIDS-related NHL, including an absolute CD4+ lymphocyte count of less than 200/mm^3; bone marrow involvement; Karnofsky performance status of less than 70%; stage IV disease; and a history of AIDS before the diagnosis of NHL. In one study, Levine and associates showed that patients with none of these poor-risk prognostic factors survived for 11.3 months, compared with 4 months for patients with any combination of poor prognostic factors.[69] At San Francisco General, the most powerful prognostic factor reported was the CD4+ lymphocyte count. Patients with CD4+ counts of 200/mm^3 or greater survived, on average, for 24 months.[59]

The prognostic importance of tumor histology and serum lactate dehydrogenase levels are not as clearly defined.[68] In an intriguing study that will require additional confirmation, Kaplan and colleagues found that the molecular characteristics of the tumors themselves may also be important predictors of clinical outcome.[70] Polyclonal proliferations without EBV DNA sequences correlated strongly with prolonged survival, chemotherapy responsiveness, and higher CD4+ cell count.

Primary CNS lymphoma portends a particularly poor outcome, with a survival time of only 2 to 3 months despite therapy.[66,67,69] Eighty percent of patients who have this devastating complication have evidence of advanced immunosuppression, as reflected by absolute CD4+ lymphocyte count of less than 50/mm^3 and a history of other AIDS-defining infections. Their poor prognosis is indicative of their depleted reserves and the likelihood of developing comorbid and life-threatening infections. In contrast, patients with AIDS-related peripheral NHL develop lymphoma with variable and often well-preserved CD4+ lymphocyte counts.[71] In such instances, the development of leptomeningeal disease is not, in itself, a poor prognostic factor.

The diagnosis of lymphoma is often obscured by the presence of constitutional symptoms related to other nonneoplastic causes. More than 80% of patients with HIV-related NHL have a history of significant weight loss, fevers, and night sweats.[59,65,68] A precipitous and unexplained rise in lactate dehydrogenase concentrations or unusual or suspicious growths occurring in the setting of a rapidly deteriorating clinical course mandate additional evaluation (eg, tissue biopsy). Assorted cultures and special stains may also be required to rule out complicating opportunistic infections. Other tests appropriate for traditional NHL can be applied to HIV-associated NHL. Patients with AIDS-related lymphoma require bone marrow biopsy and computed tomography scans of the chest, abdomen, and pelvis.

Because asymptomatic leptomeningeal disease may be present in as many as 20%, a lumbar puncture is recommended after brain imaging studies have ruled out the presence of a space-occupying CNS lesion.[66] The first dose of intrathecal chemotherapy (ie, methotrexate or cytarabine) is delivered at the time of the staging lumbar puncture, with additional doses given weekly for 1 month.[65]

Because of a high incidence of occult cardiomyopathy in this young population, a cardiac multigated acquisition (MUGA) or echocardiogram should be obtained if anthracycline-based chemotherapy is a consideration. Tests to quantify retroviral loads are commercially available, and although promising, they will require validation in prospective studies before they become part of the routine clinical evaluation of these NHL patients.

TREATMENT

The optimal therapy for AIDS-related NHL has not been determined. Bone marrow depression caused by the direct effects of HIV on marrow progenitor and stromal cells, the toxicity of myelosuppressive drugs (including antiviral drugs), and the effects of chronic infection with *Mycobac-*

terium avium complex and CMV limit patients' abilities to tolerate conventional dosed chemotherapy.[72] Retrospective studies using standard first- and second-generation lymphoma chemotherapy regimens indicate that complete responses are achieved in 17% to 56% of cases, with a 5-month median survival, compared with complete response rates of roughly 55% to 75% and median survivals of greater than 5 years for patients not infected with HIV (Table 15.2-2).[58,68,69,73–78]

Three sentinel studies employing chemotherapy dose-intensive strategies sought to achieve higher and more durable response rates. In the first, Kaplan and collaborators reported 33 patients receiving combination chemotherapy that included high doses of cyclophosphamide and cytarabine.[59] Although complete responses were seen in 58%, median survival was only 5 months. In a multivariate analysis, patients who received more than 1 g/m^2 of cyclophosphamide had a median survival of 4.6 months, compared with 12.2 months for those receiving less than 1 g/m of cyclophosphamide. In the second study, Gill and colleagues attempted to treat patients with a high-dose cytarabine-based regimen but achieved a complete response rate of only 33%.[79] The trial was stopped prematurely when 7 of 9 treated patients developed fatal opportunistic infections. In the third study, investigators from New York University employed the intense ProMACE-MOPP regimen, which also required extensive delays and dose-limiting reductions, resulting in poor complete remissions and shortened survival.[80]

These studies indicate that high-intensity chemotherapy does not necessarily translate into a better outcome. They led to a rethinking of how best to deliver chemotherapy in this compromised patient group. Levine and associates used a dose-attenuated modification of the m-BACOD regimen (less Cytoxan, Adriamycin, and methotrexate), with early CNS prophylaxis consisting of intrathecal cytarabine and initiation of AZT at completion of chemotherapy.[81] With 35 evaluable patients, complete responses were achieved in 46%. The median survival was 6.5 months for all patients and 15 months for complete responders. Hematologic toxicity was moderate, with grade IV neutropenia (absolute neutrophil count <500/mm^3) complicating only 10% of chemotherapy cycles. Despite the use of prophylactic therapy, PCP occurred in roughly 20% of patients, emphasizing the absolute need for vigilance in evaluating fevers, night sweats, and pulmonary symptoms.

On the basis of these results, Walsh and colleagues initiated a phase I trial of the m-BACOD regimen and granulocyte-macrophage colony-stimulating factor (GM-CSF) to determine the optimal dose of m-BACOD combination chemotherapy.[82] A total of 17 patients were treated at three different doses every 3 weeks in conjunction with 20 µg/kg of subcutaneous GM-CSF delivered on days +3 to +13 of each cycle. Eight (50%) of 16 evaluable patients achieved complete remission, including 5 of 8 who received standard-dose m-BACOD. In a randomized trial at San Francisco General, patients receiving standard CHOP chemotherapy

TABLE 15.2-2. *HIV-related non-Hodgkin's Lymphoma: Retrospective Study Results*

Investigation	Evaluable Patients	Predominant Chemotherapy Regimen	Complete Response (%)	Opportunistic Infections (%)	Median Survival (mo)
Knowles[58]	83	COMP + HIDAC	33	NS	5
Kaplan[59]	26	Multiple	46	48	11
Lowenthal[68]	30	Multiple	56	NS	6
Zeigler et al.[73]	66	CHOP ± MTX, VP-16, Bleo	53	33	6
Kalter[74]	14	Multiple	43	NS	NS
Bermudez[75]	12	MACOP-B, CHOP, COP	17	NS	NS
Monfardini[76]	44	CHOP; ProMACE/MOPP	23	NS	4–5
Roithmann[77]	100	CHOP	37	NS	5
Pedersen[78]	33	CHOP/HDMTX	36	NS	5

COMP + HIDAC, cyclophosphamide, vincristine, methotrexate, prednisone, high-dose cytarabine; Multiple, standard first- and second-generation regimens without a majority of patients treated with one specific therapy; CHOP, cyclophosphamide, adriamycin, vincristine, prednisone; MTX, methotrexate; VP-16, etoposide; Bleo, bleomycin; MACOP-B, methotrexate, Adriamycin, cyclophosphamide, vincristine, prednisone, bleomycin; COP, cyclophosphamide, vincristine, prednisone; ProMACE/MOPP, prednisone, methotrexate, Adriamycin, cyclophosphamide, etoposide/mechlorethamine, vincristine, prednisone, procarbazine; HDMTX, high-dose methotrexate with leucovorin rescue; NS, not specified.

coupled with GM-CSF had a significantly higher mean nadir absolute neutrophil counts, a shorter duration of severe neutropenia, and spent fewer days in the hospital than those receiving the same chemotherapy without growth factor support.[83] Complete responses were observed in 67% of control patients and 70% in GM-CSF–treated patients, without statistically significant differences in median survival. Tirelli and coworkers recently compared 18 patients treated with AZT, G-CSF, and the aggressive LNH84 regimen with 19 patients who received the same chemotherapy without G-CSF or AZT.[84] Although the G-CSF–supported cohort had less neutropenia and mucositis, less delay in drug delivered, and less febrile neutropenic fevers requiring hospitalization, there was no significant impact on the overall response rate (78% in the G-CSF group, 88% in the control group).

A prospective, randomized trial conducted by the AIDS Clinical Trial Group randomized 188 HIV-NHL patients to receive low-dose m-BACOD or standard m-BACOD plus GM-CSF support.[85] The complete response rate was 46% in the low-dose group and 50% in the standard-dose group (AIDS Clinical Trials Group 142). The median survival time was 34 weeks in the low-dose group and 31 weeks for those receiving standard-dose m-BACOD plus GM-CSF. These differences were not statistically significant. Only 21.9% of study participants receiving low-dose chemotherapy suffered neutropenia, compared with 35.9% in the standard-dose group. These results challenge the notion that higher doses of chemotherapy and supplemental growth factor support should be given routinely to all HIV-NHL patients.

Novel studies designed to take advantage of the different ways chemotherapy can be delivered were reflected in two reports. Remick and colleagues studied an oral chemotherapy regimen that achieved complete remissions in 7 (39%) of 18 patients and a median survival time of 7 months.[86] Although myelotoxicity was significant, the protocol proved convenient to deliver and less costly than standard chemotherapy given intravenously. Sparano and colleagues entered patients into a pilot study using a continuous infusion CDE regimen (cyclophosphamide, doxorubicin, and etoposide) for 96 hours.[87] Patients with small, non-cleaved cell lymphoma and those with bone marrow involvement received CNS prophylaxis consisting of intrathecal methotrexate and whole-brain radiation therapy. All patients received PCP prophylaxis during therapy. This regimen induced complete remissions in 75% of patients, and a median survival of 17 months was reported. Although patients required placement of semipermanent long-line catheters, therapy was generally well tolerated and amenable to outpatient administration with the aid of portable infusion pumps.

The clinical outcome after therapy for HIV-related NHL may depend on the underlying stage of HIV disease more than the intensity of the treatment employed.[88] The French-Italian Cooperative Study Group conducted a prospective trial using two individualized groups of patients with HIV-associated NHL.[89] Patients with a previous history of opportunistic infections and decreased performance status were treated with a low-dose CHOP chemotherapy regimen and AZT. Patients without these factors were eligible for intensive drug therapy with a slightly modified LNH84 regimen.[90] In the low-risk group, complete responses were achieved in 63% of 141 patients, which was not significantly different from that obtained from HIV-negative NHL patients (75%). With a median follow-up of 28 months, the average survival and disease-free survival times were 9 and 16 months, respectively. In contrast, the high-risk group achieved only a 14% percent complete response rate and a disappointing median survival of only 3.5 months.[91] A multivariate analysis demonstrated three factors strongly associated with shorter survival: CD4+ counts less than 100/mm^3, poor performance status, and a prior AIDS diagnosis. For patients with CD4+ counts greater than 100/mm and good performance status, the probability of survival at 2 years was 50%.

The clinical benefit of chemotherapy may also depend on the molecular characteristics of the tumor itself. Employing several different chemotherapy regimens, Kaplan found that 18 (78%) of 23 patients with polyclonal lymphoproliferations achieved complete responses.[70] Such patients were more likely to have elevated CD4+ cell counts (mean = 277/mm³) than their monoclonal counterparts (mean = 123/mm³). Patients whose tumors were negative for EBV sequences had a median survival of 9 months, but those with EBV-positive tumors survived for a median period of 3.2 months.

From these and other studies, it is apparent that the precise role of incorporating hematopoietic growth factors and antiretroviral drugs in chemotherapy protocols requires further research.[88] Although there is no consensus about what constitutes the optimal treatment approach for the AIDS-related NHL patient, current strategies seek to integrate antiretroviral therapy, meningeal prophylaxis, and infection prophylaxis into chemotherapy protocols. Kaplan suggested that for patients who are in a good-prognosis category (ie, CD4+ >200/mm³) and have no prior opportunistic infections, a standard chemotherapy regimen may be used, coupled with prophylactic growth factor support if severe neutropenia occurs (Table 15.2-3).[92] For those with a more advanced stage of HIV disease, lower-dose chemotherapy or no chemotherapy at all may be appropriate. Individuals with CD4+ cell counts between 100 and 200/mm³ should have therapy individualized according to other clinical factors such as performance status, history of prior opportunistic infections, and degree of myelosuppression at time of diagnosis. Caution must be exercised when using vincristine in this group because of the increased incidence of peripheral neuropathy due to HIV or specific antiretroviral therapy (eg, didanosine, zalcitabine, stavudine).

Experimental therapeutic strategies seek to capitalize on information garnered from studies of the etiopathogenesis of AIDS-related NHL and include the use of biologic therapies, inhibitors of growth factors or cytokines, monoclonal antibodies, and new antineoplastic agents. Ultimately, however, the key strategies will be those directed toward maintaining a significantly intact immune system to help prevent the development of cancer.

AIDS-RELATED MALIGNANCIES

Primary Central Nervous System Lymphoma

Primary CNS lymphoma occurs in 1% to 3% of all patients with AIDS, typically in the milieu of severe immunodeficiency (CD4+ <50/mm³) and prior AIDS-defining opportunistic infections.[22,69,93] Patients may have dramatic focal neurologic deficits, headaches, and seizures. However, in more than one half of the patients in one large series, the clinical presentation consisted of subtle signs and symptoms, including memory loss, confusion, and lethargy.[94] Histologically, such tumors are immunoblastic or large cell, unlike Burkitt's histology, and they are associated with EBV in virtually 100% of tested cases.[67,95]

Single and multiple contrast-enhancing lesions may be seen on computed tomography and magnetic resonance imaging. The differential diagnosis of a space-occupying cerebral mass is broad and includes toxoplasmosis and, much less commonly, fungus, tuberculosis, gummatous lesions, and gliomas.[96-100] Although it has been suggested that solitary lesions are more likely to be primary CNS lymphomas, only tissue obtained from brain parenchyma (ie, by stereotactic brain biopsy), cerebrospinal fluid (ie, cytologic analysis), or orbit (ie, aqueous tumor cytology) can reliably differentiate primary CNS lymphoma from cerebral toxoplasmosis.[100-102] At experienced centers, stereotactic brain biopsy is considered when lesions appear neuroradiographically unusual, serum toxoplasmosis titers are negative, or for patients whose clinical and radiographic findings deteriorate after 10 to 14 days of empiric antitoxoplasmosis therapy.

After a diagnosis of primary CNS lymphoma is established, a decision regarding treatment is appropriately based

TABLE 15.2-3. *Commonly used therapy regimens for systemic AIDS-related non-Hodgkin's lymphoma*

Regimen	Drugs Used	Dosage
Modified m-BACOD[81] (Each cycle, 21–28 days)	Cyclophosphamide	300 mg/m² IVPB day 1
	Doxorubicin	25 mg/m² IVPB day 1
	Vincristine	1.4 mg/m² (not to exceed 2 mg) IVP day 1
	Dexamethasone	3 mg/m² PO days 1–5
	Methotrexate	200 mg/m² IVPB day 15 (with leucovorin rescue)
CHOP[83] (Each cycle, 21–28 days)	Cyclophosphamide	750 mg/m² IVPB day 1
	Doxorubicin	50 mg/m² IVPB day 1
	Vincristine	1.4 mg/m² (not to exceed 2 mg) IVPB day 1
	Prednisone	100 mg PO days 1–5
Oral[86] (Each cycle, 42 days)	CCNU	100 mg/m² PO day 1 (cycles 1, 3, 5)
	Etoposide	200 mg/m² PO days 1–3
	Cyclophosphamide	100 mg/m² PO days 22–31
	Procarbazine	100 mg/m² PO days 22–31
CDE[87]	Cyclophosphamide	187.5 mg/m² CI days 1–4
	Doxorubicin	12.5 mg/m² CI days 1–4
	Etoposide	60 mg/m² CI days 1–4

on the patient's performance status, extent of disease, and comorbid medical conditions. Those who decline therapy usually deteriorate rapidly and die within 4 to 6 weeks of tumor progression or complicating opportunistic infections.[103] The primary therapy for this group is whole-brain radiation therapy. Several retrospective analyses suggest improved neurologic function, quality of life, and survival is to be expected with this modality.[93,94,104] In a representative study, Nisce and Metroka described 21 patients with primary CNS lymphomas, 20 of whom had prior AIDS-defining opportunistic infections.[105] The cohort was treated over 3 to 4 weeks with 30 to 40 Gy of whole-brain irradiation, with a 14-cGy boost in responding patients. Nineteen (79%) of 24 exhibited improvements in neurologic status. Seven (87.5%) of eight had marked tumor regression on repeated computed tomography scans or magnetic resonance imaging. The mean survival of 4.8 months falls within the range of 2 to 5 months that others have reported.

For the rare patient who presents with primary CNS lymphoma and CD4+ cell counts greater than 200/mm; disease limited to the brain, excluding orbit and spine; and a good performance status, multimodality therapy may be an option. Chamberlain was able to identify only four such patients, representing approximately 10% of all AIDS-related primary CNS lymphomas seen at a single institution during a 7-year period.[103] With a treatment program including whole-brain irradiation and hydroxyurea, followed by three cycles of procarbazine, lomustine, and vincristine chemotherapy, a median survival time of 13.5 months was achieved (range, 11 to 16 months). The use of single-cycle chemotherapy before or at the time of initiating radiation therapy may also improve response and outcome, and this approach is under investigation in an Eastern Cooperative Oncology Group–initiated intergroup study.

Hodgkin's Disease

More than 200 cases of Hodgkin's disease in HIV-infected patients have been reported. Nonetheless, the association of HIV infection with Hodgkin's disease remains controversial. Hessol and associates conducted an epidemiologic review of 6704 homosexual men enrolled in the San Francisco Clinic Cohort Study.[106] The authors identified an excess incidence of Hodgkin's disease in HIV-infected homosexual men. Population rate comparisons were made with data from the Surveillance, Epidemiology and End Results Cancer Registry. The excess risk of developing Hodgkin's disease attributable to HIV was 19.3 cases per 100,000 person-years. This contrasts with an excess risk of 225 cases of NHL per 100,000 person-years in the same population. European and American investigators have also noticed increasing numbers of Hodgkin's disease cases, but they suggest that the high incidence is confined principally to intravenous drug users.[107,108] In one study in which an increased incidence of Hodgkin's disease among HIV-infected patients was reported, the ratio of homosexual cases

to intravenous drug abuse cases was 1 : 3.7.[109] The debate continues, however, because several studies from large cities have not confirmed an unusually high incidence of Hodgkin's disease within a single male population between the ages of 20 and 49. The disparate findings among these studies may be partially explained by misclassification of NHL cases, because even a small misclassification rate of AIDS-related NHL could cause a spurious elevation of Hodgkin's disease rates.[110]

Regardless of the questionable effect on incidence, American and European investigators have observed a high incidence of advanced-stage disease and frequent bone marrow involvement at the time of presentation and a relative increase in mixed-cellularity or lymphocyte-depleted histology.[111,112] HIV patients with Hodgkin's disease are also less likely to obtain durable complete responses. Of 17 patients treated with conventional Hodgkin's chemotherapy regimens, only 8 achieved complete responses.[107] The median survival time was 15 months. Full doses of chemotherapy were difficult to deliver in the face of poor bone marrow reserves and frequent and recurrent opportunistic infections. Other studies employing Hodgkin's regimens have achieved complete remissions ranging from 44% to 55% and median survival times between 10.5 to 18 months.[88,113] In a preliminary report, a well-tolerated chemotherapy regimen consisting of bleomycin, vincristine, etoposide, and streptozocin achieved a complete response in 4 of 5 patients with advanced disease.[114] The major advantage of this combination was that no fever or neutropenia occurred, despite full drug doses. Clinical trials incorporating aggressive opportunistic infection prophylaxis along with other drug combinations and colony-stimulating factors are in progress.

Cervical and Anal Cancers

Cervical intraepithelial lesions associated with HPV infections occur more frequently among women with HIV infection. Several studies suggest that the incidence and severity are related to a deteriorating immune system and a decline in the absolute CD4+ cell count.[115,116] Although an excess of cervical cancer attributed to HIV disease has not been observed, in 1993, the CDC revised the classification for HIV infection to include invasive cervical cancer in HIV-infected women as an AIDS diagnosis because of the anticipated large clinical and public health impact in this population.[117]

When clinical features of invasive cervical cancer in females with and without HIV infection are compared, HIV-infected women are more likely to have clinically advanced disease at presentation, a higher recurrence after primary therapy, and an overall poorer prognosis than non–HIV-infected women.[118,119] These generalizations are best reflected in a relatively large study by Maiman and colleagues, which compared 16 seropositive women with 68 seronegative woman.[120] In this group, 15 of 16 seropositives had advanced surgical pathologic stage, and 9 of 11 evaluable patients had persistent or recurrent cervical cancer, with a mean interval from diagnosis to death of 9.2 months. Although the stage of disease did not predict the CD4+ levels, CD4+ status did influence subsequent outcome. Patients with suboptimal immune function responded poorly to therapy, and those with CD4+ cell counts greater than 500/mm³ had more favorable courses.

There is epidemiologic evidence that homosexuality and receptive anal intercourse are important risk factors for anal-rectal cancer.[121-123] An association between these tumors and HIV infection was to be expected.[124] With the spread of HIV infection, an increased proportion of anal cancers have been diagnosed among HIV-positive men, suggesting a strong association between this cancer and HIV infection. Melbye and collaborators used a link between AIDS cases and cancer registries in seven U.S. health departments and found a 40- to 80-fold excess of anal cancer after a diagnosis of AIDS compared with the general population.[125]

Surawicz and colleagues reviewed the anal findings for 512 homosexual men (ie, 299 HIV-seropositive and 213 HIV-seronegative).[126] Anal dysplasia was common in biopsy specimens from homosexual men with visible HPV-associated internal anal abnormalities. They also demonstrated HPV DNA by Southern blot analysis and polymerase chain reaction and found DNA viruses in 47 (98%) of 48 HIV-seropositive men and in 12 (86%) of 14 HIV-seronegative men. High-risk HPV serotypes (ie, 16, 19, or 45) were most commonly observed in the HIV-seropositive group. The researchers recommended resecting lesions containing recurrent high-grade dysplasia or carcinoma in situ.

Lorenz and associates reviewed the surgical experience with anal carcinoma in HIV-infected men at the University of California San Francisco.[127] They reported poor treatment outcomes and short survival times for this patient population, similar to the experience described for cervical cancer patients. Combined-modality therapy consisting of neoadjuvant chemotherapy (ie, cisplatin, bleomycin, and vincristine) and radiotherapy must be administered cautiously in this group because of the high incidence of severe mucositis.

The diagnostic guidelines for anogenital disease in HIV-positive men and women remain controversial. Several studies indicate a lower sensitivity of Papanicolaou smears for detecting squamous epithelial lesions in women and men. The CDC issued guidelines recommending that all HIV-infected women undergo Papanicolaou smear evaluations at the time of the initial pelvic examination and, if normal, 6 months later.[128] If the latter is normal, annual screening is suggested. In contrast, Maiman cites several studies that indicate a lower sensitivity of Papanicolaou smears for detecting squamous intraepithelial lesions in women and eschews Papanicolaou smears for routine cervical colposcopy.[129-132]

Information is lacking on which to base recommendations regarding how best and how frequently to screen for anal and genital neoplasia in HIV-infected persons.[133] Additional studies investigating the natural history of anogenital carcinoma and cost-benefit analyses of various screening strategies are required. There is, however, agreement that cervical cancer must be excluded in women at risk for HIV infection, especially those who complain of pelvic pain, dysuria, dyspareunia, or abnormal vaginal discharge. Anal cancer must be excluded in any HIV-infected person complaining of anorectal discomfort, bleeding, bowel irregularity, or pruritus ani.

Miscellaneous Tumors

Numerous case reports of malignancies other than Kaposi's sarcoma, NHL, Hodgkin's disease, and anogenital cancers occurring among HIV-infected adults have been published, most notably neoplasms of the lung, testes, and skin.[134] These reports usually emphasize the peculiar pathologic characteristics, advanced stage at presentation, and the poor response of these tumors to conventional therapies.[135,136] Nonetheless, population-based studies have not clearly demonstrated an increased incidence of these and other miscellaneous tumors among HIV-infected cohorts.[7,24,137,138]

Smooth muscle tumors rarely occur in children; the annual incidence is less than two cases per 10 million children.[139] Thirteen cases have been reported among the roughly 5000 children with AIDS in the United States and represent a much higher frequency than would otherwise be expected.[139-145] EBV may contribute to the pathogenesis of these tumors. McClain and colleagues, using in situ hybridization and quantitative polymerase chain reaction techniques, were able to demonstrate high levels of EBV genomes in five leiomyosarcomas and two leiomyomas from five children and one young man with AIDS.[145] Similar tumor types collected from HIV-negative controls did not contain EBV genomes.

REFERENCES

1. Gottlieb MS, Schroff R, Shanker HM, et al. *Pneumocystis carinii* pneumonia and mucosal candidiasis in previously healthy homosexual men: evidence of a new acquired cellular immunodeficiency. N Engl J Med 1981;305:1425.
2. Centers for Disease Control. Revision of the case definition of acquired immunodeficiency syndrome for national reporting. United States. MMWR 1985;34:373.
3. Gatti RA, Good RA. Occurrence of malignancy in immunodeficient diseases. Cancer 1971;28:89.
4. Penn I. Cancers complicating organ transplantation. N Engl J Med 1990;323:767.
5. Starzl TE, Naleskin MA, Porter KA, et al. Reversibility of lymphomas and lymphoproliferative lesions developing under cyclosporine therapy. Lancet 1984;1:583.
6. Shapiro R, McClain K, Frizzera G, et al. Epstein-Barr virus associated B-cell lymphoproliferative disorders following bone marrow transplantation. Blood 1988;71:1234.
7. Penn I. Cancer of the urogenital region in renal transplant recipients: analysis of 65 cases. Cancer 1988;58:611.
8. Halpert R, Fruchter RG, Sedlis A, et al. Human papillomavirus and lower genital tract neoplasia in renal transplant patients. Obstet Gynecol 1986;68:251.

9. Zulman J, Jaffe R, Talal N. Evidence that the malignant lymphoma of Sjögren's syndrome is a monoclonal B-cell neoplasm. N Engl J Med 1975;292:1.

10. Burke JS, Butler JJ, Fuller LM. Malignant lymphomas of the thyroid: a clinical pathologic study of 35 patients including ultrastructural observations. Cancer 1977;39:1587.

11. Brincker M, Wilbek E. The incidence of malignant tumors in patients with respiratory sarcoid. Br J Cancer 1974;19:247.

12. Purtilo PT. Immune deficiency predisposing to Epstein-Barr virus induced lymphoproliferative diseases: the X-linked lymphoproliferative syndrome as a model. Adv Cancer Res 1981;34:279.

13. Wong O. An industry-wide mortality study of chemical workers occupationally exposed to benzene: II. Dose-response analyses. Br J Cancer 1987;44:328.

14. Wood JS, Polissar L, Severson RK, et al. Soft tissue sarcoma and non-Hodgkin's lymphoma in relation to phenoxyherbicide and chlorinated phenol exposure in western Washington. J Natl Cancer Inst 1987;78:899.

15. Pearce NE, Sheppard RA, Smith AH, et al. Non-Hodgkin's lymphoma and farming: an expanded case-control study. Int J Cancer 1987; 39:155.

16. Kristal AR, Nasca PC, Burnett WS, Mikl J. Changes in the epidemiology of non-Hodgkin's lymphoma and selected malignancies in a population with a high incidence of acquired immunodeficiency syndrome (AIDS). Am J Epidemiol 1988;128:711.

17. Reynolds P, Sanders LD, Layefsky ME, Lemp GF. The spectrum of acquired immunodeficiency syndrome (AIDS)-associated malignancies in San Francisco, 1980–1987. Am J Epidemiol 1993;137:19.

18. Harnly ME, Swan SH, Holly EA, Kelter A, Padian N. Temporal trends in the incidence of non-Hodgkin's lymphoma and selected malignancies in a population with a high incidence of acquired immunodeficiency syndrome (AIDS). Am J Epidemiol 1988;128:261.

19. Serraino D, Salamina G, Franceshi S, La Vecchia C, Brunet JB, Ancelle-Park R. The epidemiology of AIDS-associated non-Hodgkin's lymphoma in the World Health Organization European Region. Br J Cancer 1992;66:912.

20. Irwin D, Kaplan L. Clinical aspects of HIV-related lymphoma. Curr Opin Oncol 1993;5:852.

21. Pluda JM, Venzon DJ, Tosato G, et al. Parameters affecting the development of non-Hodgkin's lymphoma in patients with severe human immunodeficiency virus infection receiving antiretroviral therapy. J Clin Oncol 1993;11:1099.

22. Pluda JM, Yarchoan R, Jaffe ES, et al. Development of non-Hodgkin's lymphoma in a cohort of patients with severe human immunodeficiency virus (HIV) infection on long-term antiretroviral therapy. Ann Intern Med 1990;113:276.

23. Ragni MV, Belle SH, Jaffe RA, et al. Acquired immunodeficiency syndrome, non-Hodgkin's lymphomas and other malignancies in patients with hemophilia. Blood 1993;81:1889.

24. Rabkin CS, Hilgartner MW, Hedberg KW, et al. Incidence of lymphomas and other cancers in HIV-infected and HIV-uninfected patients with lymphomas. JAMA 1992;267:1090.

25. Moore RD, Kessler H, Richman DD, Flexner C, Chaisson RE. Non-Hodgkin's lymphoma in patients with advanced HIV infection treated with zidovudine. JAMA 1991;265:2508.

26. Gail MH, Pluda JM, Rabkin CS, et al. Projections of the incidence of non-Hodgkin's lymphoma related to acquired immunodeficiency syndrome. J Natl Cancer Inst 1991;83:695.

27. Beral V, Peterman T, Berkelman R, et al. AIDS-associated non-Hodgkin's lymphoma. Lancet 1991;337:805.

28. Levine AM. AIDS-related malignancies: the emerging epidemic. J Natl Cancer Inst 1993;85:1382.

29. Yano T, Van Krieken HJM, Magrath IT, et al. Histogenetic correlations between subcategories of small non-cleaved cell lymphomas. Blood 1992;79:1282.

30. Pelicci PG, Knowles DM, Arlin Z, Weilzorek R, Lucia P, Dina D, Basilico C, Della-Favera R. Multiple monoclonal B-cell expression and c-myc oncogene rearrangements in AIDS-related lymphoproliferative disorders: implications for lymphomagenesis. J Exp Med 1986; 164:2049.

31. Subar M, Neri A, Inghirami G, Knowles DM, Della-Favera R. Frequent c-myc oncogene activation and infrequent presence of Epstein-Barr virus genome in AIDS-associated lymphoma. Blood 1988;72:667.

32. Ballerini P, Giadano G, Gong JZ, Tassi V, Saglio G, Knowles DM, Della-Favera R. Multiple genetic lesions in AIDS-related non-Hodgkin's lymphoma. Blood 1993;81:166.

33. Shiramizu B, Herndier B, Meaker T, Kaplan L, McGrath M. Molecular and immunophenotypic characterization of AIDS-associated non-Hodgkin's lymphoma. J Clin Oncol 1992;10:383.

34. Pelicci PG, Knowles DM, Arlin ZA, et al. Multiple monoclonal B-cell expansions and c-myc oncogene rearrangements in acquired immunodeficiency syndrome-related lymphoproliferative disorders: implications for lymphomagenesis. J Exp Med 1986;164:2049.

35. Penn I. Lymphomas complicating organ transplantation. Transplant Proc 1983;15(Suppl):2790.

36. de-The G, Gesar A, Day NE, et al. Epidemiological evidence for casual relationship between Epstein-Barr virus and Burkitt's lymphoma from Ugandan Prospective Study. Nature 1978;274:756.

37. Cleary ML, Sklar J. Lymphoproliferative disorders in cardiac recipients are multiclonal lymphomas. Lancet 1989;2:489.

38. Birx DL, Redfield RR, Tosato G. Defective regulation of Epstein-Barr virus infection in patients with acquired immunodeficiency syndrome (AIDS) or AIDS-related disorders. N Engl J Med 1986;14:874.

39. Knowles DM. Biologic aspects of AIDS-associated non-Hodgkin's lymphoma. Curr Opin Oncol 1993;5:845.

40. Goldschmidts WL, Bhatia K, Johnson JF, et al. Epstein-Barr virus genotypes in AIDS-associated lymphomas are similar to those in endemic Burkitt's lymphomas. Leukemia 1992;6:875.

41. Shibata D, Weiss LM, Nathwani BN, Brynes NK, Levine AM. Epstein-Barr virus in benign lymph node biopsies from individuals infected with the human immunodeficiency virus is associated with concurrent or subsequent development of non-Hodgkin's lymphoma. Blood 1991;77:1527.

42. Lombardi L, Newcomb EW, Della-Favera R. Pathogenesis of Burkitt's lymphoma: expansion of an activated c-myc oncogene causes the tumorigenic conversion of EBV injected human B-lymphocytes. Cell 1987;49:161.

43. Hamilton-Dutoit SJ, Pallesen G, Karkov J, Skinhoj P, Franzmann MB, Pedersen C. Identification of EBV-DNA in tumor cells of AIDS-related lymphomas by in situ hybridization. Lancet 1989;1:544.

44. Ganser A, Carlo-Stella C, Bartram CR, et al. Establishment of two Epstein-Barr virus negative Burkitt cell lines from a patient with AIDS and B-cell lymphomas. Blood 1988;72:1255.

45. Shiramizu B, Herndier B, Meeker T, et al. Molecular and immunophenotypic characterization of AIDS-associated Epstein-Barr virus negative, polyclonal lymphoma. J Clin Oncol 1992;10:383.

46. Haluska FG, Russo G, Kant J, et al. Molecular resemblance of an AIDS-associated lymphoma and endemic Burkitt lymphoma: implications for their pathogenesis. Proc Natl Acad Sci USA 1986; 86:8907.

47. Cherepakhin V, Feigal E, Kipps TJ. Immunoglobulin heavy chain variable region genes expressed in AIDS-associated monoclonal B-cell lymphomas. Blood 1992;80:116a.

48. Levine AM, Shibata D, Weiss LM, et al. Molecular characteristics of intermediate/high (I/H) grade lymphomas (NHL) arising in HIV-positive vs HIV-negative patients: preliminary data from a population (POP) based study in the County of Los Angeles. Blood 1992; 80:259a.

48. Nakajima K, Martinez-Maza O, Hirano T, et al. Indication of IL-6 (B-cell stimulatory factor-2/IFN-beta 2) production by human immunodeficiency virus. J Immunol 1989;142:531.

49. Breen EC, Rezai AR, Nakajimi K, et al. Infection with HIV is associated with elevated IL-6 levels and production. J Immunol 1990;144:480.

50. Emilie D, Coumbaras J, Raphael M, et al. Interleukin-6 production in high-grade B lymphomas: correlation with the presence of indignant immunoblasts in acquired immunodeficiency syndrome and in human immunodeficiency virus-seronegative patients. Blood 1992;80:498.

51. Karp JE, Groopman JE, Broder S. In: Devita VT, Hellman S, Rosenberg SA, eds. Corner on AIDS in cancer: principles and practice of oncology. 4th ed. Philadelphia: JB Lippincott, 1993:2093.

52. Benjamin D, Knobloch TJ, Abrams J, et al. Human B cell IL-10: B cell lines derived from patients with AIDS and Burkitt's lymphoma constitutively secrete large quantities of IL-10. Blood 1991; 78:384a.

53. Masood R, Bond M, Scadden D, et al. Interleukin-10. An autocrine B-cell growth factor for human B-cell lymphoma and their progenitors. Blood 1992;80:115a.

54. Nakamura H, Said JW, Miller CW, Koeffler HP. Mutation and protein expression of p53 in acquired immunodeficiency syndrome-related lymphomas. Blood 1993;82:920.
55. DeRe V, Carbone A, De Vita S, et al. P53 protein over expression and p53 gene abnormalities in HIV-1-related non-Hodgkin's lymphoma. Int J Cancer 1994;54:662.
56. Shibata D. Biologic aspects of AIDS-related lymphoma. Curr Opin Oncol 1994;6:503.
57. Shiramizu B, Herndier BG, McGrath BS. Identification of a common clonal human immunodeficiency virus integration site on human immunodeficiency virus-associated lymphomas. Cancer Res 1994; 54:2069.
58. Knowles DM, Chamulak GA, Subar M, et al. Lymphoid neoplasia associated with the acquired immunodeficiency syndrome (AIDS): the New York University experience with 105 patients (1981–1986). Ann Intern Med 1988;108:744.
59. Kaplan LD, Abrams DI, Feigal E, et al. AIDS associated non-Hodgkin's lymphoma in San Francisco. JAMA 1989;261:719.
60. Ioachim ML, Dorsett B, Cronin W, et al. Acquired immunodeficiency syndrome-associated lymphomas: clinical pathologic, immunologic and viral characteristics of 111 cases. Hum Pathol 1991;22:659.
61. Carbone A, Tirelli U, Vaccher E, et al. A clinicopathologic study of lymphoid neoplasms associated with human immunodeficiency virus infection in Italy. Cancer 1991;68:842.
62. Crane GA, Variakojis D, Rosen ST, et al. Cutaneous T-cell lymphoma in patients with human immunodeficiency virus infection. Arch Dermatol 1991;127:989.
63. Karcher DS, Dawkin F, Garrett CT, Shulof RS. Body cavity-based non-Hodgkin's lymphoma (NHL) in HIV-infected patients: B-cell lymphoma with unusual clinical, immunophenotypic, and genomic features. Lab Invest 1992;66:80A.
64. Knowles DM, Chamulak GA, Subar M, et al. Clinicopathologic, immunophenotypic and molecular genetic analysis of AIDS-associated lymphoid neoplasia: clinical and biologic implications. Pathol Ann 1988;22:33.
65. Levine AM. AIDS-related lymphoma. Blood 1992;80:8.
66. Gill PS, Levine AM, Meyer RR, et al. Primary central nervous system lymphoma in homosexual men: clinical, immunologic and pathologic features. Am J Med 1985;8:742.
67. MacMahon EME, Glass JD, Hayward SD, et al. Epstein-Barr virus in AIDS-related primary central nervous system lymphoma. Lancet 1991;338:969.
68. Lowenthal DA, Straus DJ, Campbell SW, et al. AIDS-related lymphoid neoplasia: the Memorial Hospital experience. Cancer 1988;61:2325.
69. Levine AM, Sullivan-Halley H, Pike PC, et al. HIV-related lymphoma: prognostic factors predictive of survival. Cancer 1991;68:2466.
70. Kaplan LD, Shiramizu B, Herndier B, et al. Influence of molecular characteristics on clinical outcome in human immunodeficiency virus-associated non-Hodgkin's lymphoma: identification of a subgroup with favorable clinical outcome. Blood 1995;85:1727.
71. Northfelt D, Volberding P, Kaplan L. Degree of immunodeficiency at diagnosis of AIDS-associated non-Hodgkin's lymphoma. Proc Am Soc Clin Oncol 1992;11:45.
72. Aboulafia DM, Mitsuyasu R. Hematologic abnormalities in AIDS. Hematol Oncol Clin North Am 1991;4:195.
73. Zeigler JL, Beckstead JA, Volberding PA, et al. Non-Hodgkin's lymphoma in homosexual men. N Engl J Med 1984;311:565.
74. Kalter SP, Riggs SA, Cabanilas F, et al. Aggressive non-Hodgkin's lymphomas in immunocompromised homosexual males. Blood 1985;66:655.
75. Bermudez MA, Grant KM, Rodvien R, Mendes F. Non-Hodgkin's lymphoma in a population with or at risk for acquired immunodeficiency syndrome: indication for intensive chemotherapy. Am J Med 1989;86:71.
76. Monfardini S, Vaccher E, Fao R, Tirelli U. AIDS-associated non-Hodgkin's lymphoma in Italy: intravenous drug users versus homosexual men. Ann Oncol 1990;1:203.
77. Roithmann S, Toledano M, Tourani JM, et al. HIV-associated non-Hodgkin's lymphomas. Clinical characteristics and outcome. The experience of the French registry of HIV-associated tumors. Ann Oncol 1991;2:289.
78. Pedersen C, Gerstoft J, Lundgre JD, et al. HIV-associated lymphoma: histopathology and association with Epstein-Barr virus genome related to clinical, immunological and prognostic factors. Eur J Cancer 1991;27:1416.
79. Gill PS, Levine AM, Krailo M, et al. AIDS-related malignant lymphoma: results of prospective treatment trials. J Clin Oncol 1987;5:1322.
80. Dugan M, Subar M, Odajnyk C, et al. Intensive multiagent chemotherapy for AIDS-related diffuse large cell lymphoma. Blood 1986;68:124a.
81. Levine AM, Wernz JC, Kaplan L, et al. Low-dose chemotherapy with CNS prophylaxis and zidovudine maintenance for AIDS-related lymphoma. A prospective multi-institutional trial. JAMA 1991;266:84.
82. Walsh C, Wernz JC, Levine A, et al. Phase I trial of m-BACOD and granulocyte-macrophage colony stimulating factor in HIV-associated non-Hodgkin's lymphoma. J Acquir Immune Defic Syndr 1993;6:265.
83. Kaplan LD, Kahn JO, Crowe S, et al. Clinical and virologic effects of recombinant human granulocyte-macrophage colony-stimulating factor in patients receiving chemotherapy for human immunodeficiency virus-associated non-Hodgkin's lymphoma: results of a randomized trial. J Clin Oncol 1991;9:929.
84. Tirrelli U, Errante D, Vaccher E, et al. Treatment of HIV-related non-Hodgkin's lymphoma (NHL) with chemotherapy (CT) and G-CSF: reduction of hospitalization and toxicity with concomitant overall reduction in cost. (Abstract 13). Proc Am Soc Clin Oncol 1993;12:53.
85. Kaplan L. ACTG 142: the results of a randomized chemical trial of low-dose chemotherapy versus full chemotherapy and cytokine in AIDS lymphoma. Second National Conference on Human Retroviruses and Related Infections, Washington, DC, Jan 29–Feb 2, 1995.
86. Remick S, McSharry JJ, Wolf BC, et al. Novel oral combination chemotherapy in the treatment of intermediate-grade and high-grade AIDS-related non-Hodgkin's lymphoma. J Clin Oncol 1993;11:1691.
87. Sparano JA, Wiernik PH, Strack M, Leaf A, Becker N, Valentine ES. Infusional cyclophosphamide, doxorubicin, and etoposide in human immunodeficiency virus and human T-cell leukemia virus type I–related non-Hodgkin's lymphoma: a highly active regimen. Blood 1993;81:2810.
88. Monfardini S. Tirelli U, Vaccher E. Treatment of acquired immunodeficiency syndrome (AIDS)-related cancer. Cancer Treat Rev 1994;20:149.
89. Gisselbrecht C, Oksenhendler E, Tirrelli U, et al. Human immunodeficiency virus-related lymphoma treated with intensive combination chemotherapy. Am J Med 1993;95:188.
90. Coiffier B, Gisselbrecht C, Herbrecht R, Tilly H, Bosly A, Brousse N. LNH-84 regimen: a multicenter study of intensive chemotherapy in 737 patients with aggressive malignant lymphoma. J Clin Oncol 1989;7:1018.
91. Tirrelli U, Errante D, Oksenhendler E, et al. Prospective study with combined low-dose chemotherapy and zidovudine in 37 patients with poor prognosis AIDS-related non-Hodgkin's lymphoma. Ann Oncol 1992;3:843.
92. Kaplan LD. Treatment of HIV-associated non-Hodgkin's lymphoma. In: Cohen PT, Sande MA, Volberding PA, eds. The AIDS knowledge base: a textbook on HIV disease from the University of California, San Francisco, and the San Francisco General Hospital. 2nd ed. New York: Little, Brown, 1994:7.
93. Goldstein JD, Dickson DW, Moser FG, et al. Primary central nervous system lymphoma in acquired immunodeficiency syndrome: a clinical and pathologic study with results of treatment with radiation. Cancer 1991;67:2756.
94. Baumgartner JE, Rachlin JR, Beckstead JH, et al. Primary central nervous system lymphoma: natural history and response to radiation therapy in 55 patients with acquired immunodeficiency syndrome. J Neurosurg 1990;73:206.
95. Meeker TC, Shiramizu B, Kaplan L, et al. Evidence for molecular subtypes of HIV-associated lymphoma: division into peripheral monoclonal, polyclonal and central nervous system lymphomas. AIDS 1991;5:669.
96. Bishburg E, Eng RHK, Slim J, et al. Brain lesions in patients with acquired immunodeficiency syndrome. Arch Intern Med 1989;149:941.
97. Ciricillo SF, Rosenblum ML. Use of CT and MR imaging to distinguish intracranial lesions and define the need to biopsy in AIDS patient. J Neurosurg 1990;73:720.
98. Horowitz HW, Valsamis MP, Wicher V, et al. Brief report: cerebrosyphilitic gumma confirmed by the polymerase chain reaction in a man with human immunodeficiency virus infection. New Engl J Med 1994;331:488.

99. Moulignier A, Mikol J, Pialoux G, Eliaszewicz M, Thurel C, Thiebaut JB. Cerebral glial tumors and human immunodeficiency virus-1 infection. More than a coincidental association. Cancer 1994;74:686.

100. Casobona J, Salas T, Salinas R. Trends and survival in AIDS-associated malignancies. Eur J Can 1993;29A:877.

101. DeAngelis LM. Primary central nervous system lymphoma: a role for adjuvant chemotherapy. J Neurooncol 1992;14:271.

102. Ciricillo SF, Rosenblum ML. Imaging of solitary lesions in AIDS. J Neurosurg 1991;74:1029.

103. Chamberlain MC. Long survival in patients with acquired immune deficiency syndrome-related primary central nervous system lymphoma. Cancer 1994;73:1728.

104. Formenti SC, Gill PS, Lean E, et al. Primary central nervous system lymphoma in AIDS: results of radiation therapy. Cancer 1989;63:1101.

105. Nisce LZ, Metroka C. Radiation therapy in patients with AIDS-related central nervous system lymphoma. JAMA 1992;267:1921.

106. Hessol NA, Katz MH, Liu JY, Buchbinder S, Rubino C, Holmberg S. Increased incidence of Hodgkin's disease in homosexual men with HIV infection. Ann Intern Med 1992;117:309.

107. Tirelli U, Errante D, Vaccher E, et al. Hodgkin's disease and HIV infection. A report of 92 patients from the GICAT (Italian Cooperative Group on AIDS and Tumors) with emphasis on prospective study with combined chemotherapy and zidovudine (AZT) in 16 patients. Proc Am Soc Clin Oncol 1992;11:44.

108. Newcomb S, Ward M, Napoli V, Kutner M. Treatment of HIV-associated Hodgkin's disease: is there a clue regarding the etiology of Hodgkin's disease? Proc Am Soc Clin Oncol 1992;11:44.

109. Monfardini S, Tirelli U, Vaccher E, Foa R, Gavosto F. Hodgkin's disease in 63 intravenous drug users infected with the human immunodeficiency virus. Ann Oncol 1991;2(Suppl 2):201.

110. Rabkin CS. Epidemiology of AIDS-related malignancies. Curr Opin Oncol 1994;6:492.

111. Serraino D, Carbone A, Francheszchi S, Tirelli U for the Italian Cooperative Group on AIDS and Tumors. Increased frequency of lymphocyte depletion and mixed cellularity subtypes of Hodgkin's disease in HIV-infected patients. Eur J Cancer 1993;29:1948.

112. Karcher D. Clinically unsuspected Hodgkin's disease presenting initially in the bone marrow of patients infected with the human immunodeficiency virus. Cancer 1993;71:1235.

113. Serrano M, Bellas C, Campo E, et al. Hodgkin's disease in patients with antibodies to human immunodeficiency virus: a study of 22 patients. Cancer 1990;65:2248.

114. Kaplan L, Kahn J, Northfelt D, Abrams D, Volberding P. Novel combination chemotherapy for Hodgkin's disease in HIV-infected individuals. Proc Am Soc Clin Oncol 1991;10:33.

115. Williams AB, Darragh TM, Vranzian K, Ochia C, Moss AR, Palefsky JM. Anal and cervical human papillomavirus infection and risk of anal and cervical intraepithelial abnormalities in human immunodeficiency virus-infected women. Obstet Gynecol 1994;83:205.

116. Sehafer A, Friedman W, Mielke M, Schwartlander R, Koch MA. The increased frequency of cervical dysplasia-neoplasia in women infected with the human immunodeficiency virus is related to the degree of immunosuppression. Am J Obstet Gynecol 1991;164:593.

117. Centers for Disease Control. 1993 Revised classification system for HIV infection and expanded surveillance case definition for AIDS among adolescents and adults. MMWR 1993;41:1.

118. Maiman M, Fruchter RG, Serur E, et al. Human immunodeficiency virus and cervical neoplasia. Gynecol Oncol 1990;38:377.

119. Mattarras R, Arieta JM, Corral J, et al. Human immunodeficiency virus-induced immunosuppression: a risk factor for human papillomavirus infection. Am J Obstet Gynecol 1991;165:42.

120. Maiman M, Fruchter RG, Guy Levis, Cuthill S, Levine P, Serur E. Human immunodeficiency virus infection and invasive cervical carcinoma. Cancer 1993;71:402.

121. Palefsky JM, Holly EA, Gonzales J, Lamborn K, Hollander H. National history of and anal cytologic abnormalities and human papillomavirus infection among homosexual men with group IV HIV disease. J Acquir Immune Defic Syndr 1992;5:1258.

122. Wexner SD, Milson JW, Dailey TH. The demographics of anal cancer are changing: identification of high risk populations. Dis Colon Rectum 1987;30:942.

123. Frisch M, Melbye M, Moller H. Trends in incidence of anal cancer in Denmark. Br Med J 1993;206:419.

124. Palefsky J, Gonzales J, Greenblatt RM, Ahn DK, Hollander H. Anal intraepithelial neoplasia and anal papillomavirus infection among homosexual males with group IV HIV disease. JAMA 1990;263:2911.

125. Melbye M, Cote TR, Kessler L, Gail M, Biggar RJ and the AIDS/Cancer Working Group. High incidence of anal cancer among AIDS patients. Lancet 1994;343:636.

126. Surawicz CM, Kirby P, Critchlow S, Sayer J, Dunpo C, Kiviat N. Anal dysplasia in homosexual men: role of anoscopy and biopsy. Gastroenterology 1993;105:659.

127. Lorenz HP, Wilson W, Leigh B, et al. Squamous cell carcinoma of the anus and HIV infection. Dis Colon Rectum 1991;34:336.

128. Centers for Disease Control and Prevention. 1993 Sexually transmitted diseases treatment guidelines. MMWR 1993;42(No RR-14):83.

129. Maiman M, Tarricone N, Viera J, et al. Coloscopic evaluation of human immunodeficiency virus seropositive women. Gynecol Oncol 1990;38:377.

130. McKinnon KJ, Ford RM, Hunter JC. High prevalence of human papillomavirus and cervical intraepithelial neoplasia in a young Australian STD population. Int J STD AIDS 1991;2:276.

131. Kell PD, Shah PM, Barton SE. Colposcopic screening in HIV seropositive women-help or hindrance? (Abstract PO B30550) Amsterdam, Netherlands Int Conf AIDS 1992:8:B96.

132. Maiman M. Cervical neoplasia in women with HIV infection. Oncol 1994;8:83.

133. Northfelt DW. Cervical and anal neoplasia and HPV infection in person with HIV infection. Oncology 1994;8:33.

134. Spina M, Tirelli U. Human immunodeficiency virus as a risk factor in miscellaneous cancers. Curr Opin Oncol 1992;4:907.

135. Karp J, Profeta G, Marantz PR, Karpel JP. Lung cancer in patients with immunodeficiency syndrome. Chest 1993;103:410.

136. Gunthel CJ, Northfelt DW. Cancers not associated with immunodeficiency in HIV-infected persons. Oncology 1994;8:59.

137. Chan TK, Aranda CP, Rom WN. Bronchogenic carcinoma in young patients at risk for acquired immunodeficiency syndrome. Chest 1993;103:862.

138. Gachupin-Garcia A, Selwyn PA, Salisbury Budner N. Population-based study of malignancies and HIV infection among injecting drug users in the New York City methadone treatment program, 1985–1991. AIDS 1992;6:843.

139. Lack EE. Leiomyosarcomas in childhood: a clinical and pathologic study of 10 cases. Pediatr Pathol 1986;6:181.

140. Chadwick EG, Connor EJ, Hanson IC, et al. Tumors of smooth muscle origin in HIV-infected children. JAMA 1990;263:3182.

141. McLoughlin LC, Nord KS, Joshi VV, DiCarlo FJ, Kane MJ. Disseminated leiomyosarcoma in a child with acquired immune deficiency syndrome. Cancer 1991;67:2618.

142. Orlow SJ, Kamino H, Lawrence RL. Multiple subcutaneous leiomyosarcomas in an adolescent with AIDS. Am J Pediatr Hematol Oncol 1992;14:265.

143. Ross JS, Del Rosario A, Bui HX, Sonbati H, Solis O. Primary hepatic leiomyosarcoma in a child with the acquired immunodeficiency syndrome. Hum Pathol 1992;23:69.

144. Van Hoeven KH, Factor SM, Kress Y, Woodruff JM. Visceral myogenic tumors: a manifestation of HIV infection in children. Am J Surg Pathol 1993;17:176.

145. McClain KL, Leach CT, Jenson HB. Association of Epstein-Barr virus with leiomyosarcomas in young people with AIDS. N Engl J Med 1995;332:12.

AIDS: Biology, Diagnosis, Treatment and Prevention, fourth edition, edited by Vincent T. DeVita, Jr., Samuel Hellman, and Steven A. Rosenberg. Lippincott–Raven Publishers, © 1997

CHAPTER 16

Central and Peripheral Nervous System Complications

Richard W. Price and Bruce J. Brew

The neurologic complications of infection with the human immunodeficiency virus (HIV-1) are both common and varied, and they contribute importantly to patient morbidity and mortality. Disorders of both the central nervous system (CNS) and the peripheral nervous system (PNS) can complicate all stages of systemic HIV-1 infection, from the period after initial infection through the end stage of severe immunosuppression. These neurologic complications can be classified in a number of ways. One classification useful for analysis of individual patients is based on neuroanatomic localization.[1,2] Table 16-1 presents such a classification, dividing conditions according to the major pattern of symptom and sign localization in the CNS and PNS and following the classic, empirically proven methods of the neurologist.

This chapter follows a second, and complementary, classification based on the underlying pathophysiology of the particular disease process, which is very often determined by the stage of systemic HIV-1 infection and resultant disturbance in immune function. Accordingly, the chapter is subdivided into sections dealing in turn with disorders known or suspected to relate to effects of HIV-1 itself on the CNS, emphasizing the AIDS dementia complex (ADC); CNS opportunistic infections and neoplasms; and CNS disorders

that are secondary to systemic illness. A fourth section considers PNS and skeletal muscle disorders. Because discussion of some of the conditions overlaps with more extensive treatment in other chapters in this book, emphasis here is on first and fourth groups and on the neurologic aspects of the second and third, particularly as they relate to diagnosis. A final section summarizes some of the general principles of diagnosis and management.

Diagnosis of the neurologic complications of HIV-1 infection and AIDS is far from an academic exercise. Rather, precise diagnosis is critical to the practical management of patients and frequently leads to specific therapy with resultant reduction of morbidity and preservation of meaningful function and quality of life. It is our impression that all too often AIDS clinicians faced with neurologic complications give up on the patient when further diagnostic and therapeutic avenues remain open and capable of preserving meaningful life.

CENTRAL NERVOUS SYSTEM CONDITIONS KNOWN OR PRESUMED TO RELATE TO EFFECTS OF HIV-1

Although it is now clear that HIV-1 can directly infect the CNS, understanding is still limited regarding the nature of this infection, including its frequency, timing, pathobiology, and relation to clinical manifestations.[3-8] Accumulating clinical and laboratory observations are beginning to clarify these issues and have allowed at least a partial definition of what may be considered overlapping phases of infection and clinical sequelae. These include CNS disorders occurring in the context of acute HIV-1 infection and seroconversion, asymptomatic infections, aseptic meningitis and headache, and ADC. These different manifestations appear to relate principally to interactions of the virus with immune defenses and subsequent outcomes involving the CNS.

Richard W. Price: Department of Neurology, San Francisco General Hospital and University of California, San Francisco, San Francisco, California. Bruce J. Brew: Department of Neurology and Centre for Immunology, St. Vincent's Hospital, Sydney, Australia, Department of Neurology and St. Paul's Hospital, University of British Columbia, Vancouver, British Columbia.

Address correspondence to Richard W. Price, Department of Neurology, Room 4M62, San Francisco General Hospital, 1001 Potrero Avenue, San Francisco, CA 94110.

TABLE 16-1. *Major neurologic complications in HIV-1–infected patients classified by neuroanatomic localization*

Brain

PREDOMINANTLY NONFOCAL

Common
　AIDS dementia complex
　Metabolic encephalopathies (alone or as exacerbating
　　influence)
　Cytomegalovirus (CMV) encephalitis (*clinical* impact
　　uncertain)
　Toxoplasmosis (encephalitic form)
Rare
　Herpes encephalitis
　Aspergillosis

PREDOMINANTLY FOCAL

Common
　Cerebral toxoplasmosis
　Primary central nervous system lymphoma
　Progressive multifocal leukoencephalopathy
Uncommon or rare
　Tuberculous brain abscess or tuberculoma
　Cryptococoma
　Varicella-zoster virus (VZV) encephalitis
　Vascular disorders

Spinal Cord

Common
　Vacuolar myelopathy (part of AIDS dementia complex)
Uncommon
　VZV myelitis (complicating herpes zoster)
　Spinal epidural or intradural lymphoma
　HTLV-I–associated myelopathy

Meninges

Common
　Cryptococcal meningitis
　Aseptic meningitis (HIV-1?)
Uncommon
　Lymphomatous meningitis (metastatic)
　Tuberculous meningitis (*M. tuberculosis*)
　Syphilitic meningitis
Rare
　Listeria monocytogenes meningitis

Peripheral Nerve and Root

Very common
　Distal sensory polyneuropathy
Common
　Autonomic neuropathy
　Herpes zoster
　Acute and chronic demyelinating neuropathies
　Nucleoside toxic neuropathies (didanosine, zalcitabine)
Uncommon
　Mononeuritis multiplex
　　Early limited form
　　Late malignant form
　CMV polyradiculopathy
　Mononeuropathy associated with aseptic meningitis
　Mononeuropathy secondary to lymphomatous meningitis

Muscle

　Polymyositis
　Noninflammatory myopathies
　Zidovudine toxic myopathy

Central Nervous System Disorders Complicating Primary HIV-1 Infection

Although a variety of CNS disorders have been noted in the context of initial HIV-1 infection and seroconversion, these reports have principally involved individual cases,[9–17] and a general picture of their incidence and natural history is not available. Nonetheless, several general principles are apparent. First, the neurologic complication usually occurs approximately 2 weeks after the primary infection illness. Second, the neurologic presentation frequently involves multiple parts of the nervous system, although one part is dominant. Third, the illness is monophasic, with the majority of patients recovering within several weeks. With respect to laboratory analysis, cerebrospinal fluid (CSF) is frequently abnormal, showing a mild mononuclear pleocytosis and modest elevation of protein. Computed tomography (CT) of the brain is usually normal, whereas the electroencephalogram (EEG) may be diffusely or focally slow. In a review of 139 published cases of primary HIV-1 infection, encephalopathy and neuropathy were each reported in 8% of cases.[18] Less specific features, such as headache, have been reported in 30% to 45% of patients.[18–20]

Meningoencephalitis of varying severity, sometimes accompanied by seizures, often occurs within 2 weeks of the primary infection illness, and, despite severe initial disability, patients usually recover within several weeks. Myelopathy occurs even less frequently but follows the same temporal pattern, with most patients making a full recovery. Cranial and peripheral neuropathies have also been reported. Some patients develop a cranial neuropathy in the context of a generalized neuropathy, whereas others suffer isolated cranial neuropathies, most commonly facial nerve palsy.

The diagnosis of these syndromes can be difficult because they are indistinguishable from other acute viral or postinfectious encephalitides, most of which never achieve specific diagnosis. In addition, there may be no background systemic illness to engender suspicion of HIV-1 infection, and even if they are present, the acute systemic manifestations of HIV-1 may be overshadowed by the prominent neurologic symptoms and signs. If the patient is not identified as a member of a high-risk group or if serologic testing is not done, there may be no clue as to the etiologic diagnosis. Moreover, in those serotested in the acute phase, anti–HIV-1 antibodies may not be detected. Immunologic assessment likewise is usually unrewarding, because T-lymphocyte subsets are often normal or include only transient elevation of the CD8-positive subset, but usually without depression of the CD4-positive subset. Consequently, acute and convalescent serologic data are needed (extended to 6 to 12 weeks or longer), and in some patients virus isolation, p24 antigen detection or polymerase chain reaction (PCR) may be required for diagnosis. The effects of zidovudine or other therapy on these conditions have not been assessed.

HIV-1 Infection and Disease of the Central Nervous System During the Asymptomatic Phase

Evidence indicates that exposure of the CNS (or at least of the leptomeninges) is common early in the course of systemic HIV-1 infection and may, in fact, be the rule. This is supported principally by studies of CSF in asymptomatic, seropositive patients. These studies have shown abnormalities of routine studies, including cell count, protein, and immunoglobulin; local synthesis of anti–HIV-1 antibodies within the CNS compartment, and isolation of virus.[11,21–28] In one instance of iatrogenic injection of HIV-1–infected leukocytes, early penetration of the brain parenchyma was also documented.[29] These observations have both biologic and practical clinical implications. They reveal that both CNS exposure and host reactions to HIV-1 occur early in infection and continue through the asymptomatic period, yet without apparent immediate clinical sequelae. These background abnormalities must be taken into account when interpreting CSF results obtained for other diagnostic purposes.

The asymptomatic phase or period of clinical latency represents a time when the biology of CNS infection appears to diverge from that of symptomatic neurologic disease. The presence of abnormal CSF has not yet been shown to confer an adverse prognosis vis-a-vis ADC or other CNS involvement. Although early controversy centered on the isolated development of ADC in the absence of systemic disease,[30] from a broad population perspective this seems to be rare. In addition, even those patients who present with ADC usually exhibit laboratory evidence of immunosuppression or minor clinical complications of declining immune defenses, even if they have not yet developed other clinical AIDS-defining diseases. Particularly compelling in this regard are the results of the Multicenter AIDS Cohort Study (MACS) and other longitudinal studies, which have shown preservation of neurologic function in infected subjects who were otherwise asymptomatic.[31–35]

These and other laboratory abnormalities beg the question of whether there are subclinical CNS abnormalities in these patients and whether these abnormalities are prognostically important with respect to subsequent neurologic disease. Pathologic studies have shown evidence of inflammatory reactions with perivascular reactions,[36] although even with PCR amplification the viral burden appears to be negligible at this stage.[37–39] Neither overt nor subclinical cognitive or motor dysfunction appears to be common. From a practical standpoint, the risk of isolated cognitive decline in asymptomatic individuals is sufficiently small as to provide no basis for disability or disqualification from work based simply on HIV-1–positive serostatus.

One exception to this absence of CNS disease in this early phase is a rare multiple sclerosis–like illness that has been reported in HIV-1–infected patients.[40,41] The presentation has included remissions and exacerbations with corticosteroid responsiveness in the setting of preserved CD4 T-lymphocyte cell counts. Although it is possible that these cases represent the concurrence of two diseases, it appears more likely that an autoimmune disease indistinguishable from multiple sclerosis is triggered by HIV-1 infection. This illness may involve pathogenetic processes similar to those that underlie immune thrombocytopenic purpura or demyelinating polyneuropathy (see later discussion) in this same group of patients.

Aseptic Meningitis and Headache

Although the seroconversion-related illness may be accompanied by headache and aseptic meningitis, these clinical problems are more common and more important later in the course of HIV-1 infection. They occur most frequently in patients undergoing progression in HIV-1 infection with dropping CD4 cell counts and clinical manifestations of the AIDS-related complex.[42,43]

Hollander and Stringari segregated aseptic meningitis into two clinical types, an acute and a chronic form.[42] Both are accompanied by meningeal symptoms, including headache, whereas meningeal signs are confined largely to the acute group. Cranial nerve palsies may also complicate the course, most often affecting cranial nerves V, VII, or VIII, with Bell's palsy sometimes recurring. The CSF shows a mononuclear pleocytosis, usually with normal glucose and slightly elevated protein. The syndrome itself is benign, although affected patients may have an overall poor prognosis with respect to progression to AIDS-defining complications. There is no evidence that these patients are either more or less likely to develop ADC than patients without headache, but population-based data are lacking. It is presumed that these aseptic meningitis syndromes relate to HIV-1 itself, because this retrovirus can be isolated from the CSF of some of these patients.[44] However, another infection could cause the meningeal inflammation and secondarily induce the entry and proliferation of HIV-1–infected cells in the meninges.

Isolated headache is a common symptom and occurs in the same clinical setting as aseptic meningitis.[45,46] Indeed, it may be difficult to segregate true aseptic meningitis, in which local inflammation causes symptoms, from this headache if it is accompanied by incidental mild pleocytosis. The cause of this type of headache is uncertain, but it can be severe and intractable. In some patients, it appears to relate to development of systemic disease such as *Pneumocystis carinii* pneumonia (PCP) and hence may be caused by systemic production of vasoactive cytokines. We have observed that low doses of amitriptyline appear to be effective in controlling these headaches in some patients, but controlled studies are lacking.

AIDS Dementia Complex

ADC, which is characterized by cognitive, motor, and behavioral dysfunction, usually develops later in the course of HIV-1 infection and is one of the most common CNS complications of late untreated HIV disease.[4,47-52] Characteristically, this syndrome manifests after patients have developed major opportunistic infections or neoplasms that define systemic AIDS. However, a small number of patients present at a time when they do not yet fulfill formal criteria for the diagnosis of AIDS on the basis of their systemic disease.[30] Recognition of this early presentation has resulted in the addition of ADC to the diagnostic criteria for AIDS.[53] However, usually such patients have already evidenced minor complications of HIV-1 infection such as lymphadenopathy, malaise, weight loss, or oral candidiasis. Only a very small number of patients who are otherwise medically well and systemically asymptomatic develop major dementia, and even they are characteristically immunosuppressed by laboratory criteria.

Classification and Terminology

The term, AIDS dementia complex, was introduced to describe a clinical syndrome rather than a clearly established, uniform etiopathogenetic disease entity.[1,4,47,48,50] It remains useful to adhere to this original intent and to conceptually segregate ADC from HIV-1 brain infection. As discussed later in this chapter, HIV-1 does clearly infect the CNS, and it probably accounts for at least one of the pathologic subtypes of ADC. However, infection and disease have not yet been demonstrated to be synonymous.

The distinct character of the cognitive changes associated with ADC, which include prominent mental slowing and inattention along with concomitant affliction of motor performance (see later discussion), underlies the classification of ADC among the subcortical dementias. This group of neurologic conditions also includes the cognitive impairments associated with Parkinson's disease, Huntington's disease, hydrocephalus, and progressive supranuclear palsy[54]. Cortical dementias, on the other hand, include Alzheimer's disease, in which memory impairment predominates, and Creutzfeldt-Jacob disease, which variously presents with aphasia, apraxia, or other focal features.[55] Although the anatomic justification for this designation remains to be fully demonstrated, it is a clinically useful distinction and emphasizes the inappropriateness of applying to AIDS patients the definitions and measurement tools that were originally targeted to Alzheimer's disease.

In coining this terminology, each of its three components was chosen for a reason. *AIDS* was included because the morbidity of the condition may be comparable to that of other AIDS-defining complications of HIV-1 infection. *Dementia* was included because acquired and persistent cognitive decline is characteristically unaccompanied by alterations in the level of alertness, and it is this cognitive impairment that is usually the most disabling manifestation. The third component, *complex,* was added because the syndrome also importantly includes impaired motor performance and, at times, behavioral change, and the syndrome therefore is not simply an isolated dementia. Myelopathy

(but not peripheral neuropathy) and organic psychosis (but not reactive anxiety or depression) are included within this term because they may coexist with or be difficult to separate from the core cognitive and motor abnormalities.

Once the diagnosis of the ADC is made, it is useful to apply a staging scheme based on functional severity in the cognitive and motor spheres.[33,50] The scheme shown in Table 16-2 relies on a relatively simple functional evaluation and provides a common vocabulary for clinical use and for comparing patients assessed by different physicians. It also provides a simple framework for correlations with laboratory studies.

An alternative terminology has been proposed by the World Health Organization (WHO) and a task force of the American Academy of Neurology (AAN).[56,57] It has both advantages and disadvantages in relation to the ADC terminology[1] and can roughly be correlated with that staging scheme. The WHO/AAN classification uses the term "HIV-1–associated cognitive/motor complex" to encompass the full constellation of the ADC. Added subcategories refer to patients with predominantly cognitive presentations (HIV-1– associated dementia) or predominantly myelopathic presentations (HIV-1–associated myelopathy) of sufficient severity to interfere with work or activities of daily living (ie, equivalent to stage 2 or greater ADC). The term "HIV-1–associated minor cognitive/motor disorder" designates patients with mild symptoms and signs and only minimal functional impairment of work or activities of daily living (stage 1 ADC). In addition to separating patients with predominant myelopathy from those with cognitive changes, this terminology restricts the term dementia to patients with a level of cognitive impairment consistent with that used in other formal definitions. It may also simplify the reporting this condition as an AIDS-defining disorder to restrict that designation to patients with HIV-1–associated dementia or HIV-1–associated myelopathy, because the requirements for this level of severity are both biologically and prognostically consistent with those of other AIDS-defining conditions. Finally, the WHO/AAN classification also does not make the implicit assumption that the disorder is a single disease entity differing only in levels of severity; rather, it allows for the possibility that milder and more severe disease may result from different processes.

Clinical Features

The clinical features of ADC are briefly summarized in Table 16-3.[48] Patients' earliest symptoms usually consist of difficulties with concentration and attention. They begin to lose track of the train of thought or of conversation, and many complain of slowness in thinking. Complex tasks become more difficult and take longer to complete, and forgetfulness and difficulty in concentration lead to missed appointments and the need to keep detailed lists outlining each day's plan. If patients require a high level of concentration or organization for their occupation or activities at

TABLE 16-2. *Staging scheme for the AIDS dementia complex (ADC)*

Stage	Characteristics
Stage 0 (Normal)	Normal mental and motor function.
Stage 0.5 (Equivocal/subclinical)	Either minimal or equivocal symptoms of cognitive or motor dysfunction characteristic of ADC, or mild signs (snout response, slowed extremity movements), but without impairment of work or capacity to perform activities of daily living (ADL). Gait and strength are normal.
Stage 1 (Mild)	Unequivocal evidence (symptoms, signs, neuropsychologic test performance) of functional intellectual or motor impairment characteristic of ADC, but able to perform all but the more demanding aspects of work or ADL. Can walk without assistance.
Stage 2 (Moderate)	Cannot work or maintain the more demanding aspects of daily life, but able to perform basic activities of self-care. Ambulatory, but may require a single prop.
Stage 3 (Severe)	Major intellectual incapacity (cannot follow news or personal events, cannot sustain complex conversation, considerable slowing of all output) or motor disability (cannot walk unassisted, requires walker or personal support, usually with slowing and clumsiness of arms as well).
Stage 4 (End-stage)	Almost vegetative. Intellectual and social comprehension and responses are at a rudimentary level. Mute or almost mute. Paraparetic or paraplegic with double incontinence.

From Sidtis JJ, Price RW. Early HIV-1 infection and the AIDS dementia complex. (Comment) Neurology 1990;40:323; and Price R, Brew B. The AIDS dementia complex. J Infect Dis 1988;158:1079.

home, ADC may be recognized early because of impaired performance. In other instances, a friend or family member may be the first to notice subtle cognitive and personality changes as the patient begins to withdraw socially and appears apathetic and uncharacteristically quiet or forgetful. Although psychologic depression is usually mild or absent in these patients, in mild cases it can be difficult to separate depression or fatigue from early ADC. Usually, dysphoria is absent. In a minority, a more agitated organic psychosis may be the presenting or predominant aspect of the illness. Such patients are irritable and hyperactive and may become overtly manic.

Although cognitive manifestations usually appear earlier than motor symptoms and continue to predominate, in those with motor dysfunction early in the course of the disease poor balance and incoordination are the most common complaints. Gait incoordination may result in more frequent tripping or falling or in a perceived need to exercise new care in walking. Usually, these patients have vacuolar myelopathy pathologically. Patients may also drop things more frequently or become slower and less precise with hand activities; this may manifest as a distinct deterioration in handwriting.

Early in the evolution of the illness, formal bedside mental status testing may be remarkably normal, although responses are usually slowed even if their content is accurate. As the disease progresses, patients begin to perform poorly on tasks requiring concentration and attention, such as word and digit reversals and serial sevens. Later, a larger array of mental status tests become abnormal, affecting multiple domains of cognition. Slowing remains a prominent feature, and afflicted individuals often appear apathetic, have poor insight, and may be indifferent to their illness.

Even if not symptomatic, motor abnormalities can usually be detected on examination early in the course of the disease. Slowing of rapid successive or alternating movements of the fingers, wrists, or feet, as well as impaired ocular motility with interruption of smooth pursuits and slowing or inaccuracy of saccades, are common early findings. Also frequent is generalized hyperreflexia, including the jaw jerk, followed later by development of pathologic release reflexes, including snout, glabellar, and, less commonly, grasp responses. As the disease evolves, ataxia, which at first affects only rapid turns or tandem gait, may become disabling, although usually as patients worsen their leg weakness increases and paraparesis limits walking. Postural tremor is not unusual, and a few patients exhibit multifocal myoclonus or even choreiform movements. Bladder and bowel incontinence are common in the late stages of disease. In the end stage, patients become almost vegetative, lying in bed mute with a vacant stare, unable to ambulate, and incontinent. However, with the exception of occasional hypersomnolence, the level of arousal is usually preserved in the absence of intercurrent illness. Characteristically, the course is also notable for the absence of distinct focal neurologic deficits (eg, aphasia, hemiparesis).

In children, the disorder has the same general features, although the course can vary somewhat and can present in either a progressive or a static form.[58,59] The progressive form is characterized by the gradual loss of previously acquired motor skills in conjunction with evolution of motor abnormalities, ranging from spastic paraparesis to quadriplegia with pseudobulbar palsy and rigidity. Acquired microcephaly is the rule. The CDC surveillance criteria and classification for childhood AIDS now include neurologic disease with one or more progressive findings. These find-

TABLE 16-3. *Clinical features of the AIDS dementia complex*

Early Manifestations

SYMPTOMS

Cognition
  Impaired concentration
  Forgetfulness
  Mental slowing
Motor
  Unsteady gait
  Leg weakness
  Loss of coordination, impaired handwriting
  Tremor
Behavior
  Apathy, withdrawal, personality change
  Agitation, confusion, hallucinations

SIGNS

Mental status
  Psychomotor slowing
  Impaired serial 7's or reversals
  Organic psychosis
Neurological examination
  Impaired rapid movements (limbs, eyes)
  Hyperreflexia
  Release reflexes (snout, glabellar, grasp)
  Gait ataxia (impaired tandem gait, rapid turns)
  Tremor (postural)
  Leg weakness

Late Manifestations: Symptoms and Signs

Mental status
  Global dementia
  Psychomotor slowing: verbal responses delayed, near or
    absolute mutism, vacant stare
  Unawareness of illness, disinhibition
  Confusion, disorientation
  Organic psychosis
Neurologic signs
  Weakness (legs more than arms)
  Ataxia
  Pyramidal tract signs (spasticity, hyperreflexia, extensor
    plantar responses)
  Urinary and fecal incontinence
  Myoclonus

Navia B, Jordan B, Price R. The AIDS dementia complex: I. Clinical features. Ann Neurol 1986; 19:517, and Price R, Brew B. The AIDS dementia complex. J Infect Dis 1988;158:1079.

ings may include (1) loss of developmental milestones or intellectual ability; (2) impaired brain growth (acquired microcephaly or brain atrophy) demonstrated on CT scan or magnetic resonance imaging (MRI); or (3) symmetric motor deficits manifested by two or more of the following: paresis, abnormal tone, pathologic reflexes, ataxia, or gait disturbance.[60]

Neuropsychologic Test Profile

Formal neuropsychologic testing can be useful in assessing patients with ADC, both in the context of clinical research

studies of epidemiology and treatment and, in some cases, for practical patient diagnosis and management.[31–33,61,62] Appropriately chosen neuropsychologic assessments target the same cardinal dysfunction sought by the AIDS-directed clinical examination and provide a formal, quantitative means of monitoring patients serially. Assessments focus on alterations in motor speed, concentration, and mental manipulation. However, the results of neuropsychologic assessments should not be used as the sole or even major criteria for diagnosis, and they do not substitute for the clinical neurologic evaluation. The results are not disease-specific and should always be interpreted in the clinical context. Some patients with ADC perform within the population norms, and some without ADC do poorly on testing for other reasons. However, with proper interpretation, such studies can provide useful ancillary data, clarifying whether the magnitude and profile of the functional deficit are consistent with the history and hence with the diagnosis of ADC and the clinical staging. This methodology is useful for assessing natural history, population functions, and responses to therapy.[4,63]

Neuroimaging Studies

Neuroimaging procedures are often essential to the evaluation of AIDS patients with CNS dysfunction. In those considered for diagnosis of ADC, neuroimaging is particularly important to rule out other conditions such as primary CNS lymphoma. In addition, neuroimaging often reveals abnormalities that are characteristic although not diagnostic. These include the almost universal finding of cerebral atrophy on either CT or MRI.[48,64–68] In some affected patients, MRI shows abnormalities in the hemispheric white matter and, less commonly, in the basal ganglia or thalamus with either patchy or diffusely increased signal, most apparent in T2-weighted images.[65,69–72] Children with AIDS-related dementia often have basal ganglia calcification in addition to atrophy.[73]

Results of metabolic imaging (eg, positron emission tomography, single-photon emission computed tomography [SPECT], MRI spectroscopy) have also been reported, although the diagnostic utility of these modalities remains to be clearly delineated.[74–83] In the case of positron emission tomography, improvements in abnormalities of cerebral glucose metabolism have been used to corroborate the therapeutic effects of antiviral treatment.[84]

Cerebrospinal Fluid

CSF examination, like neuroimaging, is used principally to exclude other diagnoses. The results need to be considered in the context of the nonspecific changes found in clinically normal HIV-1–infected individuals (discussed previously). Routine examination of the CSF of patients with ADC reveals nonspecific findings of mildly elevated protein in approximately two thirds and a mild mononuclear pleocytosis in almost one quarter.[48] When CSF findings in a group of patients with ADC were analyzed in relation to clinical severity, there appeared to be a reduction in pleocytosis with greater severity.[85] HIV-1 can be isolated directly from the CSF of many of these patients,[28] but this finding is common also in infected patients who are asymptomatic or who have aseptic meningitis. In approximately half of severely affected patients (ADC stages 3 and 4), HIV-1 p24 antigen may be detected by immunoassay in the CSF; however, in less severely affected patients (ie, those in whom laboratory diagnosis would be most helpful), p24 is infrequently detected.[85] This finding is also usually of limited practical utility because the diagnosis is most often clinically quite evident in such patients. This may also be the case with detection of HIV-1 DNA in the CSF by PCR, again because of a high false-positive rate among a wide array of HIV-1–infected individuals. Whether quantitative PCR to assess the CSF viral burden will prove to be clinically useful awaits further study.

Of perhaps greater value, certain surrogate markers of immune-cell activation have been noted to be increased in the CSF of patients with ADC, with concentrations correlating, to some extent, with clinical severity. These markers include β_2-microglobulin, a noncovalently-bound portion of the class I major histocompatibility complex, and neopterin, a product of pteridine metabolism that appears to be released by activated macrophages.[86–90] Quinolinic acid is similarly elevated[91]; this product of tryptophan metabolism can be induced by interferon-γ and perhaps by other cytokines, and it can act at the N-methyl-D-aspartate (NMDA) receptor as an endogenous excitotoxin. It has been hypothesized that quinolinic acid may contribute to CNS injury in patients with ADC.[92] Whether or not quinolinic acid is a major factor in brain injury, its elevation along with the other surrogate markers in CSF indicates that, although AIDS patients are immunosuppressed, certain immune-cell responses are upregulated as disease progresses. This occurs in both the blood and CSF compartments and reflects parallel processes in systemic and CNS disease. Because these markers may be increased by the action of cytokines, these observations suggest that cytokine-related reactions may be involved in the production of CNS injury.[51,93–102] Other markers of immune activation that may be elevated in the CSF, probably as a result of shared pathways but seemingly of less clinical utility, include as tumor necrosis factor-α, prostaglandins, interleukin-1β, and interleukin-6, among others.[87,89,90,103–108]

CSF surrogate markers may also be clinically useful, although further study is needed. Elevated levels of β_2-microglobulin, neopterin, and quinolinic acid in the CSF are not diagnostically specific; they also occur in the CSF of patients with opportunistic CNS infections and CNS lymphoma.[87,88,91] However, in the absence of such conditions, increased concentrations of these markers may be helpful in assessing mild or equivocal ADC. They may also prove useful in monitoring the effects of therapy, because zidovudine treatment lowers their concentration in CSF.[87,89]

Specialized CSF examination may also reveal abnormalities in immunoglobulin, including evidence of intrathecal IgG synthesis and presence of oligoclonal bands, but because these abnormalities are also detected in patients who do not have ADC, their diagnostic utility is uncertain.[24]

Epidemiology and Natural History

The epidemiology of ADC, including its prevalence at various stages of systemic HIV-1 infection, is not fully delineated.[51] Initial estimates were based largely on clinical case observations rather than on prospective, controlled epidemiologic investigations. However, a number of more recent studies have more clearly characterized some of the neurologic and neuropsychologic aspects of asymptomatic HIV-1 seropositivity.[31,32,35] It is now recognized that ADC develops principally in the setting of late HIV-1 infection and severe immunosuppression, and consequently its prevalence differs greatly according to the stage of infection in the group studied.[48,52,109,110] Recent prospective data from the MACS show an ADC incidence rate over a 5-year period of 7.3 cases per 100 person-years for patients with blood CD4 counts of 100 cells/mm^3 or lower, 3.0 cases for counts of 101 to 200 cells/mm^3, 1.3 to 1.7 cases for counts of 201 to 500 cells/mm^3, and 0.5 cases per 100 person-years for counts higher than 500 cells/mm^3.[110] Data from the Community Programs for Clinical Research on AIDS also document that ADC is associated with limited survival times. The 6-month cumulative mortality rate for 97 patients with stage 2, 3, or 4 ADC was 67%.[52] This was almost three times the rate for patients with PCP. In addition, the epidemiology of ADC may be undergoing modification related to the widespread early use of antiviral therapy.[111,112]

Some studies have suggested that certain risk factors for development of progressive ADC may be identified. For example, in the prospective MACS, McArthur and colleagues noted that lower hemoglobin concentration and body mass index before development of AIDS and more constitutional symptoms and older age at onset of AIDS were associated with increased subsequent progression to ADC.[109] In a multivariate analysis, lower hemoglobin concentration was the only significant factor. Brew and associates (unpublished observations) have studied patients with more advanced HIV-1 infection (CD4 count <200 cells/mm^3) and observed an increasing risk of subsequent development of ADC with increasing CSF concentrations of β_2-microglobulin and neopterin. In this more advanced population of patients, hemoglobin concentration was not a risk factor. In the future, clear identification of such risk factors may be useful in selecting patients for more rigorous secondary prophylaxis against ADC.

Neuropathology

The histopathologic abnormalities most commonly found in patients with ADC are white matter pallor and gliosis, multinucleated-cell encephalitis, and vacuolar myelopathy.[49,113–117]

Other findings include vacuolar changes in the brain, focal necrosis, and neuronal loss. These abnormalities are most prominent in the subcortical structures—the central white matter, the deep gray structures including basal ganglia and thalamus, the brain stem, and the spinal cord—with relative sparing of the cortex, at least on routine examination. It is attractive to hypothesize that this predilection underlies the subcortical character of the clinical dementia.

Vacuolar myelopathy pathologically resembles subacute combined degeneration caused by vitamin B_{12} deficiency,[118] but levels of this vitamin are usually normal in serum. Although there is a general correlation between the incidence of vacuolar myelopathy and that of other pathologic abnormalities found in the brain, it can occur in the absence of the changes associated with multinucleated cells and vice versa, and it does not correlate with the presence of productive infection in the way that multinucleation does.[119–122] These discrepancies leave open the question of whether vacuolar myelopathy is an etiopathogenetically independent process. Patients with this pathology usually manifest hyperactive deep tendon reflexes, ataxia, spasticity, or paraplegia, depending on its severity.

Etiology and Pathogenesis

Evidence from clinical observations, direct studies of brain, and animal models supports the hypothesis that ADC is caused by HIV-1 itself rather than some other pathogen. However, the mechanisms connecting the virus to brain injury remain enigmatic. Infection of the CNS by HIV has been detected by a variety of techniques, beginning with Southern blot analyses, which showed a high frequency of proviral DNA (comparable to that of lymphatic tissue) and high copy number in the brains of some patients with ADC.[123] In situ studies have also detected the presence of viral DNA and RNA within the brains of these patients.[124,125] Viral antigens have been observed in brain with the use of immunohistochemical techniques,[126–130] and HIV-1 virions have been identified by electron microscopy.[131,132] Both integrated and nonintegrated forms of the genome have been found. Strains isolated or cloned from brain have exhibited the phenotypic characteristic of macrophage-tropism[133–135] and may even share sequences conferring particular brain-tropism.[136]

Consistent with the macrophage-tropism, the principal cell type that has been identified as supporting productive HIV-1 brain infection is the macrophage and its brain counterpart with similar bone marrow origin, the microgliocyte. This appears to be a critical cell in the pathogenesis of both HIV-1 brain infection and ADC. This cell sustains productive infection and triggers cytokine pathways.[3,4,95,122,137–139] Although not an invariant finding in HIV-1–infected brains, the multinucleated cells are histologic markers of productive HIV-1 brain infection, and the multinucleation probably results from direct virus-induced cell fusion of macrophages and microglia. The role of infection of other cell types remains uncertain but has received support from more recent studies using PCR amplification in concert with in situ hybridization.[140] Neurons, vascular endothelial cells, and astrocytes may all be infected at a low level. Replication appears to be restricted in the case of astrocytes, and probably with these other cells as well; there is little output of progeny virions but, in some instances, there is expression of regulatory genes, including [141,142] Even with restricted expression, the HIV-1 genome may alter cell function.

Because of the limited productive infection in many cases[143,144] and the limited direct involvement of neuroectodermal cells in infection, a variety of indirect mechanisms of brain injury by HIV-1 are paramount. These involve toxic viral gene products and pathologic amplification of toxicity by cytokines and endogenous neurotoxic pathways. These pathogenetic theories have been extensively reviewed elsewhere.[3,93,95,99,122,145]

Management and Treatment of Central Nervous System HIV-1 Infection and the AIDS Dementia Complex

Accumulating evidence indicates that ADC can be treated and perhaps prevented, at least to some extent, by antiretroviral drug therapy. Initial anecdotal case reports[146] have been supplemented by controlled studies showing that zidovudine improves neuropsychologic performance in adult patients with HIV-1 infection, compared to placebo.[63,147] A pediatric trial of constant infusion of zidovudine resulted in striking improvement in neuropsychologic performance in a group of children with and without overt neurodevelopmental abnormalities.[148,149] Pertinent to the issue of prevention, a study of the epidemiology of ADC in the Netherlands suggested that zidovudine reduced the incidence of new cases of ADC after it was first introduced into widespread clinical practice.[112]

Unresolved issues with zidovudine include the question of optimal dosages in both prophylactic and therapeutic situations. In the absence of precise guidelines, conventional dosage (500 to 600 mg/day) is recommended in both situations. For patients who deteriorate neurologically on this regimen, the clinician may either increase the dosage to 1000 mg or more per day, thereby increasing the risk of toxicity, or switch to another antiretroviral agent such as dideoxyinosine (ddI). Although there is some suggestion of activity,[150] the efficacy of ddI in ADC is still under investigation.

The possible role of toxins in the genesis ADC underlies proposed therapies that interfere with various steps in their action. For example, the calcium channel blocker nimodipine, which blocks the toxicity of HIV-1 gp120 in neuronal cell culture,[151] has been tested in a pilot clinical trial, although without clear indication of efficacy. Other inhibitors of neurotoxic reactions are now being explored.

OPPORTUNISTIC CENTRAL NERVOUS SYSTEM INFECTIONS

A variety of infections of the CNS commonly complicate late-stage HIV-1 infection,[152–154] including most importantly

Toxoplasma gondii, Cryptococcus neoformans, JC virus (which causes progressive multifocal leukoencephalitis, or PML), and cytomegalovirus (CMV). Specific diagnosis of these and other CNS infections is important, because several of them can be effectively treated.

Cerebral Toxoplasmosis

Cerebral toxoplasmosis is the most frequent of the CNS opportunistic infections occurring in AIDS; it complicates the course of 5% to 15% of patients or more, depending on geographic origin.[110,155–163] The varying incidence relates principally to the likelihood of earlier environmental exposure to the etiologic protozoan parasite, *T gondii.* Cerebral toxoplasmosis almost invariably results from recrudescence of previously acquired infection and relates to loss of the immune defenses that maintain *T gondii* in an inactive, encysted form. One study estimated that approximately one quarter of HIV-1–infected patients with antibodies against this parasite eventually develop cerebral toxoplasmosis.[157] The incidence has declined where trimethaprim-sulfamethoxazole has been used as prophylaxis for PCP, because this regimen is also effective in reducing the development of cerebral toxoplasmosis.[164,165]

Clinical presentation of cerebral toxoplasmosis is characteristically subacute, evolving over several days from initial symptoms to presentation with neurologic deficit.[155,160] Focal cerebral dysfunction usually predominates but is often combined with or occasionally overshadowed by nonfocal, encephalitis-like symptoms and signs. Focal manifestations usually relate to hemispheric lesions and include hemiparesis, hemianesthesia, aphasia, apraxia, or seizures. Cerebellar ataxia and brain stem abnormalities are far less common. The encephalitic features include general confusion or altered consciousness with lethargy or even coma. In a minority of patients, a picture of subacute encephalitis without clear focal features predominates. Headache and fever are also relatively common. The typical patient appears ill and lethargic and exhibits lateralizing neurologic symptoms or signs.

Pathologically, the disease is characterized by a variable number of cerebral abscesses.[155,166] In the acute encephalitic form of the disease, the brain exhibits numerous small lesions, with little in the way of cellular reaction.[167] The more common, slowly developing lesions are often larger and are surrounded by mononuclear cell reaction, edema, and, at times, vascular occlusion or an element of microscopic hemorrhage. Chronic healed lesions exhibit minor fibrotic changes. Untreated disease is characterized by the presence of free forms (tachyzoites) of *T gondii;* after treatment, these are no longer seen, although encysted forms may persist.

The diagnosis of cerebral toxoplasmosis relies on ready clinical suspicion, the use of neuroimaging procedures, and therapeutic trial, with blood serology being of ancillary help.[2,155,160] In approaching AIDS patients with suspected toxoplasmosis or other focal disorders, MRI (or, less optimally,

CT scanning) is critical, both to confirm the presence of macroscopic focal disease and to determine the nature of the abnormalities.[168] A finding of multiple lesions involving the cortex or deep brain nuclei (thalamus, basal ganglia) surrounded by edema strongly favors a diagnosis of cerebral toxoplasmosis. *Toxoplasma* abscesses usually exhibit ring-like contrast enhancement on MRI and CT, but either homogeneous contrast enhancement or nonenhancing hypodense lesions may be noted in some cases. MRI is usually superior to CT for detection of *Toxoplasma* abscesses, revealing location and multiplicity of lesions.

Table 16-4 compares cerebral toxoplasmosis with the two other common causes of focal brain disease in AIDS, primary CNS lymphoma and PML, and with ADC. The most common issue in these patients is the differentiation of cerebral toxoplasmosis from primary CNS lymphoma, because the appearance of these lesions on CT or MRI may be similar. The lesions of lymphoma commonly exhibit more diffuse or less clear-cut contrast enhancement on CT; they tend to be radiologically less numerous and are more often located in the white matter adjacent to the lateral ventricles, with a tendency for subependymal extension. PML lesions are in the white matter, often at the cortical junction, and do not have mass effect. Recently, thallium SPECT imaging has been applied to the differentiation of these entities, with toxoplasmosis characterized by decreased uptake of the radionuclide and lymphoma by increased uptake.[169] This is a promising methodology but needs to be evaluated further, particularly with respect to its utility in otherwise ambiguous cases.

Toxoplasma serology is of additional help if appropriately interpreted. Because the disease is caused by reactivation of the organism, patients with cerebral toxoplasmosis rarely have negative serum IgG antibody titers.[155,157] However, these titers may be low (occasionally an apparently negative titer is positive if a more concentrated specimen, such as a 1:4 dilution, is tested), and they frequently do not rise during the course of the disease. A positive titer therefore indicates susceptibility, and a negative titer casts doubt on the diagnosis. Recently, PCR has been used to detect *T gondii* nucleic acid in tissue samples, CSF, or serum[170–173]; although promising, further work is needed before this technique can be accepted for use in routine diagnosis.

Practical diagnosis of cerebral toxoplasmosis now relies principally on a therapeutic trial of antitoxoplasmosis treatment.[2,155,160,174] Brain biopsy is reserved for treatment failures or clinically atypical patients, such as those who are seronegative or have uncharacteristic MRI or CT studies. If treated promptly, toxoplasmosis responds with clear clinical and neuroimaging improvement, usually within a few days to 1 week. If brain biopsy is done, immunoperoxidase staining considerably increases the sensitivity for detection of *T gondii,* and PCR may prove helpful as well.

Because therapy for cerebral toxoplasmosis is discussed in chapter 14.1, it is not reviewed here. However, one issue related to neurologic care in these patients is the use of corticosteroids to reduce cerebral edema. In general, corticos-

TABLE 16-4. *Differential diagnosis of four common central nervous system complications of AIDS*

Disorder	Temporal Evaluation	Alertness	Number of Lesions	Type of Lesions	Location of Lesions
Cerebral toxoplasmosis	Days	Reduced	Multiple	Spherical enhancement, mass effect	Cortex, basal ganglia
Primary CNS lymphoma	Days to weeks	Variable	1 or few	Diffuse enhancement, mass effect	Periventricular, white matter
Progressive multifocal leukoencephalitis	Weeks	Preserved	Multiple	Nonenhancing, no mass effect	White matter, adjacent to cortex
AIDS dementia complex	Weeks to months	Preserved	None, multiple or diffuse	Increased T2 signal, no enhancement or mass effect	White matter, basal ganglia

teroids should be avoided, if possible, in the treatment of any AIDS patient. This is particularly important when considering a therapeutic trial to differentiate between toxoplasmosis and CNS lymphoma. Because the latter may respond symptomatically and radiologically to corticosteroids alone, clinical or neuroimaging improvement on combination antibiotic and steroid treatment is difficult to interpret. More generally, corticosteroids intensify the impairment of immune defenses in AIDS patients, potentially worsening not only toxoplasmosis but also other systemic opportunistic infections. For these reasons, we use corticosteroids only if mass effect is sufficient to threaten brain herniation; after improvement is seen, corticosteroids are tapered rapidly.

Cryptococcal Meningitis

Cryptococcal meningitis is the most common CNS fungal infection in AIDS, eventually affecting 5% to 10% of patients.[175–180] Although it most frequently presents as a subacute meningitis with headache, nausea, vomiting, confusion, and lethargy, just as in non-AIDS patients, symptoms and signs can be remarkably mild and unspecific. Likewise, the CSF formula may be bland, with few or no cells and little or no perturbation in glucose or protein levels. Accordingly, CSF cryptococcal antigen titers should be obtained routinely, as should fungal cultures and India ink preparations in all AIDS patients at lumbar puncture. Serum cryptococcal antigen is also almost always positive[181] and may therefore serve as a screening tool in patients in whom the diagnostic suspicion is low, or if the patient refuses a spinal tap or a spinal tap should be avoided (eg, with thrombocytopenia or other bleeding diathesis). Neuroimaging is frequently negative or only nonspecifically abnormal. However, MRI may show meningitis or meningoencephalitis, dilated Virchow-Robin spaces, cyst-like structures (gelatinous pseudocysts), and granulomas (cryptococcomas) of the choroid plexuses, which suggest the diagnosis.[176]

Therapy for cryptococcal meningitis is also discussed in chapter 14.2. At present, optimal treatment is still somewhat uncertain. The overall efficacy of fluconazole is similar to that of amphotericin B.[179,182–184] In a comparison trial, amphotericin B initially led to more rapid clearing of cryptococcus from the CSF, but the differences were not significant at 8 weeks, and the advantage of amphotericin B was countered by its propensity for organ toxicity, principally renal toxicity, and by the necessity of administration through a central venous catheter with the attendant risk of infection.[179] Consequently, one recommendation is that amphotericin be used initially in more severely ill patients, such as patients who are obtunded or who have a CSF antigen titer greater than 1:256; fluconazole can be used in the remainder and after the severely affected patients improve and stabilize. The dose of fluconazole that is used is 200 to 400 mg/day (after a loading dose of 800 mg); that for amphotericin B is 0.4 to 0.8 mg/kg/day. The efficacy of 5-flucytosine is controversial in this group of patients, and it is not routinely administered.

Patients who do not respond to these regimens deserve assessment to determine the precise reason for the failure. Failure may result from continued active infection or from the residual sequelae of infection, including hydrocephalus in particular. Patients who develop hydrocephalus as the cause of persistent headache or other symptoms may require ventriculoperitoneal shunting or repeated spinal taps. Persistent cryptococcal infection may also result from poor oral absorption of fluconazole or from drug resistance. Although fluconazole levels are not generally available, they have been useful in some patients, in our experience, to demonstrate poor oral absorption and the necessity for higher than usual doses. Drug resistance to fluconazole does not appear to be common, but sensitivity testing has proven to be of some use in difficult patients. In some patients, resistance to fluconazole can be circumvented by the use of higher than usual doses of the drug.

After successful induction therapy, the relapse rate is still high, and all patients require maintenance therapy. Usually, this consists of a lower dose of the agent used for induction. For example, amphotericin may be given at a dose of 1 mg/kg one to three times per week, or fluconazole at doses of 100 to 200 mg/day.[185]

There are now data showing that fluconazole is an effective prophylactic agent against cryptococcal meningitis,[186] although the optimal dose and time to start this drug are still uncertain. There is also still the theoretical risk of the development of drug resistance as a consequence of long-term drug administration.

Progressive Multifocal Leukoencephalitis

PML is an opportunistic infection caused by JC virus, the human papovavirus,[187–191] that develops in about 4% of AIDS patients. The disease is characterized by selective demyelination. The pathologic lesions begin as small foci, most often in the subcortical white matter, which then coalesce to form larger lesions that eventually cavitate. Lesions of the hemispheres are most common, but the cerebellum and brain stem may also be affected. The microscopic appearance includes pathognomonic inclusion-bearing, swollen oligodendrocyte nuclei and bizarre pleomorphic, hyperchromatic astrocytes. The oligodendrocyte inclusions are filled with JC virus nucleocapsids, which can be identified by electron microscopy, and the demyelinating lesions are caused by the death of these cells with secondary degeneration of their myelin-forming processes. Inflammation is inconspicuous in most cases.

Like toxoplasmosis and primary CNS lymphoma, PML presents with focal neurologic deficit. However, in PML the clinical evolution is usually more protracted, and altered consciousness or other encephalitic signs are usually not present (see Table 16-4). Rather, the picture is one of worsening focal deficits, such as hemiparesis, hemianopsia, aphasia, hemisensory deficit, and ataxia. The hemispheres are more commonly involved than the posterior fossa structures. Diagnosis often can be suspected clinically, whereas neuroimaging usually helps to support the diagnosis and rule out confounding diseases.[192,193] Again, MRI is superior to CT and shows white matter lesions, often adjacent to the cortex and usually most evident on T2-weighted images. These abnormalities should correlate with clinical deficits and should not be confused with the white matter changes associated with ADC. A useful aphorism is, "In PML, the patient is worse than the scan, and in ADC, the scan looks worse than the patient." This refers particularly to focal clinical deficits, which are characteristic of PML and absent in ADC. Usually, the PML abnormalities do not enhance and are not accompanied by mass effect; importantly, the lesions of PML usually show low attenuation (black) on T1-weighted images, whereas those of the ADC most often are not seen in this sequence. Neither serum nor CSF serologies are useful in diagnosis, because positive serum titers against JC virus are found in the majority of the normal population and CSF titers are negative. Definitive diagnosis is made by brain biopsy or at autopsy. Light microscopy is usually adequate to establish the diagnosis, but occasionally immunocytochemistry or in situ hybridization may be useful. PCR of spinal fluid has been introduced and shows considerable promise, although both false-positive and false-negative results can be obtained.[194,195] Standardization of this assessment modality may provide considerable help in specific diagnosis in the future.

There is no proven effective therapy for the disease. Uncontrolled studies indicate that zidovudine, interferon-γ, or cytosine arabinoside (administered either intrathecally or intravenously) may be helpful in some cases, but further study is required.[196,197] Spontaneous sustained remission of PML in AIDS does occur and provides hope for development of new interventional strategies.[198] Currently, only optimization of antiretroviral therapy (to possibly reverse the loss of anti–JC virus defenses) and entry into ongoing clinical trials can be recommended.

Cytomegalovirus Infection

The role of CMV in the spectrum of the neurologic morbidity of HIV-1 infection remains incompletely defined, largely because antemortem diagnosis may be very difficult. Systemic CMV infection is common in AIDS patients, and evidence of minor brain CMV infection in the form of isolated inclusion-bearing cells within an occasional microglial nodule can be found at autopsy in as many as one third.[49,113,199] The contribution of this level of CMV infection to neurologic symptoms and signs in AIDS patients is uncertain; probably, it is most often minor and overshadowed by the ADC.[49] However, CMV may on occasion cause clinically overt encephalitis. In one retrospective study in which the diagnosis of CMV encephalitis was made by pathologic examination of the brain, patients most often presented with the subacute onset over weeks of a confusional state.[200] Approximately 20% had the additional finding of cranial neuropathies, and 14% had seizures. In more than half of the patients, CMV encephalitis occurred in the setting of maintenance or, less commonly, induction therapy with ganciclovir for CMV retinitis. Radiologically, periventricular inflammation on MRI scanning of the brain was seen in most patients. Hyponatremia was common. The CSF profile did not show a polymorphonuclear pleocytosis; a pleocytosis was observed in only 20%, and in those cases it was predominantly lymphocytic. Amplification of CMV DNA from the CSF by the PCR was positive in only one third of these patients, but other studies have found a higher positive yield.[201–204]

In cases in which CMV infection of the brain is highly suspected, specific antiviral therapy with the use of ganciclovir, foscarnet, or a combination of these drugs should be considered, although their efficacy in CNS CMV infection, other than in retinopathy, has not yet been adequately tested, nor have optimum doses been established. Efficacy of treatment is suggested only by anecdotal experience.

Mycobacterial Infections

Although *Mycobacterium tuberculosis* is not strictly an opportunistic pathogen, CNS infection with this organism is more common and perhaps more severe in certain groups of HIV-1–infected individuals. The development of tuberculosis is also influenced by socioeconomic factors, and it predominantly affects persons with inadequate health care and living conditions, including intravenous drug abusers, rather than those in middle and upper income groups, including many whose risk factors for AIDS are homosexuality or transfusion.[205-207] Even among AIDS patients with systemic tuberculosis, CNS involvement appear to be uncommon, although, if it is present, it may be more aggressive in these patients. Clinical presentations can include meningitis, acute abscess, and indolent, chronic tuberculoma.[208,209] Diagnosis in some cases may be difficult and may require brain biopsy; as in other infections, PCR detection of nucleic acid in blood or spinal fluid, or at brain biopsy in the obtained specimen, may strengthen the diagnosis.[210] Although systemic atypical mycobacteria, especially *Mycobacterium avium-intracellulare,* commonly infect AIDS patients, they only very rarely cause overt clinical CNS disease. Even though organisms have been detected on occasion in the CSF or even in brain, they have not been shown to infiltrate the brain parenchyma or to cause clinical symptoms and signs.[211]

Varicella-Zoster Virus and Herpes Simplex Virus Infections

Although unusual, varicella-zoster virus (VZV) and, to a lesser extent, herpes simplex virus (HSV-1 and HSV-2) have been reported to cause CNS disease in AIDS patients. VZV infections are of several types: (1) multifocal direct brain infection affecting principally the white matter and partially mimicking PML[212-214]; (2) cerebral vasculitis, which may involve medium-sized vessels, characteristically occurring in the setting of ophthalmic herpes zoster and causing contralateral hemiplegia,[215,216] or may involve smaller vessels, associated at times with meningeal reaction and causing multifocal infarcts in brain or spinal cord; (3) myelopathy complicating herpes zoster and (4) ventriculitis.[217,220] Both HSV-1 and HSV-2 have been identified in brains of some AIDS patients, but the clinical correlates of these infections in AIDS patients have not yet been wholly delineated.[218,219]

Syphilis

The influence of HIV-1 infection on the course, diagnosis, and treatment of syphilis is controversial.[221-228] There is some evidence that syphilis may have a more aggressive course, with neurologic complications occurring at an earlier time, and that the complications may be atypical. Patients have been described who presented with meningovascular syphilis and cerebral gummata after seemingly adequate treatment for primary syphilis.[229] In addition to meningovascular syphilis, a polyradiculopathy has also been emphasized.[230] However, such treatment failures have been known for a considerable time, and unusually short times to progression have been recorded in the absence of HIV-1 infection. Both diagnosis and therapeutic monitoring of neurosyphilis in patients infected with HIV-1 can be problematic, because it can be difficult to know which process is responsible for CSF abnormalities. Moreover, neurosyphilis can occur despite a negative CSF result on the VDRL test or even on the fluorescent treponemal antibody absorption test. From a practical viewpoint, clinical suspicion should be high in these patients, and, if neurosyphilis is suspected, full-dose treatment (eg, 1 to 2 million units of intravenous penicillin for 10 days) should be given, and benzathine penicillin should not be relied on.

Other Infections

Although unusual, cerebral aspergillus and *Nocardia, Candida,* and *Listeria* CNS infections have all been reported in AIDS patients.[231-243] These are usually agonal complications, and they can be taken as evidence that host defenses other than those typically impaired by HIV-1 infection are involved in protecting the brain against these organisms. Because susceptibility is increased by neutropenia, an increased incidence may be anticipated in the setting of therapies that depress the bone marrow. Diagnosis is difficult and depends on identification of the organism in the brain by biopsy, in CSF, or outside the brain; these complications usually follow well established infection elsewhere. *Strongyloides stercoralis* hyperinfection has also been reported as a complication of HIV-1 disease.[244]

OPPORTUNISTIC CENTRAL NERVOUS SYSTEM NEOPLASMS

The CNS of AIDS patients is also subject to the development of opportunistic neoplasms, and in particular to lymphomas, which either arise in the brain itself or metastasize from extraneural sites. Although Kaposi's sarcoma involving the brain has been reported,[245] it is so exceedingly rare that it does not warrant general consideration in differential diagnosis of brain disease.

Primary Central Nervous System Lymphoma

Primary CNS lymphomas of B-cell origin are opportunistic neoplasms that complicate the course of AIDS in approximately 5% of patients; this estimate, however, includes lymphomas noted only incidentally at autopsy.[110,246-253] The incidence of primary CNS lymphoma in non-AIDS patients is increasing,[252,253] and our own recent experience suggests that this may also be the case in AIDS patients, perhaps because of their increased longevity and the efficacy of both prophylactic and therapeutic measures against various opportunistic infections. Patients with primary brain lymphomas present with progressive focal or multifocal neurologic deficits similar to those seen with toxoplasmosis or PML. The tempo of disease evolution is usually somewhere between those of these other two diseases, with patients presenting after several days to a few weeks of progressive symptoms (see Table 16-4). These symptoms may include change of personality or behavior, hemiparesis, dysphasia, and other indications of hemispheral dysfunction. Headache is relatively common, but fever and constitutional symptoms are absent except in the case of systemic infection. Because of the deep location of the lymphoma, some patients may appear dull and apathetic, with gait disturbance but few lateralizing signs; in such cases, ADC may be a principal differential diagnosis.

Neuroradiologic studies are most important in evaluation of these patients, and both MRI and CT usually are able to detect symptomatic lesions. Once again, MRI is the more sensitive of these two methods. Characteristically, primary CNS lymphoma tumors are microscopically multicentric, but they often show only one or two lesions on MRI or CT scan. Their location is characteristically deep in the brain, adjacent to the lateral ventricles, and often in the white rather than the gray matter; MRI may show characteristic subependymal extension. On CT scan, the lesions may enhance after contrast administration, but often such enhancement is weak or absent or assumes a diffuse rather than a ring-like pattern. Mass effect is present, but there may be little surrounding edema. CSF cytology is frequently negative or equivocal, and definitive diagnosis therefore almost always relies on brain biopsy. Most often, brain biopsy is undertaken after a trial of antitoxoplasmosis therapy fails to result in clinical improvement. However, the decision to proceed with biopsy can be accelerated if the lesion or lesions have the characteristic appearance and periventricular distribution of lymphoma and if blood toxoplasmosis serology is negative. Clinicians familiar with CNS lymphoma can often predict the correct diagnosis and accelerate the decision to proceed with biopsy. Thallium SPECT may also prove useful in supporting the diagnosis of lymphoma and early biopsy.[169] The use of stereotaxic biopsy techniques has increased the access to these tumors and reduced the morbidity of biopsy.

The current standard therapy for lymphoma in AIDS patients consists of whole-brain irradiation and administration of corticosteroids.[250,249,250] If the latter are used, these patients should also receive PCP prophylaxis. At present, there is no defined role for systemic chemotherapy. Aggressive chemotherapy has become the treatment of choice for primary CNS lymphoma in non-AIDS patients,[253] and it may eventually become so in AIDS patients as well. However, primary CNS lymphomas characteristically occur late in the course of HIV-1 infection, at a time when systemic disease is advanced and patients are more vulnerable to the toxic effects of cytoreductive drugs. Their bone marrow reserve is limited, and tolerance for chemotherapy is reduced, both by HIV-1 itself and often by the use of zidovudine. Chemotherapy may also preclude the continued chronic use of concurrent zidovudine, ganciclovir, or other therapies. Moreover, these patients most often die of other HIV-1–related complications rather than lymphoma, and most often within a time frame before the recurrence that characterizes lymphoma in non-AIDS patients.[246,249] Overall, primary CNS lymphomas in AIDS patients respond relatively well to radiation therapy, and many patients can remain "cured" for the remainder of their lives. Because early treatment decreases morbidity, the diagnosis should be pursued with vigor and treatment should be advocated. On the other hand, these patients are usually in a poor prognostic group because of the presence of systemic disease, and their overall survival time is short. It is possible that corticosteroids or other therapeutic measures may accelerate systemic disease in these patients, but this is difficult to judge.

Metastatic Lymphoma

Systemic lymphoma complicating HIV-1 infection may secondarily involve the CNS. The incidence of metastatic CNS spread is as high as 40%.[250,254–257] Unlike primary brain lymphomas, metastatic lymphomas most frequently involve the meninges or dura rather than the brain parenchyma. The presentation therefore involves cranial nerve palsies, headaches, spinal epidural cord compression, or increased intracranial pressure rather than with hemiparesis or other hemispheral signs. However, metastatic parenchymal brain disease or multifocal disease appearing simultaneously in both the brain and systemic organs can also occur, and in some cases the course may be fulminant. Otherwise, the clinical and diagnostic features resemble those of non-AIDS lymphomas. Because systemic lymphomas often occur early in HIV-1 infection rather than late, like the primary CNS lymphomas, some patients may be able to tolerate systemic and intrathecal chemotherapy along with whole-brain irradiation. Aggressive chemotherapy may therefore be warranted, depending on the stage of HIV-1 infection and immunosuppression.

OTHER CENTRAL NERVOUS SYSTEM DISORDERS: COMPLICATIONS OF SYSTEMIC DISEASES

Cerebrovascular Complications

Some HIV-1–infected patients experience transient neurologic deficits that are unrelated to an underlying opportunistic infection or neoplasm.[258–260] In approximately half of these patients, no cause is found although a vascular pathogenesis is suspected.[261] Preliminary clinical data suggest that such events are uncommon, although in one autopsy study as many as 20% of patients had evidence of small areas of infarction.[113,262] Despite these pathologic data, few patients with transient deficits appear to progress to a clinically significant stroke. Before these deficits are diagnosed as being related to HIV-1, other causes such as meningovascular syphilis and thrombotic thrombocytopenic purpura must be excluded. In addition, Gray and colleagues[220] pointed out that patients with advanced HIV-1 infection and transient neurologic deficits may have evidence of herpes zoster vasculitis of the cerebral vessels, although it is not known how commonly this occurs. The pathogenesis of HIV-1 vascular disorders is completely unknown, but they may resemble the vascular complications noted in cancer patients and may include nonbacterial thrombotic endocarditis. It is also possible that anticardiolipin antibodies and protein S deficiency, both of which have been demonstrated in HIV-1–infected patients,[263,264] may play a role. Another speculation is that changes may relate directly to HIV-1 infection of blood vessels.[265,266] Treatment is empiric and currently follows practices used in similarly affected patients without HIV-1 infection. Less common, but more severe, are agonal vascular events, including cerebral hemorrhage from thrombocytopenia and cerebral infarction from more aggressive nonbacterial thrombotic endocarditis and cerebral venous occlusion.

Metabolic and Nutritional Diseases

Patients with AIDS are subject to a constellation of metabolic brain disorders as a result of their complex systemic illnesses, particularly if they are acutely ill. These include encephalopathies related to hypoxia and pulmonary disease, hepatic failure, bacterial or fungal sepsis, disseminated intravascular coagulation, and, less commonly, renal failure. Likewise, toxic encephalopathies may relate to various medications with CNS side effects. Such metabolic and toxic influences can exacerbate or unmask ADC, leading to abrupt functional deterioration. Wernicke's disease and other nutritional disorders may occur in these patients and should be prevented or treated promptly with appropriate supplements.[267–269] The diagnostic approach and treatment of these disorders parallels that in patients without HIV infection.

Seizures

Seizures may occur in patients with HIV-1 infection as a result of various underlying opportunistic infections and neoplasms and also perhaps in relation to ADC or direct HIV-1 infection of the brain.[266,270–273] Seizures should lead to careful clinical and neuroimaging evaluation (preferably MRI) for focal opportunistic disease. In the absence of a definable cause, even a single seizure should probably be treated with chronic anticonvulsant therapy. Both phenytoin and carbamazepine are reasonable first-line drugs in these patients, although drug rashes are common, particularly with phenytoin. Valproic acid is probably the next line of therapy for such intolerant patients.

DISORDERS OF PERIPHERAL NERVOUS SYSTEM AND MUSCLE

Peripheral Neuropathies

Peripheral neuropathies are common, cause considerable morbidity, and may complicate HIV-1 infection at each of its stages.[274] During the earliest stage, at or near the time of seroconversion, a variety of neuropathies have been described, although their incidence appears to be low. These have included brachial plexopathy, mononeuritides involving either peripheral or cranial nerves, and polyneuropathy.[10,14,15,17] Each appears to be self-limiting with good general recovery. These neuropathies probably have a postinfectious, autoimmune pathogenesis.

Apparently much more common is the development of demyelinating neuropathies during the asymptomatic or latent phase of HIV-1 infection.[275,276] These resemble Guillain-Barré syndrome or, more commonly, the chronic inflammatory demyelinating polyneuropathy seen in other contexts, except that the CSF often exhibits an uncharacteristic mild pleocytosis. These patients are usually otherwise well. The pathophysiology of their neuropathy probably parallels that of the disorder in other settings and has an autoimmune basis. These patients respond favorably to plasmapheresis or corticosteroids, and plasmapheresis is now recommended as the treatment of choice.[277] Intravenous immunoglobulin infusion may provide an alternative therapy.[278]

In the setting of early symptomatic HIV-1 infection, and more commonly with AIDS, several other neuropathies have been described. It is in the AIDS-related complex phase of infection, when CD4+ T-lymphocyte counts are not yet severely depressed, that uncomplicated herpes zoster most often develops, although more invasive VZV infection of the CNS occurs later (see previous discussion). It is during this late stage that the more severe infectious neuropathies related to CMV occur.[274,279–281] The most distinct of these is an ascending polyradiculopathy[282]; this disorder deserves particular attention because it apparently can be arrested if recognized and treated promptly. The syndrome is clinically subacute and fulminating in onset and course and involves painful ascending sensory-motor neuropathy with early bladder and bowel impairment. The CSF characteristically contains a high percentage of polymorphonuclear leukocytes, a finding that otherwise is rare in AIDS patients except in the setting of acute bacterial meningitis. Although CMV can be cultured from CSF, this often takes time, and patients should be started on ganciclovir on the basis of clinical suspicion alone.[283] If there is evidence of previously treated CMV infection elsewhere, the issue of drug resistance and the need to change or combine anti-CMV drugs should be addressed.

Mononeuritis multiplex has also been described in AIDS patients[280,284] and may be divided into two general groups.[280,284] The first is a more benign mononeuritis that occurs earlier and possibly relates to a vasculitis. This condition is less aggressive and may be self-limiting; plasmapheresis or immunoglobulin therapy may be helpful. The second condition is more aggressive, subacutely involving major nerves or roots, and leads to progressive paralysis and death in some. There is accumulating evidence that this second type of mononeuritis multiplex may relate to CMV infection of peripheral nerve.[274,279–281,284] It therefore may be justified to treat these patients with ganciclovir or foscarnet, although there is only anecdotal evidence of effectiveness. Cranial mononeuritides may also complicate the aseptic meningitis[285] that is presumably related to HIV-1 infection; likewise, cranial neuropathies and radiculopathies may be caused by metastatic systemic lymphoma or lymphomatous meningitis, as previously described.

The most common neuropathy in AIDS patients is a distal, predominantly sensory axonal neuropathy.[110,122,275,286–288] This is usually a late complication of HIV-1 infection and occurs in the setting of AIDS. Characteristically, the sensory symptoms far exceed either sensory or motor dysfunction. The incidence of this disorder is uncertain, but probably it is very common in mild form. A variant is a less frequent, but clinically important, sensory polyneuropathy in which patients experience severe "burning feet" symptoms, clinically reminiscent of severe alcoholic or diabetic neuropathy. Even in these patients, sensory loss and motor weakness are usually relatively mild but the painful paresthesias and burning may cause sufficient disability to prevent walking. The pathogenesis of this disorder is uncertain, but it may be related to cytokine dysregulation, either alone or in concert with HIV-1 infection of nerve or dorsal root ganglia.[122,288] Treatment is symptomatic, with administration of tricyclic antidepressants or, if there is a tic-like component to the pain, carbamazepine or phenytoin. Narcotic analgesics may be helpful and may be needed in some patients.

Several of the nucleoside antiretroviral drugs, including ddI, dideoxycyttidine (ddC), and dideoxythymidine (d4T), have peripheral neurotoxicity as a major, dose-related side effect.[289–293] The pathogenesis is not fully established but may relate to an effect of these drugs on the mitochondrial DNA polymerase of dorsal root ganglia. Symptoms usually begin with pain in the feet, described as aching, burning, or bruise-like. Such symptoms should provide warning to discontinue the drug. Although patients may continue to worsen for a few weeks, a phenomenon termed "coasting," usually the condition is reversible if recognized early. A frequent practical issue relates to whether symptoms of neuropathy relates to HIV disease or to these treatments. In some patients, drug discontinuation may be needed to determine association.

Autonomic neuropathy has also been reported in AIDS patients, often in conjunction with the more general sensory polyneuropathy.[274,294,295] The clinical features have ranged from postural hypotension to cardiovascular collapse in the setting of invasive procedures such as lung biopsy.

Myopathies

Myopathies of various types may also occur at several stages of HIV-1 infection, although they are less common and have not been as well characterized and classified as the neuropathies.[296–302] The wide range of presentations extends from asymptomatic creatine kinase elevation to progressive and severe proximal weakness. Some patients present with a typical polymyositis picture, with proximal weakness and inflammatory muscle biopsy.[296] These patients may respond to corticosteroids or other immunomodulatory therapies. Less clear cut are the myopathies without inflammatory changes, some of which show nemaline rods on biopsy. Simpson has reported that some of these patients also may respond to corticosteroids.[296] Treatment with intravenous gamma globulin may provide an alternative avenue of therapy without further compromise of the immune system. There is also some controversy as to whether the wasting syndrome may, at times, relate to a primary myopathy.[303,304]

Confounding the diagnostic and therapeutic spectrum is the fact that zidovudine causes a toxic myopathy.[305–313] This occurs after prolonged exposure and may be less likely with current recommended doses than with the higher doses used earlier. It is thought to result from an effect of the drug on muscle mitochondrial DNA polymerase. Characteristically, this myopathy presents with wasting of the buttock and thigh muscles and is associated with proximal leg weakness more than arm weakness. Serum creatine kinase is usually elevated. Diagnosis of zidovudine-related myopathy and its differentiation from the other myopathies occurring in HIV-1–infected patients may be difficult. Muscle biopsy can be helpful if it shows mitochondrial abnormalities, either "ragged red fibers" by light microscopy or abnormal mitochondrial morphology by electron microscopy. There is some controversy regarding how common these findings are and how essential for diagnosis. Not all patients exhibit these changes, and if zidovudine is still thought to be responsible for a patient's myopathy, it may be necessary to withdraw the drug and see whether there is clinical and laboratory (creatine kinase level) improvement. The latter may take several weeks or even a few months to become evident. In the absence of clearer guidelines, we have usually evaluated these patients fully with muscle biopsy and, lacking a clear diagnosis, switched them to ddI or ddC (if not otherwise contraindicated) for at least 2 to 3 months.

GENERAL APPROACH TO DIAGNOSIS AND MANAGEMENT OF NERVOUS SYSTEM COMPLICATIONS

The approach to the diagnosis of CNS disease in patients with HIV-1 infection or AIDS follows that of neurologic diagnosis in general but takes into account the particular vulnerabilities of these patients. The steps involved are outlined in Table 16-5. It is critical to establish a diagnosis of systemic HIV-1 infection (by serologic or virologic confir-

TABLE 16-5. *Diagnosis of neurologic disease in patients with HIV-1 infection or AIDS: approach and methods*

Diagnosis and staging of HIV-1 infection
  Serostatus, virus identification (antigen, culture, polymerase chain reaction)
  Systemic disease record, immune status, serum surrogate markers, CD4+ T-lymphocyte count
Neurologic history
  Temporal profile of evolution
  Provisional anatomic localization
  Functional severity
Neurologic examination
  Refined anatomic localization
Neuroimaging (magnetic resonance imaging, computed tomography; less commonly, myelography, angiography)
  Refined anatomic localization
  Preliminary or presumptive etiological diagnosis
Analysis of cerebrospinal fluid
  Presence of host response (cells, protein, surrogate markers)
  Etiologic diagnosis (culture, cytology)
Neuropsychologic testing
  Quantitation and confirmation of deficit, staging the AIDS dementia complex
Electrodiagnosis (electroencephalography, evoked potentials, electromyelography, nerve conduction)
  Physiologic diagnosis and localization
Therapeutic trial
  Focal brain lesions: targeted to toxoplasmosis
  Withdrawal of potential toxin (eg, zidovudine for myopathy)
Tissue biopsy
  Diagnosis of focal brain lesions: lymphoma, progressive multifocal leukoencephalitis
  Diagnosis of neuropathies, myopathies

mation) in order to confirm the arena of diagnosis, especially in patients who first present with neurologic disease. In addition, it is important to establish the "stage" of HIV-1 infection in each patient, because the probabilities of neurologic differential diagnosis vary with the changing immunologic and virologic status. The CD4 count is probably the most useful laboratory index in this regard. In the early phase of infection, when the patient is asymptomatic but seropositive and the CD4 count is higher than 500 cells/mm^3, neurologic diseases related to autoimmunity occur (eg, demyelinating polyneuropathies). However, neurologic disorders are still relatively uncommon in these individuals, and differential diagnosis must also take into account diseases occurring in the general population or in the particular risk groups (eg, endocarditis or intoxication in the case of drug abusers). In the late phase of HIV-1 infection, when the CD4 count is lower than 250 cells/mm^3 and even more so after the count falls below 50 cells/mm^3, severe immunosuppression ensues, and AIDS-related complications are so common as to clearly predominate. An additional consideration in the late phase of HIV-1 infection is that patients may develop more than one neurologic disease; usually, these occur sequentially, and repeated evaluations may be needed as new symptoms or signs develop or if there is progression of old symptoms in the face of seemingly adequate therapy.

As in the non-AIDS patient, the approach to specific neurologic diagnosis begins with the careful neurologic history. This establishes the background setting of the illness, its temporal profile, and an initial impression of its anatomic localization. The tempo of neurologic disease is a critical factor in differential diagnosis, separating acute events (vascular episodes or seizures) from those with slower evolution

over days (toxoplasmosis) or weeks (ADC or PML). The neurologic examination serves to refine anatomic localization and uncover additional asymptomatic abnormalities. Anatomic-physiologic diagnosis distinguishes among diffuse brain disease with concomitant depressed alertness (eg, metabolic encephalopathies), diffuse brain disease with preserved alertness (eg, ADC), focal brain diseases (eg, cerebral toxoplasmosis, primary CNS lymphoma, PML), meningitides (eg, aseptic or cryptococcal meningitis), myelopathies, peripheral neuropathies, and myopathies (see Table 16-1).

Neuroimaging studies add further precision to anatomic localization and also narrow the range of possible underlying pathologic processes. ADC, for example, is typically marked by cerebral atrophy, at times accompanied by white matter abnormalities by MRI, whereas the predominantly focal brain diseases show mass lesions (toxoplasmosis, primary lymphoma) or demyelination (PML). Spinal MRI is usually negative in vacuolar myelopathy. Electrodiagnosis by EEG or evoked potentials may also be helpful to delineate and localize physiologic dysfunction in seizures, metabolic encephalopathies, or myelopathies. Similarly, nerve conduction studies and electromyography can refine diagnosis of neuromuscular disorders by providing information regarding the anatomy (neuropathy versus myopathy) or type (eg, demyelinating versus axonal neuropathies) of disease.

Examination of the CSF provides a direct view of inflammatory reactions in the meninges and can precisely diagnose invading organisms (eg, HIV-1, cryptococcus) or neoplasms. CSF surrogate markers may be helpful in confirming the presence of disease. In certain cases, tissue biopsy may be needed. Brain biopsy may be necessary before therapy, as in primary CNS lymphoma or tuberculosis, or it may be done to establish prognosis, as with PML. Nerve or muscle biopsy may be needed to further differentiate axonal from demyelinating neuropathy or polymyositis from zidovudine myopathy.

In some cases, biopsy can be avoided by the use of a therapeutic trial. Focal brain lesions with surrounding edema and mass effect are usually managed with a trial of antitoxoplasmosis therapy and only biopsied if such therapy fails—unless there is reason to consider *T gondii* infection unlikely (compliance with trimethaprim-sulfamethoxazole prophylaxis, negative serology, single or few lesions centered in the periventricular white matter). Similarly, drug toxicities may be diagnosed by clinical improvement after their discontinuation.

In general, traditional serologic studies are of limited use, because most infections relate to reactivated latent infection or ubiquitous organisms to which most HIV-1–infected patients exhibit antibodies, whether or not they are suffering active CNS infection. Moreover, antibody titers do not reliably rise in association with active infection. However, the presence of antibodies can be used as an index of susceptibility, as in the case of *T gondii* or CMV infection.

These clinical and laboratory evaluations, if pursued with a background understanding of the spectrum of neurologic disorders affecting patients with HIV-1 infection, allow exact neurologic diagnosis in the most patients. This is an important and often fruitful exercise with gratifying relief of morbidity and prevention of death.

REFERENCES

1. Price R, Worley J. Management of neurologic complications of HIV-1 infection and AIDS. In: Sande M, Volberding P, eds. Medical management of AIDS. Philadelphia: WB Saunders, 1995:261.
2. Simpson DM, Tagliati M. Neurologic manifestations of HIV infection [published erratum appears in Ann Intern Med 1995;122:317]. (Review) Ann Intern Med 1994;121:769.
3. Price R. Understanding the AIDS dementia complex (ADC): the challenge of HIV and its effects on the central nervous system. In: Price R, Perry S, eds. HIV, AIDS and the brain. New York: Raven Press, 1994:1.
4. Price R. Management of AIDS dementia complex and HIV-1 infection of the nervous system. AIDS 1995;9(A):S221.
5. Price R, Brew B, Sidtis J, et al. The brain in AIDS: central nervous system HIV-1 infection and AIDS dementia complex. Science 1988;239:586.
6. Achim C, Schrier R, Wiley C. Immunopathogenesis of HIV encephalitis. Brain Pathol 1991;1:177.
7. Wiley C, Budka H. HIV-induced CNS lesions. Brain Pathol 1991;1:153.
8. Wiley CA, Achim C. Human immunodeficiency virus encephalitis is the pathological correlate of dementia in acquired immunodeficiency syndrome [published erratum appears in Ann Neurol 1995;37:140]. Ann Neurol 1994;36:673.
9. Tindall B, Cooper D. Primary HIV infection: host responses and intervention strategies. AIDS 1991;5:1.
10. Brew B, Perdices M, Darveniza P, et al. The neurological features of early and "latent" human immunodeficiency virus infection. Aust N Z J Med 1989;19:700.
11. Ho D, Sarngadhara M, Resnick L, et al. Primary human T lymphotropic virus type III infection. Ann Intern Med 1985;103:880.
12. Denning D, Anderson J, Rudge P, et al. Acute myelopathy associated with primary infection with human immunodeficiency virus. Br Med J 1987;294:143, 1987.
13. Piette A, Tusseau F, Vignon D, et al. Letter to the editor. Lancet 1986;1:852.
14. Wiselka M, Nicholson K, Ward S, et al. Acute infection with human immunodeficiency virus associated with facial nerve palsy and neuralgia. J Infect 1987;15:189.
15. Hagberg L, Malmval B, Svennerholm L, et al. Guillain-Barre syndrome as an early manifestation of HIV central nervous system infection. Scand J Infect Dis 1987;18:591.
16. Carne C, Smith A, Elkington S, et al. Acute encephalopathy coincident with seroconversion for anti HTLV-III. Lancet 1985;2:1206.
17. Calabrese L, Proffitt M, Levin K, et al. Acute infection with the human immunodeficiency virus (HIV) associated with acute brachial neuritis and exanthematous rash. Ann Intern Med 1987;107:849.
18. Clark SJ, Saag MS, Decker WD, et al. High titers of cytopathic virus in plasma of patients with symptomatic primary HIV-1 infection. N Engl J Med 1991;324:954.
19. Gaines H, von Sydow M, Pehrson PO, et al. Clinical picture of primary HIV-1 infection presenting as a glandular-fever–like illness. Lancet 1988;297:1363.
20. Rabeneck L, Popovic M, Gartner S, et al. Acute HIV-1 infection presenting with painful swallowing and esophageal ulcers. JAMA 1990;263:2318.
21. Resnick L, diMarzo-Veronese F, Schupbach J, et al. Intra-blood-brain-barrier synthesis of HTLV-III–specific IgG in patients with neurologic symptoms associated with AIDS or AIDS-related complex. N Engl J Med 1985;313:1498.
22. Resnick L, Berger J, Shapshak P, et al. Early penetration of the blood-brain-barrier by HIV. Neurology 1988;38:9.
23. Goudsmit J, Wolters E, Bakker M, et al. Intrathecal synthesis of antibodies to HTLV-III in patients without AIDS or AIDS related complex. Br Med J 1986;292:1231.
24. Marshall D, Brey R, Cahill W, et al. Spectrum of cerebrospinal fluid findings in various stages of human immunodeficiency virus infection. Arch Neurol 1988;45:954.
25. McArthur J, Cohen B, Farzadegan H, et al. Cerebrospinal fluid abnormalities in homosexual men with and without neuropsychiatric findings. Ann Neurol 1988;23(Suppl):S34.
26. Elovaara I, Iivanainen M, Valle S, et al. CSF protein and cellular profiles in various stages of HIV infection related to neurological manifestations. J Neurol Sci 1987;78:331.
27. Elovaara I, Nykyri E, Poutiainen E, et al. CSF follow-up in HIV-1 infection: intrathecal production of HIV-specific and unspecific IgG, and beta-2-microglobulin increase with duration of HIV-1 infection. Acta Neurol Scand 1993;87:388.
28. Ho D, Rota T, Schooley R, et al. Isolation of HTLV-III from cerebrospinal fluid and neural tissues of patients with neurologic syndromes related to the acquired immunodeficiency syndrome. N Engl J Med 1985;313:1493.
29. Davis LE, Hjelle BL, Miller VE, et al. Early viral brain invasion in iatrogenic human immunodeficiency virus infection. Neurology 1992;42:1736.
30. Navia B, Price R. The acquired immunodeficiency syndrome dementia complex as the presenting or sole manifestation of human immunodeficiency virus infection. Arch Neurol 1987;44:65.
31. Selnes O, Miller E, McArthur J, et al. No evidence of cognitive decline during the asymptomatic stages. Neurology 1990;40:204.
32. Miller E, Selnes O, McArthur J, et al. Neuropsychological performance in HIV-1–infected homosexual men: the Multicenter AIDS Cohort Study (MACS). Neurology 1990;40:197.
33. Sidtis JJ, Price RW. Early HIV-1 infection and the AIDS dementia complex. (Comment) Neurology 1990;40:323.
34. Selnes OA, Miller EN. Asymptomatic HIV-1 infection and aviation safety. (Letter; comment) Aviat Space Environ Med 1993;64:172.
35. Selnes OA, Galai N, Bacellar H, et al. Cognitive performance after progression to AIDS: a longitudinal study from the Multicenter AIDS Cohort Study. Neurology 1995;45:267.
36. Gray F, Lescs MC, Keohane C, et al. Early brain changes in HIV infection: neuropathological study of 11 HIV seropositive, non-AIDS cases. J Neuropathol Exp Neurol 1992;51:177.
37. Boni J, Emmerich BS, Leib SL, et al. PCR identification of HIV-1 DNA sequences in brain tissue of patients with AIDS encephalopathy. Neurology 1993;43:1813.
38. Bell J, Busuttil A, Ironside J, et al. Human immunodeficiency virus and the brain: investigation of viral load in pre-AIDS individuals. J Infect Dis 1993;168:919.
39. Donaldson Y, Bell J, Ironside J, et al. Redistribution of HIV outside the lymphoid system with onset of AIDS. Lancet 1994;343:382.

40. Berger J, Sheremata W, Resnick L, et al. Multiple sclerosis-like leukoencephalopathy revealing human immunodeficiency virus infection. Neurology 1989;39:324.

41. Gray F, Chimelli L, Mohr M, et al. Fulminating multiple sclerosis-like leukoencephalopathy revealing human immunodeficiency virus infection. Neurology 1991;41:105.

42. Hollander H, Stringari S. Human immunodeficiency virus-associated meningitis: clinical course and correlations. Am J Med 1987;83:813.

43. Hollander H, McGuire D, Burack JH. Diagnostic lumbar puncture in HIV-infected patients: analysis of 138 cases. Am J Med 1994;96:223.

44. Levy J, Shimabukuro J, Hollander H, et al. Isolation of AIDS-associated retroviruses from cerebrospinal fluid and brain of patients with neurological symptoms. Lancet 1985;2:586.

45. Goldstein J. Headache and acquired immunodeficiency syndrome. Neurol Clin 1990;8:947.

46. Brew BJ, Miller J. Human immunodeficiency virus-related headache. Neurology 1993;43:1098.

47. Price R, Sidtis J, Brew B. AIDS dementia complex and HIV-1 infection: a view from the clinic. Brain Pathol 1991;1:155.

48. Navia B, Jordan B, Price R. The AIDS dementia complex: I. Clinical features. Ann Neurol 1986;19:517.

49. Navia B, Cho E-W, Petito C, et al. The AIDS dementia complex: II. Neuropathology. Ann Neurol 1986;19:525.

50. Price R, Brew B. The AIDS dementia complex. J Infect Dis 1988;158:1079.

51. Price RW. Understanding the AIDS dementia complex (ADC): the challenge of HIV and its effects on the central nervous system. (Review) Res Publ Assoc Res Nerv Ment Dis 1994;72:1.

52. Neaton J, Wentworth D, Rhane F, et al. Methods of studying interventions: considerations in choice of a clinical endpoint for AIDS clinical trials. Stat Med 1994;13:2107.

53. Centers for Disease Control. Revision of the CDC surveillance case definition for acquired immunodeficiency syndrome. MMWR 1987;36:3S.

54. Cummings J, Benson D. Subcortical dementia: review of an emerging concept. Arch Neurol 1984;41:874.

55. Navia B, The AIDS dementia complex. New York: Oxford University Press, 1990:181.

56. Nomenclature and research case definitions for neurologic manifestations of human immunodeficiency virus-type 1 (HIV-1) infection: report of a working group of the American Academy of Neurology AIDS Task Force. (See comments) (Review) Neurology 1991;41:778.

57. World Health Organization. 1990 World Health Organization consultation on the neuropsychiatric aspects of HIV-1 infection. AIDS 1990;49:935.

58. Epstein LG, Sharer LR, Joshi VV, et al. Progressive encephalopathy in children with acquired immune deficiency syndrome. Ann Neurol 1985;17:488.

59. Belman A, Ultmann M, Horoupian D, et al. Neurological complications in infants and children with acquired immune deficiency syndrome. Ann Neurol 1985;18:560.

60. Centers for Disease Control. Classification system for human immunodeficiency virus (HIV) infection in children under 13 years of age. MMWR 1987;36:225.

61. Tross S, Price R, Navia B, et al. Neuropsychological characterization of the AIDS dementia complex: a preliminary report. AIDS 1988;2:81.

62. Sidtis JJ. Evaluation of the AIDS dementia complex in adults. (Review) Res Publ Assoc Res Nerv Ment Dis 1994;72:273.

63. Sidtis JJ, Gatsonis C, Price RW, et al. Zidovudine treatment of the AIDS dementia complex: results of a placebo-controlled trial. AIDS Clinical Trials Group. Ann Neurol 1993;33:343.

64. Post M, Berger JR, Quencer RM. Asymptomatic and neurologically symptomatic HIV-seropositive individuals: prospective evaluation with cranial MR imaging. Radiology 1991;178:131.

65. Post M, Tate L, Quencer R, et al. CT, MR, and pathology in HIV encephalitis and meningitis. AJR Am J Roentgenol 1988;151:373.

66. Petty RK. Recent advances in the neurology of HIV infection. (Review) Postgrad Med J 1994;70:393.

67. Dal Pan GJ, McArthur JH, Aylward E, et al. Patterns of cerebral atrophy in HIV-1–infected individuals: results of a quantitative MRI analysis. Neurology 1992;42:2125.

68. Gelman B, Guinto FJ. Morphometry, histopathology, and tomography of cerebral atrophy in the acquired immunodeficiency syndrome. Ann Neurol 1992;31:32.

69. Jakobsen J, Gyldensted C, Brun B, et al. Cerebral ventricular enlargement relates to neuropsychological measures in unselected AIDS patients. Acta Neurol Scand 1989;79:59.

70. Moeller AA, Backmund HC. Ventricle brain ratio in the clinical course of HIV infection. Acta Neurol Scand 1990;81:512.

71. Jarvik J, Hesselink J, Kennedy C, et al. Acquired immunodeficiency syndrome: magnetic resonance patterns of brain involvement with pathologic correlation. Neurology 1988;45:731.

72. Power C, Kong PA, Crawford TO, et al. Cerebral white matter changes in acquired immunodeficiency syndrome dementia: alterations of the blood-brain barrier. Ann Neurol 1993;34:339.

73. Belman AL, Lantos G, Horoupian D, et al. AIDS: calcification of the basal ganglia in infants and children. Neurology 1986;36:1192.

74. Rottenberg DA, Moeller JR, Strother SC, et al. The metabolic pathology of the AIDS dementia complex. Ann Neurol 1987;22:700.

75. Jarvik JG, Lenkinski RE, Grossman RI, et al. Proton MR spectroscopy of HIV-infected patients: characterization of abnormalities with imaging and clinical correlation. Radiology 1993;186:739.

76. Kuni CC, Rhame FS, Meier MJ, et al. Quantitative I-123-IMP brain SPECT and neuropsychological testing in AIDS dementia. Clin Nucl Med 1991;16:174.

77. Masdeu JC, Yudd A, Van Heertum RL, et al. Single-photon emission computed tomography in human immunodeficiency virus encephalopathy: a preliminary report. (See comments) J Nucl Med 1991;32:1471.

78. Menon DK, Ainsworth JG, Cox IJ, et al. Proton MR spectroscopy of the brain in AIDS dementia complex. J Comput Assist Tomogr 1992;16:538.

79. O'Connell RA, Sireci S, Jr, Fastov ME, et al. The role of SPECT brain imaging in assessing psychopathology in the medically ill. Gen Hosp Psychiatry 1991;13:305.

80. Pohl P, Vogl G, Fill H, et al. Single photon emission computed tomography in AIDS dementia complex. J Nucl Med 1988;29:1382.

81. Pohl P, Riccabona G, Hilty E, et al. Double-tracer SPECT in patients with AIDS encephalopathy: a comparison of ^{123}I-IMP with 99Tcm-HMPAO. Nucl Med Commun 1992;13:586.

82. Schwartz RB, Komaroff AL, Garada BM, et al. SPECT imaging of the brain: comparison of findings in patients with chronic fatigue syndrome, AIDS dementia complex, and major unipolar depression. AJR Am J Roentgenol 1994;162:943.

83. Bottomley PA, Hardy CJ, Cousins JP, et al. AIDS dementia complex: brain high-energy phosphate metabolite deficits. Radiology 1990;176:407.

84. Brunetti A, Berg G, Di Chiro G, et al. Reversal of brain metabolic abnormalities following treatment of AIDS dementia complex with 3'-azido-2',3'-dideoxythymidine (AZT, zidovudine): a PET-FDG study. J Nucl Med 1989;30:581.

85. Brew BJ, Paul MO, Nakajima G, et al. Cerebrospinal fluid HIV-1 p24 antigen and culture: sensitivity and specificity for AIDS-dementia complex. J Neurol Neurosurg Psychiatry 1994;57:784.

86. Sonnerborg A, von Stedingk L, Hannsson L, Strannegard OO. Elevated neopterin and beta-2 microglobulin levels in blood and cerebrospinal fluid occur early in HIV-1 infection. AIDS 1989;3:277.

87. Brew B, Bhalla R, Paul M, et al. Cerebrospinal fluid neopterin in human immunodeficiency virus type 1 infection. Ann Neurol 1990;28:556.

88. Brew B, Bhalla R, Fleisher M, et al. Cerebrospinal fluid B2 microglobulin in patients infected with human immunodeficiency virus. Neurology 1989;39:830.

89. Brew BJ, Bhalla RB, Paul M, et al. Cerebrospinal fluid beta 2-microglobulin in patients with AIDS dementia complex: an expanded series including response to zidovudine treatment. AIDS 1992;6:461.

90. Griffin DE, McArthur JC, Cornblath DR. Neopterin and interferon-gamma in serum and cerebrospinal fluid of patients with HIV-associated neurologic disease. Neurology 1991;41:69.

91. Heyes M, Brew B, Martin A, et al. Increased cerebrospinal fluid concentrations of the excitotoxin quinolinic acid in HIV infection and AIDS dementia complex. Ann Neurol 1991;29:202.

92. Heyes MP, Saito K, Crowley JS, et al. Quinolinic acid and kynurenine pathway metabolism in inflammatory and non-inflammatory neurological disease. Brain 1992;115:1249.

93. Price R, Brew B, Sidtis J, et al. The brain in AIDS: central nervous system HIV-1 infection and AIDS dementia complex. Science 1988;239:586.

94. Tyor WR, Glass JD, Griffin JW, et al. Cytokine expression in the brain during the acquired immunodeficiency syndrome. Ann Neurol 1992;31:349.

95. Price R. The cellular basis of central nervous system HIV-1 infection and the AIDS dementia complex: introduction. J Neuro-AIDS 1995;1:1.

96. Achim CL, Heyes MP, Wiley CA. Quantitation of human immunodeficiency virus, immune activation factors, and quinolinic acid in AIDS brains. J Clin Invest 1993;91:2769.

97. Benos DJ, McPherson S, Hahn BH, et al. Cytokines and HIV envelope glycoprotein gp120 stimulate Na+/H+ exchange in astrocytes. J Biol Chem 1994;269:13811.

98. Blumberg BM, Gelbard HA, Epstein LG. HIV-1 infection of the developing nervous system: central role of astrocytes in pathogenesis. (Review) Virus Res 1994;32:253.

99. Epstein LG, Gendelman HE. Human immunodeficiency virus type 1 infection of the nervous system: pathogenetic mechanisms. (See comments) (Review) Ann Neurol 1993;33:429.

100. Gendelman HE, Genis P, Jett M, et al. An experimental model system for HIV-1–induced brain injury. (Review) Adv Neuroimmunol 1994;4:189.

101. Lipton SA. Neuronal injury associated with HIV-1 and potential treatment with calcium-channel and NMDA antagonists. (Review) Dev Neurosci 1994;16:145.

102. Wesselingh SL, Power C, Glass JD, et al. Intracerebral cytokine messenger RNA expression in acquired immunodeficiency syndrome dementia. Ann Neurol 1993;33:576.

103. Gallo P, Sivieri S, Rinaldi L, et al. Intrathecal synthesis of interleukin-10 (IL-10) in viral and inflammatory diseases of the central nervous system. J Neurol Sci 1994;126:49.

104. Gallo P, Laverda AM, De Rossi A, et al. Immunological markers in the cerebrospinal fluid of HIV-1–infected children. Acta Paediatr Scand 1991;80:659.

105. Gallo P, Pagni S, Giometto B, et al. Macrophage-colony stimulating factor (M-CSF) in the cerebrospinal fluid. J Neuroimmunol 1990;29:105.

106. Gallo P, Piccinno MG, Krzalic L, et al. Tumor necrosis factor alpha (TNF alpha) and neurological diseases: failure in detecting TNF alpha in the cerebrospinal fluid from patients with multiple sclerosis, AIDS dementia complex, and brain tumours. J Neuroimmunol 1989;23:41.

107. Griffin D, Wesselingh S, McArthur J. Elevated central nervous system prostaglandins in human immunodeficiency virus-associated dementia. Ann Neurol 1994;35:592.

108. Grimaldi LM, Martino GV, Franciotta DM, et al. Elevated alpha-tumor necrosis factor levels in spinal fluid from HIV-1 infected patients with central nervous system involvement. (See comments) Ann Neurol 1991;29:21.

109. McArthur JC, Hoover DR, Bacellar H, et al. Dementia in AIDS patients: incidence and risk factors. Multicenter AIDS Cohort Study. Neurology 1993;43:2245.

110. Bacellar H, Munoz A, Miller EN, et al. Temporal trends in the incidence of HIV-1–related neurologic diseases: multicenter AIDS Cohort Study, 1985–1992. Neurology 1994;44:1892.

111. Portegies P, Enting RH, de Gans J, et al. Presentation and course of AIDS dementia complex: 10 years of follow-up in Amsterdam, The Netherlands. AIDS 1993;7:669.

112. Portegies P, de Gans JîAL JM, Derix M, et al. Declining incidence of AIDS dementia complex after introduction of zidovudine treatment. Br Med J 1989;299:819.

113. Petito C, Cho E-S, Lemann W, et al. Neuropathology of acquired immunodeficiency syndrome (AIDS): an autopsy review. J Neuropathol Exp Neurol 1986;45:635.

114. Budka H. Neuropathology of human immunodeficiency virus infection. (Review) Brain Pathol 1991;1:163.

115. Rosenblum M. Infection of the central nervous system by the human immunodeficiency virus type 1: morphology and relation to syndromes of progressive encephalopathy and myelopathy in patients with AIDS. Pathol Annu 1990;25:117.

116. Gray F, Haug H, Chimelli L, et al. Prominent cortical atrophy with neuronal loss as correlate of human immunodeficiency virus encephalopathy. Acta Neuropathol (Berl) 1991;82:229.

117. Masliah E, Achim CL, Ge N, et al. Cellular neuropathology in HIV encephalitis. (Review) Res Publ Assoc Res Nerv Ment Dis 1994;72:119.

118. Petito C, Navia B, Cho E, et al. Vacuolar myelopathy pathologically resembling subacute combined degeneration in patients with acquired immunodeficiency syndrome (AIDS). N Engl J Med 1985;312:874.

119. Dal Pan GJ, Glass JD, McArthur JC. Clinicopathologic correlations of HIV-1–associated vacuolar myelopathy: an autopsy-based case-control study. Neurology 1994;44:2159.

120. Petito CK, Vecchio D, Chen YT. HIV antigen and DNA in AIDS spinal cords correlate with macrophage infiltration but not with vacuolar myelopathy. J Neuropathol Exp Neurol 1994;53:86.

121. Rosenblum M, Scheck A, Cronin K, et al. Dissociation of AIDS-related vacuolar myelopathy and productive human immunodeficiency virus type 1 (HIV-1) infection of the spinal cord. Neurology 1989;39:892.

122. Tyor W, Wesselingh S, Griffin J, et al. Unifying hypothesis for the pathogenesis of HIV-associated dementia complex, vacuolar myelopathy, and sensory neuropathy. J Acquir Immune Defic Syndr 1995;9:379.

123. Shaw G, Harper M, Hahn B, et al. HTLV-III infection in brains of children and adults with AIDS encephalopathy. Science 1985;227:177.

124. Koenig S, Gendelman H, Orenstein J, et al. Detection of AIDS virus in macrophages in brain tissue from AIDS patients with encephalopathy. Science 1986;233:1089.

125. Stoler M, Eskin T, Benn S, et al. Human T-cell lymphotropic virus type III infection of the central nervous system: preliminary in situ analysis. JAMA 1986;256:2360.

126. Wiley C, Schrier R, Nelson J, et al. Cellular localization of human immunodeficiency virus infection within the brains of acquired immune deficiency patients. Proc Natl Acad Sci USA 1986;83:7089.

127. Gabuzda D, Ho D, De La Monte S, et al. Immunohistochemical identification of HTLV-III antigen in brains of patients with AIDS. Ann Neurol 1986;20:289.

128. Vazeux R, Brousse N, Jarry A, et al. AIDS subacute encephalitis: identification of HIV-infected cells. Am J Pathol 1987;126:403.

129. Pumarole-Sune T, Navia B, Cordon-Cardo C, et al. HIV antigen in the brains of patients with the AIDS dementia complex. Ann Neurol 1987;21:490.

130. Michaels J, Price R, Rosenblum M. Microglia in the human immunodeficiency virus encephalitis of acquired immune deficiency syndrome: proliferation, infection and fusion. Acta Neuropathol 1988;76:373.

131. Epstein LG, Sharer LR, Cho ES, et al. HTLV-III/LAV-like retrovirus particles in the brains of patients with AIDS encephalopathy. AIDS Res 1984;1:447.

132. Gyökey F, Melnick J, Györkey P. Human immunodeficiency virus in brain biopsies of patients with AIDS and progressive encephalopathy. J Infect Dis 1987;155:870.

133. O'Brien W, Genetic and biologic basis of HIV-1 neurotropism, In: Price R, Perry S, eds. HIV, AIDS and the brain. New York: Raven Press, 1994:47.

134. Sharpless N, O'Brien W, Verdin E, et al. Human immunodeficiency virus type 1 tropism for brain microglial cells is determined by a region of the env glycoprotein that also controls macrophage tropism. J Virol 1992;66:2588.

135. Westervelt P, Trowbridge D, Epstein L, et al. Macrophage tropism determinants of HIV-1 in vivo. J Virol 1992;66:2577.

136. Power C, McArthur JC, Johnson RT, et al. Demented and nondemented patients with AIDS differ in brain-derived human immunodeficiency virus type 1 envelope sequences. J Virol 1994;68:4643.

137. Dickson D, Lee S. Microglia and HIV-related CNS neuropathology: an update. J Neuro-AIDS 1996;1:57.

138. Dickson DW, Lee SC, Hatch W, et al. Macrophages and microglia in HIV-related CNS neuropathology. (Review) Res Publ Assoc Res Nerv Ment Dis 1994;72:99.

139. Dickson DW, Mattiace LA, Kure K, et al. Microglia in human disease, with an emphasis on acquired immune deficiency syndrome. (Review) Lab Invest 1991;64:135.

140. Nuovo G, Gallery F, MacConnel P, Braun A. In situ detection of polymerase chain reaction–amplified HIV-1 nucleic acids and tumor necrosis factor-α RNA in the central nervous system. Am J Pathol 1994;144:659.

141. Tornatore C, Chandra R, Berger JR, et al. HIV-1 infection of subcortical astrocytes in the pediatric central nervous system. Neurology 1994;44:481.

142. Saito Y, Sharer L, Epstein L, et al. Overexpression of *nef* as a marker for restricted HIV-1 infection of astrocytes in postmortem pediatric central nervous system tissues. Neurology 1994;44:474.

143. Brew B, Rosenblum M, Cronin K, et al. The AIDS dementia complex (ADC) and human immunodeficiency virus type 1 (HIV-1) brain infection: clinical virological correlations. Ann Neurol 1995;38:563.

144. Glass JD, Wesselingh SL, Selnes OA, et al. Clinical-neuropathologic correlation in HIV-associated dementia. Neurology 1993; 43:2230.

145. Lipton SA, Gendelman HE. Seminars in medicine of the Beth Israel Hospital, Boston: dementia associated with the acquired immunodeficiency syndrome. (Review) N Engl J Med 1995;332:934.

146. Yarchoan R, Berg G, Brouwers P, et al. Response of human immunodeficiency virus associated neurological disease to 3'-azido-3'-deoxythymidine. Lancet 1987;1:132.

147. Schmitt F, Bigleg J, McKinnis R, et al. Neuropsychological outcome of azidothymidine (AZT) in the treatment of AIDS and AIDS-related complex: a double blind, placebo-controlled trial. N Engl J Med 1988;319:1573.

148. Pizzo P, Eddy J, Fallon J, et al. Effect of continuous intravenous infusion of zidovudine (AZT) in children with symptomatic HIV infection. N Engl J Med 1988;319:889.

149. Brouwers P, Moss H, Wolters P, et al. Effect of continuous-infusion zidovudine therapy on neuropsychologic functioning in children with symptomatic human immunodeficiency virus infection. J Pediatr 1990;116:980.

150. Yarchoan R, Mitsuya H, Thomas R, et al. In vivo activity against HIV and favorable toxicity profile of 2', 3' dideoxyinosine. Science 1989;245:412.

151. Dreyer E, Kaiser P, Offermann J, et al. HIV-1 coat protein neurotoxicity prevented by calcium channel antagonists. Science 1990;248:364.

152. Brew B, Sidtis J, Petito C, et al., The neurological complications of AIDS and human immunodeficiency virus infection. In: Plum F, ed. Advances in contemporary neurology. Philadelphia: FA Davis, 1988:1.

153. Snider W, Simpson D, Nielson S, et al. Neurological complications of acquired immune deficiency syndrome: analysis of 50 patients. Ann Neurol 1983;14:403.

154. McArthur JC. Neurologic manifestations of AIDS. (Review) Medicine (Baltimore) 1987;66:407.

155. Navia B, Petito C, Gold J, et al. Cerebral toxoplasmosis complicating the acquired immune deficiency syndrome: clinical and neuropathological findings in 27 patients. Ann Neurol 1986;19:224.

156. Haverkos H. Assessment of therapy for *Toxoplasma* encephalitis. Am J Med 1987;82:907.

157. Grant I, Gold J, Rosenblum M, et al. *Toxoplasma gondii* serology in HIV-infected patients: the development of central nervous system toxoplasmosis in AIDS. AIDS 1990;4:519.

158. Climent C, DeVinatea ML, Lasala G, et al. Geographical pathology profile of AIDS in Puerto Rico: the first decade. Mod Pathol 1994;7:647.

159. Kennedy PG, Kennedy D, Love C, et al. Neurological features of HIV-related disease in Glasgow. Scott Med J 1989;34:433.

160. Luft BJ, Hafner R, Korzun AH, et al. Toxoplasmic encephalitis in patients with the acquired immunodeficiency syndrome. Members of the ACTG 077p/ANRS 009 Study Team. N Engl J Med 1993;329:995.

161. New LC, Holliman RE. Toxoplasmosis and human immunodeficiency virus (HIV) disease. (Review) J Antimicrob Chemother 1994; 33:1079.

162. Wang F, So Y, Vittinghoff E, et al. Incidence, proportion of and risk factors for AIDS patients diagnosed with HIV dementia, central nervous system toxoplasmosis, and cryptococcal meningitis. J Acquir Immune Defic Syndr 1995;8:75.

163. Gray F, Geny C, Lionnet F, et al. Neuropathologic study of 135 adult cases of acquired immunodeficiency syndrome (AIDS) (in French). Ann Pathol 1991;11:236.

164. Gallant JE, Moore RD, Chaisson RE. Prophylaxis for opportunistic infections in patients with HIV infection. (Review) Ann Intern Med 1994;120:932.

165. Mallolas J, Zamora L, Gatell JM, et al. Primary prophylaxis for *Pneumocystis carinii* pneumonia: a randomized trial comparing cotrimoxazole, aerosolized pentamidine and dapsone plus pyrimethamine. AIDS 1993;7:59.

166. Falangola MF, Reichler BS, Petito CK. Histopathology of cerebral toxoplasmosis in human immunodeficiency virus infection: a comparison between patients with early-onset and late-onset acquired immunodeficiency syndrome. Hum Pathol 1994;25:1091.

167. Gray F, Gherardi R, Wingate E, et al. Diffuse "encephalitic" cerebral toxoplasmosis in AIDS: report of four cases. J Neurol 1989;236:273.

168. Jarvik J, Hasselink J, Kennedy C, et al. Acquired immunodeficiency syndrome: magnetic resonance patterns of brain involvement with pathologic correlation. Arch Neurol 1988;45:731.

169. Ruiz A, Ganz WI, Post MJ, et al. Use of thallium-201 brain SPECT to differentiate cerebral lymphoma from *Toxoplasma* encephalitis in AIDS patients. AJNR Am J Neuroradiol 1994;15:1885.

170. Johnson JD, Butcher PD, Savva D, et al. Application of the polymerase chain reaction to the diagnosis of human toxoplasmosis. J Infect 1993;26:147.

171. Dupouy-Camet J, de Souza SL, Maslo C, et al. Detection of *Toxoplasma gondii* in venous blood from AIDS patients by polymerase chain reaction. J Clin Microbiol 1993;31:1866.

172. Ostergaard L, Nielsen AK, Black FT. DNA amplification on cerebrospinal fluid for diagnosis of cerebral toxoplasmosis among HIV-positive patients with signs or symptoms of neurological disease. Scand J Infect Dis 1993;25:227.

173. Schoondermark-van de Ven E, Galama J, Kraaijeveld C, et al. Value of the polymerase chain reaction for the detection of *Toxoplasma gondii* in cerebrospinal fluid from patients with AIDS. Clin Infect Dis 1993;16:661.

174. Cohm J, McMeeking A, Cohen W, et al. Evaluation of the policy of empiric treatment of suspected *Toxoplasma* encephalitis in patients with the acquired immunodeficiency syndrome. Am J Med 1989;86:521.

175. Saag MS. Cryptococcosis and other fungal infections (histoplasmosis, coccidiodomycosis). In: Sande M, Volberding P, eds. The medical management of AIDS, 4th ed. Philadelphia, WB Saunders, 1995:437.

176. Andreula CF, Burdi N, Carella A. CNS cryptococcosis in AIDS: spectrum of MR findings. J Comput Assist Tomogr 1993;17:438.

177. Dismukes WE. Management of cryptococcosis. (Review) Clin Infect Dis 1993;17:S507.

178. Powderly WG. Cryptococcal meningitis and AIDS. (Review) Clin Infect Dis 1993;17:837.

179. Saag MS, Powderly WG, Cloud GA, et al. Comparison of amphotericin B with fluconazole in the treatment of acute AIDS-associated cryptococcal meningitis: The NIAID Mycoses Study Group and the AIDS Clinical Trials Group. (See comments) N Engl J Med 1992;326:83.

180. Sugar AM. Overview: cryptococcosis in the patient with AIDS. (Review) Mycopathologia 1991;114:153.

181. Chuck S, Sande M. Infections with *Cryptococcus neoformans* in the acquired immunodeficiency syndrome. N Engl J Med 1989;321:794.

182. Stern J, Hartman B, Sharkey P, et al. Oral fluconazole therapy for patients with acquired immunodeficiency syndrome and cryptococcosis: experience with 22 patients. Am J Med 1988;85:477.

183. Larsen R, Leal M, Chan L. Fluconazole compared with amphotericin B plus flucytosine for cryptococcal meningitis in AIDS: a randomized trial. Ann Intern Med 1988;85:481.

184. Sugar A, Saunder C. Oral fluconazole as suppressive therapy of disseminated cryptococcosis in patients with the acquired immunodeficiency syndrome. Am J Med 1988;85:481.

185. Powderly WG, Saag MS, Cloud GA, et al. A controlled trial of fluconazole or amphotericin B to prevent relapse of cryptococcal meningitis in patients with the acquired immunodeficiency syndrome: The NIAID AIDS Clinical Trials Group and Mycoses Study Group. (See comments) N Engl J Med 1992;326:793.

186. Quagliarello VJ, Viscoli C, Horwitz RI. Primary prevention of cryptococcal meningitis by fluconazole in HIV-infected patients. Lancet 1995;345:548.

187. Richardson E. Progressive multifocal leukoencephalopathy. In: Vinken P, Bruyn G, eds. Handbook of clinical neurology. Amsterdam: Elsevier, 1978:307.

188. Padgett B, Walker D, Zu Rhein G, et al. JC papovavirus in progressive multifocal leukoencephalopathy. J Infect Dis 1976;133:868.

189. Houff S, Major E, Katz D, et al. Involvement of JC virus-infected mononuclear cells from the bone marrow and spleen in the pathogenesis of progressive multifocal leukoencephalopathy. N Engl J Med 1988;318:301.

190. Schmidbauer M, Budka H, Shah K. Progressive multifocal leukoencephalopathy (PML) in AIDS and in the pre-AIDS era. Acta Neuropathol 1990;80:375.

191. Berger J, Kaszovitz B, Donovan Post M, et al. Progressive multifocal leukoencephalopathy in association with human deficiency virus infection: a review of the literature with a report of sixteen cases. Ann Intern Med 1987;107:78.

192. Krupp L, Lipton R, Swerdlow M, et al. Progressive multifocal leukoencephalopathy: clinical and radiographic features. Ann Neurol 1985;17:344.

193. Mark A, Atlas S. Progressive multifocal leukoencephalopathy in patients with AIDS: appearance on MR images. Radiology 1989; 173:517.

194. Weber T, Turner RW, Frye S, et al. Specific diagnosis of progressive multifocal leukoencephalopathy by polymerase chain reaction. J Infect Dis 1994;169:1138.

195. Weber T, Turner RW, Frye S, et al. Progressive multifocal leukoencephalopathy diagnosed by amplification of JC virus-specific DNA from cerebrospinal fluid. AIDS 1994;8:49.

196. Conway B, Halliday W, Brunham R. Human immunodeficiency virus-associated progressive multifocal leukoencephalopathy: apparent response to 3'-azido-3'deoxythymidine. Rev Infect Dis 1990; 12:479.

197. Portegies P, Algra P, Hollak C, et al. Response to cytarabine in progressive multifocal leukoencephalopathy in AIDS. Lancet 1991; 1:680.

198. Berger J, Mucke L. Prolonged survival and partial recovery in AIDS-associated progressive multifocal leukoencephalopathy. Neurology 1988;38:1060.

199. Vinters H, Kwok M, Ho H, et al. Cytomegalovirus in the nervous system of patients with the acquired immunodeficiency syndrome. Brain 1989;112:245.

200. Holland NR, Power C, Mathews VP, et al. Cytomegalovirus encephalitis in acquired immunodeficiency syndrome (AIDS). Neurology 1994;44:507.

201. Cinque P, Vago L, Brytting M, et al. Cytomegalovirus infection of the central nervous system in patients with AIDS: diagnosis by DNA amplification from cerebrospinal fluid. J Infect Dis 1992; 166:1408.

202. Gozlan J, Salord JM, Roullet E, et al. Rapid detection of cytomegalovirus DNA in cerebrospinal fluid of AIDS patients with neurologic disorders [published erratum appears in J Infect Dis 1993; 167:995]. J Infect Dis 1992;166:1416.

203. Wolf DG, Spector SA. Diagnosis of human cytomegalovirus central nervous system disease in AIDS patients by DNA amplification from cerebrospinal fluid. J Infect Dis 1992;166:1412.

204. Weber T, Beck R, Stark E, et al. Comparative analysis of intrathecal antibody synthesis and DNA amplification for the diagnosis of cytomegalovirus infection of the central nervous system in AIDS patients. J Neurol 1994;241:407.

205. Sunderam G, McDonald R, Maniatias T, et al. Tuberculosis as a manifestation of the acquired immunodeficiency syndrome (AIDS). JAMA 1986;256:362.

206. Guarner J, Del Rio C, Slade B. Tuberculosis as a manifestation of the acquired immunodeficiency syndrome (letter). JAMA 1986; 256:3092.

207. Bishburg, E, Sunderam G, Reichman L, et al. Central nervous system tuberculosis with the acquired immunodeficiency syndrome and its related complex. Ann Intern Med 1986;105:210.

208. Dube MP, Holtom PD, Larsen RA. Tuberculous meningitis in patients with and without human immunodeficiency virus infection. Am J Med 1992;93:520.

209. Berenguer J, Moreno S, Laguna F, et al. Tuberculous meningitis in patients infected with the human immunodeficiency virus. (See comments) N Engl J Med 1992;326:668.

210. Folgueira L, Delgado R, Palenque E, et al. Polymerase chain reaction for rapid diagnosis of tuberculous meningitis in AIDS patients. Neurology 1994;44:1336.

211. Jacob CN, Henein SS, Heurich AE, et al. Nontuberculous mycobacterial infection of the central nervous system in patients with AIDS. South Med J 1993;86:638.

212. Horten B, Price R, Jimenez D. Multifocal varicella-zoster virus leukoencephalitis temporally remote from herpes zoster. Ann Neurol 1981;9:251.

213. Ryder JW, Croen K, Kleinschmidt-DeMasters BK, et al. Progressive encephalitis three months after resolution of cutaneous zoster in a patient with AIDS. Ann Neurol 1986;19:182.

214. Morgello S, Block G, Price R, et al. Varicella-zoster virus leukoencephalitis and cerebral vasculopathy. Arch Pathol Lab Med 1988;112:173.

215. Hilt D, Bucholz D, Krumholz A, et al. Herpes zoster ophthalmicus and delayed contralateral hemiparesis caused by cerebral angiitis: diagnosis and management approaches. Ann Neurol 1983;14:543.

216. Eidelberg D, Sotrel A, Horopian D, et al. Thrombotic cerebral vasculopathy associated with herpes zoster. Ann Neurol 1986;19:7.

217. Devinsky O, Cho E, Petito C, et al. Herpes zoster myelitis. Brain 1991;114:1181.

218. Levy R, Bredesen D, Rosenblum M. Neurological manifestations of the acquired immunodeficiency syndrome (AIDS): experience at UCSF and review of the literature. J Neurosurg 1985;62:475.

219. Rhodes R. Histopathology of the central nervous system in the acquired immunodeficiency syndrome. Hum Pathol 1987;18:636.

220. Gray F, Belec L, Lescs MC, et al. Varicella-zoster virus infection of the central nervous system in the acquired immune deficiency syndrome. (Review) Brain 1994;117:987.

221. Berger J. Neurosyphilis in human immunodeficiency virus type 1-seropositive individuals. Arch Neurol 1991;48:700.

222. Johns D, Tierney M, Felsenstein D. Alteration in the natural history of neurosyphilis by concurrent infection with the human immunodeficiency virus. N Engl J Med 1987;316:1569.

223. Berry C, Hooton T, Collier A, et al. Neurologic relapse after benzathine penicillin therapy for secondary syphilis in a patient with HIV infection. N Engl J Med 1987;316:1587.

224. Katz D, Berger J. Neurosyphilis in acquired immunodeficiency syndrome. Arch Neurol 1989;46:895.

225. Davis L. Neurosyphilis in the patient infected with human immunodeficiency virus. Ann Neurol 1990;27:211.

226. Lukehart S, Hook E, Baker-Zander S. Invasion of the central nervous system by *Treponema pallidum*: implications for the diagnosis and treatment. Ann Intern Med 1988;109:855.

227. Gordon SE, Eaton ME, George R, et al. The response of symptomatic neurosyphilis to high-dose intravenous penicillin G in patients with human immunodeficiency virus infection. N Engl J Med 1994;331:1469.

228. Simon R. Neurosyphilis. Neurology 1994;44:2228.

229. Horowitz HW, Valsamis MP, Wicher V, et al. Brief report: cerebral syphilitic gumma confirmed by the polymerase chain reaction in a man with human immunodeficiency virus infection. N Engl J Med 1994;331:1488.

230. Lanska M, Lanska D, Schmidley J. Syphilitic polyradiculopathy in an HIV-positive man. Neurology 1988;38:1297.

231. Carrazana EJ, Rossitch E Jr, Morris J. Isolated central nervous system aspergillosis in the acquired immunodeficiency syndrome. Clin Neurol Neurosurg 1991;93:227.

232. Decker CF, Parenti DM. Invasive aspergillosis in patients with HIV infection: report of two patients and a review of the literature. (Review) J Acquir Immune Defic Syndr 1991;4:603.

233. Khoo SH, Denning DW. Invasive aspergillosis in patients with AIDS. (Review) Clin Infect Dis 1994;19(Suppl 1):S41.

234. Pursell KJ, Telzak EE, Armstrong D. Aspergillus species colonization and invasive disease in patients with AIDS. (Review) Clin Infect Dis 1992;14:141.

235. Kim J, Minamoto GY, Grieco MH. Nocardial infection as a complication of AIDS: report of six cases and review. (Review) Rev Infect Dis 1991;13:624.

236. LeBlang SD, Whiteman ML, Post MJ, et al. CNS *Nocardia* in AIDS patients: CT and MRI with pathologic correlation. J Comput Assist Tomogr 1995;19:15.

237. Long PF. A retrospective study of *Nocardia* infections associated with the acquired immune deficiency syndrome (AIDS). (Letter; review) Infection 1994;22:362.

238. Miralles GD. Disseminated *Nocardia farcinica* infection in an AIDS patient. Eur J Clin Microbiol Infect Dis 1994;13:497.

239. Bruinsma-Adams IK. AIDS presenting as *Candida albicans* meningitis: a case report [Published erratum appears in AIDS 1991, vol 5, following page 1547]. (Letter) AIDS 1991;5:1268.

240. Manfredi R, Mazzoni A, Cavicchi O, et al. Invasive mycotic and actinomycotic oropharyngeal and craniofacial infection in two patients with AIDS. 1994;Mycoses 1994;37:209.

241. Berenguer J, Solera J, Diaz MD, et al. Listeriosis in patients infected with human immunodeficiency virus. (Review) Rev Infect Dis 1991;13:115.
242. da Silva LJ, Resende MR, de Abreu WB, et al. Listeriosis and AIDS: case report and literature review. (Review) Rev Inst Med Trop Sao Paulo 1992;34:475.
243. Decker CF, Simon GL, DiGioia RA, et al. *Listeria monocytogenes* infections in patients with AIDS: report of five cases and review. (Review) Rev Infect Dis 1991;13:413.
244. Harcourt-Webster JN, Scaravilli F, Darwish AH. *Strongyloides stercoralis* hyperinfection in an HIV positive patient. J Clin Pathol 1991;44:346.
245. Shapshak P, Sun NC, Resnick L, et al. HIV-1 propagates in human neuroblastoma cells. J Acquir Immune Defic Syndr 1991;4:228.
246. So Y, Beckstead J, Davis R. Primary central nervous system lymphoma in acquired immune deficiency syndrome: a clinical and pathological study. Ann Neurol 1986;20:566.
247. Levine AM. Non-Hodgkin's lymphomas and other malignancies in the acquired immune deficiency syndrome. (Review) Semin Oncol 1987;14(Suppl 3):34.
248. Meeker TC, Shiramizu B, Kaplan L, et al. Evidence for molecular subtypes of HIV-associated lymphoma: division into peripheral monoclonal, polyclonal and central nervous system lymphoma. AIDS 1991;5:669.
249. Baumgartner JE, Rachlin JR, Beckstead JH, et al. Primary central nervous system lymphomas: natural history and response to radiation therapy in 55 patients with acquired immunodeficiency syndrome. J Neurosurg 1990;73:206.
250. Formenti SC, Gill PS, Lean E, et al. Primary central nervous system lymphoma in AIDS: results of radiation therapy. Cancer 1989;63:1101.
251. Remick S, Diamond C, Migliozzi J, et al. Primary central nervous system lymphoma in patients with and without the acquired immune deficiency syndrome: a retrospective analysis and review of the literature. Medicine (Baltimore) 1990;69:345.
252. DeAngelis L. Primary CNS lymphoma: a new clinical challenge. Neurology 1991;41:619.
253. DeAngelis L, Yaholom J, Heineman M. Primary CNS lymphoma: combined treatment with chemotherapy and radiotherapy. Neurology 1990;40:80.
254. Engstrom J, Lowenstein D, Bredesen D. Cerebral infarctions and transient neurologic deficits associated with acquired immunodeficiency syndrome. Am J Med 1989;86:528.
255. Berger JR, Flaster M, Schatz N, et al. Cranial neuropathy heralding otherwise occult AIDS-related large cell lymphoma. J Clin Neuro-Ophthalmol 1993;13:113.
256. Bomfim da Paz R, Kolmel HW. Meningitis with Burkitt like B-cell lymphoma in HIV infection. J Neurooncol 1992;13:73.
257. Enting RH, Esselink RA, Portegies P. Lymphomatous meningitis in AIDS-related systemic non-Hodgkin's lymphoma: a report of eight cases. J Neurol Neurosurg Psychiatry 1994;57:150.
258. Engstrom JW, Lowenstein DH, Bredesen DE. Cerebral infarctions and transient neurologic deficits associated with acquired immunodeficiency syndrome. Am J Med 1989;86:528.
259. Moriarty DM, Haller JO, Loh JP, et al. Cerebral infarction in pediatric acquired immunodeficiency syndrome. Pediatr Radiol 1994;24:611.
260. Philippet P, Blanche S, Sebag G, et al. Stroke and cerebral infarcts in children infected with human immunodeficiency virus. Arch Pediatr Adolesc Med 1994;148:965.
261. Mizusawa H, Hirano J, Llena J, et al. Cerebral lesions in acquired immune deficiency syndrome (AIDS). Acta Neuropathol 1988;76:451.
262. Maclean C, Flegg P, Kilpatrick D. Anti-cardiolipin antibodies and HIV infection. Clin Exp Immunol 1990;81:263.
263. Yankner B, Skolnik P, Shoukimas G, et al. Cerebral granulomatous angiitis associated with isolation of human T lymphotropic virus type III from the central nervous system. Ann Neurol 1986;20:362.
264. Bissuel F, Berruyer M, Causse X, et al. Acquired protein S deficiency: correlation with advanced disease in HIV-1 infected patients. J Acquir Immune Defic Syndr 1992;5:484.
265. Cho E, Sharer L, Peress N, et al. Intimal proliferation of leptomeningeal arteries and brain infarcts in subjects with AIDS. J Neuropathol Exp Neurol 1987;46:385.
266. Wong M, Suite N, Labar D. Seizures in human immunodeficiency virus infection. Arch Neurol 1990;47:640.
267. Boldorini R, Vago L, Lechi A, et al. Wernicke's encephalopathy: occurrence and pathological aspects in a series of 400 AIDS patients. Acta Biomed 1 Ateneo Parmense 1992;63:43.
268. Schwenk J, Gosztonyi G, Thierauf P, et al. Wernicke's encephalopathy in two patients with acquired immunodeficiency syndrome. J Neurol 1990;237:445.
269. Vanpaesschen, W, Bodian C, Maker H. Metabolic abnormalities and new-onset seizures in human immunodeficiency virus-seropositive patients. Epilepsia 1995;36:146.
270. So Y, Holtzman D, Abrams D, et al. Peripheral neuropathy associated with acquired immunodeficiency syndrome: prevalence and clinical features from a population based survey. Arch Neurol 1988;45:945.
271. Bartolomei F, Pellegrino P, Dhiver C, et al. Epilepsy seizures in HIV infection: 52 cases (in French). (Review) Presse Med 1991;20:2135.
272. Holtzman D, Kaku D, So Y. New onset seizures associated with human immunodeficiency virus infection: causation and clinical features in 100 cases. Am J Med 1989;87:173.
273. Van Paesschen W, Bodian C, Maker H. Metabolic abnormalities and new-onset seizures in human immunodeficiency virus-seropositive patients. Epilepsia 1995;36:146.
274. Simpson DM, Olney RK. Peripheral neuropathies associated with human immunodeficiency virus infection. (Review) Neurol Clin 1992;10:685.
275. Cornblath D, McArthur J. Predominantly sensory neuropathy in patients with AIDS and AIDS-related complex. Neurology 1988;38:794.
276. Cornblath D. Treatment of the neuromuscular complications of human immunodeficiency virus infection. Ann Neurol 1988;23(Suppl):S88.
277. Cornblath D, Chaudhry V, Griffin J. Treatment of chronic inflammatory demyelinating polyneuropathy with intravenous immunoglobulin. Ann Neurol 1991;30:104.
278. Eidelberg D, Sotrel A, Vogel H, et al. Progressive polyradiculopathy in acquired immune deficiency syndrome. Neurology 1986;36:912.
279. Fuller GN. Cytomegalovirus and the peripheral nervous system in AIDS. (Review) J Acquir Immune Defic Syndr 1992;5:S33.
280. Said G, Lacroix C, Chemouilli P, et al. CMV neuropathy in AIDS: a clinical and pathological study. Ann Neurol 1991;29:139.
281. Roullet E, Assuerus V, Gozlan J, et al. Cytomegalovirus multifocal neuropathy in AIDS: analysis of 15 consecutive cases. Neurology 1994;44:2174.
282. Miller R, Storey J, Greco C. Ganciclovir in the treatment of progressive AIDS-related polyradiculopathy. Neurology 1990;40:569.
283. Fuller G, Gill S, Guilloff R, et al. Ganciclovir treatment of lumbosacral polyradiculopathy in AIDS. Lancet 1990;335:48.
284. So Y, Olney R. The natural history of mononeuropathy multiplex and simplex in patients with HIV infection. (Abstract) Neurology 1991;41(Suppl):374.
285. Miller R, Parry G, Lang W, et al. AIDS-related inflammatory polyradiculoneuropathy: successful treatment with plasma exchange. (Abstract) Neurology 1986;36:206.
286. Miller R, Parry G, Pfaeffl W, et al. The spectrum of peripheral neuropathy associated with ARC and AIDS. Muscle Nerve 1988;11:857.
287. Lipkin W, Parry G, Kiprov D, et al. Inflammatory neuropathy in homosexual men with lymphadenopathy. Neurology 1985;35:1479.
288. Griffin JW, Wesselingh SL, Griffin DE, et al. Peripheral nerve disorders in HIV infection: similarities and contrasts with CNS disorders. (Review) Res Publ Assoc Res Nerv Ment Dis 1994;72:159.
289. Berger AR, Arezzo JC, Schaumburg HH, et al. 2′,3′-dideoxycytidine (ddC) toxic neuropathy: a study of 52 patients. Neurology 1993;43:358.
290. Browne MJ, Mayer KH, Chafee SB, et al. 2′,3′-didehydro-3′-deoxythymidine (d4T) in patients with AIDS or AIDS-related complex: a phase I trial. J Infect Dis 1993;167:21.
291. Kieburtz KD, Seidlin M, Lambert JS, et al. Extended follow-up of peripheral neuropathy in patients with AIDS-related complex treated with dideoxyinosine. J Acquir Immune Defic Syndr 1992;5:60.
292. Meng TC, Fischl MA, Boota AM, et al. Combination therapy with zidovudine and dideoxycytidine in patients with advanced human immunodeficiency virus infection: a phase I/II study. (See comments] Ann Intern Med 1992;116:13.
293. Simpson DM, Tagliati M. Nucleoside analogue-associated peripheral neuropathy in human immunodeficiency virus infection. (Review) J Acquir Immune Defic Syndr 1995;9:153.

294. Craddock C, Pasvol G, Bull R, et al. Cardiorespiratory arrest and automatic neuropathy in AIDS. Lancet 1987;2:16.

295. Welby SB, Rogerson SJ, Beeching NJ. Autonomic neuropathy is common in human immunodeficiency virus infection. J Infect 1991;23:123.

296. Bailey RO, Turok DI, Jaufmann BP, et al. Myositis and acquired immunodeficiency syndrome. Hum Pathol 1987;18:749.

297. Illa I, Nath A, Dalakas M. Immunocytochemical and virological characteristics of HIV-associated inflammatory myopathies: similarities with seronegative polymyositis. Ann Neurol 1991;29:474.

298. Gherardi RK. Skeletal muscle involvement in HIV-infected patients. (Review) Neuropathol Appl Neurobiol 1994;20:232.

299. Manji H, Harrison MJ, Round JM, et al. Muscle disease, HIV and zidovudine: the spectrum of muscle disease in HIV-infected individuals treated with zidovudine. J Neurol 1993;240:479.

300. Simpson DM, Bender AN. Human immunodeficiency virus-associated myopathy: analysis of 11 patients. Ann Neurol 1988;24:79.

301. Nordstrom DM, Petropolis AA, Giorno R, et al. Inflammatory myopathy and acquired immunodeficiency syndrome. Arthritis Rheum 1989;32:475.

302. Wrzolek MA, Sher JH, Kozlowski PB, et al. Skeletal muscle pathology in AIDS: an autopsy study. Muscle Nerve 1990;13:508.

303. Berger JR, Pall L, Winfield D. Effect of anabolic steroids on HIV-related wasting myopathy. South Med J 1993;86:865.

304. Miller RG, Carson PJ, Moussavi RS, et al. Fatigue and myalgia in AIDS patients. Neurology 1991;41:1603.

305. Chalmers A, Greco C, Miller R. Prognosis in AZT myopathy. Neurology 1991;41:1181.

306. Dalakas M, Illa I, Pezeshkpour G, et al. Mitochondrial myopathy caused by long term zidovudine therapy. N Engl J Med 1990;322:1098.

307. Arnaudo E, Dalakas M, Shanske S, et al. Depletion of muscle mitochondrial DNA in AIDS patients with zidovudine-induced myopathy. Lancet 1991;337:508.

308. Dalakas MC, Leon-Monzon ME, Bernardini I, et al. Zidovudine-induced mitochondrial myopathy is associated with muscle carnitine deficiency and lipid storage. Ann Neurol 1994;35:482.

309. Damati G, Lewis W. Zidovudine causes early increases in mitochondrial ribonucleic acid abundance and induces ultrastructural changes in cultured mouse muscle cells. Lab Invest 1994;71:879.

310. Mhiri C, Baudrimont M, Bonne G, et al. Zidovudine myopathy: a distinctive disorder associated with mitochondrial dysfunction. Ann Neurol 1991;29:606.

311. Modica-Napolitano JS. AZT causes tissue-specific inhibition of mitochondrial bioenergetic function. Biochem Biophys Res Commun 1993;194:170.

312. Peters BS, Winer J, Landon DN, et al. Mitochondrial myopathy associated with chronic zidovudine therapy in AIDS. Q J Med 1993;86:5.

313. Simpson DM, Citak KA, Godfrey E, et al. Myopathies associated with human immunodeficiency virus and zidovudine: can their effects be distinguished? Neurology 1993;43:971.

AIDS: Biology, Diagnosis, Treatment and Prevention, fourth edition, edited by Vincent T. DeVita, Jr., Samuel Hellman, and Steven A. Rosenberg. Lippincott–Raven Publishers, © 1997

CHAPTER 17

Oral Disease in Human Immunodeficiency Infection

John S. Greenspan and Deborah Greenspan

Understanding of the nature, significance, and management of the numerous oral and pharyngeal expressions of disease associated with HIV infection has grown in parallel with the AIDS epidemic. Oral candidiasis and the oral lesions of Kaposi's sarcoma (KS) were among the earliest features of AIDS[1,2] to be described in homosexual and bisexual men, and in the ensuing 14 years, a growing body of literature and clinical experience have reinforced and confirmed these early descriptions.[3–5]

SIGNIFICANCE OF ORAL DISEASE

The mouth and pharynx are easily examined. The oral lesions are for the most part clearly visible, and many can be diagnosed on clinical features alone. If the HIV status is unknown or HIV testing is difficult, as occurs in many developing areas of the world, certain oral lesions provide strong indication of HIV infection. Oral candidiasis, hairy leukoplakia, and other oral lesions are indicators of progression to AIDS. They parallel the decline in CD4 T-cell counts in this regard and are also independent indicators of prognosis. It is therefore not surprising that certain of these lesions, notably oral candidiasis and hairy leukoplakia, feature in all classification,[6,7] staging,[8,9] and prognosis[10,11] systems in use.[12,13] These observations alone mandate thorough oral examination at every stage in the diagnosis and care of all HIV-positive patients and emphasize the importance of these lesions in HIV prevention and intervention.[12] However, the presence of oral lesions or their development also

John S. Greenspan, Department of Stomatology and Oral AIDS Center, School of Dentistry, Room S612, Box 0422, University of California, San Francisco, CA 94143-0422.

Deborah Greenspan, Department of Stomatology and Oral AIDS Center, School of Dentistry, Room S612, Box 0422, University of California, San Francisco, CA 94143-0422.

are widely used as entry criteria and end points for prophylaxis, treatment, and vaccine trials. Moreover, certain oral lesions, notably those representing herpes simplex and Epstein-Barr virus (EBV) infections, may act as cofactors or risk modifiers that modulate the progress and outcome of HIV infection.[13]

ROLE OF DENTISTRY

HIV-infected patients should receive regular dental examinations and care of the same standard and at least the same frequency as the general population. Such care should be provided in general dental practice. Referral to dental and other specialists, such as periodontitis, oral and maxillofacial surgeons, endodontists, and oral medicine specialists should be based on the clinical needs of the patient. HIV status is not a reason to alter dental treatment, and dental care in this population is not associated with delayed healing or other complications.[14] As with all patients, timely attention to oral and dental disease can dramatically improve the quality of life, nutritional status, speech, and appearance. Early attention to developing oral mucosal and periodontal disease and to oral hygiene preventive measures can obviate much suffering and save much expense. To this end, many AIDS primary care providers have developed close and effective working relationships with members of the dental health care team.

EPIDEMIOLOGY

Many studies attest to the frequency of oral disease in those with HIV infection. In three San Francisco cohorts of homosexual and bisexual men—the San Francisco City Clinic Cohort Study, the San Francisco General Hospital Study, and the San Francisco Men's Health Study—a cross sectional analysis revealed a point prevalence of oral mucosal lesions of about 28% among those who were HIV positive, but the prevalence was low among HIV-negative men.[15] Similar results have been found in numerous other studies, including those of women.[16,17] Most studies show that hairy leukoplakia and pseudomembranous candidiasis are the commonest lesions in HIV-infected persons and AIDS patients (11% to 96%), with higher prevalence and incidence figures reported as the CD4 count falls and the disease progresses. Several studies have emphasized that HIV-infected individuals with oral candidiasis or hairy leukoplakia progress to AIDS more rapidly than matched controls without these lesions.[11,18–21] The incidence of oral candidiasis increases with time since seroconversion from 4% at 1 year to 26% at 5 years, and for hairy leukoplakia, the respective numbers are 9% and 42%.[22] Oral lesions are more common in those who smoke.[23] However, HIV salivary gland disease appears to be associated with slower progression to AIDS (Fig. 17-1).[24]

CLASSIFICATION

The latest set of definitions and diagnostic criteria for the oral lesions of HIV infection are those provided by the EEC Working Group[25] and the U.S. Oral AIDS Collaborative Group.[26] One classification of oral lesions is shown in Table 17-1.[26]

MUCOSAL IMMUNITY

Although the very high frequency and significance of the oral lesions have been studied extensively, far less is known about their pathogenesis. Normal immunologic and other host defense systems serve to neutralize microorganisms and their toxins, prevent adherence of potentially pathogenic organisms to epithelial cells, and contribute to the maintenance of the latent phase of many viruses. The elements involved include T lymphocytes of several types, B cells, and

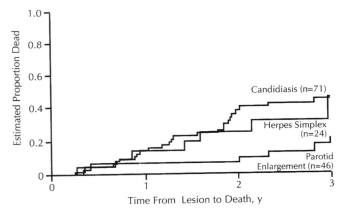

FIG. 17-1. Parotid enlargment in HIV-infected children denotes a better prognosis. (Katz MH, Mastrucci MT, Leggott PJ, Westenhouse J, Greenspan JS, Scott GB. Prognostic significance of oral lesions in children with perinatally acquired human immunodeficiency virus infection. Am J Dis Child 1993;147:45.)

TABLE 17-1. *Classification of oral lesions*

Neoplastic lesions
  Kaposi's sarcoma
  Non-Hodgkin's lymphoma
  Hodgkin's lymphoma

Fungal lesions
  Candidiasis
    Pseudomembranous
    Erythematous
    Angular cheilitis
  Histoplasmosis
  Cryptococcocosis
  Penicillinosis
  Other

Bacterial lesions
  Periodontal disease
  Necrotizing stomatitis
  Tuberculosis
  Mycobacterium avian complex
  Bacillary angiomatosis
  Other

Viral lesions
  Herpes simplex
  Chicken pox
  Herpes zoster
  Cytomegalovirus
  Hairy leukoplakia

Autoimmune or idiopathic lesions
  Salivary gland disease
  Aphthous ulcers
  Abnormal pigmentation
  Other

plasma cells with their antibody products. The latter are predominantly of the IgA class in the mouth, but IgG and IgM are also involved. Langerhans' cells, dendritic cells of several classes, and macrophages are also vital components.

Nonimmunologic mechanisms include the continual shedding of keratinocytes; keratinocyte products, including cytokines; and a number of antimicrobial components of saliva. The delicate balance between the multitude of potentially pathogenic microorganisms within the mouth and this complex homeostatic mechanism can readily be tipped even in the otherwise healthy individual. In HIV infection, progressive loss of CD4 cells and HIV disturbance of lymphoid architecture and function are well documented.[27] However, surprisingly little is known of the effects of HIV infection on the host response and of the nature of the events leading to oral opportunistic infections.

FUNGAL INFECTIONS

Candidiasis

Oral and pharyngeal candidiasis are among the commonest oral features of HIV disease. Although often asymptomatic, all three of the forms of oral and pharyngeal candidiasis described here can cause soreness, burning, dysgeusia, and dysphagia.

The three forms of candidiasis are pseudomembranous (ie, thrush), erythematous, and angular cheilitis. In pseudomembranous candidiasis (Fig. 17-2), soft, creamy white, removable plaques can be seen on any oral or pharyngeal mucosal surface, often at multiple sites. They are readily removed, and sometimes the underlying mucosa is red. Erythematous candidiasis (Fig. 17-3) is much more subtle and consists of smooth, flat, red areas on the palate, dorsal

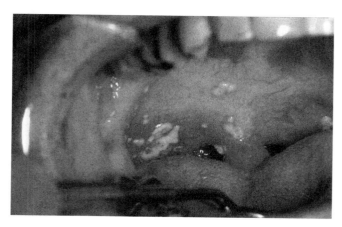

FIG. 17-2. Pseudomembranous candidiasis, palate. See also Color Figure 17-2.

tongue, and other oropharyngeal locations. Pseudomembranous and erythematous candidiasis are equally predictive of the development of AIDS,[28] making the subtle red lesion of oral candidiasis an important diagnosis. In angular cheilitis, cracks and fissures appear at the corners of the mouth and are often painful.

Although in current clinical practice HIV is the predominant predisposing factor for these lesions, several others must be considered. These include systemic and local steroid therapy, antibiotics, poorly controlled diabetes, anemia, reduced salivary flow as occurs in Sjögrens syndrome, radiation therapy involving the salivary glands, and drugs that interfere with salivary function. Candidiasis is also seen in the newborn (ie, neonatal thrush) and as denture stomatitis on mucosal surfaces occluded by plastic denture material.

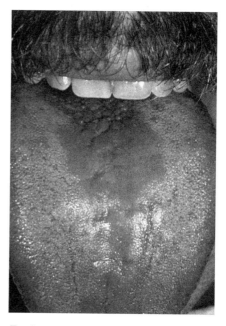

FIG. 17-3. Erythematous candidiasis of the dorsal tongue. See also Color Figure 17-3.

The pathogenesis of mucosal candidiasis may involve the upregulation of genes controlling virulence factors, expressed, for example, through switching of phenotypes; the emergence of virulent strains within the patient's preexisting flora; and new infection with virulent strains or species.[29] A disturbing development is the emergence of azole-resistant strains of *Candida* and related fungi.[30]

Diagnosis of oropharyngeal candidiasis is based on clinical appearance and may be confirmed using smears taken from lesions and examined by one of several techniques, including potassium hydroxide preparation, Gram stain, or periodic acid–Schiff(PAS) stain. These reveal fungal hyphae and blastospores. Culture may be of use to identify the causative organism. This method is less valuable in diagnosis, because a significant proportion of the healthy population and an even greater number of those with HIV infection carry *Candida* in the mouth in the absence of oral lesions. The predominant organism is *Candida albicans*, but several other species can be found, including *C krusei* and *C glabrata*. *C krusei* exhibits primary resistance to fluconazole, and *C glabrata* and *C albicans* are being reported as developing secondary resistance.

Topical and systemic routes can be used for the treatment of oral candidiasis.[31] Nystatin is available in several formulations, including nystatin vaginal tablets (100,000 units) that are dissolved slowly in the mouth three to four times each day for 14 days; nystatin pastilles (Mycostatin, 200,000 units), taken as one or two pastilles dissolved in the mouth four to five times each day for 14 days; nystatin suspension (100,000 units/mL), used as 5 to 10 mL of a mouth rinse three to five times each day for 14 days. Clotrimazole is available as an oral troche (Mycelex); a 10-mg troche dissolved in the mouth five times each day for 14 days. Oral systemic agents include 200 mg of ketoconazole (Nizoral) taken daily; fluconazole (Diflucan), with 200 mg taken on the first day, followed by 100 mg daily; and 200 mg of itraconazole (Sporanox) taken each day for 14 days.

Determination of which systemic antifungal to use may be influenced by the possibility of interactions with the patient's other medications, and it should be remembered that adequate gastric acidity is required for the absorption of ketoconazole. The topical oral agents nystatin pastille, nystatin suspension, and clotrimazole oral troche contain sweeteners that can contribute to dental caries if used frequently and for prolonged periods. However, oral candidiasis usually recurs, often many times, and use of these topical medications should be accompanied by the use of a daily fluoride mouth rinse. Factors to be taken into consideration when choosing an antifungal drug include the likelihood of patient compliance, concomitant medications, and cost effectiveness. Systemic agents require once-daily dosing, and response to therapy may occur after 2 days. Topical oral agents require multiple daily dosing, the flavor may not be palatable, and response times may be a little slower. If oral candidiasis does not respond to fluconazole, other azoles can be tried, including itraconazole. Amphotericin B can be used as a topical mouth rinse, although this is not an indication approved by the U.S. Food and Drug Administration.

Other Fungal Infections

Some cases of oral lesions of histoplasmosis are seen, and there are rare case reports of oral cryptococcosis,[32] penicillinosis,[33] and geotrichosis.[34] Histoplasmosis[35] and cryptococcosis may present as unusual nonhealing ulcers, and penicillinosis and geotrichosis may resemble erythematous candidiasis.

BACTERIAL INFECTIONS

Periodontal Disease

Some individuals with HIV infection develop troublesome periodontal disease. Although some cases are expressions of the same chronic process that is seen in the general population, a few persons present with conditions that seem to be more specifically associated with HIV infection.[36]

The first of these, known as linear gingival erythema, is a striking bright red linear band of intense erythema at the gingival margin that is not associated with plaque and does not respond to conventional plaque removal procedures. Linear gingival erythema does not appear to be an inflammatory gingivitis, but it may result from capillary dilatation caused perhaps by cytokine defects. This condition may or may not be the precursor to a more severe HIV-associated periodontitis now known as necrotizing ulcerative periodontitis.[37] In this often rapid-onset and progressive condition (Fig. 17-4), necrosis of the gingival soft tissue resembling necrotizing ulcerative gingivitis (ie, trench mouth) extends into the tooth-supporting tissues and causes bleeding, pain, halitosis, and rapid loss of alveolar bone, with loosening of teeth and their loss if the condition is left untreated. In rare cases, the necrosis may extend beyond the tooth-supporting tissues, with resultant soft tissue loss and bone exposure and

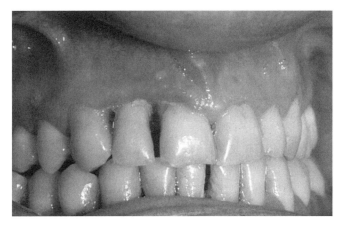

FIG. 17-4. Necrotizing ulcerative periodontitis of the maxilla. See also Color Figure 17-4.

sequestration in the alveolus and palate (ie, necrotizing stomatitis). This complication resembles cancrum oris or noma.[38]

Several epidemiologic studies indicate that the prevalence of these conditions is much lower than oral candidiasis or hairy leukoplakia. However, in patients with significant loss of CD4 cells and HIV-related diseases, the prevalence of periodontal complications rises to almost 10%.[39] Smoking predisposes patients to these forms of periodontal disease.[23] Other factors involved in the pathogenesis may include loss of cell-mediated local immune response, polymorph defects or hyperresponsiveness,[40] and changes in the bacterial flora. The latter possibility has been investigated extensively,[41] but the flora appears to be similar to that seen in chronic inflammatory periodontal disease in the general population. Although these data may reflect methodologic limitations, there is no evidence to support the hypothesis that a single pathogenic organism or a small number of such organisms are the cause of these conditions.

There is a fairly straightforward protocol for the management of these HIV-related periodontal diseases.[42] Linear gingival erythema usually responds to careful oral hygiene and the use of twice-daily chlorhexidine mouth rinses. Management of necrotizing periodontal diseases involves local irrigation with povidone-iodine, combined with meticulous root planing, curettage, and removal of necrotic tissue and debris. These office procedures are supplemented by the home use of povidone-iodine irrigation, chlorhexidine mouth rinses twice daily, and antibiotics. Antibiotics that have been found to be useful, notably metronidazole, amoxicillin-clavulanate (Augmentin), and clindamycin, are effective against a wide range of the putatively causative microorganisms in these conditions. For rare cases in which alveolar and adjoining bone is exposed, a combination of the local and antimicrobial measures described, along with careful observation of the sequestration process, may obviate the need for extensive surgical intervention.

Other Bacterial Infections

A few case reports describe oral ulcers secondary to disseminated mycobacterial infections of[43] and *Mycobacterium avium* complex. Similarly, bacillary angiomatosis[44] has presented with oral mucosal papules, which can be confused clinically with KS sarcoma. Biopsy and appropriate culture is necessary to establish the diagnosis.

VIRAL DISEASES

Herpes Simplex

Primary and recurrent herpes simplex infections occur in HIV-positive patients. Primary herpetic gingivostomatitis may occur in adults who have not previously been exposed to herpes simplex virus, and rare examples of apparently recurrent herpetic gingivostomatitis are also seen. More commonly, recurrent herpes is seen as herpes labialis and as intraoral herpes simplex. The latter appears as vesicles that ulcerate on keratinized mucosa such as the palate and gingiva. Atypical lesions may occur on the dorsal tongue, appearing as slit-like or dendritic ulcers that are usually painful (Fig. 17-5). Treatment with acyclovir may be indicated for lesions that persist beyond 7 to 10 days. Rare instances of acyclovir resistance have been reported.[45] These cases may respond to foscarnet.

Varicella-Zoster

Chicken pox and herpes zoster can involve the oral mucosa and perioral skin. In herpes zoster infections, there is marked unilateral distribution of vesicles that break down to form ulcers; these can occur on any mucosal surface including the vermilion border. The orofacial lesions follow the distribution of one or more branches of the trigeminal nerve. The prodrome may involve pain referred to one or more teeth. Prompt treatment with acylovir is indicated.

Cytomegalovirus

Oral mucosal ulcers associated with cytomegalovirus (CMV) infection[46] are usually associated with systemic CMV disease, although there are a few case reports of oral lesions that were the presenting or only features of CMV infection. The ulcers of CMV infection can be confused with aphthous ulcers, and the diagnosis is based on biopsy and immunohistochemistry results. After diagnosis of the oral lesions, the patient should be evaluated for the presence of CMV disease.

Hairy Leukoplakia

The EBV lesion hairy leukoplakia is notable for several reasons. Our description of this lesion in 1984 in homosexual men[47] was the first and noticed its association with the development of AIDS. This prognostic significance has been confirmed by several studies.[11,18] It is the first lesion associated with fully replicative EBV infection of epithelial cells,[48,49] because in nasopharyngeal and associated upper aerodigestive tract carcinomas, portions of EBV DNA are found, not the entire virion.

Hairy leukoplakia does not appear to be premalignant, and its pathogenesis may involve infection of tongue epithelial cells by multiple EBV strains. The development of defective EBV and recombinant strains may occur.[49] The clinical appearance is of white, corrugated thickening of the lateral tongue (Figs. 17-6 and 17-7) and occasionally of flat lesions of other oral and pharyngeal sites.[50] The thickening results from hyperparakeratosis, acanthosis, and swelling of EBV-infected prickle cells. It has been speculated that reduced loss of surface epithelium may be related to delayed apoptosis and that this may explain the histologic and clinical appearances. The source of the EBV is unclear. Although it does not appear to be latent EBV infection of the cycling basal cell layer, there is dispute about whether EBV infects the epithelium from the saliva, perhaps originating from a salivary gland or other mucosal site of latency and shedding, or whether EBV is carried into the epithelium by B cells.

Although originally described exclusively in association with HIV infection, hairy leukoplakia is almost as prevalent among renal transplant patients[51] and has been described in patients who are immunosuppressed as part of a wide range of other organ transplant procedures or for other reasons. The diagnosis can be made on clinical appearance, but biopsy, followed by EBV in situ hybridization can be employed. Noninvasive cytologic and in situ hybridization approaches are also useful, employing epithelial cells scraped from the lesion. Hairy leukoplakia may be superinfected with *Candida*, and

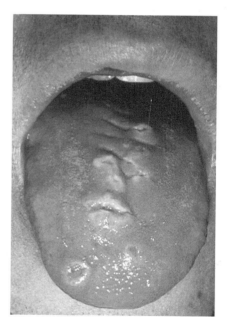

FIG. 17-5. Herpes simplex on the dorsal tongue. See also Color Figure 17-5.

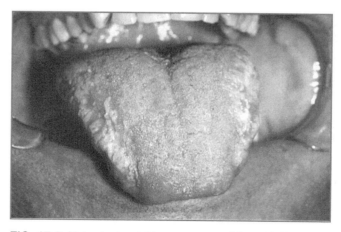

FIG. 17-6. Hairy leukoplakia appears as bilateral thickening of the tongue. See also Color Figure 17-6.

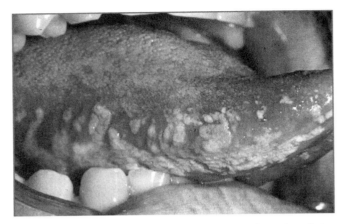

FIG. 17-7. Hairy leukoplakia of the tongue. See also Color Figure 17-7.

although that organism can be eliminated with antifungal medication, the hairy leukoplakia lesion persists.

Hairy leukoplakia can be treated with herpes zoster doses of acyclovir, and although the lesion may disappear, it usually returns some time after treatment is discontinued. Hairy leukoplakia has been reported as disappearing in individuals taking Gancyclovin and foscarnet.[52] Topical agents, including Retin-A and podophyllin,[53] have been reported as eliminating hairy leukoplakia, but after treatment is stopped, the lesion returns.

Human Papillomavirus Lesions

Human papillomavirus lesions include papilliferous and flat warts. Spiky, cauliflower, and flat warts can be seen on any mucosal surface (Fig. 17-8) and can be removed surgically or with the laser. Recurrences and multiple lesions are common. The flat warts may represent focal epithelial hyperplasia and contain HPV types 13 or 32. Unusual HPV types have been identified, notably HPV 7, previously found only in butcher's warts of skin.[54] We have described warts with atypia[55] that contain previously undescribed HPV types. Malignant transformation has yet to be seen in HIV-infected patients.

NEOPLASMS

Kaposi's Sarcoma

The oral lesions of KS[56] are similar to those seen on the skin. Small, flat, red or purplish areas of the mucosa, including the gingiva, represent the early stage (Fig. 17-9). As the lesions grow, they may become nodular and interfere with oral function and esthetics. Extensive lesions of the gingiva may make oral hygiene difficult, leading to secondary infection with pain, bleeding, and ulceration.

Confirmation of the clinical diagnosis of oral lesions is based on histopathologic analysis. The differential diagnosis includes pyogenic granuloma, hemangioma, hematoma, and bacillary angiomatosis. In patients with already diagnosed skin KS, biopsy may not be necessary. It is not clear why oral lesions are so common in this disease, and it is interesting to speculate on the possibility of oral transmission of the recently described KS-associated herpes virus, HHV8.[57]

Treatment of small lesions may be indicated to prevent their growth. Successful treatment modalities include localized chemotherapy with vinblastine for small, flat palatal lesions and surgical excision for small, localized nodular lesions on the gingiva and buccal mucosa. There are case reports of the use of a sclerosing agent (ie, sodium tetradecyl sulfate) for the treatment of small intraoral lesions.[58] Radiation therapy may be needed for extensive, bulky lesions. However, radiation therapy may be accompanied by the development of mucositis. There appears to be a better response to therapy of lesions involving the gingiva if oral hygiene is good and when, if appropriate, dental scaling and polishing are done before commencement of therapy.

Non-Hodgkin's Lymphoma

Oral non-Hodgkin's lymphoma manifests as a swelling or nonhealing ulcer.[56] These lesions may occur on the retromolar pad, dorsal surface of the tongue, gingiva, and buccal or palatal mucosa (Fig. 17-10). Diagnosis is based on biopsy

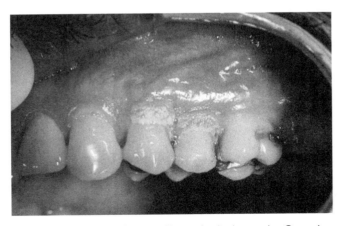

FIG. 17-8. Wart on the maxillary gingival margin. See also Color Figure 17-8.

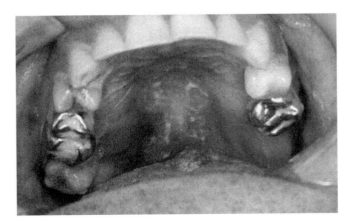

FIG. 17-9. Kaposi's sarcoma of the palate. See also Color Figure 17-9.

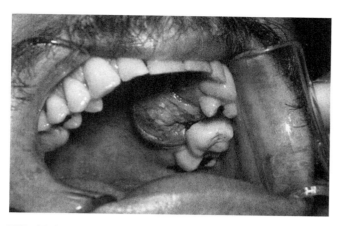

FIG. 17-10. Lymphoma of the palate. See also Color Figure 17-10.

results, and the differential diagnosis of swellings includes KS, fibroma, mycobacterial infections, and a large range of other neoplasms. The ulcers may be confused with long-standing aphthous ulcers, deep fungal infections, and CMV ulcers. Multifocal ulcerative lymphoma has been described as has an example of lymphoma that regressed and then reappeared.[59] The oral lymphomas show the same distribution of phenotypes as AIDS lymphomas at other locations. Treatment of oral non-Hodgkin's lymphoma follows the same approaches as are used for this disease at other sites.

One case of Hodgkin's lymphoma of the gingiva has been described.[60] Although squamous cell carcinomas occur occasionally in individuals who are HIV positive, several epidemiologic studies show no excess incidence of the disease in this population, and the association is probably coincidental.

NONNEOPLASTIC LESIONS

Aphthous ulcers

Oral ulcers often are a troublesome feature of HIV infection.[61,62] Many of them probably represent a form of recurrent aphthous ulceration. The cause of this condition remains unknown, although immune defects have been implicated.

These ulcers, which are usually surrounded by a red halo, may be single or multiple. They are painful and may interfere significantly with eating, speaking, and swallowing. These ulcers are found on the movable (nonkeratinized) oral mucosa of the soft palate, buccal and labial mucosa, oropharynx, and lateral and ventral tongue. Three varieties are seen. The major form consists of one or more ulcers, often 1 cm or larger in diameter, and if associated with HIV infection, they may not heal for weeks if left untreated. The minor form consists of several smaller ulcers that usually heal within 7 to 10 days, but they recur in weeks or months. Some persons are never without them. The rarest form, herpetiform ulcers, consists of larger numbers of tiny ulcers, which may coalesce. There is some suggestion that aphthous ulcers, particularly the major

and herpetiform varieties, may be more common in association with HIV infection. They also seem to be more severe and last longer in this population.

Diagnosis of these ulcers usually is based on history, clinical appearance, and location. However, large, persistent ulcers may require biopsy to exclude lymphoma, deep fungal or mycobacterial infections, atypical herpes simplex lesions, and cytomegalovirus disease.

Aphthous ulcers usually respond to topical steroids. Useful preparations include 0.05% fluocinonide ointment (Lidex), mixed half and half with Orabase; 0.05% clobetasol ointment (Temovate), mixed half and half with Orabase; and dexamethasone elixir (0.5 mg/5 mL), used as a mouth rinse and expectorated; all are used three times each day. There are case reports and small-scale studies indicating a possible role for thalidomide in the treatment of large, long-standing aphthous ulcers,[63,64] although this is not an FDA approved use. Colchicine has also been used for the management of such large ulcers.[65]

Salivary Gland Disease

Dry mouth and salivary gland enlargement occur in HIV-infected persons. In many cases, the xerostomia results from the side effects of medications, including ddI, antidepressants, antianxiety medications, antihistamines, and many others. However, there remains a group of patients with xerostomia, salivary gland enlargement, or both, who appear to have an HIV-associated disease of the salivary glands variously known as HIV–salivary gland disease,[66] benign lymphoepithelial cysts of the salivary glands, and CD8 lymphocytosis syndrome.[67] In this condition, there occurs an apparently benign infiltration of the salivary glands, predominantly the parotid gland, by CD8 lymphocytes. Other organs may also be affected. The condition is found in children and adults, and there is evidence that it confers a slightly improved prognosis.[24]

CONCLUSION

The global HIV epidemic presents enormous ongoing challenges at all levels of health care, from the individual provider to national and international public health agencies. Oral health is a vital component of all aspects of the battle against AIDS.[68]

ACKNOWLEDGMENT

This work was supported by grant PO1-DE-07946, from the USPHS, NIH, and NIDR.

REFERENCES

1. Gottlieb MS, Schroff R, Schantez HM. *Pneumocystis carinii* pneumonia and mucosal candidiasis in previously healthy homosexual men: evidence of a new acquired cellular immunodeficiency. N Engl J Med 1981;305:1425.

2. Murray HW, Hillman AD, Rubin BY, et al. Patients at risk for AIDS-related opportunistic infections. N Engl J Med 1985;313:1504.

3. Greenspan D, Greenspan JS, Pindborg JJ, Schiodt M. AIDS and the mouth. Copenhagen: Munksgaard, 1990.

4. Greenspan JS, Greenspan D. Oral manifestations of HIV infection: proceedings of the 2nd International Workshop on the Oral Manifestations of HIV Infection, January 31–February 3 1993, San Francisco, California. Carol Stream, IL: Quintessence Publishing Company, 1995.

5. Glick M. Dental management of patients with HIV. Carol Stream, IL: Quintessence Publishing Company, 1994.

6. Centers for Disease Control and Prevention. Classification system for HIV-associated disease. MMWR 1986;35:334.

7. Centers for Disease Control and Prevention. 1993 revised classification system for HIV infection and expanded surveillance case definition for AIDS among adolescents and adults. MMWR 1993;41:1.

8. Montaner JSG, Lee TN, Le N, Craib KJP, Schechter MT. Application of the World Health Organization system for HIV infection in a cohort of homosexual men in developing a prognostically meaningful staging system. AIDS 1992;6:719.

9. Royce RA, Luckmann RS, Fusaro RE, Winkelstein WJ. The natural history of HIV-1 infection: staging classifications of disease. AIDS 1991;5:355.

10. Saah AJ, Munoz A, Kuo V, et al. Predictors of the risk of development of acquired immunodeficiency syndrome within 24 months among gay men seropositive for human immunodeficiency virus type 1: a report from the Multicenter AIDS Cohort Study. Am J Epidemiol 1992;135:1147.

11. Katz MH, Greenspan D, Westenhouse J, et al. Progression to AIDS in HIV-infected homosexual and bisexual men with hairy leukoplakia and oral candidiasis. AIDS 1992;6:95.

12. Agency for Health Care Policy Research. Evaluation and management of early HIV infection. Rockville, MD, US Public Health Service: 1994.

13. Youle MS, Gazzard BG, Johnson MA, et al. Effects of high-dose oral acyclovir on herpesvirus disease and survival in patients with advanced HIV disease: a double-blind placebo-controlled study. AIDS 1994;8:641.

14. Glick M, Abel SN, Muzyka BC, DiLorenzo M. Dental complications after dental treatment of patients with AIDS. J Am Dent Assoc 1994;125:296.

15. Feigal DW, Katz MH, Greenspan D, et al. The prevalence of oral lesions in HIV-infected homosexual and bisexual men: three San Francisco epidemiological cohorts. AIDS 1991;5:519.

16. Shiboski CH, Hilton JF, Greenspan D, et al. HIV-related oral manifestations in two cohorts of women in San Francisco. J Acquir Immune Defic Syndr 1994;7:964.

17. Ramirez-Amador V, Reyes-Teran G, Ponce-de-Leon S, Ponce-de-Leon S. Oral lesions of HIV infection in Mexico city. In: Greenspan JS, Greenspan D, eds. Oral manifestations of HIV infection: proceedings of the 2nd International Workshop on the Oral Manifestations of HIV Infection, January 31–February 3 1993, San Francisco, California. Carol Stream, IL: Quintessence Publishing Company, 1995:73.

18. Greenspan D, Greenspan JS, Hearst NG, et al. Relation of oral hairy leukoplakia to infection with the human immunodeficiency virus and the risk of developing AIDS. J Infect Dis 1987;155:475.

19. Greenspan D, Greenspan JS, Overby G, et al. Risk factors for rapid progression from hairy leukoplakia to AIDS: a nested case control study. J Acquir Immune Defic Syndr 1991;4:652.

20. Moniaci D, Greco D, Flecchia G, Raiteri R, Sinicco A. Epidemiology, clinical features and prognostic value of HIV-1 related oral lesions. J Oral Pathol Med 1990;19:477.

21. Nielsen H, Bentsen KD, Hojtved L, et al. Oral candidiasis and immune status of HIV-infected patients. J Oral Pathol Med 1994;23:140.

22. Lifson AR, Hilton JF, Westenhouse JL, et al. Time from seroconversion to oral candidiasis or hairy leukoplakia among homosexual and bisexual men enrolled in three prospective cohorts. AIDS 1994;8:73.

23. Swango PA, Kleinman DV, Konzelman JL. HIV and periodontal health: a study of military personnel with HIV. J Am Dent Assoc 1991;122:49.

24. Katz MH, Mastrucci MT, Leggott PJ, Westenhouse J, Greenspan JS, Scott GB. Prognostic significance of oral lesions in children with perinatally acquired human immunodeficiency virus infection. Am J Dis Child 1993;147:45.

25. EC-Clearinghouse on Oral Problems Related to HIV infection and WHO Collaborating Centre on Oral Manifestations of the Immunodeficiency Virus. Classification and diagnostic criteria for oral lesions in HIV infection. J Oral Pathol Med 1993;22:289.

26. Greenspan JS, Barr CE, Sciubba JJ, Winkler JR, USA Oral AIDS Collaborative Group. Oral manifestations of HIV infection: definitions, diagnostic criteria and principles of therapy. Oral Surg Oral Med Oral Pathol 1992;73:142.

27. Panteleo G, Graziosi C, Fauci A. The immunopathogenesis of human immunodeficiency virus infection. N Engl J Med 1993; 328:327.

28. Dodd CL, Greenspan D, Katz MH, Westenhouse JL, Feigal DW, Greenspan JS. Oral candidiasis in HIV infection: pseudomembranous and erythematous candidiasis show similar rates of progression to AIDS. AIDS 1991;5:1339.

29. Agabian N, Miyasaki SH, Kohler G, White TC. Candidiasis and HIV infection: virulence as an adaptive response. In: Greenspan JS, Greenspan D, eds. Oral manifestations of HIV infection: proceedings of the 2nd International Workshop on the Oral Manifestations of HIV Infection, January 31–February 3 1993, San Francisco, California. Carol Stream,IL: Quintessence Publishing Company, 1995:85.

30. Rex JH, Rinaldi MG, Pfaller MA. Resistance of *Candida* species to fluconazole. Antimicrob Agents Chemother 1995;39:1.

31. Greenspan D. Treatment of oral candidiasis in HIV infection. Oral Surg Oral Med Oral Pathol 1994;78:211.

32. Kuruvilla A, Humphrey DM, Emka P. Coexistent oral cryptococcosis and Kaposi's sarcoma in acquired immunodeficiency syndrome. Cutis 1992;49:260.

33. Borradori L, Schmit JC, Stetzkowski M, Dussoix P, Saurat JH, Filthuth I. *Penicilliosis marneffei* infection in AIDS. J Am Acad Dermatol 1994;31:843.

34. Heinic GS, Greenspan D, MacPhail LA, Greenspan JS. Oral *Geotrichum candidum* infection in association with HIV infection. Oral Surg Oral Med Oral Pathol 1992;73:726.

35. Heinic G, Greenspan D, MacPhail LA, et al. Oral *Histoplasma capsulatum* in association with HIV infection: a case report. J Oral Pathol Med 1992;21:85.

36. Lamster I, Grbic J, Fine J, et al. A critical review of periodontal disease as a manifestation of HIV infection. In: Greenspan JS, Greenspan D, eds. Oral manifestations of HIV infection: proceedings of the 2nd International Workshop on the Oral Manifestations of HIV Infection, January 31–February 3 1993, San Francisco, California. Carol Stream, IL: Quintessence Publishing Company, 1995:247.

37. Glick M, Muzyka BC, Salkin LM, Lurie D. Necrotizing ulcerative periodontitis: a marker for immune deterioration and a predictor for the diagnosis of AIDS. J Periodontol 1994;65:393.

38. Soubry R, Taelman H, Banyangiliki V, Ladner J, Van de Perre P. Necrotizing periodontal disease in HIV-1 infected patients: a four year study in Kigali, Rwanda. In: Greenspan JS, Greenspan D, eds. Oral manifestations of HIV infection: proceedings of the 2nd International Workshop on the Oral Manifestations of HIV Infection, January 31–February 3 1993, San Francisco, California. Carol Stream, IL: Quintessence Publishing Company, 1995:60.

39. Masouredis CM, Katz MH, Greenspan D, et al. Prevalence of HIV-associated periodontitis and gingivitis in HIV-infected patients attending an AIDS clinic. J Acquir Immune Defic Syndr 1992;5:479.

40. Ryder MI, Winkler JR, Weintreb RN. Elevated phagocytosis, oxidative burst and F actin formation in PMNs from individuals with intraoral manifestations of HIV infection. J Acquir Immune Defic Syndr 1988;1:346.

41. Zambon JJ, Reynolds H, Smutko J, et al. Are unique bacterial pathogens involved in HIV-associated periodontal diseases? In: Greenspan JS, Greenspan D, eds. Oral manifestations of HIV infection: proceedings of the 2nd International Workshop on the Oral Manifestations of HIV Infection, January 31–February 3 1993, San Francisco, California. Carol Stream, IL: Quintessence Publishing Company, 1995:257.

42. Palmer GD. Periodontal therapy for patients with HIV infection. Oral manifestations of HIV infection: proceedings of the 2nd International Workshop on the Oral Manifestations of HIV Infection, January 31–February 3 1993, San Francisco, California. Carol Stream, IL: Quintessence Publishing Company, 1995.

43. Fowler CB, Nelson JF, Henley DW, Smith BR. Acquired immune deficiency syndrome presenting as a palatal perforation. Oral Surg Oral Med Oral Pathol 1989;67:313.

44. Levell NJ, Bewley AP, Chopra S, et al. Bacillary angiomatosis with cutaneous and oral lesions in an HIV-infected patient from the U.K. Br J Dermatol 1995;132:113.

45. MacPhail LA, Greenspan D, Schiodt M, et al. Acyclovir-resistant, foscarnet-sensitive oral herpes simplex type 2 lesion in a patient with AIDS. Oral Surg Oral Med Oral Pathol 1989;67:427.

46. Heinic GS. Oral cytomegalovirus infection in association with HIV infection: a review. In: Greenspan JS, Greenspan D, eds. Oral manifestations of HIV infection: proceedings of the 2nd International Workshop on the Oral Manifestations of HIV Infection, January 31–February 3 1993, San Francisco, California. Carol Stream,IL: Quintessence Publishing Company, 1995:225.

47. Greenspan D, Greenspan JS, Conant M, Petersen V, Silverman S Jr, DeSouza Y. Oral "hairy" leucoplakia in male homosexuals: evidence of association with both papillomavirus and a herpes-group virus. Lancet 1984;2:831.

48. Greenspan JS, Greenspan D, Lennette ET, et al. Replication of Epstein-Barr virus within the epithelial cells of "hairy" leukoplakia, an AIDS-associated lesion. N Engl J Med 1985;313:1564.

49. Raab-Traub N, Walling DM. Epstein-Barr virus strain variation and expression in oral hairy leukoplakia. In: Greenspan JS, Greenspan D, eds. Oral manifestations of HIV infection: proceedings of the 2nd International Workshop on the Oral Manifestations of HIV Infection, January 31–February 3 1993, San Francisco, California. Carol Stream,IL: Quintessence Publishing Company, 1995:159.

50. Greenspan D, Greenspan JS. The significance of oral hairy leukoplakia. Oral Surg Oral Med Oral Pathol 1992;73:151.

51. King GN, Healy CM, Glover MT, Kwan JTC, Williams DM, Thornhill MH. Prevalence and risk factors associated with leukoplakia, hairy leukoplakia, erythematous candidiasis, and gingival hyperplasia in renal transplant recipients. Oral Surg Oral Med Oral Pathol 1994;78:18.

52. Albrecht H, Stellbrink H-J, Brewster D, Greten H. Resolution of oral hairy leukoplakia. AIDS 1994;8:1014.

53. Lozada-Nur F, Costa C. Retrospective findings of the clinical benefits of podophyllum resin 25% solution on hairy leukoplakia. Oral Surg Oral Med Oral Pathol 1992;73:555.

54. Greenspan D, de Villiers EM, Greenspan JS, DeSouza YG, zur Hausen H. Unusual HPV types in the oral warts in association with HIV infection. J Oral Pathol 1988;17:482.

55. Regezi JA, Greenspan D, Greenspan JS, Wong E, MacPhail LA. HPV-associated epithelial atypia in oral warts in HIV+ patients. J Cutan Pathol 1994;21:217.

56. Ficarra G, Eversole R. HIV-related tumors of the oral cavity. Crit Rev Oral Biol Med 1994;5:159.

57. Chang Y, Cesarman E, Pessin MS, et al. Identification of herpesvirus-like DNA sequences in AIDS-associated Kaposi's sarcoma. Science 1994;266:1865.

58. Lucatorto FM, Sapp JP. Treatment of oral Kaposi's sarcoma with a sclerosing agent in AIDS patients. Oral Surg Oral Med Oral Pathol 1993;75:192.

59. Dodd CL, Greenspan D, Schiodt M, et al. Unusual oral presentation of non-Hodgkin's lymphoma in association with HIV infection. Oral Surg Oral Med Oral Pathol 1992;73:603.

60. Laskaris G, Stergiou G, Kittas C, Scully C. Hodgkin's disease involving the gingiva in AIDS. Eur J Cancer 1992;28B:39.

61. MacPhail LA, Greenspan D, Feigal DW, Lennette ET, Greenspan JS. Recurrent aphthous ulcers in association with HIV infection: description of ulcer types and analysis of T-cell subsets. Oral Surg Oral Med Oral Pathol 1991;71:678.

62. MacPhail LA, Greenspan D, Greenspan JS. Recurrent aphthous ulcers in association with HIV infection: diagnosis and treatment. Oral Surg Oral Med Oral Pathol 1992;73:283.

63. Oldfield EC. Thalidomide for severe aphthous ulceration in patients with human immunodeficiency virus (HIV) infection. Am J Gastroenterol 1994;89:2276.

64. Paterson DL, Georghiou PR, Allworth AM, Kemp RJ. Thalidomide as treatment of refractory aphthous ulceration related to human immunodeficiency virus infection. Clin Infect Dis 1995;20:250.

65. Ruah CB, Stram JR, Chasin WD. Treatment of severe recurrent aphthous stomatitis with colchicine. Arch Otolaryngol Head Neck Surg 1988;114:671.

66. Schiødt M, Dodd CL, Greenspan D, Greenspan JS. HIV-associated salivary gland disease. In: Greenspan JS, Greenspan D, eds. Oral manifestations of HIV infection: proceedings of the 2nd International Workshop on the Oral Manifestations of HIV Infection, January 31–February 3 1993, San Francisco, California. Carol Stream,IL: Quintessence Publishing Company, 1995:145.

67. Itescu S, Dalton J, Zhang HZ, Winchester R. Tissue infiltration in a CD8 lymphocytosis syndrome associated with human immunodeficiency virus-1 infection has the phenotypic appearance of an antigenically driven response. J Clin Invest 1993;91:2216.

68. Kleinman DV. Building the capacity for the response of the dental profession to the global HIV pandemic: a case study in international collaboration. J Public Health Dent 1994;54:234.

AIDS: Biology, Diagnosis, Treatment and
Prevention, fourth edition, edited by Vincent T.
DeVita, Jr., Samuel Hellman, and Steven A.
Rosenberg. Lippincott–Raven Publishers, © 1997

CHAPTER 18

Gastrointestinal Manifestations of Human Immunodeficiency Virus Infection

Donald P. Kotler

Gastrointestinal (GI) symptoms are exceedingly common in patients with acquired immunodeficiency syndrome (AIDS), as they are in other immune deficiency states.[1-3] The GI tract, like other mucous membranes, is inherently vulnerable to pathogens because of the lack of a strong physical barrier. Intimate contact with the external (luminal) environment is essential for solute absorption. An elaborate defense has evolved to protect the GI tract, including a multicompartmental immune system. The immune defenses of the various mucous membranes are linked as a common mucosal immune system.[4]

GI involvement in cases of human immunodeficiency virus (HIV) infection and AIDS may be significant on several levels. Epidemiologic studies imply that HIV infection is efficiently transmitted through rectal mucosa.[5] Bidirectional transmission is likely. Evidence from several laboratories indicates that cellular reservoirs for HIV exist in the intestines. Alterations in bowel habits associated with "nonspecific" inflammation are common in HIV-infected persons without AIDS, and are related to the expression of HIV genome and protein antigens in tissue.[6,7] The development of opportunistic GI infections contributes to debilitation and a terminal course. Chronic diarrhea has been associated with shortened survival,[8,9] diminished quality of life, and increased use of health care resources.[10]

The aim of this chapter is to discuss the effects of HIV infection and AIDS on the GI tract. Mucosal immunity and the results of studies localizing HIV to the intestine are discussed. Specific infectious and neoplastic complications are reviewed. Diagnosis and management of these complica-

tions, which have variable and overlapping clinical expressions, are organized as a group of clinical syndromes.

MUCOSAL IMMUNITY AND IMMUNE DEFICIENCY

Normal Mucosal Immunity

The systemic and mucosal immune systems function, in large part, independently, although they share a common embryologic heritage and homologous structures and functions. However, the defense of all mucous membranes are combined as a common mucosal immune system. The mucosal immune system has an afferent limb, which is composed of lymphoid follicles in the tonsils, intestinal lamina propria (ie, Peyer's patches and other mucosal lymphoid follicles), and mesentery, and an efferent system composed of diffuse collections of cells in the lamina propria and epithelial compartments.[11] The epithelium overlying mucosal lymphoid follicles and Peyer's patches contains specialized cells (ie, M cells) that allow penetration of particulate antigens.[12] The liver also contains components of the mucosal immune system.

Lymphoid follicles are the sites of luminal antigen uptake and presentation. Epithelial cells also can present antigens.[13] Sensitized B- and T-lymphocyte precursors then migrate to mesenteric lymph nodes and distant sites, where they proliferate and differentiate. B cells and helper T cells return to the intestine, but suppressor T cells localize to the spleen.[14] Several elegant studies have demonstrated the distinctive trafficking patterns of gut-associated lymphocytes.[15] Normal and disease-associated homing of lymphocytes to the intestine is mediated by the expression of specific adhesion molecules on the lymphoid cell surface, which interact with receptors on high endothelial venules in the mucosa and skin.[16]

Donald P. Kotler, Gastrointestinal Division, Department of Medicine, St. Luke's-Roosevelt Hospital Center, 421 West 113th Street, New York, NY 10025.

The intestinal mucosa contains a diversity of immunologically active cells. The proportion of mucosal helper T lymphocytes to suppressor T lymphocytes is approximately the same in mucosa and peripheral blood.[17] B lymphocytes comprise about 10% of the mononuclear cells in the lamina propria. Plasma cells also are an important constituent of the cell population. Macrophages are the major form of phagocytic cell in the lamina propria, although eosinophils and mast cells also are found in mucosal biopsies from healthy individuals.[18] Extravascular neutrophils are not normal inhabitants of the lamina propria.

Mononuclear cells also course through the epithelium. The phenotypic composition of the intraepithelial mononuclear cell population is different from the lamina propria. The major cell type found is the CD8+ T cell, and the normal helper to suppressor ratio is about 0.05.[19] The proportion of γ/δ lymphocytes in the epithelium is higher than in other body compartments.[20] Intraepithelial macrophages are another important cell type. Occasional mast cells or eosinophils may be seen in normal epithelium, but neutrophils in the epithelium is indicative of a pathologic process.

The mucosa contains elements of humoral (ie, secretory) and cell-mediated immunity. The antibody system in the intestine produces mainly secretory IgA, although substantial quantities of IgM are normally made.[21] Secretory IgA binds and excludes foreign luminal antigens from the body. Secretory IgA does not have Fc receptors and does not activate complement by the classic pathway. Most secreted IgA exists in dimeric form linked by a peptide (ie, J piece). IgA is actively secreted from the epithelial cell after binding to a glycoprotein of epithelial cell origin (ie, secretory component), which protects the antibody from degradation in the lumen. Hepatic bile also contains secretory IgA. Cell-mediated immune reactions in the GI tract are similar to reactions in other body compartments.

Mucosal immune function is highly coordinated. The mucosa is uninflamed despite its proximity to many potential pathogens. The processes of immune suppression and immune activation (ie, contrasuppression) are finely regulated, limiting the intensity, extent, and duration of an immune reaction and thereby protecting the integrity of the mucous membrane.[22] As with systemic immune function, cell signaling is accomplished through the activities of cytokines and chemokines. In addition to lymphoid cells, epithelial cells produce and secrete cytokines,[23] which add further specificity to the immune response. Epithelial proliferation[24] and cellular function,[25] particularly ion and water transport, also are modulated by cytokines.

Mucosal immune function is integrated with systemic immunity. The most striking interaction is the active suppression of systemic immune responses to previously encountered luminal antigens (ie, tolerance).[26] Potential adverse responses to inadvertent systemic introduction of foreign antigens, such as food antigens, are limited by tolerance.

Other, nonimmunologic factors promote the defense of the GI tract.[27] Gastric acid is antiseptic, and salivary, pan-creatic, and biliary secretions contain specific antiinfective factors. Secreted mucus is a lubricant, a diffusion barrier for particulate materials, and a scaffold to which IgA, lysozyme, and other proteins attach.[28] Intestinal motility is an important factor in maintaining low intraluminal bacterial counts in the upper intestine, and a stable pattern of colonic flora also contributes to homeostasis.[29] The normal enteric bacterial flora serve physiologic functions, such as fermentation of unabsorbed carbohydrates and salvage of metabolizable carbons, as well as a defensive function by suppressing the proliferation of potential pathogens. This property is illustrated by *Clostridium difficile*, a bacteria in the intestines of many healthy persons that may cause a colitis during therapy with broad-spectrum antibiotics.[30]

Mucosal Immunity in HIV Infection

Mucosal immunity in HIV-infected patients has received little study. Clinical and experimental observations suggest that homologous defects exist in the mucosal and systemic immune systems. Early studies of mucosal biopsies, using immunohistochemical techniques, demonstrated decreases in the CD4+ lymphocyte population in blood and intestinal mucosa, although the number of mucosal CD8+ lymphocytes increased.[31-33] In one study, peripheral blood helper T cell numbers were decreased in healthy homosexual men, and the number of mucosal helper T cells and cells bearing surface antigens of a cytotoxic cell phenotype were normal.[31] Later studies suggest that the CD4+ lymphocyte population in lamina propria decreases disproportionately at an early stage of disease,[34,35] but the CD4+ population in lymphoid aggregates falls at a slower rate.[35] Another study, using flow cytometric analysis of isolated mucosal lymphocytes, found increased expression of the killer cell markers Leu-7 and Leu-11a (CD16).[36] Although functional activity of the killer cells was not assessed, deficient killer cell activity in peripheral blood lymphocytes has been demonstrated repeatedly.[37] Alterations in the state of lymphoid cell differentiation[38] or specific lymphoid subsets[39] have been reported. Electron microscopic studies have demonstrated evidence of activation of intraepithelial lymphocytes in AIDS patients.[40] Flow cytometric studies showed increased cell membrane expression of DR antigen in lamina propria and intraepithelial mononuclear cells from rectal mucosa, implying cell activation.[36] However, a decrease in the number of activated T cells was associated with villus atrophy in duodenal biopsies.[41]

An immunohistologic study demonstrated depletion of plasma cells containing IgA in mucosal biopsies from AIDS patients and a decrease in salivary IgA secretion.[42] The numbers of plasma cells containing IgM were increased in several patients, implying a defect in T-lymphocyte–directed gene rearrangement in plasma cell precursors (ie, switching). A second study confirmed the depletion of IgA plasma cells but found a deficiency in IgM plasma cells as well.[43] In contrast to evidence of decreased secretory immunity, serum

IgA concentrations often are elevated in HIV-infected persons. One study has suggested that the IgA in serum is of gut origin.[44] IgA also is commonly found in immune complexes[45] and has been shown to possess rheumatoid factor–like activity.[46] In contrast to the immunohistochemical studies, two studies of oral vaccination have shown preservation of intestinal antibody responses in HIV-infected subjects,[47–48] and cell-mediated immune reactions against HIV antigens were shown in lamina propria mononuclear cells.[49]

HIV INFECTION AND THE GASTROINTESTINAL TRACT

Several investigators have found evidence of HIV in the GI tract. Using the polymerase chain reaction (PCR) technique, evidence of HIV DNA can be found in mucosal homogenates or in isolated mononuclear cells in almost all patients.[7] In situ hybridization studies demonstrated HIV-1 RNA in lymphocytes and macrophages in intestinal lamina propria in a subset of AIDS patients.[50,51] Other studies have shown HIV DNA in intestinal cells, including the crypt epithelium and enterochromaffin cells.[52–54] HIV core antigen (p24) has been localized by immunohistologic techniques to various cell types in the GI tract.[7,55–57] Primary intestinal cell lines and colonic tumor epithelial cell lines can be productively infected with HIV.[58–61] Because intestinal cell lines containing and not containing CD4 antigen can be infected, the mode of infection probably is different from infection of CD4+ lymphocytes. There is evidence that infection of epithelial cells occurs by interaction with cell membrane galactosyl ceramide, as in other cell types.[62] In vitro studies demonstrated apparent endocytosis of HIV by an epithelial cell line.[63] Experimental infection of intestinal cell lines and fetal intestinal explants were shown to affect epithelial cell proliferation and cell function.[64,65] In contrast, a clinical study of HIV-infected patients showed hyporegenerative atrophy and decreased brush border enzyme activity, which was less severe in patients receiving zidovudine (AZT).[66]

Animal studies indicate that intestinal cells are reservoirs for retroviruses. Infection of intestinal crypt epithelium by a feline retrovirus isolate produced an acquired immunodeficiency associated with diarrhea and wasting.[67] Monkeys experimentally infected with simian immunodeficiency virus developed diarrhea and malnutrition associated with malabsorption.[68] One variant of SIV was shown to produce a hyperacute syndrome associated with severe enteropathy and rapid deterioration leading to death within a few weeks.[69]

DISEASE COMPLICATIONS

Infections

Many infections threaten immunocompromised patients. The GI pathogens found in AIDS patients are listed in (Table 18-1).

TABLE 18-1. *Gastrointestinal pathogens in AIDS patients*

PARASITES

Cryptosporidium parvum
Enterocytozoon bieneusi
Septata intestinalis
Isospora belli
Giardia lamblia
Entameba histolytica
*Blastocystis hominis**
Cyclospora sp.

BACTERIA

Salmonella sp.
Shigella sp.
Campylobacter sp.
Enteroadherent bacteria
Helicobacter pylori
Mycobacterium tuberculosis
Mycobacterium avium complex
Clostridium difficile

VIRUSES

Cytomegalovirus
Herpes simplex
Human immunodeficiency virus
Adenovirus
Epstein-Barr virus
Human papillomavirus
Hepatitis B
Hepatitis C
Hepatitis D

FUNGI

Candida albicans
Torulopsis glabrata
Histoplasma capsulatum
Coccidiodes imitis
Cryptococcus neoformans
Actinomyces sp.

*Uncertain pathogenetic potential.

Viruses

HIV

The potential role of HIV as an enteric pathogen is ill defined. A prospective study of HIV-infected subjects with GI or proctologic symptoms demonstrated significant correlations between altered bowel habits and histologic evidence of intestinal injury, which was independent of the presence of enteric pathogens.[6] Mucosal HIV p24 contents, determined by quantitative ELISA, were highest in non-AIDS patients in Walter Reed classes 3 and 4. The expression of p24 correlated with altered bowel habits and histologic alterations. Other results demonstrated elevated tissue contents of the cytokines, tumor necrosis factor, and interleukin-1 and lesser elevations of the inflammatory mediators, prostaglandin E_2 and leukotriene B_4, adding biochemical evidence in support of mucosal inflammation.

In a companion study, qualitative and quantitative histopathologic studies were performed on rectal biopsies from HIV-infected patients and controls, and the findings were correlated with disease stage.[70] Mucosal cellularity and the numbers of lymphocytes and degranulating eosinophils were maximal in Walter Reed class 3 and 4 patients. Mucosal lymphoid cellularity correlated with mucosal p24 content. The increased lymphoid cellularity occurred in the face of falling CD4+ lymphocyte counts in peripheral blood. Diffuse nodular lymphoid hyperplasia in intestinal mucosa has been reported by others.[71] The results of several studies suggest that cytokine production and secretion are altered in mucosa,[72–74] but one study found no evidence of mucosal cytokine alterations.[75] One study showed high levels of apoptosis in lamina propria cells.[76] Such a finding is of great potential importance, because apoptosis is thought to be an important mechanism of CD4+ lymphocyte depletion.[77]

Although these studies provide no insight into the precise pathogenic mechanism of the colonic inflammation and immune depletion, the results strongly suggest that inflammation and HIV expression in mucosa are related. Other studies also have found an association between mucosal HIV expression and inflammation.[78] An HIV-associated inflammatory bowel disease could be an important factor in the pathogenesis of the immunodeficiency and a factor in disease transmission.

Cytomegalovirus

Cytomegalovirus (CMV) infection is common in AIDS, and evidence of CMV infection was found in up to two thirds of autopsies in early studies.[79] Disseminated CMV infection is a progressive disease and frequently contributes to mortality. Serologic evidence of infection is extremely common worldwide and almost invariably present in patients from groups at high risk for the development of AIDS.[80] CMV infects many cell types, including epithelial cells in mucous membranes, such that CMV may be shed in secretions. It is likely that sexually promiscuous persons are infected with multiple strains of the virus.

The primary viral infection is not a significant clinical illness in most cases, although a mononucleosis-like syndrome has been observed. The infection then enters a latent phase, which is lifelong in most immunocompetent persons. In the HIV-infected patient with diminished T-cell function, repeated episodes of viral reactivation occur, as demonstrated by intermittent virus shedding and the reappearance by anti-CMV IgM antibodies in the serum.[81] Reactivations become more frequent and prolonged over time, until persistent reactivation and dissemination occur and lead to widespread tissue injury.

Several GI syndromes have been associated with CMV, including esophageal ulcers, esophagitis, gastritis, isolated intestinal ulcers, terminal ileitis, intestinal perforation, focal or diffuse colitis, hepatitis, pancreatitis, sclerosing cholangitis, and unexplained wasting. The clinical approach is based on the usual evaluation of presenting signs and symptoms, and the diagnosis is made by biopsy and histologic analysis. Evaluation is limited by the lack of an appropriate "gold standard" with high positive and negative predictive values.[82]

The key histopathologic feature of CMV infection is the intracellular inclusion (Fig. 18-1). A large argyrophilic nuclear inclusion is often surrounded by a clear halo. The cytoplasm is markedly enlarged and may contain numerous small, granular, basophilic inclusions. Inclusions are seen most often in endothelial cells but occasionally are seen in crypt epithelial cells. CMV inclusions are found in multiple cell types in inflamed, ulcerated tissues. In most cases, inclusions are found in the lamina propria. In one case associated with intestinal perforation, inclusions were seen throughout the bowel wall.[83] When inclusions are rare or atypical, immunohistologic or in situ hybridization techniques may be helpful.[84,85] PCR has been claimed as the most sensitive technique for diagnosing CMV infection,[82] although the positive predictive value, the specificity of the technique, is uncertain. Other available diagnostic techniques generally are less useful. The presence of anti-CMV IgG is nonspecific, and some patients with disseminated infection lack serum IgM or even serum IgG anti-CMV. Viral culture is of little value, because normal individuals may intermittently shed CMV,[86,87] and some patients with widespread disease have negative culture results.

Several agents capable of inhibiting CMV replication are available. The most widely studied is ganciclovir.[88,89] Clinical benefit from ganciclovir therapy in patients with serious CMV infection includes clinical stabilization, repletion of body mass, and prolonged survival.[90–92] Ganciclovir is administered intravenously using an induction regimen followed by maintenance therapy. The drug has hematologic toxic effects, the most relevant of which is neutropenia. In most cases, a chronically indwelling intravenous catheter must be placed. Despite the potential problems, patients have been treated for as long as 4 years with reasonable comfort and good functional performance. An oral form of ganciclovir has been approved for use.

Foscarnet is an antiviral agent with activity against CMV and HIV. Evidence of clinical benefit has been reported.[93,94] Like ganciclovir, foscarnet must be given by intravenous infusion. Immune globulins with high-titer antibodies to CMV have been developed, but no data support their efficacy in AIDS patients with GI disease.[95]

Herpes Simplex Virus

Herpes simplex virus infections are common in HIV-infected persons and may cause esophagitis or proctitis. However, the major clinical syndrome in AIDS is a slowly spreading, painful, shallow, clean-based perianal or perineal ulcer.[96] Herpesvirus is readily cultured from the ulcerated surface. These ulcers respond favorably to acyclovir. A propensity for herpes simplex virus to produce perforation or fistulization was shown in two case reports, one in an immunocompromised patient without AIDS.[97,98]

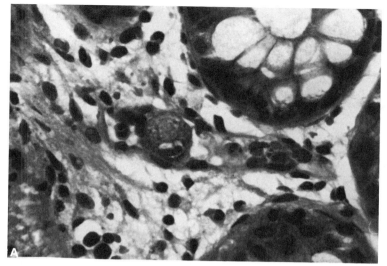

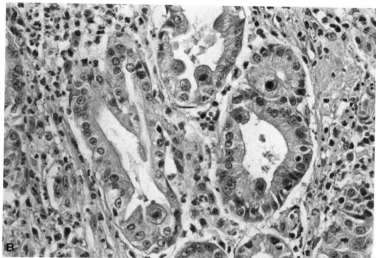

FIG. 18-1. (**A**) Intranuclear and cytoplasmic inclusions of cytomegalovirus (CMV) in an endothelial cell in the lamina propria of the colon (hematoxylin & eosin [H&E] stain; original magnification ×600). (**B**) CMV inclusion bodies in gastric epithelial cells (H&E stain; original magnification ×250).

Epstein-Barr Virus

There has been surprisingly little study of Epstein-Barr virus (EBV) in the GI tract, despite its prevalence in other epithelia.[99] Diverse GI symptoms are common in patients with sustained serologic evidence of EBV reactivation.[100] EBV has been found in lesions of oral hairy leukoplakia.[101] EBV genome also has been found in a small percentage of B-cell lymphomas.[102] It is possible that EBV plays a pathologic role in the GI tract.

Adenovirus

Adenoviruses are occasionally isolated from rectal swabs or biopsies from AIDS patients with diarrheal disorders.[103] The patients may be clinically stable or have progressive disease. A diarrheal syndrome attributed to adenovirus has been described, with cytoplasmic inclusion bodies seen in superficial epithelial cells that are identified as adenovirus with electron microscopy.[104]

Other Viruses

A single report identified a number of novel enteric viruses, including astroviruses and picornaviruses, in HIV-infected subjects.[105] Isolation of these viruses, but not others such as rotavirus or Norwalk agent, was significantly more common in patients with diarrhea than in those without diarrhea. The role of these viruses in producing diarrhea is undefined.

Parasites

Cryptosporidium parvum

Cryptosporidium is the most widely recognized enteric pathogen in patients with AIDS. The illness has a worldwide distribution and is responsible for 5% to 10% of cases of severe diarrhea in American AIDS patients. *Cryptosporidium* is a cause of "slim disease," a wasting syndrome described in African AIDS patients.[106,107] The parasite may infect immunocompetent and immunodeficient persons.[108] As many as one third of control subjects had serologic evidence of cryptosporidial infection in one study.[109] Prolonged shedding of cysts may occur after clinical resolution,[110] even in immunocompetent hosts, and evidence of latent infection in the GI tract has been reported.[111] Cryptosporidiosis has been implicated in traveler's diarrhea and in outbreaks of diarrheal disease in day care centers.[112] Contamination of municipal water supply systems has been observed.

Cryptosporidiosis usually is chronic and protracted in AIDS patients. A biologic gradient between intensity of infection and intestinal involvement has been reported.[113] Spontaneous remissions occur infrequently and may be related to a temporal rise in CD4+ lymphocyte counts,[114,115] sometimes associated with AZT therapy.[115] The positive effect of AZT suggests a direct T-cell influence on cryptosporidiosis, although the effects on cytotoxic cells, suppressor cells, and antibodies are unclear. Protracted disease occurs despite the presence of antibodies in stool, suggesting a prominent role of delayed hypersensitivity in the control of cryptosporidia.[116]

There is little host specificity,[117] and bidirectional infection between humans and animals has been reported.[118] Chronic intestinal cryptosporidiosis has occurred in agammaglobulinemic patients without AIDS,[119] suggesting that secretory immunodeficiency may promote chronicity, as has been shown in a murine model of giardiasis.[120]

After ingestion and excystation of the oocysts, the sporozoite invades the epithelial cell, possibly by specific receptor binding,[121] and occupies an extracytoplasmic site beneath the brush border.[122] Cycles of asexual division with autoinfection occur, as does sexual division with production and fecal excretion of thick-walled oocysts. Destruction of epithelial cells with villus atrophy and inflammation results from the infection.

There is considerable variation in disease localization, clinical severity, and the course of cryptosporidiosis in AIDS.[123] Most patients have diffuse small intestinal disease without or with mild colonic involvement. A smaller percentage have ileocolitis with preserved jejunal structure and function. A small percentage have isolated ileitis. Some patients with AIDS have massive secretory diarrhea, reminiscent of cholera. The most severe clinical form of the disease is biliary and pancreatic infection, associated with pancreatitis, sclerosing cholangitis, or (acalculous) cholecystitis.[124] Isolated cases of cryptosporidiosis in gastric, respiratory epithelium or nasal epithelium[125] or invading the lamina propria have been reported.[126,127]

Cryptosporidiosis can be diagnosed by special examination of stool specimens or intestinal aspirates. Several methods of concentration and staining of the oocysts have been described,[128] although several cases have been seen with negative stool examinations but cryptosporidial involvement on biopsy. The cryptosporidia are readily seen in intestinal biopsies (Fig. 18-2). The infection may be patchy, especially in the colon.

The therapeutic options for cryptosporidiosis are limited. Many antibiotics have been tried. Spiramycin, a macrolide antibiotic available in Europe and Canada (Rhone Poulenc), may improve symptoms and occasionally causes clearance of the parasite in stool samples, but it demonstrated no objective benefit in controlled trials. Immune bovine colostrum suppressed cryptosporidial infection in a child with a congenital agammaglobulinemia and in a few AIDS patients.[129–131] Some studies found a positive clinical effect of paromomycin (Humatin) in some patients.[132] Azithromycin also demonstrates clinical effectiveness in some patients (Soave R: personal communication, 1994).

Treatment of diarrhea due to cryptosporidiosis may be difficult. Diet modification may be helpful in patients with clinically mild disease. A lactose-free, low-fat diet with calorie-rich fluid supplements containing extra protein may be well tolerated. Standard formulas containing substantial quantities of long-chain fats and high concentrations of sugar often cause bloating and worsen diarrhea. Hydrophilic bulking agents generally are unhelpful. Opiates such as diphenoxylate, paregoric, or tincture of opium may be effective, although the amount required sometimes causes excessive sedation, and escalating doses may be required.

A subset of patients with AIDS have severe secretory diarrhea with fluid losses of up to 15 L/day. Rapid volume depletion with azotemia and electrolyte abnormalities may occur. The disease resembles cholera clinically. A secretory enterotoxin was detected in an experimental model of cryptosporidiosis,[133] but it has not been reported in clinical infections. Diminished diarrheal volume may occur during treatment with indomethacin or the phenothiazines, chlorpromazine (Thorazine) or trifluoperazine (Stelazine), which inhibit chloride secretion by crypt epithelial cells. Therapy with the somatostatin analog, octreotide, may be successful in some cases, although controlled trials have given disparate results.[134,135] Despite these approaches, parenteral fluids often are required to maintain adequate hydration.

Microsporidiosis

Microsporidia are protozoa only recently recognized to infect humans, although they are known to cause disease in other animals.[136] The first case of microsporidiosis reported was in 1985, and the illness has been seen worldwide.[136,137] An electron microscopic study of small intestinal biopsies from patients with AIDS and unexplained diarrhea revealed 20 cases of microsporidiosis.[138] Since that time, several hundred cases have been reported, and the infection is increasingly recognized.

Microsporidia are characterized by the presence of a coiled polar tubule with an intracellular extrusion apparatus.[139] Cellular infection occurs through extrusion of the polar filament, followed by ejection of the sporoplasm through the hollow tube. Two species have been identified in intestinal biopsies from AIDS patients, *Enterocytozoon bieneusi*,[140] and *Septata intestinalis*.[141] Although *E bieneusi*

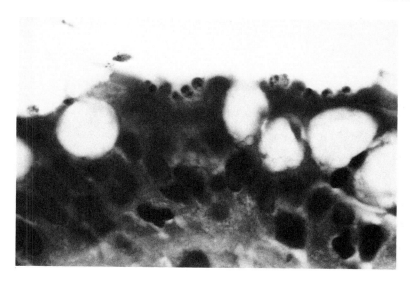

FIG. 18-2. Localization of cryptosporidia along the luminal membrane of villus epithelial cells (hematoxylin & eosin stain; original magnification ×1000).

infection is limited to enterocytes, *S intestinalis* produces disseminated disease.[141] Spores of *S intestinalis* can be found in epithelial cells in the urinary sediment. Autopsy studies also localized the organism to the kidney and the liver.

The prevalence of microsporidial infection in different population groups ranges from 2% to 50%.[142-148] The prevalence in our laboratory has remained constant since 1988 at about one third of cases of chronic diarrhea with weight loss. One report identified *E bieneusi* in an immunocompetent individual with a self-limited diarrheal illness.[149] This observation implies that human infection may be widespread and could be a significant cause of community-acquired or traveler's diarrhea. One prospective study of HIV-infected patients with and without diarrhea found a prevalence for microsporidiosis of more than 20% for each group by electron microscopy.[148] Follow-up showed that some patients remained clinically stable despite persistent infection.[150] These results suggest that *E bieneusi* is a common infection in humans and that infection may not necessarily be associated with diarrhea.

The mode of transmission of *E bieneusi* infection has not been defined, although it is likely to be by the oral route. Little is known about immunity to *E bieneusi* infection. Several studies have examined the development of symptomatic microsporidiosis as a function of the level of immunodeficiency and found that patients typically have severe depletion of CD4 lymphocyte counts (<50 cell/mm^3).[143,151] The one study finding similar rates of infection in patients with and without diarrhea also found much higher CD4 lymphocyte counts.[149]

Clinically, infection with microsporidia resembles infection with cryptosporidia, other diffuse small intestinal diseases, or short bowel syndrome. Microscopically, partial villus atrophy and crypt hyperplasia are seen and are associated with xylose malabsorption and diminished specific activities of brush border disaccharidases, implying a pathogenic role for this organism.[139,152] Electron microscopic studies have shown that the infection may vary along the

length of the small intestine, with the jejunum being more heavily infested than the duodenum.[153] A few reports documented microsporidia in colonic epithelial cells.[149,154] Microsporidiosis also has been associated with cholangiopathy.[155]

Previously, diagnosis required electron microscopy. Later studies showed that light microscopy augmented by special stains can provide a high positive predictive value for the diagnosis. Prominent cytopathic changes in villus epithelial cells, especially in the upper villus, is a clue to the diagnosis (Fig. 18-3). The supranuclear regions contain globular inclusions (ie, meronts and sporonts) that may deform the nucleus (see Fig. 18-3). The fully developed spores erupt through the luminal membrane, destroying the cell. The ability to identify microsporidial spores has advanced rapidly, and several techniques promise to provide a sensitive and specific diagnosis.[156-159] PCR reaction techniques have been developed and may be of clinical and investigative use.[160]

There is no known effective therapy for *E bieneusi*. Studies are being performed using albendazole (Smith-Kline Beecham Pharmaceuticals, Philadelphia, PA).[161] Albendazole has been shown to be effective therapy for *S intestinalis*.[162] Nutritional therapy is based on diet modification to decrease the fat and lactose content. Elemental diets may be well tolerated. Parenteral nutrition has been used in some patients.

Microsporidiosis is an important and newly recognized pathogen. The organism may be a significant cause of enteric disease in patients with AIDS in the United States and elsewhere and in infectious diarrhea in general. Further studies are needed to enhance the diagnostic and therapeutic armamentarium.

Isospora belli

Isospora belli is a coccidium closely related to cryptosporidial organism. It has been reported frequently in

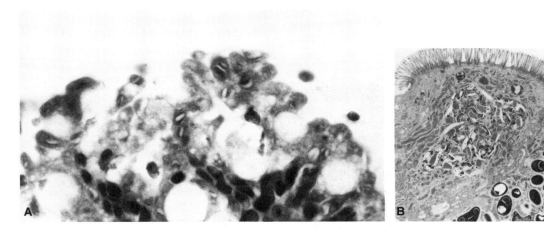

FIG. 18-3. (A) Developing forms of microsporidia located in an area of cell necrosis and sluffing at the villus tip. (hematoxylin & eosin; original magnification × 600). **(B)** Transmission electron micrograph demonstrates a developing sporont in the cell on the left and maturing spores on the right (original magnification × 8000).

AIDS patients from Haiti and West Africa.[163-165] The symptoms of isosporiasis are similar to those of cryptosporidiosis. Because oocysts may be scarce in stool specimens,[164,165] the diagnosis may be easily missed. On biopsy, *Isospora* organisms are found in the apical cytoplasm of villus epithelial cells and produce partial villus atrophy and crypt hyperplasia (Fig. 18-4). A case of disseminated isosporiasis with extensive infection in the mesenteric lymph nodes and other organs has been reported.[166] Isosporiasis has been associated with acalculous cholecystitis, and it probably is a cause of cholangiopathy.[167] Successful disease suppression with improved intestinal function has been reported with trimethoprim sulfa at various dosages[165] but does not occur in every patient. Because diarrhea recurs after discontinuation of therapy, chronic therapy with trimethoprim sulfa, trimethoprim alone, or pyrimethamine plus folinic acid are necessary.

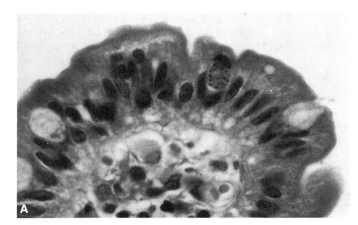

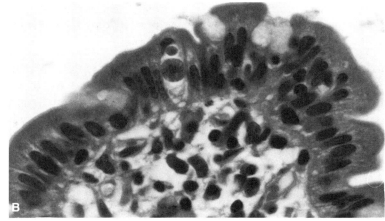

FIG. 18-4. (A) Microgametocyte form of isospora and **(B)** Merozoite form of isospora (hematoxylin & eosin stain; original magnification × 600).

Giardia lamblia

Enteric infection with *Giardia lamblia* is an important problem in many parts of the world. Giardiasis was diagnosed commonly in sexually active homosexual men during the 1970s and early 1980s and was a frequent cause of the "gay bowel syndrome."[168] The infection is acquired during ingestion of cysts in contaminated water or through sexual activity that includes oral-anal contact. The organism elicits a strong immune response, but the infection may not be eradicated completely because of temporal alterations in giardial antigens.[169]

Giardiasis is not a common cause of acute diarrhea in AIDS. Cysts are seen occasionally in stool specimens, or trophozoites are identified in intestinal biopsies (Fig. 18-5). Mucosal structure may be normal because injury of the small intestine in giardiasis is T-cell mediated.[170] The serum antibody response to acute giardial infection was lower in HIV-seropositive persons than in seronegatives.[171] In the absence of intestinal injury, *Giardia* may affect nutrient absorption by local effects on brush border proteins, bile salt deconjugation in the lumen, or other mechanisms. Drug therapy with quinacrine or metronidazole is indicated if cysts or trophozoites are found, although other causes of diarrhea should be suspected.

Amebiasis

Intestinal infection with *Entamoeba histolytica* is another common infection of homosexual males[172] and a cause of gay bowel syndrome. Like giardiasis, amebiasis is not a common cause of severe illness in HIV-infected patients, despite frequent shedding of organisms in the stool. The virulence of strains of *E histolytica* is related to specific zymogens, which are not present in all isolates,[173] and many isolates probably represent commensal organisms. Although metronidazole therapy should be prescribed, the possibility of coexisting pathogens should be kept in mind.

Other parasites have been reported, including *Strongyloides stercoralis* (Fig. 18-6), which may produce a hyper-

infection syndrome.[174] Several AIDS patients have been diagnosed as having *Cyclospora* infection. *Cyclospora* are protozoal parasites resembling cryptosporidia, but they are larger.[175] *Blastocystis hominis,* which is thought by some to be an enteric pathogen,[176] has been found in many HIV-seropositive persons with diarrhea, although the pathogenic potential is unknown.

Bacteria

Mycobacteria

Systemic infections with *Mycobacterium avium* complex (MAC) and *Mycobacterium tuberculosis* are common in AIDS patients.[177] Extrapulmonary tuberculosis often is an early complication of AIDS. The major GI manifestation is granulomatous hepatitis, although isolated ulcers of the intestine, especially the ileum, have been observed.

MAC occurs with high prevalence in AIDS patients. The infection usually occurs late in the course of AIDS. MAC rarely causes infections in immunocompetent persons, because it is less virulent than *M tuberculosis*. It is acquired orally or possibly by an aerosol route. Atypical mycobacteria may be cultured from the water supplies in urban areas.[178]

MAC is a systemic infection with widespread tissue distribution and usually is most prominent in the liver, spleen, mesenteric lymph nodes, bone marrow, and intestinal mucosa (Fig. 18-7). Organomegaly often occurs. Intraabdominal lymphadenopathy is prominent on ultrasound or computed tomography (CT) examination, but MAC must be differentiated from other infections and neoplasms.

The intestinal lesion of MAC is the result of mucosal and submucosal infiltration with macrophages containing intracellular organisms that are not lysed, possibly because of a local deficiency of interferon-γ.[179] The cellular infiltration blocks intramucosal lymphatic flow and produces fat malabsorption with exudative enteropathy. The infection is a pathophysiologic counterpart to Whipple's disease.[180] Severe cases are characterized by villus atrophy and impaired absorption of sugars and amino acids.

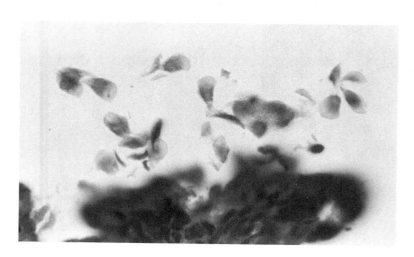

FIG. 18-5. Trophozoites of giardia adjacent to villus cells (hematoxylin & eosin stain; original magnification × 800).

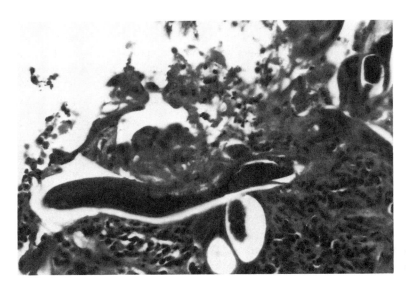

FIG. 18-6. Larval forms of *Strongyloides* in a patient with a hyperinfection syndrome (hematoxylin & eosin; original magnification × 400).

The major clinical syndrome in patients with disseminated MAC is fever, progressive wasting and debilitation, with or without diarrhea.[177] The fever and constitutional symptoms may respond promptly to therapy with prostaglandin synthesis inhibitors. Diagnosis is accomplished by culture or biopsy (Fig. 18-8). An enlarged left supraclavicular node (ie, Virchow's node) may contain MAC (Kotler DP: personal observation) and is a clue to intraabdominal disease. Occasionally, nodes undergo liquefaction necrosis and produce a mycobacterial peritonitis. It is important to diagnose this complication, because the clinical presentation may mimic an acute abdominal crisis. Intestinal obstruction or perforation also may result from advanced MAC infection.[181,182] Blood cultures may become positive before local symptoms develop, and bacteremia usually is sustained.[183] Histologic demonstration of acid-fast bacilli in intestinal or liver tissue is straightforward.

Molecular hybridization techniques are being developed to allow species identification on tissue sections. Colonization of the GI tract may be detected by stool acid-fast stains, but the association between colonization and tissue invasion is uncertain.[184]

The treatment of *M tuberculosis* in HIV-infected and noninfected patients generally is similar and includes multidrug regimens. The optimal length of treatment needed is unknown. Some clinicians continue antituberculosis therapy indefinitely, but other studies indicate that standard regimens are adequate for HIV-infected patients.

MAC is less responsive to therapy than is *M tuberculosis*. Early trials failed to show benefit of single-drug or two-drug regimens, and later studies demonstrated clinical benefit of three- to five-drug regimens.[185,186] Successful prophylactic regimens have been reported.

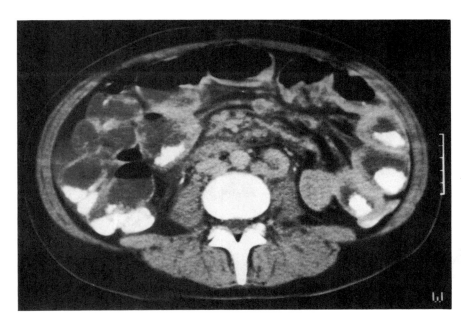

FIG. 18-7. Computed tomography scan of the abdomen demonstrates mesenteric lymphadenopathy, tethering of the mesentery, and thickening of the bowel wall in a patient with *Mycobacterium avium* complex.

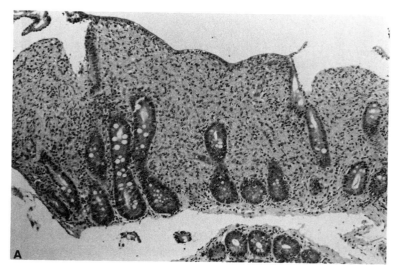

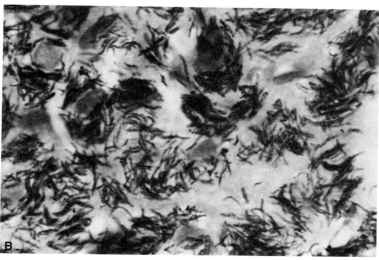

FIG. 18-8. (A) Massive infiltration of the jejunum with *Mycobacterium avium* complex (hematoxylin & eosin; original magnification × 250). (B) Acid-fast stain, demonstrating intracellular bacilli. The characteristic beaded appearance of the bacilli can be detected (Ziehl-Neelsen stain; original magnification × 1000).

Other mycobacterial species have been found on occasion, with variable clinical consequences based on their sensitivity to antibiotics.[187] A few patients have had a MAC-like intestinal lesion in which the foamy macrophages contained gram-positive bacilli rather than acid-fast organisms. Some of these cases may represent infection with *Rhodococcus equus*, a complication previously reported in AIDS.[188] The foamy macrophages seen in Whipple's disease also contain gram-positive, non–acid-fast rods, although sequencing studies using the short arm of ribosomal RNA indicate that the Whipple's bacillus is an *Actinomyces* species.[189]

Bacterial Enteritides

Bacterial enteritides in HIV-infected persons include *Salmonella, Shigella,* and *Campylobacter* infections.[190–193] The incidence of serious disease is higher than in the general population. One study found a high incidence of *Campylobacter*-like organisms, but their presence did not correlate with clinical symptoms.[194] Enhanced susceptibility could be related to achlorhydria, which is found in a proportion of AIDS patients.[195] Classic studies demonstrated the relation between gastric acidity and the infective dose of various enteric pathogens.[196]

Bacterial enteritides in AIDS may have a chronic, relapsing course, often with bacteremia. The presentation resembles "enteric fever," with abdominal pain, distension, and a diarrheal syndrome varying from ileocolitis to proctocolitis. The diagnosis is straightforward with routine evaluation. Blood cultures should be part of the workup of suspected infectious diarrhea with fever in an HIV-infected patient. Patients respond to antibiotic therapy with parenteral agents.

An unusual feature of bacterial enteritides in AIDS is the tendency for clinical and microbiologic relapse.[193] It is possible that disease recurs because of impaired intracellular killing in macrophages. The intracellular reservoir may protect the organisms against lysis. Quinolones, such as ciprofloxacin, are thought to be bacteriocidal to intracellular organisms,[197] although the drug was unable to eliminate the carrier state after *Salmonella* infections in a non-AIDS treatment group.[198] Further studies are needed to determine if complete eradication of the enteric bacterial pathogens in AIDS is possible or if chronic therapy will continue to be needed.

Antibiotic-associated colitis, related to elaboration of *Clostridium difficile* toxin is a common occurrence in AIDS patients who receive prolonged courses of broad-spectrum antibiotics. Clindamycin therapy and prolonged hospitalization have been identified as risk factors for the development of colitis, suggesting the existence of nosocomial transmission.[199,200] The clinical syndrome is similar in AIDS and non-AIDS patients.[200] Suspicion should be raised by the clinical situation, and the diagnosis is confirmed by stool toxin assay. Treatment with vancomycin or metronidazole is as effective in AIDS as in non-AIDS patients. Residual symptoms can be managed with oral cholestyramine (Questran), which binds the bacterial toxin. Surveillance against recurrent colitis may be necessary for patients who require chronic antibiotic therapy.

Enteropathogenic Bacterial Infection

A syndrome of chronic diarrhea and malabsorption associated with bacteria adherent to epithelial cells has been recognized.[201–206] The infection is localized to the terminal ileum, cecum, and colon and occurs in patients with severe CD4+ lymphocyte depletion. The histopathologic findings are similar to those seen in infants with enteropathogenic *Escherichia coli* infection.[207] Treatment with broad-spectrum antibiotics may lead to clinical improvement. It is unclear if the same mechanism applies in AIDS patients or if the immunodeficiency renders the mucosa vulnerable to "nonpathogens." Alternatively, the problem may result from a community-acquired, low-grade intestinal infection that cannot be cleared because of the severity of the immune deficit.

Fungi

Candida albicans

Candidiasis is a common opportunistic infection occurring in more than 80% of AIDS patients. Early clinical observations associated the occurrence of thrush, not related to antibiotic use or other immune impairment, with an increased risk of progression to AIDS within 6 months.[208] The most commonly detected species is *Candida albicans,* which is part of the normal enteric flora. However, infection by *Torulopsis glabrata* has been reported and may be a cause of a treatment failure.[209] Candidiasis in AIDS is predominantly a mucosal disease, which differs from what is seen in other states of immune derangement such as uncontrolled diabetes mellitus or drug-induced leukopenia. In those circumstances, tissue invasion and septicemia are common. Systemic candidiasis in AIDS patients usually is associated with idiopathic or drug-induced neutropenia.

Other Fungi

The luminal GI tract, liver, spleen, and mesenteric lymph nodes may be involved by histoplasmosis, coccidioidomycosis, or other fungal infections.[210–211] Systemic fungal infections in AIDS usually are rapidly progressive diseases. Although the fungi are not primary enteric pathogens, visceral dissemination and involvement of the luminal GI tract may occur. Typically, there is a chronic febrile illness with constitutional symptoms. Suspicion should be aroused by a history of residence in an endemic area. The diagnosis is made by culture or examination of tissue samples, using special stains (Fig. 18-9). Treatment with antifungal agents must be continued for months and perhaps indefinitely.

Actinomycotic infection of esophageal ulcers also has been described.[212] Disseminated pneumocystosis in patients receiving aerosolized pentamidine as prophylaxis against *Pneumocystis carinii* pneumonia has been reported.[213]

Neoplasms

Kaposi's Sarcoma

The diagnosis of Kaposi's sarcoma (KS) in young homosexual males in 1981 was one of the earliest observations indicating a new disorder of immune function.[214] The lesion is indistinguishable histopathologically from the classic KS that occurs in elderly men, endemic forms of KS found in Africa, or the form that occurs during immunosuppressive therapy. KS in AIDS is demographically limited, being more common in white homosexual males than in other persons with AIDS,[215] suggesting the presence of a separate cofactor for this complication. Evidence of a novel herpesvirus has been isolated from KS lesions from HIV-positive and HIV-negative patients.[216]

Visceral involvement with KS is more common in AIDS than in classic KS.[217] Lesions in the GI tract are common and often asymptomatic, but they may cause a swallowing disorder, luminal obstruction, intussusception, disturbed motility from neural involvement, or lymphatic blockade with exudative enteropathy. Severe bleeding is uncommon, and perforation is rare. Severe diarrhea is not a common finding in uncomplicated KS, and patients with diarrhea should be evaluated for other pathogens.

The diagnosis of KS can be made by visual inspection and confirmed by biopsy. Endoscopic biopsy may be falsely negative because of the submucosal location of the tumor.[218] KS is responsive to chemotherapy or radiation therapy, but no treatment is needed in asymptomatic cases. Obstructive lesions can be treated effectively by laser ablation.[219]

Lymphoma

An increasing incidence of extranodal, high-grade non-Hodgkin's B-cell lymphomas in young men was noticed in the early 1980s.[220] The development of lymphoma later was

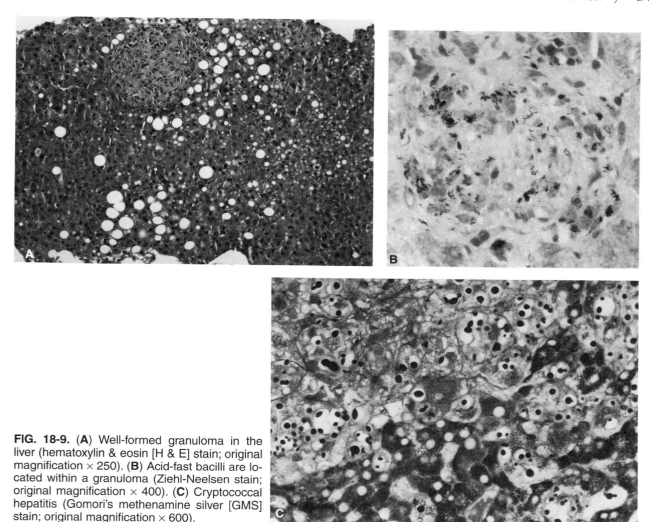

FIG. 18-9. **(A)** Well-formed granuloma in the liver (hematoxylin & eosin [H & E] stain; original magnification × 250). **(B)** Acid-fast bacilli are located within a granuloma (Ziehl-Neelsen stain; original magnification × 400). **(C)** Cryptococcal hepatitis (Gomori's methenamine silver [GMS] stain; original magnification × 600).

shown to be related to HIV infection. B-cell lymphomas have a special predilection for the central nervous system and the GI tract. EBV virus genomes have been identified in some of these tumors,[102] suggesting a possible etiologic role. Lymphoproliferative disease involving T cells has been seen in some HIV-infected persons and appears to be related to coexisting infection with HTLV-I, a T-lymphotropic oncogenic retrovirus.[221]

GI lymphomas in AIDS patients are biologically aggressive, especially the Burkitt's lymphoma subtype. However, the lesions may respond to combination chemotherapy. There are few long-term survivors, however, because of the underlying immunodeficiency.

Other Cancers

Sporadic reports of patients with carcinomas in the GI tract have been published. These include carcinomas of the tongue, esophagus, stomach, colon, and anus. In some cases, tumors are biologically aggressive, with widespread hematogenous dissemination and short survival times. The relation of these tumors to AIDS is uncertain, but they may be related to infection with a cocarcinogenic agent or the loss of immune surveillance against developing tumors.

CLINICAL SYNDROMES

Disorders of Food Intake

Oral candidiasis is the most commonly encountered complication in HIV-seropositive patients. Clinically, the infection presents as erosions or plaques on the gingiva, palate, hypopharynx, and esophagus (Fig 18-10). Isolated involvement of the esophagus has been reported.[222] Bronchial, gastric, and intestinal mucosae are not involved grossly or microscopically. The most common complaints are sore

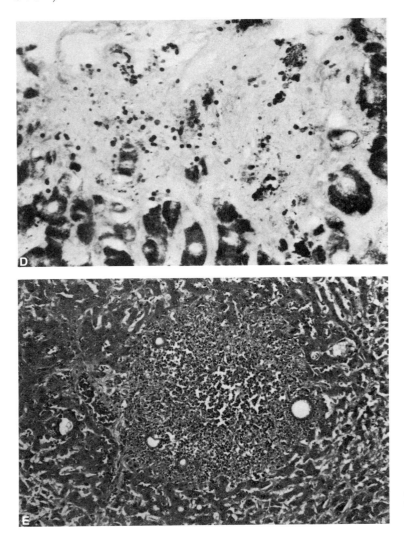

FIG. 18-9. (D) Histoplasmosis of the liver (GMS stain; original magnification × 600). **(E)** Cocciodomycosis of the liver (H&E stain; original magnification × 400).

throat and odynophagia, sometimes with choking or aspiration, plus a mild to moderate substernal discomfort. Food intake is decreased, and the oral cavity may become more sensitive to temperature and acidity.

In most cases, the diagnosis can be made by inspection and confirmed by a response to treatment. On radiologic examination, plaques with or without erosions is seen. Culture, biopsy, or brush cytology can be used to confirm the diagnosis. A cytology brush for the esophagus has been developed that avoids possible contamination by oral secretions.[223]

Candidiasis can be successfully treated with topical or systemic agents. Topical therapies often are sufficient for oral candidiasis and include nystatin and clotrimazole troches (Mycelex). Esophageal candidiasis usually requires systemic therapy using azoles, such as ketoconazole (Nizoral), fluconazole (Diflucan), or itraconazole (Sporonox). Fluconazole is associated with a higher response rate than is ketoconazole.[224] Resistance to azole therapy may develop.[225] Ketoconazole and fluconazole occasionally are associated

with abnormal liver function tests. A potential problem with treatment is decreased bioavailability; ketoconazole absorption is optimal at an acid pH, but many AIDS patients are achlorhydric.[195,226] Administration of an acidifying agent may improve effectiveness. The infection becomes resistant to oral therapy in a small percentage of cases[226] and must then be treated with intravenous amphotericin.

Oral hairy leukoplakia is a whitish, verrucous excrescence occurring mainly along the sides of the tongue[227] that has been mistaken for candidiasis. EBV virus has been found in the lesions by molecular hybridization studies and electron microscopic examinations.[101] The diagnosis is made by inspection and confirmed, if necessary, by biopsy. Acyclovir or ganciclovir therapy achieves resolution.[228]

Painful ulcers of the oral cavity, hypopharynx, or esophagus may cause significant impairment of food intake. The most common causes are viral and idiopathic, although ulcerating neoplasms and mycobacterial or fungal infections are seen rarely. Small aphthous ulcers in the oral cavity are common and may resolve spontaneously or after adminis-

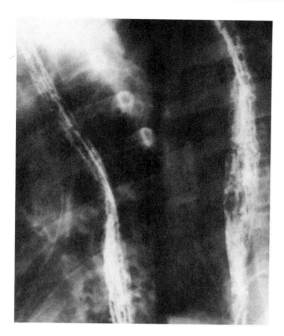

FIG. 18-10. Two views of a barium swallow demonstrate mucosal plaques due to candidiasis.

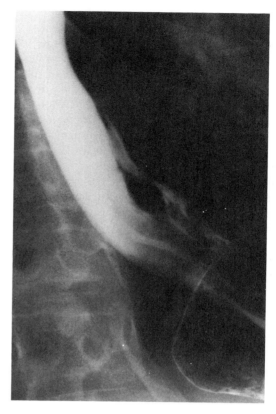

FIG. 18-11. Barium esophagogram demonstrates an idiopathic ulcer that is undermining the superior edge and tracking submucosally to the gastric cardia.

tration of topical steroids. Acute necrotizing ulcerative gingivitis is a focal, destructive process of uncertain etiology that may extend to the bone.[229] The most common virus-associated ulcer is caused by CMV infection and occurs in the oral cavity or esophagus. The lesions usually appear as erosions or shallow coalescing ulcerations with abundant intracellular viral inclusions. Occasionally, CMV esophagitis assumes a pseudotumor appearance.[230] The lesion responds to ganciclovir therapy.

Many esophageal ulcers have no etiologic agent identified. The ulcers are atypical in their large size and in the extensively undermining of the mucosa (Fig 18-11). The ulcers typically are refractory to therapy against gastric acid secretion, and the pain may respond poorly to opiates. Progressive malnutrition is the usual result in untreated cases. Biopsies show inflamed granulation tissue, sometimes with rare CMV inclusions. Ganciclovir therapy does not bring symptomatic relief or healing, although viral inclusions disappear. The presence of HIV in esophageal ulcers has been demonstrated by RNA in situ hybridization and by the detection of an HIV core protein, p24, in cells in the ulcer.[231–232] Viral particles suggestive of HIV were seen in transient esophageal ulcers associated with primary HIV infection.[233] However, evidence of HIV also can be seen in other lesions, such as CMV esophagitis.[234] One study also found evidence of EBV-infected cells in esophageal ulcers.[235]

Corticosteroids have produced symptomatic relief, weight gain, and ulcer healing in a substantial proportion of patients.[232,236–239] Therapy has been administered by oral, parenteral, and intralesional routes. Despite the potential hazards of steroid therapy, clinical experience has demonstrated

that the treatment can be administered with relative safety. Prophylaxis against tuberculosis, herpesviruses, fungi, or other pathogens should be considered if corticosteroids are used. Studies of the use of thalidomide in esophageal ulcers are ongoing.

Neoplasms such as KS or lymphoma may affect food intake by interfering with mastication or swallowing. These lesions may respond to a variety of therapies.

In many cases, food intake is diminished in the absence of pathologic lesions. The causes are diverse but fall into several general categories. Organic neurologic diseases may interfere with the initiation or coordination of eating. More diffuse lesions such as HIV-associated encephalitis cause anorexia through alterations in consciousness, damage to neurons involved in appetite behavior, or the release of cytokines, such as tumor necrosis factor, which reversibly suppress food intake.[240] Secondary anorexia is a common feature of systemic infections and malabsorptive illnesses because of the release of inhibitory factors acting at the level of the central nervous system.[241–242] Alterations in taste, anorexia, and nausea are common side effects of medications. Psychosocial factors such as depression, isolation, poverty, and debilitation itself may lead to inadequate intake. Such considerations are an important part of clinical therapeutics in AIDS.

Dyspepsia

Nausea and dyspepsia are common symptoms of AIDS patients but rarely dominate the clinical picture. These symptoms may result from a variety of pathologic processes. The stomach may be involved by disseminated infections such as CMV, MAC, and fungus or by tumors such as KS, lymphoma, and adenocarcinoma. Symptomatic gastritis due to *Helicobacter pylori* has been found but is not common, possibly because of frequent antibiotic use by AIDS patients.[243] Some medications, such as nonsteroidal antiinflammatory agents, promote gastric ulceration and produce dyspepsia. However, symptomatic peptic ulcer disease is uncommon in AIDS patients, possibly because of decreased gastric acid secretion.[195,244] Achlorhydria may alter drug absorption or lead to increased bacterial colony counts in the stomach and upper small intestine, potentially decreasing nutrient absorption. However, not all studies have confirmed achlorhydria in these patients.[245] Dyspepsia is caused by a low-grade pancreatitis in some patients and may precede the development of biliary tract disease.

The treatment of dyspeptic complications depends on their exact nature. Symptomatic *H pylori* in an AIDS patient is treated in a manner similar to the infection in other symptomatic patients. Diagnosis of CMV or MAC infection is an indication for systemic antiinfective therapy. Widespread or ulcerating KS is an indication for systemic chemotherapy, as is lymphoma.

Diarrhea and Wasting

Diarrhea and weight loss are common problems for AIDS patients, occurring in as many as 80% of cases in some series. Altered bowel habits also are common in HIV-infected persons without AIDS and may even be present in patients referred to as asymptomatic.[246,247] Symptoms are associated with small intestinal injury and malabsorption or with enterocolitis (Table 18-2). Although early studies reported large numbers of patients with unexplained diarrhea, an infectious agent can be found in most comprehensively evaluated AIDS patients.[142,248] In contrast, diarrhea is unexplained in most HIV-infected patients without AIDS.

Nutrient malabsorption is an extremely common occurrence in AIDS. In many cases, it is clinically occult and involves fat[249] or vitamin B_{12}.[51] A subset of AIDS patients have severe malabsorption associated with histologic evidence of small intestine injury. Many cases are caused by cryptosporidiosis, isosporiasis, or microsporidiosis. The intestinal injury appears similar to tropical sprue and includes partial villus atrophy and crypt hyperplasia. Total villus atrophy, as occurs in celiac disease, is rare. Malabsorption also may occur as a result of MAC infection. Severe malabsorption is not a feature of giardiasis. CMV infection produces a diffuse disease in the lamina propria but rarely causes severe injury to the villus epithelium. Although adherent bacteria may be responsible for some

TABLE 18-2. *Causes of diarrhea and wasting*

MALABSORPTIVE DISEASES
Cryptosporidiosis
Isosporiasis
Microsporidiosis
Giardiasis
Mycobacterium avium complex infection
Bacterial adherence

ENTEROCOLITIS
Cytomegalovirus infection
Mycobacterium avium complex infection
Mycobacterium tuberculosis
Cryptosporidiosis
Adenovirus infection
Salmonella sp. infection
Shigella sp. infection
Campylobacter sp. infection
Fungal infections
Human immunodeficiency virus infection
Clostridium difficile toxin

cases of ileal dysfunction, there is little evidence to implicate bacterial overgrowth as a cause for intestinal injury, despite reports of alterations in the upper intestinal flora.[250] Although intraluminal bacterial colony counts may be somewhat elevated as a result of hypochlorhydria or achlorhydria, unpublished series have shown most AIDS patients to have jejunal colony counts within the normal range (Kapembwa M: personal communication; Kotler DP: personal observations).

Some HIV-infected patients have severe intestinal dysfunction without an etiologic agent found after comprehensive evaluation.[8,9,70,142–144,251–254] It is possible that HIV or another unidentified pathogen is responsible for the damage. However, the report of clinical improvement in response to a gluten-free diet[255] suggests that other pathogenic mechanisms are possible.

There are several causes of enterocolitis in patients with AIDS. CMV colitis is diagnosed frequently and produces a progressive disease that may result in bowel infarction and perforation. MAC produces a infiltrative disease without specific findings in the colon. Disseminated *M tuberculosis* also has been found in the GI tract and causes focal ulcerations, especially in the ileocecal region. Some patients with cryptosporidiosis have ileitis or ileocolitis and present with symptoms of severe proctocolitis without significant malabsorption. Fungal infection may involve the bowel. Adenovirus also may cause a persistent colitis. Other causes of enterocolitis or proctocolitis include *Salmonella*, *Shigella*, and *Campylobacter* infections and antibiotic-associated colitis.

Clinical differentiation of malabsorptive from colitic disease is important to focus the diagnostic evaluation, although the possibility of multiple coexisting diseases may require a comprehensive workup (Table 18-3). An algorithmic approach may be used (Fig 18-12). Important information often can be obtained from the patient's history. The

TABLE 18-3. *Clinical differentiation of malabsorptive and colitic diarrhea*

Characteristic	Malabsorption	Colitis
Stool frequency (number/24 h)	3–8	3–30
Stool volumes (24 h)	750–10,000 mL	250–1000 mL
Stool volume (per BM)	Variable, often large	Small
Regularity of BM	Variable	Regular
Formed stools	Rarely	Never
Occult blood in stools	No	Yes
Fecal leukocytes	No	Yes
Tenesmus	No	Sometimes
Fever	No	Yes
Debility	Yes	Yes
Appetite	Fair–good	Fair–poor

BM, bowel movement.

symptoms related to small intestinal infection are those of malabsorption and are similar to symptoms in patients with tropical sprue or short bowel syndrome. Enterocolitic diseases produce typical symptoms of colitis, often associated with fever, anorexia, progressive weight loss, and extreme debilitation.

Optimal diagnostic techniques vary with the specific pathogen. The diagnosis of cryptosporidiosis is made from stool or tissue biopsies. Isosporiasis also can be diagnosed by stool examination or tissue biopsy. The diagnosis of microsporidiosis is more difficult, because spores are not easily identified in stool specimens, although several techniques have been published. In some cases the presence of microsporidia in intestinal biopsies can be suggested by histopathologic features on light microscopy. The diagnosis of CMV infection is made by histologic examination of tissue biopsies (see Fig. 18-1). Acid-fast bacilli can be seen on stool examination, and their presence suggests possible intestinal involvement with MAC. Mucosal abnormalities on barium x-ray films or thickening of the intestinal wall plus enlargement of mesenteric and retroperitoneal nodes on CT scans are characteristic of MAC. Diagnosis by biopsy (see Figs. 18-8 and 18-9) often can be made in 1 day, compared with mycobacterial cultures, which may take as long as 6 weeks to become positive.

Maintenance of nutritional status and fluid balance are important clinical tasks, especially for patients with malabsorption. Studies of food intake in patients with malabsorption, with or without AIDS, have shown that decreased intake contributes significantly to the negative caloric balance and that adaptive hyperphagia does not occur. Oral rehydration solutions are hypocaloric and may promote wasting if used excessively. A low-fat, lactose-free diet supplemented with medium-chain triglycerides may be beneficial. Standard polymeric formula diets generally are tolerated poorly, but elemental diets may lead to less diarrhea. Palatability is a problem with elemental diets, but therapy may lead to weight stabilization or gain (Kotler DP: personal observations). In refractory cases, parenteral hydration and nutrition may be employed and have been shown to improve nutritional status.[256]

Nutritional support is less effective in patients with enterocolitis associated with systemic infections than in patients with malabsorptive diseases due to the associated metabolic derangements. Anorexia may be mediated in the central nervous system by cytokines. In the study cited previously, total parenteral nutrition resulted in weight gain due entirely to an increase in body fat content, while body cell mass was progressively depleted.[256] Although nutritional support may slow the rate of protein depletion, the key to successful therapy is proper diagnosis and treatment of the specific disease complication. Ganciclovir treatment of CMV colitis led to body mass repletion in the absence of formal nutritional support.[90]

Anorectal Diseases

The anorectal region may be affected by ulcers, masses, warts, infections, and hemorrhoids. Anorectal ulcers may arise from stratified squamous epithelium in the anal canal, perianal and perineal skin, or rectal mucosa. Herpes simplex virus type II is a common cause of anorectal ulceration. The primary lesion occurs at the pectinate line. Large, shallow, spreading perianal ulcers are recognized more commonly. A proctitis may occur, but it is more common in non HIV-infected subjects. Most cases respond to therapy with acyclovir or ganciclovir. Herpes simplex virus resistant to acyclovir has been demonstrated in patients with refractory ulcerations. The use of foscarnet may bring resolution.[257] CMV also can cause anorectal ulcerations. The diagnosis is established by biopsy. Ganciclovir therapy may achieve clinical resolution.

A variety of classic venereal diseases can produce anorectal ulcerations. Epidemiologic studies in Africa suggest strongly that genital ulceration promotes the transmission of HIV infection.[258] Diagnosis and therapy of *Neisseria gonorrhea* proctitis is similar in AIDS and non-AIDS patients. Syphilis may have an atypical presentation in HIV-infected subjects, and serologic diagnosis may be problematic.[259] Dark-field examination or fluorescent antibody discloses the *Treponema palladium* spirochete. Prolonged intravenous antibiotic therapy is required. *Chlamydia*

Diagnostic Algorithm for Diarrhea and Wasting in AIDS

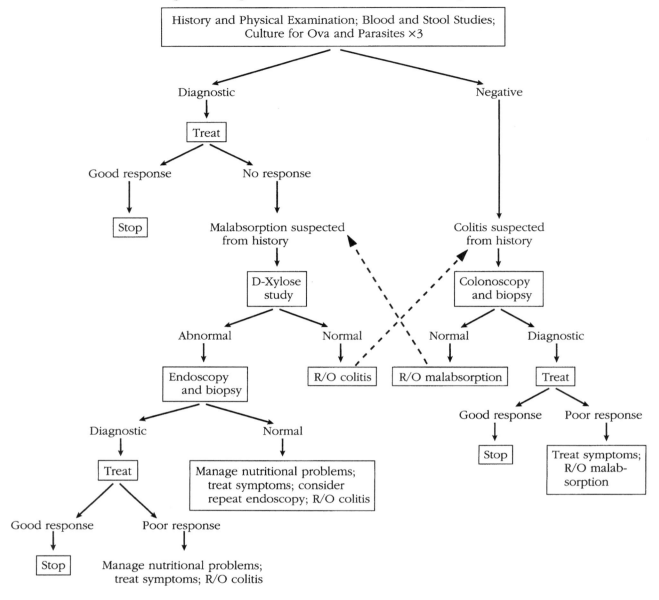

FIG. 18-12. Diagnostic algorithm for diarrhea and wasting in AIDS. (Adapted from Hecker LM, Kotler DP. Gastrointestinal manifestations in AIDS. In: Conn RB, ed. Current diagnosis. Philadelphia: JB Lippincott, 1991.)

species are the most prevalent sexually transmitted diseases in sexually active groups, and the risk of infection rises with the level of sexual activity.[260] Definitive diagnosis is made by cell culture. The standard therapy is oral tetracycline or doxycycline. The frequency of chancroid, caused by *Haemophilus ducreyi,* in HIV-infected patients is unknown. The diagnosis usually is suggested on clinical grounds and confirmed after infection with *T pallidum* is excluded. Therapy with trimethoprim-sulfamethoxazole or sulfa alone may be successful.

Rectal spirochetosis has been recognized in homosexual men with or without HIV infections.[261] The infection usually

is asymptomatic and an incidental finding on evaluation (Fig 18-13).

Idiopathic ulcers of the anorectal region, similar to those occurring in the esophagus are seen in AIDS patients. CMV, herpes simplex virus, human papillomavirus, acid-fast bacilli, fungi, and bacteria must be excluded by culture or histologic studies. The pathogenesis of the ulceration is unknown. Intralesional or systemic corticosteroids produce a prompt clinical response but have a variable effects on healing.

The incidence of anogenital neoplasms is increased in AIDS patients, as it is in immunosuppressed renal transplant recipients.[262] KS and lymphoma are the most common neoplasms, characterized by mass lesions or ulcers. Epidermoid cancers, including squamous cell and cloacagenic cancers, occur in anal skin and rectal glands, respectively. Although these cancers rarely metastasize in immunocompetent persons, they may do so in patients with AIDS. For these lesions, management after diagnostic biopsy includes excision, chemotherapy, or laser photocoagulation. Laser therapy of rectal KS also is effective and may cause dramatic regression of bulky disease.

The role of papillomavirus, the etiologic agent of condyloma acuminata (ie, common venereal warts), in anorectal cancers is unclear.[263] Specific serotypes of papillomaviruses are suspected as being cofactors in carcinogenesis in the anogenital region, particularly of squamous cell carcinomas of the cervix or anus.[264] Leukoplakia of the anal canal is thought to be an intermediate form of the lesion and is a common finding in HIV-infected homosexual men.[265] The incidence of squamous cell carcinoma of the anus was known to be increased in homosexual men before the recognition of AIDS.[266]

Hemorrhoids are common in HIV-infected persons. The factors predisposing these patients to hemorrhoids may have predated the HIV infection. Severe diarrhea or proctitis may promote thrombosis, ulceration, and secondary infection. Fleshy skin tags, resembling those seen in Crohn's disease, are commonly seen and are related to underlying inflammation.

Other Syndromes

Hemorrhage

GI hemorrhage is not a common consequence of AIDS, but serious or life-threatening bleeding does occur.[267–268] Bleeding may result from the same conditions occurring in the non-HIV–infected patient, as well as from the tumors and ulcers seen in AIDS patients. Episodes of massive arterial hemorrhage have occurred in patients with acute or chronic intestinal ulcers and those with rapidly progressive KS.

The clinical presentation of GI hemorrhage in an AIDS patient is the same as in a non-AIDS patient, and the basic concepts of diagnosis and treatment also are the same. Bleeding lesions may be visualized by endoscopy and controlled locally while diagnostic material is obtained. Angiographic localization of obscure lesions and pharmacologic control may be successful. If bleeding is related to a discrete ulcer, surgical excision may be indicated, but surgery is less appropriate for patients with widespread disease. Proper management of bleeding neoplasms involves effective local control followed by systemic chemotherapy.

Surgical Complications

Disease complications requiring consideration of emergent surgical intervention occur in patients with AIDS. Perforated viscus occurs in AIDS, but the cause may be a solitary ulcer, CMV infection[269] or tumor[270] rather than peptic ulcer disease or diverticulitis. Malignant obstruction usually results from KS or lymphoma rather than adenocarcinoma. KS or lymphoma also may be the leading edge in an intussusception. Some patients with peritonitis have had only mild fibrinous exudate found at laparotomy.[271] The clinical appearance of appendicitis, cholecystitis, or generalized peritonitis are the same in AIDS and non-AIDS patients. Appendicitis typically responds well to surgery. Laparoscopic approaches have been successfully applied to the treatment of symptomatic gallbladder disease in HIV infection.

Although the physical findings of the acute abdomen are not significantly affected by the presence of AIDS, the laboratory evaluation differs markedly from expected findings. Elevated leukocyte counts with early forms in the circulation may not be present, especially if there is preexisting leukopenia or prior treatment with myelosuppressive drugs. Isotopic imaging studies such as an indium-labeled white blood cell study or gallium scan may be falsely negative in the presence of severe leukopenia. Imaging studies such as a CT scan with luminal contrast

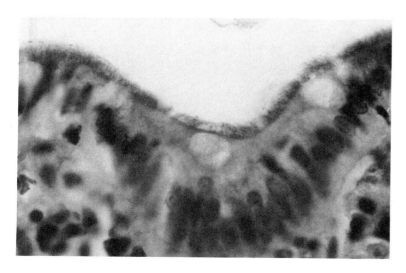

FIG. 18-13. Spirochetes are located along the luminal membrane of rectal crypt epithelial cells, giving it a shaggy appearance (hematoxylin & eosin stain; original magnification × 800).

may be particularly valuable in detecting extraluminal collections of pus or fluid.

Although the indications for surgery are the same for AIDS and non-HIV–infected patients, the expected outcomes may differ. The surgeon can anticipate the possibility of unusual pathogens, prolonged recovery times, and impaired wound healing. The incidence of postoperative complications and mortality is high in several series,[272–274] but this results in part from the seriousness of the underlying illness and other complications, and the immunodeficiency itself may not be an important independent risk factor. Complete recovery after major abdominal surgery is possible for AIDS patients and may be followed by prolonged survival.[275]

Hepatobiliary Diseases

Liver dysfunction in AIDS patients may be related to preexisting hepatic diseases, infectious or neoplastic disease complications, or drug toxicity. Three distinct clinical syndromes have been recognized: diffuse hepatocellular injury, granulomatous hepatitis, and sclerosing cholangitis (Fig 18-14). Many other patients with abnormal liver function tests have macrovesicular or microvesicular fatty infiltration or other nonspecific changes.

Diffuse hepatitis is most commonly a result of drug toxicity or of hepatitis C[276] or hepatitis D infection.[277] Acute hepatitis B infection is uncommon because of prior exposure in most patients, and it may be clinically mild, because hepatocyte injury is produced by the immune reaction. Autoimmune chronic active hepatitis and chronic hepatitis B infections also are clinically mild syndromes in HIV-seropositive persons.

Granulomatous hepatitis in AIDS is related to mycobacterial or fungal diseases or drug toxicity (Fig 18-9). *P carinii* may cause a hepatitis and other evidence of disseminated disease in patients receiving aerosol drug prophylaxis.[278] Isolated cases of cryptosporidia or microsporidia affecting the liver have been reported.[270] Fever and constitutional symptoms are prominent. Liver function tests demonstrate progressive elevations in the levels of alkaline phosphatase and γ-glutamyl transpeptidase, but bilirubin concentrations are less affected. Liver biopsy reveals granulomas, which may be poorly formed. Giant cells are seen only rarely. Special stains can presumptively identify the causative organisms, although mycobacterial and fungal cultures of the liver should be obtained routinely.

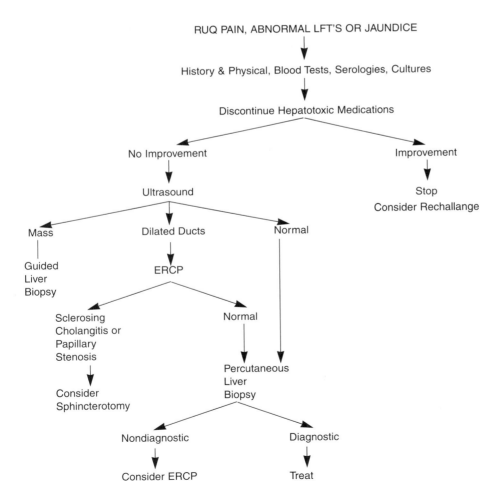

FIG. 18-14. Algorithm for diagnosing hepatobiliary disease in AIDS. ERCP, endoscopic retrograde cholangiopancreatography. (Adapted from Hecker LM, Kotler DP. Gastrointestinal manifestations in AIDS. In: Conn RB, ed. Current diagnosis. Philadelphia: JB Lippincott, 1991.)

Peliosis hepatis has been described in AIDS patients.[280] Unlike the syndrome in non-AIDS patients, the lesion in AIDS patients is caused by infection with a *Rickettsia*-like organism related to the organisms than causes cat-scratch fever.[281,282]

A syndrome of sclerosing cholangitis recognized in AIDS patients[124,283] resembles the non-AIDS variety. The lesion in AIDS patients often is associated with cryptosporidial, microsporidial, or CMV infections. The pathogenetic mechanisms underlying sclerosing cholangitis in AIDS and the non-AIDS variety are unknown. Patients present with a nonspecific abdominal complaints and progressive cholestasis. Endoscopic retrograde examination demonstrates single or multiple areas of narrowing and dilatation of the intrahepatic or extrahepatic ducts, with mucosal ulceration in many cases (see Fig 18-13). The short-term results of endoscopic decompression are variable. In a few long-term cases, progressive jaundice and liver failure developed.

Pancreatic Diseases

Pancreatic diseases in AIDS patients have received little attention. The pancreas may be affected as part of a systemic

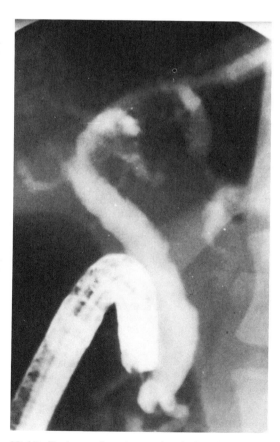

FIG. 18-15. Endoscopic retrograde cholangiogram demonstrates irregularities of the intrahepatic and extrahepatic bile ducts.

complication caused by CMV, MAC, fungal infection, KS, or lymphoma.[284] Pancreatic involvement often is not recognized premortem. Some AIDS patients have presented with an acute pancreatitis. The disease, which is clinically mild in most cases, is associated with abdominal pain, nausea, vomiting, and elevations in serum amylase and lipase concentrations. In some cases, a medication such as trimethoprim sulfa or didanosine (Videx) can be implicated, but no etiologic agent can be found in others. Intravenous pentamidine therapy for *Pneumocystis* pneumonia has been associated with hypoglycemia due to selective damage to beta cells in the islets of Langerhans.[285] A few patients have become insulin-requiring diabetics after pentamidine therapy. Hyperlipidemic pancreatitis has been observed in a few patients receiving intravenous lipids. There are no reports of chronic pancreatitis occurring as a specific complication of AIDS. Pancreatic insufficiency is an uncommon cause of fat malabsorption in AIDS patients.[286]

REFERENCES

1. Connolly GM, Shanson D, Hawkins DDA, et al. Non-cryptosporidial diarrhoea in human immunodeficiency virus (HIV) infected patients. Gut 1989;30:195.
2. Rene E, Marche C, Requier B, et al. Intestinal infections in patients with acquired immunodeficiency syndrome: a prospective study in 132 patients. Dig Dis Sci 1989;34:773.
3. Horowitz S, Lorenzsonn VW, Olsen WA, Albrecht R, Hong R. Small intestinal disease in T cell deficiency. J Pediatr 1974;85:457.
4. Bienenstock J. The mucosal immunological network. Ann Allergy 1984;53:535.
5. Berkelman RB, Heyward WL, Stehr-Green JK, Curran JW. Epidemiology of human immunodeficiency virus infection and acquired immunodeficiency syndrome. Ann Intern Med 1989;86:761.
6. Kotler DP, Reka S, Clayton F. Intestinal mucosal inflammation associated with human immunodeficiency virus infection. Dig Dis Sci 1993;38:1119.
7. Kotler DP, Reka S, Borcich A, Cronin WJ. Detection, localization and quantitation of HIV-associated antigens in intestinal biopsies from HIV-infected patients. Am J Pathol 1991;139:823.
8. Greenson J, Belitsos P, Yardley J, Bartlett J. AIDS enteropathy: occult enteric infections and duodenal mucosal alterations in chronic diarrhea. Ann Intern Med 1991;114:366.
9. Ehrenpreis ED, Ganger DR, Kochvar GT, Patterson BK, Craig RM. D-Xylose malabsorption: characteristic finding in patients with AIDS wasting syndrome and chronic diarrhea. J Acquir Immune Defic Syndr 1992;5:1047.
10. Lubeck DP, Bennett CL, Mazonson PD, Fifer SK, Fries JF. Quality of life and health service use among HIV-infected patients with chronic diarrhea. J Acquir Immune Defic Syndr 1993;6:478.
11. Hodges JR, Wright R. Normal immune responses in the gut and liver. Clin Sci 1982;63:339.
12. Wolf JL, Bye WA. The membranous epithelial (M) cell and the mucosal immune system. Ann Rev Med 1984;35:95.
13. Bland PW, Warren JG. Antigen presentation by epithelial cells of the small intestine: kinetics, antigen specificity and blocking by anti-Ia antisera. Immunology 1986;58:1.
14. Richman LK, Graeff AS, Yarchoan R, Strober W. Simultaneous induction of antigen-specific IgA helper T cells and IgG suppressor T cells in the murine Peyer's patch after protein feeding. J Immunol 1981;126:2079.
15. Guy-Grand D, Griscelli C, Vassalli P. The mouse gut lymphocyte, a novel type of T cell: nature, origin and trafficking in normal and graft-vs-host conditions. J Exp Med 1978;148:1661.
16. Schmitz M, Nunoz D, Butcher EC. Selective recognition of mucosal lymphoid high endothelium by intraepithelial leukocytes. Gastroenterology 1988;94:576.

17. Selby WS, Janossy G, Goldstein G, Jewell DP. T lymphocyte subsets in human intestinal mucosa: the distribution and relationship to MHC-derived antigens. Clin Exp Immunol 1981;44:453.
18. Marsh MN, Hinde J. Inflammatory component of celiac sprue mucosa. I. Mast cells, basophils and eosinophils. Gastroenterology 1985;89:92.
19. Selby WS, Janossy G, Bofill M, Jewell DP. Lymphocyte subpopulations in the human small intestine: the findings in normal mucosa and in the mucosa of patients with adult celiac disease. Clin Exp Immunol 1983;52:219.
20. Bonneville M, Janeway CA, Ito K, Haser W, Ishida I, Nakanishi N, Tonegawa S. Intestinal intraepithelial lymphocytes are a distinct set of gamma-delta T cells. Nature 1988;336:479.
21. Tomasi TB Jr, Tan EM, Solomon A, Prendergast RA. Characteristics of an immune system common to certain external secretions. J Exp Med 1965;121:101.
22. Green DR, Gold J, St. Martin S, Gershon R, Gershon RK. Microenvironmental immunoregulation: possible role of contrasuppressor cells in maintaining immune responses in gut-associated lymphoid tissues. Proc Natl Acad Sci USA 1982;79:889.
23. Radema SA, Van Deventer SJH, Cerami A. Interleukin-1B is expressed predominantly by enterocytes in experimental colitis. Gastroenterology 1991;100:1180.
24. Clemmens MJ, McNurlan MA. Regulation of cell proliferation and differentiation by interferons. Biochem J 1985;226:345.
25. Chang EB, Musch W, Mayer L. Interleukins 1 and 3 stimulate anion secretion in chicken intestine. Gastroenterology 1990;98:1518.
26. Kagnoff MF. Oral tolerance. Ann N Y Acad Sci 1982;392:248.
27. Walker WA. Host defense mechanisms in the gastrointestinal tract. Pediatrics 1976;57:901.
28. Edwards PAW. Is mucus a selective barrier for macromolecules? Br Med Bull 19;34:55.
29. Zubrzycki L, Spaulding EH. Studies on the stability of the normal fecal flora. J Bacteriol 1962;83:968.
30. Bartlett JG, Chang T, Taylor NS, Onderdonk AB. Colitis induced by *Clostridium difficile*. Rev Infect Dis 1979;1:370.
31. Rodgers VD, Fassett R, Kagnoff MF. Abnormalities in intestinal mucosal T cells in homosexual populations including those with the lymphadenopathy syndrome and acquired immunodeficiency syndrome. Gastroenterology 1986;90:552.
32. Ellakany S, Whiteside TL, Schade RR, van Thiel DH. Analysis of intestinal lymphocyte subpopulations in patients with acquired immunodeficiency syndrome (AIDS) and AIDS-related complex. Am J Clin Pathol 1987;87:356.
33. Budhraja M, Levandoglu H, Kocka F, Manghorn M, Sherer M. Duodenal mucosal T cell subpopulation and bacterial cultures in acquired immune deficiency syndrome. Am J Gastroenterol 1987;82:427.
34. Lim SG, Corder A, Lee CA, Johnson MA, Elia C, Poulter LW. Loss of mucosal CD4 lymphocytes is an early feature of HIV infection. Clin Exp Immunol 1993;92:448.
35. Clayton F, Reka S, Kotler DP. Preferential depletion of rectal lamina propria CD4+ lymphocytes. Abstract. Tenth International Conference on AIDS. 1994 (in press).
36. Kotler DP, Francisco A, Goldie P, Paderon H, Comer GM, Ramey WG. Preservation of natural killer cell phenotypes in rectal mucosa in AIDS. (Abstract) Gastroenterology 1985;88:1455A.
37. Bekesi JG, Tsang P, Lew F, Roboz JP, Teirstein A, Selikoff IJ. Functional integrity of T, B, and natural killer cells in homosexual subjects with prodromata and in patients with AIDS. Ann N Y Acad Sci 1984;437:28.
38. Schneider T, Ullrich R, Bergs C, Schmidt W, Riecken EO, Zeitz M. Abnormalities in subset distribution, activation and differentiation of T cells isolated from large intestine biopsies in HIV infection. Clin Exp Immunol 1994;95:430.
39. Lim SG, Condez A, Poulter LW. Mucosal macrophage subsets of the gut in HIV: decrease in antigen-presenting cell phenotype. Clin Exp Immunol 1993;92:442.
40. Weber JR, Dobbins WO. The intestinal and rectal epithelial lymphocyte in AIDS. Am J Surg Pathol 1986;10:627.
41. Ulrich R, Zeitz M, Heise W, et al. Mucosal atrophy is associated with loss of activated T cells in the duodenal mucosa of human immunodeficiency virus (HIV)-infected patients. Digestion 1990;46:302.
42. Kotler DP, Tierney AR, Scholes JV. Intestinal Plasma Cell alterations in the acquired immunodeficiency syndrome. Dig Dis Sci 1987;32:129.
43. Trajman A, Belo M, Oliviera A, Madi K, Elia C. Quantitative and qualitative changes in intestinal immunoglobulin-bearing plasma cell in jejunal mucosa of 52 HIV-infected patients. Braz J Med Biol Res 1994;27:1215.
44. Quesnal A, Moja P, Lucht F, Touraine JL, Pozzetto B, Genin C. Is there IgA of gut mucosal origin in the serum of HIV1 infected patients? Gut 1994;35:803.
45. Jackson S, Dawson LM, Kotler DP. IgA$_1$ is the major immunoglobulin component of immune complexes in the acquired immune deficiency syndrome. J Clin Immunol 1988;8:64.
46. Jackson S, Tarkowski A, Collins JE, Dawson LM, Schroheniher RE, Kotler DP, Koopman WJ. Occurrence of polymeric immunoglobulin A1 rheumatoid factor in the acquired immune deficiency syndrome. J Clin Immunol 1988;9:390.
47. Eriksson E, Kilander A, Hagberg L, Norkrans G, Holmgren J, Czerinsky C. Intestinal antibody responses to oral vaccination in HIV-infected individuals. AIDS 1993;7:1087.
48. Lewis DJM, Gilks CF, Ojoo S, et al. Immune response following oral administration of cholera toxin B subunit to HIV-1-infected UK and Kenyan subjects. AIDS 1994;8:779.
49. DiMassimo AM, Placido R, Bach S, Anastasi AM, Colizzi V, et al. Cytotoxic activity of intestinal lamina propria lymphocytes on human immunodeficiency virus (HIV) infected cells. Immunology 1992;76:117.
50. Fox CH, Kotler DP, Tierney AR, Wilson CS, Fauci AS. Detection of HIV-1 RNA in intestinal lamina propria of patients with AIDS and gastrointestinal disease. J Infect Dis 1989;159:467.
51. Harriman GR, Smith PD, McDonald KH, et al. Vitamin B$_{12}$ malabsorption in patients with the acquired immunodeficiency syndrome. Arch Intern Med 1989;149:2039.
52. Nelson JA, Wiley CA, Reynolds-Kohler C, et al. Human immunodeficiency virus detected in bowel epithelium from patients with gastrointestinal symptoms. Lancet 1988;2:259.
53. Mathijs JM, Hing M, Grierson J, Dwyer DE, et al. HIV infection of rectal mucosa. Lancet 1988;1:1111.
54. Bigornia E, Simon DE, Weiss LM, et al. Detection of HIV-1 protein and genomic sequences in enterochromaffin cells of HIV-1 seropositive patients. Am J Gastroenterol 1992;87:1624.
55. Jarry A, Cortez A, Rene E, et al. Infected cells and immune cells in the gastrointestinal tract of AIDS patients. An immunohistochemical study of 127 cases. Histopathology 1990;16:133.
56. Ullrich R, Zeitz M, Heise M, L'age M, Hoffken G, Rieken EO. Small intestinal structure and function in patients infected with human immunodeficiency virus (HIV): evidence for HIV-induced enteropathy. Ann Intern Med 1989;111:15.
57. Heise C, Dandekar S, Kumar P, Duplantier R, Donovan R, Halstead CH. Human immunodeficiency virus infection of enterocytes and mononuclear cells in human jejunal mucosa. Gastroenterology 1991;100:1521.
58. Moyer MP, Huot RI, Ramirez A Jr, Joe S, Meltzer MS, Gendelman HE. Infection of human gastrointestinal cells by HIV-1. AIDS Res Hum Retroviruses 1990;66:1409.
59. Adachi A, Koenig S, Gendelman HE, et al. Productive, persistent infection of human colorectal cell lines with human immunodeficiency virus. J Virol 1987;61:209.
60. Omary MB, Brenner DA, de Grandpre LY, Roebuck KA, Richman DR, Kagnoff MF. HIV-1 infection and expression in human colonic cells: infection and expression in CD4+ and CD4− cell lines. AIDS 1991;5:275.
61. Fantini J, Yahi N, Delezay O, Gonzalez-Scarano F. GalCer, CD26 and HIV infection of intestinal epithelial cells. AIDS 1994;8:1347.
62. Callebaut C, Krust B, Jacotot E, Hovanessian AG. T-cell activation antigen, CD26, as a cofactor for entry of HIV in CD4+ cells. Science 1993;262:2045.
63. Bourinbaiar AS, Phillip DM. Transmission of human immunodeficiency virus from monocytes to epithelia. J Acquir Immune Defic Syndr 1991;4:55.
64. Batman PA, Fleming SC, Sedgwick PM, MacDonald TT, Griffin GE. HIV infection of human fetal intestinal explant cultures induces epithelial cell proliferation. AIDS 1994;8:161.
65. Asmuth DM, Hammer SM, Wanke CA. Physiological effects of HIV infection on human intestinal epithelial cells: an in vitro model for HIV enteropathy. AIDS 1994;8:205.
66. Ullrich R, Heise W, Bergs C, L'Age M, Riecken E-O, Zeitz M. Effects of zidovudine treatment on the small intestinal mucosa in patients in-

fected with the human immunodeficiency virus. Gastroenterology 1992;102:1489.

67. Hoover EA, Mullins JI, Quackenbush SL, et al. Experimental transmission and pathogenesis of immunodeficiency syndrome in cats. Blood 1987;70:1880.

68. Stone JD, Heise CC, Miller CJ, Halsted CH, Dandekar S. Development of malabsorption and nutritional complications in simian immunodeficiency virus–infected rhesus macaques. AIDS 1994;8:1245.

69. Kodama T, Mori K, Kawahara T, Ringer DJ, Desroziers RC. Analysis of simian immunodeficiency virus sequence variation in tissues of rhesus macaques with simian AIDS. J Virol 1993;67:6522.

70. Clayton F, Reka S, Cronin WJ, Torlakovic E, Sigal SH, Kotler DP. Rectal mucosal pathology varies with human immunodeficiency virus antigen content and disease stage. Gastroenterology 1992;103:919.

71. Levendoglu H, Rosen Y. Nodular lymphoid hyperplasia of gut in HIV infection. Am J Gastroenterol 1992;87:1200.

72. Reka S, Kotler DP. Detection and localization of HIV RNA and TNF mRNA in rectal biopsies from patients with AIDS. Cytokine 1993;5:305.

73. Reka S, Garro ML, Kotler DP. Variation in the expression of HIV, RNA and cytokine mRNA in rectal mucosa during the progression of HIV infection. Lymphokine Cytokine Res 1994;13:391.

74. McGowan I, Radford-Smith G, Jewell DP. Cytokine gene expression in HIV-infected intestinal mucosa. AIDS 1994;8:1569.

75. Snijders F, van Deventer JH, Bartelsman JFW, et al. Diarrhea in HIV-infected patients: no evidence of cytokine-mediated inflammation in jejunal mucosa. AIDS 1995;9:367.

76. Reka S, Kotler DP. Apoptosis in rectal mucosa lamina propria: variation with disease stage. (Abstract) J Invest Med 1995;43:290A.

77. Groux H, Torpier G, Monte D, Mouton Y, Capron A, Ameisin JC. Activation-induced death by apoptosis in CD4+ T cells from HIV-infected asymptomatic individuals. J Exp Med 1992;175;331.

78. Hing M, Goldschmidt C, Mathijs JM, Cunningham AL, Cooper DA. Chronic colitis associated with human immunodeficiency virus infection. Med J Aust 1992;156:683.

79. Reichert CM, O'Leary TJ, Levens DL, et al. Autopsy pathology in the acquired immune deficiency syndrome. Am J Pathol 1983;112:357.

80. Drew WL, Mintz L, Miner RC, Sands M, Ketterer B. Prevalence of cytomegalovirus infection in homosexual men. J Infect Dis 1981;143:188.

81. Lange M, Klein EB, Kornfield H, et al. Cytomegalovirus isolation from healthy homosexual men. JAMA 1984;252:1908.

82. Goodgame RW, Genta RM, Estrada R, Demmler G, Buffone G. Frequency of positive tests for cytomegalovirus in AIDS patients: endoscopic lesions compared with normal mucosa. Am J Gastroenterol 1993;88:338.

83. Genta RM, Bleyzer I, Cate TR, Tandon AK, Yoffe B. In situ hybridization and immunohistochemical analysis of cytomegalovirus-associated ileal perforation. Gastroenterology 1993;104:1822.

84. Rotterdam H. Tissue diagnosis of selected AIDS-related opportunistic infections. Am J Surg Pathol 1987;11(Suppl):3.

85. Martin DC, Katzenstein DA, Yu GSM, et al. Cytomegalovirus viremia detected by molecular hybridization and electron microscopy. Ann Intern Med 1984;100:222.

86. Culpepper-Morgan J, Kotler DP, Tierney AR, Scholes JV. Evaluation of diagnostic criteria for disseminated cytomegalovirus infection in the acquired immune deficiency syndrome. Am J Gastroenterol 1987;82:1264.

87. Clayton F, Klein EB, Kotler DP. Correlation of in situ hybridization with histology and viral culture in AIDS patients with cytomegalovirus colitis. Arch Pathol Lab Med 1989;113:124.

88. Koretz SH, Buhles WC, Brewin A, et al. Treatment of serious cytomegalovirus infections using 9-(1,3-dihydroxy-2-propoxy-methyl) guanine in patients with AIDS and other immunodeficiencies. N Engl J Med 1986;314:801.

89. Dieterich DT, Kotler DP, Busch D, et al. Ganciclovir treatment of cytomegalovirus colitis in AIDS: a randomized, double-blind, placebo-controlled multicenter trial. J Infect Dis 1992;167:278.

90. Kotler DP, Tierney AR, Altilio D, Wang J, Pierson RN Jr. Body mass repletion during ganciclovir therapy of cytomegalovirus infections in patients with the acquired immunodeficiency syndrome. Arch Intern Med 1989;149:901.

91. Kotler DP, Culpepper-Morgan J, Tierney AR, Klein EB. Treatment of disseminated cytomegalovirus infection with 9-(1,3-dihydroxy-2-propoxymethyl) guanine: evidence of prolonged survival in patients

with the acquired immunodeficiency syndrome. AIDS Res 1987;2:299.

92. Dieterich DT, Chachoua A, Lafleur F, Worrell C. Ganciclovir treatment of gastrointestinal infections caused by cytomegalovirus in patients with AIDS. Rev Infect Dis Suppl 1988;10:S532.

93. Weber JN, Thom S, Barrison I, et al. Cytomegalovirus colitis and esophageal ulceration in the context of AIDS: clinical manifestations and preliminary report of treatment with foscarnet. Gut 1987;28:482.

94. Dieterich DT, Poles M, Dicker M, Tepper R, Lew E. Foscarnet treatment of cytomegalovirus gastrointestinal infections in acquired immunodeficiency syndrome patients who have failed ganciclovir induction. Am J Gastroenterol 1993;88:542.

95. Snydman DR, Werner BG, Heinze-Lacey B, et al. Use of cytomegalovirus immune globulin to prevent cytomegalovirus disease in renal-transplant recipients. N Engl J Med 1987;317:1049.

96. Siegel FP, Lopez C, Hammer GS, et al. Severe acquired immunodeficiency in male homosexuals manifested by chronic perianal ulcerative herpes simplex lesions. N Engl J Med 1981;305:1439.

97. Wasselle JA, Sedgwick JH, Dawson PJ, Fabri PJ. Intestinal herpes simplex infection presenting with intestinal perforation. Am J Gastroenterol 1992;87:1475.

98. Cirillo NW, Lyon DT, Schuller AM. Tracheoesophageal fistula complicating herpes esophagitis in AIDS. Am J Gastroenterol 1993;88:587.

99. Sixbey JW, Nedrud JG, Raab-Traub N, Hanes RA, Pagano JS. Epstein-Barr virus replication in oropharyngeal epithelial cells. N Engl J Med 1984;310:1225.

100. Lipscomb H, Tatsumi E, Harada S, et al. Epstein-Barr virus and chronic lymphadenomegaly in male homosexuals with acquired immunodeficiency syndrome (AIDS). AIDS Res 1983;1:59.

101. Greenspan JS, Greenspan D, Lennette ET, et al. Replication of Epstein-Barr virus within the epithelial cells of oral "hairy" leukoplakia, an AIDS-associated lesion. N Engl J Med 1985;313:1564.

102. Knowles DN, Inghirami G, Ubriaco A, Della-Favera R. Molecular genetic analysis of three AIDS-associated neoplasms of uncertain lineage demonstrates their B-cell derivation and the possible pathogenetic role of Epstein-Barr virus. Blood 1989;73:792.

103. Horowitz MS, Valdarrama G, Hatcher V, et al. Characteristics of adenovirus isolates from AIDS patients. Ann N Y Acad Sci 1984;437:161.

104. Janoff EN, Orenstein JM, Manischewitz JF, Smith PD. Adenovirus colitis in the acquired immunodeficiency syndrome. Gastroenterology 1991;100:976.

105. Grohmann GS, Glass RI, Pereira HG, et al. Enteric viruses and diarrhea in HIV-infected patients. N Engl J Med 1993;329:14.

106. Sewankambo N, Mugerwa RD, Godgame RD, et al. Enteropathic AIDS in Uganda. An endoscopic, histologic and microbiologic study. AIDS 1987;1:9.

107. Serwadda D, Mugerwa RD, Sewankambo NK, et al. Slim disease: a new disease in Uganda and its association with HTLV-III infection. Lancet 1985;2:849.

108. Current WL, Reese NC, Ernst JV, et al. Human cryptosporidiosis in immunocompetent and immunodeficient persons: studies of an outbreak and experimental transmission. N Engl J Med 1985;308:1252.

109. Unger BLP, Soave R, Fayer R, Nash TE. Enzyme immunoassay detection of immunoglobulin M and G antibodies to *Cryptosporidium* in immunocompetent and immunocompromised persons. J Infect Dis 1986;153:570.

110. Jokiph L, Jokiph AMM. Timing of symptoms and oocyst excretion in human cryptosporidiosis. N Engl J Med 1986;315:1643.

111. Zar F, Geiseler PJ, Brown VA. Asymptomatic carriage of Cryptosporidium in the stool of a patient with acquired immunodeficiency syndrome. J Infect Dis 1985;151:195.

112. Alpert G, Bell LM, Kirkpatrick CE, et al. Outbreak of cryptosporidiosis in a day-care center. Pediatrics 1986;77:152.

113. Genta RM, Chappell CL, White AC, Kimball KT, Goodgame RW. Duodenal morphology and intensity of infection in AIDS-related intestinal cryptosporidiosis. Gastroenterology 1993;105:1769.

114. Flanigan T, Whalen C, Turner J, Soave R, Havlir D, Kotler DP. *Cryptosporidium* infection and CD4 counts. Ann Intern Med 1992;116:840.

115. Greenberg R, Bank S, Siegal FP. Resolution of intestinal cryptosporidiosis after treatment of AIDS with AZT. Gastroenterology 1989;97:1327.

116. Cozon G, Biron F, Jeannin M, Cannella D, Revillard J-P. Secretory IgA antibodies to *Cryptosporidium parvum* in AIDS patients with chronic cryptosporidiosis. J Infect Dis 1994;169:696.
117. Tzipori S, Angus KW, Campbell I, Grey EW. *Cryptosporidium*: evidence for a single-species genus. Infect Immun 1980;30:884.
118. Tzipori S, Angus KW, Campbell I, et al. Experimental infection of lambs with *Cryptosporidium* isolated from a human patient with diarrhoea. Gut 1982;23:71.
119. Sloper KS, Dourmashkin RR, Bird RB, et al. Case report: chronic malabsorption due to cryptosporidiosis in a child with immunoglobulin deficiency. Gut 1982;23:80.
120. Snider DP, Gordon J, McDermott MR, Underdown BJ. Chronic *Giardia muris* infection in anti-IgM-treated mice. I. Analysis of immunoglobulin and parasite-specific antibody in normal and immunoglobulin-deficient animals. J Immunol 1985;134:4153.
121. Thea DM, Pereira MEA, Sterling C, Kotler DP, Keusch GT. Isolation and partial purification of a lectin on the surface of the sporozoite of *Cryptosporidium*. J Parasitol 1992;78:886.
122. Marcial MA, Madara JL. *Cryptosporidium* localization, structural analysis of absorptive cell-parasite membrane interactions in guinea pigs, and suggestion of protozoan transport by M cells. Gastroenterology 1986;90:583.
123. Clayton FC, Heller TH, Reka S, Kotler DP. Variation in the distribution of cryptosporidiosis in AIDS. Am J Clin Pathol 1994;102:420.
124. Cello JP. Acquired immunodeficiency syndrome cholangiopathy: spectrum of disease. Am J Med 1989;86:539.
125. Giang TT, Pollack G, Kotler DP. Cryptosporidiosis of the nasal mucosa in a patient with AIDS. AIDS 1994;8:555.
126. Gross TL, Wheat J, Bartlett M, O'Connor KW. AIDS and multiple system involvement with cryptosporidium. Am J Gastroenterol 1986;81:456.
127. Ma P, Villanueva TG, Kaufman D, et al. Respiratory cryptosporidiosis in acquired immune deficiency syndrome. JAMA 1984;252:1298.
128. Casemore DP, Armstrong M, Sands RL. Laboratory diagnosis of cryptosporidiosis. J Clin Pathol 1985;38:1337.
129. Tzipori S, Roberton D, Chapman C. Remission of diarrhoea due to cryptosporidiosis in an immunodeficient child treated with hyperimmune bovine colostrum. Br Med J 1986;293:1276.
130. Ungar BLP, Ward DJ, Fayer R, Quinn CA. Cessation of *Cryptosporidium*-associated diarrhea in an acquired immunodeficiency syndrome patient after treatment with hyperimmune bovine colostrum. Gastroenterology 1990;98:486.
131. Nord J, Ma P, DiJohn D, Tzipori S, Tacket CO. Treatment with bovine hyperimmune colostrum of cryptosporidial diarrhea in AIDS patients. AIDS 1990;4:581.
132. White AC, Chappell CL, Hayat CS, Kimball KT, Flanigan TP, Goodgame RW. Paromomycin for cryptosporidiosis in AIDS: a prospective double-blind trial. J Infect Dis 1994;170:419.
133. Guarino A, Canani RB, Pazio E, Terracciano L, Albano F, Mazzeo M. Enteroxic effect of stool supernatant of *Cryptosporidium*-infected calves on human jejunum. Gastroenterology 1994;106:28.
134. Simon DM, Cello JP, Valenzuela J, et al. Multicenter trial of octreotide in patients with refractory acquired immunodeficiency syndrome-associated diarrhea. Gastroenterology 1995;108:1753.
135. Garcia Compean D, Jimenez JR, De La Garza FG, et al. Octreotide therapy of large volume refractory AIDS-associated diarrhea: a randomized controlled trial. AIDS 1994;8:1563.
136. Canning EU, Lom J. The microsporidia of vertebrates. New York: Academic Press, 1986.
137. Dobbins WO III, Weinstein WM. Electron microscopy of the intestine and rectum in acquired immunodeficiency syndrome. Gastroenterology 1985;88:738.
138. Orenstein JM, Chiang J, Steinberg W, Smith P, Rotterdam H, Kotler DP. Intestinal microsporidiosis as a cause of diarrhea in HIV-infected patients: a report of 20 cases. Hum Pathol 1990;21:475.
139. Canning EU, Hollister WS. Microsporidia of mammals—widespread pathogens or opportunistic curiosities? Parasitol Today 1987;3:267.
140. Canning EU, Hollister WS. *Enterocytozoon bieneusi* (Microspora): prevalence and pathogenicity in AIDS patients. Trans R Soc Trop Med 1990;84:181.
141. Orenstein JM, Dieterich DT, Kotler DP. Systemic dissemination by a newly recognized microsporidia species in the acquired immunodeficiency syndrome. AIDS 1992;6:1143.
142. Kotler DP, Orenstein JM, Prevalence of intestinal microsporidiosis in HIV-infected individuals for gastroenterological evaluation. Am J Gastroenterol 1994;89:1998.
143. Kotler DP, Francisco A, Clayton F, Scholes J, Orenstein JM. Small intestinal injury and parasitic disease in AIDS. Ann Intern Med 1990;113:444.
144. Greenson J, Belitsos P, Yardley J, Bartlett J. AIDS enteropathy: occult enteric infections and duodenal mucosal alterations in chronic diarrhea. Ann Intern Med 1991;114:366.
145. Swenson J, MacLean JD, Kokoskin-Nelson E, Szabo J, Lough J, Gill MJ. Microsporidiosis in AIDS patients. Can Commun Dis Rep 1993;19:13.
146. Cotte L, Rabodonirina M, Piens A, Perreard M, Mofon M, Trepo C. Prevalence of intestinal protozoans in French patients infected with HIV. J Acquir Immune Defic Syndr 1993;6:1024.
147. Molina JM, Sarfati C, Beauvais B, et al. Intestinal microsporidiosis in human immunodeficiency virus-infected patients with chronic unexplained diarrhea: prevalence and clinical and biologic features. J Infect Dis 1993;167:217.
148. Rabeneck L, Gyorkey F, Genta R, Gyorkey P, Foote L, Risser JMH. The role of microsporidia in the pathogenesis of HIV-related chronic diarrhea. Ann Intern Med 1993;119:895.
149. Sandfort J, Hannamen A, Stark D, Gelderblom H, Rof B. *Enterocytozoon bieneusi* in a patient not infected with HIV. Presented at Microsporidiosis and Cryptosporidiosis in Immunodeficient Patients meeting, Ceska Budejovice, Czech Republic, September 29–October 1, 1993.
150. Rabeneck L, Genta RM, Gyorkey F, Clarridge JE, Gyorkey P, Foote LW. Observations on the pathological spectrum and clinical course of microsporidiosis in men infected with the human immunodeficiency virus: follow-up study. Clin Infect Dis 1995;20:1229.
151. Eeftinck Schattenkerk JKM, van Gool T, van Ketel RJ, et al. Clinical significance of small-intestinal microsporidiosis in HIV-1 infected individuals. Lancet 1991;337:895.
152. Kotler DP, Reka S, Chow K, Orenstein JM. Effects of enteric parasitoses and HIV infection upon small intestinal structure and function in patients with AIDS. J Clin Gastroenterol 1993;16:10.
153. Orenstein JM, Tenner M, Kotler DP. Localization of infection by the microsporidian *Enterocytozoon bieneusi* in the gastrointestinal tract of AIDS patients with diarrhea. AIDS 1992;6:195.
154. Gourley WK, Swedo JL. Intestinal infection by microsporidia *Enterocytozoon bieneusi* of patients with AIDS: an ultrastructural study of the use of human mitochondria by a protozoan. (Abstract) Lab Invest 1988;58:35A.
155. Pol S, Romana CA, Richard S, Amouyal P, Desportes-Livage I, Carnot F, Pays JF, Berthelot P. Microsporidia infection in patients with human immunodeficiency virus and unexplained cholangitis. N Engl J Med 1993;328:95.
156. van Gool J, Hollister JS, Eeftinck Schattenkerk J, et al. Diagnosis of *Enterocytozoon bieneusi* microsporidiosis in AIDS patients by recovery of spores from faeces. Lancet 1990;336:697.
157. Orenstein JM, Zierdt W, Zierdt C, Kotler DP. Identification of microsporidial spores in stool and duodenal fluid from AIDS patients. Lancet 1990;336:1127.
158. Weber R, Bryan RT, Owen RL, Wilcox CM, Gorelkin L, Visvesvara GS. Improved light-microscopical detection of microsporidia spores in stool and duodenal aspirates. N Engl J Med 1992;326:161.
159. Bryan RT, Weber R, Stewart JM, Angritt P, Visvesvara GS. New manifestations and simplified diagnosis of human microsporidiosis. Am J Trop Med Hyg 1991;45:133.
160. Zhu X, Wittner M, Tanowitz H, Kotler DP, Cali A, Weiss LM. Small subunit rRNA sequence of *Enterocytozoon bieneusi* and its potential diagnostic role with use of the polymerase chain reaction. J Infect Dis 1993;168:1570.
161. Dieterich DT, Lew E, Kotler DP, Poles M, Orenstein JM. Treatment with albendazole for intestinal disease due to *Enterocytozoon bieneusi* in patients with AIDS. J Infect Dis 1994;169:173.
162. Orenstein JM, Dieterich DT, Kotler DP. Albendazole as a treatment for disseminated microsporidiosis due to *Septata intestinalis* in AIDS patients. AIDS 1993;7(Suppl 3):S40.
163. Malebranche R, Arnoux E, Guerin JM, et al. Acquired immunodeficiency syndrome with severe gastrointestinal manifestations in Haiti. Lancet 1983;1:873.

164. DeHovitz JA, Pape JW, Boncy M, Johnson WD Jr. Clinical manifestation of *Isospora belli* infection in patients with the acquired immunodeficiency syndrome. N Engl J Med 1986;315:87.

165. Soave R, Johnson WD Jr. Cryptosporidium and *Isospora belli* infections. J Infect Dis 1988;157:225.

166. Restropo C, Macher AM, Radany EH. Disseminated extraintestinal isosporiasis in a patient with acquired immunodeficiency syndrome. Am J Clin Pathol 1987;87:536.

167. Benator DA, French AL, Beaudet LM, Levy CS, Orenstein JM. *Isospora belli* infection associated with acalculous cholecystitis in a patient with AIDS. Ann Intern Med 1994;121:663.

168. Kazal HL, Sohn N, Carasco JI, Robilotti JS Jr, Delaney WE. The gay bowel syndrome: clinico-pathological correlations in 260 patients. Ann Clin Lab Sci 1976;6:184.

169. Nash TE, Agrawal A, Adam RD, Conrad JT, Merritt JW Jr. Antigenic variation in *Giardia lamblia*. J Immunol 1988;141:636.

170. Stevens D, Frank D, Mahmoud AAF. Thymus dependency of host resistance to *Giardia muris* infection in nude mice. J Immunol 1978;120:680.

171. Janoff EN, Smith PD, Blaser MJ. Acute antibody responses to *Giardia lamblia* are depressed in patients with human immunodeficiency virus-1 infection. J Infect Dis 1988;157:798.

172. Schmerin MJ, Gelston A, Jones TC. Amebiasis. An increasing problem among homosexuals in New York City. JAMA 1977;238:1386.

173. Allason-Jones E, Mindel A, Sargeaunt P, Williams P. *Entamoeba histolytica* as a commensal parasite in homosexual men. N Engl J Med 1986;315:353.

174. Maayan S, Wormser GP, Widerhorn J, Sy ER, Kim YH, Ernst JA. *Strongyloides stercoralis* hyperinfection in a patient with the acquired immunodeficiency syndrome. Am J Med 1987;83:945.

175. Ortega YR, Sterling CR, Gilman RH, Cama VA, Diaz F. Cyclospora species—a new protozoan pathogen of humans. N Engl J Med 1993;328:1308.

176. Russo AR, Stone SL, Taplin ME, et al. Presumptive evidence for *Blastocystis hominis* as a cause of colitis. Arch Intern Med 1988;148:1064.

177. Young LS, Interlied CB, Berlin OG, Gottlieb MS. Mycobacterial infections in AIDS patients, with an emphasis on the *Mycobacterium avium* complex. Rev Infect Dis 1986;8:1024.

178. Goslee S, Wolinsky E. Water as a source of potentially pathogenic mycobacteria. Am Rev Respir Dis 1976;113:287.

179. Murray HW, Rubin BY, Masur H, Roberts RB. Impaired production of lymphokines and immune (gamma) interferon in the acquired immunodeficiency syndrome. N Engl J Med 1984;310:883.

180. Roth RI, Owen RL, Keren DF, Volberding PA. Intestinal infection with *Mycobacterium avium* in acquired immunodeficiency syndrome (AIDS): histological and clinical comparison with Whipple's disease. Dig Dis Sci 1985;30:497.

181. Cappell MS, Hassan T, Rosenthal S, Mascarenhas M. Gastrointestinal obstruction due to *Mycobacterium avium-intracellulare* associated with the acquired immunodeficiency syndrome. Am J Gastroenterol 1992;87:1823.

182. Friedberg KA, Draguesku JO, Kiyabu M, Valenzuela JE. Intestinal perforation due to *Mycobacterium tuberculosis* in HIV-infected individuals: report of two cases. Am J Gastroenterol 1993;88:604.

183. Wong B, Edwards FF, Kiehn TE, et al. Continuous high-grade *Mycobacterium avium-intracellulare* bacteremia in patients with the acquired immune deficiency syndrome. Am J Med 1985;78:35.

184. Havlik JA, Metchock B, Thompson SE, Barrett K, Rimland D, Horsburgh CR. A prospective evaluation of *Mycobacterium avium* complex colonization of the respiratory and gastrointestinal tracts of persons with human immunodeficiency virus infection. J Infect Dis 1993;168:1045.

185. Chiu J, Nussbaum J, Bozzette S, et al. Treatment of disseminated *Mycobacterium avium* complex infection in AIDS with amikacin, ethambutol, rifampin and ciprofloxacin. Ann Intern Med 1990;113:358.

186. Agins BD, Berman DS, Spicehandler D, El-Sadr W, Simberkoff MS, Rahal JJ. Effect of combined therapy with ansomycin, clofazimine, ethambutol, and isoniazid for *Mycobacterium avium* infection in patients with AIDS. J Infect Dis 1989;159:784.

187. Hirschel B, Chang HR, Mach N, et al Fatal infection with a novel, unidentified *Mycobacterium* in a man with the acquired immunodeficiency syndrome. N Engl J Med 1990;323:109.

188. Wang HH, Tollerud D, Danar D, et al. Another Whipple-like disease in AIDS? N Engl J Med 1986;314:1577.

189. Relman DA, Schmidt TM, MacDermott RP, Falkow S. Identification of the uncultured bacillus of Whipple's disease. N Engl J Med 1992;327:293.

190. Smith PD, Macher AM, Bookman MA, et al. *Salmonella typhimurium* enteritis and bacteremia in the acquired immunodeficiency syndrome. Ann Intern Med 1985;102:207.

191. Baskin DH, Lax JD, Barenberg D. *Shigella* bacteremia in patients with acquired immune deficiency. Am J Gastroenterol 1987;82:338.

192. Pasternak J, Bolivar R, Hopfer RL, et al. Bacteremia caused by *Campylobacter*-like organisms in two male homosexuals. Ann Intern Med 1984;101:339.

193. Nelson MR, Shanson DC, Hawkind DA, Gazzard BG. *Salmonella, Campylobacter*, and *Shigella* in HIV-seropositive patients. AIDS 1992;6:1495.

194. Laughon BE, Druckman DA, Vernon A, et al. Prevalence of enteric pathogens in homosexual men with and without acquired immunodeficiency syndrome. Gastroenterology 1988;94:984.

195. Lake-Bakaar G, Quadros E, Beidas S, et al. Gastric secretory failure in patients with the acquired immunodeficiency syndrome (AIDS) Ann Intern Med 1988;1:502.

196. Hornick RB, Musik SI, Wenzel R, et al. The Broad St. pump revisited: response of volunteers to ingested cholera vibrios. Bull N Y Acad Med 1971;47:1181.

197. Easmon CSF, Crane JP. Uptake of ciprofloxacin by macrophages. J Clin Pathol 1985;38:442.

198. Neill MA, Opal SM, Heelan J, et al. Failure of ciprofloxacin to eradicate convalescent fecal excretion after acute salmonellosis: experience during an outbreak in health care workers. Ann Intern Med 1991;114:195.

199. Hutin Y, Molina JM, Casin I, et al. Risk factors for *Clostridium difficile*-associated diarrhoea in HIV-infected patients. AIDS 1993;7:1441.

200. Lu SS, Schwartz JM, Simon DM, Brandt LJ. *Clostridium difficile*-associated diarrhea in patients with HIV infection: a prospective controlled study. Am J Gastroenterol 1994;89:1226.

201. Kotler DP, Orenstein JM. Diarrhea and malabsorption due to enterocyte-adherent bacterial infection in a patient with AIDS. Ann Intern Med 1993;119:127.

202. Kotler DP, Giang TT, Thiim M, Nataro JP, Sordillo EM, Orenstein JM. Chronic bacterial enteropathy in patients with AIDS. J Infect Dis 1995;171:552.

203. Orenstein JM, Kotler DP. Diarrheagenic bacterial enteritis in AIDS: a light and electron microscopic study. Hum Pathol 1995;26:481.

204. Mayer HB, Wanke CA. Enteroaggregative *Escherichia coli* as a possible cause of diarrhea in an HIV-infected patient. (Letter) N Engl J Med 1995;332:273.

205. Thea DM, St Louis ME, Atido U, et al. A prospective study of diarrhea and HIV-1 infection among 429 Zairian infants. N Engl J Med 1993;329:1696.

206. Pavia AT, Long EG, Ryder RW, et al. Diarrhea among African children born to human immunodeficiency virus 1-infected mothers: clinical, microbiologic and epidemiologic features. Pediatr Infect Dis 1992;11:996.

207. Nataro JP, Kaper JB, Levine MM. Plasmid-mediated factors conferring diffuse and localized adherence of enteropathogenic *Escherichia coli*. Infect Immun 1985;48:378.

208. Klein RS, Harris CA, Small CB, et al. Oral candidiasis in high risk patients as the initial manifestation of the acquired immunodeficiency syndrome. N Engl J Med 1984;311:354.

209. Tom W, Aaron J. Esophageal ulcers caused by *Torulopsis glabrata* in a patient with AIDS. Am J Gastroenterol 1987;82:766.

210. Johnson PC, Khardorf N, Najjar AF, Butt F, Mansell PW, Sarosi GA. Progressive disseminated histoplasmosis in patients with acquired immunodeficiency syndrome. Am J Med 1988;85:152.

211. Bronnimann DA, Adam RD, Galgiani JN, et al. Coccidioidomycosis in the acquired immunodeficiency syndrome. Ann Intern Med 1987;106:372.

212. Poles MA, McMeeking AA, Scholes JV, Dieterich DT. Actinomyces infection of a cytomegalovirus esophageal ulcer in two patients with acquired immunodeficiency syndrome. Am J Gastroenterol 1994;89:1569.

213. Dieterich DT, Lew EA, Bacon DJ, Pearlman KI, Scholes JV. Gastrointestinal pneumocystosis in HIV-infected patients on aerosolized pentamidine: report of five cases and literature review. Am J Gastroenterol 1992;87:1763.
214. Friedman-Kien AE, Laubenstein LJ, Marmor M, et al. Kaposi's sarcoma and *Pneumocystis carinii* pneumonia among homosexual men—New York and California. MMWR 1981;30:250.
215. Beral V, Peterman TA, Berkelman RL, et al. Kaposi's sarcoma among persons with AIDS: a sexually transmitted infection? Lancet 1990;335:123.
216. Chang Y, Cesarman E, Pessin MS, Lee F, Culpepper J, Knowles DM, Moore PS. Identification of herpesvirus-like DNA sequences in AIDS-associated Kaposi's sarcoma. Science 1994;266:1865.
217. Saltz RK, Kurtz RC, Lightdale CJ. Kaposi's sarcoma: gastrointestinal involvement and correlation with skin findings and immunologic function. Dig Dis Sci 1984;29:817.
218. Friedman SL, Wright TL, Altman DF. Gastrointestinal Kaposi's sarcoma in patients with acquired immunodeficiency syndrome: endoscopic and autopsy findings. Gastroenterology 1985;98:102.
219. Winkler WP, Kotler DP, McCray RS. Nd:YAG laser palliation of Kaposi's sarcoma. (Abstract) Gastroenterol Endosc 1989;35:98A.
220. Ziegler JL, Beckstead JA, Volberding PA, et al: non-Hodgkin's lymphoma in 90 homosexual men: relation to generalized lymphadenopathy and the acquired immunodeficiency syndrome. N Engl J Med 1984;311:565.
221. Harper ME, Kaplan MH, Marsell LM, et al. Concomitant infection with HTLV-I and HTLV-III in a patient with T8 lymphoproliferative disease. N Engl J Med 1987;315:1073.
222. Farman J, Tavitian A, Rosenthal LE, Schwartz GE, Raufman JP. Focal esophageal candidiasis in acquired immunodeficiency syndrome (AIDS). Gastrointest Radiol 1986;11:213.
223. Rosario MT, Raso CL, Comer GM, Clain DJ. Transnasal brush cytology for the diagnosis of *Candida* esophagitis in the acquired immunodeficiency syndrome. Gastrointest Endosc 1989;35:102.
224. Laine L, Dretler RH, Conteas CN, et al. Fluconazole compared with ketoconazole for the treatment of *Candida* esophagitis in AIDS. Ann Intern Med 1992;117:655.
225. Baily GG, Perry FM, Denning DW, Mandal BK. Fluconazole-resistant candidosis in an HIV cohort. AIDS 1994;8:787.
226. Lake-Bakaar G, Tom W, Lake-Bekaar D, et al. Gastropathy and ketoconazole malabsorption in the acquired immunodeficiency syndrome. Ann Intern Med 1988;109:471.
227. Alessi E, Berti E, Cusini M, et al. Oral hairy leukoplakia. J Am Acad Dermatol 1990;22:79.
228. Newman C, Polk F. Resolution of oral hairy leukoplakia during therapy with 9-(1,3-dihydroxy-2-propoxymethyl) guanine (DHPG). Ann Intern Med 1987;107:348.
229. Winkler JR, Murray PA. Periodontal disease, a potential oral expression of AIDS may be a rapidly progressive periodontitis. Calif Dent Assoc J 1987;15:20.
230. Laguna F, Garcia-Samaniego J, Alonso MJ, Alvarez I, Gonzalez-Lahoz JM. Pseudotumoral appearance of cytomegalovirus esophagitis and gastritis in AIDS patients. Am J Gastroenterol 1993;88:1108.
231. Kotler DP, Wilson CS, Haroutounian G, Fox CH. Detection of HIV-1 RNA in solitary esophageal ulcers in two patients with the acquired immunodeficiency syndrome. Am J Gastroenterol 1989;84:313.
232. Kotler DP, Reka S, Orenstein JM, Fox CF. Chronic idiopathic esophageal ulceration in the acquired immunodeficiency syndrome: characterization and treatment with corticosteroids. J Clin Gastroenterol 1992;15:284.
233. Rabenek L, Boyko WJ, McLean DM, McLeod WA, Wong KK. Unusual esophageal ulcers containing enveloped virus-like particles in homosexual men. Gastroenterology 1986;90:1881.
234. Wilcox CM, Schwartz DA, Coffield I, Zaki SR. Evaluation of idiopathic esophageal ulcers (IEU) for human immunodeficiency virus (HIV) by polymerase chain reaction (PCR): is HIV an esophageal pathogen? (Abstract) Gastroenterology 1992;1–2:A712.
235. Kitchen VS, Helbert M, Francis MD, et al. Epstein-Barr virus-associated oesophageal ulcers in AIDS. Gut 1990;31:1223.
236. Bach MC, Howell DA, Valenti AJ, Smith TJ, Winslow DL. Aphthous ulceration of the gastrointestinal tract in patients with the acquired immunodeficiency syndrome. Ann Intern Med 1990;112:465.
237. Dretler RH, Rausher DB. Giant esophageal ulcer healed with steroid therapy in an AIDS patient. Rev Infect Dis 1989;11:768.
238. Wilcox CM, Schwartz DA. A pilot study of oral corticosteroid therapy for idiopathic esophageal ulcerations associated with human immunodeficiency virus infection. Am J Med 1992;93:131.
239. Wilcox CM, Schwartz DA. Comparison of two corticosteroid regimens for the treatment of HIV-associated idiopathic esophageal ulcer. Am J Gastroenterol 1994;89:2163.
240. Tracey KJ, Wei H, Manogue KR. Cachectin/tumor necrosis factor induces cachexia, anemia and inflammation. J Exp Med 1988;167:1211.
241. Fong Y, Moldawer LL, Marono M, et al (1989): Cachectin/TNF or IL-1 alpha induces cachexia with redistribution of body proteins. Am J Physiol 256:R659.
242. Sclafani A, Koopmans HS, Vasselli J, Reivhman M. Effects of intestinal bypass surgery on appetite, food intake, and body weight in obese and lean rats. Am J Physiol 1978;234:E389.
243. Marano BJ, Smith F, Bonanno CA. *Helicobacter pylori* prevalence in acquired immunodeficiency syndrome. Am J Gastroenterol 1993;88:687.
244. Herzlich BC, Schiano TD, Moussa Z, Zimbalist E, Panagopoulos G, Nawabi I. Decreased intrinsic factor secretion in AIDS: relation to parietal cell acid secretory capacity and vitamin B_{12} malabsorption. Am J Gastroenterol 1992;87:1781.
245. Shaffer RT, LaHatte LJ, Kelly JW, et al. Gastric acid secretion in HIV-1 infection. Am J Gastroenterol 1992;87:1777.
246. May GR, Gill MJ, Church DL, Sutherland LR. Gastrointestinal symptoms in ambulatory HIV-infected subjects. Dig Dis Sci 1993;38:1388.
247. Hoover DR, Saah AJ, Bacellar H, et al. Signs and symptoms of "asymptomatic" HIV-1 infection in homosexual men. J Acquir Immune Defic Syndr 19936:66.
248. Smith PD, Lane C, Gill VJ, et al. Intestinal infections in patients with acquired immunodeficiency syndrome (AIDS). Ann Intern Med 1988;108:328.
249. Gillin JS, Shike M, Alcock N, et al. Malabsorption and mucosal abnormalities of the small intestine in the acquired immunodeficiency syndrome. Ann Intern Med 1985;102:619.
250. Batman PA, Miller AR, Forster SM, Harris JR, Pinching AJ, Griffin GE. Jejunal enteropathy associated with human immunodeficiency virus infection: quantitative histology. J Clin Pathol 1989;42:275.
251. Griffin GE, Miller A, Batman P, et al. Damage to jejunal intrinsic autonomic nerves in HIV infection. AIDS 1988;2:379.
252. Cummings AG, LaBrooy JT, Stanley DP, et al. Quantitative histologic study of enteropathy associated with HIV infection. Gut 1990;31:317.
253. Mathan MM, Griffin GE, Miller A, et al. Ultrastructure of the jejunal mucosa in human immunodeficiency virus infection. J Pathol 1990;161:119.
254. Kotler DP, Gaetz HP, Klein EB, Lange M, Holt PR. Enteropathy associated with the acquired immunodeficiency syndrome. Ann Intern Med 1984;101:421.
255. Quinones-Galvan A, Lifshitz-Guinzberg A, Ruiz-Arguelles GJ. Gluten-free diet for AIDS-associated enteropathy. Ann Intern Med 1990;113:806.
256. Kotler DP, Tierney AR, Wang J, Pierson RN Jr. Effect of home total parenteral nutrition on body composition in AIDS. J Parenter Enteral Nutr 1990;14:454.
257. Chatis PA, Miller CH, Schrager LE, Crumpacker CS. Successful treatment with foscarnet of an acyclovir-resistant mucocutaneous infection with herpes simplex virus in a patient with acquired immunodeficiency syndrome. N Engl J Med 1989;320:297.
258. Simonsen JN, Cameron W, Galinya MN, et al. Human immunodeficiency virus infection among men with sexually transmitted disease. N Engl J Med 1988;319:274.
259. Hicks CB, Benson PM, Lupton GP, Tramont EC. Seronegative secondary syphilis in a patient infected with the human immunodeficiency virus (HIV) with Kaposi sarcoma. Ann Intern Med 1987;107:492.
260. Sulaiman MZ, Foster J, Pugh SF. Prevalence of *Chlamydia trachomatis* infection in homosexual men. Genitourin Med 1987;63:179.
261. Jones JM, Miller JN, George WL. Microbiological and biochemical characterization of spirochetes isolated from the feces of homosexual males. J Clin Microbiol 1986;24:1071.
262. Penn I. Cancers of the anogenital region in renal transplant recipients. Cancer 1986;58:611.
263. Palefsky JM, Holly EA, Gonzales J, Lamborn K, Hollander H. Natural history of anal cytologic abnormalities and papillomavirus infection among homosexual men with group IV HIV disease. J Acquir Immune Defic Syndr 1992;5:1258.

264. DePalo G, Rilke F, Zur Hausen H, eds. Herpes and papilloma viruses: their role in the carcinogenesis of the lower genital tract, vol 2. New York: Raven Press, 1988.

265. Frazer IH, Medley G, Crapper RM, Brown TC, Mackay IR. Association between anorectal dysplasia, human papilloma virus and human immunodeficiency virus infection in homosexual men. Lancet 1986;2:657.

266. Cooper HS, Patchefsky AJ, Marks G. Cloacogenic carcinoma of the anorectum in homosexual men: an observation of four cases Dis Colon Rectum 1979;22:557.

267. Parente F, Cernuschi M, Valsecchi L, Musicco M, Lazzarin A, Bianchi Porro G. Acute upper gastrointestinal bleeding in patients with AIDS: a relatively uncommon condition associated with reduced survival. J Br Soc Gastroenterol 1991;32:987.

268. Cappell MS, Geller AJ. The high mortality of gastrointestinal bleeding in HIV-seropositive patients: a multivariate analysis of risk factors and warning signs of mortality in 50 consecutive patients. Am J Gastroenterol 1992;87:815.

269. Frank D, Raicht RF. Intestinal perforation associated with cytomegalovirus infection in patients with acquired immune deficiency syndrome. Am J Gastroenterol 1984;79:201.

270. Biggs BA, Crow SM, Lucas CR, et al. AIDS related Kaposi's sarcoma presenting as ulcerative colitis and complicated by toxic megacolon. Gut 1987;28:1302.

271. Kuhlman JE, Fishman EK. Acute abdomen in AIDS: CT diagnosis and triage. Radiographics 1990;10:621.

272. Scannell KA. Surgery and human immunodeficiency virus disease. J Acquir Immune Defic Syndr 1989;2:43.

273. Robinson G, Wilson SE, Williams RA. Surgery in patients with acquired immunodeficiency syndrome. Arch Surg 1987;122:170.

274. Wexner SD, Smithy WB, Milsom JW, Dailey TH. The surgical management of anorectal diseases in AIDS and pre-AIDS patients. Dis Colon Rectum 1986;29:719.

275. Schneider PA, Abrams DI, Rayner AA, Hohn DC. Immunodeficiency associated thrombocytopenic purpura. Arch Surg 1987;122:1175.

276. Martin P, DiBisceglie AM, Kassianides C, et al. Rapidly progressive non-A non-B hepatitis in patients with human immunodeficiency virus infection. Gastroenterology 1989;97:1559.

277. Soloman RE, Kaslow RA, Phair JP, et al. Human immunodeficiency virus and hepatitis delta virus in homosexual men: a study of four cohorts. Ann Intern Med 1988;108:51.

278. Hagopian WA, Huseby JS. *Pneumocystis* hepatitis and choroiditis despite successful aerosolized pulmonary prophylaxis. Chest 1989;96:949.

279. Terada S, Reddy R, Jeffers LJ, Cali A, Schiff ER. Microsporidian hepatitis in the acquired immunodeficiency syndrome. Ann Intern Med 1987;107:61.

280. Czapar CA, Weldon-Linne CM, Moore DM, Rhone DP. Peliosis hepatitis in the acquired immunodeficiency syndrome. Arch Pathol Lab Med 1986;110:611.

281. Perkocha LA, Geahan SM, Benedict Yen TS, et al. Clinical and pathological features of Bacillary peliosis hepatitis in association with HIV infection. N Engl J Med 1990;323:1581.

282. Adal KA, Cockrell CJ, Petri WA. Cat scratch disease, bacillary angiomatosis and other infections due to *Rochalimaea*. N Engl J Med 1994;330:1509.

283. Benhamou Y, Caumes E, Gerosa Y, et al. AIDS-related cholangiopathy: critical analysis of a prospective series of 26 patients. Dig Dis Sci 1993;38:1113.

284. Schwartz MS, Brandt LJ. The spectrum of pancreatic disorders in patients with the acquired immunodeficiency syndrome. Am J Gastroenterol 1989;84:459.

285. Bouchard P, Sai P, Reach G, et al. Diabetes mellitus following pentamidine-induced hypoglycemia in humans. Diabetes 1982;31:40.

286. Kapembwa MS, Fleming SC, Griffin GE, Caun K, Pinching AJ, Harris JRW. Fat absorption and exocrine pancreatic function in human immunodeficiency virus infection. Q J Med 1990;74:49.

AIDS: Biology, Diagnosis, Treatment and Prevention, fourth edition, edited by Vincent T. DeVita, Jr., Samuel Hellman, and Steven A. Rosenberg. Lippincott–Raven Publishers, © 1997

CHAPTER 19 Noninfectious Organ-Specific Complications of HIV Infection

19.1 Dermatologic Complications of HIV Infection

Bijan Safai

The cutaneous manifestations of human immunodeficiency virus (HIV) infection are extensive, encompassing malignancies (eg, Kaposi's sarcoma, lymphoma), a variety of bacterial, viral, and fungal infections, and noninfectious complications. This chapter considers the noninfectious cutaneous manifestations of HIV infection.

The noninfectious cutaneous disorders are numerous (Table 19.1-1) and may occur in all stages of HIV infection. Subtle findings, such as dry skin or telangiectasias, or severe reactions, such as an exacerbation of psoriasis or extensive seborrheic dermatitis, may be the first clues to the presence of HIV infection. As HIV infection progresses, these conditions occur with greater frequency and severity.[1,2]

Although none of the disorders reported in this group have been linked directly to an infectious agent, these conditions may result in part from an abnormal host response to infectious agents other than HIV.

SEBORRHEIC DERMATITIS

Seborrheic dermatitis is a common skin condition characterized by erythematous, scaly patches of skin. It is most often seen in the malar region, nasolabial fold, eyebrows, scalp, chest, and behind the ears. The prevalence of seborrheic dermatitis in the general population is reported to be 3%.[3] Among HIV-infected persons, the prevalence of seborrheic dermatitis ranges from 7% to 50%,[4-9] making this dermatitis the most common noninfectious skin disorder associated with HIV.

Features of HIV-Associated Seborrheic Dermatitis

The incidence and the severity of HIV-associated seborrheic dermatitis are closely related to the stage of HIV infection

Bijan Safai, Department of Dermatology, New York Medical College, Valhalla, NY 10595.

and, as a result, are inversely correlated with the absolute CD4+ helper T cells.[7] In a larger series,[10] the incidence of seborrheic dermatitis was reported to be 4.7% for patients classified as Walter Reed stage 1, with an upward rise to 26.7% for those with stage 6 disease. In another report,[11] seborrheic dermatitis was seen in 15 (83%) of 18 patients with acquired immunodeficiency syndrome (AIDS) and in 5 (42%) of 12 patients with AIDS-related complex (ARC), and it was more severe in the former group.

Most cases of HIV-associated seborrheic dermatitis have an ordinary clinical presentation. However, atypical features such as thick greasy scales on the scalp and face and involvement of the axillae, groin, genitalia, and perianal areas have been described.[11,12] Histologically, HIV-associated seborrheic dermatitis is usually identical to non-HIV–infected cases, although distinct features such as parakeratosis, keratinocyte necrosis, lymphoid clusters at the dermoepidermal junction, and a perivascular plasma cell infiltrate have been reported.[13]

Etiology

The cause of seborrheic dermatitis in persons with or without HIV infection remains unclear. The incidence of seborrheic dermatitis is increased in many neurologic disorders such as Parkinson's disease, epilepsy, poststroke encephalopathy, and central nervous system (CNS) malignancies.[11-14] Seborrheic dermatitis occurs with greater frequency in patients with AIDS-associated dementia.[15] A dysfunction in neurohormonal regulation with increased sebum production has been proposed to explain the association of seborrheic dermatitis and neurologic disorders.

The yeast-line fungus *Pityrosporum* (*P ovale, P orbiculare*), commonly found on the skin, is thought to play a role in the pathogenesis of seborrheic dermatitis. In one series,[13] excessive *Pityrosporum* organisms were found in only a

TABLE 19.1-1. *Noninfectious cutaneous manifestations of HIV infection in nine groups of patients*

Characteristics	Affected Patients								
	1[7]*	2[4]	3[2]	4[5]	5[10]	6[142]	7[11]	8[6]	9[173]
Total patients	222	117	150	100	516	1124	30	59	40
Cutaneous finding	N (%)	N (%)	N (%)	N (%)	N (%)	N (%)	N (%)	N (%)	N (%)
Seborrheic dermatosis	11 (5)	37 (32)	28 (19)	49 (49)	41 (8)	122 (11)	30 (67)	21 (36)	
Xerosis and asteatosis	11 (5)		6 (4)	23 (23)					
Xerosis and ichthyosis		36 (31)							
Ichthyosis	3 (1)								
Psoriasis	3 (1)	1 (1)	5 (3)	5 (5)					
Papular eruption		2 (2)			12 (2)	22 (2)			
Telangiectasia	2 (1)								25 (62)
Yellow nails		10 (9)				12 (1)			
Erythroderma	2 (1)								
Hair disease			2 (1)						
Drug rash						22 (2)			

*Refers to text reference number.

minority of biopsy specimens from AIDS patients with seborrheic dermatitis. However, in another study,[16] a correlation between the severity of clinical disease and the number of *Pityrosporum* organisms was observed on Giemsa-stained smears. Two patients treated with a 2% concentration of ketoconazole, a topical antifungal agent, exhibited rapid clearing and a reduction in the number of *Pityrosporum* organisms per keratinocyte. Additional evidence suggesting a role for *Pityrosporum* in seborrheic dermatitis comes from a report in which 22% of patients taking oral ketoconazole had seborrheic dermatitis, compared with 36% of those not using the drug.[4] However, the absence of pityrospora in many other HIV-associated seborrheic dermatitis cases suggests that *Pityrosporum* yeasts are not the cause of seborrheic dermatitis but that their presence may aggravate this common skin condition.

Treatment

Seborrheic dermatitis is much more difficult to treat in patients with HIV infection than in non-HIV–infected individuals. There is a poor response to topical corticosteroids and other conventional modalities. In one series, topical ketoconazole was helpful in 25% of cases.[7] In general, as the condition of the patient worsens, the seborrheic dermatitis becomes more severe and refractory to treatment. Skin care and a combination of topical corticosteroids and topical imidazoles have been helpful in controlling seborrheic dermatitis.

PSORIASIS

Psoriasis is a common skin disorder seen in 1% to 2% of the general population and affecting persons of both sexes and all ages. Available data do not indicate an increased prevalence of psoriasis among HIV-infected individuals. In a series of more than 1000 HIV-infected individuals, psoriasis was found only in 13 (1%).[17] Another report described psoriasis in 8 (2%) of 400 patients.[7] However, in smaller series, a prevalence of 3% to 5% has been reported.[2,5,12] Psoriatic arthritis appears to be more prevalent among HIV-infected individuals (1.7%) than non-HIV–infected persons (0.5%).[18]

Features of HIV-Associated Psoriasis

Although the prevalence of psoriasis in HIV-seropositive persons is similar to that in the general population, there appears to be a strong correlation between the initial onset of psoriasis and HIV infection. Psoriasis has been reported as the first clinical manifestation of HIV infection,[4,7] and the development of eruptive psoriasis or a sudden exacerbation of preexisting disease in any person at risk of HIV should suggest the possibility of HIV infection.[17,19] More commonly, psoriasis is first noticed at some point after HIV seroconversion.[17,19,20] Psoriasis is reported to become more severe as the degree of immunodeficiency increases.[21]

The clinical features of psoriasis in HIV-infected individuals are often atypical. The lesions may be guttate (similar to the lesions characteristic of a psoriatic flair associated with streptococcal infection) and may appear on the groin, axillae, scalp, palms, and soles. Severe onychodystrophy and palmar or plantar keratoderma are often seen. Extensive exfoliative psoriasis with generalized erythroderma has also been reported.[17]

The histopathology of psoriasis in HIV-infected persons is different to some degree from those of HIV-negative individuals. Features such as fewer Monro's abscesses (ie, accumulation of pyknotic neutrophil nuclei within the epidermis), irregular acanthosis, slight spongiosis, and less suprapapillary thinning of the epidermis are reported to be more characteristic of HIV-associated psoriasis. A moderate perivascular and diffuse mononuclear infiltrate that may contain abundant macrophage and occasional multinucleated giant cells is also observed.[15] There are fewer T cells but significantly higher numbers of plasma cells in the dermal infiltrates of HIV-infected individuals.[22] This histologic appearance may also share features of HIV-associated seborrheic dermatitis. In one study, all 13 AIDS patients with psoriasis also had seborrheic dermatitis. The investigators concluded that, rather than representing two distinct entities, there is a spectrum of disease, with seborrheic dermatitis being the least and psoriasis the most severe presentation.[17] HIV RNA transcripts have been demonstrated in 5 of 15 psoriatic lesions by the in situ hybridization technique; HIV RNA transcripts have not been found in normal-appearing skin of HIV-positive patients with psoriasis or in psoriatic skin of normal control.[23]

In other study interferon-γ has been shown to stimulate monocyte-macrophages to produce and release large amounts of neopterin, which is decreased after cyclosporine treatment of psoriasis. HIV-positive patients have increased levels of serum interferonγ, suggesting its possible role in the pathogenesis of HIV-associated psoriasis.[24]

Etiology

It is likely that HIV-associated psoriasis shares features with common psoriasis, in which there is a genetically influenced host response. Human leukocyte antigen (HLA) loci studies indicate an association of HLA class I molecules (eg, HLA-B13, -Bw16, -Bw17, -Bw37) and psoriasis. CD8+ suppressor T cells can interact with cells bearing class I molecules, but CD4+ T cells are restricted to interactions with cells bearing HLA class I molecules. This suggests an interaction between CD8+ cells and a putative psoriatic antigen and may in part account for the onset and severity of psoriasis in HIV infection, in which there is usually a predominance of CD8+ cells.[25] Peripheral arthritis has been reported in 32% of HIV-infected men and correlated with the presence of HLA-B27.[26] HLA-CV6 and other major histocompatibility antigens associated with psoriasis are less commonly found in patients developing the psoriasis of HIV infection.[27]

It is also possible that the T-cell stimulation and increased cytokine activity seen in HIV infection may play a role in the pathogenesis of HIV-associated psoriasis. For example, increased levels of interferon-α and interferon-γ have been reported in patients with AIDS,[24,28–30] and both cytokines have been shown to exacerbate psoriasis.[31,32]

Streptococcal infections may influence the development of psoriasis in HIV-infected persons. It is well documented that streptococcal pharyngitis can trigger the onset of guttate psoriasis, and monoclonal antibodies to streptococcal antigens have been found to cross-react with skin antigens.[33] In one series, 5 of 13 AIDS patients with psoriasis had skin or throat cultures that were positive for streptococcal infection.[17] Multiple courses of antibiotic therapy, however, have produced little or no improvement. Complete remission occurred for a group of patients treated with trimethoprim-sulfamethoxazole (TMP-SMX).[28]

Treatment

Most therapeutic modalities used in the treatment of severe forms of psoriasis have immunosuppressive effects, including ultraviolet light B (UVB), psoralen plus ultraviolet light A (PUVA), corticosteroids, methotrexate, and cyclosporine.[17,19,34,35] The use of methotrexate in the first reported cases of HIV-associated psoriasis led to worsening immune function and poor outcomes and is contraindicated for this group of patients. Phototherapy has been effective in the treatment of psoriasis, but it exacerbates Kaposi's sarcoma in some HIV-infected persons.[17] Conventional treatments such as tar and topical corticosteroids have been largely ineffective.

Zidovudine has successfully treated the psoriasis of some patients with HIV infection.[17,36–38] In all cases, the condition relapsed after the medication was discontinued.[35,37] The mechanism of action of zidovudine in these cases is unknown, but it is postulated that the drug may act against a putative psoriasis retrovirus.[13] Limited disease usually responds well to routine topical therapy, including topical tar, anthralin, and corticosteroids. Extensive disease responds to UVB and PUVA therapy. The fear of HIV activation and the possible immunosuppressive effects of phototherapy remain.[34,39] In a small study, 5 patients were treated with PUVA for two courses each of 4 weeks, spaced 2 months apart. These cases are reported to have remained stable, with no sign of progression of HIV.[35] Cyclosporine, although immunosuppressive, has been successfully used in the treatment of psoriatic arthritis and severe skin psoriasis.[40]

The retinoid etretinate, which does not affect the immune system, may be useful in treating some psoriatic cases.[17] Cimetidine has been effective for resistant forms of psoriasis.[41,42] In some patients with advanced HIV disease, the psoriasis has disappeared completely.[42,43]

REITER'S SYNDROME

Reiter's syndrome consists of the classic triad of urethritis, conjunctivitis, and an additive oligoarticular arthritis, involving mainly the large joints of the lower extremity. The skin manifestations include keratoderma blennorrhagica (ie, acral, pustular, keratotic lesions with onychodystrophy), circinate balanitis, and painless oral ulcers.[17]

Reiter's syndrome is more prevalent among patients with HIV infection than the general population.[44–47] In a series of 101 patients with AIDS, 10 persons were found to have Reiter's syndrome.[45] Reiter's syndrome has been reported in 1.7% to 10% of HIV-infected individuals, compared with a prevalence of 0.06% among healthy men 20 to 29 years of age.[44,45,48] The onset of Reiter's syndrome occurs before or at the same time when symptoms of HIV infection appear. Articular symptoms may be the first manifestation of HIV infection and can precede the onset of immunodeficiency by 14 months. Joint involvement is characterized predominantly by severe, persistent arthritis involving primarily one large joint of the lower extremities and occasionally the sacroiliac joint.[45]

Features of HIV-Associated Reiter's Syndrome

Organisms known to trigger Reiter's syndrome are rarely identified in HIV-infected persons.[44] HLA-B27 has been reported in 15 (71%) of 21 persons with HIV-associated complete or incomplete Reiter's syndrome. Considerable overlaps exist among Reiter's syndrome, psoriatic arthritis, and psoriasis.[26,49]

In a review of 36 patients with Reiter's syndrome and HIV infection, nine had keratoderma blennorrhagica.[45] However, keratoderma is also seen in AIDS-associated psoriasis and acquired ichthyosis without any accompanying arthritic symptoms.[7] The differential diagnosis also includes syphilis and *Trichophyton rubrum* infection, which can produce a similar clinical picture.

Treatment

As with the treatment of psoriasis in patients with HIV infection, immunosuppressive therapies for Reiter's syndrome were associated with increased morbidity.[19,44] There is also a poor response to conventional therapy. The use of oral etretinate and topical corticosteroids has been described as an effective treatment for the arthropathy and the cutaneous lesions of Reiter's syndrome in HIV-associated cases.[50,51]

ACQUIRED ICHTHYOSIS

Acquired ichthyosis has been associated with a number of conditions, such as lymphoma, carcinoma, classic Kaposi's sarcoma, leprosy, and sarcoidosis.[4,52] In patients with HIV infection, acquired ichthyosis has been described as severe and involving the lower extremities.[4,15] Acquired ichthyosis is reported in 23% to 30% of HIV-infected patients.[4,53,54] It may be related to malnutrition, poor hygiene, immunologic deficit, or chronic illness. The prevalence or the severity of acquired ichthyosis does not correlate with the degree of immune suppression, and the association is assumed to be more complex and perhaps not directly related to the HIV infection.[52,55] Treatment has focused on controlling symptoms with the use of keratolytic agents such as lactic acid and urea compounds.[15]

PORPHYRIA CUTANEA TARDA

Porphyria cutanea tarda (PCT), although rare, is the most common of the porphyric diseases. The defect in porphyrin metabolism is a decrease in hepatic uroporphyrin decarboxylase activity, which leads to an increase in metabolic precursors.[56] Clinical manifestations consist of cutaneous photosensitivity as the major symptom, facial hypertrichosis, and generalized hyperpigmentation. Lesions are typically found on sun-exposed areas of skin and range from small white plaques to fluid-filled vesicles and bullae that may erode and heal slowly.

Features of HIV-Associated Porphyria Cutanea Tarda

Several reports[56-69] strongly suggest a close association between HIV infection and the development of porphyria cutanea tarda. Two brothers with hemophilia developed porphyria cutanea tarda shortly after they became HIV seropositive.[57] In 8 of 9 other cases, the symptoms of porphyria cutanea tarda heralded a rapid progression to AIDS.[56,58-61] Clinical presentation of PCT may occur before the diagnosis or later in the course of the HIV infection.[62,63] The onset of skin manifestations of PCT usually coincides with deterioration of the immune function.[64] Urinary excretion of increased levels of porphyrin was reported for patient with HIV infection.[65,66] Underlying liver dysfunction associated with alcohol ingestion or hepatitis B virus infection may affect the porphyrin metabolism.[67]

Although PCT and HIV may coexist by chance, the increasing incidence of this disorder among HIV-infected individuals suggests that HIV or an associated factor triggers the development of PCT in predisposed cases.[68,69] The role of HIV infection in the development of porphyria cutanea tarda remains unclear. However, the close temporal association between HIV infection and the onset of porphyric symptoms suggests a cause and effect association. Viral hepatitis, alcohol ingestion, use of certain drugs, and altered hormonal metabolism are known to exacerbate porphyria cutanea tarda. An increase in estrogens, observed in some patients with HIV infection, has been proposed as one possible factor.[56]

Abnormal porphyrin metabolism has been demonstrated in patients with HIV infection.[60] It is speculated that anemia, commonly seen in HIV infection, can lead to an upregulation of porphyrin biosynthesis. A correlation was made between immune activation, as measured by increased urine neopterin levels, and increased levels of urinary porphyrin and its precursors. Further investigation is needed to clarify the relation between HIV infection and porphyria cutanea tarda.

Treatment

Avoidance of ultraviolet light is the most simple and effective therapeutic modality. Phlebotomy has led to improvement of skin lesions in three cases,[51,60] but this therapy has obvious limitations in patients with HIV disease. The antimalarial Plaquenil (hydroxychloroquine sulfate) was used in one patient without benefit.[58]

ACUTE AND CHRONIC PHOTOSENSITIVITY

Increased photosensitivity has been observed in patients with HIV infection. It may result in increased pigmentation, especially in black patients. Two similar case reports describe HIV-seropositive patients who developed severe generalized erythroderma, which began in sun-exposed areas. In neither case was a photosensitizing agent identified.[70,71] Another report describes a patient with HIV infection and extreme sensitivity to UVB who developed granuloma annular restricted to sun-exposed areas.[72]

Lichenoid photodermatitis has been observed in patients with HIV infection. Blacks are disproportionately affected.[73] Several light-induced pathologic changes in skin have been observed among HIV-infected person.[74]

The relation between HIV infection and the photosensitivity reaction appears to be more than conjectural and requires further investigation. It is speculated that an immune response to certain photoproducts may cause the generalized reactions described in these cases.

PAPULAR AND FOLLICULAR ERUPTIONS IN HIV INFECTION

Several reports have described papular and follicular eruptions in patients with HIV infection, but because of the lack of uniformity in the terminology used, it is uncertain whether the conditions described represent distinct clinical entities or a spectrum of one disease process. In most instances, these eruptions are clinically and histologically nonspecific.[75] The shared features include pruritus; localization of the eruption to the head and neck, upper trunk, and proximal extremities; a perivascular or perifollicular inflammatory infiltrate; a noninfectious cause; and difficulty in treating the condition effectively. However, some conditions may respond to topical antipruritic, topical corticosteroids, and UV light treatment. These conditions include acute and chronic papular eruption, chronic follicular eruption (including HIV-associated eosinophilic folliculitis), pruritus, and prurigo nodularis.

Papular Eruptions

Transient maculopapular eruptions occur most frequently on the face and trunk and usually heals within 4 to 6 weeks. Histologically, a lymphoplasmacytic angiitis is repeatedly observed in many of these cases. In a series of 219 HIV-positive cases, 41 (12.2%) were reported to have transient papular eruptions.[76]

A more chronic eruption, often pruritic, has also been described among patients with AIDS and ARC.[4,77,78] The eruption consists of multiple, discrete, 2- to 5-mm skin-colored papules distributed over the head, neck, and upper truck. The histologic features are nonspecific. No correlation has been found between the severity of the eruption and the stage of HIV infection.

A chronic papulofollicular eruption also occurs in HIV-infected individuals. The eruption consists of follicular papules, usually occurring on the limbs and trunk. A perifollicular neutrophilic infiltrate has been observed histologically. No evidence of bacterial or fungal elements has been reported. Treatment with antibiotics has not been effective.[1,10,79]

Eosinophilic Pustular Folliculitis

Eosinophilic pustular folliculitis is a chronic pruritic, culture-negative folliculitis that is unresponsive to systemic antibiotic therapy.[80] It is a rare disorder, which is being observed with increased frequency in patients with HIV infection.[80–84] The eruption is characterized by multiple urticarial, pruritic, follicular papules, 1 to 4 mm in diameter and scattered on the trunk, face, neck, and proximal extremities. The papules may coalesce to form erythematous plaques. The main histologic feature is a neutrophilic and eosinophilic infiltrate of the hair follicle.[80,83,84]

In addition to the previously reported cases of HIV-associated eosinophilic pustular folliculitis, one report used to term HIV-associated eosinophilic folliculitis to describe the same condition in 13 additional patients.[80] Of all the patients described in these reports, 19 had AIDS at the time of onset and 3 had ARC. In one study, eosinophilic pustular folliculitis was associated with CD4+ counts less than 250 to 300/mm^3, making the entity a manifestation of late-stage HIV infection.[80] A relatively peripheral eosinophilia (>6%) was seen in 15 of the 19 reported HIV associated cases. An elevated serum IgE level has also been reported.[80] Leukocytosis has been observed in some of these cases. The differential diagnosis most commonly includes acne vulgaris, rosacea, and staphylococcal folliculitis.

Etiology

The cause of these disorders remains obscure. One group of researchers postulated that the eruption might represent an aberrant immunologic response to common skin antigens such as a dermatophyte or the mite *Demodex folliculorum*, which has been seen in histologic sections of eosinophilic pustular folliculitis.[83] No other pathogens have been found despite multiple cultures and serologic tests.[80,83]

Treatment

Topical corticosteroids have been largely palliative in controlling these conditions. The size and number of lesions, as well as the pruritus, decreased in six patients treated with UVB phototherapy.[84] However, the condition recurred on discontinuation of the treatment. The use of the antihistamines astemizole and cetirizine has been moderately effective in some cases.[80,85]

Other Pruritic Eruptions

Other papular eruptions have been described in HIV-infected individuals, but nonspecific clinical and histologic features prevent definitive diagnosis.[76,86–89]

Pruritus without skin eruptions frequently occurs in HIV-infected individuals on the extensor surfaces of the arms before it becomes widespread.[90] In some cases, pruritus is the first sign of HIV infection. Pruritus and prurigo nodularis are mostly seen in Haitians and in patients with AIDS in Central Africa.

Inflammatory follicular and pruritic papules may be secondary to a severe reaction to insect bites[91] or caused by a localized *Staphylococcus aureus* infection.[92]

HIV-ASSOCIATED AUTOIMMUNE AND HYPERIMMUNE CONDITIONS

Sicca Syndrome

Sicca syndrome has been seen in HIV-infected persons, but it seems to be different from Sjögren's syndrome, because most cases are men with different HLA types, have no autoantibodies, and show inflammatory infiltrates of salivary glands.[93]

Vitiligo

Vitiligo has been associated with HIV infections. It is, however, unclear whether it is caused by the autoantibodies produced as a result of HIV infection or it is unrelated to HIV.[94]

Bullous Pemphigoid

Bullous pemphigoid has been associated with HIV infection. Patients present with severe pruritus and antibodies to the basement membrane zone of skin.[95,96]

Other forms of blistering skin disorders have also been reported in HIV patients.[97] Vesiculopustular eruption has been the first manifestation of primary HIV infection.[98] Antinuclear antibodies and some of the clinical features of systemic lupus erythematosus (SLE) may been seen in HIV-infected persons, but true SLE has not been reported.[99,100]

Atopic Dermatitis

Atopic dermatitis may be exacerbated by HIV infection.[102] Dermatosis associated with markedly elevated serum IgE concentrations has responded to zidovudine treatment.[102]

Thrombocytopenic Purpura

Thrombocytopenic purpura is one of the most common autoimmune phenomenon observed in HIV patients and may be the presenting sign of HIV infection.[103] It is characterized by bruising, nonpalpable petechia and hemorrhage.[104,105]

Cutaneous Leukocytoclastic Vasculitis and Polyarteritis Nodosa

Cutaneous leukocytoclastic vasculitis has been associated with HIV infection.[106-110] It is unknown whether HIV is the primary antigen causing vasculitis[111] or some other antigen such as cytomegalovirus (CMV) is responsible. HIV antigen has not been isolated from the vasculitic tissue infiltrates.[112] Polyarthritis nodosa[113] and erythema elavatum diatinum have been reported in the HIV setting.[114]

Other Autoimmune and Hyperimmune Conditions

Erythema multiforme, Stevens-Johnson syndrome, and toxic epidermal necrolysis have been reported in HIV-infected individuals.[115-118] In most cases, the etiologic agent is drugs, not just HIV infection alone. Erythema multiform has been the primary HIV-related symptom at the time of seroconversion.[118]

INTERFACE DERMATITIS

Interface dermatitis is a histologic entity showing vacuolization and necrosis of basal keratinocytes and a dense inflammatory infiltrate at the dermoepidermal junction. This entity is thought to be specific to HIV disease and clinically may manifest as maculopapular eruptions, erythroderma, blister formation, or erythema multiform.[119]

ERYTHRODERMA

Erythroderma is a rare condition among HIV-infected individuals. It is usually caused by an exacerbation of other skin disorders, such as atopic dermatitis, hyper eosinophilic syndrome, psoriasis, photosensitive dermatitis, and cutaneous T-cell lymphoma.[120-124]

PITYRIASIS RUBRA PILARIS

Pityriasis rubra pilaris (PRP) has been reported with increasing frequency among HIV-infected individuals.[125-129] In some cases, rapid clearing has been observed after zidovudine therapy.[127-131] Patients have presented with follicular papules with elongated spines and comedo-like lesions.[125] Most patients simultaneously developed severe cystic acne (ie, acne conglobata).[126-128] The lesions are located on the back, flanks, and proximal extremities.

Orthokeratotic plugs and perifollicular mucinous degeneration have been seen on histologic examination.[125] One case of PRP has been reported in a HIV-positive child. It is thought that PRP and acne conglobata occur in a more virulent form in HIV-infected persons.

SKIN CHANGES IN HIV-ASSOCIATED NUTRITIONAL DISORDERS

HIV-associated weight loss and skin changes usually results from malabsorption or enterocolitis, producing wasting and the so-called slim disease of Africa.

GRANULOMA ANNULAR

Granuloma annular is characterized by erythematous or flesh-colored papules seen in an annular ring-shaped grouping. Although there have been a number of reported cases,[132-135] it is difficult to make a strong association with HIV infection, because granuloma annular is a common dermatosis. In an HIV-infected patient, granuloma annular disappeared after 4 weeks of zidovudine therapy.[134] This suggests a possible association between the development of granuloma annular and HIV infection or the resulting immune dysfunction. In two other cases, the absolute number of helper T cells was 40 and 72, evidence of severe cellular immune impairment.[133,134]

Localized and generalized granuloma annular conditions have been observed in HIV patients. However, the duration was just a few months. Perforating granuloma annular[133] and reactive perforating collagenosis have also been reported.[136]

Sometimes, the atypical generalized form of granuloma annular is clinically indistinguishable from the papular eruption of AIDS and from the HIV-associated lichenoid granulomatous papular dermatosis.[137,138] Skin biopsy and histologic examination may be helpful in differentiating these entities. The histology of granuloma annular in HIV-infected cases is similar to that in non-HIV–infected cases, showing a focally altered collagen surrounded by a palisading granuloma. However, suppressor T cells are seen in AIDS-associated granuloma annular, in contrast to the helper T-cell infiltrate in non-HIV–infected cases.[133]

NAILS AND HAIR CHANGES

Yellow discoloration of the nails (not associated with any infectious agent) is reported among persons with advanced HIV infection and *Pneumocystis carinii* pneumonia.[139] In one report, 4 of 8 patients had yellow discoloration of the distal portion of the nails,[139] and in another report, 10 of 117 patients had yellow nail syndrome. The yellow nail syndrome was initially described in association with pulmonary disease and lymphedema.

Although referred to as yellow nail syndrome, the cases described in HIV-infected persons may not fulfill the diagnostic criteria for yellow nail syndrome, which includes the absence of cuticles and a distinctive onychodystrophy.[140,141] Many conditions other than HIV infection, such as diabetes, drugs reactions, and the use of zidovudine and nail polish, can cause a yellow discoloration of the nail plate.

Numerous abnormalities of the hair, from alopecia to hypertrichosis, have been reported in patients with HIV infection.[142,143] A diffuse thinning of the hair may be the most common abnormality observed.[144] In some cases, an underlying inflammatory cell infiltrate of the scalp has been reported.[145]

For at least 50% of the black patients with AIDS, hair curl is lost, and the scalp hair gradually straightens. In one case, the hair changes were noticed 6 months before the diagnosis of AIDS.[146] Sudden premature graying is also seen.[147] Elongation of eyelashes may result from increased levels of prolactin.

ADVERSE CUTANEOUS DRUG REACTIONS

The incidence of adverse skin drug reactions is very high in HIV disease. Many drugs, especially antimicrobial agents, cause reactions in AIDS patients. These drugs singly or in combination cause skin eruptions.[148] The pathogenesis of this increased incidence is not understood, but immunodeficiency and underlying infection, such as with CMV or Epstein-Barr virus (EBV), may play a role. Reactivity to

ampicillin and amoxicillin is mostly reported in patients with primary EBV or CMV mononucleosis.[149]

Trimethoprim-Sulfamethoxazole and Other Sulfonamides

TMP-SMX is the combination drug choice for the prophylaxis and treatment of *Pneumocystis carinii* pneumonia. Sulfonamides are also most effective therapy for prophylaxis and treatment of CNS toxoplasmosis. Intravenous use of TMP-SMX caused exanthematous eruptions in 50% to 60% of HIV-infected patients. The eruptions appeared 1 to 2 weeks after the start of therapy.[150,151]

Desensitization has been successful for TMP-SMX, dapsone, and sulfadiazine.[152–156] The recommended prophylactic treatment for *Pneumocystis carinii* pneumonia includes daily low-dose TMP-SMX, weekly sulfadoxine-pyrimethamine (eg, Fansidar), and monthly aerosolized pentamidine. Pentamidine can cause maculopapular, pruritic skin eruptions in one fifth of the treated HIV-infected patients.[157] Fansidar is known to cause erythema multiform and toxic epidermal necrolysis.[158] These drugs are reported to cause severe erythema multiform and toxic epidermal necrolysis.[159,160] Fourteen of the 80 reported cases of toxic epidermal necrolysis from France were HIV positive and had taken sulfa drugs.[161] A mortality rate of 21% was reported for these 14 cases.

The likelihood of toxic effects from this drug is much higher in patients with HIV infection than in background populations. Skin eruptions, the most common toxic manifestation, were reported in 18 of 35 patients with AIDS who were treated with high doses of the drug (trimethoprim, 20 mg/kg/day), a frequency 10 times higher than for non-AIDS patients.[150] The eruption has been described as a generalized erythematous, maculopapular rash occurring 8 to 12 days into treatment. Fever is often associated with the rash. Six patients with AIDS taking standard doses of a sulfonamide developed toxic epidermal necrolysis. The patients recovered after discontinuation of the medication. All patients had fever and mucosal lesions.[142]

Zidovudine

Patients taking zidovudine have had increased pigmentation of the fingernails and toenails, resulting in a bluish discoloration.[162] The discoloration progressed distally, starting at the base of the fingernail. This side effect was most commonly seen in patients receiving high-dose zidovudine (1200 mg/day). The nail changes consisted of a longitudinal, brown-black streak of hyperpigmentation in the nail plate in almost 40% of zidovudine-treated cases.[163] This is more common in blacks than Caucasian or Latino patients; it was noticed 4 to 8 weeks after starting the drug. The hyperpigmentation is caused by increased melanogenesis in the nail matrix.[164] Longitudinal nail dyschromia is reported in HIV patients independent of zidovudine therapy.[165]

Hypertrichosis and increased growth of eyelashes have occurred in zidovudine-treated patients,[166,167] as well as in some persons never exposed to drugs.[168,169] Other reactions to zidovudine include acne, urticaria, hyperpigmentation, vasculitis, and pruritus.[106]

Foscarnet (trisodium phosphonoformate) is reported to cause painful penile ulcers in almost 30% of HIV-positive CMV retinitis patients within 8 to 12 weeks after starting high doses of the drug.[170] Methotrexate and corticosteroids used for the treatment of HIV-associated psoriasis, vasculitis, and non-Hodgkin's lymphoma have caused the sudden appearance and proliferation of Kaposi's sarcoma.[171]

Systemic reactions to zidovudine have been observed in HIV-infected persons. These include fever, leukopenia, thrombocytopenia, hepatitis, and nephritis.[172] The decision to discontinue a given drug usually depends on the severity of the adverse reactions, the indication for the treatment, and available alternative choices. In some cases, the eruption subsides while treatment is continued.

Glucan-Induced Keratoderma

Glucan is an oligosaccharide derived from the inner cell wall of the yeast *Saccharomyces cerevisiae,* and it is used as an immune system stimulant. Keratoderma has been reported in 6 of 20 patients with AIDS or ARC who were treated with this immunostimulant. Thick, yellow hyperkeratosis of the palms and soles, with fissuring of the skin, developed during the first 2 weeks of therapy. The condition is symmetric and resolves over 2 to 4 weeks after treatment. There were no pustules or nail changes suggestive of the keratoderma blennorrhagica that is seen in HIV-associated psoriasis or Reiter's syndrome.[173] The mechanism of this unusual reaction to the yeast antigen is unknown.

BANAL SKIN FINDINGS IN HIV-INFECTED PATIENTS

Along with the severe cutaneous manifestations, a few mild cutaneous signs and symptoms are commonly reported in patients with HIV infection.

Xerosis

Dry and cracking skin (ie, erosis and steatosis) is reported in some of the large series.[5,7] The dry skin is often pruritic. Antihistamines are ineffective in controlling the pruritus,[15] and the treatment should be directed toward the underlying xerosis.

Telangiectasia

Although not frequently reported in the larger series, telangiectasia has been observed in HIV-infected individuals.[174] Linear telangiectasias of the anterior chest were reported in one study[175] to occur in 25 (62%) of 40 HIV-seropositive homo-

sexual men. The incidence increased as the stage of HIV infection advanced. Histologic studies showed dilated vessels and a perivascular infiltrate. The anterior chest telangiectasia described was thought to be distinct from the condition in any other disease. No cause has been identified, but a disregulation of hormonal metabolism may be involved.

MISCELLANEOUS CONDITIONS

Other skin disorders affect HIV patients that may not be related to HIV infection. These include eruptive dysplastic nevi,[176] Grover's acantholytic dermatosis,[148,177] pitted keratolysis,[178] lichen planus,[143] panniculitis,[143] Kawasaki's disease,[179,180] and Dupuytren's contracture.[181]

REFERENCES

1. Lim W, Sadick N, Gupta A, et al. Skin diseases in children with HIV infection and their association with degree of immunosuppression. Int J Dermatol 1990;29:24.
2. Sindrup JH, Weismann K, Petersen CS, et al. Skin and oral mucosal changes in patients infected with human immunodeficiency virus. 1988;68:440.
3. Johnson M-LT, Roberts J. Prevalence of dermatological diseases among persons 1–74 years of age: United States. Publication No. (PHS) 79-1660. Washington, DC: U.S. Government Printing Office, 1977.
4. Goodman DS, Teplitz ED, Wishner A, et al. Prevalence of cutaneous disease in patients with acquired immunodeficiency syndrome (AIDS) or AIDS-related complex. J Am Acad Dermatol 1987;17:210.
5. Coldiron BM, Bergstresser PR. Prevalence and clinical spectrum of skin disease in patients infected with human immunodeficiency virus. Arch Dermatol 1989;125:357.
6. Matis WL, Triana A, Shapiro R, et al. Dermatologic findings associated with human immunodeficiency virus infection. J Am Acad Dermatol 1987;17:746.
7. Kaplan MH, Sadick N, McNutt NS, et al. Dermatologic findings and manifestations of acquired immunodeficiency syndrome (AIDS). J Am Acad Dermatol 1987;16:485.
8. Garbe C, Husak R, Orfanos CE. HIV-associated dermatoses and their prevalence in 456 HIV-infected patients. Relation to immune status and its importance as a diagnostic marker. Hautarzt 1994;45:623.
9. Smith KJ, Skelton HG, Yeager J, et al. Cutaneous findings in HIV-1 positive patients: a 42 month prospective study. Military Medical Consortium for the Advancement of Retroviral Research (MMCARR). J Am Acad Dermatol 1994;31:746.
10. Alessi E, Cusini M, Zerroni R. Mucocutaneous manifestations in patients infected with human immunodeficiency virus. J Am Acad Dermatol 1988;19:290.
11. Mathes BM, Douglas MC. Seborrheic dermatitis in patients with acquired immunodeficiency syndrome. Am Acad Dermatol 1985;13:947.
12. Eisenstat BA, Wormer GP. Seborrheic dermatitis and butterfly rash in AIDS. N Engl J Med 1984;311:189.
13. Soeprono FF, Schinella RA, Cockerell CJ, et al. Seborrheic-like dermatitis of acquired immunodeficiency syndrome. J Am Acad Dermatol 1986;14:242.
14. Binder RL, Jonelis FJ. Seborrheic dermatitis in neuroleptic-induced parkinsonism. Arch Dermatol 1983;119:473.
15. Sadick NS, Mcnutt NS, Kaplan MH. Papulosquamous dermatotses of AIDS. J Am Acad Dermatol 1990;22:1270.
16. Groisser D, Bottone EJ, Lebwohl M. Association of *Pityrosporum orbiculare* (*Malasseziz furfur*) with seborrheic dermatitis is patients with acquired immunodeficiency syndrome (AIDS). J Am Acad Dermatol 1989;20:770.
17. Duvic M, Johnson TM, Rapini RP et al. Acquired immunodeficiency syndrome-associated psoriasis and Reiter's syndrome. Arch Dermatol 1987;123:1622.
18. Calabrese LH, et al. Rheumatic symptoms and human immunodeficiency virus infection. The influence of clinical and laboratory variables in a longitudinal cohort study. Arthritis Rheum 1991;34:257.

19. Johnson TM, Duvic M, Rapini RP. AIDS exacerbates psoriasis. N Engl J Med 1985;313:1415.
20. Lazar AP, Roenigk HH. AIDS and psoriasis. Cutis 1987;39:347.
21. Obuch ML, et al. Psoriasis and human immunodeficiency virus infection. J Am Acad Dermatol 1992;27:667.
22. Horn TD, et al. Characterization of the dermal infiltrate in human immunodeficiency virus-infected patients with psoriasis. Arch Dermatol 1990;126:1462.
23. Mahoney SE, at al. Human immunodeficiency virus transcripts identified in HIV-related psoriasis and Kaposi's sarcoma lesions. J Clin Invest 1991;88:175.
24. Fuchs D, et al. Interferon-gamma concentrations are increased in sera from individuals infected with the human immunodeficiency virus. J Acquir Immune Defic Syndr 1989;2:158.
25. Baadsgaard O, Fisher GJ, Voorhees JJ, Cooper KD. Interactions of epidermal cels and T cells in inflammatory skin diseases. J Am Acad Dermatol 1990;23:1312.
26. Reveille JD, et al. Human immunodeficiency virus-associated psoriasis, psoriatic arthritis, and Reiter's syndrome: a disease continuum? Arthritis Rheum 1990;33:1574.
27. Kaplan MH, et al. Antipsoriatic effects of zidovudine in human immunodeficiency virus-associated psoriasis. J Am Acad Dermatol 1989;20:76.
28. Espinoza LR, Berman A, Vasey FB, et al. Psoriatic arthritis and acquired immunodeficiency syndrome. Arthritis Rheum 1988;31:1034.
29. Eyster ME, Goedert JJ, Poon MC, Preble OT. Acid-labile alpha interferon: a possible preclinical marker for the acquired immunodeficiency syndrome in hemophilia. N Engl J Med 1983;309:583.
30. Fuchs D, Hausen A, Reibnegger G et al. Urinary neopterin in the diagnosis of acquired immunodeficiency syndrome. Eur J Clin Microbiol 1984;3:70.
31. Baker BS, Griffiths CEM, Fry L, Valdimarsson H. Psoriasis and interferon. Lancet 1986;2:342.
32. Quesada JR, Gutterman JV. Psoriasis and alpha-interferon. Lancet 1986;1:1466.
33. Swerlick RA, Cunningham MW, Hall NK. Monoclonal antibodies cross-reactive with group A streptococci and normal and psoriatic skin. J Invest Dermatol 1986;87:367.
34. Noonan FP, Kripke ML, Pedersen GM, et al. Suppression of contact hypersensitivity in mice by ultraviolet irradiation is associated with defective antigen presentation. Immunology 1981;43:527.
35. Ranki A et al. Effect of PUVA on immunologic and virologic findings in HIV-infected patients. J Am Acad Dermatol 1991;24:404.
36. Kaplan MH, Sadick NS, Wieder J, et al. Antipsoriatic effects of zidovudine in human immunodeficiency virus-associated psoriasis. J Am Acad Dermatol 1989;20:76.
37. Ruzicka T, Froschl M, Hohenleutner U, et al. Treatment of HIV-induced retinoid-resistant psoriasis with zidovudine. Lancet 1987;2:1469.
38. Duvic M, Crane MM, Conant M, Mahoney SE, Reveille JD, Lehrman SN. Zidovudine improves psoriasis in human immunodeficiency viru–positive males. Arch Dermatol 1994;130:447.
39. Stanely SK, et al. Induction of expression of human immunodeficiency virus in a chronically infected promonocytic cell line by ultraviolet radiation. AIDS Res Hum Retroviruses 1989;5:375.
40 Allen BR. Use of cyclosporin for psoriasis in HIV-positive patient. Lancet 1992;339:686.
41. Stashower ME, Yeager JK, Smith KJ, Skelton HG, Wanger KF. Cimetidine as therapy for treatment-resistant psoriasis in a patient with acquired immunodeficiency syndrome. Arch Dermatol 1993;129:848.
42. Colebunders R, et al. Psoriasis regression in terminal AIDS. Lancet 1992;339:1110.
43. Duvic M, et al. Remission of AIDS-associated psoriasis. Lancet 1987;2:627.
44. Winchester R, Bernstein DH, Fischer HD, et al. The co-occurrence of Reiter's syndrome and acquired immunodeficiency syndrome. Ann Intern Med 1987;106:19.
45. Kaye BR. Rheumatologic manifestations of infection with human immunodeficiency virus (HIV). Ann Intern Med 1989;111:158.
46. Berman A, Espinosa LR, Diaz JD, et al. Rheumatic manifestations of human immunodeficiency virus infection. Am J Med 1988;85:59.
47. Vaughan Jones, SA, McGibbon DH. Reiter's disease in a homosexual HIV-positive male. Clin Exp Dermatol 1994;19:430.
48. Solomon G, et al. Arthritis, psoriasis and related syndromes associated with HIV infection. (Abstract) Arthritis Rheum 1988;31(Suppl 2):S12.
49. Lin RY. Reiter's syndrome and human immunodeficiency virus infection. Dermatologica 1988;176:39.
50. Belz J, Breneman DL, Nordlund JJ, Solinger A. Successful treatment of a patient with Reiter's syndrome and acquired immunodeficiency syndrome using etretinate. J Am Acad Dermatol 1989;20:898.
51. Richman TB, Kerdel FA. Reiter's syndrome. (Letter) Arch Dermatol 1988;124:1007.
52. Brenner S. Acquired ichthyosis in AIDS. Cutis 1987;39:421.
53. Valle S-L. Dermatologic findings related to HIV infection in high-risk individuals. J Am Acad Dermatol 1987;17:951.
54. Coldiron BM, Bergstesser PR. Prevalence and clinical spectrum of skin disease in patients infected with the human immunodeficiency virus. Arch Dermatol 1989;125:357.
55. Young L. Steinman HK. Acquired ichthyosis in a patient with AIDS and Kaposi's sarcoma. J Am Acad Dermatol 1987;16:395.
56. Wissel PS, Sordillo P, Anderson KE, et al. Porphyria cutanea tarda associated with the acquired immune deficiency syndrome. Am J Hematol 1987;25:107.
57. Hogan D, Card RT, Ghadially, et al. Human immunodeficiency virus infection and porphyria cutanea tarda. J Am Acad Dermatol 1989;20:17.
58. Reynaud P, Goodfellow K, Svec F. Porphyria cutanea tarda as initial presentation of the acquired immunodeficiency syndrome in two patients. (Letter) J Infect Dis 1990;161:1032.
59. Lobata MN, Berger TG. Porphyria cutanea tarda associated with the acquired immunodeficiency syndrome. Arch Dermatol 1988;124:1009.
60. Conrad ME. AIDS and porphyria cutanea tarda. (Letter) Am J Hematol 1988;28:207.
61. Nip-Sakamoto CJ, Wong RHW, Izumi AK. Porphyria cutanea tarda and AIDS. Cutis 1989;44:470-471.
62. Lafeuillade A, et al. Porphyria cutanea tarda associated with HIV infection. AIDS 1990;4:924.
63. Blauvelt A, et al. Porphyria cutanea tarda and human immunodeficiency virus infection. Int J Dermatol 1992;31:474.
64. Conlan MG, Hoots WK. Porphyria cutanea tarda in association with human immunodeficiency virus infection in a hemophiliac. J Am Acad Dermatol 1992;26:857.
65. Fuchs D, Artner-Dworzak E, Hausen A, et al. Urinary excretion of porphyrins is increased in patients with HIV-1 infection. AIDS 1990;4:341.
66. el Sayed F, Viraben R, Bazex J, Gorguet B. Porphyria cutanea tarda and HIV-1 infection: 2 new cases. Ann Dermatol Venereol 1993;120:455.
67. Boisseau AM, et al. Porphyria cutanea tarda associated with human immunodeficiency virus infection. A study of four cases and review of the literature. Dermatologica 1991;182:155.
68. Russel MG, Lustermans FA, Wuite J, van Pelt J. Porphyria cutanea tarda in a patient with AIDS. Neth J Med 1992;41:68.
69. Soriano E, Catala MT, Lacruz J, Campayo A, Lopez Aldeguer J, Perello A. Porphyria cutanea tarda and human immunodeficiency virus infection. Rev Clin Esp 1993;192:120.
70. Toback AC, Longley J, Cardullo AC, et al. Severe chronic photosensitivity in association with acquired immunodeficiency syndrome. J Am Acad Dermatol 1986;15:1056.
71. Herman LE, Kurban AK. Erythroderma as a manifestation of the AIDS-related complex. J Am Acad Dermatol 1987;17:507.
72. Cohen PR, Grossman ME, Silvers DN, DeLeo VA. Generalized granuloma annulare located on sun-exposed areas in a human immunodeficiency virus-seropositive man with ultraviolet B photosensitivity. Arch Dermatol 1990;126:830.
73. Berger TG, Dhar A. Lichenoid photoeruptions in human immunodeficiency virus infection. Arch Dermatol 1994;130:609.
74. Gregory N, DeLeo VA. Clinical manifestations of photosensitivity in patients with hum an immunodeficiency virus infection. (Editorial) Arch Dermatol 1994;130:630.
75. Smith KJ, et al. Papular eruption of human immunodeficiency virus disease. A review of the clinical histologic, and immunohistochemical findings in 48 cases. Am J Dermatopathol 1991;13:445.
76. James WD, Redfield RR, Lupton GP, et al. A papular eruption associated with human T cell lymphotropic virus type III disease. J Am Acad Dermatol 1985;13:563.
77. Warner LC, Fisher BK. Cutaneous manifestations of the acquired immunodeficiency syndrome. Int J Dermatol 1986;25:337.
78. Hira SK, Wadhawan d, Kamanga J, et al. Cutaneous manifestations of human immunodeficiency virus in Lusaka, Zambia. J Am Acad Dermatol 1988;19:451.

79. Barlow RJ, Schulz EJ. Necrotizing folliculitis in AIDS related complex. Br J Dermatol 1987;116:581.
80. Rosenthal D, LeBoit PE, Klumpp L, Berger TG. Human immunodeficiency virus-associated eosinophilic folliculitis. Arch Dermatol 1991;127:206.
81. Takematsu H, Nakamura K, Igarashi M, Tagami H. Eosinophilic pustular folliculitis. Arch Dermatol 1985;121:917.
82. Jenkins, D, Fisher BK, Chalvardjian A, Adam P. Eosinophilic pustular folliculitis in a patients with AIDS. Int J Dermatol 1988;27:34.
83. Soeprono FF, Schinella RA. Eosinophilic pustular folliculitis in patients with acquired immunodeficiency syndrome. J Am Acad Dermatol 1986;14:1020.
84. Buchness MR, Lim HW, Hatcher VA, et al. Eosinophilic pustular folliculitis in the acquired immunodeficiency syndrome. N Engl J Med 1988;318:1183.
85. Harris DWS, et al. Eosinophilic pustular folliculitis in an HIV-positive man: response to cetirizine. Br J Dermatol 1992;126:392.
86. Hevia O, et al. Pruritic papular eruption of the acquired immunodeficiency syndrome. A clinicopathologic study. J Am Acad Dermatol 1991;24:231.
87. Colebunders R, et al. Generalized papular pruritic eruption in African patients with human immunodeficiency virus infection. AIDS 1987;1:117.
88. Pardo RJ, et al. UVB phototherapy of the pruritic papular eruption of the acquired immunodeficiency syndrome. J Am Acad Dermatol 1992;26:423.
89. Ansary MA, et al. A colour atlas of AIDS in the tropics. London: Wolfe, 1989:28.
90. Liautaud B, Pape JW, DeHovitz JA, et al. Pruritic skin lesions. Arch Dermatol 1989;125:629.
91. Sundharam JA. Pruritic skin eruption in the acquired immunodeficiency syndrome: arthropod bites. Arch Dermatol 1990;126:539.
92. Scully M, Berger TG. Pruritus, Staphylococcus aureus, and human immunodeficiency virus infection. Arch Dermatol 1990;126:684.
93. Itescu S. Brancato LJ, Winchester R. A sicca syndrome in HIV infection: association with HLA-DR5 and CD8 lymphocytosis. Lancet 1989;2:466.
94. Duvic M, et al. Human immunodeficiency virus-asssociated vitiligo. Expression of autoimmunity with immunodeficiency. J Am Acad Dermatol 1987;17:656.
95. Kinloch-de-Loes S, et al. Bullous pemphigoid antibodies, HIV-1 infection and pruritic papular eruption. AIDS 1991;5:451.
96. Levy PM, Balavoine J-F, Salomon D, et al. Ritodrine-responsive bullous pemphigoid in a patient with AIDS-related complex. Br J Dermatol 1986;114:635.
97. Bull RH, Fallowfield ME, Marsden RA. Autoimmune blistering diseases associated with HIV infection. Clin Exp Dermatol 1994;19:47.
98. Grange A, Saiag P, Winter C, Marinho E, Delzant G. Vesiculo-pustular cutaneous eruption disclosing primary infection by HIV virus. Ann Dermatol Venereol 1992;119:872.
99. Aguilar JL, Berman A, Espinoza LR, et al. Autoimmune phenomena in human immunodeficiency virus infection. Am J Med 1988;1988;85:283.
100. Kopelman RG, Zolla-Pazner S. Association of human immunodeficiency virus infection and autoimmune phenomena. Am J Med 1988;84:82.
101. Parkin JM, Eales L-J, Galazka AR, et al. Atopic manifestations in the acquired immune deficiency syndrome: response to recombinant interferon gamma. Br Med J 1987;294:1185.
102. Lin RY, Chronic diffuse dermatitis and hyper-IgE in HIV infection. Acta Derm Venereol (Stockh) 1988;68:486.
103. Abrams DI, AIDS-related conditions. In: Pinching AJ, ed. AIDS and HIV Infection. Clin Immunol Allergy 1986;6:581.
104. Kim HC, et al. Immune thrombocytopenia in hemophiliacs infected with HIV and their response to splenectomy. Arch Intern Med 1989;149:1685.
105. Plantanias LC, et al. Thrombotic thrombocytopenic purpura as the first manifestation of HIV infection. Am J Med 1989;87:699.
106. Torres RA, et al. Zidovudine-induced leukocytoclastic vasculitis. Arch Intern Med 1992;152:850.
107. Velji AM. Leukocytoclastic vasculitis associated with positive HTLV-III serologic findings. JAMA 1986;256:2196.
108. Chren MM, et al. Leukocytoclastic vasculitis in a patient infected with HIV. J Am Acad Dermatol 1989;21:1161.
109. Walker MM, Griffiths CEM, Leonard JN, et al. Dermatological conditions associated with HTLV-III virus infection. Br J Dermatol 1986;115(Suppl 30):16.
110. Weismann K, Petersen CS, Sondergaard J, et al. Skin signs in AIDS. Copenhagen: Munksgaard, 1988.
111. Farthing CF, Staughton RCD, Rowland Payne CME. Skin disease in homosexual patients with acquired immune deficiency syndrome (AIDS) and lesser forms of human T cell leukemia virus (HTLV III) disease. Clin Exp Dermatol 1985;10:3.
112. Calabrese LH, et al. Systemic necrotizing vasculitis and the human immunodeficiency virus (HIV): an important etiologic relationship. Arthritis Rheum 1988;31(Suppl 2):S35.
113. Borleffs JC, Lamme TM, Beek FJ, Kater L. Polyarteritis nodosa in a patient with AIDS. Neth J Med 1993;43:215.
114. LeBoit PE, Cockerell CJ. Nodular lesions of erythema elevatum diutinum in patients infected with the human immunodeficiency virus. J Am Acad Dermatol 1993;28:919.
115. Rzany B. Mockenhaupt M, Stocker U, Hamouda O, Schopf E. Incidence of Stevens-Johnson syndrome and toxic epidermal necrolysis in patients with the acquired immunodeficiency syndrome in Germany [see comments]. (Letter) Arch Dermatol 1993;129:1059.
116. Schlienger RG, Haefeli WE, Bircher A, Leib SL, Luscher TF. Drug-induced Stevens-Johnson syndrome in a patient with AIDS. Schweiz Rundsch Med Prax 1993;83:888.
117. Dukes CS, Sugarman J, Cegielski JP, Lallinger GJH, Mwakyusa DH. Severe cutaneous hypersensitivity reactions during treatment of tuberculosis in patient with HIV infection in Tanzania. Trop Geogr Med 1992;44:308.
118. Lewis DA, Brook MG. Erythema multiforme as a presentation of human immunodeficiency virus seroconversion illness. Int J STD AIDS 1992;3:56.
119. Rico MJ, Kory WP, Gould EW, et al. Interface dermatitis in patients with the acquired immunodeficiency syndrome. J Am Acad Dermatol 1987;16:1209.
120. Herman LE, Kurban AK. Erythroderma as a manifestation of the AIDS-related complex. J Am Acad Dermatol 1987;17:507.
121. May LP, et al. Hypereosinophilic syndrome with unusual cutaneo us manifestations in two men with HIV infection. J Am Acad Dermatol 1990;23:202.
122. Harper ME, et al. Concomitant infection with HTLV-1 and HTLV-II in a patient with T8 lymphoproliferative disease. N Engl J Med 1986;315:1073.
123. Janier M, et al. Pseudo-Sezary syndrome with CD8 phenotype in a patient with AIDS. Ann Intern Med 1989;110:738.
124. Janniger CK, et al. Erythroderma as the initial presentation of the acquired immunodeficiency syndrome. Dermatologic 1991;183:143.
125. Blauvelt A, et al. Pityriasis rubra pilaris and HIV infection. J Am Acad Dermatol 1991;24:703.
126. Auffret N Quint L, Domart P, Dubertret L, Lecam JY, Binet O. Pityriasis rubra pilaris in a patient with human immunodeficiency virus infection [see comments]. J Am Acad Dermatol 1992;27:260.
127. Martin AG, Weaver CC, Cockerell CJ, Berger TG. Pityriasis rubra pilaris in the setting of HIV infection: clinical behaviour and association with explosive cystic acne. Br J Dermatol 1992;126:617.
128. Le Bozec P, et al. Pityriasis rubra pilaris in a patient with acquired immunodeficiency syndrome. Ann Dermatol Venereol 1991;118:862.
129. Menni S, Brancaleone W, Grimalt R. Pityriasis rubra pilaris in a child seropositive for the human immunodeficiency virus. J Am Acad Dermatol 1992;27:1009.
130. Perrin C, Durant JM, Lacour JP, Michiels JF, Dellamonica P, Ortonne JP. Horny perifollicular mucinosis. An atypical pityriasis rubra pilaris-like eruption associated with HIV infection. Am J Dermatopathol 1993;15:358.
131. Resnick SD, Murrell DF, Woosley JT. Pityriasis rubra pilaris, acne conglobata, and elongated follicular spines: an HIV-associated follicular syndrome [see comments]? (Letter) J Am Acad Dermatol 1993;29:283.
132. Bakos L, Hampe S, da Rocha JL, et al. Generalized granuloma annulare in a patient with acquired immunodeficiency syndrome (AIDS) 1987;17:844.
133. Huerter CJ, Bass J, Bergfeld WF, Tubbs RR. Perforating granuloma annulare in a patient with acquired immunodeficiency syndrome. Arch Dermatol 1987;123:1217.
134. Leenutaphong V, Erckenbrecht, Zuleger S, Plewig G. Remission of human immunodeficiency virus-associated generalized granuloma

annulare under zidovudine therapy. (Letter) J Am Acad Dermatol 1988;19:1126.

135. Pennys NS, Hicks B. Unusual cutaneous lesions associated with acquired immunodeficiency syndrome. J Am Acad Dermatol 1985;13:845-852.

136. Bank DE, et al. Reacting perforating collagenosis in a setting of double disaster: acquired immunodeficiency syndrome and end-stage renal disease. J Am Acad Dermatol 1989;21:371.

137. Jones SK, Haman RRM. Atypical granuloma annulare in patients with the acquired immunodeficiency syndrome. J Am Acad Dermatol 1989;20:299.

138. Viraben R, Dupre R. Lichenend granulomatous papular dermatosis associated with human immunodeficiency virus infection: an immunohistochemical study. J Am Acad Dermatol 1988;18:1140.

139. Chernosky ME, Finley VK. Yellow nail syndrome in patients with acquired immunodeficiency disease. J Am Acad Dermatol 1985;13:731.

140. Scher RK. Acquired immunodeficiency syndrome and yellow nails. (Letter) J Am Acad Dermatol 1988;18:758.

141. Haas A, Dover JS. Yellow nail syndrome and acquired immunodeficiency disease. J Am Acad Dermatol 1986;14:845.

142. Pennys NS. Skin manifestations of AIDS. London: Dunitz, 1990.

143. Sadick NS. Clinical and laboratory evaluation of AIDS trichopathy. Int J Dermatol 1993;32:33.

144. Rippis GE, Becker B, Scott G. Hypertrophic lichen planus in three HIV-positive patients: a histologic and immunological study. J Cutan Pathol 1994;21:52.

145. Valle S-L. Dermatologic findings related to HIV infection in high-risk individuals. J Am Acad Dermatol 1987;17:951.

146. Friedman-Kien AE, DeVita VT, Krigel R, et al. A color atlas of AIDS. Philadelphia: WB Saunders, 1989.

147. Kinchelow T, Schmidt U, Ingato S. Changes in the hair of black patients with AIDS. (Letter) J Infect Dis 1988;157:394.

148. Farthing CF, Brown SE, Staughton RCD. A colour atlas of AIDS and HIV disease. 2nd ed. London: Wolfe, 1988.

149. Wignants H, et al. Multiple drug reactions in a patient with AIDS. Lancet 1989;2:1455.

150. Greenberger RG, Patterson R. Management of drug allergy in patients with acquired immunodeficiency syndrome. J Allergy Clin Immunol 1987;79:484.

151. Gordin FM, Simon GL Wofsy CB, Mills J. Adverse reactions to trimethoprim-sulfamethoxazole in patients with the acquired immunodeficiency syndrome. Ann Intern Med 1984;100:495-499.

152. Matsuyasu R, et al. Cutaneous reaction to trimethoprim- sulfamethoxazole in patients with AIDS and Kaposi's sarcoma. N Engl J Med 1983;308:1535.

153. Moreno JN, et al. Oral desensitization to sulfadiazine and trimethoprim-sulfamethoxazole (TMP-SMX) in 4 patients with AIDS. N Engl J Med 1983;308:340.

154. Tenant-Flowers M, et al. Sulfadiazine desensitization in patients with AIDS and cerebral toxoplasmosis. AIDS 1991;5:322.

155. Torgovnick J, Arsura A. Desensitization to sulfonamides in patients with HIV infection. Am J Med 1990;88:548.

156. Shafer RW, et al. Successful prophylaxis of Pneumocystis pneumonia with trimethoprim-sulfamethoxazole in AIDS patients with previous allergic reactions. J Acquir Immune Defic Syndr 1990;2:389.

157. Metroka CE, et al. Desensitization to dapsone in HIV-positive patients. JAMA 1992;267:512.

158. Berger TG, et al. Aerosolized pentamidine and cutaneous findings. Ann Intern Med 1989;110:1035.

159. Raviglione MC, et al. Fatal toxic epidermal necrolysis during prophylaxis with pyrimethamine and sulfadoxine in a human immunodeficiency virus-infected person. Arch Intern Med 1988;148:2683.

160. Roujeau JC, et al. Toxic epidermal necrolysis. J Am Acad Dermatol 1990;23:1039.

161. Porteous DM, Berger TG. Severe cutaneous drug reactions (Stevens-Johnson syndrome and toxic epidermal necrolysis) in human immunodeficiency virus infection. Arch Dermatol 1991;127:740.

162. Saiag P, et al. Drug-induced toxic epidermal necrolysis (Lyell's syndrome) in patients infected with the human immunodeficiency virus. J Am Acad Dermatol 1992;26:5676.

163. Furth PA, Kazakis AM. Nail pigmentation changes associated with azothymidine (zidovudine). (Letter) Ann Intern Med 1987;107:350.

164. Don PC, et al. Nail dyschromia associated with zidovudine. Ann Intern Med 1990;112:145.

165. Greenberger RG, Berger TG. Nail and mucocutaneous hyperpigmentation with azidothymidine therapy. J Am Acad Dermatol 1990;22:237.

166. Gallais V, et al. Acral hyperpigmented macules and longitudinal melanonychia in AIDS patients. Br J Dermatol 1992;126:387.

167. Klutman NE, Hinthorn DR. Excessive growth of eyelashes in a patient with AIDS being treated with zidovudine. N Engl J Med 1991;324:1896.

168. Sahai J, et al. Zidovudine-associated hypertrichosis and nail pigmentation in an HIV-infected patient. AIDS 1991;5:1395.

169. Kaplan MH, et al. Acquired trichomegaly of the eyelashes: a cutaneous marker of acquired immunodeficiency syndrome. J Am Acad Dermatol 1991;25:801.

170. Van der Piju JW, et al. Foscarnet and penile ulceration. Lancet 1990;335:286.

171. Gill PS, et al. Clinical effects of glucocorticoids on Kaposi 's sarcoma related to the acquired immunodeficiency syndrome. Ann Intern Med 1989;110:937.

172. Kovacs JA, Masur H. *Pneumocystis carinii* pneumonia: therapy and prophylaxis. J Infect Dis 1988;158:254.

173. Duvic M, Reisman M, Finley V, et al. Glucan-Induced Keratoderma in acquired immunodeficiency syndrome. Arch Dermatol 1987;123:751.

174. MacFarlane DF, Gregory N. Telangiectases in human immunodeficiency virus-positive patients. Cutis 1994;53:79.

175. Fallon T, Abell E, Kingsley L, et al. Telangiectasias of the anterior chest in homosexual men. Ann Intern Med 1986;105:679.

176. Duvic M, Lowe L, Rapini RP, et al. Eruptive dysplastic nevi associated with human immunodeficiency virus infection. Arch Dermatol 1989;125:397.

177. Muhlemann MF, Anderson MG, Paradinas FJ, et al. Early warning skin signs in AIDS and persistent generalised lymphadenopathy. Br J Dermatol 1986;114:419.

178. Weismann K, Petersen CS, Sondergaard J, et al. Skin signs in AIDS. Copenhagen: Munksgaard, 1988.

179. Viraben R, Dupre A. Kawasaki disease associated with HIV infection. Lancet 1987;1:1430.

180. Bezold LI, Bricker JT. Acquired Heart disease in children. Curr Opin Cardiol 1994;9:121.

181. Bower M, Nelson M, Gaxxard BG. Dupuytren's contractures on patients infected with HIV. Br Med J 1990;300:164.

AIDS: Biology, Diagnosis, Treatment and
Prevention, fourth edition, edited by Vincent T.
DeVita, Jr., Samuel Hellman, and Steven A.
Rosenberg. Lippincott–Raven Publishers, © 1997

19.2

Noninfectious Pulmonary Complications of Human Immunodeficiency Virus Infection

Stewart J. Levine and James H. Shelhamer

Noninfectious disorders represent an important cause of lung disease in patients infected with the human immunodeficiency virus (HIV).[1] These noninfectious pulmonary complications include neoplastic processes (eg, Kaposi's sarcoma, non-Hodgkin's lymphoma), interstitial pneumonitis (ie, nonspecific and lymphocytic interstitial pneumonitis), and inflammatory airway disorders. This chapter reviews the pathology, clinical and radiographic presentation, diagnosis, natural history, and treatment of these noninfectious pulmonary complications of HIV infection.

NEOPLASTIC PULMONARY COMPLICATIONS OF HIV INFECTION

Kaposi's Sarcoma

Kaposi's sarcoma, the most common malignancy complicating the acquired immunodeficiency syndrome (AIDS), is frequently a multifocal disease involving the skin, mucocutaneous membranes, lymph nodes, and visceral organs, most commonly the respiratory and gastrointestinal systems.[2-6] Despite earlier fluctuations, the incidence of Kaposi's sarcoma as an initial AIDS-defining diagnosis in the United States has remained relatively constant for the period from 1988 to 1991 at approximately 2 cases per 100 person-years.[7] Similarly, the incidence of Kaposi's sarcoma in Canada has been stable from 1987 to 1991 at 1.06 to 1.14 cases per 100,000 persons.[8]

AIDS-related Kaposi's sarcoma preferentially occurs in homosexual or bisexual men.[2,3] Women who acquire HIV

Stewart J. Levine, Critical Care Medicine Department, National Institutes of Health, Clinical Center, Building 10, Room 7D43, 10 Center Drive MSC 1662, Bethesda, MD 20892-1662.

James H. Shelhamer, Critical Care Medicine Department, National Institutes of Health, Clinical Center, Building 10, Room 7D43, 10 Center Drive MSC 1662, Bethesda, MD 20892-1662.

infection by sexual contact with bisexual men also appear to be at increased risk for developing Kaposi's sarcoma, but it is uncommon in pediatric AIDS patients.[9] Consistent with the epidemiology of Kaposi's sarcoma, which is suggestive of a sexually transmitted etiologic agent, a Kaposi's sarcoma–associated herpesvirus (KSHV) has been identified in AIDS-related and classic Kaposi's sarcoma cases, as well as in the Kaposi's sarcoma that occurs in HIV-negative homosexual men.[10,11]

Other suggested etiologic factors have included genetic cofactors (ie, HLA-DR5, HLA-DQ1) and HIV-related immunosuppression.[2,3,12] For example, the HIV Tat protein may initiate the transformation of spindle cells by enhancing the expression of interleukin-6 and oncostatin-M receptors, both of which are growth factors for Kaposi's sarcoma. HIV Tat protein also promotes the growth of Kaposi's sarcoma cells.[9,12,13] Production of angiogenic growth factors and cytokines by Kaposi's sarcoma cells and by HIV-infected CD4+ cells may also contribute to the pathogenesis of Kaposi's sarcoma lesions.[9]

Pathology

Pulmonary involvement by AIDS-related Kaposi's sarcoma has been reported in 6% to 35% of autopsies of patients with Kaposi's sarcoma, although some series have reported frequencies as high as 40% to 75%.[4,5,14-17] Although pulmonary Kaposi's sarcoma is generally found in patients with previously documented cutaneous, nodal, or visceral disease, isolated intrathoracic lesions have been reported in approximately 11% of cases.[4,5,18-25] Pulmonary Kaposi's sarcoma can progress despite limited or stable extrapulmonary disease.[26]

Intrathoracic Kaposi's sarcoma can involve the pulmonary parenchyma, airways, pleura, or mediastinal lymph nodes.[15,18,19,23,27-29] Pulmonary parenchymal involvement is multifocal and follows interstitial lymphatic pathways along bronchovascular bundles, interlobular septa, and the pleura.[15,16,21–23] Although tumor cells frequently completely dissect into and thicken the walls of airways and blood vessels, they generally do not compress these structures.[20,21,27] Disease progression may result in the formation of nodular masses that have a peribronchial or perivascular distribution.[16,22,23,27] Advanced parenchymal lesions may obliterate alveolar spaces, with resulting radiographic consolidation.[21,23]

Submucosal lesions of the trachea and bronchi have an appearance similar to that of cutaneous lesions and appear grossly as erythematous, irregular, macular, or papular lesions.[15,27,30,31] Multiple discrete lesions may be distributed throughout the tracheobronchial tree, but they are frequently located at the carinas of segmental orifices.[18,31] Endobronchial lesions correlate histologically with extensive submucosal infiltration by Kaposi's sarcoma cells that secondarily entrap and obliterate mucosal glandular structures and denude the columnar epithelium.[27,32] Infrequently, extensive endobronchial tumor masses can compromise the luminal integrity of the tracheobronchial tree or the upper airway.[16,20,33]

Pleural Kaposi's sarcoma involves only the visceral pleura, with resultant plaque formation secondary to infiltrating tumor cells.[23,27] The pleural surface, however, is not disrupted, and concomitant pleural effusions frequently exist.[18,23,26,27] Hilar or mediastinal lymph node involvement by Kaposi's sarcoma may result in gross adenopathy or only in microscopic evidence of tumor infiltration.[23] Pleural or hilar and mediastinal lymph node involvement can occur independently, without associated pulmonary parenchymal lesions.[23]

The histopathology of Kaposi's sarcoma reveals a vascular tumor composed of interstitial linear and nodular accumulations of plump to elongated spindle cells within an extracellular network of reticulin fibers.[6,16,18,22,26,34] These spindle cells form numerous vascular clefts that are filled with erythrocytes. The lesions of Kaposi's sarcoma are associated with various degrees of acute and chronic hemorrhage, as evidenced by extravasated erythrocytes and hemosiderin-laden macrophages.[16,18,22,26] An inflammatory infiltrate composed of lymphocytes and plasma cells is often present and may vary in intensity from scarce to so extensive that the classic spindle cell lesions are almost completely obscured.[15,16,22,26,35] An early form of Kaposi's sarcoma may be characterized by lesions that have an extensive inflammatory component with nonspecific, plump mesenchymal cells and few spindle cells. Consequently, sampling of this inflammatory type of lesion may result in an incorrect diagnosis of an organizing interstitial pneumonitis rather than Kaposi's sarcoma.[15,21]

Parenchymal interstitial and intraalveolar hemorrhage, which may be extensive, often is associated with Kaposi's sarcoma lesions.[15,16,21,36] Pulmonary hemorrhage occurs secondary to extravasation of erythrocytes from foci of Kaposi's sarcoma, especially in patients with underlying defects in hemostasis. Pulmonary hemosiderosis may also occur.[21] Focal lymphoid infiltrates in areas unassociated with Kaposi's sarcoma lesions also have been reported.[21]

Clinical Presentation

The clinical signs and symptoms of pulmonary Kaposi's sarcoma are often nonspecific and may be difficult to differentiate from those of AIDS-related opportunistic infections. Dyspnea and cough are the most common clinical manifestations and may be present in 100% of patients.[18,22,26,27,32] Fever and sputum production are not characteristic of pulmonary Kaposi's sarcoma and should alert the clinician to the possibility of an opportunistic infection.[15,18,19,22,26,32,37] Wheezing occurred in 18% of 11 patients in one study; it represented airways obstruction secondary to endobronchial disease or pulmonary edema caused by obstruction of lymphatic vessels.[24] Hemoptysis has occurred in 11% to 18% of cases and may represent extensive intraalveolar hemorrhage or bleeding from endobronchial lesions.[16,21,27,29] However, in one series of pulmonary Kaposi's sarcoma in Africa, hemoptysis occurred in 81% of individuals, perhaps reflecting increased disease severity due to late presentation.[38] The development of stridor is a sign of laryngeal or tracheal obstruction by Kaposi's sarcoma lesions and may be exacerbated by secondary hemorrhage and intraluminal thrombus formation.[27,33] Hoarseness suggests vocal cord lesions.[37] The presence of focal wheezing, stridor, or hemoptysis, especially in the setting of previously documented cutaneous Kaposi's sarcoma, should alert the clinician to the possibility of endobronchial or mucosal lesions. Pleuritic chest pain may suggest the presence of underlying pleural disease and has been reported for 9% to 30% of cases.[27]

The physical examination of patients with pulmonary Kaposi's sarcoma is often nonrevealing. In one series of 19 patients with pulmonary Kaposi's sarcoma, 16% had evidence of bilateral crackles on lung auscultation, and all other patients had normal breath sounds.[18] Decreased breath sounds and dullness to percussion may suggest a pleural effusion associated with Kaposi's sarcoma. Because the physical examination often yields nonspecific findings, it is important to document the presence of cutaneous or mucocutaneous Kaposi's sarcoma lesions, which can serve as markers for possible lung involvement. For example, palatal lesions were detected in 77% of African patients with pulmonary Kaposi's sarcoma, and in a London series, oral lesions were found in 95% of patients with pulmonary Kaposi's sarcoma.[38,39] Similarly, in two series involving 39 patients with pulmonary Kaposi's sarcoma, only one individual with localized endobronchial disease did not have concomitant cutaneous lesions.[39,40] It is uncommon to have isolated endobronchial disease without concomitant mucocutaneous disease. However, the extent or stability of cutaneous lesions cannot be used as a marker for the severity of tracheobronchial Kaposi's sarcoma, because patients with stable or limited cutaneous disease have been found to have progressive or extensive pulmonary involvement.[26]

Although arterial blood gas determinations and pulmonary function test results are frequently abnormal in the setting of pulmonary Kaposi's sarcoma, neither can be used to definitively differentiate Kaposi's sarcoma from opportunistic infections. Arterial blood gases usually reveal the presence of mild to moderate hypoxemia and an increased alveolar to arterial oxygen gradient (PAO_2–PaO_2).[18,27,32,41,42] The response of the PAO_2–PaO_2 to exercise testing varies.[42] Results of pulmonary function testing may be consistent with the presence of parenchymal or endobronchial disease. The diffusing capacity for carbon monoxide is frequently abnormal in patients with parenchymal Kaposi's sarcoma, with reported mean values ranging from 41% to 72% of predicted in four studies involving 66 patients.[39–43] Air flow obstruction, as evidenced by a forced expiratory volume in 1 second to forced vital capacity (FEV_1/FVC) ratio of less than 75%, has been reported in 50% to 100% of patients with endobronchial Kaposi's sarcoma who did not have a concomitant history of cigarette smoking or atopic disease.[43]

Significant airflow obstruction has been found to correlate with the extent of endobronchial disease.[39,40] For example, two series involving 39 patients found significant reductions in FEV_1, FVC, and peak expiratory flow rates in patients with extensive endobronchial disease compared with patients with localized disease.[39,40] Decreases in lung volumes, consistent with the presence of a restrictive pulmonary process, have been found in approximately 30% of patients.[27,42]

The radiographic manifestations of pulmonary Kaposi's sarcoma correlate well with the anatomic and histologic distribution of disease.[18,21,23,26,27,34,41,44,45] Parenchymal pulmonary involvement is characterized by patchy, multifocal, bilateral, perihilar infiltrates that are interstitial, alveolar, or mixed alveolar-interstitial. These infiltrates often radiate from abnormal hilar masses (Fig. 19.2-1).[44,45]

Computed tomography (CT) reveals perivascular and peribronchial extension of Kaposi's sarcoma lesions consistent with the histopathologic progression of disease along interstitial lymphatic pathways, with secondary involvement of alveolar spaces (Fig. 19.2-2).[44] These lesions are characteristically multiple, bilateral, and flame-shaped or nodular in appearance, with ill-defined margins, and they radiate out from the pulmonary hilum along bronchovascular bundles.[46] Several studies, however, have not described this perihilar distribution but instead observed diffusely distributed interstitial, alveolar, or alveolar-interstitial infiltrates.[21,26,32,34,41] In these studies, interstitial infiltrates had a reticular or reticulonodular appearance, consistent with tumor involvement of the pulmonary interstitium and interlobular septa. With disease progression, these alveolar-interstitial infiltrates coalesced into large, poorly defined areas of nodular parenchymal opacification or consolidation.[23,34,41]

Multiple pulmonary nodules and nodular-appearing alveolar infiltrates ranging in size from 0.5 to 3 cm in diameter are also common; they were found in 24% of 167 patients in ten series (see Fig. 19.2-2).[21,42,44] One case report described multiple cavitary nodules that were thought to represent tumor necrosis.[47] Focal, unilateral alveolar infiltrates, which may be associated with segmental consolidation, have been reported in 5% of patients. Occlusion of lobar orifices by endobronchial Kaposi's sarcoma mass lesions with secondary lobar atelectasis is rare.[20] Chest radiographs were normal for 10% of 204 patients in 10 series and corresponded with endobronchial involvement or small parenchymal lesions that ranged in size from microscopic foci to 7 mm nodules at autopsy.[18,23,26,27,32,34,38–40,44,45]

The extent of radiographic disease does not appear to accurately predict the extent of endobronchial disease.[23,38,40] For example, chest radiographs of patients with extensive tracheobronchial disease have appeared normal. Kaposi's sarcoma lesions also can be obscured by concomitant infectious processes.[38,40]

Unilateral or bilateral hilar or mediastinal lymphadenopathy, consistent with lymphatic involvement, has been described in 39% of 91 patients in six series.[41,44] However, one study of 24 patients found mediastinal adenopathy on only 2% of chest radiographs, although CT scans revealed spotty or 1+ adenopathy in 63% of patients.[44] Axillary lymphadenopathy visualized by CT was a common finding in one series, and internal mammary lymph node enlargement was also reported.[46] CT radiographic evidence of chest wall and bone disease has been reported, with involvement of the sternum and thoracic spine and evidence of soft tissue mass lesions and diffuse infiltrative lesions involving the subcutaneous fat and skin.[46]

Nonloculated pleural effusions are a common radiographic finding. Pleural effusions, often bilateral and of various sizes, were detected in 45% of 167 cases in 10 series.[17,21,41,44] Parenchymal infiltrates were associated with pleural effusions in 90% of cases in one series involving 21 patients.[17] Thoracocentesis typically yields serous, serosanguineous, or frankly hemorrhagic exudative fluid.[18,21,26,27,32,41] Cytologic examination typically does not reveal any abnormalities predictive of Kaposi's sarcoma, and pleural biopsies are nondiagnostic, revealing normal pleura or reactive mesothelial cells.[18,21,26,27,32,41] Pulmonary Kaposi's sarcoma has resulted in bilateral chylous pleural effusions, which can be massive and represent sequelae of thoracic duct disruption by mediastinal disease.[48] A case of spontaneous pneumothorax complicating pleural Kaposi's sarcoma has been reported.[49]

Magnetic resonance imaging may also provide evidence of Kaposi's sarcoma. Pulmonary Kaposi's sarcoma lesions have irregularly increased signal intensity in T1-weighted images, markedly reduced signal intensity in T2-weighted images, and contrast enhancement along perivascular and peribronchial pathways after gadolinium administration.[50] Enhancement of lesions after gadolinium administration may be related to the angiomatous nature of the tumor.

Radionuclide scintigraphy, although not specific, may provide evidence suggesting pulmonary Kaposi's sarcoma. Because pulmonary Kaposi's sarcoma often does not label with ^{67}Ga citrate, a negative study result for a patient with typical radiographic abnormalities and known Kaposi's sarcoma may be compatible with pulmonary involvement.[32,49,51,52] Even though pulmonary Kaposi's sarcoma occasionally may take up ^{67}Ga citrate, a positive study result

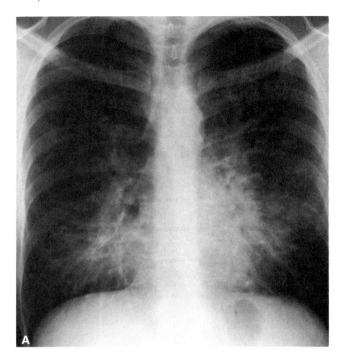 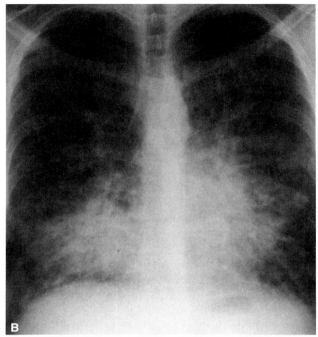

FIG. 19.2-1. (A) Typical chest radiographic manifestations of pulmonary Kaposi's sarcoma in a patient with bilateral patchy perihilar alveolar-interstitial infiltrates. **(B)** Follow-up chest radiograph after 1 month revealed progressive pulmonary Kaposi's sarcoma complicated by acute intra-alveolar hemorrhage. (Radiographs courtesy of Irwin Feuerstein, MD)

is more likely to indicate the presence of an opportunistic infection or another neoplastic process, such as lymphoma.[32,53] Thallium 201 scintigraphy may be useful in identifying pulmonary Kaposi's sarcoma, because the lesions appear to be thallium avid.[53–55]

Diagnosis

Invasive diagnostic procedures, such as fiberoptic bronchoscopy or open lung biopsy, are necessary to definitively establish the diagnosis of pulmonary Kaposi's sarcoma, because clinical and radiographic findings are nonspecific and thoracocentesis and pleural biopsy are nondiagnostic. The utility of fiberoptic bronchoscopy in establishing the diagnosis of pulmonary Kaposi's sarcoma varies and depends on the type of pulmonary manifestation. Inspection of the tracheobronchial tree alone may be sufficient for a presumptive diagnosis if characteristic erythematous, irregular, flat, or slightly raised lesions, often at airway branch points, are visualized.[18,27,37,54] These lesions have correlated with histologic evidence of Kaposi's sarcoma at autopsy.[32] Endobronchial lesions typical of Kaposi's sarcoma have been found in 9% of 585 patients with AIDS who underwent fiberoptic bronchoscopy.[21,39,40] In three series involving 70 patients with mucocutaneous Kaposi's sarcoma, 44% were found to have endobronchial lesions typical of Kaposi's sarcoma.[31,39,45] When endobronchial biopsies have been attempted, the reported yields have been extremely variable, probably reflecting the

submucosal location of this lesion. In eight small studies, the yield of endobronchial biopsy ranged from 0% to 83%, with an overall yield of 60%.[18,21,27,30,31,56–58]

Because a presumptive diagnosis of endobronchial Kaposi's sarcoma is almost always adequate and because cases of excessive bleeding have been reported after attempts at endobronchial biopsy, this procedure is not used in this setting. However, a careful visual examination of the nasal mucosa, oropharynx, larynx, and trachea should be performed, because these areas are potential sites of involvement.

If endobronchial lesions are not identified, histologic examination of the pulmonary parenchyma is necessary to establish the diagnosis. Unfortunately, the yield of transbronchial biopsy is low. This may reflect a sampling error due to the multifocal nature of Kaposi's sarcoma and the requirement for large pieces of tissue for pathologic examination, because crush artifact, hemorrhage, and granulation tissue can mimic the lesions of Kaposi's sarcoma.[26] In 10 small series involving 79 patients, transbronchial biopsies yielded a diagnosis of Kaposi's sarcoma for only 17% of cases.[14,18,22,26,28,31,36,58–60] Clinicians should be aware of the possibility of significant pulmonary hemorrhage after transbronchial biopsy in patients with pulmonary Kaposi's sarcoma.[24]

Bronchoalveolar lavage (BAL) cannot establish the diagnosis of pulmonary Kaposi's sarcoma. Although hemosiderin-laden macrophages in BAL fluid consistent with occult pulmonary hemorrhage has been reported for 70% of patients in a series of 23 individuals with pulmonary Kaposi's

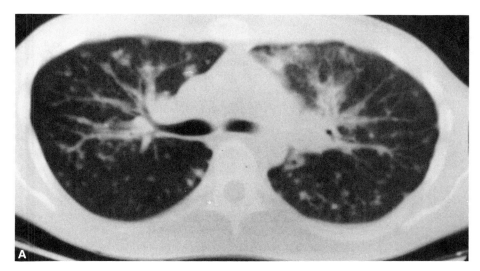

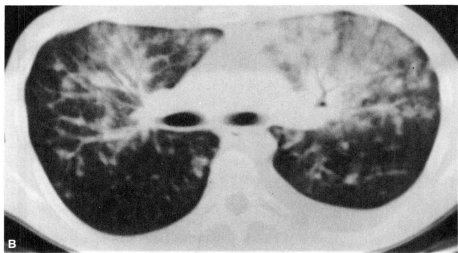

FIG. 19.2-2. Chest CT scans corresponding to Figure 19.2-1. (**A**) Bilateral parenchymal nodules, as well as interstitial and alveolar infiltrates radiating from abnormal hilar masses. (**B**) Progressive pulmonary Kaposi's sarcoma with increased air space disease secondary to acute intra-alveolar hemorrhage. (CT scans courtesy of Irwin Feuerstein, MD)

sarcoma, this was a nonspecific finding that was duplicated for pneumonia secondary to *Pneumocystis carinii* and bacterial infections.[61] Although BAL and transbronchial biopsy are of limited utility in establishing the diagnosis of pulmonary Kaposi's sarcoma, these procedures can provide important diagnostic information for patients with known pulmonary involvement in whom a concomitant opportunistic infection is suspected because of a change in respiratory symptoms or radiographic infiltrates.

If fiberoptic bronchoscopy is nondiagnostic, an open lung biopsy may be necessary to establish the diagnosis.[14,26,62–64] The advantage of an open lung biopsy is that it provides the pathologist with a larger piece of tissue for examination, minimizing the likelihood of crush artifact or sampling error.[14,26] However, even open lung biopsy is not 100% sensitive, and it, too, may be subject to sampling errors because of the focal nature of the lesions.[18,26,54] In one series of nine patients, open lung biopsy had a sensitivity of only 56%.[18] Thoracoscopic lung biopsy has also been used to establish the diagnosis of pulmonary Kaposi's sarcoma and offers the advantage of being less invasive than an open lung biopsy.[65]

Natural History

Pulmonary Kaposi's sarcoma is often a late or terminal manifestation of AIDS, with most studies reporting a life expectancy of less than 1 year after diagnosis of the tumor, although instances of prolonged survival have been reported.[18,41,54] The median survival time after the diagnosis of pulmonary Kaposi's sarcoma ranged from 1.1 to 12 months in six studies involving 185 patients.[18,27,32,38–40,66] Concurrent opportunistic pulmonary infections (eg, *P carinii*, cytomegalovirus, fungi) were present in 48% of 85 patients at the time of death and were associated with diminished survival.[18,27,32,66]

Progressive pulmonary Kaposi's sarcoma without concurrent pulmonary disorders may also result in respiratory failure and death.[15] For example, 40% of patients in four reports involving 70 patients died secondary to progressive hypoxemia resulting from extensive pulmonary Kaposi's sarcoma.[26,27,32,66] Other factors that may contribute to respiratory failure in patients with pulmonary Kaposi's sarcoma include alveolar hemorrhage and upper airway obstruction secondary to large endobronchial tumor masses. Factors predictive of decreased survival have included CD4 cell counts less than 300/mm^3, systemic B symptoms, pleural effusion, absence of cutaneous disease, previous opportunistic infection, neutropenia, anemia and absence of radiographic response to therapy.[12,38,66]

Therapy

Therapeutic modalities for pulmonary Kaposi's sarcoma include cytotoxic chemotherapy regimens, radiation therapy, and immunomodulatory therapy (ie, interferon-α).[3] Unfortunately, none of these regimens have been effective in achieving a long-term cure. However, therapeutic interventions may afford palliation and prolong survival.[3] Systemic chemotherapy has been used in patients with progressive pulmonary disease, and external radiation therapy and neodymium-doped yttrium-aluminum-garnet (Nd:YAG) laser surgery has been used to alleviate obstructing intraluminal lesions.[20,41] However, systemic chemotherapeutic regimens can induce bone marrow suppression and neutropenia, which may place these patients at increased risk for infectious complications.[66]

Liposomal daunorubicin has been used to target cytotoxic therapy to Kaposi's sarcoma lesions, producing a high frequency of tumor regression and improvement of the quality of life.[67] Although only limited information exists regarding the efficacy of this agent in pulmonary Kaposi's sarcoma, all three patients reported in the literature have had partial responses.[67,68] Granulocyte colony-stimulating factor has been used to limit the myelosuppression associated with this agent.[68]

Although most pleural effusions secondary to Kaposi's sarcoma do not require intervention, effusions that are large or produce symptoms may necessitate intermittent therapeutic thoracocentesis, chest tube drainage, or pleural sclerosis.[54] However, in one series, neither systemic chemotherapy nor chest tube thoracostomy with tetracycline sclerosis was effective in controlling the pleural effusions of Kaposi's sarcoma.[17]

Non-Hodgkin's Lymphoma

HIV-infected patients are at increased risk for developing non-Hodgkin's lymphomas.[69–71] Non-Hodgkin's lymphoma is the second most common malignancy complicating AIDS and, in contrast to Kaposi's sarcoma, does not appear to be confined to any particular risk group for HIV infection.[72–74] Non-Hodgkin's lymphoma is considered an AIDS-defining illness by the Centers for Disease Control (CDC) when an HIV-seropositive patient develops an intermediate- or high-grade lymphoma of B-cell origin.[72] AIDS-associated non-Hodgkin's lymphoma is characterized by an aggressive pattern of behavior, with high-grade histologic features and advanced stage of disease at the time of presentation.[73–78] There is a predilection for dissemination and involvement of extranodal sites of disease, especially the central nervous system (CNS), gastrointestinal system, and bone marrow. Intrathoracic involvement is uncommon; it has been

reported in 9% of 504 patients in 12 series.[74–85] However, in one series of 35 patients with AIDS-related lymphomas, 31% had biopsy-proven thoracic involvement.[85] Although the pulmonary parenchyma is the most common intrathoracic site of disease, pleural and mediastinal lesions have also been reported. Intrathoracic disease may represent the primary site of involvement.[76,86]

Pathology

AIDS-associated non-Hodgkin's lymphoma is most frequently of B-cell lineage and can be categorized into three aggressive histopathologic groups: large cell immunoblastic, large noncleaved cell, and small noncleaved cell Burkitt's or non-Burkitt's type.[69,71,72] Although low-grade cell types have also been reported in HIV-infected patients, it is not clear whether these represent a manifestation of AIDS.[72] Although uncommon, large cell non-Hodgkin's T-cell lymphomas localized to or involving the lung have also been reported.[87,88]

The pathogenesis of AIDS-associated non-Hodgkin's lymphoma has yet to be fully elucidated. Possible mechanisms include underlying immunosuppression, chronic antigenic stimulation leading to dysregulated T-cell and B-cell function, cellular transformation secondary to latent Epstein-Barr virus (EBV) expression, and MYC oncogene translocation and dysfunction leading to B-cell transformation.[12,89] For example, polyclonal stimulation of B-cell populations by EBV infection, with subsequent MYC gene activation, may mediate the malignant transformation of B-cell clones into non-Hodgkin's lymphoma.

Because not all cases of AIDS-associated non-Hodgkin's lymphomas contain EBV sequences or proteins, other viruses or oncogenes may be also play an important pathogenic role.[69,89] For example, CD4+ T lymphoblasts from an AIDS-associated acute T-cell lymphoma have been documented to express HIV p24 antigens and to contain monoclonally integrated HIV-1 within the tumor genome.[88] This suggests that HIV-1 may contribute to malignant transformation. One report documented a subgroup of AIDS-related lymphomas characterized by body-cavity involvement (eg, pleura, pericardium, peritoneum) in which EBV and KSHV were identified without MYC gene rearrangement, suggesting an etiologic role for this newly identified herpesvirus.[90]

Clinical Manifestations

Only limited information regarding the pulmonary manifestations of AIDS-related non-Hodgkin's lymphoma has been reported. Pulmonary symptoms are often nonspecific and include dyspnea, cough, and chest pain, although patients may be completely asymptomatic.[76,81,86] Nonspecific extrapulmonary B symptoms, such as fever, weight loss, or night sweats, are common. Physical examination of the thorax may be unrevealing or reveal ronchi or findings consistent with a pleural effusion. The superior vena cava syndrome has been reported in a patient who presented with a large anterior mediastinal mass.[76] Generalized or focal extrapulmonary lymphadenopathy may also be present.

The radiographic manifestations of thoracic involvement by non-Hodgkin's lymphoma are varied. In one small series, 91% of patients had multiple sites of involvement, with pleural effusions representing the most common intrathoracic manifestation.[85] Although most often bilateral in location, unilateral pleural effusions have been observed at the time of presentation.[54,74,80,85] Pleural masses, which can extend into the chest wall, have also been reported.[85] Pulmonary parenchymal non-Hodgkin's lymphoma can appear as noncavitary nodular lesions, reticulonodular infiltrates consistent with interstitial lung disease, or alveolar infiltrates.[85] Noncavitary nodular lesions are often multiple and range in size from 0.5 to 3 cm in diameter, although a single 7-cm parenchymal nodule has been reported in a patient with isolated pulmonary disease (Fig. 19.2-3).[81,86] Reticulonodular infiltrates may suggest the presence of lymphangitic involvement.[72] However, diffuse infiltrates may accompany nodular non-Hodgkin's lesions and indicate concurrent opportunistic infection, such as *P carinii* pneumonia.[81] Hilar or mediastinal lymphadenopathy is uncommon in AIDS-related non-Hodgkin's lymphoma and was reported in only 27% of patients in one small series.[81,85,86] When present, hilar adenopathy may be unilateral in location.[85]

Diagnosis

The antemortem diagnosis of AIDS-related pulmonary non-Hodgkin's lymphoma is extremely difficult. For example, although an autopsy series documented pulmonary involvement in eight cases, only three of the patients had been diagnosed before death.[91] Despite the limited amount of information that is available regarding the utility of fiberoptic bronchoscopy in this setting, it appears to be an extremely poor diagnostic method. In three series reporting seven cases of pulmonary non-Hodgkin's lymphoma, transbronchial biopsy results were falsely negative in all cases.[28,81,86] Consequently, open lung biopsy is often necessary to establish the diagnosis. No information is available regarding the use of transbronchial or percutaneous needle aspiration in this setting. Thoracocentesis should be performed if a pleural effusion exists, and the specimen should be sent for cytologic analysis, which may yield the diagnosis.

Natural History

The prognosis for patients with AIDS-associated non-Hodgkin's lymphoma is generally poor, with reported median survival times of less than 1 year, although longer survival times have been reported in several recent series.[72,74,75,77,78,80,92] However, survival may be prolonged if a complete response to multidrug chemotherapeutic regimens is achieved.[78,80] Poor prognostic indicators include the presence of *P carinii* pneumonia, a prior diagnosis of AIDS, extranodal lesions, CD4 T-cell counts of less than 100 cells/mm^3, and a low Karnofsky performance score.[77,78]

AIDS patients with lymphoma are at increased risk for pulmonary disease compared with their counterparts without lymphoma.[82] These patients can develop AIDS-related opportunistic infections, such as *P carinii* pneumonia, as well as bacterial and fungal (eg, *Aspergillus*) pneumonias secondary to chemotherapy-related neutropenia.[74,78,82,84,91] Prophylactic therapy for *P carinii* pneumonia should be administered to all patients with AIDS-related non-Hodgkin's lymphoma.

Three of four patients in one series of pulmonary non-Hodgkin's lymphoma developed catheter-related *Staphylococcus aureus* bacteremia, which was associated with a fatal diffuse pneumonitis in one patient.[81] Besides opportunistic infections, these patients may also develop interstitial pneumonitis secondary to cytotoxic chemotherapeutic agents.[82,84]

Hodgkin's Disease

Whether the incidence of Hodgkin's disease is elevated among AIDS patients is controversial, but its natural history in this setting appears to be significantly altered from that of non-HIV–infected patients.[74,93] AIDS-related Hodgkin's disease is characterized by advanced stage (stage III or IV), common occurrence of B symptoms, and extranodal involvement, typically of the bone marrow.[69,70,74,93–95]

Hodgkin's disease may disseminate in a random, noncontiguous pattern, and widespread disease may occur without hilar or mediastinal lymphadenopathy.[69,74] Mixed cellularity is the most frequently reported histology in HIV-seropositive patients.[93] Pulmonary parenchymal involvement, which may appear radiographically as lobar infiltrates, may also occur without associated hilar or mediastinal lymphadenopathy.[96,97] It appears that hilar or mediastinal adenopathy occurs infrequently in AIDS-related Hodgkin's disease, even in patients with nodular sclerosing histologic subtypes.[70,74,94–97]

Although the morphologic characteristics are similar in classic and AIDS-related Hodgkin's disease, AIDS-related lesions display high-grade histopathologic features.[69] AIDS-related Hodgkin's disease has an aggressive clinical course marked by progressive disease, concurrent opportunistic infections, and poor survival.[69,70,74,94,95]

Bronchogenic Carcinoma

During the past several years, multiple reports have described the development of bronchogenic carcinoma in HIV-seropositive patients, but it is unclear whether there exists a causal or coincidental association between these two disorders. Although the clinical manifestations of bronchogenic carcinoma appear to be altered by HIV infection, it is controversial as to whether the incidence of pulmonary neoplasms is actually increased.[98,99] For example, a retrospective analysis of the tumor registry at Bellevue Hospital in New York failed to reveal an increased number of cases or a change in age distribution of bronchogenic carcinoma when groups from the pre-AIDS era (1976–1979) were

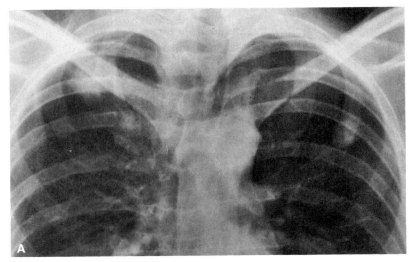

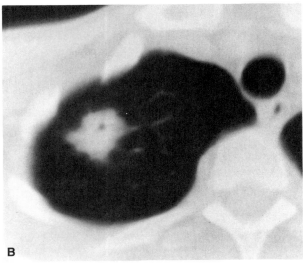

FIG. 19.2-3. Chest radiograph (**A**) of a patient with pulmonary non-Hodgkin's lymphoma who presented with bilateral upper lobe nodular mass lesions. (**B**) The corresponding chest CT scan of the right upper lobe nodular lesion. (Courtesy of Irwin Feuerstein, MD)

compared with those in the AIDS era (1987–1990).[98] Nevertheless, bronchogenic carcinoma may represent an underappreciated cause of pulmonary disease in HIV patients, as evidenced by the finding that 22% of HIV-seropositive patients with focal radiographic abnormalities at San Francisco General Hospital were reported to have bronchogenic carcinoma diagnosed by percutaneous transthoracic needle biopsy.[100]

Pathology

Bronchogenic carcinoma in HIV-positive individuals is most commonly of the non-small cell type, with adenocarcinomas representing the most common histology.[99,101–103] Other histologic types of non-small cell bronchogenic carcinomas in HIV-positive patients include epidermoid, bronchoalveolar, large cell anaplastic, mixed small and large cell, and adenosquamous carcinomas.[99,102,104] Small cell carcinomas and mesotheliomas have also been reported in HIV-positive patients.[99,102,104,105]

Clinical Manifestations

The natural history of bronchogenic carcinoma in HIV-infected individuals appears to be altered compared with HIV-negative patients. HIV-positive patients have developed bronchogenic carcinoma at an earlier age than HIV-negative patients, with a reported median age ranging from 38 to 48 years in six series.[101–103,105–107] HIV-positive individuals also have more extensive radiographic abnormalities, are more likely to present with pleural effusions, and more likely to have a more fulminant course and significantly shortened survival compared with sex-matched, HIV-negative controls.[107] Bronchogenic carcinoma in HIV-positive individuals also appears to have a male predominance, to be more common in intravenous drug abusers, and to be associated with cigarette smoking.[99,101–103,105,107] An association between extant adenocarcinoma and radiographic evidence of tuberculosis has also been suggested.[102] However, there appears to be no association between CD4+ counts and the development of lung carcinoma, suggesting that bronchogenic carcinoma can occur as an early manifestation of HIV infection.[100,103,105,106]

The clinical and radiographic manifestations of bronchogenic carcinoma in HIV-positive patients do not appear to differ from those of individuals who are HIV negative.[103,104,106] Symptoms commonly include cough, chest pain, hemoptysis, and dyspnea, although HIV-positive patients have been reported to have less hypoxemia on admission than non-HIV–positive patients.[106,107] Radiographic manifestations commonly include hilar or peripheral masses and parenchymal nodular lesions.[103] Other common radiographic manifestations are mediastinal adenopathy, atelectasis secondary to hilar mass lesions, cavitary lesions, pleural effusions, and pleura-based masses or pleural thickening.[101,103,104] Pleural disease appears to be frequently associated with adenocarcinomas in HIV-positive patients and reflects the advanced stage of these tumors.[103] However, none of these clinical or radiographic manifestations is specific for bronchogenic carcinoma.

Bronchogenic carcinoma must be included in the differential diagnosis of HIV-positive patients with pulmonary disease who are undergoing an evaluation for other, more common HIV-related infectious or neoplastic disorders. In particular, invasive procedures to obtain tissue for histologic evaluation should be considered in the workup of HIV-positive patients with focal parenchymal mass or nodular lesions. Diagnostic modalities that may be helpful in the evaluation of patients with suspected bronchogenic carcinoma include fiberoptic bronchoscopy with transbronchial biopsies, percutaneous fine-needle aspiration, mediastinoscopy, open lung biopsy, thoracentesis, and pleural biopsy.[100,106,107] Clinicians should be suspicious for concomitant infectious processes, such as *P carinii* pneumonia or tuberculosis, which have been described in the setting of bronchogenic carcinoma.[101]

Natural History

HIV-positive patients frequently present with advanced-stage disease (stage III or IV) and have a fulminant course, with shortened survival times compared with HIV-negative patients.[99,100,103,105,107] Consequently, these patients are frequently not candidates for curative resection and are often treated with combination chemotherapy, radiation therapy, or both modalities.[102,107] Median survival times in two series were reported as 1 and 3 months, with all 26 patients having died by 10 months.[102,105] However, individual patients in other series have survived for as long as 17 months.[99,102]

INTERSTITIAL PNEUMONITIS

Lymphocytic Interstitial Pneumonitis

Lymphocytic interstitial pneumonitis (LIP) and pulmonary lymphoid hyperplasia (PLH) are important, potentially treatable causes of pulmonary disease in children with AIDS. LIP has been reported in as many as 43% to 48% of non-

hemophiliac infants and children with AIDS and in 40% of pediatric AIDS patients who died or required lung biopsy for the diagnosis of pulmonary disease.[108–111] The presence of biopsy-proven LIP in an HIV-seropositive patient younger than 13 years of age is considered diagnostic of AIDS by CDC criteria.[112]

In contrast to the situation in children, LIP infrequently complicates AIDS in adults and does not represent an AIDS-defining illness. The frequency of LIP in adult AIDS patients with pulmonary disease is estimated to be less than 1% to 2%, and only a few cases have been reported in the medical literature.[113] LIP in adults does not appear to be restricted to any particular AIDS risk group; however, black patients may be more predisposed than whites.[54] The diagnosis of adult LIP may precede or follow the diagnosis of AIDS.[54]

Pathology

Although PLH and LIP were originally considered distinct disorders in pediatric patients, the term PLH/LIP complex is currently used to describe what is thought to represent a continuum or spectrum of pulmonary lymphoid lesions.[114,115] PLH and LIP are benign lymphocytic infiltrative disorders that differ in the predominant pattern and location of lymphoid aggregates.[114] In PLH, nodular lymphoid aggregates are localized to the bronchial mucosa and the adjacent interalveolar septa in a distribution corresponding to that of bronchial-associated lymphoid tissue (BALT).[108,114] These nodules are diffusely distributed throughout the pulmonary parenchyma and usually are 0.5 to 2 mm in diameter.[108] Larger nodules, which can be 5 mm in diameter, may contain germinal centers and a thick-walled venule, consistent with hyperplastic BALT.[108,114] Microscopically, these nodules are composed of aggregates of mature and immature lymphocytes and some plasma cells.[108,109]

LIP is characterized histologically by diffuse infiltration of the alveolar septa and peribronchiolar areas by lymphocytes, plasma cells, plasmacytoid lymphocytes, and immunoblasts.[115] LIP characteristically does not cause destruction of the pulmonary vasculature or airways; however, alveolar consolidation secondary to lymphocytic infiltration has been observed in some adult cases.[116–118] LIP has not resulted in interstitial fibrosis in children or adults.[119]

Features of PLH and LIP are often found concurrently in a biopsy specimen, consistent with the hypothesis that these disorders represent a spectrum of the lymphocytic infiltrative process.[108,109,115] The degree of lymphoid infiltration in the PLH/LIP complex may range from mild to severe.[116]

Extrapulmonary sites of lymphoid infiltration have been documented in children and adults with PLH/LIP, suggesting that this process is part of a systemic, polyclonal B-cell lymphoid hyperplasia.[115,118] These extrapulmonary sites have included the liver, colon, thymus, spleen, kidneys, bone marrow, nasopharynx, skeletal muscle, and the parotid, adrenal, and salivary glands (with associated sicca syndrome). A diffuse, infiltrative CD8 lymphocytosis syndrome has been described in adult HIV-infected patients.[120] This syndrome is characterized by a CD8 lymphocytosis with lymphocytic infiltration of the salivary and lacrimal glands and pulmonary parenchyma resulting in sicca symptoms and LIP. Lymphocytic infiltrations of the liver, gastric mucosa, renal interstitium, and thymus also occurred. This disorder was associated with HLA-DR5, black race, and improvement after zidovudine therapy, which suggested that it represented a genetically predetermined host immune response to HIV infection.

Bronchiolitis obliterans has been associated with LIP and may complicate more severe cases.[119] For example, in one study, bronchiolitis obliterans was detected in 8 of 16 adult patients with LIP.[121] Histologically, bronchiolitis obliterans is characterized by loose myxoid connective tissue occluding respiratory bronchioles with distal atelectasis and changes consistent with endogenous lipoid pneumonia.[119] Other unusual disorders reported in the setting of LIP include transformation into Kaposi's sarcoma, development of multiple vascular leiomyomas, and a lymphocytic arteritis resembling the plexiform lesions of primary pulmonary hypertension.[119]

Studies aimed at classifying the cell type of origin in PLH/LIP have yielded variable results.[14] The cellular composition of the lymphocytic infiltrates (ie, lymphocytes, plasma cells, plasmacytoid lymphocytes, and immunoblasts) is consistent with B-cell hyperplasia.[115,122] Immunoperoxidase staining for κ and λ immunoglobulin light chains has revealed the lymphoid infiltrates to be polyclonal.[115,116,123,124] Mixed B-cell and T-cell proliferation has been reported in a pediatric patient, with a predominance of OKT8+ cells.[123] Immunoperoxidase staining of cells from another pediatric LIP patient revealed a predominance of T8 and T11 cells, with occasional T4 and B cells.[125] Immunohistologic staining of lung biopsy specimens from two adults with LIP revealed T lymphocytes, with equal numbers of helper and suppressor T cells in one case and essentially only suppressor cells in the other.[14,54,126] Monoclonal antibody staining of LIP tissue from two children and one adult patient revealed polyclonal lymphocyte populations with a predominance of T cells over B cells and a predominance of suppressor T cells over helper T cells.[119]

Although the pathogenesis of AIDS-associated PLH/LIP remains to be definitively determined, some evidence suggested an etiologic role for EBV or HIV, or both.[14,54,115] For example, in two separate studies involving adult and pediatric patients, all those with LIP had serologic evidence of recrudescent or primary EBV infection, compared with control subjects who were more likely to have evidence of prior EBV infection.[127,128] EBV DNA was detected in the lungs of 80% of 15 patients with LIP in two other studies, along with elevations in levels of antibodies to EBV capsid antigen.[108,125] EBV DNA has also been detected in peribronchiolar lymphocytic infiltrates, peripheral blood lymphocytes, and saliva from an infant with AIDS.[114,123] Consequently, the pathogenesis of the PLH/LIP complex may represent an atypical response to EBV infection by an immune system altered by HIV infection.[115] This theory is supported by the

finding that EBV can activate B cells in a independent, direct fashion, without T cells or macrophages.

Other evidence has suggested that LIP may represent a sequela of pulmonary infection by HIV. Prior studies have found HIV antigen and IgG antibody in BAL specimens from LIP patients, as well as HIV RNA (by in situ hybridization) within pulmonary lymphocytes and macrophages.[129–131] These HIV-infected cells may be capable of inciting an inflammatory infiltrative pulmonary process by the release of cytokines or toxic viral products. For example, HIV proviral DNA has been detected by polymerase chain reaction techniques in alveolar fibroblasts and macrophages from patients with LIP.[132] In this study, HIV-infected alveolar macrophages and fibroblasts were selectively killed in vitro by CD8 HIV-specific cytotoxic T lymphocytes, which suggested the involvement of cell-mediated cytotoxicity in the pathogenesis of LIP. This may also explain the predominance of suppressor-cytotoxic T lymphocytes in lung biopsy specimens from some patients with LIP. Although earlier studies suggested that identification of HIV in BAL fluid or tissue specimens may be specific for LIP, other studies have reported the culture of HIV from BAL fluid from AIDS patients without LIP.[133,134] In one of these studies, however, HIV p24 antigen was detected by immunoassay only from a patient with LIP.[134]

Clinical Presentation

Pediatric PLH/LIP is a subacute or chronic disorder that is characterized by the insidious development of pulmonary disease that can potentially result in respiratory failure. Cough is the most common pulmonary symptom in this age group, occurring in all 11 patients in one study, but fever and dyspnea are uncommon.[108,122] Failure to thrive was reported in all 21 patients in three series.[108,110,122] The physical examination is remarkable for the absence of tachypnea or adventitial lung sounds, but digital clubbing, salivary gland enlargement, and generalized lymphadenopathy are characteristic findings.[108] Fever, tachypnea, and adventitial lung sounds are more likely to represent an infectious process rather than the PLH/LIP complex.[108]

Arterial blood gas analysis generally reveals mild to moderate hypoxemia, with mean PAO_2-PaO_2 gradients ranging from 24 to 40 mm Hg in two studies.[108,135] Although serum lactate dehydrogenase levels may be elevated compared with levels in healthy controls, they are significantly lower than the levels found in the setting of *P carinii* pneumonia.[108] Hypergammaglobulinemia in excess of that found in *P carinii* pneumonia is also common.[108] Chest radiographs reveal a diffuse pattern of 1- to 5-mm nodules associated with an underlying interstitial pulmonary infiltrate.[108] With disease progression, these nodules increase in size, and there is concomitant widening of the hilum and superior mediastinum, suggesting lymphadenopathy.[108,114,135] Gallium scans may reveal a diffuse pattern of uptake within the lungs that is indistinguishable from that observed in *P carinii* pneumonia.[114] CT radiographic evidence of bronchiectasis complicating pediatric LIP was reported in 13% of cases in one series.[136]

The clinical manifestations of adult LIP are remarkable for the insidious development of pulmonary disease. Presenting complaints are often nonspecific and have included dyspnea, nonproductive cough, fever, and weight loss.[117,118,126,137] Physical examination often reveals bilateral inspiratory crackles on lung auscultation, as well as diffuse lymphadenopathy.[118,124,137] Severe immunologic abnormalities consistent with AIDS, such as an inverted T4 : T8 ratio, decreased T4 count, and polyclonal hyperimmunoglobulinemia, are common.[118,121] Arterial blood gas values may be normal or may reveal hypoxemia, increased PAO_2-PaO_2, and mild hypocapnia.[117,118,126,137] Pulmonary function tests may disclose restrictive impairments on spirometric testing and reductions in the diffusing capacity for carbon monoxide, which have been reported to be as low as 28% of predicted values.[118,126,137] Chest radiographs characteristically reveal diffuse reticulonodular interstitial infiltrates, with nodules up to 5 mm in diameter (grade I).[118,119,121,126,137] In later-stage disease, single or multiple patchy areas of alveolar consolidation may be associated with diffuse reticulonodular infiltrates (grade II).[118,119,121,126,137] In one study of 16 patients with LIP, 56% had combined reticulonodular interstitial and patchy alveolar infiltrates, and the remainder had isolated interstitial infiltrates.[121] In this study, the nodules were as large as 5 mm in diameter. Radiographic evidence of mediastinal and hilar lymph node enlargement has also been reported.[137] Gallium 67 scans of adult patients with LIP have shown areas of increased activity within the pulmonary parenchyma.[126,137]

Diagnosis

Histologic examination of the pulmonary parenchyma is necessary to establish a definitive diagnosis of LIP. Although a large sample of pulmonary parenchyma is better suited to establishing this diagnosis, transbronchial biopsies may be adequate if there is evidence of an interstitial lymphocytic and plasma cell infiltration.[117,121,126,130,137,138] In five small studies involving 10 adult patients, transbronchial biopsies established the diagnosis of LIP in 50% of cases.[117,126,130,137,139] Open lung biopsy may be necessary if transbronchial biopsy fails to establish a diagnosis. Because LIP in adults is often an indolent process that may not require specific therapy, the role of diagnostic procedures, such as fiberoptic bronchoscopy, often is to exclude the presence of an opportunistic infection, which can have similar clinical and radiographic manifestations. This is important in patients with an established diagnosis of LIP who experience a change in symptoms or radiographic infiltrates, especially if immunosuppressive therapy (eg, corticosteroids) is being administered.

For pediatric patients, an open lung biopsy is often necessary to establish a definitive histologic diagnosis of PLH/LIP complex.[54] In an attempt to avoid invasive diagnostic procedures in this patient population, it has been suggested that PLH/LIP complex can be discriminated from opportunistic infections, such as *P carinii* pneumonia, on the basis of characteristic clinical and radiographic manifestations.[114] BAL, which has been effective for the diagnosis of *P carinii* pneumonia in pediatric AIDS patients, should be considered to exclude the possibility of an infectious process if the diagnosis of PLH/LIP is established on clinical grounds alone.[54,140]

Natural History and Therapy

The natural history of PLH/LIP in children ranges from spontaneous resolution to slowly progressive pulmonary disease.[54,114] The typical course of pediatric PLH/LIP is characterized by the indolent development of hypoxemia, digital clubbing, and worsening radiographic infiltrates. Frank tachypnea and severe hypoxemia leading to respiratory failure may occur late in the course of disease.[114,141] Because of the variable course of PLH/LIP, therapy often is not required immediately and may be reserved until clinical evidence of disease progression occurs, such as worsening hypoxemia (PaO_2 >60 mm Hg).[141] Frequent and careful monitoring of disease activity is necessary in managing all patients.

If therapy is required, corticosteroids may be used, although limited data exist regarding their efficacy in this setting. In one study, all five patients experienced improvements in oxygenation and radiographic infiltrates after at least 3 months of therapy (prednisone, 2 mg/kg/day for 2 to 4 weeks until the PaO_2 increased by 20 mm Hg, followed by 0.5 to 0.75 mg/kg on alternate days).[135] Neither the rate nor the severity of opportunistic infections increased, but all patients received intravenous γ-globulin. The 10 patients who did not receive corticosteroid therapy developed finger clubbing and progressive nodular infiltrates, and nine had progressive hypoxemia. Termination of corticosteroids in one patient was associated with worsening hypoxemia. Although relapses have been reported after termination of corticosteroids, stable remissions after discontinuation of long-term corticosteroid therapy have also been described.[114,125] Intravenous γ-globulin has not been efficacious for this disorder, and no data are available regarding antiretroviral therapy for pediatric PLH/LIP.[54,114,135]

The prognosis for children with PLH/LIP is generally more favorable than for other pediatric AIDS patients. In five series involving 22 patients, 95% were alive at the conclusion of the follow-up periods, which ranged from 6 months to 5.5 years.[108–110,122,124] These patients appear to be less likely to develop opportunistic infections.[108,125] Progression of PLH/LIP to frank lymphoma has not been a feature of pediatric PLH/LIP, although there has been one case of an infant who developed CNS lymphoma.[54,125] Pediatric PLH/LIP has been found rarely to progress to a polyclonal B-cell lymphoproliferative disorder (PBLD).[142] PBLD is characterized by a polyclonal B-cell nodular infiltration of nodal and extranodal sites that is thought to represent an intermediate portion of the spectrum of lymphoproliferative disorders, between PLH/LIP complex and malignant lymphoma.

Adult LIP has a variable course that ranges from mild, stable disease to more severe pneumonitis resulting in significant dyspnea. The characteristic natural history of adult LIP is that of an insidious, chronic process with stable clinical manifestations that often does not require specific therapy. Spontaneous improvement of disease manifestations has also been reported.[117,118,138] When progressive dyspnea necessitates the institution of therapy, corticosteroids have been used with various results.[138] Although improvement of symptoms, hypoxemia, and radiographic infiltrates has occurred with oral prednisone therapy, relapses have been reported after discontinuation of therapy.[126] Adult LIP generally does not progress to respiratory failure or death, and most patients eventually succumb to other HIV-related complications, especially opportunistic infections.[54,126,137,138] Consequently, corticosteroids should probably be withheld unless severe dyspnea or hypoxemia occurs. Only limited and conflicting data are available regarding the role of antiretroviral therapy in this setting. Two patients were reported to improve after zidovudine therapy, but another patient did not respond to zidovudine or high-dose acyclovir.[139,143] As in pediatric LIP/PLH, progression to lymphoma does not appear to occur.[121]

Nonspecific Interstitial Pneumonitis

Nonspecific interstitial pneumonitis (NIP) is a frequent but usually self-limited cause of pulmonary dysfunction in adult AIDS patients.[115] NIP has been documented in 5% to 38% of 240 AIDS patients in two series and was the cause of pneumonitis in 11% to 32% of patients with pulmonary disease.[42,144] NIP occurred in 8% of 23 asymptomatic HIV-infected patients without *P carinii* pneumonia in a prospective study.[145] Little information exists regarding NIP complicating pediatric HIV infections. Although early reports described desquamative interstitial pneumonitis (DIP) as a distinct entity, a later reappraisal found concurrent processes, such as LIP and *Aspergillus* and *Pneumocystis* infections, in these patients.[109,114,115] Consequently, it is unclear whether DIP in pediatric patients occurs secondary to other pulmonary disorders or represents a primary response to HIV or other infectious agents.[116]

Pathology

The histopathology of NIP is characterized by mild interstitial infiltration with lymphocytes and plasma cells.[144] Moderate edema, fibrin deposition, alveolar lining cell hyperplasia, and alveolar septal thickening are common.[144] Hyaline membranes, consistent with endothelial-epithelial damage, and interstitial lymphoid aggregates may also be present.[144] Histopathologic findings in asymptomatic patients with NIP are characterized by perivascular and peribronchial lymphocytic interstitial infiltrates and aggregates without associated edema, fibrin deposition, hyaline membranes, or alveolitis.[145]

The cause of NIP is unclear. Although it has been suggested that NIP might represent an inflammatory response to HIV or EBV, no data exist to support this hypothesis.[144] In one report, in situ hybridization studies of 10 patients failed to demonstrate the presence of HIV.[144] However, another study found that only 1 of 11 patients with NIP was receiving zidovudine, compared with 7 of 12 patients without pulmonary disease, which suggests a possible etiologic role for HIV.[145] In many patients, NIP may be a consequence of prior pulmonary infections, concurrent pulmonary Kaposi's sarcoma, or exposure to potentially toxic recreational or therapeutic drugs.[144,146] However, NIP has also been documented in patients without any of these possible causes.[144]

Clinical and Radiographic Presentation

The clinical presentation of NIP is nonspecific and may be indistinguishable from that of other pulmonary complications of HIV infection, such as opportunistic infections.[144] Disease manifestations are characteristically mild, and patients are asymptomatic or complain of fever or cough.[144,145] Physical examination may reveal diffuse, bilateral rales.[146] Arterial blood gas determinations characteristically reveal mild to moderate widening of the PAO_2–PaO_2 gradient, which ranged from 11 to 32 mm Hg in 24 patients in two studies.[144,145] Exercise testing may reveal abnormal widening of the PAO_2–PaO_2.[42] Pulmonary function testing of 14 patients in two series revealed normal mean diffusing capacities ranging from 82% to 85% of predicted values, although individual patients had values as low as 66% of predicted.[42,145]

Radiographic manifestations are also often mild and nonspecific. Chest radiographs reveal diffuse interstitial infiltrates or are normal.[42,144,146,147] These interstitial infiltrates may be subtle or coarse in appearance and occasionally are unilateral or associated with pleural effusions.[118] Chest radiographs were normal for 44% to 100% of patients in three studies but normal for only 1 of 7 patients in another series.[42,144,145,147]Ga citrate scans were commonly normal or revealed mild 1+ pulmonary uptake; however, two patients had 2+ or 3+ pulmonary uptake.[145]

Natural History

The natural history of NIP is characterized by a chronic, indolent course that commonly stabilizes or resolves without specific therapy.[42,144] Patients can be completely asymptomatic, with only histopathologic evidence of subclinical disease.[145] Although NIP can result in ongoing lung injury, it does not result in respiratory failure or death, and its mild manifestations usually do not justify the institution of immunosuppressive therapy. The clinical relevance of NIP is that its clinical presentation may be identical to that of an AIDS-related opportunistic infections, such as *P carinii* pneumonia, that requires the institution of specific antimicrobial therapy.[144] The role of diagnostic procedures in this setting is to exclude the presence of other potentially treatable pulmonary infections rather than document NIP. As in

LIP, fiberoptic bronchoscopy is indicated to rule out an opportunistic infection when a patient with known NIP has a change in symptoms or radiographic infiltrates.

Lymphocytic Alveolitis

Analysis of BAL cell populations from AIDS patients by various investigators have revealed increases in the proportion and number of lymphocytes consistent with lymphocytic alveolitis.[148–150] Subtyping studies revealed these cells to be CD8+ cytotoxic T lymphocytes that were capable of recognizing and killing HIV-infected alveolar macrophages.[151,152] In one report, a CD8+ cytotoxic lymphocytic alveolitis affected 72% of 22 HIV-infected patients without pulmonary infections or neoplasms, suggesting that it is a common finding in this setting.[152] Sixty-seven percent of these patients had pulmonary symptoms (ie, nonproductive cough and dyspnea on exertion), and 36% had diffuse interstitial infiltrates that reflected the degree of lymphocytosis. Moreover, 85% had abnormal pulmonary function test results with a decreased diffusing capacity for carbon monoxide or abnormal widening of the PAO_2–PaO_2 gradient with exercise. Another study found a significant correlation between the number and cytotoxic activity of CD8+/D44+ T lymphocytes against alveolar macrophages and the clearance of aerosolized technetium-labeled DTPA, which suggested disruption of the alveolar epithelium.[153] Open lung biopsy in four of the patients disclosed a diffuse lymphocytic infiltration involving lymphatic vascular channels but sparing the alveolar septa. Consequently, the investigators suggested that lymphocytic alveolitis might represent part of the spectrum of HIV-related pulmonary lymphoid infiltrative disorders, a spectrum that includes PLH/LIP and NIP.[152,153]

INFLAMMATORY AIRWAY DISORDERS

Lymphocytic Bronchiolitis

Inflammatory disorders of the airways have been described in HIV-infected patients. Lymphocytic bronchiolitis has been described in an adult patient with AIDS-related complex who presented with dyspnea, cough, diffuse micronodular infiltrates, mild obstructive and restrictive spirometric abnormalities, and a severely decreased carbon monoxide diffusing capacity.[154] BAL revealed a cytotoxic-suppressor T-cell lymphocytosis, and transbronchial biopsy revealed an intense peribronchiolar infiltration with lymphocytes and plasma cells. The patient was observed expectantly, without a change in disease manifestations. In a study of 33 patients with lymphocytic alveolitis, 8 had spirometric evidence of small airways disease and 3 of 4 patients who underwent open lung biopsy had bronchiolitis.[152] Lymphocytic bronchiolitis may represent part of the spectrum of HIV-related pulmonary lymphoid infiltrative processes and contribute to the airways obstruction that has been documented in some AIDS patients.

Bronchiolitis Obliterans Organizing Pneumonia

At least three cases of corticosteroid-responsive bronchiolitis obliterans organizing pneumonia (BOOP) have been reported in HIV-positive patients.[155,156] All patients had AIDS-related complex or AIDS and had presented with an acute respiratory distress or a subacute illness.[156] Clinical manifestations include fever, nonproductive cough, dyspnea, bibasilar dry crackles, and hypoxemia. Chest radiographs may reveal focal or progressive bilateral alveolar infiltrates. Fiberoptic bronchoscopy with BAL and transbronchial biopsies are typically nondiagnostic in this setting, and an open or thoracoscopic lung biopsy is required to establish the diagnosis. Lymphocytic alveolitis has been detected by BAL in a patient with BOOP. It is important to establish the diagnosis of BOOP, because this is a corticosteroid-responsive disorder, although some cases are resistant to therapy.

Bronchiectasis

CT radiographic evidence of bronchiectasis has been documented in adult AIDS patients. In most cases, bronchiectasis appeared to be a consequence of pyogenic infection and had an accelerated clinical course.[157] Other disorders associated with the development of bronchiectasis included *P carinii* pneumonia, LIP, and NIP.[157]

PULMONARY HYPERTENSION

Several reports have described primary pulmonary hypertension in AIDS patients. Although pulmonary hypertension has been identified in HIV-seropositive individuals with potential risk factors for secondary pulmonary hypertension, such as hemophilia, intravenous drug abuse, or infectious pulmonary processes, cases have been identified in individuals without these risk factors and without concomitant pulmonary disease.[158–162] Even in the setting of a history of intravenous drug abuse, no evidence of granulomatous inflammation secondary to foreign body microemboli were observed, and characteristic plexogenic pulmonary arterial lesions were detected.[162] Although it has been hypothesized that an HIV-associated vasculitis might be responsible for the development of primary pulmonary hypertension, no evidence of vasculitic lesions was found, and attempts to localize HIV-1 infection to the vascular endothelium by electron microscopy, immunohistochemistry, in situ hybridization, and polymerase chain reaction have been unsuccessful.[161,162] It remains unclear whether the development of primary pulmonary hypertension is associated with HIV infection or represents a coincidental finding.

CONCLUSIONS

Noninfectious pulmonary manifestations of HIV infection represent a spectrum of malignant and nonmalignant diseases. The accurate diagnosis of these disorders is important for three reasons. First, specific therapy may be indicated in some clinical settings. Second, the short-term and long-term prognoses may be significantly altered. Third, these processes are frequently indistinguishable from infectious pulmonary complications of HIV infection that may require specific and immediate antimicrobial therapy.

REFERENCES

1. Murray JF, Garay SM, Hopewell PC, et al. Pulmonary complications of the acquired immunodeficiency syndrome: an update. Report of the Second National Heart, Lung and Blood Institute Workshop. Am Rev Respir Dis 1987;135:504.
2. Steis RG, Longo DL. Clinical, biologic and therapeutic aspects of malignancies associated with the acquired immunodeficiency syndrome: part 1. Ann Allergy 1988;60:310.
3. Krown SE. AIDS-associated Kaposi's sarcoma: pathogenesis, clinical course and treatment. AIDS 1988;2:71.
4. Guarda LA, Luna MA, Smith JL, et al. Acquired immunodeficiency syndrome: Postmortem findings. Am J Clin Pathol 1984;81:549.
5. Niedt GW, Schinella RA. Acquired immunodeficiency syndrome: clinicopathologic study of 56 autopsies. Arch Pathol Lab Med 1985;109:727.
6. Safai B, Johnson KD, Myskowski PL, et al. The natural history of Kaposi's sarcoma in the acquired immunodeficiency syndrome. Ann Intern Med 1985;103:744.
7. Munoz A, Schrager LK, Bacellar H, et al. Trends in the incidence of outcomes defining acquired immunodeficiency syndrome (AIDS) in the Multicenter AIDS Cohort Study: 1985–1991. Am J Epidemiol 1993;137:423.
8. Montaner JSG, Le T, Hogg R, et al. The changing spectrum of AIDS index diseases in Canada. AIDS 1994;8:693.
9. Tappero JW, Conant MA, Wolfe SF, Berger TG. Kaposi's sarcoma: etiology, pathogenesis, histology, clinical spectrum, staging criteria and therapy. J Am Acad Dermatol 1993;28:371.
10. Moore PS, Chang Y. Detection of herpesvirus-like DNA sequences in Kaposi's sarcoma in patients with and those without HIV infection. N Engl J Med 1995;332:1227.
11. Roizman B. New viral footprints in Kaposi's sarcoma. N Engl J Med 1995;332:1181.
12. Levine AM. AIDS-related malignancies: the emerging epidemic. J Natl Cancer Inst 1993;85:1382.
13. Ensoli B, Barillari G, Salahuddin SZ, et al. Tat protein of HIV-1 stimulates growth of cells derived from Kaposi's sarcoma lesions of AIDS patients. Nature 1990;345:84.
14. Travis WD, Lack EE, Ognibene FP, et al. Lung biopsy interpretation in the acquired immunodeficiency syndrome: experience of the National Institutes of Health with literature review. Prog AIDS Pathol 1989;1:51.
15. Case records of the Massachusetts General Hospital: case 1—1990. N Engl J Med 1990;320:43.
16. Nash G, Flefiel S. Pathologic features of the lung in the acquired immune deficiency syndrome: an autopsy study of seventeen homosexual males. Am J Clin Pathol 1984;81:6,1984.
17. O'Brien RF, Cohn DL. Serosanguineous pleural effusions in AIDS-associated Kaposi's sarcoma. Chest 1989;96:460.
18. Garay SM, Belenko M, Fazzini E, Schinella R. Pulmonary manifestations of Kaposi's sarcoma. Chest 1987;91:39.
19. Bach MC, Bagwell SP, Fannin, JP. Primary pulmonary Kaposi's sarcoma in the acquired immunodeficiency syndrome: a cause of persistent pyrexia. Am J Med 1988;85:274.
20. Nathan S, Vaghaiwalla R, Mohsenifar Z. Use of Nd:YAG laser in endobronchial Kaposi's sarcoma. Chest 1990;98:1299.
21. Fouret PJ, Touboul JL, Mavaud CM, et al. Pulmonary Kaposi's sarcoma in patients with acquired immune deficiency syndrome: a clinicopathological study. Thorax 1981;42:162.
22. Purdy LJ, Colby TV, Yousem SA, Battifora H. Pulmonary Kaposi's sarcoma: premortem histologic diagnosis. Am J Surg Pathol 1986;10:301.
23. Davis SD, Henschke CL, Chamides BK, Westcott JL. Intrathoracic Kaposi sarcoma in AIDS patients: radiographic pathologic correlation. Radiology 1987;163:495.
24. Kornfield H, Axelrod JL. Pulmonary presentation of Kaposi's sarcoma in a homosexual patient. Am Rev Respir Dis 1983;127:248.
25. Roux FJ, Bancal C, Dombret MC, et al. Pulmonary Kaposi's sarcoma revealed by a solitary nodule in a patient with acquired immunodeficiency syndrome. Am J Respir Crit Care Med 1994;149:1041.
26. Ognibene FP, Steis RG, Macher AM, et al. Kaposi's sarcoma causing pulmonary infiltrates and respiratory failure in the acquired immunodeficiency syndrome. Ann Intern Med 1985;102:471.
27. Meduri GU, Stover DE, Lee M, et al. Pulmonary Kaposi's sarcoma in the acquired immune deficiency syndrome: clinical, radiographic and pathologic manifestations. Am J Med 1986;81:11.
28. Marchevsky A, Rosen MJ, Chrystal G, Kleinerman J. Pulmonary complications of the acquired immunodeficiency syndrome: a clinicopathologic study of 70 cases. Hum Pathol 1985;16:659.
29. Misra DP, Sunderrajan EV, Hurst DJ, Maltby JD. Kaposi's sarcoma of the lung: radiography and pathology. Thorax 1982;37:155.
30. Pitchenik AE, Fischl MA, Saldana MJ. Kaposi's sarcoma of the tracheobronchial tree: clinical, bronchoscopic, and pathologic features. Chest 1985;87:122.
31. Hamm PG, Judson MA, Aranda CP. Diagnosis of pulmonary Kaposi's sarcoma with fiberoptic bronchoscopy and endobronchial biopsy: a report of five cases. Cancer 1987;59:807.
32. Kaplan LD, Hopewell PC, Jaffe J, et al. Kaposi sarcoma involving the lung in patients with the acquired immunodeficiency syndrome. J Acquir Immune Defic Syndr 1988;1:23.
33. Greenberg JE, Fischl MA, Berger JR. Upper airway obstruction secondary to acquired immunodeficiency syndrome-related Kaposi's sarcoma. Chest 1985;88:638.
34. Sivit CJ, Schwartz AM, Rockoff SD. Kaposi's sarcoma of the lung in AIDS. Radiologic-pathologic analysis. AJR Am J Roentgenol 1987;148:25.
35. Santucci M, Pimpinelli N, Moretti S, Giannotti B. Classic and immunodeficiency-associated Kaposi's sarcoma. Arch Pathol Lab Med 1988;112:1214.
36. Nash G, Flegiel S. Kaposi's sarcoma presenting as pulmonary disease in the acquired immunodeficiency syndrome: diagnosis by lung biopsy. Hum Pathol 1984;15:999.
37. Ognibene FP, Shelhamer JH. Kaposi's sarcoma. Clin Chest Med 1988;9:459.
38. Pozniak AL, Latif AS, Neill P, Houston S, Chen K, Robertson V. Pulmonary Kaposi's sarcoma in Africa. Thorax 1992;47:730.
39. Mitchell DM, McCarty M, Fleming J, Moss FM. Bronchopulmonary Kaposi's sarcoma in patients with AIDS. Thorax 1992;47:726.
40. Miller RF, Tomlinson MC, Cottril CP, Donald JJ, Spittle MF, Semple SJG. Bronchopulmonary Kaposi's sarcoma in patients with AIDS. Thorax 1992;47:721.
41. Gill PS, Akil B, Colletti P, et al. Pulmonary Kaposi's sarcoma: clinical findings and results of therapy. Am J Med 1989;87:57.
42. Stover DE, White DA, Romano PA, et al. Spectrum of pulmonary diseases associated with the acquired immune deficiency syndrome. Am J Med 1985;78:429.
43. Stover DE, Meduri GU. Pulmonary function tests. Clin Chest Med 1988;9:473.
44. Naidich DP, Tarras M, Garay SM, et al. Kaposi's sarcoma: CT-radiographic correlation. Chest 1989;96:723.
45. Zibrak JD, Silvestri RC, Costello P, et al. Bronchoscopic and radiologic features of Kaposi's sarcoma involving the respiratory system. Chest 1986;90:476.
46. Wolff SD, Kuhlman JE, Fishman EK. Thoracic Kaposi's sarcoma in AIDS: CT findings. J Comput Assist Tomogr 1993;17:60.
47. Lai KK. Pulmonary Kaposi's sarcoma presenting as diffuse reticular nodular infiltrates with cavitary lesions. South Med J 1990;83:1096.
48. Pandya K, Lal C, Tuchschmidt J, et al. Bilateral chylothorax with pulmonary Kaposi's sarcoma. Chest 1988;94:1316.
49. Floris C, Sulis ML, Turno R, et al. Pneumothorax in pleuropulmonary Kaposi's sarcoma related to acquired immunodeficiency syndrome. Am J Med 1989;87:123.
50. Khalil AM, Carette MF, Cadranel JL, Mayaud ChM, Akoun GM, Bigot JM. Magnetic resonance imaging findings in pulmonary Kaposi's sarcoma: a series of 10 cases. Eur Respir J 1994;7:1285.
51. Woolfenden JM, Carrasquillo JA, Larson SM, et al. Acquired immunodeficiency syndrome: Ga-67 citrate imaging. Radiology 1987;162:383.

52. Kramer EL, Sanger JJ, Garay SM, et al. Gallium-67 scans of the chest in patients with acquired immunodeficiency syndrome. J Nucl Med 1987;28:1107.

53. Golden JA, Sollitto RA. The radiology of pulmonary disease: chest radiography, computed tomography and gallium scanning. Clin Chest Med 1988;9:481.

54. White DA, Matthay RA. Noninfectious pulmonary complications of infection with the human immunodeficiency virus. Am Rev Respir Dis 1989;140:1763.

55. Lee VW, Rosen MP, Baum A, et al. AIDS-related Kaposi sarcoma: findings on thallium 201 scintigraphy. AJR Am J Roentgenol 1988;151:1233.

56. Lau K, Av J, Rubin A, et al. Kaposi's sarcoma of the tracheobronchial tree. Chest 1986;89:158.

57. Au JP, Krauthammer M, Lau K, Rubin A. Kaposi's sarcoma presenting with endobronchial lesions. Heart Lung 1986;15:411.

58. Hanson PJV, Harcourt-Webster JN, Gazzard BG, Collins JV. Fiberoptic bronchoscopy in diagnosis of bronchopulmonary Kaposi's sarcoma. Thorax 1987;42:269.

59. Stover DE, White DA, Romano PA, Gellene RA. Diagnosis of pulmonary disease in acquired immune deficiency syndrome. Am Rev Respir Dis 1984;130:659.

60. Griffiths MH, Kocjan G, Miller RF, Godfrey-Faussett P. Diagnosis of pulmonary disease in human immunodeficiency virus infection: role of transbronchial biopsy and bronchoalveolar lavage. Thorax 1989; 44:554.

61. Hughes-Davies L, Kocjan G, Spittle MF, Miller RF. Occult alveolar haemorrhage in bronchopulmonary Kaposi's sarcoma. J Clin Pathol 1992;45:536.

62. Pass HI, Potter D, Shelhamer J, et al. Indications for and diagnostic efficacy of open-lung biopsy in the patient with acquired immunodeficiency syndrome. Ann Thorac Surg 1986;41:307.

63. McKenna RJ, Campbell A, McMunrey MJ, Mountain CF. Diagnosis for interstitial lung disease in patients with acquired immunodeficiency syndrome: a prospective comparison of bronchial washing, alveolar lavage, transbronchial lung biopsy, and open-lung biopsy. Ann Thorac Surg 1986;41:318.

64. Fitzgerald W, Bevelaqua FA, Garay SM, Aranda CP. The role of open lung biopsy in patients with the acquire immunodeficiency syndrome. Chest 1987;91:659.

65. Hill ADK, Darzi A, Menzies-Gow N, Riordan JF. Thoracoscopic biopsy in the diagnosis of pulmonary Kaposi's sarcoma. J Laparoendosc Surg 1993;3:571.

66. Cadranel JL, Kammoun S, Chevret S, et al. Results of chemotherapy in 30 AIDS patients with symptomatic pulmonary Kaposi's sarcoma. Thorax 1994;49:958.

67. Presant CA, Scolaro M, Kennedy P, et al. Liposomal daunorubicin treatment of HIV-associated Kaposi's sarcoma. Lancet 1993;341:1242.

68. Schurmann D, Dormann A, Gruenwald T, Rif B. Successful treatment of AIDS-related pulmonary Kaposi's sarcoma with liposomal daunorubicin. Eur Respir J 1994;7:824.

69. Knowles DM, Chadburn A. The neoplasms associated with AIDS. In: Joshi W, ed. Pathology of AIDS and other manifestations of HIV infection. New York: Igaku-Shoin, 1990:83.

70. Safai B, Lynfield R, Lowenthal DA, Koziner B. Cancers associated with HIV infection. Anticancer Res 1987;7:1055.

71. Raphael BG, Knowles DM. Acquired immunodeficiency syndrome-associated non-Hodgkin's lymphoma. Semin Oncol 1990;17:361.

72. Levine AM. Lymphoma in acquired immunodeficiency syndrome. Semin Oncol 1990;104:12.

73. Kaplan MH, Susin M, Pahwa SG, et al. Neoplastic complications of HTLV-III infection: lymphomas and solid tumors. Am J Med 1987;82:389.

74. Knowles DM, Chamulak GA, Subar X, et al. Lymphoid neoplasia associated with the acquired immunodeficiency syndrome. Ann Intern Med 1988;108:744.

75. Ziegler JL, Beckstead JA, Volberdini PA, et al. Non-Hodgkin's lymphoma in 90 homosexual men: relation to generalized lymphadenopathy and the acquired immunodeficiency syndrome. N Engl J Med 1984;311:565.

76. Levine AM, Meyer PR, Begandy MK, et al. Development of B-cell lymphoma in homosexual men: clinical and immunologic findings. Ann Intern Med 1984;100:7.

77. Kaplan LD, Abrams DI, Feigal E, et al. AIDS-associated non-Hodgkin's lymphoma in San Francisco. JAMA 1989;261:719.

78. Bermudez MA, Grant KM, Rodvien R. Non-Hodgkin's lymphoma in a population with or at risk for acquired immunodeficiency syndrome: indications for intensive chemotherapy. Am J Med 1989;86:71.

79. Levine AM, Gill PS, Meyer PR, et al. Retrovirus and malignant lymphoma in homosexual men. JAMA 1985;254:1921,1985.

80. Lowenthal DA, Straus DJ, Campbell SW, et al. AIDS-related lymphoid neoplasia: the Memorial Hospital experience. Cancer 1988;61:2325.

81. Polish LB, Cohn DL, Ryder JW, et al. Pulmonary non-Hodgkin's lymphoma in AIDS. Chest 1989;96:1321.

82. Sourour MS, Stover DE, Fels AOS. Pulmonary disease in AIDS patients with lymphoma. Am Rev Respir Dis 1987;131:A168.

83. Kalter SP, Riggs SA, Cabanillas F, et al. Aggressive non- Hodgkin's lymphomas in immunocompromised homosexual males. Blood 1985;66:655.

84. Ioachim HL, Cooper MC, Hellman GC. Lymphomas in men at high risk for acquired immune deficiency syndrome. Cancer 1985;56:2831.

85. Sider L, Weiss AJ, Smi MD, VonRoenn JH, Glassroth J. Varied appearance of AIDS-related lymphoma in the chest. Radiology 1989;171:629.

86. Poelzleitner D, Huebsch P, Mayerhofer S, et al. Primary pulmonary lymphoma in a patient with the acquired immune deficiency syndrome. Thorax 1989;44:4138.

87. Colebunders R, Mertens V, Blot K, et al. Pulmonary T-cell lymphoma in a patient with the acquired immunodeficiency syndrome. Clin Infect Dis 1993;16:188.

88. Herndier BG, Shiramizu BT, Jewett NE, Aldape KD, Reyes GR, McGrath MS. Acquired immunodeficiency syndrome-associated T-cell lymphoma: evidence for human immunodeficiency virus type 1-associated T-cell transformation. Blood 1992;79:1768.

89. Irwin DH, Kaplan LD. Pulmonary manifestations of acquired immunodeficiency syndrome-associated malignancies. Semin Respir Infect 1993;8:139.

90. Cesarman E, Chang Y, Moore PS, Said JW, Knowles DM. Kaposi's sarcoma-associated herpesvirus-like DNA sequences in AIDS-related body-cavity-based lymphomas. N Engl J Med 1995;332:1186.

91. Loureiro C, Gill PS, Meyer PR, et al. Autopsy findings in AIDS-related lymphoma. Cancer 1988;62:735.

92. Monfardini S, Tirelli U, Vaccher E. Treatment of acquired immunodeficiency syndrome (AIDS)-related cancer. Cancer Treat Rev 1994;20:149.

93. Bernstein L, Hamilton AS. The epidemiology of AIDS-related malignancies. Curr Opin Oncol 1993;5:822.

94. Prior E, Goldberg AF, Conjalka MS, et al. Hodgkin's disease in homosexual men: an AIDS-related phenomenon? Am J Med 1986;81:1085.

95. Unger PD, Strauchen JA. Hodgkin's disease in AIDS complex patients: report of four cases and tissue immunologic marker studies. Cancer 1986;58:821.

96. Scheib RG, Siegel RS. Atypical Hodgkin's disease and the acquired immunodeficiency syndrome. Ann Intern Med 1985;102:554.

97. Schoeppel SL, Hoppe RT, Dorfman RF, et al. Hodgkin's disease in homosexual men with generalized lymphadenopathy. Ann Intern Med 1985;102:68.

98. Chan TK, Aranda CP, Rom WN. Bronchogenic carcinoma in young patients at risk for acquired immunodeficiency syndrome. Chest 1993;103:862.

99. Fraire AE, Awe RJ. Lung cancer in association with human immunodeficiency virus infection. Cancer 1992;70:432.

100. Gruden JF, Klein JS, Webb WR. Percutaneous transthoracic needle biopsy in AIDS: analysis in 32 patients. Radiology 1993;189:567.

101. Fishman JE, Schwartz DS, Sais GJ, Flores MR, Sridhar KS. Bronchogenic carcinoma in HIV-positive patients: findings on chest radiographs and CT scans. AJR Am J Roentgenol 1995;164:57.

102. Vaccher E, Tirelli U, Spina M, et al. Lung cancer in 19 patients with HIV infection. Ann Oncol 1993;4:85.

103. White CS, Haramati LB, Elder KH, Karp J, Belani CP. Carcinoma of the lung in HIV-positive patients: findings on chest radiographs and CT scans. AJR Am J Roentgenol 1995;164:593.

104. Braun MA, Killam DA, Remick SC, Ruckdeschel JC. Lung cancer in patients seropositive for human immunodeficiency virus. Radiology 1990;175:341.

105. Sridhar KS, Flores MR, Raub WA, Saldana M. Lung cancer in patients with human immunodeficiency virus infection compared with historic control subjects. Chest 1992;102:1704.

106. Tenholder MF, Jackson HD. Bronchogenic carcinoma in patients seropositive for human immunodeficiency virus. Chest 1993;104:1049.

107. Karp J, Profeta G, Marantz PR, Karpel JP. Lung cancer in patients with immunodeficiency syndrome. Chest 1993;103:410.

108. Rubinstein A, Morecki R, Silverman B, et al. Pulmonary disease in children with acquired immune deficiency syndrome and AIDS-related complex. J Pediatr 1986;108:498,1986.

109. Joshi W, Oleske JM, Minnefor AB, et al. Pathologic pulmonary findings in children with the acquired immunodeficiency syndrome: a study of ten cases. Hum Pathol 1985;16:241.

110. Scott GB, Buck BE, Leterman JG, et al. Acquired immunodeficiency syndrome in infants. N Engl J Med 1984;310:76.

111. Jason JM, Stehr-Green J, Holman RC, et al, for the Hemophilia-AIDS Collaborative Study Group. Human immunodeficiency virus infection in hemophilic children. Pediatrics 1988;82:565.

112. Centers for Disease Control. Classification system for human immunodeficiency virus (HIV) infection in children under 13 years of age. MMWR 1987;36:225.

113. Cohn DL, Stover DE, O'Brien RF, et al. Pulmonary complications of AIDS. Advances in diagnosis and treatment. Am Rev Respir Dis 1988;138:1051.

114. Rubinstein A, Morecki R, Goldman H. Pulmonary diseases in infants and children. Clin Chest Med 1988;9:507.

115. Joshi W, Oleske JM. Pulmonary lesions in children with the acquired immunodeficiency syndrome: a reappraisal based on data in additional cases and follow-up study of previously reported cases. Hum Pathol 1986;17:641.

116. Joshi W. Pathology of acquired immunodeficiency syndrome in children. In: Joshi W, ed. Pathology of AIDS and other manifestations of HIV infection. New York: Igaku-Shoin, 1990:239.

117. Grieco MH, Chinoy-Acharya P. Lymphocytic interstitial pneumonia associated with the acquired immune deficiency syndrome. Am Rev Respir Dis 1985;131:952.

118. Solal-Celigny P, Couderc LJ, Herman D, et al. Lymphoid interstitial pneumonitis in acquired immunodeficiency syndrome-related complex. Am Rev Respir Dis 1985;131:956,1985.

119. Saldana MJ, Mones JM. Pulmonary pathology in AIDS: atypical *Pneumocystis carinii* infection and lymphoid interstitial pneumonia. Thorax 1994;49(Suppl):S46.

120. Itescu S, Brancato LJ, Buxbaum J, et al. A diffuse infiltrative CD8 lymphocytosis syndrome in human immunodeficiency virus infection: a host immune response associated with HLA-DR5. Ann Intern Med 1990;112:3.

121. Oldham SAA, Castillo M, Jacobson FL, et al. HIV associated lymphocytic interstitial pneumonia: radiologic manifestations and pathologic correlation. Radiology 1989;170:83.

122. Joshi W, Oleske JM, Minnefor AB, et al. Pathology of suspected acquired immune deficiency syndrome in children: a study of eight cases Pediatr Pathol 1984;2:71.

123. Fackler JC, Nagel JE, Adler WH, et al. Epstein-Barr virus infection in a child with acquired immunodeficiency syndrome. Am J Dis Child 1985;139:1000.

124. Boccon-Gibod L, Sacre JP, Just J, et al. Lymphoid interstitial pneumonia in children with AIDS or AIDS-related complex. Pediatr Pathol 1986;5:238.

125. Kornstein MJ, Pietra GG, Hoxie JA, Conley ME. The pathology and treatment of interstitial pneumonitis in two infants with AIDS. Am Rev Respir Dis 1986;133:1196.

126. Morris JC, Rosen MJ, Marchevsky A, Teirstein AS. Lymphocytic interstitial pneumonia in patients at risk for the acquired immune deficiency syndrome. Chest 1987;91:63.

127. Katz BZ, Berkman AB, Shapiro ED. Serologic evidence of active Epstein-Barr virus infection in Epstein-Barr virus-associated lympho-

proliferative disorders of children with acquired immunodeficiency syndrome. J Pediatr 1992;120:228.

128. Kramer MR, Saldana MJ, Ramos M, Pithcenik AE. High titers of Epstein-Barr virus antibodies in adult patients with lymphocytic interstitial pneumonitis associated with AIDS. Respir Med 1992;86:49.

129. Ziza JM, Brun-Vezinet F, Venet A, et al. Lymphadenopathy associated virus isolated from bronchoalveolar lavage fluid in AIDS-related complex with lymphoid interstitial pneumonitis. N Engl J Med 1985;313:183.

130. Resnick L, Pitchenik AE, Fisher E, Croney R. Detection of HTLV-III/LAV-specific IgG and antigen in bronchoalveolar lavage from two patients with lymphocytic interstitial pneumonitis associated with AIDS-related complex. Am J Med 1987;82:553.

131. Chayt KJ, Harper ME, Marselle LM, et al. Detection of HTLV-III RNA in lungs of patients with AIDS and pulmonary involvement. JAMA 1986;256:2356.

132. Plata F, Garcia-Pons F, Ryter A, et al. HIV-1 infection of lung alveolar fibroblasts and macrophages in humans. AIDS Res Hum Retroviruses 1990;6:979.

133. Dean NC, Golden JA, Evans LA, et al. Human immunodeficiency virus recovery from bronchoalveolar lavage fluid in patients with AIDS. Chest 1988;93:1176.

134. Linneman CC, Baughman RP, Frame PT, Floyd R. Recovery of human immunodeficiency virus and detection of p24 antigen in bronchoalveolar lavage fluid from adult patients with AIDS. Chest 1989;96:64.

135. Rubinstein A, Bernstein LJ, Charytan M, et al. Corticosteroid treatment for pulmonary lymphoid hyperplasia in children with the acquired immune deficiency syndrome. Pediatr Pulmonol 1988;4:13.

136. Amorosa JK, Miller RW, Laraya-Cuasay L, et al. Bronchiectasis in children with lymphocytic interstitial pneumonia and acquired immune deficiency syndrome. Pediatr Radiol 1992;22:603.

137. Lin RY, Gruber PJ, Saunders R, Perla EN. Lymphocytic interstitial pneumonitis in adult HIV infection. NY State J Med 1988;88:273,1988.

138. Teirstein AS, Rosen MJ. Lymphocytic interstitial pneumonia. Clin Chest Med 1988;9:467.

139. Bach MC. Zidovudine for lymphocytic interstitial pneumonia associated with AIDS. Lancet 1987;2:796.

140. Bye MR, Bernstein L, Shah K, et al. Diagnostic bronchoalveolar lavage in children with AIDS. Pediatr Pulmonol 1987;3:425.

141. Rubinstein A. Pediatric AIDS. Curr Probl Pediatr 1986;16:364.

142. Joshi W, Kauffman S, Oleske JM, et al. Polyclonal polymorphic B-cell lymphoproliferative disorder with prominent pulmonary involvement in children with acquired immune deficiency syndrome. Cancer 1987;59:1455.

143. Helbert M, Stoneham C, Mitchell D, Pinching AJ. Zidovudine for lymphocytic interstitial pneumonitis in AIDS. Lancet 1987;2:1333.

144. Suffredini AF, Ognibene FP, Lack EE, et al. Nonspecific interstitial pneumonitis: a common cause of pulmonary disease in the acquired immunodeficiency syndrome. Ann Intern Med 1987;107:7.

145. Ognibene FP, Masur H, Rogers P, et al. Nonspecific interstitial pneumonitis without evidence of *Pneumocystis carinii* in asymptomatic patients infected with human immunodeficiency virus. Ann Intern Med 1988;109:874.

146. Ramaswamy G, Jagadha V, Tchertkoff V. Diffuse alveolar damage and interstitial fibrosis in acquired immunodeficiency syndrome patients without concurrent pulmonary infection. Arch Pathol Lab Med 1985;109:408.

147. Simmons JT, Suffredini AF, Lack EE, et al. Nonspecific Interstitial pneumonitis in patients with AIDS. Radiologic features. AJR Am J Roentgenol 1987;149:265,1987.

148. White DA, Gellene RA, Gupta S, et al. Pulmonary cell populations in the immunosuppressed patient: bronchoalveolar lavage findings during episodes of pneumonitis. Chest 1985;88:352.

149. Wallace JM, Barbers RG, Oishi JS, Prince H. Cellular and T-lymphocyte subpopulation profiles in bronchoalveolar lavage fluid from patients with acquired immunodeficiency syndrome and pneumonitis. Am Rev Respir Dis 1984;130:786.

150. Young KR, Rankin JA, Naegel GP, et al. Bronchoalveolar lavage cells and proteins in patients with the acquired immunodeficiency syndrome: an immunologic analysis. Ann Intern Med 1985; 103:522.

151. Plata F, Autran B, Pedroza Marans L, et al. AIDS virus specific cytotoxic T lymphocytes in lung disorders. Nature 1987;328:348.

152. Guillon JM, Autran B, Denis M, et al. Human immunodeficiency virus-related lymphocytic alveolitis. Chest 1988;94:1264.

153. Meignan M, Guillon JM, Denis M, et al. Increased lung epithelial permeability in HIV-infected patients with isolated cytotoxic T-lymphocytic alveolitis. Am Rev Respir Dis 1990;141:1241.

154. Ettensohn DB, Mayer KH, Kessimian N, Smith PS. Lymphocytic bronchiolitis associated with HIV infection. Chest 1988;93:201.

155. Allen JN, Wewers MD. HIV-associated bronchiolitis obliterans organizing pneumonia. Chest 1989;96:197.

156. Leo YS, Pitchon HE, Messler G, Meyer RD. Bronchiolitis obliterans organizing pneumonia in a patient with AIDS. Clin Infect Dis 1994;18:921.

157. McGuinness G, Naidich DP, Garay S, Leitman BS, McCauley DI. AIDS associated bronchiectasis: CT features. J Comput Assist Tomogr 1993;17:260.

158. Coplan NL, Shimony RY, Ioachim HL, et al. Primary pulmonary hypertension associated with human immunodeficiency viral infection. Am J Med 1990;89:96.

159. Himelman RB, Dohrmann M, Goodman P, et al. Severe pulmonary hypertension and cor pulmonale in the acquired immunodeficiency syndrome. Am J Cardiol 1989;64:1396.

160. Martos A, Carratala J, Cabellos C, Rodriguez P. AIDS and primary pulmonary hypertension. Am Heart J 1993;125:1819.

161. Mette SA, Palevsky HI, Pietra GG, et al. Primary pulmonary hypertension in association with human immunodeficiency virus infection. A possible viral etiology for some forms of hypertensive pulmonary arteriopathy. Am Rev Respir Dis 1992;145:1196.

162. Speich R, Jenni R, Opravil M, Pfab M, Russi EW. Primary pulmonary hypertension in HIV infection. Chest 1991;100:1268.

AIDS: Biology, Diagnosis, Treatment and Prevention, fourth edition, edited by Vincent T. DeVita, Jr., Samuel Hellman, and Steven A. Rosenberg. Lippincott–Raven Publishers, © 1997

19.3

Renal Complications

Jeffrey B. Kopp and James E. Balow

As might be expected of an infectious agent with protean manifestations, human immunodeficiency virus (HIV) infection is associated with a wide range of renal and metabolic disturbances. This chapter reviews the fluid and electrolyte disorders, acute renal failure, tubulointerstitial disease, and glomerular lesions seen in patients with HIV infection. Several excellent reviews[1-6] are also available.

HIV-1 IN URINE

Urine does not contain infectious HIV, although proviral HIV sequences can be detected by polymerase chain reaction (PCR) methods, and viral RNA can be detected by reverse transcriptase–PCR in urine cell pellets.[7-9] The Centers for Disease Control and Prevention has recommended that universal precautions do not apply to urine unless visible blood is present.[10] Nevertheless, in view of the potential for urine to transmit other pathogens (eg, cytomegalovirus), body substance isolation procedures are recommended to reduce nosocomial transmission of all infectious agents.[11]

The urine of HIV-infected patients may contain antibodies directed against HIV-1 antigens even when the serum does not contain antibodies.[12] Whether this is caused by a compartmentalized response of the mucosal immune system or indicates recognition of HIV peptides or unrelated antigens remains to be determined, as does the relevance of this finding to the pathogenesis of genitourinary pathology.

FLUID AND ELECTROLYTE DISORDERS

Hyponatremia is the most common electrolyte disorder in HIV-infected patients.[2,13,14] Gastrointestinal salt losses from diarrhea, with only water repletion, is a frequent cause; management with volume repletion using appropriate crystalloid is generally straightforward. Another cause of hyponatremia is adrenal insufficiency, which may result from adrenal infection (ie, involvement with cytomegalovirus, mycobacteria, or *Cryptococcus* is common but rarely affects function) or from adrenal tumors. Adrenal insufficiency in HIV-1–infected patients may be caused by the acquired glucocorticoid resistance of uncertain pathogenesis.[15] Patients with adrenal insufficiency typically manifest hyponatremia, hyperkalemia, and renal sodium wasting. The syndrome of inappropriate antidiuretic hormone (SIADH) is another uncommon cause of hyponatremia and typically results from infections or mass lesions in the brain or lungs. SIADH is associated with euvolemic hyponatremia and is managed primarily by water restriction and vasopressin antagonists (eg, demeclocycline).

Other electrolyte disturbances, such as hypokalemia, hyperkalemia, hypernatremia, hypocalcemia (primarily due to hypoalbuminemia), and hyperuricemia (primarily from volume depletion) occur relatively commonly in acquired immunodeficiency syndrome (AIDS) patients.[1,2] Typically, these occur as complications of opportunistic infections, tumors, or treatment.

ACUTE RENAL FAILURE

Acute renal failure appears commonly during the course of HIV infection. The major causes are summarized in Table 19.3-1. *Prerenal azotemia* is the most frequent cause of acute renal failure and often stems from saline depletion or sepsis. *Renal azotemia* is most often caused by nephrotoxic drugs or glomerular diseases. Acute renal failure associated with infectious interstitial nephritis has been described, and the organisms responsible include adenovirus,[16] BK virus (member of the *Polyomavirus* family),[17,18] and a microsporidian of the genus *Encephalitozoon*.[19] *Postrenal azotemia* (ie, obstruction) may be intrinsic, as occurs with tubular precipitation of acyclovir[20] or sulfadiazine,[21] or extrinsic, resulting from ureteral

Jeffrey B. Kopp, Kidney Disease Section, NIDDK, National Institutes of Health, Building 10, Room 3N-112, Bethesda, MD 20892.

James E. Balow, Kidney Disease Section, NIDDK, National Institutes of Health, Building 10, Room 9N-222, Bethesda, MD 20892.

TABLE 19.3-1. *Acute renal failure in patients with HIV infection*

Classification	Etiology
Prerenal azotemia	Intravascular volume depletion (e.g., vomiting, diarrhea, glucocorticoid deficiency)
	Capillary leak (e.g., sepsis, hypoalbuminemia, therapy with interleukin-2, interferon-α, or interferon-γ)
	Hypotension (e.g., sepsis, HIV cardiomyopathy)
	Decreased renal blood flow (e.g., nonsteroidal antiinflammatory drugs)
Renal azotemia	Acute tubular necrosis (e.g., ischemia, sepsis, antimicrobials, radiographic contrast, rhabdomyolysis)
	Interstitial nephritis (e.g., penicillins, ciprofloxacin, nonsteroidal antiinflammatory drugs, adenovirus, BK virus, microsporidia)
	Rapidly progressive nephritic syndrome (e.g., immune complex glomerulonephritis, thrombotic thrombocytopenic purpura)
Postrenal azotemia	Tubular obstruction (e.g., sulfadiazine, acyclovir, tumor lysis)
	Ureteral and pelvic obstruction (e.g., lymphoma)
	Ureteral obstruction (e.g., stone, fungus ball, blood clot, sloughed papilla)

compression. In HIV-infected patients, acute renal failure with a creatinine concentrations greater than 6 mg/dL is most commonly caused by sepsis (75%) and rarely by postrenal causes; when dialysis treatment is instituted, recovery is similar to that seen in patients without HIV infection.[22]

Careful attention to drug pharmacology is essential in treating AIDS patients because of the probability of multisystem complications and the frequent need for multidrug regimens.[23] Renal and electrolyte complications of drugs commonly used in AIDS patients are summarized in Table 19.3-2. Trimethoprim-sulfamethoxazole can produce mild azotemia through its competition for tubular secretion of creatinine, but rarely does it cause a true depression of glomerular filtration rate. Nephrotoxic agents, particularly radiographic contrast dye, aminoglycosides, amphotericin B, pentamidine, and foscarnet, are common causes of azotemia.[23,24] Allergic reactions may occur with increased frequency in HIV-infected patients, producing interstitial nephritis with drugs such as ciprofloxacin that otherwise are associated with a low rate of nephrotoxicity.[25]

Acid-base disturbances are relatively common in HIV-infected patients. Metabolic acidosis can be caused by chronic diarrhea or renal tubular acidosis related to nephro-

toxic drugs. Lactic acidosis type B (ie, no tissue hypoxia) has been described in HIV-1 infected patients.[26]

Zidovudine induces a myopathy characterized by mitochondrial abnormalities. This represents a possible mechanism to explain the increased lactate production.[27] The HIV protease inhibitor indinavir has been associated with nephrolithiasis in approximately 4% of patients treated (Merck, Prescribing Information, unpublished data). The renal stones are more common at higher drug doses and are composed largely of indinavir. Preventive measures include maintaining a high urine volume. Nephrolithiasis has not been reported with the other currently-available protease inhibitors, saquinavir and ritonavir.

URINARY TRACT INFECTIONS AND INTERSTITIAL NEPHRITIS

Symptomatic urinary tract infections are common, occurring in 20% of men and women with HIV-1 infection.[28] The most common organisms are *Pseudomonas* and *Escherichia coli*, and infections with *Klebsiella, Serratia, Enterobacter,* and *Staphylococcus epidermidis* are seen less frequently. Atypical pathogens and agents particularly associated with chronic

TABLE 19.3-2. *Renal complications of drugs commonly used in HIV patients*

ANTIBACTERIAL AND ANTIPROTOZOAL AGENTS

Aminoglycosides	Acute renal failure, magnesium wasting
Ciprofloxacin	Allergic interstitial nephritis
Pentamidine	Rhabdomyolysis, azotemia, acute renal failure
Rifampin	Acute renal failure, Fanconi's syndrome, renal tubular acidosis, nephrogenic diabetes insipidus, interstitial nephritis, glomerulonephritis
Sulfa drugs	Azotemia without a change in the glomerular filtration rate, sulfadiazine crystal-induced obstructive nephropathy, allergic interstitial nephritis

ANTIFUNGAL AGENTS

Amphotericin	Azotemia, acute renal failure, potassium and magnesium wasting, distal renal tubular acidosis, nephrocalcinosis

ANTIVIRAL AGENTS

Acyclovir	Acyclovir crystal-induced obstructive nephropathy
Dideoxyinosine	Hypokalemia, hyperuricemia, Fanconi's syndrome
Foscarnet	Acute renal failure, nephrogenic diabetes insipidus
Zidovudine	Rhabdomyolysis, lactic acidosis
Indinavir	Nephrolithiasis

pyelonephritis include *Acinetobacter, Nocardia, Histoplasma, Cryptococcus, Candida, Mycobacteria (M tuberculosis* and *M avium* complex), and *Pneumocystis carinii.*

Other causes of chronic tubulointerstitial nephritis in the patient with HIV-1 infection include nephrotoxic antibiotics, nonsteroidal antiinflammatory drugs, and nephrocalcinosis, which is often related to amphotericin B therapy and chronic infection with *M avium* complex or *P carinii.*[29]

GLOMERULAR DISEASES

The first reports of glomerular disease occurring in AIDS patients emanated from New York and Miami in 1984.[30–32] These reports described several glomerular lesions, especially mesangial hyperplasia and focal segmental glomerulosclerosis (FSGS). Approximately 10% to 15% of HIV-infected patients develop glomerular disease, manifested by the nephrotic syndrome or, less commonly, the nephritic syndrome. FSGS is the most common glomerular lesion, particularly in black patients, and is also called HIV-associated nephropathy (Table 19.3-3).[33–38] These patients typically present with heavy proteinuria, often with the nephrotic syndrome, and progress to end-stage renal failure over a matter of months.[39] The size of the kidneys appears normal or even diffusely increased by ultrasound, which is unusual for end-stage renal failure but can also be seen in diabetic and amyloid nephropathies.

FSGS is defined as a focal lesion (ie, affecting some glomeruli) and a segmental lesion (ie, involving only portions of affected glomeruli), as illustrated in Fig. 19.3-1. Glomerular features that are present in some but not all cases and that tend to differentiate HIV-associated FSGS from idiopathic FSGS include the following: striking hyperplastic or degenerative changes in glomerular epithelial

TABLE 19.3-3. *Kidney pathology in HIV patients with clinical evidence of renal disease*

COMMON RENAL LESIONS
Acute tubular necrosis
Mesangial hyperplasia
Focal segmental glomerulosclerosis
Interstitial nephritis
Nephrocalcinosis
Parenchymal and collecting system viral, bacterial, fungal, and protozoal infections

OTHER RENAL LESIONS
Minimal change nephropathy
Postinfectious glomerulonephritis
IgA nephropathy
Membranous nephropathy
Membranoproliferative glomerulonephritis
Thrombotic microangiopathy or hemolytic uremic syndrome
Kaposi's sarcoma
Lymphoma, infiltrative
Carcinoma, renal cell or metastatic

cells, glomerular collapse, and tubuloreticular aggregates in glomerular endothelial cells. Glomerular hyalinosis is less frequently seen than idiopathic FSGS. Tubular features that are typical of HIV-associated FSGS include cystic dilatation and atrophy of tubules and cast formation. A focal mononuclear cell infiltrate frequently resides within the interstitium.[36,40–43]

Persons of African descent are clearly at increased risk for FSGS, whether idiopathic,[44] heroin-associated,[45] or HIV-associated.[46,47] The basis for this susceptibility remains to be elucidated, but it seems likely to be in part genetic. Patient series with few African Americans (eg, from the National Institutes of Health,[48] from San Francisco in the initial but not subsequent report,[49,50] from Germany,[51] and from Italy[52]) have found few or no cases of FSGS. Patient series from France[53] and Brazil[54] in which significant numbers of black patients were included have confirmed the role of FSGS in this population, suggesting that genetic factors may be more important than environmental factors.

The pathogenesis of HIV-associated FSGS remains unclear. It is unknown whether the observed pathology is a consequence of direct infection of intrinsic renal cells by HIV-1, a consequence of the viral products or cytokines released by HIV-infected lymphocytes and monocytes located in kidney or elsewhere, or a consequence of opportunistic infection. It has been demonstrated in vitro that HIV-1 infects glomerular endothelial cells readily, mesangial cells poorly or not at all, and glomerular epithelial cells not at all.[55,56] It has been reported that the p24 nucleocapsid protein is present in renal tubular epithelial cells and that viral nucleic acid is present in glomerular parietal and visceral epithelial cells in patients with HIV-associated FSGS.[57] Other groups, however, have reported difficulty localizing HIV-1 antigens[58,59] or RNA in kidney.[60] Although HIV proviral DNA can be identified within microdissected kidney fragments by PCR,[61] the cellular source has yet to be established. Patients with HIV-associated nephropathy and chronic renal failure have an increased prevalence of HIV-1 viremia, as assessed by viral culture, compared with patients without renal disease.[62] It is unclear whether this finding reflects the additional immunosuppressive effects of uremia or whether increased viral burden is a risk factor of or marker for the development of HIV-associated nephropathy. A link has been proposed between renal infection with *Mycoplasma fermentans* and HIV-associated nephropathy, but these findings await general confirmation.[63,64]

Perhaps the best evidence that opportunistic infection is not required for the development of HIV-associated FSGS derives from studies in mice transgenic for a *gag-pol* deleted HIV genome. These mice develop renal disease that resembles HIV-associated FSGS in histology and outcome, suggesting that particular HIV gene products are sufficient to produce this characteristic renal histopathology.[65–67]

Other than FSGS, a variety of glomerular lesions occur in HIV-infected patients and are particularly seen in white patients (see Table 19.3-2 and Fig. 19.3-1).[51–53] These include

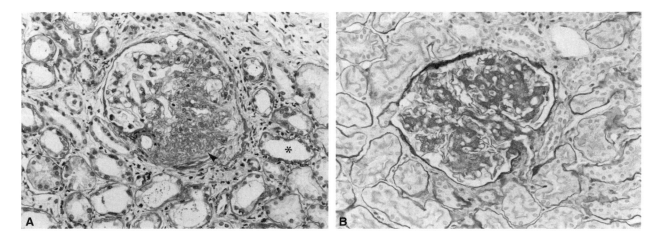

FIG. 19.3-1. Glomerular pathology in HIV–infected patients. (**A**) Kidney from a patient with HIV-associated FSGS showing segmental glomerulosclerosis (*arrow*) and dilated tubules lined by atrophic tubular epithelial cells (*). Electron microscopy showed glomerular epithelial cell foot process fusion, foam cells, and scanty subendothelial deposits within the segmentally sclerotic lesion (not shown). (**B**) Kidney from a patient with HIV-associated membranoproliferative glomerulonephritis shows diffuse increase in mesangial matrix and increase in glomerular cell number. The tubules and interstitium are normal. Immunofluorescent analysis showed deposits of IgG, IgM and C3. On electron microscopy, mesangial and subendothelial deposits were present, together with tubuloreticular inclusions within glomerular endothelial cells (not shown). Both sections were stained with PAS.

minimal change disease,[36,37,68] membranous nephropathy[36,57,69] (including a focal and segmental variant of membranous nephropathy[70]), other forms of proliferative glomerulonephritis (including the postinfectious form),[30,31,36,49,57] mesangial hyperplasia (particularly in children),[37] IgA nephropathy,[71,72] lupus-like proliferative glomerulonephritis,[53] membranoproliferative glomerulonephritis,[73,74] and thrombotic microangiopathy.[48,75–78] In some forms of immune complex glomerulonephritis, HIV antigens have been identified within the kidney.[79]

EVALUATION AND TREATMENT OF CHRONIC RENAL DISEASE IN THE HIV PATIENT

Glomerular disease in the HIV patient may appear at any stage of infection, including the asymptomatic seropositive phase and in AIDS. There has been also a report of mesangial proliferative glomerulonephritis complicating acute HIV infection.[80] The typical presentation of a patient with HIV-associated FSGS includes nephrotic-range proteinuria (>3.5 g/day) and unusually rapid progression of renal insufficiency, often reaching end-stage renal disease in a matter of months.[39] Ultrasound frequently reveals enlarged and echogenic kidneys, as are also seen in patients with diabetic and amyloid nephropathy.[81] There is no evidence that monitoring urinary protein excretion in the asymptomatic patient offers any benefit. Although microalbuminuria is more common in HIV-infected patients, it is unclear whether this identifies a population at risk for functionally significant renal disease.[82,83] There are no established guidelines indicating which HIV patient with heavy proteinuria should be considered for renal biopsy, but many nephrologists do not obtain a biopsy for a patient with a prototypical course as described previously, particularly if the patient is black and therefore at particular risk for FSGS. Among the other glomerular lesions, mesangial hyperplasia,[84] membranous nephropathy, and thrombotic microangiopathy[78] have the potential to respond to therapy. A renal biopsy should be considered if these diagnoses are significant possibilities, based on the clinical presentation and the urinalysis findings.

The treatment of HIV-associated nephropathy is not well defined. Case reports have suggested improvement with antiviral therapy (ie, zidovudine), and data have been presented suggesting a slowed rate of renal function decline in treated patients compared with historical controls[85,86] or nonrandomized controls.[87] Corticosteroid therapy appeared beneficial in an initial study of four patients,[88] and a multicenter, randomized trial is in progress (Kalajian M: personal communication). Angiotensin converting enzyme inhibitors have been shown to reduce proteinuria in various renal diseases, and a case report extends these findings to HIV-associated nephropathy. There was no effect on serum creatinine, suggesting that the beneficial effect may reflect decreased intraglomerular hydraulic pressure.[89]

HIV-infected patients with end-stage renal disease should be considered for chronic dialysis, although this is not be the right choice for every patient. Initially, it was suggested that dialysis was ineffective at prolonging survival of patients with AIDS for more than a few months.[33,90] Survival has improved somewhat in recent years, with median survival ranging from 6 to 14 months for patients with end-stage renal disease and AIDS and a median survival of greater than 1 year for patients with end-stage renal disease and asymptomatic HIV infection.[91–93] The median survival exceeds 3 years for patients with end-stage renal disease in the absence of HIV infection.

ACKNOWLEDGMENT

The authors wish to thank Dr. Howard Austin for critical review of the manuscript, and Drs. Andrew Abraham and Paul Kimmel, George Washington University Medical Center, for sharing the renal biopsy slide shown in Figure 19.3-1A.

REFERENCES

1. Bourgoignie JJ. Renal complications of human immunodeficiency virus type 1. Kidney Int 1990;37:1571.
2. Glassock RJ, Cohen AH, Danovitch G. Human immunodeficiency virus infection and the kidney. Ann Intern Med 1990;112:35.
3. Schoenfeld P, Feduska NJ. Acquired immunodeficiency syndrome and renal disease: report of the National Kidney Foundation—National Institutes of Health Task Force on AIDS and Kidney Disease. Am J Kidney Dis 1990;16:14.
4. Ortiz-Butcher C. The spectrum of kidney diseases in patients with human immunodeficiency virus infection. Curr Opin Nephrol Hyperten 1993;2:355.
5. Strauss J, Zilleruelo G, Abitbol C. Human immunodeficiency virus nephropathy. Pediatr Nephrol 1993;7:220.
6. Rappaport J, Kopp JB, Klotman PE. Host-virus interactions and the molecular regulation of HIV-1: role in the pathogenesis of HIV-associated nephropathy. Kidney Int 1994;46:16.
7. Skolnik PR, Kosloff BR, Bechtel LJ. Absence of infectious HIV-1 in the urine of seropositive viremic subjects. J Infect Dis 1989;160:1056.
8. Li JJ, Huang YQ, Poiesz BJ. Detection of HIV-1 in urine cell pellets from HIV-1 seropositive individuals. J Clin Microbiol 1992;30:1051.
9. VedBrat SS, Shepherd LP, Pierce PF. Higher incidence of infectious HIV in body fluids detected by PCR analysis of their coculture supernatants. Biomed Lett 1994;49:191.
10. Centers for Disease Control. Update: universal precautions for prevention of transmission of human immunodeficiency virus, hepatitis B virus, and other bloodborne pathogens in health-care settings. MMWR 1988;37:377.
11. Lynch P, Cummings MJ, Roberts PL. Implementing and evaluating a system of generic infection precautions: body substance isolation. Am J Infect Control 1990;18:1.
12. Urnovitz HB, Clerici M, Shearer GM. HIV-1 antibody serum negativity with urine positivity. Lancet 1993;342:1458.
13. Peter SA. Electrolyte disorders and renal dysfunction in acquired immunodeficiency syndrome patients. J Natl Med Assoc 1991;83:889.
14. Tang WW, Kaptein EM, Feinstein EI. Hyponatremia in hospitalized patients with the acquired immunodeficiency syndrome and the AIDS-related complex. Am J Med 1993;94:169.
15. Norbiato G, Bevilacqua M, Vago T. Cortisol resistance in acquired immunodeficiency syndrome. J Clin Endocrinol Metab 1992;74:608.
16. Green WR, Greaves WL, Frederick WR. Renal infection due to adenovirus in a patient with human immunodeficiency virus infection. Clin Infect Dis 1994;18:989.
17. Smith RD, Linnemann C, Anderson P. ESRD due to polyomavirus interstitial nephritis in an HIV(+) patient. J Am Soc Nephrol 1993;4:287.
18. Vallbracht A, Lÿ94hler J, Gossman J. Disseminated BK type polyomavirus infection in an AIDS patient associated with central nervous system disease. Am J Pathol 1993;143:29.
19. Aarons EJ, Woodrow D, Hollister WS. Reversible renal failure caused by a microsporidian infection. AIDS 1994;8:1119.
20. Sawyer MH, Webb DE, Balow JE. Acyclovir induced renal failure: clinical course and histology. Am J Med 1988;84:1067.
21. Simon DI, Brosius FC, Rothstein DM. Sulfadiazine crystalluria revisited. The treatment of *Toxoplasma* encephalitis in patients with acquired immunodeficiency syndrome. Arch Intern Med 1990;150:2379.
22. Rao TKS, Friedman EA. Outcome of severe acute renal failure in patients with acquired immunodeficiency syndrome. Am J Kidney Dis 1995;25:390.
23. Berns JS, Cohen RM, Stumacher RJ. Renal aspects of therapy for human immunodeficiency virus and associated opportunistic infections. J Am Soc Nephrol 1991;1:1061.
24. Lachaal M, Venuto R. Nephrotoxicity and hyperkalemia in patients with acquired immunodeficiency syndrome treated with pentamidine. Am J Med 1989;87:260.
25. Lucena MI, Marquez M, Velasco JL. Acute renal failure attributable to ciprofloxacin in a patient with the acquired immunodeficiency syndrome. Arch Intern Med 1995;155:114.
26. Cattha G, Arieff AI, Cummings G. Lactic acidosis complicating the acquired immunodeficiency syndrome. Ann Intern Med 1993;118:37.
27. Gopinath R, Hutcheon M, Cheema-Dhadli S. Chronic lactic acidosis in a patient with acquired immunodeficiency syndrome and mitochondrial myopathy: biochemical studies. J Am Soc Nephrol 1992;3:1212.
28. Kaplan MS, Wechsler M, Benson MC. Urologic manifestations of AIDS. Urology 1987;30:441.
29. Feuerstein IM, Francis P, Raffeld M. Widespread visceral calcifications in disseminated Pneumocystis carinii infection: CT characteristics. J Comput Assist Tomogr 1990;14:149.
30. Gardenswartz MH, Lerner CW, Seligson G. Renal disease in patients with AIDS: a clinicopathologic study. Clin Nephrol 1984;21:197.
31. Rao TKS, Filippone EJ, Nicastri AD. Associated focal and segmental glomerulosclerosis in the acquired immunodeficiency syndrome. N Engl J Med 1984;310:669.
32. Pardo V, Aldana M, Colton RM. Glomerular lesions in the acquired immunodeficiency syndrome. Ann Intern Med 1984;101:429.
33. Rao TK, Friedman EA, Nicastri AD. The types of renal disease in the acquired immunodeficiency syndrome. N Engl J Med 1987;316:1062.
34. Pardo V, Meneses R, Ossa L. AIDS-related glomerulopathy: occurrence in specific risk groups. Kidney Int 1987;31:1167.
35. Bourgoignie JJ, Meneses R, Ortiz C. The clinical spectrum of renal disease associated with human immunodeficiency virus. Am J Kidney Dis 1988;12:131.
36. D'Agati V, Suh J-I, Carbone L. Pathology of HIV-associated nephropathy: a detailed morphologic and comparative study. Kidney Int 1989;35:1358.
37. Strauss R, Abitbol C, Zilleruelo G. Renal disease in children with the acquired immunodeficiency syndrome. N Engl J Med 1989;321:625.
38. Humphreys MH. Human immunodeficiency virus-associated glomerulosclerosis. Kidney Int 1995;48:311.
39. Langs C, Gallo G, Schact RG. Rapid renal failure in AIDS-associated focal glomerulosclerosis. Arch Intern Med 1990;150:287.
40. Chander P, Soni A, Suri A. Renal ultrastructural markers in AIDS-associated nephropathy. Am J Pathol 1987;126:513.
41. Alpers CE, Harawi S, Rennke HG. Focal glomerulosclerosis with tubuloreticular inclusions: possible predictive value for acquired immunodeficiency syndrome. Am J Kidney Dis 1988;12:240.
42. Chander P, Agarwal A, Soni A. Renal cytomembranous inclusions in idiopathic renal disease as predictive markers for the acquired immunodeficiency syndrome. Hum Pathol 1988;19:1060.
43. Bourgoignie JJ, Pardo V. The nephropathology in human immunodeficiency virus infection. Kidney Int 1991;35:S19.
44. Bakir AA, Bazilinski NG, Rhee HL. Focal segmental glomerulosclerosis. A common entity in nephrotic black adults. Arch Intern Med 1989;149:1802.
45. Cunningham EE, Brentjens JR, Zielezny MA. Heroin nephropathy. A clinicopathologic and epidemiologic study. Am J Med 1980;68:47.
46. Bourgoignie JJ, Ortiz-Interian C, Green DF. Race, a cofactor in HIV-1–associated nephropathy. Transplant Proc 1989;21:3899.
47. Cantor ES, Kimmel PL, Bosch JP. Effect of race on expression of acquired immunodeficiency syndrome-associated nephropathy. Arch Intern Med 1991;151:125.
48. Balow JE, Macher AM, Rook AH. Paucity of glomerular disease in acquired immunodeficiency syndrome. (Abstract) Kidney Int 1986;29:178.
49. Mazbar SA, Schoenfeld PY, Humphreys MH. Renal involvement in patients infected with HIV: experience at San Francisco General Hospital. Kidney Int 1990;37:1325.
50. Frassetto L, Schoenfeld P, Humphreys M. The increasing incidence of human immunodeficiency virus associated nephropathy at San Francisco General Hospital. Am J Kidney Dis 1991;18:655.

51. Brunkhorst R, Brunkhorst U, Eisenbach GM. Lack of clinical evidence for a specific HIV-associated glomerulopathy in 203 patients with HIV infection. Nephrol Dial Transplant 1992;7:87.

52. Casanova S, Mazzucco G, Barbiano di Belgiojoso G. Pattern of glomerular involvement in human immunodeficiency virus-infected patients: an Italian study. Am J Kidney Dis 1995;26:446.

53. Nochy D, Gloz D, Dosquet P. Renal disease associated with HIV infection: a multicentric study of 60 patients from Paris hospitals. Nephrol Dial Transplant 1993;8:11.

54. Lopes GS, Marques LPJ, Rioja LS. Glomerular disease and human immunodeficiency virus infection in Brazil. Am J Nephrol 1992;12:281.

55. Green DF, Resnick L, Bourgoignie JJ. HIV infects endothelial and mesangial but not epithelial cells. Kidney Int 1992;41:956.

56. Alpers C, McClure J, Burstein SL. Human mesangial cells are resistant to productive infection by multiple strains of human immunodeficiency virus types 1 and 2. Am J Kidney Dis 1992;19:126.

57. Cohen AH, Sun NCJ, Shapshak P. Demonstration of human immunodeficiency virus in renal epithelium in HIV-associated nephropathy. Mod Pathol 1989;2:125.

58. Barbiano di Belgiojoso G, Genderini A, Vago L. Absence of HIV antigens in renal tissue from patients with HIV-associated nephropathy. Nephrol Dial Transplant 1990;5:489.

59. Nadasdy T, Hanson-Painton O, Davis L. Conditions affecting the immunohistochemical detection of HIV in fixed and embedded renal and nonrenal tissues. Mod Pathol 1992;5:283.

60. Pardo F, Shapshak P, Yoshioka M. HIV associated nephropathy: direct renal invasion or indirect glomerular involvement? FASEB J 1991;15:A907.

61. Kimmel PL, Ferriera-Centeno A, Farkas-Szallazi T. Viral DNA in microdissected renal biopsy tissue from HIV infected patients with nephrotic syndrome. Kidney Int 1993;43:1347.

62. Kimmel PL, VedBrat SS, Pierce PF. Prevalence of viremia in human immunodeficiency virus-infected patients with renal disease. Arch Intern Med 1995;155:1578.

63. Bauer FA, Wear DJ, Angritt P. *Mycoplasma fermentans* (incognitus strain) infection in the kidneys of patients with acquired immunodeficiency syndrome and associated nephropathy: a light microscopic, immunohistochemical, and ultrastructural study. Hum Pathol 1991;22:63.

64. Ainsworth JG, Katseni V, Hourshid S. *Mycoplasma fermentans* and HIV-associated nephropathy. J Infect 1994;29:323.

65. Dickie P, Felser M, Eckhaus M. HIV-associated nephropathy in transgenic mice expressing HIV-1 genes. Virology 1991;185:109.

66. Kopp JB, Klotman ME, Adler SH. Progressive glomerulosclerosis and enhanced renal accumulation of basement membrane components in mice transgenic for HIV-1 genes. Proc Natl Acad Sci USA 1992;89:1577.

67. Kopp JB, Klotman PE. Animal models of lentiviral-associated renal disease. In: Berns J, Kimmel P, eds. Contemporary issues in nephrology. New York: Churchill Livingstone, 1995:381.

68. Singer DRJ, Jenkins AP, Gupta S. Minimal change nephropathy in the acquired immune deficiency syndrome. Br Med J 1985;291:868.

69. Guerra IL, Abraham AA, Kimmel PL. Nephrotic syndrome associated with chronic persistent hepatitis B in an HIV antibody positive patient. Am J Kidney Dis 1987;17:380.

70. Bass PS, Garrett PJ, Ellison DW. AIDS presenting as focal segmental membranous glomerulopathy. J Clin Pathol 1993;47:179.

71. Jindal K, Trillo A, Bishop G. Crescentic IgA nephropathy as a manifestation of human immune deficiency virus infection. Am J Nephrol 1991;11:147.

72. Kimmel PL, Phillips TM, Ferreira-Centeno A. Idiotypic IgA nephropathy in patients with human immunodeficiency virus infection. N Engl J Med 1992;327:702.

73. Kim KK, Factor SM. Membranoproliferative glomerulonephritis and plexogenic pulmonary arteriopathy in a homosexual man with acquired immunodeficiency syndrome. Hum Pathol 1987;18:1293.

74. de Chadar-vian J-P, Lischner HW, Karmazin N. Pulmonary hypertension and HIV infection: new observations and review of the syndrome. Mod Pathol 1994;7:685.

75. Charasse C, Michelet C, Le Tulzo Y. Thrombotic thrombocytopenic purpura with the acquired immunodeficiency syndrome: a pathologically documented case report. Am J Kidney Dis 1991;17:80.

76. Thompson C, Damon L, Ries C. Thrombotic microangiopathies in the 1980s: clinical features, response to treatment, and the impact of the human immunodeficiency virus epidemic. Blood 1992;80:1890.

77. Frem GJ, Rennke HG, Sayegh MH. Late renal allograft failure secondary to thrombotic microangiopathy-human immunodeficiency virus nephropathy. J Am Soc Nephrol 1994;4:1643.

78. Ucar A, Fernandez JF, Byrnes JJ. Thrombotic microangiopathy and retroviral infections: a 13-year experience. Am J Hematol 1994;45:304.

79. Kimmel PL, Phillips TM, Ferreira-Centeno A. HIV-associated immune renal disease. Kidney Int 1993;44:1327.

80. del Rio C, Soffer O, Widell JL. Acute human immunodeficiency virus infection temporally associated with rhabdomyolysis, acute renal failure, and nephrosis. Rev Infect Dis 1990;12:282.

81. Schaffer R, Schwartz G, Becker J. Renal ultrasound in acquired immune deficiency syndrome. Radiology 1984;153:511.

82. Luke DR, Sarnoski TP, Dennis S. Incidence of microalbuminuria in ambulatory patients with acquired immunodeficiency syndrome. Clin Nephrol 1992;38:69.

83. Busch HW, Riechman S, Heyern P. Albuminuria in HIV-infected patients. AIDS Res Hum Retroviruses 1994;10:717.

84. Appel RG, Neill J. A steroid-responsive nephrotic syndrome in a patient with human immunodeficiency virus infection. Ann Intern Med 1990;113:892.

85. Michel C, Dosquet P, Ronco P. Nephropathy associated with infection by human immunodeficiency virus: a report on 11 cases including 6 treated with zidovudine. Nephron 1992;62:434.

86. Ifudu O, Rao TKS, Tan CC. Zidovudine improves prognosis in HIV-associated nephropathy. (Abstract) J Am Soc Nephrol 1993;4:277.

87. Ahmed U, Kloser P, Miller MA. Does zidovudine slow the progression of HIV nephropathy? (Abstract) J Am Soc Nephrol 1993;4:269.

88. Smith MC, Pawar R, Carey JT. Effect of corticosteroid therapy on human immunodeficiency virus-associated nephropathy. Am J Med 1994;97:145.

89. Burns GD, Matute R, Onyema D. Response to inhibition of angiotensin-converting enzyme in human immunodeficiency virus-associated nephropathy: a case report. Am J Kidney Dis 1994;23:441.

90. Ortiz C, Meneses R, Jaffe D. Outcome of patients with human immunodeficiency virus on maintenance hemodialysis. Kidney Int 1988;34:248.

91. Feinfeld DA, Kaplan R, Dressler R. Survival of human immunodeficiency virus-infected patients on maintenance dialysis. Clin Nephrol 1989;32:221.

92. Kimmel PL, Umana WO, Simmens SJ. Continuous ambulatory peritoneal dialysis and survival of HIV infected patients with end-stage renal disease. Kidney Int 1993;44:373.

93. Tebben JA, Rigsby MO, Selwyn PA. Outcome of HIV infected patients on continuous ambulatory peritoneal dialysis. Kidney Int 1993;44:191.

AIDS: Biology, Diagnosis, Treatment and Prevention, fourth edition, edited by Vincent T. DeVita, Jr., Samuel Hellman, and Steven A. Rosenberg. Lippincott–Raven Publishers, © 1997

19.4

Hematologic Complications of Human Immunodeficiency Virus Infection

John P. Doweiko and Jerome E. Groopman

The first human retroviruses were discovered in the late 1970s.[1] Before that, the concept of organisms carrying their genome as RNA with DNA as an intermediate between genome and protein was implausible. Infection with human immunodeficiency virus-1 (HIV-1) has advanced from an obscure syndrome in the 1980s to a major public health problem.

The retroviruses capable of infecting human share several features.[1-3] They have common modes of transmission, there is a characteristic quiescent phase within target cells, and the neutralizing humoral immune response to these viruses is relatively insubstantial. HIV is a member of the *Lentivirinae* subfamily of retroviruses. The viral particle consists of a "shell" composed of four nucleocapsid "core" proteins: p24, p17, p9, and p7. Surrounding this is a lipid bilayer of cellular and viral origin, in the middle of which are embedded glycoproteins of viral and host-cell origin.

Within the shell of core proteins is contained the genome of HIV-1, consisting of a single strand of RNA and preformed reverse transcriptase. The genome of HIV-1 is more complex that of other retroviruses.[1,2] It contains the three "standard" genes characteristic of retroviruses (ie, *gag, pol,* and *env*) and six other genes not encountered within other retroviruses. Certain genes of HIV-1 are error prone, particularly reverse transcriptase and the envelope genes. Because of this propensity to mutate in vivo, HIV-1 becomes a quasispecies com-posed of viral variants.[4-6] This allows extensive genomic variation to develop from a single infecting event.

The CD4 antigen may be the sole high-affinity cellular receptor for HIV-1.[2,7] This protein is highly concentrated on helper T cells and monocytes, designating these cells as the major targets of the infection.[2,3,7,8] Other cells also express surface CD4 antigen, rendering them vulnerable to infection by HIV-1.[9] These include fibroblasts and related cells such as glial cells, and the stromal reticular cells of the bone marrow.[2,7] Data indicate that cells may be infected through routes other than the CD4 antigen.[2,7]

Some strains of HIV-1 preferentially infect monocytes, and others display selectivity for CD4 lymphocytes.[2] This is important to the evolution of the intricate syndrome that results from the viral infection. The two major sequelae of HIV-1 infection are degradation of cellular immunity and an ultimately detrimental cytokine response.

Early in the HIV infection, HIV tropism for monocytes and macrophages predominates.[10] Although HIV assembles almost exclusively on the plasma membrane of CD4 lymphocytes, it can assemble and accumulate within cytoplasmic vacuoles of monocytes and macrophages where it remains hidden from the immune system.[8] This permits these cells to serve as reservoirs for the virus. In nonlymphoid tissues, such as the central nervous system, local infection is predominately sustained by cells of monocytic lineage.[10,11] Moreover, infection of monocytic cells is important to the propagation of infection throughout the body, particularly to the central nervous system.[12]

Cells of monocytic lineage are central to the complex network of growth factors and cytokines that sustains and regulates the hematopoietic and immune systems. Infection of these cells is responsible in large part for one of the major sequelae of this viral infection: an ultimately detrimental

John P. Doweiko, Department of Medicine, Division of Hematology and Oncology, Division of Infectious Disease, Deaconess Hospital, Harvard Medical School, 1 Autumn Street K-6, Boston, MA 02215.

Jerome E. Groopman, Department of Medicine, Harvard Medical School and Division of Hematology and Oncology, New England Deaconess Hospital, 110 Francis Street 4-A, Boston, MA 02215.

cytokine response. Infection of cells of monocytic origin by HIV-1 results in a cytokine response that is deleterious because it accelerates the HIV infection and promotes tissue injury.[12] Levels of inflammatory cytokines in the serum increase as the viral infection progresses.[13]

Progression of HIV-1 infection is associated with a shift toward more lymphocytotropic variants of the virus.[10] This is important to the cellular immune dysfunction that is characteristic of AIDS.[12] From the onset of the infection, there is a constant production of viral particles, with upward of 1 billion viral particles produced each day, and almost one third of the total viral burden is turned over within 2 days.[14,15] There is an attempt to balance this with production of new CD4 lymphocytes, but the destructive capacity of HIV-1 for these cells eventually exceeds the replicative capacity of the body, resulting in progressive deterioration of cellular immunity.[14,16]

Some of those infected with HIV-1 do not succumb to the infection as rapidly as do others. In long-term survivors, the viral burden in the plasma and peripheral blood mononuclear cells is less by several orders of magnitude than in less fortunate patients with similar duration of disease.[17,18] These long-term survivors seem to have a vigorous viral-inhibitory CD8 lymphocyte response and a stronger neutralizing antibody response than is typically seen.[17]

SPECIFIC CYTOPENIAS IN PATIENTS WITH HIV INFECTION

Infection with HIV-1 is associated with suppression of hematopoiesis.[18–22] The hematologic perturbations encountered with HIV-1 infection are responsible for some of the morbidity, and these processes hinder therapy directed toward the primary viral infection and secondary infectious and neoplastic complications.[23,24] The need to reduce doses or interrupt therapy because of poor hematologic tolerance may cause emergence of drug-resistant organisms and progression of infections or neoplasms.[23,24]

Anemia

The most common cytopenia associated with HIV-1 infection is anemia. The degree of anemia increases as the HIV-1 infection advances. Although 10% to 20% are anemic at the time of presentation, 70% to 80% eventually become anemic with progression of the infection.[25–29] The major cause of anemia in HIV-infected patients is impaired erythropoiesis.

The anemia is typically normochromic and normocytic and associated with an inappropriately low reticulocyte count.[30] Macrocytosis is unusual and tends to occur in those treated with zidovudine.[30,31] Iron stores are normal or elevated, and there is typically a decrease in serum iron along with a parallel decrease in the total iron-binding capacity that is characteristic of the "anemia of chronic disease." Serum ferritin levels are often increased,[30] and the levels tend to parallel the severity and duration of the infection with HIV-1.[32–34]

Although decreases in serum B_{12} levels are found in about 20% of HIV-infected patients,[25,30,35] it is not clear to what extent, if any, these low levels cause or contribute to the cytopenias of HIV.[35–37] Patients usually do not have other manifestations of B_{12} deficiency and typically do not improve markedly with parenteral repletion.[30,36] The low B_{12} levels seem to result from altered serum transport of the vitamin,[223,254] but there may be abnormal absorption with advanced HIV infection.[35]

Although some patients are Coombs' test positive, this is usually nonspecific and not a cause or major contributing factor to the anemia. Sensitive assays show that 2% to 44% of asymptomatic HIV-infected patients are direct Coombs' test positive, as are 60% to 70% with AIDS-related complex (ARC) and up to 85% of those with AIDS.[25,30] Although these antibodies may be reactive with specific minor antigens on erythrocytes,[25,26,30] they most commonly result from nonspecific binding of antiphospholipid antibodies or deposition of immune complexes on erythrocytes.[25,26,30] Immune hemolysis is rare.[25,30]

Paraproteinemia may occur in as many as one half of HIV-infected patients.[30] The peripheral smear may demonstrate rouleaux and dimerization, or co-migration of these proteins during electrophoresis may result in the appearance of a monoclonal protein.[30] However, a polyclonal pattern on electrophoresis is more common, and the paraproteinemia does not cause or contribute to the cytopenias seen with HIV-1 infection.[30]

Neutropenia

Granulocytopenia tends to occur concomitantly with anemia.[33] Although 10% to 30% of those with ARC may be neutropenic, this may progress to about three fourths of those with AIDS.[25–28,33] A review of the peripheral smear reveals a variable deficiency of neutrophils, lymphocytes, and perhaps monocytes; atypical lymphocytes may be seen. Vacuolization of the monocytes is a typical finding, and hypolobulation of the neutrophils may occur and may imitate a left shift.[33,39]

Impaired myelopoiesis is the major cause of the leukopenia associated with HIV-1 infection.[33,40–43] Myelotoxic medications may exacerbate this problem, and concurrent use of these drugs may be synergistic in this regard. Although about one third of patients have antibodies on the circulating neutrophils, their presence does not correlate with the incidence or severity of the neutropenia.[30]

Thrombocytopenia

Etiology

Although anemia and granulocytopenia tend to occur concomitantly, with a severity that parallels the course of the HIV-1 infection, thrombocytopenia can occur independently of other cytopenias and at all stages of HIV infection.[28,33,44] Some degree of thrombocytopenia may occur in 30% to

60% of HIV-infected patients.[23,25–27,38,43,45] By itself, thrombocytopenia is not prognostic of the HIV infection.[46]

The causes of thrombocytopenia that occurs with HIV infection include reduced bone marrow production and immune and nonimmune destruction. Reduction in the productive capacity of megakaryocytes that occurs with HIV infection leads to a lack of a compensatory megakaryocytopoiesis in HIV-infected patients to counter peripheral cell destruction.[47,48] HIV-1 may directly suppress platelet production in that megakaryocytes are potential targets of infection by the virus.[49] HIV-1 indirectly suppresses platelet production by exposing or altering antigens on the surface of the megakaryocyte, which renders them targets of antiplatelet antibodies.[44,50] Alterations in cytokines and growth factors during the HIV infection that modify platelet production.[47,48]

Peripheral destruction of platelets is an important contributing cause of thrombocytopenia. Infections and fevers that occur with HIV infection decrease the lifespan of circulating platelets. Other causes of nonimmune destruction of circulating platelets are the syndromes of hemolytic uremia and thrombotic thrombocytopenia purpura, which occur more commonly in HIV-infected patients.[44,51,52]

Immune destruction of platelets is the major cause of thrombocytopenia of HIV patients. Most HIV-infected patients have antibodies coating the platelets.[50,53,54] Although some of these may be the result of nonspecific binding of immune complexes, molecular mimicry between the gp160/120 antigen of HIV-1 and gpIIb/IIIa of platelets may lead to production of more specific antibodies to the platelet surface.[49,50,53,55,56] The presence of antibodies on the surface of the platelets does not correlate well with the platelet count because of defective reticuloendothelial clearance in HIV-infected patients.[57–59]

Treatment for HIV-Associated Thrombocytopenia

There are no well-controlled, prospectively randomized trials of the various treatment options for HIV-associated thrombocytopenia.[30] Spontaneous remissions may occur in 10% to 20% of patients.[32,60] A sudden elevation in the platelet count, however, may indicate deterioration of the immune system and herald the onset of AIDS.[44,60] In those who have a sustained decrease in platelet counts, therapy is not always necessary, because the incidence of significant bleeding episodes is low despite low platelet counts.[61–63] It is, however, difficult to predict the risk of bleeding based solely on the platelet count.[64]

In those with thrombocytopenia associated with HIV infection, administration of zidovudine may result in elevations of platelet counts in a minimum of 30% of patients within 12 weeks of initiation of therapy.[31,44,48,60] Although some studies have shown a dose-response association, this has not been demonstrated in other studies.[31] Other nucleoside reverse transcriptase inhibitors have not been shown to have this effect. Similar to the effects of zidovudine, dapsone may elevate platelet counts in a minority of patients within 3 weeks of initiating therapy.[54] Although the mechanism of zidovudine is not clear, dapsone may act through a reduction in phagocyte-mediated cytotoxicity.[54]

Corticosteroids elevate platelet counts in 40% to 80% of patients with HIV-associated immune thrombocytopenia; long-term remissions occur in only 10% to 20% after such therapy.[44] Although chronic, low-dose steroids may be effective in maintaining an acceptable platelet count,[58] side effects preclude their use. No controlled trials have demonstrated any adverse effects of short-term steroid use on HIV infection.[58]

Patients who have failed the treatment modalities previously described have been tried on other therapies. Vincristine and anabolic steroids have an overall response rate of about only 10%.[65,66] High-dose ascorbate (2 to 4 g/day) over several months has been shown in small studies to increase platelet counts in those with HIV-associated immune thrombocytopenia; the mechanism and durability of the response are uncertain.[44] Interferons, particularly interferon-α (IFN-α), have been shown in controlled trial to have some efficacy in those with zidovudine-resistant, HIV-1–related thrombocytopenia.[30,67] One potential mechanism by which IFN-α restores platelet production may be by increasing levels of interleukin-6 (IL-6),[173] a cytokine with tropic effects on megakaryocytes.

Infusions of γ-globulins offer the potential for a rapid elevation in platelet counts, with an acute response rate of 70% to 90%[44,68,69]; the median response duration is only 3 weeks. Sustained remissions from a single course of such therapy occur in fewer than 10% of patients.[44] A similar response is offered by anti-D (anti-Rh) antibody, which produces a short-term response rate of 75%,[70] with sustained remissions in fewer than 10% of patients. As with γ-globulin infusions, readministration is effective in elevating the platelet counts in those who initially responded.[44,71,72] Unlike γ-globulin, however, the response may take as long as 3 weeks to occur, and there may be some hemolysis; anti-D antibody is not effective with splenectomized patients or in those who are Rh negative.[70] Immune globulin infusions and anti-D antibody may work by increasing production of thrombopoietic cytokines, such as IL-6, from cells of the reticuloendothelial system rather than by decreasing platelet destruction.[73]

When other therapies fail, splenectomy needs to be considered. This procedure has a short-term response rate of 60% to 100%, and durable responses occur in 40% to 60% of patients.[44] No studies have demonstrated any detrimental effects of splenectomy on HIV progression.[64,74,75] This procedure can, however, result in artificial elevations in CD4 counts because of peripheral lymphocytosis.[74] Consequently, splenectomized patients may develop opportunistic infections at higher levels of CD4 cells than otherwise expected.[74]

A compromise to splenectomy is offered by low-dose splenic irradiation.[54,76] Small, uncontrolled studies have demonstrated a short-term response rate of 70%, with durable responses occurring in about 40% of patients.[76] The total doses are about 900 to 1000 cGy administered over the course of a month. Some degree of splenic function is maintained by low-dose irradiation.[77]

MARROW ABNORMALITIES WITH HIV INFECTION

The bone marrow in most HIV patients exhibits morphologic aberrations.[19,21,78] The incidence increases with progression of HIV infection.[25,79] None of the marrow abnormalities seen with HIV infection, however, are specific for the disease.[21,23,80,81]

The most common morphologic demonstration encountered is hypercellularity of the marrow.[82–84] This occurs in 50% to 60% of cases and is caused by absolute hyperplasia of one or more of the nonlymphoid cell lines.[79] The myeloid to erythroid cell ratio tends to remain close to normal or exhibits a mild myeloid hyperplasia.[81] Because much of the hypercellularity may not represent effective hematopoiesis, the marrow cellularity correlates neither with the peripheral blood counts nor with the stage of HIV infection.[30,81,83,84] Hypocellularity of the marrow is rare, occurring in fewer than 5% of cases, and is usually a manifestation of advanced HIV infection.[23,25,27] In the end stages of HIV infection, atrophy or necrosis of the marrow may occur.[81]

Dysplasia of at least one cell line occurs in more than 70% of HIV-infected patients.[27,39,82] This dysplasia is similar to that of myelodysplastic syndromes, and it is usually indistinguishable from the latter on morphologic criteria alone.[27,85] Dysplasia of the granulocyte series is the most common occurrence, with vacuolization of the granulocyte precursors in the marrow and in the peripheral neutrophils.[86] Erythrocytic dysplasia is somewhat less common, seen in 50% to 60% of HIV-infected patients, and dysplasia of the megakaryocytes occurs in about one third of HIV-infected patients.[82] In general, the degree and frequency of dysplastic changes in the marrow increase with progression of the HIV-1 infection and with concurrent opportunistic infections.[26]

Less common aberrations in the bone marrow include lymphoid aggregates and increased numbers of lymphocytes in the marrow. These conditions are encountered in about 20% of patients and occur despite the peripheral lymphopenia that is characteristic of HIV infection.[26,39] A similar proportion of those with advanced HIV infection have focal or diffuse increases in reticulin deposition in the marrow.[25,26] In general, marrow fibrosis increases in incidence and severity with the progression of the HIV-1 infection and with marrow involvement by fungal or mycobacterial organisms.[30] Other nonspecific morphologic changes that may be seen in the marrow include increases in eosinophils and plasma cells and histiocytic erythrophagocytosis.[25,87]

CAUSES OF CYTOPENIAS IN PATIENTS WITH HIV INFECTION

Hematopoietic Alterations Due to HIV

The hematologic abnormalities that occur during the course of HIV infection mostly result from ineffective hematopoiesis. A compounding factor is peripheral cell destruction. In a few of those with significant splenomegaly, sequestration may further compound the problem.

Hematopoiesis is a process that is constitutive and inducible. Constitutive hematopoiesis is largely under the direction of the colony-stimulating factors,[88] and inducible hematopoiesis is more within the realm of action of other cytokines and interleukins that modulate hematopoiesis during situations of altered demand.[89,900] These cytokines are released from the marrow fibroblasts, endothelial cells, T cells, and monocytes in response to a multitude of stimuli.[88,89]

The hematologic perturbations that occur in association with HIV infection may be a direct result of HIV-1 on stem cells and the marrow stromal cells. The alterations in growth factors and cytokines that occur as a result of HIV infection contribute to hematopoietic abnormalities. Other factors that merit recognition are opportunistic infections, neoplasms invading the marrow, and myelosuppressive medications.

Hematopoietic Alterations Due to Tumor, Infection, or Medications

HIV infection is associated with the development of lymphomas, Kaposi's sarcoma, and squamous cell carcinomas. The incidence of neoplasms that occur with HIV infection are likely to increase as the infectious complications of AIDS are better controlled. The bone marrow is affected in about one third of those with AIDS-related lymphomas.[91] The extent of replacement of the marrow by these malignant cells does not correlate well with the peripheral blood counts.[91] The antineoplastic drugs needed to treat these tumors are myelosuppressive, and the dose reductions that may be needed to preserve hematopoietic function hinder therapy of the tumor.

The medications used to treat HIV infection and the opportunistic infections that occur with AIDS cause disease-stage and dose-dependent suppression of hematopoiesis.[24,30] All of the dideoxynucleoside analogs can inhibit hematopoiesis at sufficiently high doses; zidovudine is the major offender.[25,92,93] Other myelosuppressive drugs include pentamidine, trimethoprim, sulfonamides, ganciclovir, acyclovir, and pyrimethamine.[92] Medications that are not typically associated with decreases in hematopoiesis may have this effect when given to persons with altered hematopoietic potential, as occurs with HIV infection. The concurrent administration of myelosuppressive medications synergistically potentiates bone marrow suppression.

Several opportunistic infections that result from HIV-induced immunosuppression may cause or contribute to marrow failure. Mycobacterial infections (ie, *Mycobacterium avium complex*, disseminated *M tuberculosis*, and atypical forms) and fungal infections (ie, *Cryptococcus* and *Histoplasmosis*) are important causes of reduced hematopoietic potential. The marrow may reveal a disseminated mycobacterial or fungal infection long before other indications of the infection become apparent in an HIV-infected host.[85,94] Special stains and cultures of the marrow for these organisms are helpful and may be positive before peripheral blood cultures turn positive.[85,94] Small studies have shown that marrow examination or cultures are positive for mycobacteria or fungi for at least 75% of patients who are subsequently found to have these infections.[85,95]

The most common morphologic manifestation of these infections of the marrow is diffuse infiltration with loose aggregates and clusters of macrophages.[32,96] The ability to detect involvement of the bone marrow by mycobacteria and fungi correlates with the number of macrophages in the marrow.[32] Although these cells may organize into granulomas, the tendency to do so is less with immunosuppression.[30] Pseudo-Gaucher cells may also be seen as a manifestation of such infections.[97]

Opportunistic infections of the marrow by viruses other than HIV-1 are important causes of marrow failure. Cytomegalovirus and parvovirus have special significance, and hepatitis viruses B and C merit recognition as causes of marrow suppression in an HIV-infected patient.[98,99]

Cytomegalovirus may cause suppression of hematopoiesis and autoimmune destruction of blood cells.[30,100] This virus can infect bone marrow progenitor cells, rendering them less responsive to colony-stimulating factors.[100] The infected cells may serve as reservoirs of latent cytomegalovirus within the marrow, causing further problems with advancing immunosuppression.[100] Cytomegalovirus can infect the bone marrow stromal cells, interfering with their hematopoietic supporting functions largely by decreasing local growth factor production by these cells.[100] Despite the hematologic problems that cytomegalovirus may cause, it does not cause distinctive histologic changes of the marrow.[30,100] It is best cultured from the buffy coat of the blood and not from the marrow itself.[100]

HIV-positive patients may be infected with parvovirus B-19, which may result in marrow suppression. These patients do not have the manifestations of Fifth's disease that is seen in immunologically normal patients.[101] The major hematopoietic target of parvovirus B19 is the erythroid progenitor.[102] This is the only permissive cell of the hematopoietic system for the virus. Morphologically, such an infection results in giant pronormoblasts[101] that are associated with erythroblastopenia, which can persist in those who are unable to make antibodies to the virus.[102] Parvovirus also has an inhibitory effect on myeloid and megakaryocyte progenitors that may result in various degrees of neutropenia or thrombocytopenia.[101,102] Treatment of parvovirus B19 infection in those who are unable to make antibodies to the infection includes intravenous γ-globulin, which results in a reduction in serum viral concentrations and recovery of erythropoiesis.[101] Simultaneous infection with parvovirus B19 and HIV-1 does not preclude a response to erythropoietin.[101]

Human herpesvirus-6 is the etiologic agent of another viral exanthem of childhood, roseola. Infection usually occurs in the first 3 years of life and then establishes latency.[103] The primary target of this virus is the CD4 lymphocyte, as well as cells of monocytic lineage.[103,104] Immunosuppression may result in the loss of latency. The subsequent exposure of marrow precursor cells to this virus inhibits their ability to respond to growth factors, and infection of lymphocytes causes further suppression of T-cell function.[103,104]

COLONY-STIMULATING FACTORS AND HIV INFECTION

The colony-stimulating factors include granulocyte colony-stimulating factor (G-CSF), macrophage colony-stimulating factor (M,-CSF), granulocyte-macrophage colony-stimulating factor (GM-CSF), interleukin-3 (IL-3), stem cell factor, and erythropoietin.[89,105] These are glycoproteins that regulate the passage of hematopoietic cells into the cell cycle and into the processes of terminal maturation.[106] Their major activity is to suppress apoptosis.[107,108] The major sources of colony-stimulating factors are T and B lymphocytes, natural killer cells (NK) cells, vascular endothelial cells, smooth muscle cells, and fibroblasts.[89,90] The monocyte, an important primary target for infection by HIV-1, is central to the network of cytokines, interleukins, and growth factors that support and regulate hematopoiesis.[89,90]

Production of G-CSF, GM-CSF, and M-CSF increases during the early phases of HIV infection.[22] This increase is stimulated by the effects of IL-1 and other inflammatory cytokines on cells within the bone marrow that produce these growth factors. T cells, monocytes, and fibroblasts are important components of the marrow and are targets of HIV infection. When infected, their ability to make growth factors progressively diminishes.[109] With advancing HIV infection, the increasing levels of inflammatory cytokines that occur alters the receptors on target cells to make them less responsive to growth factors.[110,111]

The pharmacokinetics of growth factors depend on the dose, amount of glycosylation, and the route of administration. Exogenous administration of growth factors offers the potential of ameliorating some of the adverse effects of HIV infection on hematopoiesis. With the exception of erythropoietin, the potentials of growth factors have been investigated in uncontrolled studies only.[112] Administration of growth factors permits the administration of myelosuppressive medications without dose reduction or interruption of therapy.[24]

Granulocyte Colony-Stimulating Factor

G-CSF is produced by activated monocytes, stimulated endothelial cells, and fibroblasts. Exogenous administration of G-CSF results in a sustained, dose-dependent rise in the circulating neutrophil counts.[40,88] High doses may result in modest elevations of monocytes and lymphocytes.[88] The relative and absolute elevation in neutrophil count is caused by an increase in the number of divisions of neutrophil precursors in the marrow and a decrease in their maturation time.[113] In vitro, G-CSF augments neutrophil function.[40,114]

Granulocyte-Monocyte Colony-Stimulating Factor

GM-CSF is produced primarily by stimulated fibroblasts and endothelial cells, although the growth factor is also produced by T cells. Administration of this growth factor, as with G-CSF, results in a dose-dependent elevation in neutrophils. The kinetic basis of the elevation in neutrophils differs from that of G-CSF in that GM-CSF prolongs the circulating half-life of neutrophils rather than decreasing the production time, as does G-CSF.[88,115] Unlike, G-CSF, it also results in a significant elevation in eosinophils and monocytes.[41,42,116,117]

GM-CSF and G-CSF have different effects on HIV-infected cells.[40,105,118] Although G-CSF does not seem to alter HIV replication in cells that are targets for the growth factor, GM-CSF can stimulate HIV replication in vitro in infected cells of monocytic lineage.[116,117,119,120] Moreover, activation of monocytes by HIV infection induces them to produce GM-CSF themselves and to stimulate T cells, endothelial cells, and fibroblasts to produce this growth factor, and this augments HIV replication in the monocytes.[89,90] When GM-CSF is administered in conjunction with zidovudine, the result is enhanced antiviral effects because of an increase in the concentration of the active drug within monocytes.[116,117,119,121] This effect has been shown only for zidovudine, and because of this, GM-CSF should be administered concomitantly with zidovudine in HIV-infected patients.[118]

Erythropoietin

Most HIV-infected patients with anemia have adequate erythropoietic capacity but are unable to augment this during times of demand, in large part because of relatively inadequate erythropoietin levels.[30] Inappropriately low endogenous levels (<500 mU/mm^3) of serum erythropoietin are seen in 75% of AIDS patients, regardless of the medications they are on.[24,122] In addition to a production problem, the cytokines that are produced in response to the HIV infection, such as IL-1 and tumor necrosis factor-α (TNF-α), blunt the normal exponential elevation between the hematocrit and serum erythropoietin levels.[123]

In placebo-controlled trials, exogenous administration of erythropoietin increased the hematocrit and improved the quality of life for patients with AIDS.[122,124] The elevation in erythrocyte counts was dose dependent.[23,24] Initial concerns about stem cell exhaustion or lineage diversion did not occur.[24] Erythropoietin neither promoted nor prevented HIV replication.[24,118] Despite these promising results, not all patients respond to the administration of erythropoietin. The benefits are principally seen in those with baseline erythropoietin levels of less than 500 mU/mm^3.[24] About 25% of patients on zidovudine do not have a significant elevation in the hematocrit with concurrent administration of erythropoietin.[24] Opportunistic infections render patients relatively resistant to the effects of exogenous erythropoietin.[125]

Administration of erythropoietin offers an alternative to transfusions and their potential morbidity. Transfusions may be immunosuppressive;[126,127] they have been shown to decrease the ratio of CD4 to CD8 lymphocytes and decrease NK cell numbers.[128] The time to progression to AIDS is shorter in those who are transfused.[24,30,129] There is the risk of

exposure to new infectious agents with transfusions[24] and a risk of transfusion reactions despite immunodeficiency due to allosensitization.[24,81]

Stem Cell Factor

Stem cell factor (ie, Kit ligand) is a multipotential growth factor that is produced by marrow cells.[130] It acts on cells of myeloid, lymphoid, and mast cell lineage.[130] For optimal stimulatory effects, it acts in synergy with other colony-stimulating factors.[89,130,131] When administered to HIV-infected patients, stem cell factor increases hematopoiesis in a dose-dependent fashion.[132] It has not been shown to alter HIV expression.[132]

Interleukin-3

IL-3 is a growth factor produced by activated T cells. It has direct effects on granulocytes, monocytes, and mast cells and indirect stimulatory effects on erythroid production and T lymphocytes.[133] Administration results in a dose-dependent increase in circulating granulocytes, erythrocytes, and platelets.[133]

The loss of T cells that is characteristic of advancing HIV infection reduces the endogenous IL-3 levels.[61,121,134–136] This may cause or contribute to the myelosuppression that occurs with HIV infection.[121] Although some researchers have found IL-3 to potentiate HIV expression in monocytes in vitro, others have found no consistent effects on viral activity.[137] Like GM-CSF, it may augment the antiviral effects of zidovudine by elevating the intracellular levels of the active form of the drug.[7,80,121,138]

BONE MARROW PROGENITOR CELLS IN HIV INFECTION

Results of studies on HIV infection of bone marrow progenitor cells have been somewhat conflicting.[25,79] Although there are data indicating progenitor cells to be targets of HIV infection, other findings have revealed that CD34+ bone marrow progenitor cells are infrequently infected with the virus.[19,20,139–143] Some investigators have shown that progenitor cells in the marrow and peripheral blood[83,144,145] are decreased with HIV infection,[27,36,186] but others have found no significant differences in the numbers of these cells in HIV-infected patients compared with normal patients.[141,148] Although some studies have revealed RNA and protein products of HIV-1 in committed myeloid and erythroid progenitor cells,[33,49] others have shown that HIV-1 DNA is not present in these cells.[148]

Reconciliation of these ostensibly conflicting results is possible by considering several factors. It is only a minority of CD34+ progenitor cells within the bone marrow that are also positive for CD4 and therefore only the minority of progenitor cells that are major targets for HIV-1.[50,143,149–151] However, the progenitor cells of HIV-1–infected patients may have defective activity without being directly affected by productive infection.[19,152]

The presence or absence of accessory cells within the marrow cultures is also a factor. T cells, monocytes, and fibroblasts are important components of the bone marrow stroma and influence hematopoiesis through the production of growth factors.[33,38,109] These cells are targets for HIV and may serve as reservoirs of virus within the bone marrow.[19,153] When infected with HIV-1, these cells are less able to make growth factors.[33,38] Because the major function of growth factors may be to prevent apoptosis, the deficiency in local production permits marrow progenitor cells to undergo this process.[152] These cells also may produce inhibitors of hematopoiesis, such as transforming growth factor-β (TGF-β), platelet factor-4, interferons, and TNF-α.[89,154–157] In vitro depletion of marrow cultures of these cells increases hematopoiesis.[153,156,158]

There are differences in cytopathogenicity of different strains of HIV-1.[142,148] Some strains have been shown to impair hematopoiesis in a dose-dependent manner.[142,147] These may alter the ability of progenitor cells to proliferate and differentiate with little cytopathogenicity.[24,159–161]

Protein products of HIV-1 can directly inhibit marrow progenitor cells. The gp120 and gp160 envelope proteins of HIV-1 have been shown to cause a dose-dependent decrease in viable CD34+ cell counts through a direct cytotoxic effect.[21,151,162] Indirectly, gp120 can suppress hematopoiesis by inducing other cells to produce TNF-α and other cytokines that inhibit hematopoiesis.[156] Other studies have shown that protein products of the *tat* and *nef* genes cause suppression of hematopoiesis directly[19] or indirectly by causing other marrow mononuclear cells to produce inhibitors of hematopoiesis such as TGF-β and TNF-α.[21,110,156]

Antibodies to gp120 can have suppressive effects on the bone marrow[44,50,163] by adversely altering the ability of the progenitor cells to proliferate in response to growth factors.[158] At least with respect to megakaryocytes, HIV-1 infection induces alterations in surface antigens that render them potential targets of antiplatelet and anti–HIV-1 antibodies.[47,48,56] The presence of antiretroviral drugs may influence the results of detecting of HIV-1 in marrow progenitors.[148,164] Taken together, the data indicate that HIV-1 has indirect and direct effects on the marrow progenitor cells that decreases their potential to differentiate and proliferate.

OTHER CYTOKINES AND INTERLEUKINS

Interleukin-1

IL-1 is one of the primary mediators of the acute-phase response.[165] This cytokine is produced largely by cells of monocytic lineage[165–167] but also is produced by dendritic cells, B and T lymphocytes, NK cells, fibroblasts, and vascular endothelial cells.[1] IL-1 causes fever and anorexia, and contributes to a catabolic state.[166] It induces secretion of colony-stimulating factors by accessory cells in the marrow,

particularly G-CSF, M-CSF, and GM-CSF,[89,168] and also IL-6.[165,168] In this way, it enhances hematopoiesis.[89,165] Prolonged secretion of IL-1, however, induces secretion of TNF-α and other inflammatory cytokines that suppress hematopoietic activity.[155,165,168] In vivo and in vitro, levels of IL-1 tend to increase with progression of HIV-1 infection.[111,157,166,169]

Interleukin-2

IL-2 is a primary growth factor for T cells[89,90] and secondarily stimulates proliferation and differentiation of B cells.[105] IL-1 and TNF-α are the major stimuli for production of IL-2 by T cells, and these cytokines also increase the T-cell membrane IL-2 receptor numbers and binding capacity.[89,90,105]

IL-2 can indirectly decrease hematopoiesis by its ability to induce synthesis of IFN-γ by other cells.[89] More importantly, production of IL-2 during the chronic inflammatory state of HIV infection augments replication of HIV-1 in infected cells.[7,80,170,171] In this way, production of this cytokine directly upregulates HIV-1 production and indirectly contributes to the suppression of hematopoiesis that is characteristic of advancing HIV-1 infection.

Interleukin-6

HIV infection is associated with increased production of IL-6 primarily by monocytes in response to interaction of gp160 antigen with the CD4 receptors of these cells.[172,173] IL-6 may also be produced by stimulated B cells, T cells, and fibroblasts.[89,90,105,131,168] Circulating neutrophils and eosinophils and vascular endothelial cells have been shown to produce this cytokine in the presence of HIV-1.[172,174] HIV-1 Tat protein has been shown to directly and indirectly upregulate IL-6 expression.[110]

Interleukin-6 can act in synergy with IL-3 to enhance hematopoiesis.[57,62,89,175–177] In this regard the elevated levels of IL-6 that occur with advancing HIV-1 infection[157,169] would be expected to upregulate hematopoiesis.[173] This cytokine, however, also induces hepatocytes to produce acute-phase proteins,[173] primarily IL-1, and this directly and indirectly downregulates the hematopoietic potential.[65,131,161,178] IL-6 also can upregulate HIV-1 production by infected cells[7,80,170,178] and may cause T-cell proliferation, thereby expanding the pool of HIV-infected cells.[131]

Interferons

The interferons are a family of cytokines that are produced by leukocytes (eg, IFN-α), fibroblasts (eg, IFN-β), and cells of lymphocyte and monocytic lineage (eg, IFN-γ).[13] The latter may be produced by cytotoxic T lymphocytes on contact with target cells that present HIV antigens.[13]

Serum interferon levels tend to increase with progression of HIV infection.[140,179,180] Interferons in general and INF-α in particular inhibit marrow progenitor cells.[180–182] This effect may be mediated by inducing secretion of other cytokines such as TNF-α and IL-1 from marrow monocytes and T cells.[2,7,80,155,168,183]

Tumor Necrosis Factor

TNF-α (ie, cachectin) is produced by stimulated monocytes and macrophages,[80,90,168] T lymphocytes,[13] stimulated B cells,[184] and vascular endothelial cells.[167] Although it is not produced constitutively by HIV-infected cells, it can be produced in response to diverse stimuli concurrent with the HIV infection.[166,167,185] The Tat protein of HIV-1 may activate TNF-α genes in vitro.[111,169] In particular, cytotoxic T lymphocytes are capable of producing TNF-α on contact with target cells presenting HIV-1 antigens.[13] Monocytes and macrophages are capable of producing TNF-α after contact with gp120,[156] and this does not require the presence of live virus.[156] In this capacity, TNF-α or IFN-γ may act through ceramide as a second messenger. HIV-1 binding to surface receptors stimulates the hydrolysis of plasma membrane sphingomyelin to ceramide, initiating a molecular cascade that results in transcriptional activation of HIV-1 provirus.[11] HIV-1 Tat protein may activate expression of the TNF-α gene in vitro.[111,169]

TNF-α levels are elevated in the sera of HIV-infected patients[156,166,169,186] and rise progressively with the disease. In vitro, TNF-α can maintain HIV expression in chronically infected cells.[7,80,168,187,188] TNF-α is therefore important to the autocrine and paracrine regulation of HIV infection.[115]

TNF-α can act as a positive or negative regulator of hematopoiesis.[156,167,189] It can alter the production of growth factors by marrow stromal cells and modulate the expression of cell surface receptors for growth factors on cells that are targets of HIV infection.[89,155,156,167,189] The concentration of TNF-α is important to the quantitative effect on hematopoiesis.[189,190] Low concentrations stimulate IL-3 and GM-CSF–induced colony formation, but high levels inhibit the actions of these growth factors.[89,155] TNF-α also has differential effects on various hematopoietic cell lines; the same concentration of TNF-α that stimulates growth of committed granulocyte and monocyte progenitor cells inhibits erythroid growth.[190] There are at least two receptors for TNF-α, a 55-kd and a 75-kd receptor, and these seem to use different signaling pathways and result in different effects on hematopoiesis. Although the inhibitory effects of TNF-α on progenitor cells involves p55 and p75, the p55 receptor alone mediates the stimulatory effects on progenitors.[189,190] TNF-α indirectly suppresses hematopoiesis by inducing the production of IL-1 by monocytes.[89,155]

Transforming Growth Factor-β

TGF-β is a stimulatory growth factor for some cell lines, fibroblasts in particular, but it is a potent inhibitor of hematopoietic proliferation.[21,154,191,192] It has a reversible, suppressive effect on marrow progenitors.[154] It acts on early cells in hematopoiesis in a multipotential and nonlineage specific fashion.[154] It may act through downregulation of cell surface Kit expression and downmodulation of IL-1 receptors.[191]

Levels of TGF-β increase progressively as infection with HIV-1 advances.[193] The Tat protein of HIV-1 upregulates production of this cytokine in a direct and indirect manner.[110] Moreover, TGF-β is capable of inducing its own synthesis.[193]

In addition to its effects on hematopoiesis, TGF-β is a potent endogenous immunosuppressive factor.[193] It downregulates activity of B cells, T cells, monocytes, and macrophages.[193] Its overall effect is to augment the immunosuppression and hematosuppression characteristic of HIV-1 infection.[193-195] Moreover, TGF-β enhances HIV-1 expression in infected cells.[196]

THE HEMATOPOIETIC MICROENVIRONMENT AND HIV INFECTION

The bone marrow stroma consists of cellular and acellular components that provide a structural framework for organizing hematopoiesis into a nonrandom distribution that is confined to the marrow cavities.[197-199] Adhesion events among hematopoietic cells, the stromal cells, and the extracellular matrix are important to the regulation of hematopoiesis.[200] In addition to providing sites of attachment for hematopoietic cells, the marrow stromal cells produce growth factors and cytokines that regulate hematopoiesis.[197,199-201]

The cytokines that are released in response to infection with HIV-1, particularly IL-1 and TNF-α, alter the adhesion molecules on the marrow stromal cells.[202] These alterations in the attachment events between the marrow stromal cells and hematopoietic cells[27,202] may suppress hematopoiesis.

HIV infection of accessory cells within the marrow adversely alters hematopoiesis.[203,204] Monocytes and lymphocytes within the marrow are important cellular components of the bone marrow stroma and regulate hematopoiesis by their capacity to locally produce growth factors, particularly GM-CSF and IL-3.[205] During the early phases of infection by HIV-1, lymphocytes and monocytes within the bone marrow may increase production of these growth factors, and this may partially explain the marrow hypercellularity commonly seen during this stage of HIV infection.[79,205] With the progression of HIV infection, these cells produce increasing levels of IL-1 and IL-2,[3,155,168,205] which decrease the hematopoietic potential[27,89,155,165,168] and upregulate HIV replication within these and other cells in the bone marrow.[80,155,170,187] These cells may also serve as a reservoir for HIV within the bone marrow.[206,207]

Nonhematopoietic cells within the bone marrow are also important to the structure and function of the bone marrow microenvironment. A major component of the stroma is the reticulum cell (ie, fibroblast). This accounts for 60% to 70% of the volume of the marrow framework.[134] The marrow reticulum cell is a target of HIV infection.[9,19,73,83,153,208,209] When infected with HIV-1, these cells are less able to support hematopoiesis in vitro[206-210] because of an impaired ability to secrete growth factors.[211] HIV-infected marrow stromal cells also may secrete factors that inhibit hematopoiesis.[158,194] Medications used to treat the HIV infection, such as zidovudine, have the potential to inhibit the growth and development of the stromal cells and hematopoietic cells.[164]

The endothelial cells that line the marrow sinusoids are important to the structure of the marrow. These cells are important to the homing of circulating hematopoietic cells and regulate the migration of marrow cells into the circulation. They also secrete growth factors. These cells are targets for HIV infection.[172,211] When infected by HIV-1, they undergo alterations in surface receptors, and their ability to secrete growth factors is hindered, which adversely alters their ability to support hematopoiesis. These cells also may serve as reservoirs of HIV-1 within the bone marrow.[211]

COAGULATION ABNORMALITIES IN HIV INFECTION

Clotting disorders are encountered in patients with HIV infection.[212] The most common of these is caused by the lupus anticoagulant, which is one of several antibodies to acidic phospholipids that can occur as a result of the abnormal immune responses characteristic of HIV infection. The incidence approaches 20% to 66% of HIV-infected patients.[213–217] Titers tend to increase with active opportunistic infections.[38,217]

The antiphospholipid antibodies include the lupus anticoagulant and nonspecific antibodies that may give positive test results for the Venereal Disease Research Laboratory (VDRL) and anticardiolipin antibody assays. These antibodies tend to cause abnormalities of in vitro tests of coagulation.[30] Most commonly seen is an elevation of the activated partial thromboplastin time that does not correct with one to one mixing of normal and patient plasma. The prothrombin time may be prolonged to a mild degree in about 10% of patients who have the lupus anticoagulant. Also abnormal are the dilute thromboplastin inhibition assay result and the viper venom clotting time. Once thought to be clinically insignificant, the lupus anticoagulant in HIV-infected patients may be associated with major thromboembolic phenomena.[218]

Thromboembolic events may also occur as a result of reduced levels of active protein S. This peptide is the cofactor for protein C, acting to localize active protein C to the phospholipid surface. Mean total and free protein S levels are statistically lower in HIV-infected patients with or without thromboses than in healthy male controls.[219] The levels of free and total protein S do not correlate with CD4 counts, stage of HIV infection, p24 antigen levels, or use of antiretroviral medications.[219] Protein S binds to C4b-binding protein, and increases in C4b-binding protein with the chronic inflammatory state encountered with HIV infection results in greater binding of protein S by C4b-binding protein so less is available to prevent abnormal thrombotic events.[219] Another mechanism that may cause or contribute to lower levels of active protein S in HIV-infected patients is the higher incidence of anti–protein S antibodies in these patients. These antibodies bind protein C, decreasing the unbound and active forms of the protein.[220]

Several of the opportunistic viral infections that result from the immunosuppression induced by HIV may cause or contribute to the prothrombotic state characteristic of HIV infection. Quiescent endothelial cells have control mechanisms that restrict expression of procoagulant phospholipids to areas of vascular injury.[221] Cytomegalovirus and herpes simplex types 1 and 2 can convert vascular endothelial cells from a noncoagulative to a procoagulative phenotype.[221] The mechanism includes alterations in the surface phospholipids to those that activate the coagulation system.[221]

Other abnormalities in coagulation that may occur with HIV infection include isolated deficiencies in prothrombin levels[222] and abnormal platelet aggregation.[221] The hypoalbuminemia that occurs with advancing HIV infection may cause fibrin polymerization and fibrinolytic defects.[212]

REFERENCES

1. Gallo RC. Human retroviruses. A decade of discovery and link with human disease. J Infect Dis 1991;164:235.
2. Greene WC. The molecular biology of human immunodeficiency virus type I infection. N Engl J Med 1991;321:308.
3. Gendelman HE, Baca LM, Turpin JA. Interactions between interferon and the human immunodeficiency virus. J Exp Pathol 1990;5:53.
4. Torbett BE, Healy PA, Shao LE, Mosier DE, Yu J. HIV-1 infection is latent in primary and transformed bone marrow stromal cells. (Abstract 1904) Blood 1994;84:480a.
5. O'Brien WA. Viral determinants of cellular tropism. Pathobiology 1992;60:225.
6. Ball JK, Holmes EC, Whitwell H, Desselberger U. Genomic variation of human immunodeficiency virus type 1 (HIV-1): molecular analyses of HIV-1 in sequential blood samples and various organs obtained at autopsy. J Gen Virol 1994;75:67.
7. Merigan TC, Katzenstein DA. Relation of pathogenesis of human immunodeficiency virus infection to various strategies for its control. Rev Infect Dis 1991;13:292.
8. Orenstein JM. Ultrastructural pathology of human immunodeficiency virus infection. Ultrastruct Pathol 1992;16:179.
9. Joling P, Bakker LJ, van Wichen DF, et al. Binding of HIV-1 to human follicular dendritic cells. Adv Exp Med Biol 1993;329:455.
10. Poli G, Pantaleo G, Fauci AS. Immunopathogenesis of human immunodeficiency virus infection. Clin Infect Dis 1993;17(Suppl 1):S224.
11. Rivas CI, Golde DW, Vera JC, Kolesnick RN. Involvement of the sphingomyelin pathway in autocrine tumor necrosis factor signaling for human immunodeficiency virus production in chronically infected HL-60 cells. Blood 1994;83:2191.
12. Chiodi F, Keys B, Albert J, et al. Human immunodeficiency virus type 1 is present in the cerebrospinal fluid of a majority of infected individuals. J Clin Microbiol 1992;30:1768.
13. Jassoy C, Harrer T, Rosenthal T, et al. Human immunodeficiency virus type 1-specific cytotoxic T lymphocytes release gamma interferon, tumor necrosis factor alpha (TNF-alpha), and TNF-beta when they encounter their target antigens. J Virology 1993;67:2844.
14. Ho DD, Neumann AU, Perelson AS, Chen W, Leonard JM, Markowitz M. Rapid turnover of plasma virions and CD4 lymphocytes in HIV-1 infection. Nature 1995;373:123.
15. Wei X, Ghosh SK, Taylor ME, et al. Viral dynamics in human immunodeficiency virus type 1 infection. Nature 1995;373:117.
16. Baltimore D. Lessons from people with nonprogressive HIV infection. N Engl J Med 1995;332:259.
17. Cao Y, Qin L, Zhang L, Safrit J, Ho D. Virologic and immunologic characterization of long-term survivors of human immunodeficiency virus type-1 infection. N Engl J Med 1995;322:201.
18. Pantaleo G, Menzo S, Vaccarezza M, et al. Studies in subjects with long-term nonprogressive human immunodeficiency virus infection. N Engl J Med 1994;332:209.

19. Louache F, Henri A, Bettaieb A, et al. Role of human immunodeficiency virus replication in defective in vitro growth of hematopoietic progenitors. Blood 1992;80:2991.

20. Re MC, Furlini G, Zauli G, La Placa M. Human immunodeficiency virus type 1 (HIV-1) and human hematopoietic progenitor cells. Arch Virol 1994;137:1.

21. Zauli G, Davis BR, Re MC, Visani G, Furlini G, LaPlaca M. Tat protein stimulates production of transforming growth factor-beta 1 by marrow macrophages: a potential mechanism for human immunodeficiency virus-1-induced hematopoietic suppression. Blood 1992;80:3036.

22. Re MC, Furlini G, Zauli G, La Placa M. Human immunodeficiency virus type 1 (HIV-1) and human hematopoietic progenitor cells. Arch Virol 1994;137:1.

23. Mir N, Costello C, Luckitt J, Lindley R. HIV disease and bone marrow changes: a study of 60 cases. Eur J Haematol 1989;42:339.

24. Miles SA. Hematopoietic growth factors in HIV infection. Hematopoiet Ther Index Rev 1991;1:1.

25. Scadden DT, Zon LI, Groopman JE. Pathophysiology and management of HIV-associated hematologic disorders. Blood 1989;74:1455.

26. Zon LI, Arkin C, Groopman GE. Hematologic manifestations of the human immunodeficiency virus (HIV). Br J Haematol 1987;66:251.

27. Ganser A. Abnormalities of hematopoiesis in the acquired immunodeficiency syndrome. Blut 1988;56:49.

28. Jacobson MA, Peiperl L, Volberding PA, Porteous D, Toy PTCY, Feigal D. Red cell transfusion therapy for anemia in patients with AIDS and ARC. Transfusion 1990;30:133.

29. Spivak JL, Barnes DC, Fuchs E, Quinn TC. Serum immunoreactive erythropoietin in HIV infected patients. JAMA 1989;261:3104.

30. Aboulafia DM, Mitsuyasu RT. Hematologic abnormalities in AIDS. Hematol Oncol Clin North Am 1991;5:195.

31. Richman DD, Fischl MA, Grieco MH, Gottlieb MS, Volberding PA, Laskin OL. The toxicity of azidothymidine (AZT) in the treatment of patients with AIDS and AIDS-related complex. N Engl J Med 1987;317:192.

32. Castella A, Croxson TS, Mildvan D, Sitt DH, Zalushy R. The bone marrow in AIDS: a histologic, hematologic and microbiologic study. Am J Clin Pathol 1985;84:425.

33. Zon LI, Groopman JE. Hematologic manifestations of the human immune deficiency virus (HIV). Semin Hematol 1988;25:208.

34. Gupta S, Inman A, Licorish K. Serum ferritin in acquired immune deficiency syndrome. J Clin Lab Immunol 1986;20:11.

35. Harriman GR, Smith PD, Horne MK, et al. Vitamin B_{12} malabsorption in patients with acquired immunodeficiency syndrome. Arch Intern Med 1989;149:2039.

36. Remacha AF, Riera A, Cadafalch J, et al. Vitamin B_{12} abnormalities in HIV-infected patients. Eur J Haematol 1991; 47:60.

37. Beach RS, Mantero-Atienza E, Shor-Posner G, et al. Specific nutrient abnormalities in asymptomatic HIV-1 infection. AIDS 1991;6:701.

38. Abrams DI, Kiprov DD, Goedert JJ, Sarngadharan MG, Gallo R, Volberding PA. Antibodies to human T-lymphotropic virus type III and development of the acquired immunodeficiency syndrome in homosexual men presenting with immune thrombocytopenia. Ann Intern Med 1986;104:47.

39. Treacy M, Lai L, Costello C. Peripheral blood and bone marrow abnormalities in patients with human immunodeficiency virus related disease. Br J Haematol 1987;65:289.

40. Miles SA, Mitsuyasu RT, Moreno J, et al. Combined therapy with recombinant granulocyte colony-stimulating factor and erythropoietin decreases hematologic toxicity from zidovudine. Blood 1991;77:2109.

41. Groopman JE, Mitsuyasu RT, DeLeo JM, Oette D, Golde DW. Effect of recombinant human granulocyte-macrophage colony-stimulating factor on myelopoiesis in the acquired immunodeficiency syndrome. N Engl J Med 1987;317:593.

42. Davey RT Jr, Davey VJ, Metcalf JA, et al. A phase I/II trial of zidovudine, interferon-alpha, and granulocyte-macrophage colony-stimulating factor in the treatment of human immunodeficiency virus type I infection. J Infect Dis 1991;164:43.

43. Murphy MF, Metcalfe P, Waters AH, et al. Incidence and mechanism of neutropenia and thrombocytopenia in patients with human immunodeficiency virus infection. Br J Haematol 1987;66:337.

44. Stricker RB. Hemostatic abnormalities in HIV disease. Hematol Oncol Clin North Am 1991;5:249.

45. Perkocha LA, Rodgers GM. Hematologic aspects of human immunodeficiency virus infection: laboratory and clinical considerations. Am J Hematol 1988;29:94.

46. Holzman RS, Walsh CM, Karpatkin S. Risk for the acquired immunodeficiency syndrome among thrombocytopenic and nonthrombocytopenic homosexual men seropositive for the human immunodeficiency virus. Ann Intern Med 1987;106:383.

47. Zauli G, Re MC, Gugliotta L, et al. Lack of compensatory megakaryocytopoiesis in HIV-1–seropositive thrombocytopenic individuals compared with immune thrombocytopenic purpura patients. AIDS 1991;5:345.

48. Ballem PJ, Belzberg A, Devine DV, et al. Kinetic studies of the mechanisms of thrombocytopenia in patients with human immunodeficiency virus infection. N Engl J Med 1992;327:1779.

49. Dominguez A, Gamallo G, Garcia R, Lopez-Pastor A, Pena JM, Vazquez JJ. Pathophysiology of HIV related thrombocytopenia: an analysis of 41 patients. J Clin Pathol 1994;47:999.

50. Louache F, Bettaieb A, Henri A, et al. Infection of megakaryocytes by human immunodeficiency virus in seropositive patients with immune thrombocytopenic purpura. Blood 1991;78:1697.

51. Leaf AN, Laubenstein LH, Raphael B, Hochster H, Baez L, Karpatkins S. Thrombotic thrombocytopenic purpura associated with human immunodeficiency virus type 1 (HIV-1 infection. Ann Intern Med 1988;109:194.

52. Thompson CE, Damon LE, Ries CA, Linker CA. Thrombotic micro-angiopathies in the 1980s: clinical features, response to treatment, and the impact of the human immunodeficiency virus epidemic. Blood 1992;80:1890.

53. Bettaieb A, Fromont P, Louache F, et al. Presence of cross-reactive antibody between human immunodeficiency virus (HIV) and platelet glycoproteins in HIV-related immune thrombocytopenic purpura. Blood 1992;80:162.

54. Durand JM, Lefevre P, Hovette P, Issifi S, Mongin M. Dapsone for thrombocytopenic purpura related to human immunodeficiency virus infection. Am J Med 1991;90:675.

55. Stanworth DR, Solder B, Lewin IV, Nayyar S. Related epitopes in HIV viral coat protein and human IgG. Lancet 1989;1:1458.

56. Gonzalez-Conejero R, Rivera J, Rosillo MC, Cano A, Rodriguez T, Vicente V. Antibodies against platelet glycoproteins Ib/IX and IIb/IIIa, and antibodies cross-reactive between HIV and platelet surface antigens in HIV seropositive narcotic addicts. (Abstract 1909) Blood 1994;84:481a.

57. Bender BS, Quinn TC, Spivak JL. Homosexual men with thrombocytopenia have impaired reticuloendothelial system Fc receptor specific clearance. Blood 1987;70:392.

58. Karpatkin S. Immunologic thrombocytopenic purpura in HIV-seropositive homosexuals, narcotic addicts and hemophiliacs. Semin Hematol 1988;25:219.

59. Baldwin GC, Fleischmann J, Chung Y, et al. Human immunodeficiency virus causes mononuclear phagocyte dysfunction. Proc Natl Acad Sci USA 1990;87:3933.

60. Walsh C, Kriegel R, Lennette E, Karpatkin S. Thrombocytopenia in homosexual patients. Ann Intern Med 1985;103:542.

61. Takatsuki F, Okano A, Suzuki C, et al. Interleukin 6 perfusion stimulates reconstitution of the immune and hematopoietic systems after 5-fluorouracil treatment. Cancer Res 1990;50:2885.

62. Hill RJ, Warren MK, Levin J. Stimulation of thrombopoiesis in mice by human recombinant interleukin-6. J Clin Invest 1990;85:1242.

63. Luikart S, MacDonald M, Herzan D. Ability of twice daily granulocyte-macrophage colony-stimulating factor (GM-CSF) to support dose escalation of etoposide (VP-16) and carboplatin (CBDCA) in extensive small cell lung cancer (SCLC). (Abstract) Proc Am Soc Clin Oncol 1991;10:825a.

64. Cazzola M, Ponchio L, Beguin Y, et al. Subcutaneous erythropoietin for treatment of refractory anemia in hematologic disorders: results of a phase I/II clinical trial. Blood 1991;79:29.

65. Ahn YS. Efficacy of danazol in hematologic disorders. Acta Haematol 1990;84:122.

66. Miller KD, Gralnick HR, Ricke ME. Hematologic problems in patients with AIDS and ARC: the NIH experience. (Abstract) Blood 1987;70:124a.

67. Marroni M, Gresele P, Landonio G, Lazzarin A, Coen M, Vezza R, et. Interferon-alpha is effective in the treatment of HIV-1-related, severe, zidovudine-resistant thrombocytopenia. A prospective, placebo-controlled, double-blind trial. Ann Intern Med 1994;121:423.

68. Beard J, Savidge GF. High-dose intravenous immunoglobulin and splenectomy for the treatment of HIV-related immune thrombocytopenia in patients with severe haemophilia. Br J Haematol 1988;68:303.

69. Pollak AN, Jaminis J, Green D. Successful intravenous immune globulin therapy for human immunodeficiency virus-associated thrombocytopenia. Arch Intern Med 1988;148:695.

70. Oskenhendler E, Bierling P, Brossard Y, M, et al. Anti-Rh immunoglobulin therapy for human immunodeficiency virus-related immune thrombocytopenia. Blood 1989;71:1499.

71. Biniek R, Malessa R, Brochmeyer NH, Luboldt W. Anti-Rh(D) immunoglobulin for AIDS-related thrombocytopenia. Lancet 1986;2:627.

72. Than S, Oyaizu N, Pahwa RN, Kalyanaraman VS, Pahwa S. Effect of human immunodeficiency virus type-1 envelope glycoprotein gp120 on cytokine production from cord-blood T cells. Blood 1994;84:184.

73. Louache F, Canque B, Marandin A, Rosenswaig M, Coulombel L, Gluckman JC. HIV-1 infection of human bone marrow stromal cells and hematopoiesis. (Abstract 1921) Blood 1994;84:484a.

74. Transfusion Safety Study Group. Splenectomy and HIV-1 progression. (Abstract 1922) Blood 1994;84:484a.

75. Zambello R, Trentin L, Agostini C, et al. Persistent polyclonal lymphocytosis in human immunodeficiency virus-1-infected patients. Blood 81:1993:3015.

76. Calverley DC, Jones GW, Kelton JG. Splenic radiation for corticosteroid-resistant immune thrombocytopenia. Ann Intern Med 1992;116:977.

77. Gold E, Chadha M, Culliney B, Zalusky R. Failure of splenic irradiation to treat HIV-associated immune thrombocytopenia. (Abstract 2787) Blood 1994;84.

78. Calenda V, Chermann JC. The effects of HIV on hematopoiesis. Eur J Haematol 1992;48:181.

79. Sugiura K, Oyaizu N, Pahwa R, Kalyanaraman V, Pahwa S. Effect of human immunodeficiency virus-1 envelope glycoprotein on in vitro hematopoiesis of umbilical cord blood. Blood 1992;80:1463.

80. Rosenberg ZF, Fauci AS. Immunopathogenic mechanisms of HIV infection: cytokine induction of HIV expression. Immunol Today 1990;11:176.

81. Perkocha LA, Rodgers GM. Hematologic aspects of human immunodeficiency virus infection. Am J Hematol 1988;29:94.

82. Goasguen JE, Bennett JM. Classification and morphologic features of myelodysplastic syndromes. Semin Oncol 1992;19:4.

83. Stutte HJ, Muller H, Falk S, Schmidt S. Pathophysiological mechanisms of HIV-induced defects in hematopoiesis: pathology of the bone marrow. Res Virol 1990;141:195.

84. Karcher DS, Frost AR. The bone marrow in human immunodeficiency virus (HIV)-related disease. Morphology and clinical correlation. Am J Clin Pathol 1991;95:63.

85. Zarabi CM, Thomas R, Adesokan A. Diagnosis of systemic histoplasmosis in patients with AIDS. South Med J 1992;85:1171.

86. Candido A, Rossi P, Menichella G, et al. Indicative morphological myelodysplastic alterations of bone marrow in overt AIDS. Haematologica 1990;75:327.

87. Abrams DI, Chinn EK, Lewis BJ, Volberding PA, Conant MA, Townsend RM. Hematologic manifestations in homosexual men with Kaposi's sarcoma. Am J Clin Pathol 1984;81:13.

88. Lieschke GJ, Burgess AW. Granulocyte colony-stimulating factor and granulocyte-macrophage colony-stimulating factor (first of two parts). N Engl J Med 1992;327:28.

89. Brach MA, Herrmann F. Hematopoietic growth factors: interactions and regulation of production. Acta Haematol 1991;86:128.

90. Sieff CA. Biological and clinical aspects of the hematopoietic growth factors. Annu Rev Med 1990;41:483.

91. Levine AM. Acquired immunodeficiency-related lymphoma. Blood 1992;80:8.

92. Pluda JM, Mitsuya H, Yarchoan R. Hematologic effects of AIDS therapies. Hematol Oncol Clin North Am 1991;5:229.

93. Bhalla K, Birkhofer M, Li GR, et al. 2'-Deoxycytidine protects normal human bone marrow progenitor cells in vitro against the cytotoxicity of 3'-azido-3'-deoxythymidine with preservation of antiretroviral activity. Blood 1989;74:1923.

94. Poropatich CO, Labriola AM, Tuazon CU. Acid-fast smear and culture of respiratory secretions, bone marrow and stools as predictors of disseminated *Mycobacterium avium* complex infection. J Clin Microbiol 1987;25:929.

95. Neubauer MA, Bodensteiner DC. Disseminated histoplasmosis in patients with AIDS. South Med J 1992;85:1166.

96. Cohen RJ, Samoszuk MK, Busch D, Lagios MA. Occult infections with *M. intracellulare* in bone marrow biopsy specimens from patients with AIDS. N Engl J Med 1983;308:1475.

97. Solis OC, Belmonte AH, Ramaswamy G. Pseudo-Gaucher cells in *Mycobacterium avium-intracellulare* infection in the acquired immune deficiency syndrome (AIDS). Am J Clin Pathol 1986;85:233.

98. Zeldis JB, Farraye FA, Steinberg HN. In vitro hepatitis B virus suppression of erythropoiesis is dependent on the multiplicity of infection and is reversible with anti-HBs antibodies. Hepatology 1988;8:755.

99. Zeldis JG, Boender PJ, Hellings JA, Steinberg H. Inhibition of human hemopoiesis by non-A, non-B hepatitis virus. J Med Virol 1989; 27:34.

100. Maciejewski JP, Bruening EE, Donahue RE, Mocarski ES, Young NS, St. Jeor SC. Infection of hematopoietic progenitor cells by human cytomegalovirus. Blood 1992;80:170.

101. Frickhofen N, Abkowitz JL, Safford M, et al. Persistent B19 parvovirus infection in patients infected with human immunodeficiency virus type 1 (HIV-1): a treatable cause of anemia in AIDS. Ann Intern Med 1990;113:926.

102. Pont J, Puchhammer-Stockl E, Chott A, et al. Recurrent granulocytic aplasia as clinical presentation of a persistent parvovirus B19 infection. Br J Haematol 1992;80:160.

103. Flamand L, Gosselin J, Stefanescu I, Ablashi D, Menezes J. Immunosuppressive effect of human herpesvirus 6 on T-cell functions: suppression of interleukin-2 synthesis and cell proliferation. Blood 1995;85:1263.

104. Carrigan DR, Knox KK. Human herpesvirus 6 (HHV-6) isolated from bone marrow: HHV-6 bone marrow suppression in bone marrow transplant patients. Blood 1994;84:3307.

105. Ohmann AB, Babink LA, Harland R. Cytokine synergy with viral cytopathic effects and bacterial products during the pathogenesis of respiratory tract infections. Clin Immunol Immunopathol 1991;60:153.

106. Gabrilove J. The development of granulocyte colony-stimulating factor in its various clinical applications. Blood 1992;80:1382-1385.

107. Williams GT, Smith CA, Spooncer E, Dexter TM, Taylor DR. Haemopoietic colony stimulating factors promote cell survival by suppressing apoptosis. Nature 1990;343:76.

108. Yu H, Bauer B, Lipke GK, Phillips RL, van Zant G. Apoptosis and hematopoiesis in murine fetal liver. Blood 1993;81:373.

109. Re MC, Zauli G, Furlini G, Giovannini M, et al. GM-CSF production by CD4+ T-lymphocytes is selectively impaired during the course of HIV-1 infection. A possible indication of a preferential lesion of a specific subset of peripheral blood CD4+ T-lymphocytes. Microbiologica 1992;15:265.

110. Gibellini D, Zauli G, Re MC, et al. Recombinant human immunodeficiency virus type-1 (HIV-1) Tat protein sequentially up-regulates IL-6 and TGF-beta 1 mRNA expression and protein synthesis in peripheral blood monocytes. Br J Haematol 1994;88:26126.

111. Buonaguro L, Barillari G, Chang HK, et al. Effects of the human immunodeficiency virus type 1 Tat protein on the expression of inflammatory cytokines. J Virol 1992;66:7159.

112. Lieschke GJ, Burgess AW. Granulocyte colony-stimulating factor and granulocyte-macrophage colony-stimulating factor (Second of two parts). N Engl J Med 1991;327:99.

113. Lord BI, Molineux G, Pojda Z, Sousa LM, Mermod J-J, Dexter TM. Myeloid cell kinetics in mice treated with recombinant interleukin-3, granulocyte colony stimulating factor (CSF), or granulocyte-macrophage CSF in vivo. Blood 1991;77:2154.

114. Lindemann A, Herrmann F, Oster W, et al. Hematologic effects of recombinant human granulocyte colony-stimulating factor in patients with malignancy. Blood 1989;74:2644.

115. Lord BI, Gurney H, Chang J, Thatcher N, Crowther D, Dexter M. Haemopoietic cell kinetics in humans treated with rGM-CSF. Int J Cancer 1992;50:26.

116. Pluda JM, Yarchoan R, Smith PD, et al. Subcutaneous recombinant granulocyte-macrophage colony-stimulating factor used as a single agent and in an alternating regimen with azidothymidine in leukopenic patients with severe human immunodeficiency virus infection. Blood 1990;76:463.

117. Perno CF, Yarchoan R, Cooney DA, et al. Replication of human immunodeficiency virus in monocytes. J Exp Med 1989;169:933.

118. Perno CF, Cooney DA, Gao W-Y, Hao Z, et al. Effects of bone marrow stimulatory cytokines on human immunodeficiency virus replication and the antiviral activity of dideoxynucleosides in cultures of monocyte/macrophages. Blood 1992;80:995.

119. Hammer SM, Gillis JM, Pinkston P, Rose R. Effect of zidovudine and granulocyte-macrophage colony-stimulating factor on human immunodeficiency virus replication in alveolar macrophages. Blood 1990;75:1215.

120. Baldwin GC, Gasson JC, Quan SG, Fleischmann J, Weisbart R, Oette D. Granulocyte-macrophage colony-stimulating factor enhances neutrophil function in acquired immunodeficiency syndrome patients. Proc Natl Acad Sci USA 1988;85:2763.

121. Schuitemaker H, Kootstra NA, van Oers MHJ, van Lambalgen R, Tersmette M, Miedema F. Induction of monocyte proliferation and HIV expression by IL-3 does not interfere with anti-viral activity of zidovudine. Blood 1990;76:1490.

122. Fischl M, Galpin JE, Levine JD, et al. Recombinant human erythropoietin for patients with AIDS treated with zidovudine. N Engl J Med 1990;322:1488.

123. Erslev A. Erythropoietin. N Engl J Med 1991;324:1339.

124. Lyman SD, Williams DE. Biological activities and potential therapeutic uses of Steel factor. A new growth factor active on multiple hematopoietic lineages. Am J Pediatr Hematol Oncol 1991;14:1.

125. Miles SA, Golde DW, Mitsuyasu RT. The use of hematopoietic hormones in HIV infection and AIDS-related malignancies. Hematol Oncol Clin North Am 1991;5:267.

126. Blajchman MA, Bardosy L, Carmen R, Sastry A, Singal DP. Allogeneic blood transfusion-induced enhancement of tumor growth: two animal models showing amelioration by leukodepletion and passive transfer using spleen cells. Blood 1993;81:1880.

127. Brunson ME, Alexander JW. Mechanisms of transfusions-induced immunosuppression. Transfusion 1990;30:651.

128. Kaplan J, Sarnaik S, Gitlin J, et al. Diminished helper/suppressor lymphocyte ratios and natural killer activity in recipients of repeated blood transfusions. Blood 1984;64:308.

129. Blumberg BS, Hann H-WL, Mildvan D, Mathur V, Lustbader E, London WT. Iron and iron binding proteins in persistent generalized lymphadenopathy and AIDS. Lancet 1984;1:347.

130. McNeice IK, Langley KE, Zsebo KM. Recombinant human stem cell factor synergizes with GM-CSF, G-CSF, IL-3 and Epo to stimulate human progenitor cells of the myeloid and erythroid lineages. Exp Hematol 1991;19:226.

131. Birx DL, Redfield RR, Tencer K, Fowler A, Burke DS, Tosato G. Induction of interleukin-6 during human immunodeficiency virus infection. Blood 1990;76:2303.

132. Miles SA, Lee K, Hutlin L, Zsebo KM, Mitsuyasu RT. Potential use of human stem cell factor as adjunctive therapy for human immunodeficiency virus-related cytopenias. Blood 1991;78:3200.

133. Guba SC, Stella G, Turka LA, et al. Regulation of interleukin 3 gene induction in normal human T cells. J Clin Invest 1989;84:1701.

134. Bruno E, Miller ME, Hoffman R. Interacting cytokines regulate in vitro human megakaryocytopoiesis. Blood 1989;73:671.

135. Briddell RA, Bruno E, Cooper RJ, Brandt JE, Hoffman R. Effect of c-kit ligand on in vitro human megakaryocytopoiesis. Blood 1991;78:2854.

136. Briddell RA, Hoffman R. Cytokine regulation of the human burst-forming unit-megakaryocyte. Blood 1990;76:516.

137. Scadden DT, Levine JD, Hammer S, McGrath J, Bresnahan J, Young DC. Recombinant human IL-3 for cytopenias in AIDS: a phase I study. (Abstract) Blood 1992;10(Suppl 1):515a.

138. Koyanagi Y, O'Brien WA, Zhao JQ, Golde DW, Gasson JC, Chenn ISY. Cytokines alter production of HIV-1 from primary mononuclear phagocytes. Science 1988;241:1673.

139. Fischl M, Galpin JE, Levine JD, et al. Human recombinant erythropoietin therapy for AIDS patients treated with AZT: a double-blind, placebo-controlled clinical study. N Engl J Med 1990;322:1488.

140. Kornbluth RS, Oh PS, Munis JR, Cleveland PH, Richman DD. The role of interferons in the control of HIV replication in macrophages. Clin Immunol Immunopathol 1990;54:200.

141. Neal T, Holland HK, Villinger F, et al. CD34+progenitors are not infected by HIV-1 in the majority of asymptomatic seropositive patients. (Abstract 1920) Blood 1994;84;484a.

142. Cen D, Zauli G, Szarnicki R, Davis BR. Effect of different human immunodeficiency virus type-1 (HIV-1) isolates on long-term bone marrow haemopoiesis. Br J Haematol 1993;85:596.

143. Louache F, Debili N, Marandin A, Coulombel L, Vainchenker W. Expression of CD4 by human hematopoietic precursors. Blood 1994;84:3344.

144. Zauli G, Re MC, Giovannini M, et al. Effect of human immunodeficiency virus type 1 on CD34+ cells. Ann N Y Acad Sci 1991;628:273.

145. Brizzi MF, Porcu P, Porteri A, Pegoraro L. Haematologic abnormalities in the acquired immunodeficiency syndrome. Haematologica 1990;75:454.

146. Bagnara GP, Zauli G, Giovannini M, Re MC, Furlini G, LaPlaca M. Early loss of circulating hematopoietic progenitor in human immunodeficiency virus I infected cells. Exp Hematol 1990;18:426.

147. Re MC, Zauli G, Furlini G, et al. The impaired number of circulating granulocyte/macrophage progenitors (CFU-GM) in human immuno-

148. Molina JM, Scadden DT, Sakaguchi M, Fuller B, Woon A, Groopman JE. Lack of evidence for infection of or effect on growth of hematopoietic progenitor cells after in vivo or in vitro exposure to human immunodeficiency virus. Blood 1990;76:2476.

149. Zucker-Franklin D, Cao Y. Megakaryocytes of human immunodeficiency virus-infected individuals express viral RNA. Proc Natl Acad Sci USA 1989;86:5595.

150. Kouri YH, Borkowsky W, Nardi M, Karpatkin S, Basch RS. Human megakaryocytes have a CD-4 molecule capable of binding human immunodeficiency virus-1. Blood 1993;81:2664.

151. Arock M, Dedenon A, Le Goff L, et al. Specific ligation of the HIV-1 viral envelope protein gp120 on human CD34+ bone marrow-derived progenitors. Cell Mol Biol 1994;40:319.

152. Re MC, Zauli G, Gibellini D, et al. Uninfected haematopoietic progenitor (CD34+) cells purified from the bone marrow of AIDS patients are committed to apoptotic cell death in culture. AIDS 1993;7:1049.

153. Watanabe J, Ringler DJ, Nakamura M, DeLong PA, Letvin NL. Simian immunodeficiency virus inhibits bone marrow hematopoietic progenitor cell growth. J Virol 1990;64:656.

154. Axelrod AA. Some hematopoietic negative regulators. Exp Hematol 1990;18:143.

155. Merrill JE, Koyanagi Y, Chen IS. Interleukin-1 and tumor necrosis factor alpha can be induced from mononuclear phagocytes by human immunodeficiency virus type I binding to the CD4 receptor. J Virol 1989;63:4404.

156. Maciejewski JP, Weichold FF, Young NS. HIV-1 suppression of hematopoiesis in vitro mediated by envelope glycoprotein and TNF-alpha. J Immunol 1994;153:4303.

157. Berman MA, Zaldivar F Jr, Imfeld KL, Kenney JS, Sandborg CI. HIV-1 infection of macrophages promotes long-term survival and sustained release of interleukins 1 alpha and 6. AIDS Res Hum Retroviruses 1994;10:529.

158. Donahue RE, Johnson MM, Zon LI, Clark SC, Groopman JE. Suppression of in vitro haematopoiesis following human immunodeficiency virus infection. Nature 1987;326:200.

159. Blumberg N, Heal MJ. Transfusion and recipient immune function. Arch Pathol Lab Med 1989;113:246.

160. Steinberg HN, Crumpacker CS, Chatis PA. In vitro suppression of normal human bone marrow progenitor cells by human immunodeficiency virus. J Virol 1991;65:1765.

161. Folks TM, Kessler SW, Orenstein JM, Justement JS, Jaffe ES, Fauci AS. Infection and replication of HIV-1 in purified progenitor cells of normal human bone marrow. Science 1988;242:919.

162. Zauli G, Re MC, Furlini G, Giovannini M, La Placa M. Human immunodeficiency virus type 1 envelope glycoprotein gp120-mediated killing of human haematopoietic progenitors (CD34+ cells). J Gen Virol 1992;73:417.

163. Donahue RE, Johnson MM, Zon LI, Clark SC, Groopman JE. Suppression of in vitro haematopoiesis following human immunodeficiency virus infection. Nature 1987;326:200.

164. Abraham NG, Chertkov JL, Staudinger R, et al. Long-term bone marrow stromal and hemopoietic toxicity to AZT: protective role of heme and IL-1. Exp Hematol 1993;21:263.

165. Fibbe WE, Willems R. The role of Interleukin-1 in hematopoiesis. Acta Haematol 1991;86:148.

166. Molina JM, Scadden DT, Burn R, Dinarello CA, Groopman JE. Production of tumor necrosis factor alpha and interleukin 1 beta by monocytic cells infected with human immunodeficiency virus. J Clin Invest 1989;84:733.

167. Valentin A, Albert J, Svenson SB, Asjo B. Blood-derived macrophages produce IL-1, but not TNF-alpha, after infection with HIV-1 isolates from patients at different stages of disease. Cytokine 1992;4:185.

168. Reuben JM, Gonik B, Li S, Loo L, Turbin J. Induction of cytokines in normal placental cells by the human immunodeficiency virus. Lymphokine Cytokine Res 1991;10:195.

169. Dolei A, Serra C, Arca MV, et al. Mutual interactions between HIV-1 and cytokines in adherent cells during acute infection. Arch Virol 1994;134:157.

170. Tsunetsugy-Yokota Y, Honda M. Effect of cytokines on HIV release and IL-2 receptor alpha expression in monocyte cell lines. J Acquir Immune Defic Syndr 1990;3:511.

171. Kovacs JA, Baseler M, Dewar RJ, et al. Increases in CD-4 lymphocytes with intermittent courses or interleukin-2 in patients with

human immunodeficiency virus infection. N Engl J Med 1995;332:567.

172. Segal GM, Ey FS, Bestwick R, Hodges W, Bagby GC. Paracrine induction of interleukin-6 (IL-6) gene expression in human vascular endothelial cells (ECs) infected by HIV-1. Blood 1992;81:1071.

173. Zauli G, Re MC, Gugliotta L, Furlini G, La Placa M. The elevation of circulating platelets after IFN-alpha therapy in HIV-1 seropositive thrombocytopenic patients correlates with increased plasma levels of IL-6. Microbiologica 1993;16:27.

174. Melani C, Mattia GF, Silvani A, et al. Interleukin-6 expression in human neutrophil and eosinophil peripheral blood granulocytes. Blood 1993;81:2744.

175. Ishibashi T, Kimura H, Uchida T, Kariyone S, Friese P, Burstein SA. Human interleukin 6 is a direct promotor of maturation of megakaryocytes in vitro. Proc Natl Acad Sci USA 1989;86:5953.

176. Williams N, De Giorgio T, Banu N, Withy R, Hirano T, Kishimoto T. Recombinant interleukin 6 stimulates immature murine megakaryocytes. Exp Hematol 1990;18:69.

177. Kimura H, Ishibashi T, Uchida T, Muruyama Y, Friese P, Burstein SA. Interleukin 6 is a differentiation factor for human megakaryocytes in vitro. Eur J Immunol 1990;20:1927.

178. Fauci AS. Cytokine regulation of HIV expression. Lymphokine Res 1990;94:527.

179. Michaelis B, Levy JA. HIV replication can be blocked by recombinant human interferon beta. AIDS 1989;3:27.

180. Francis ML, Meltzer MS, Gendelman HE. Interferons in the persistence, pathogenesis and treatment of HIV infection. AIDS Res Hum Retroviruses 1991;8:199.

181. Mansan KF, Zidar B, Shadduck RK. Interferon-induced aplasia: evidence for T-cell mediated suppression of hematopoiesis and recovery after treatment with horse antihuman thymocyte globulin. Am J Hematol 1985;19:401.

182. Ganser A, Carlo-Stella C, Greher J, Volkers B, Hoelzer D. Effect of recombinant interferons alpha and gamma on human bone marrow-derived megakaryocytic progenitor cells. Blood 1987;70:1173.

183. Collart MA, Belin D, Vassalli J-D, de Kossodo S, Vassalli P. Gamma interferon enhances macrophage transcription of the tumor necrosis factor/cachectin, interleukin 1, and urokinase genes, which are controlled by short-lived repressors. J Exp Med 1986;164:2113.

184. Boue F, Wallon C, Goujard C, Barre-Sinoussi F, Galamaud P, Delfraissy J-F. HIV induces IL-6 production by human B lymphocytes. Role of IL-4. J Immunol 1992;148:3761.

185. Shalaby MR, Espevik T, Rice GC, et al. The involvement of human tumor necrosis factors-alpha and -beta in the mixed lymphocyte reaction. J Immunol 1988;141:499.

186. Means FT, Krantz SB. Progress in understanding the pathogenesis of the anemia of chronic disease. Blood 1992;80:1639.

187. Mabondzo A, Le Naour R, Raoul H, et al. In vitro infection of macrophages by HIV. Res Virol 1991;142:205.

188. Carlo-Stella C, Ganser A, Hoelzer D. Defective in vitro growth of the hematopoietic progenitor cells in the acquired immunodeficiency syndrome. J Clin Invest 1987;80:286.

189. Rusten LS, Jacobsen FW, Lesslauer W, Loetscer H, Smeland EB, Jacobsen SEW. Bifunctional effects of tumor necrosis factor alpha (TNF-α) on the growth of mature and primitive human hematopoietic progenitor cells: involvement of p55 and p75 TNF receptors. Blood 1994;83:3152.

190. Rusten LS, Jacobsen SEW. Tumor necrosis factor (TNF)-α directly inhibits human erythropoiesis in vitro: role of p55 and p75 TNF receptors. Blood 1995;85:989.

191. Dubois CM, Ruscetti RW, Stankova J, Keller JR. Transforming growth factor-beta regulates c-kit message stability and cell-surface protein expression in hematopoietic progenitors. Blood 1994;83:3138.

192. Bonewald LF, Dallas SL. Role of active and latent transforming growth factor beta in bone formation. J Cell Biochem 1994;55:350.

193. Kekow J, Wachsman W, McCutchan JA, Cronin M, Carson DA, Lotz M. Transforming growth factor beta and noncytopathic mechanisms of immunodeficiency in human immunodeficiency virus infection. Proc Natl Acad Sci USA 1990;87:8321.

194. Leiderman IZ, Greenberg ML, Adelsberg BR, Siegal FP. A glycoprotein inhibitor of in vitro granulopoiesis associated with AIDS. Blood 1987;70:1267.

195. Canque B, Gluckman JD. MIP-1 alpha is induced by and it inhibits HIV infection of blood-derived macrophages. (Abstract 1907) Blood 1994;84:480a.

196. Lazdins JK, Klimkait T, Alteri E, et al. TGF-beta: upregulator of HIV replication in macrophages. Res Virol 1991;142:239.

197. McGinnes K, Quesniaux V, Hitzler J, Paige C. Human B-lymphopoiesis is supported by bone marrow-derived stromal cells. Exp Hematol 1991;19:294.

198. Johnson A, Dorshkind K. Stromal cells in myeloid and lymphoid long term bone marrow cultures can support hematopoiesis and modulate the production of hematopoietic growth factors. Blood 1986;68:1348.

199. Lichtman M. The ultrastructure of the hemopoietic environment: a review. Exp Hematol 1981;9:391.

200. Tavassoli M, Hardy CL. Molecular basis of homing of intravenously transplanted stem cells to the marrow. Blood 1990;76:1059.

201. Yang Y-C, Schickwann T, Wong GG, Clark SC. Interleukin-1 regulation of hematopoietic growth factor production by human stromal fibroblasts. J Cell Physiol 1988;134:292.

202. Simmons PJ, Masinovsky B, Longenecker BM, Berenson R, Torok-Storb B, Gallatin WM. Vascular cell adhesion molecule-1 expressed by bone marrow stromal cells mediates the binding of hematopoietic progenitor cells. Blood 1992;80:388.

203. Bagby GC, Rigas D, Bennett RM, Vandenbark AA, Garewal HS. Interaction of lactoferrin, monocytes and T lymphocyte subsets in the regulation of steady state granulopoiesis in vitro. J Clin Invest 1981;68:56.

204. Ganser A, Ottmann OG, von Briesen H, Volkers B, Rubsamen-Waigmann H, Hoelzer D. Changes in the hematopoietic progenitor cell compartment in the acquired immunodeficiency syndrome. Res Virol 1990;141:185.

205. Platzer E. Human hematopoietic growth factors. Eur J Haematol 1989;42:1.

206. Scadden DT, Zeira M, Woon A, et al. Human immunodeficiency infection of human bone marrow stromal fibroblasts. Blood 1990;76:317.

207. Anonymous. Human immunodeficiency virus infection of human bone marrow stromal fibroblasts. (Editorial) Dis Markers 1991;9:57.

208. Neil JC, Onions DE. Feline leukaemia viruses: molecular biology and pathogenesis. Anticancer Res 1985;5:49.

209. Linenberger ML, Abkowitz J. Studies in feline lone-term marrow culture: hematopoiesis on normal and feline leukemia virus infected stromal cells. Blood 1992;80:651.

210. Chehimi J, Prakash K, Shanmugam V, Jackson SJ, Bandyopadhyay S, Starr SE. In-vitro infection of peripheral blood dendritic cells with human immunodeficiency virus-1 causes impairment of accessory functions. Adv Exp Med Biol 1993;329: 521.

211. Moses A, Nelson J, Bagby GC. CD34+ bone marrow microvascular endothelial cells are consistently infected by HIV-1 in patients with AIDS. (Abstract 1903) Blood 1994;84:479a.

212. Toulon P, Blanche P, Bachmeyer D, Gorin I, Sereni D, Sicard D. Thromboembolism and HIV infection. Protein S deficiency and hypoalbuminemia as risk factors for thrombosis. (Abstract 1910) Blood 1994;84:481a.

213. Cohen AJ, Phillips TM, Kessler CM. Circulating coagulation inhibitors in the acquired immunodeficiency syndrome. Ann Intern Med 1986;104:175.

214. Gold JE, Haubenstock A, Zalusky R. Lupus anticoagulant and AIDS. N Engl J Med 1986;314:1252.

215. Bloom EJ, Abrams DI, Rodgers GM. Lupus anticoagulant in the acquired immunodeficiency syndrome. JAMA 1986;256:491.

216. Cohen H, Mackie IJ, Anagnostopoulos N, Savage GF. Lupus anticoagulant, anticardiolipin antibodies, and human immunodeficiency virus in haemophilia. J Clin Pathol 1989;42:629.

217. Cohen AJ, Philips TM, Kessler CM. Circulating coagulant inhibitors in the acquired immunodeficiency syndrome. Ann Intern Med 1986;104:175.

218. Cappell MS, Simon T, Tiku M. Splenic infarction associated with anticardiolipin antibodies in a patient with acquired immunodeficiency syndrome. Dig Dis Sci 1993;38:1152.

219. Stahl CP, Sideman CS, Spira TJ, Haff ED, Hixon GJ, Evatt BL. Protein S deficiency in men with long-term human immunodeficiency virus infection. Blood 1993;81:1801.

220. Lafeuillade A, Sorice M, Griggi T, Pellegrino P, Geoffroy M, Profizi N. Role of autoimmunity in protein S deficiency during HIV-1 infection. Infection 1994;22:201.

221. Herstein L, Cappacino A, Cappacino H. Platelet function and bound antibodies in AIDS-ARC patients with thrombocytopenia. (Abstract) Blood 1987;70:118a.

AIDS: Biology, Diagnosis, Treatment and
Prevention, fourth edition, edited by Vincent T.
DeVita, Jr., Samuel Hellman, and Steven A.
Rosenberg. Lippincott–Raven Publishers, © 1997

CHAPTER 20

Pediatric Human Immunodeficiency Virus Infections

Brigitta U. Mueller and Philip A. Pizzo

Human immunodeficiency virus type 1 (HIV-1) infection is often more accelerated in children, and in some infants, symptoms can manifest during the first few months of life. Because many organs, especially the brain, are not yet mature, the impact of an infection can have devastating consequences on growth and development in children. Pediatric HIV infection should be considered a family disease, because it affects parents and their children. The burden of caring for these children and their parents not infrequently becomes the responsibility of grandparents, who may bear to witness to the suffering and loss of two younger generations. Children without family providers may be placed in foster homes or adopted, and these surrogate parents have to take on the task of caring for a child through a difficult and often painfully shortened period. If only one child in the family is infected, siblings have to cope with the sickness and the premature loss of their brother or sister and sometimes with the lack of support and understanding provided by their social networks, such as school or neighborhood.

Emphasis should be placed on treating HIV infection as a chronic condition, and therapy should include antiretroviral agents and seek to preserve normal development. If possible, the pediatric patient should be allowed to participate in normal childhood activities, such as kindergarten and school, and if feasible, the care of the infected parent should be coordinated with the child's care.

HISTORY AND EPIDEMIOLOGY

A syndrome of immunodeficiency leading to opportunistic infections in children was observed in 1982,[1] and the first

Brigitta U. Mueller and Philip A. Pizzo, Pediatric Branch, Division of Clinical Sciences, National Cancer Institute, Building 10, Room 13N240, 10 Center DR MSC 1928, Bethesda, MD 20892-1928.

descriptions of children with HIV-1 infection or the acquired immunodeficiency syndrome (AIDS) were published in 1983.[2-4] It was the observation of AIDS cases in infants who had received a blood transfusion that led to the recognition of this mode of transmission.[2,5] The initial definition of AIDS in children younger than 13 years of age has undergone several revisions, and the current version attempts to delineate the differences in clinical and laboratory manifestations that differentiate children and adults.[6-8]

As of December 1994, a total of 6209 children younger than 13 years of age had been reported to the Centers for Disease Control and Prevention (CDC) as meeting the definition for AIDS, and more than one half of these children have already died.[9] More than 80% of these children were 5 years of age or younger at the time of diagnosis, and almost 90% had acquired their infection through their mothers. Another 1965 adolescents between 13 and 19 years of age have been reported with AIDS, and their number is increasing every year.

Worldwide, it is estimated that about 1.5 million children are infected with HIV-1 and that a cumulative total of 5 million children will have developed clinical AIDS by the year 2000. More than 10 million children are expected to be orphaned during the 1990s because their caretakers will have died of AIDS.[10] HIV-2 infection is most prevalent in West Africa, where between 1% and 2% of the population are infected. Cases of HIV-2 infection in children have been described, but the mother-to-infant transmission rate appears to be much lower than for HIV-1.[11] Of considerable concern is the fact that heterosexual HIV transmission to women of childbearing age is increasing significantly on a worldwide basis.[12]

HIV-1 infection is the seventh leading cause of death in children in the United States, and in some cities, such as Newark and New York, AIDS has become the first or second leading cause of death in black or Hispanic children between 1 and 4 years of age.[13,14] HIV infection and AIDS are the sixth leading cause of death in young persons between 15 and 24 years of age.[15] Infant mortality in Africa is projected to be more than 4% higher than it would have been without AIDS, and by the mid-1990s, the increase in childhood mortality due to AIDS will start to negate the public health progress achieved during the last decades through better nutrition and immunization programs.[16]

In the United States, a disproportionate number of HIV-infected children and adolescents belong to minority groups, with fewer than 20% of children younger than 13 years of age or female adolescents between 13 and 19 years of age meeting the criteria for AIDS being of Caucasian origin.[9] More than one half of the children and almost two thirds of the female teenagers with AIDS are of African-American heritage. Although 47% of the male adolescents are white, this largely reflects the population of infected hemophiliacs, and the statistic is expected to change as a greater proportion of minority teenagers become infected through sexual activity or drug-related behavior.

TRANSMISSION AND PREVENTION

Vertical transmission, which is transmission from an infected mother to her child, accounts for 89% of all cases of pediatric HIV-1 infection, and in the future, it will be the route of transmission for virtually all children who become infected with HIV-1.[9] However, not all children born to HIV-infected mothers will become infected. The transmission rate ranges from 13% in Europe to about 45% in African countries.[17–19] Several studies have suggested that breast-feeding may increase the risk for infection by an additional 15%.[20–22] However, because the risks associated with the use of contaminated water used to prepare powdered infant formulas outweighs the risk for HIV infection from breast milk, the World Health Organization recommends that women in developing nations whose water supplies are unsafe continue to breast-feed their infants.[23–25] Breast-feeding by HIV-infected mothers is not recommended in the United States or other industrialized nations where safe oral infant formulas are available. The rate of vertical transmission of HIV-2 is much lower (0% to 2%), and if the mother is infected with HIV-1 and HIV-2, HIV-1 is preferentially transmitted.[19,26–29]

Although HIV-1 has not been demonstrated to infect germ cells, it has been found in trophoblastic and villous Hofbauer cells, in amniotic fluid, and in fetal organ tissues during the first trimester of pregnancy.[30–35] Overall, it appears that only about one fourth to one third of infants who become vertically infected acquire HIV during the intragestational period. Two thirds to three fourths of these infants appear to have become infected during labor and delivery. This hypothesis is based mainly on two observations. First, it has become evident from studies in twins that the first-born infant, whether delivered vaginally or by cesarean section, has a substantially higher risk of becoming infected with HIV than the second born.[36] In a multicenter study of 148 evaluable sets of twins born to HIV-infected women, it

was demonstrated that 35% of first-born twins delivered vaginally and 16% of the first-born babies delivered by cesarean section were infected, compared with 15% and 8%, respectively, of second-born twins.[37] This may occur because the first-born twin has been exposed to the infectious cervical secretions for a longer period and, by the process of delivery, has "cleaned out" the birth canal for the second baby, who is usually also delivered more rapidly. Second, of those infants ultimately shown to be infected with HIV-1, only about 25% have positive virus blood cultures or polymerase chain reaction (PCR) results during the first 48 hours of life, suggesting that they were infected before birth, but the remaining 75% produce positive virus cultures or PCR results within the first 2 to 3 months of life, suggesting that they became infected during the intrapartum period.[38,39]

An unsolved but important question is why 75% of the children born of HIV-infected mothers never develop infection. Several factors contribute to this risk, and perhaps the most important is the level of maternal viremia. Factors that contribute to the risk of vertical transmission include the state of the mother's health (eg, women with lower CD4 counts, who often have a higher virus burden or detectable p24 antigen, are more likely to transmit HIV), the maternal virus phenotype (eg, syncytium-inducing virus may be more readily transmitted than non–syncytium-inducing virus), the presence or absence of maternal neutralizing antibodies, and the presence of a concurrent infection of the placenta or the maternal cervical canal.[40–42] Several investigators have suggested that some infants may have been exposed but not infected with HIV, based on the presence of antibodies against virus-specific epitopes in the absence of demonstrable evidence of infection.[43] The report of a 5-year-old child who appeared to have cleared his HIV infection, demonstrated by virus culture and PCR during the first month of life, has raised the possibility, that, albeit rare, it may be possible to recover from or be insusceptible to infection with HIV.[44] However, the limited data available on this single reported case, coupled with the incomplete homology of the virus isolate, has not dismissed the possibility of laboratory contamination and pseudoinfection.

Perhaps the best support for the association of virus burden with vertical transmission was the report that the perinatal transmission rate was decreased by 67% when HIV-seropositive mothers received zidovudine during pregnancy and delivery and the infant was treated for the first 6 weeks of life.[45] In this double-blind, placebo-controlled study (ACTG 076), the mothers were treated with oral zidovudine or placebo starting at 14 to 34 weeks of gestation and received intravenous zidovudine or placebo during labor and delivery, and their infants then received oral zidovudine or placebo for the first 6 weeks of life. The stunning results of this trial suggest that HIV-1 transmission and infection can be reduced by an agent that lowers the maternal-infant virus burden. However, the women who entered this study were relatively healthy and had minimal prior exposure to zidovudine. It is unknown how well this approach may work in women with more advanced disease and higher virus burden or in those with prior zidovudine exposure and potentially drug-resistant virions.

Although this approach was effective, it is unclear whether the entire treatment program or simply components of the regimen are necessary for efficacy. Moreover, this approach is expensive and certainly not suitable for developing nations. Accordingly, studies investigating nonpharmacologic approaches, such as vaginal washings during labor and delivery, are underway. The fact that vertical transmission can be significantly reduced has underscored the importance of identifying infected or high-risk women who might benefit from this intervention. Consequently, the United States Public Health Service has recommended that all pregnant women in the United States be counseled about the importance of HIV screening.

Transmission of HIV-1 through blood products has become rare in industrialized countries and accounted for only 6% of new AIDS cases in children who were reported in 1995, compared with 19% in 1985.[9,46,47] The decrease reflects more rigorous screening of donors and donated units, as well as improved manufacturing techniques for coagulation factor concentrates.[48,49] However, the screening of blood products may be less common or sophisticated in developing countries, as evidenced within the last several years by a newly discovered HIV epidemic in Romanian children.[50,51]

A growing concern is the transmission of HIV-1 through sexual contacts among adolescents and older children.[15] Thirty-three percent of male adolescents 13 to 19 years of age with AIDS and 41% with HIV infection (not AIDS) reported sex with another man as their exposure risk; 2% of the male and 47% of the female adolescents with AIDS were exposed through heterosexual contact.[9] Sexually acquired HIV infection in adolescents is strongly associated with other sexually transmitted diseases.[52,53] In sexually active teenage girls, susceptibility to HIV and other sexually transmitted diseases may be increased because of the immature epithelium of the cervical canal. Unfortunately, high risk behaviors, including unprotected sex, remain common in adolescents, and the use of illicit drugs potentiates this problem. Inner-city or runaway youth are even more likely to become infected.[54,55] Knowledge about HIV infection and the associated risk factors for transmission varies among adolescents, and although a nationwide effort has been made to incorporate AIDS education into school programs, the adolescents that are most at risk for infection may not be attending school.[56,57]

The risk for casual transmission among children has been studied extensively and appears to be extremely small. Common contacts, such as occur in households, schools, and day care centers, have not been associated with transmission of HIV-1.[58] Only six cases have been reported in the United States involving children or adolescents; one occurred after biting, and five had documented exposure to blood or body fluids.[59,60] The risk of transmission during sports is extremely low, and the American Academy of Pediatrics, the World Health Organization, the National Collegiate Athletic Association, and National Football League have issued guidelines regarding HIV infection and sports. HIV-infected athletes are permitted to participate in competitive sports but should be counseled about the theoretical risk of HIV transmission, especially during injury-prone activities such as wrestling, boxing, or football.[61]

DEFINITION AND DIAGNOSIS

The definition of AIDS in children under the age of 13 years has undergone several revisions; the latest was in 1994.[8] The most current definition takes into account the age-dependent decline in CD4 counts (Table 20-1) and differentiates mild, moderate, and severe degrees of clinical symptoms (Table 20-2). As shown in Table 20-3, this new classification system ranges from a stage with no clinical or immunologic impairment (N0) to one of severe clinical and immunologic suppression (C3).

A child older than 18 months of age can be reliably diagnosed with a positive enzyme-linked immunoassay and confirmatory test (eg, Western blot, indirect fluorescent antibody test).[8] However, the diagnosis of HIV infection in infants is complicated by the fact that maternal antibodies are transmitted through the placenta and are measurable in the child for a median of 13.3 months (range, 10.4 to 15.6).[62] A child younger than 18 months of age who is known to be HIV seropositive or who is born to an HIV-infected mother is considered to be infected if the child has positive results on two separate determinations (excluding cord blood) from one or more of the following HIV detection tests: HIV culture, HIV PCR, or HIV antigen (p24),[8] or the child meets the criteria for an AIDS diagnosis based on the 1987 AIDS surveillance case definition.[7]

Virus culture and PCR can identify 30% to 50% of infected infants shortly after birth and almost 100% by 3 to 6 months of age.[39,63,64] Unfortunately, many children are still only identified as being HIV-infected when they present with their AIDS-defining illness, often a fatal episode of *Pneumocystis carinii* pneumonia (PCP), underscoring the importance of screening and early identification of potentially HIV-infected infants.[65]

MORBIDITY, MORTALITY, AND PROGNOSTIC FACTORS

Virtually all children who are born to HIV-infected women appear normal at birth, even if they were infected intragestationally. Although a putative embryopathy was described several years ago in HIV-infected children, this association has not been sustained.[66-69] HIV-infected children may manifest the stigmata of poor maternal health, drug or alcohol use, or social deprivation leading to failure to thrive.[17,70]

After birth and the immediate perinatal period, a trimodal rate of disease progression is observed in vertically

TABLE 20-1. *Immunologic categories based on age-Ssecific CD4+ T-lymphocyte counts and percentage of total lymphocytes*

	Age of Child					
	<12 Months		1–5 Years		6–12 Years	
Immunologic category	(cells/mm³)	(%)	(cells/mm³)	(%)	(cells/mm³)	(%)
1: No evidence of suppression	≥1500	(≥25)	≥1000	(≥25)	≥500	(≥25)
2: Evidence of moderate suppression	750–1499	(15–24)	500–999	(15–24)	200–499	(15–24)
3: Severe suppression	<750	(<15)	<500	(<15)	<200	(<15)

infected children. Approximately one third of these children become symptomatic within the first few months of life and are considered "rapid progressors." Presumably, these are largely the children who become infected intragestationally. Approximately 70% of vertically infected children are "less rapid progressors," becoming symptomatic within the first several years of life. These children presumably acquired their infection during the intrapartum period and, overall, have a more rapid rate of disease progression than adults. A small percentage of children with vertically acquired infection do not develop evidence of disease progression until after 8 to 10 years of age, behaving more like "adult equivalents."[71–75]

Advances in supportive care and antiretroviral therapy have improved the quality and duration of life of HIV-infected infants and children. For example, in the early days of the pandemic, it was estimated that 50% of HIV-infected children would die by the age of 36 months.[17,73,76] Since then, survival time has more than doubled. In a study from New York City, the survival trends for children reported with AIDS before August 1987 (the time of the first revision of the CDC classification system) were compared with the survival for children diagnosed later.[77] The overall rate of children surviving more than 12 months after birth increased from 32% to 65%. Mortality is highest when AIDS-related symptoms (eg, PCP, encephalopathy) emerge during the first year of life (*P* <0.001).[71–73,76] In contrast, a later onset of symptoms or specific disease manifestations (eg, lymphocytic interstitial pneumonitis) has been reported to be correlated with a better prognosis.[73]

An absolute CD4 count below 500 cells/mm³ in untreated infants is strongly correlated with rapid progression of disease, and the presence of a very low CD4 count (<21% of the lower limit of normal for age, which is equivalent to 50 cells/mm³ in adults) is significantly associated with an increased risk of death within 2 years.[72,78] Serum p24 antigen levels are often positive in HIV-infected neonates and children and have been used widely as surrogate markers.[64] We evaluated a cohort of 35 matched pairs of children to determine whether p24 antigen had a prognostic value in predicting disease progression.[79] Although children who had been taken off therapy because of disease progression had at that time a significantly higher p24 antigen level (difference is not sustained, if corrected for entry level), there was no predictive pattern 45 days before

stopping therapy. If CD4 counts and p24 antigen were compared, p24 antigen did not add any predictive value to the CD4 counts.[78]

CLINICAL AND LABORATORY MANIFESTATIONS

Although children and adults have many similarities in the clinical manifestations of HIV infection, there are several differences in the rate of disease progression and relative properties of patients who develop specific symptom complexes (see Table 20-2). Recurrent bacterial infections and encephalopathy are typical and often early manifestations of HIV disease in children, but severe opportunistic infections occur mainly in children with advanced impairment of the immune system. In children and adults, HIV infection is associated with a progressive destruction of the lymph node architecture, with the loss of the filtering capability and "leaking" of viral particles into the peripheral circulation, demonstrated by an increase in viremia at later stages of disease.[80–84] The severe impairment of cellular and humoral immune functions predisposes the infected host to the occurrence of opportunistic infections and neoplasms.

Immunologic Abnormalities

The progressive loss of CD4-positive lymphocytes is a hallmark of the course of HIV disease in children. However, the number of lymphocytes and their subgroups undergo age-related changes in children.[85–88] The percentage of CD4 cells decreases with age (especially during the first 24 months of life), and the CD8 percentage increases, resulting in a decrease in the CD4/CD8 ratio.[88] CD4 percentages and CD4/CD8 ratios become significantly lower in HIV-infected children than in noninfected children of HIV-seropositive mothers after the age of 12 months.[89] Accordingly, age-dependent changes in the CD4 count and percentage have been incorporated into the definition of AIDS in children and into the recommendations for PCP prophylaxis and initiation of antiretroviral therapy (see Table 20-1).[8,90]

In children, apoptosis of T cells occurs normally at a high rate in the thymus. Autopsy studies of HIV-infected children reveal extensive thymic involvement, including thymitis and premature involution, but the role of apoptosis in the progressive loss of CD4 cells remains to be elucidated.[91]

TABLE 20-2. *Clinical categories for children with HIV infection*

CATEGORY N: NOT SYMPTOMATIC

Children who have no signs or symptoms considered to be the result of HIV infection or who have only one of the conditions listed in category A

CATEGORY A: MILDLY SYMPTOMATIC

Children with *two or more* of the conditions listed but none of the conditions listed in categories B and C:
  Lymphadenopathy (≥0.5 cm at more than two sites; bilateral = one site)
  Hepatomegaly
  Splenomegaly
  Dermatitis
  Parotitis
  Recurrent or persistent upper respiratory infection, sinusitis, or otitis media

CATEGORY B: MODERATELY SYMPTOMATIC

Children who have symptomatic conditions other than those listed for category A or C that are attributed to HIV infection. Examples of conditions in clinical category B *include but are not limited to* the following:
  Anemia (<8 g/dL), neutropenia (<1000 cells/mm^3), or thrombocytopenia (<100,000/mm^3) persisting ≥30 days
  Bacterial meningitis, pneumonia, or sepsis (single episode)
  Candidiasis, oropharyngeal thrush, persisting (>2 months) in children >6 months of age
  Cardiomyopathy
  Cytomegalovirus infection, with onset before 1 month of age
  Diarrhea, recurrent or chronic
  Hepatitis
  Herpes simplex virus (HSV) stomatitis, recurrent (more than two episodes within 1 year)
  HSV bronchitis, pneumonitis, or esophagitis with onset before 1 month of age
  Herpes zoster (ie, shingles) involving at least two distinct episodes or more than one dermatome
  Leiomyosarcoma
  Lymphoid interstitial pneumonia (LIP) or pulmonary lymphoid hyperplasia complex
  Nephropathy
  Nocardiosis
  Persistent fever (lasting >1 month)
  Toxoplasmosis, onset before 1 month of age
  Varicella, disseminated (complicated chickenpox)

CATEGORY C: SEVERELY SYMPTOMATIC

  Children who have any condition listed in the 1987 surveillance case definition for acquired immunodeficiency syndrome (with the exception of LIP),[7] including:
  Serious bacterial infections, multiple or recurrent (ie, any combination of at least 2 culture-confirmed infections within a 2-year period, of the following types: septicemia, pneumonia, meningitis, bone or joint infection, or abscess of an internal organ or body cavity (excluding otitis media, superficial skin or mucosal abscesses, and indwelling catheter-related infections)

Candidiasis, esophageal or pulmonary (eg, bronchi, trachea, lungs)
Coccidiomycosis, disseminated (at site other than or in addition to lungs or cervical or hilar lymph nodes)
Cryptococcosis, extrapulmonary
Cryptosporidiosis or isosporidiosis with diarrhea persisting >1 month
Cytomegalovirus disease with onset of symptoms at age >1 month (at a site other than liver, spleen, or lymph nodes)
Encephalopathy (at least one of the following progressive findings present for at least 2 months in the absence of a concurrent illness other than HIV infection that could explain the findings: failure to attain or loss of developmental milestones or loss of intellectual ability, verified by standard developmental scales or neuropsychological tests; impaired brain growth or acquired microcephaly demonstrated by head circumference measurements or brain atrophy demonstrated by computerized tomography or magnetic resonance imaging (serial imaging is required for children <2 years of age); acquired symmetric motor deficit manifested by two or more of the following: paresis, pathologic reflexes, ataxia, or gait disturbances
Herpes simplex virus infection causing a mucocutaneous ulcer that persists for >1 month or bronchitis, pneumonitis, or esophagitis for any duration affecting a child >1 month of age
Histoplasmosis, disseminated (at site other than or in addition to lungs or cervical or hilar lymph nodes)
Kaposi's sarcoma
Lymphoma, primary, in brain
Lymphoma, small, non-cleaved cell (eg, Burkitt's) or immunoblastic or large cell lymphoma of B-cell or unknown immunologic phenotype
Mycobacterium tuberculosis, disseminated or extrapulmonary
Mycobacterium, other species or unidentified species, disseminated (at a site other than or in addition to lungs, skin, or cervical or hilar lymph nodes)
Mycobaterium avium complex or *Mycobacterium kansasii,* disseminated (at site other than or in addition to skin, lungs or cervical or hilar lymph nodes)
Pneumocystis carinii pneumonia
Progressive multifocal leukoencephalopathy
Salmonella (nontyphoid) septicemia, recurrent
Toxoplasmosis of the brain with onset >1 month of age
Wasting syndrome in the absence of a concurrent illness other than HIV infection that could explain the following findings: persistent weight loss >10% of baseline or downward crossing of at least two of the following percentile lines on the weight-for-age chart in a child ≥1 year of age or >5th percentile on weight-for-height chart on two consecutive measurements ≥30 days apart plus chronic diarrhea (ie, at least two loose stools per day for ≥30 days) or documented fever (for ≥30 days, intermittent or constant)

Adapted from Centers for Disease Control and Prevention. Revised classification system for human immunodeficiency virus infection in children less than 13 years of age. MMWR 1994;43:1.

TABLE 20-3. *Pediatric human immunodeficiency virus classification*

Immunologic Categories	Clinical Categories, Based on Signs and Symptoms			
	N (None)	A (Mild)	B (Moderate)	C (Severe)
1: No evidence of suppression	N1	A1	B1	C1
2: Moderate suppression	N2	A2	B2	C2
3: Severe suppression	N3	A3	B3	C3

Activated CD4 cells may be more easily infected. It has been demonstrated that CD4 and CD8 cells coexpressing CD38 and HLA-DR (ie, markers of cell activation) are increased in HIV-infected children compared with healthy controls.[92]

T-cell function is also impaired in HIV-infected children, although a difference between children with factor-associated and those with vertically acquired HIV infection has been described.[93–95] In one study, HIV-1 *Gag*-specific cytotoxic T lymphocyte (CTL) responses were detected in most pediatric hemophiliacs, but only a few vertically infected children were able to mount an adequate CTL response.[93] The degree of T-cell impairment depends on the stage of disease, with an early loss of CTL response to the *Pol* protein occurring even in clinically asymptomatic children, followed by the added inability to respond to the *Gag* protein during clinically symptomatic stages.[96] Production of type 1 cytokines (ie, interferon-γ and interleukin-2) are significantly decreased, and type 2 cytokines (ie, interleukin-4 and interleukin-10) are increased in HIV-infected children compared with uninfected control subjects.[94] In our own group, patients with functional defects of helper T cells (measured by response to recall antigens, allogeneic HLA, and phytohemagglutinin) had a history of more opportunistic and bacterial infections compared with HIV-infected children with functionally intact helper T cells.[97] CTL activity against viral antigens, including *Env*, *Gag-Pol*, and *Nef*, can be detected in peripheral blood lymphocytes of as many as 25% of uninfected children born to HIV-infected mother, possibly indicating a mechanism of protection against infection.[43]

Some degree of hypergammaglobulinemia, the result of nonspecific B-cell stimulation, occurs in most children, mainly with increases in IgG and IgA concentrations, although a small subgroup of children may present with hypogammaglobulinemia.[89,98] In a group of 47 HIV-infected children, we found an abnormality in at least one subclass in 83%, but this could not be correlated with the frequency of bacterial infections.[99] Other immune abnormalities include altered monocyte and neutrophil function, sometimes reversible with antiretroviral therapy.[100–105]

Nonspecific Findings

A common nonspecific finding in HIV-infected children is failure to thrive. In a study of 35 HIV-positive hemophiliacs, a decrease of more than 15 percentile points in height or weight for age was a predictive marker for children who developed symptoms of AIDS.[106] Impairment of linear growth and weight gain are most probably related to the chronic infection, but other causes, such as endocrine deficiencies or malnutrition, should be considered.[106–110] Loss of energy and increased fatigue often limit the activity level of HIV-infected children. Older children may suffer from depression, and children of all age groups may be afflicted by pain from several sources, such as chronic pancreatitis or *Mycobacterium avium* complex (MAC) infection. Because medical or psychologic interventions may improve the quality of life significantly, it is imperative to investigate behavioral changes that may be treatable.[111–113]

Encephalopathy and Peripheral Neuropathy

One of the most devastating aspects of childhood HIV infection is encephalopathy. Over time, neuroencephalopathy may ultimately occur in 40% to 90% of HIV-infected children.[114–119] In 1993, 115 cases or 15% of all pediatric AIDS patients had encephalopathy as their indicator disease.[9] Encephalopathy in children can be the very first symptom of HIV infection, or as in adults, it may be a manifestation of end-stage disease. HIV-related encephalopathy in children is characterized by motor or cognitive deficits, and neurodevelopment deterioration can be progressive, static, or subacute.[120] Some children develop a painful spastic paraparesis, and others present with behavioral abnormalities or problems with school performance. A marked discrepancy has been found between receptive and expressive language faculties.[121] Expressive language appears to be significantly more impaired than receptive language, a difference observed in encephalopathic and in putatively "nonencephalopathic" HIV-infected children. Seizures or focal neurologic deficits are rarely part of HIV encephalopathy and should always lead to a search for a focal abnormality.[115]

HIV-1 can be detected in fetal brain tissue, and an HIV-associated meningoencephalitis has been described in a newborn child.[122,123] It is presumed that children who present at a very early age with progressive encephalopathy have been infected in utero. Typical findings of HIV-associated encephalopathy in children include cortical atrophy, increased ventricular size, calcifications in the basal ganglia, and abnormalities of the frontal white matter (Fig. 20-1).[124] These abnormalities are usually more severe in children with more advanced stages of encephalopathy. DeCarli and

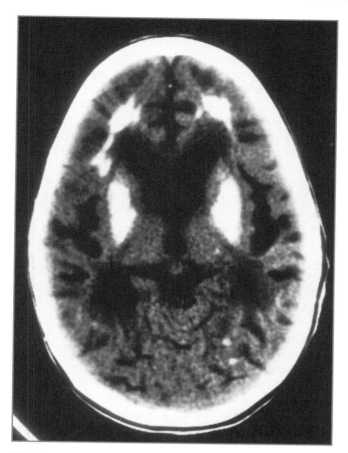

FIG. 20-1. Computed tomography scan of the head of a child with vertically acquired HIV infection. Marked atrophy and basal ganglia calcifications are manifestations of HIV-associated encephalopathy.

colleagues found a striking correlation between the appearance of intracerebral calcifications and the route of transmission and degree of encephalopathy.[119] Calcifications are almost exclusively seen in children with vertically acquired disease, supporting the hypothesis of an intrauterine infection, similar to other intrauterine pathogens that result in intracerebral calcifications (eg, cytomegalovirus infection, toxoplasmosis).

Quinolinic acid is a neurotoxin that has been found to be significantly elevated in the cerebrospinal fluid (CSF) of children with encephalopathy compared with HIV-infected children without central nervous system disease.[125] Although this is a nonspecific inflammatory marker, it has been shown to decrease during therapy with zidovudine, the only dideoxynucleoside that penetrates to a significant degree into the central nervous system. Other markers (ie, neurotoxins) that appear to correlate with encephalopathy include neopterin, platelet-activating factor and certain cytokines (eg, interleukin-1b, interferon-γ).[126–128] These toxins presumably overstimulate the N-methyl-D-aspartate (NMDA) receptors in the brain, resulting in an increase in neuronal calcium ions, which stimulates the cells to release glutamate. This leads to

further excitation and injury, possibly through the generation of free radicals.[128]

Autopsy findings include dystrophic calcifications of blood vessels in the basal ganglia and cerebral white matter, as well as a subacute encephalitis with microglial nodules and multinucleated giant cells.[116] Although HIV can be demonstrated with in situ hybridization techniques, most of the infection appears restricted to glial cells or macrophages. Because of its reversibility, it is presumed that many of the manifestations of encephalopathy result from toxic cytokine production from infected macrophages.[129] This may explain the clinical observation that steroids and antiviral agents may have a beneficial effect on encephalopathy.[130] Abnormalities of small and large intracerebral vessels are not uncommon, and strokes or fatal hemorrhages, sometimes caused by the rupture of an aneurysm, can occur.[116,131,132]

Spinal corticospinal tract degeneration can be observed in HIV-infected children and can affect the myelin, axon, or both.[115,116] It is presumed that HIV infection interferes with the normal myelination of the spinal cord. Other spinal cord lesions are less common in children than in adults, but a vacuolar myelopathy has been described.[133] Peripheral neuropathy in HIV-infected children is most commonly a side effect of the treatment with antiretroviral agents (eg, zalcitabine, stavudine).[134] It manifests with tingling or numbness in hands and feet. Often, the first symptom that is appreciated by parents or caregivers can be an impairment in fine motor functions (eg, tying of shoe laces).

Opportunistic infections of the central nervous system usually are less common in children than in adults. Cerebral toxoplasmosis with or without ocular involvement is observed as a congenital infection in the very young child or as a newly acquired infection in older adolescents but is exceedingly rare in the other age groups.[135–137] The incidence of fungal disease, especially with *Cryptococcus neoformans* or *Coccidioides mitis,* varies regionally but is also relatively low in the pediatric population.[135–138] Cytomegalovirus can cause a devastating and often unrelenting encephalitis in HIV-infected individuals.[139,140]

Malignancies of the central nervous system can occur in HIV-infected children but appear to be less common than in adults. High-grade B-cell lymphomas, which often manifest with focal neurologic findings or seizures, are the most common cause of a mass lesion in the central nervous system.[141] The radiologic appearance and therapeutic approaches are not different from those of adults.

Infections

Bacterial and viral infections are common in childhood, and to some extent, their manifestation in HIV-infected children represents the far end of the normal spectrum. Recurrent serious bacterial infections, such as meningitis, sepsis, and pneumonia, are characteristic for HIV infection in children and have been included in the CDC definition AIDS in children (see Table 20-3).

Bacterial Infections

The most common bacterial organisms causing infections in the HIV-infected child are *Streptococcus pneumonia*, *Haemophilus influenzae*, and *Staphylococcus aureus*, especially in the presence of a central venous catheter.[142–146] In addition to *Salmonella* spp., there has been an increase in the frequency of *Pseudomonas* spp. infections in children and adults with HIV infection.[147]

Mycobacterial Infections

The number of HIV-infected children in the United States who are infected with *Mycobacterium tuberculosis* is still relatively small, but as the number of infected adults grows, more children will be infected.[148–152] The diagnosis of *M tuberculosis* infection is difficult in the HIV-infected child (as in adults) because of the anergy that is frequently associated with AIDS, leading to a negative Mantoux test despite infection.[153] Gastric lavage appears to be more sensitive than bronchoalveolar lavage to diagnose mycobacterial disease in children.[154]

Treatment of *M tuberculosis* in children is also complicated by the lack of suitable pediatric formulations of several effective drugs, but it should include isoniazid, rifampin, and during the first 2 months, pyrazinamide.[153] If multidrug-resistant *M tuberculosis* is suspected, initial therapy should include a minimum of 4 to 5 drugs.

Infection with the *Mycobacterium avium* complex (MAC) occurs in almost 20% of HIV-infected children with CD4 counts below 50 cells/mm^3, and it manifests with nonspecific symptoms such as night sweats, weight loss, and low-grade fevers.[155] Treatment usually consists of three or more drugs, such as clarithromycin or azithromycin, ethambutol, rifampin or amikacin (or both), ciprofloxacin, and clofazimine. Although intervention can reduce symptoms and prolong life, the infection is only suppressed and ultimately progresses.[156,157] Studies of adults have demonstrated that the onset of MAC symptoms and infection can be delayed if rifabutin prophylaxis is initiated when the absolute CD4 count falls below 100 cells/mm^3.[158] Although controlled clinical trials using children have not been performed, it has been demonstrated that rifabutin is safe in children, and its use for prophylaxis of MAC infection is recommended.[156,159]

Viral Infections

Viral infections, especially with herpesviruses, contribute to morbidity and mortality in HIV-infected children. As in adults, cytomegalovirus (CMV) infection can result in disseminated or localized infections, including esophagitis, hepatitis, pneumonitis, and enterocolitis.[139,140,160,161] The incidence of CMV retinitis appears to be lower in children than in adults, but diagnosis can be difficult in young children, making routine ophthalmologic evaluations important, especially in children with a CD4 count less than 100 cells/mm^3. First-line therapy usually consists of ganciclovir (5 mg/kg given twice daily) or foscarnet (60 mg/kg given three times daily).

Primary chickenpox, (caused by varicella zoster virus (VZV), may be unusually severe in immunocompromised children and can recur as shingles or chronic varicella in HIV-infected patients, often presenting with very few, atypical lesions.[162,163] Prompt initiation of therapy with intravenous acyclovir (1500 mg/m^2/day divided into three doses) is usually effective, and foscarnet may be used for recurrent, presumably resistant cases. An oral agent, BVAraU, is being evaluated in children with chronic VZV infections. To decrease morbidity and epidemiologic sequel, specific hyperimmune globulin (VZIG) or intravenous immunoglobulin (IVIG) should be administered to immunosuppressed children (and HIV-infected parents) within 72 hours after the exposure to a patient with VZV infection.[164] Mild herpes simplex infections (eg, oral ulcers) can be treated with oral acyclovir, but more severe infections (eg, esophagitis) should be treated intravenously with acyclovir (750 mg/m^2/day divided into three doses). Primary or reactivated Epstein-Barr virus infection can cause impressive lymphadenopathy, with or without concurrent lymphocytic interstitial pneumonitis or parotitis, and sometimes gives rise to a polyclonal lymphoproliferative syndrome.[165–168]

Infection with the measles virus has been associated with a high mortality rate for HIV-infected children, and it can occur without the typical rash and result in a fatal giant cell pneumonia.[169–172] Infection with respiratory syncytial virus or adenovirus, alone or together, can also result in rapid and sometimes fatal respiratory compromise, as well as in chronic or persistent viral shedding or infection.[173]

Fungal Infections

Oral candidiasis and esophagitis are common in HIV-infected children. Fungemia with *Candida* spp. has emerged as an increasing problem associated with the use of indwelling catheters.[174] *Aspergillus* spp. can cause an exit site or tunnel infection around an indwelling central line, and we have observed at least one infant with perinatally acquired HIV infection and associated myelodysplastic syndrome who developed fatal pulmonary aspergillosis. Other fungal infections are much less common in children than in adults with HIV infection.[138] Coccidiomycosis and infection with *Histoplasma capsulatum* or *Cryptococcus neoformans* are rare in young children, but they may be seen in the older child, especially if living in an endemic area.[175–178]

Parasitic Infections

PCP was the AIDS indicator disease in 38% of the pediatric cases reported to the CDC in 1993 and is the major cause of death in HIV-infected children younger than 1 year of age.[9,65] Although *P carinii* can be transmitted transplacentally, infection is rare in the newborn period.[179] The peak incidence of PCP occurs between 3 and 6 months of age, presumably representing primary infection.[179,180] Unfortunately, PCP has been associated with a mortality rate of 39% to 65% for infants, with a median survival after the diagnosis of PCP as short as 1 month.[73,181,182] In 1989, with improved diagnosis, prophylaxis, and treatment, 42% of the children, compared with 19% before 1987, were still alive 12 months after the diagnosis of PCP.[65,77]

Most children with PCP present with an acute illness, with hypoxemia, and without a "typical" radiographic picture.[183,184] The diagnosis is usually made by obtaining an induced sputum (which can be done by experienced therapists even in very young children) or by performing a bronchoalveolar lavage, and only rarely is an open lung biopsy necessary.[185,186] Treatment with high-dose intravenous trimethoprim-sulfamethoxazole (TMP-SMX; eg, 20 mg/kg/day as trimethoprim) or pentamidine (4 mg/kg/day) and early adjunctive treatment with steroids follows the same guidelines as in adults.[187]

In 1994, the CDC updated guidelines for PCP prophylaxis in infants and children, taking into account the age-dependent levels of the CD4 cell numbers.[65] These guidelines recommend that PCP prophylaxis should be given during the first year of life (starting at 6 weeks of age) to all children who are born to HIV-infected mothers, regardless of CD4 counts. After the first year of life, prophylaxis should be administered if the child has had a prior episode of PCP or if the CD4 count falls below an age-appropriate threshold: less than 500 cells/mm^3 for children between 12 months and 6 years of age and less than 200 cells/mm^3 for children older than 6 years of age or a CD4 percentage of less than 15%, regardless of the absolute count.[65] The recommended regimen for prophylaxis is TMP-SMX with 150 mg of TMP/m^2/day and 750 mg/m^2/day of SMX given orally in divided doses twice daily during three consecutive days per week or on a Monday, Wednesday, Friday schedule.[188] Alternative regimens, if TMP-SMX is not tolerated, include oral dapsone (2 mg/kg/day) or aerosolized pentamidine. However, breakthrough infections can occur with every regimen, most commonly with intravenous pentamidine.[189-191]

Toxoplasma gondii is common in adults with HIV infection but only rarely seen in children.[137] Protozoal infections of the gastrointestinal tract, caused by *Cryptosporidia*, *Isospora belli*, *Microsporidia*, or *Giardia* often present difficult diagnostic and therapeutic problems and can be associated with a intractable diarrhea, posing problems for child care settings.[192,193]

Pulmonary Manifestations

The lung is commonly involved in pediatric HIV disease.[194,195] Lymphocytic interstitial pneumonitis is seen almost exclusively in the pediatric patient with HIV infection, and although no longer considered to be an indicator for severe clinical disease, it is included in the CDC definition of AIDS-defining diseases for children younger than 13 years of age.[8] The incidence of lymphocytic interstitial pneumonitis is difficult to assess, but it may affect as many as 50% of the HIV-infected children.[196] A diffuse, interstitial, often reticulonodular infiltrative process is typically observed, sometimes with hilar or mediastinal lymphadenopathy.[197] Rarely, bronchiectases can develop and be associated with secondary infections, including *Pseudomonas* spp.[198] On biopsy, peribronchiolar lymphoid aggregates or a diffuse lymphoid infiltration of the alveolar septa and peribronchiolar areas can be observed.[199,200] The cause of lymphocytic interstitial pneumonitis is poorly understood, but coinfection of HIV and Epstein-Barr virus has been implicated. Clinically, a child may be asymptomatic with only radiologic changes or can become severely compromised with exercise intolerance or even with oxygen dependency and the need for high-dose steroid therapy.[197]

Other lung pathologies range from infectious to neoplastic diseases. Although our ability to diagnose pulmonary disease with noninvasive measures has improved markedly, in certain circumstances, it is still necessary to perform a fine-needle aspirate or an open lung biopsy.

Cardiovascular Problems

The incidence of cardiomyopathy in HIV-infected children has been reported to be between 14% and 93% and may be more likely to occur with advancing stage of HIV disease.[73,201,202] These wide differences probably result from the fact that some estimates were based on the prospective monitoring of children with echocardiograms and ultrasound studies, and others were based on cardiac evaluations that were performed in the presence of clinical symptoms.

The most common findings on physical examination include symptoms of congestive heart failure, including hepatosplenomegaly, tachypnea, tachycardia, and a S3 gallop. On electrocardiography, signs of left or right (or both) ventricular dysfunction, as well as T-wave abnormalities, can be demonstrated.[203,204] Progressive left ventricular dysfunction, often combined with an increase in ventricular afterload, is the most common abnormality found on echocardiography and Doppler studies.[205] Hemodynamic abnormalities and dysrhythmias can lead to sudden death.[202,204] Treatment for cardiomyopathy in HIV-infected children is the same as for noninfected children and usually responds well to therapy.

The cause of cardiomyopathy in children with HIV infection is not fully defined. HIV-1 RNA and DNA have been demonstrated in the cardiac tissue of some children, but the typical changes of viral myocarditis or endocarditis are rarely observed.[82,206,207] Although zidovudine is known to cause a reversible myopathy of skeletal muscle, its contribution to cardiomyopathy is more controversial. Lipshultz and colleagues were not able to define any positive or negative effects of zidovudine on cardiac function in children.[205] In patients treated at the Pediatric Branch of the National Cancer Institute (NCI), Domanski and associates noticed a significant increase in the incidence of decreased ejection fraction and cardiomyopathy in children who had ever been treated with zidovudine compared with those receiving didanosine.[208]

An arteriopathy affecting various organs, including cardiac and cerebral vessels, has been described in several HIV-infected children.[209] In the brain, this can lead to the formation of giant aneurysms, resulting in neurologic and endocrinologic deficits or even sudden death from hemorrhage.[132]

Gastrointestinal Tract Abnormalities

Asymptomatic, unilateral or bilateral enlargement of the parotid glands is seen in some HIV-infected children and may be part of a lymphoproliferative disorder that also involves the lungs (ie, lymphocytic interstitial pneumonitis).[210] The concurrent elevation of the serum amylase reflects an increase in the salivary component.

Oropharyngeal or esophageal infections, especially with *Candida* spp. or herpes simplex virus, are a common problem in children. In the younger child, it is sometimes difficult to establish the diagnosis of esophagitis, but a decrease in appetite or weight loss should always prompt a careful evaluation. Antifungal therapy with one of the azoles or, in refractory cases, with amphotericin B, is usually successful and can improve the quality of life significantly, although repeated courses of therapy may be necessary.[138]

Dysfunction of the digestive tract is a frequent problem in children with AIDS, resulting in a failure to gain weight or in weight loss.[211] As with adults, several organisms have been associated with chronic diarrhea syndromes, including *Cryptosporidia*, *Microsporida*, *Salmonella*, *Shigella*, mycobacteria, and several viruses, especially rotavirus and adenovirus.[212–214] Some investigators have attributed the diarrheal syndrome to HIV infection of the gastrointestinal tract.[215] Primary or secondary disaccharide intolerance can also contribute to the chronic diarrhea in these children.[216,217]

Hepatobiliary abnormalities have been described in children and adults and can represent a diagnostic and therapeutic challenge. A clinical syndrome characterized by cholestasis and hepatitis may be the first manifestation of vertically acquired HIV disease in some children, even before a significant decline in the CD4 count has occurred.[218,219] Chronically elevated transaminases have been found in as many as 20% of infants perinatally exposed to HIV infection and may be correlated with poor outcome.[220] Although infectious hepatitis can be caused by hepatitis A, B, or C, MAC, or several noninfectious agents such as didanosine, rifabutin, and dapsone, the specific cause of the transaminitis commonly remains undefined.

Although uncommon in children, the frequency of pancreatitis in HIV-infected children is notable and can be caused by drugs (eg, didanosine, zalcitabine, pentamidine) or infections (CMV, MAC).[221–224] Pancreatitis may become chronic and be associated with persistently elevated amylase levels and intermittent symptoms. The management of these patients is complicated by the fact that they often need to take drugs for the treatment of other problems, such as MAC infection, that are only available in oral form and the observation that even total parenteral nutrition is not easily tolerated.[225,226]

Renal Manifestations

Renal disease in children with HIV infection is predominantly characterized by focal glomerulosclerosis or mesangial hyperplasia. In one study, 12 of 155 children between the ages of 7 months and 8 years were found to have proteinuria, five of whom developed severe renal failure within a year of diagnosis.[227] This nephrotic syndrome is often resistant to the treatment with steroids, but cyclosporins may induce a remission.[228] An IgA nephritis has been observed in a few HIV-infected children and adults who presented with recurrent gross hematuria.[229,230]

Hematopoietic System Disorders

The most common hematologic disorder observed in HIV-infected children is anemia, which occurs in 16% to 94%, depending on the severity of HIV disease, the age group, and the use of antiretroviral therapy.[76,231–234] Bone marrow aspirate or biopsy may show lymphoid aggregates, some degree of dysplasia, or an ineffective erythropoiesis. Pure red cell aplasia secondary to acute or persistent B19 parvovirus infection has been described in some HIV-infected children and should be considered when the red blood cell production rate is less than expected for the degree of anemia.[235–237] Hemolytic anemia as part of a hemolytic-uremic syndrome, an autoimmune process, or a virus-associated hemophagocytic syndrome has been seen in HIV-infected children and can be difficult to treat.[233,238] Subcutaneous or intravenous erythropoietin has been successfully used to treat anemia in some HIV-infected children.[239]

A white blood cell count of less than 3000 cells/mm^3 is observed in 26% to 38% of untreated pediatric patients, and neutropenia, defined as an absolute neutrophil count of less than 1500 cells/mm^3, occurs in 43%.[240,241] These conditions can result from infection with HIV or opportunistic pathogens such as MAC or CMV, or they can be the result of agents that have myelosuppressive effects, including zidovudine. Treatment with subcutaneous granulocyte colony-stimulating factor at doses between 1 and 20 μg/kg/day has been effective in treating many HIV-infected children with neutropenia.[242]

In our patient population at the NCI, we have found a platelet count of less than 50,000 cells/mm^3 in 19% of our patients, and thrombocytopenia has also been described in HIV-infected infants.[243–245] Treatment often provides only a temporary rise in platelet counts, but some children have improved on adequate antiretroviral therapy. Other treatment options include IVIG, anti-D, or a short course of steroids.[246,247]

Deficiency of the vitamin K–dependent factors II, VII, IX, and X is common in HIV-infected children and can result in a coagulopathy that is relatively easy to correct.

Disseminated intravascular coagulopathy (DIC) has been described as a complication of fulminant infectious conditions, but there are no data to indicate that this complication occurs more frequently in HIV-infected individuals. However, a coagulopathy that is caused by the presence of a lupus-like anticoagulants is more frequent in HIV-infected children.

Problems of the Endocrine System

Failure to thrive or grow is commonly observed in children with HIV infection, often with no definable endocrine cause.[109,248] At the Pediatric Branch of the NCI, we are evaluating insulin-like growth factor 1 and recombinant growth hormone to determine whether they can favorably influence linear growth, weight gain, and immunologic function in HIV-infected children. Dysregulation of thyroid function appears to be more common than expected in HIV-infected children[248a] and, if persistent, can easily be corrected.[249] In a study of 9 children with AIDS and failure to thrive, there was one case of primary hypothyroidism, six cases of deficient nocturnal TSH increase, and one child with growth hormone deficiency.[109] Adrenal insufficiency may be caused by CMV infection of the adrenal gland.[250] We have observed at least one child with severe salt craving who required therapy with fluorocortisol.

Ophthalmologic Manifestations

As in adults, ocular pathologies are more common in children with very low CD4 counts. Retinitis caused by infection with CMV is the most common ocular disorder. Unfortunately, because young children may not complain of visual changes, the retinitis is frequently far advanced at the time of diagnosis. Regular ophthalmologic examinations, with sedation if necessary, should therefore be routine part of the care of HIV infected children, especially when their CD4 counts fall below an age-equivalent of 100 cells/mm^3. The course and treatment of CMV retinitis is not different from that of adults. The first-line therapy is ganciclovir (5 mg/kg twice daily for induction and once daily for maintenance) or foscarnet (60 mg/kg three times daily for induction therapy and 90 mg/kg daily for maintenance). For some patients with retinitis that is refractory to ganciclovir or foscarnet, their combination may prove beneficial.[251]

Chorioretinitis due to *Toxoplasma gondii* is rare in children and, when it is observed, is most likely caused by a reactivation of a congenital infection. This condition may or may not be associated with intracerebral lesions, and it is usually treated with pyrimethamine and sulfadiazine. An alternative treatment, especially for isolated ocular findings, is atavoquone, which we used successfully in a 14-year-old hemophiliac patient with AIDS.[252] Other pathologies that have been described in children include HIV-related cotton-wool spots, necrotizing herpetic retinopathy, and lesions thought to be caused by *P carinii* infection.[253]

Two drugs that are frequently used in the treatment of HIV infection and related opportunistic infections, didanosine and rifabutin, have been associated with ocular abnormalities. Didanosine can cause a peripheral depigmentation of the retina, which may affect dark adaptation.[254] Rifabutin has been associated with a reversible anterior uveitis in adults and in a few children with HIV infection, especially if they were also receiving fluconazole.[255]

Cutaneous Lesions

Cutaneous manifestations are common and can have infectious, inflammatory, or drug-related causes (Table 20-4).[256-25] Some diseases are more common in children and therefore more prevalent in HIV-infected children as well.[259,260] Children can have primary infection with VZV and may present with dermatomal zoster (ie, shingles) or a chronic or recurrent disease that can range from papular to verrucous or pyoderma-like lesions. Patients with chronic varicella may also pose an infectious risk and often require prolonged and repetitive courses of antiviral therapy (eg, acyclovir, foscarnet).[261]

The most common neoplastic disease of the skin in adults, Kaposi's sarcoma, is exceedingly rare in children.[261] Only 25 cases with Kaposi's sarcoma were reported to the CDC through 1993.[9] However, we observed a 2.5-year-old child with a CD30+ (Ki-1) lymphoma with an indolent waxing and waning course typical for lymphomatoid papillomatosis for almost 18 months.[262] It is likely that a spectrum of such unusual malignancies and lymphoproliferative disorders will be observed during the years ahead.

Malignancies

Cancer is the AIDS defining illness in only 2% of children, compared with 14% of the adults.[9,263] The most common malignancy in HIV-infected children is non-Hodgkin's lymphoma, manifesting as a systemic disease or as a primary central nervous system tumor. Kaposi's sarcoma is rare in children.[141,264-268] Some of these tumors appear to follow a much less aggressive course than expected, and if rapid growth necessitates chemotherapy, these children can tolerate cytotoxic agents fairly well when appropriate supportive care is provided. We initiate chemotherapy with therapeutic intent in children who have an adequate performance status, and our preliminary experience in treating 8 children has been promising. A lymphoproliferative syndrome, sometimes associated with Epstein-Barr virus infection, occurs more commonly. We have seen several children with cystic mediastinal masses that, when biopsied, were found to be polyclonal lymphoproliferative processes with a mixture of B and T cells.

In contrast to adults, an increased incidence of leiomyomas and leiomyosarcomas, soft tissue tumors that were not previously associated with immunodeficiency, has been reported.[266,269] An apparent correlation with Epstein-Barr virus infection was established in HIV-infected children with smooth muscle tumors and in patients who developed leiomyomatous tumors after organ transplantation.[270,271]

TREATMENT

The care of HIV-infected children is complex and includes antiretroviral therapy, prophylaxis for opportunistic infections, management of acute problems, and intervention on the child's behalf with school officials, day care centers, the legal system, or insurance companies. Because the standards of care are still evolving, collaboration between the child's primary health care provider and an HIV treatment center is important. Information about possible enrollment into clinical trials can be obtained by calling 1-800-TRIALS-A (AIDS Clinical Trial Group [ACTG]) or 1-301-402-0696 (Pediatric Branch, NCI).

The question of when to initiate antiretroviral therapy in children has been a topic of discussion and is still not definitively determined. The new definition of AIDS in children has not resulted in new guidelines, but it is anticipated that they will not be very different from the ones previously proposed by the National Pediatric HIV Resource Center.[272] An HIV-infected child with normal age-adjusted CD4 counts who is asymptomatic (N0) or has only lymphadenopathy, hepatomegaly, or hypergammaglobulinemia (A1) does not need antiretroviral therapy. However, symptomatic children, regardless of their CD4 count, or children with a significantly decreased CD4 count for age should receive treatment. For the infant younger than 12 months of age with proven infection (ie, HIV culture or PCR positive on two occasions), it is preferable to initiate therapy when the CD4 percentage falls below 30% or the absolute CD4 count below 1750 cells/mm^3. In the child between 1 and 6 years of age, therapy should be initiated if the CD4 percentage falls below 25% or the absolute CD count below 750 cells/mm^3. This is purposefully above the level for the initiation of PCP prophylaxis and should be based on at least two different measurement of CD4 counts within a 2-week interval.

Three agents are approved for the use in HIV-infected children: zidovudine, didanosine and the combination of lamivudine and zidovudine. Although the labeling still indicates that the indication for didanosine is failure of therapy with zidovudine, this will change in the near future based on new results from ACTG 152, a trial comparing zidovudine monotherapy to didanosine monotherapy to the combination of these two agents. The zidovudine arm was found to be less active and more toxic than the other arms (ie, didanosine alone or together with zidovudine therapies that had comparable efficacy rates).

Monitoring of the HIV-infected child includes many of the same laboratory tests used in adults, but in addition, it should include careful documentation of growth and developmental parameters. Regular ophthalmologic examinations, especially of the child with very low CD4 counts (ie, for CMV retinitis) or those receiving therapy with didano-

sine (ie, for retinal depigmentation), should be part of the routine of young children who are unable to call attention to visual impairments. However, because of the limited number of effective drugs, a change in antiretroviral therapy should only be made when objective signs of treatment failure or toxicity are observed.[272]

Antiretroviral Therapy

Zidovudine

Zidovudine (2',3'-azidothymidine) is well absorbed orally (about 65%) and is the only available agent that penetrates to a significant degree into the CSF (approximately 24%), an important feature for the treatment of children with encephalopathy. However, zidovudine has a short plasma half-life of about 1 hour.[273,274] Pharmacokinetic parameters for children older than 12 months of age are similar to adults.[275] Zidovudine does cross the placenta and can be measured in amniotic fluid, cord blood, and fetal organs, and it has been successfully used to decrease the rate of transmission from mother to fetus (ACTG 076).[45,276,277] Pharmacokinetics in newborns whose mothers had been treated with oral zidovudine during pregnancy until delivery demonstrated that the elimination of zidovudine and its main metabolite was markedly prolonged during the first 24 to 36 hours of life, with a mean serum half-life after maternal ingestion of 14.4 ± 7.5 hours.[276,278] Pharmacokinetics of zidovudine administered to infants born to seropositive mothers were linear in 23 asymptomatic children younger than the age of 3 months within a dose range of 2 to 4 mg/kg, and no side effects were observed.[277,279,280]

In May 1990, zidovudine was approved for the use in children with symptomatic HIV infection. One of the first studies of zidovudine, beginning in 1986, evaluated a continuous infusion schedule of zidovudine, designed to maintain a minimal constant level of 1 mm, the inhibitory concentration in vitro. This was achieved with all four dose levels between 0.5 and 1.8 mg/kg/hour and a steady-state CSF to plasma ratio of 0.24 ± 0.07 was maintained.[241] Improvement in neurodevelopmental status was demonstrated after 6 months in all 13 children who had presented with encephalopathy, and follow-up examination after a year of treatment indicated that these patients had maintained their gains in IQ points and improvements in general cognitive functioning.[241,281] Improvement in the degree of cerebral atrophy as measured by CT scan and a decrease in CSF protein, an nonspecific marker for HIV-related encephalopathy, were also observed.[282] We are evaluating a larger group of children with moderate to severe encephalopathy who had progressed on full dose (120 to 180 mg/m^2 every 6 hours) oral therapy with zidovudine and have determined that more than one half of these patients have some improvements in neurodevelopmental function when switched to a continuous infusion route of delivery, some with dramatic results.

TABLE 20-4. *Common dermatologic manifestations in HIV-Infected children*

Etiology	Manifestation	Comment
Infections		
Bacterial	Impetigo	Perioral infection, caused by *S aureus*. Chronic varicella can mimic impetiginous lesions.
	Cellulitis	Anywhere, including exit site of indwelling catheters or around G-tubes; mainly caused by *S epidermidis* and *S aureus*
	Folliculitis	Often difficult to treat; sometimes underlying allergic component with eosinophilic infiltrate and bacterial superinfection (mainly *S aureus* and *S pyogenes*). Gianotti-Crosti syndrome, associated with HIV or hepatitis, has been described.
	Folliculitis	Disseminated infection with *M. avium* complex is rarely associated with folliculitis; other atypical mycobacteria can cause exit site infections.
Viral	Mucocutaneous herpes	Herpes simplex virus (HSV), in children mostly type I; when HSV type 2 is found in anogenital area, suspect child abuse.
	Shingles	Varicella zoster virus (VZV) can present with typical dermatomal or multidermatomal distribution and vesicular appearance but may also present with atypical, relatively indolent, and scattered lesions (chronic varicella).
	Mollusca contagiosa	Common in children, can disseminate, and is very resistant to therapeutic interventions
	Rash	Any other childhood infection (eg, measles, parvovirus)
	Warts, condyloma acuminata	Caused by human papillomavirus; flat warts (often on forehead) or common warts (mainly on hands and feet). Condyloma acuminata can be indicator of child abuse.
	Diaper rash	Can be caused by cytomegalovirus infection with chronic urinary shedding
Fungal	Thrush, Cheilosis	Very common, may interfere with eating, sometimes resistant to many antifungal agents
	Diaper rash	Common, caused by Candida spp.
	Tinea capitis or corporis	Infection with dermatophytes can lead to regional hair loss and chronic nail infections (can also be caused by *C albicans*)
	Exit site infection	Rarely caused by Aspergillus spp.
Parasitic	Scabies	Norwegian scabies with heavy infestation possible. Very contagious!
	Lice	In children, commonly found in eye lashes and around hair follicles.
Inflammatory disorders	Atopic dermatitis	Often accompanied by severe pruritus; lesions superinfected; typical in infants and children: facial and extensor distribution
	Seborrhoic dermatitis	Nasolabial folds, eyebrows and retroauricular area
	Drug eruptions	Rash very common, sometimes evolving into fixed drug reactions or Stevens-Johnson syndrome
	Sweet syndrome	Dermatophilic leukocyte infiltration has rarely been observed in children receiving granulocyte colony-stimulating factor
Nutritional deficiencies	Zinc deficiency	Relatively common, leading to dry skin, thin hair, and alopecia
	Vitamin A deficiency	Dry skin and mucosal surfaces
Noninflammatory drug-related changes	Blue nails, hypertrichosis	Caused by zidovudine; nail discoloration mainly in African-American children; hypertrichosis of eye lashes may need intervention
	Mouth ulcers	Caused by zalcitabine
	Changes in skin color	Clofazimine causes a gray-orange tint of whole integument
Neoplasms	Kaposi's sarcoma	Rare; only described in a few Haitian children or older hemophiliacs
	Ki-1 lymphoma (lymphomatoid papillomatosis?)	Cutaneous non-Hodgkin's lymphoma that can follow a relatively indolent, waxing-and-waning course for months

A multicenter trial of oral zidovudine in a dosage of 180 mg/m² every 6 hours in children with advanced HIV disease achieved similar results.[283] There was a marked improvement in weight gain, cognitive function, and serum and CSF concentrations of p24 antigen. Similar to observations in HIV-infected adults, an increase of CD4 counts was demonstrated after the first 12 weeks of treatment but not maintained after 24 weeks. Hematologic toxicities, anemia in 26%, and neutropenia in 48% of the children were the main reasons for lowering the dose, but only 3 of 88 children had to stop zidovudine because of hematologic problems. Because the hematologic toxicity of zidovudine is dose related, there have been attempts to use lower doses in adults and children with HIV infection. A study comparing an oral dose of zidovudine of 180 mg/m² every 6 hours with 90 mg/m² every 6 hours (ACTG 128) demonstrated that the lower dose was as beneficial but less toxic in children who did not have encephalopathy at the time of entry into the study (Brouwers P, personal communication). If a child appears to benefit from high-dose zidovudine but experiences dose-limiting neutropenia, granulocyte colony-stimulating factor can be given subcutaneously to maintain the white blood cell count.[242]

Zidovudine should not be used alone as first-line single-drug therapy because of the superiority of regimens containing didanosine. When employed, certain doses of zidovudine are recommended:

0 to 2 weeks of age: 2 mg/kg/dose orally every 6 hours
2 to 4 weeks of age: 3 mg/kg/dose orally every 6 hours
4 weeks to 13 years: 90 mg/m2/dose orally every 6 hours for children without encephalopathy; 120 to 180 mg/m2/dose orally every 6 hours or 360 to 480 mg/m2/24 hours as continuous intravenous infusion for children with encephalopathy.

Didanosine

Didanosine (2′,3′-dideoxyinosine) was approved simultaneously for use in symptomatic children and adults in the autumn of 1991. In children, it has a plasma half-life of about 1 hour, a high interpatient variability in the area under the time curve, a low penetration rate into CSF, and a lower and more variable oral absorption rate (19 ± 17%) than in adults.[284] A phase I-II study of 43 children with symptomatic HIV infection, 16 of whom had previously been treated with zidovudine, was conducted through the Pediatric Branch of the NCI.[240] At the dose levels studied (ie, 60, 120, 180, 360, or 540 mg/m² divided into three daily oral doses), improvements in clinical and immunologic parameters occurred in previously treated and untreated patients. The median level of serum p24 antigen decreased significantly, with a significant correlation with plasma levels of didanosine. Patients with a CD4 count above 200 cells/mm³ were more likely to show an increase after 24 weeks of treatment than the patients with lower counts. This increase was sustained even after years of therapy in children who entered the trial with CD4 counts greater than 100 cells/mm³ (Fig. 20-2).[285]

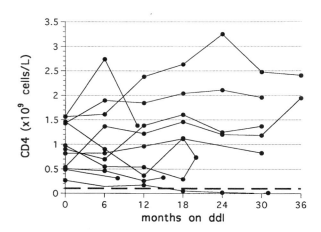

FIG. 20-2. CD4 counts during prolonged therapy with didanosine (ddI). Shown is a group of children between 2 and 6 years of age who entered the study with CD4 counts greater than 100 cells/mm³.

Therapy with didanosine is generally well tolerated, but several side effects have been seen in a few children. Similar to adults, a reversible pancreatitis develops in about 7% of children, but unlike adults, peripheral neuropathy appears to be rare.[222,285] In a French study of children who had previously been treated with zidovudine and then received didanosine at daily doses of 120 or 270 mg/m², liver function abnormalities developed in 5 of 34 children, and 1 child died of unexplained hepatocellular failure, suggesting the possibility for liver toxicity.[286] Peripheral retinal depigmentation has been described in children receiving didanosine, especially at dosages above 270 mg/m² per day.[287] Because these retinal lesions are located in the periphery, they usually do not affect central vision, but a slight constriction of the peripheral field was observed in one child.

Other Reverse Transcriptase Inhibitors

Zalcitabine (2′,3′-dideoxycytidine) has not been studied extensively in children. The plasma half-life is less than 1 hour, with a bioavailability of 54%. Penetration into CSF is lower than for zidovudine.[134] In a pilot study performed by the Pediatric Branch of the NCI, 15 children with symptomatic HIV infection were treated at four different dosage levels (ie, 0.015, 0.02, 0.03, and 0.04 mg/kg given orally every 6 hours).[134] An alternating schedule of zalcitabine for 7 days followed by 21 days of zidovudine (180 mg/m² every 6 hours orally) was used. Two thirds of the patients experienced a rise in CD4 counts and a decrease in p24 antigen levels. No hematologic toxicity was observed, but a rash developed in three patients at the highest dose level, and mouth sores were seen in 9 of 15 patients. Four children who presented initially with encephalopathy improved behaviorally.[134] Although zalcitabine is a very potent drug in vitro, the associated toxicities and its poor penetration into CSF make it more suitable for use in combination, for example, with zidovudine.

Lamivudine (2'-deoxy-3'-thiacytidine) has been evaluated in 89 children by the Pediatric Branch of the NCI in collaboration with the Los Angeles Children's Hospital since April 1992 and was approved in November 1995 in combination with zidovudine for the treatment of HIV-infected children and adults. Antiviral activity was demonstrated by a significant decrease in p24 antigenemia and quantitative viral measurements (Lewis L, personal communication). The drug was generally well tolerated, and children often reported an increase in appetite and energy level. Except for hyperactivity at the highest dose level, which was possibly drug related, no significant toxicities were encountered. Studies of lamivudine combined with zidovudine, didanosine, or both agents have been underway since early 1994 and have demonstrated that these combinations are tolerable for patients who have not been extensively pretreated.

Stavudine (2',3'-didehydro-2',3'-dideoxythymidine) has been evaluated in 37 children with HIV infection and appeared to be well tolerated. Bioavailability was between 61% and 78%, and a variable penetration into CSF was observed[289].

Combination Therapy

Combination therapy for the treatment of HIV-infected children is being pursued to develop regimens that are more potent, especially by using agents that act on different steps in the HIV life cycle; more tolerable, by using lower dosages; or more capable of delaying or preventing the emergence of resistant HIV-1 isolates. Several combination regimens employing dideoxynucleosides (eg, zidovudine plus zalcitabine, zidovudine plus didanosine) alone or in conjunction with nonnucleoside reverse transcriptase inhibitors (eg, zidovudine plus didanosine plus nevirapine) have been conducted.[134,288] As new agents are developed that act on different parts of the HIV life cycle, new combination regimens will become possible. For example, studies of protease inhibitors combined with dideoxynucleosides are being explored in children.

Other Investigational Therapies

In addition to agents that suppress or alter the HIV life cycle, strategies to improve or booster the immune system are also being explored in children. These include the use of interleukin-2 in combination with reverse transcriptase inhibitors and the co-administration of growth hormone or insulin-like growth factor combined with dideoxynucleosides.

Supportive Care and Immunizations

The Academy of Pediatrics recommends routine immunizations with some modifications for all seropositive children, whether they are infected or not.[164,289] Live virus vaccines (eg, oral poliovirus) or live bacterial vaccines (eg, bacillus Calmette-Guérin) should not be given to patients with HIV infection, with the exception of measles, mumps, and rubella vaccination, because the risk for severe measles in immunocompromised children appears much higher than the risk associated with the vaccination.[172] However, prior immunization does not necessarily provide complete protection, as evidenced by the occurrence of pertussis in previously immunized HIV-infected children.[290]

Because of the dysgammaglobulinemia and, rarely, hypogammaglobulinemia that occur in HIV-infected children, coupled with their heightened frequency of serious bacterial infections, the administration of IVIG has been studied in asymptomatic and symptomatic children with HIV infection.[291,292] In a group of children who did not receive any antiretroviral treatment, children with a CD4 count of 200 cells/mm^3 or higher appeared to benefit from monthly IVIG.[293] A study evaluating children receiving antiretroviral therapy did not find a statistically significant difference between children who received IVIG and children treated with placebo (ie, albumin), as long as they were also receiving PCP prophylaxis with TMP-SMX. Because of the limited benefit and the potential risk for the transmission of infectious agents, we restrict the use of IVIG to patients with hypogammaglobulinemia or with a history of recurrent infections with encapsulated organisms despite TMP-SMX prophylaxis.[292,294]

Antimicrobial prophylaxis has been recommended for several organisms. Of these, PCP prophylaxis can be considered a standard of care. Prophylaxis for MAC is also strongly recommended for high-risk patients (eg, with a CD4 count <100 cells/mm^3).

CONCLUSION AND GOALS

During the past dozen years, frustration and progress have characterized the evolution of knowledge of HIV infection and AIDS in children. Although new and more effective antiretroviral agents are needed, considerable progress has been made in drug development for children, with most drugs now being developed simultaneously for children and adults. Although studies of adult patients have reflected only modest gains with dideoxynucleosides, the progress in children has been more gratifying. Significant improvements in weight gain and growth velocity, reversal of neurodevelopmental deficits, and sustained improvements in CD4 counts have been observed in children treated with reverse transcriptase inhibitors. Children with AIDS are living longer, with an improved quality of life. Nonetheless, AIDS remains an inevitably fatal disease, and new agents and therapeutic strategies are essential.

Perhaps the most stunning result in clinical AIDS research was the recognition that a significant amount of HIV transmission could be prevented with the ACTG 076 regimen. However, many questions about the optimal and necessary components of this preventive strategy remain to be defined. Moreover, the need for less expensive and cumbersome schedules is evident, especially for the developing countries that are shouldering the major burden of the AIDS pandemic. Coupled with these preventive strategies, sustained efforts at education and behavioral modification are necessary to reduce the high-risk behaviors that continue to fuel the pandemic. Nowhere are these efforts more necessary than in the adolescent population. Ultimately, the course of AIDS rests on how successful we are in educating children and adolescents about this disease.

REFERENCES

1. Centers for Disease Control. Unexplained immunodeficiency and opportunistic infections in infants—New York, New Jersey, California. MMWR 1982;31:665.
2. Ammann AJ, Cowan MJ, Wara DW, et al. Acquired immunodeficiency in an infant: possible transmission by means of blood products. Lancet 1983;1:956.
3. Oleske J, Minnefor A, Cooper R, et al. Immune deficiency syndrome in children. JAMA 1983;249:2345.
4. Rubinstein A, Sicklick M, Gupta A, et al. Acquired immunodeficiency with reversed T4/T8 ratios in infants born to promiscuous and drug-addicted mothers. JAMA 1983;249:2350.
5. Church JA, Isaacs H. Transfusion associated acquired immune deficiency syndrome in infants. J Pediatr 1984;105:731.
6. Centers for Disease Control. Revision of the case definition of acquired immunodeficiency syndrome for national reporting—United States. MMWR 1985;34:373.
7. Centers for Disease Control. Revision of the CDC surveillance case definition for acquired immunodeficiency syndrome. MMWR 1987;36 (Suppl 1s):1S.
8. Centers for Disease Control and Prevention. Revised classification system for human immunodeficiency virus infection in children less than 13 years of age. MMWR 1994;43:1.
9. Centers for Disease Control and Prevention. U.S. HIV and AIDS cases reported through December 1994. HIV AIDS Surveill Rep 1995;6:1.
10. Mann JM. AIDS-the second decade: a global perspective. J Infect Dis 1992;165:245.
11. The HIV Infection in Newborns French Collaborative Study Group. Comparison of vertical human immunodeficiency virus type 2 and human immunodeficiency virus type 1 transmission in the French prospective cohort. Pediatr Infect Dis J 1994;13:502.
12. Centers for Disease Control and Prevention. Update: AIDS among women—United States, 1994. MMWR 1995;44:81.
13. Gayle JA, Selik RM, Chu SY. Surveillance for AIDS and HIV infection among black and Hispanic children and women of childbearing age, 1981–1989. MMWR CDC Surveill Summ 1990;39:23.
14. Chu SY, Buehler JW, Oxtoby MJ, Kilbourne BW. Impact of the human immunodeficiency virus epidemic on mortality in children, United States. Pediatrics 1991;87:806.
15. Lindegren ML, Hanson C, Miller K, Byers RH Jr, Onorato I. Epidemiology of human immunodeficiency virus infection in adolescents, United States. Pediatr Infect Dis J 1994;13:525.
16. Chin J, Remenyi MA, Morrison F, Bulatao R. The global epidemiology of the HIV/AIDS pandemic and its projected demographic impact in Africa. World Health Stat Q 1992;45:220.
17. Blanche S, Rouzioux C, Guihard Moscato M-L, et al. A prospective study of infants born to women seropositive for human immunodeficiency virus type 1. N Engl J Med 1989;320:1643.
18. Ryder RW, Nsa W, Hassig SE, et al. Perinatal transmission of the human immunodeficiency virus type 1 to infants of seropositive women in Zaire. N Engl J Med 1989;320:1637.
19. Adjorlolo-Johnson G, De Cock KM, Ekpini E, et al. Prospective comparison of mother-to-child transmission of HIV-1 and HIV-2 in Abidjan, Ivory Coast. JAMA 1994;272:462.
20. De Martino M, Tovo P-A, Tozzi AE, et al. HIV-1 transmission through breast-milk: appraisal of risk according to duration of feeding. AIDS 1992;6:991.
21. Ruff AJ, Halsey NA, Coberly J, Boulos R. Breast-feeding and maternal-infant transmission of human immunodeficiency virus type 1. J Pediatr 1992;121:325.
22. Nicoll A, Newell M-L, Van Praag E, Van de Perre P, Peckham C. Infant feeding policy and practice in the presence of HIV-1 infection. AIDS 1995;9:107.
23. Van de Perre P, Simonon A, Hitimana D-G, et al. Infective and anti-infective properties of breast milk from HIV-1 infected women. Lancet 1993;341:914.
24. Ryder RW, Manzila T, Baende E, et al. Evidence from Zaire that breast-feeding by HIV-1-seropositive mothers is not a major route for perinatal HIV-1 transmission but does decrease morbidity. AIDS 1991;5:709.
25. World Health Organization. Global program on AIDS. Consensus statement from the WHO/UNICEF consultation on HIV transmission and breast-feeding. Wkly Epidemiol Rec 1992;67:177.
26. De Cock KM, Adjorlolo G, Ekpini E, et al. Epidemiology and transmission of HIV-1. Why there is no HIV-2 pandemic. JAMA 1993;270:2083.
27. De Cock KM, Zadi F, Adjorlolo G, et al. Retrospective study of maternal HIV-1 and HIV-2 infections and child survival in Abidjan, Cote d'Ivoire. Br Med J 1994;308:441.
28. Andreasson PA, Dias F, Naucler A, et al. A prospective study of vertical transmission of HIV-2 in Bissau, Guinea-Bissau. AIDS 1993;7:989.
29. Poulsen AG, Kvinesdal BB, Aaby P, et al. Lack of evidence of vertical transmission of human immunodeficiency virus type 2 in a sample of the general population in Bissau. J Acquir Immune Defic Syndr 1992;5:25.
30. Lewis SH, Reynolds-Kohler C, Fox HE, Nelson JA. HIV-1 in trophoblastic and villous Hofbauer cells, and haematological precursors in eight-week fetuses. Lancet 1990;335:565.
31. Jovaisas E, Koch KA, Schäfer A, Stauber M, Löwenthal D. LAV/HTLV-III in 20-week fetus. Lancet 1985;2:1129.
32. Sprecher S, Soumenkoff G, Puissant F, Degueldre M. Vertical transmission of HIV in 15-week fetus. Lancet 1986;2:288.
33. Mundy DC, Schinazi RF, Gerber AR, Nahmias AJ, Randall HW Jr. Human immunodeficiency virus isolated from amniotic fluid. Lancet 1987;2:459.
34. Mano H, Chermann J-C. Fetal human immunodeficiency virus type 1 infection of different organs in the second trimester. AIDS Res Hum Retroviruses 1991;7:83.
35. Courgnaud V, Laure F, Brossard A, et al. Frequent and early in utero HIV-1 infection. AIDS Res Hum Retroviruses 1991;7:337.
36. Goedert JJ, Duliege AM, Amos CI, Felton S, Biggar RJ, The International Registry of HIV-exposed Twins. High risk of HIV-1 infection for first-born twins. Lancet 1991;338:1471.
37. Duliege A-M, Amos CI, Felton S, Biggar RJ, The International Registry of HIV-Exposed Twins, Goedert JJ. Birth order, delivery route, and concordance in the transmission of human immunodeficiency virus type 1 from mothers to twins. J Pediatr 1995;126:625.
38. De Rossi A, Ometto L, Mammano F, Zanotto C, Giaquinto C, Chieco-Bianchi L. Vertical transmission of HIV-1: lack of detectable virus in peripheral blood cells of infected children at birth. AIDS 1992;6:1117.
39. McIntosh K, Pitt J, Brambilla D, et al. Blood culture in the first 6 months of life for the diagnosis of vertically transmitted human immunodeficiency virus infection. The Women and Infants Transmission Study Group. J Infect Dis 1994;170:996.
40. St. Louis ME, Kamenga M, Brown C, et al. Risk for perinatal HIV-1 transmission according to maternal immunologic, virologic, and placental factors. JAMA 1993;269:2853.
41. Borkowsky W, Krasinski K, Cao Y, et al. Correlation of perinatal transmission of human immunodeficiency virus type 1 with maternal viremia and lymphocyte phenotypes. J Pediatr 1994;125:345.
42. Thomas PA, Weedon J, Krasinski K, et al. Maternal predictors of perinatal human immunodeficiency virus transmission. The New York City Perinatal HIV Transmission Collaborative Study Group. Pediatr Infect Dis J 1994;13:489.
43. De Maria A, Cirillo C, Moretta L. Occurrence of human immunodeficiency virus type 1 (HIV-1)-specific cytolytic T cell activity in apparently uninfected children born to HIV-1-infected mothers. J Infect Dis 1994;170:1296.
44. Bryson YJ, Pang S, Wei LS, Dickover R, Diagne A, Chen ISY. Clearance of HIV infection in a perinatally infected infant. N Engl J Med 1995;332:833.

45. Connor EM, Sperling RS, Gelber R, et al. Reduction of maternal-infant transmission of immunodeficiency virus type 1 with zidovudine treatment. N Engl J Med 1994;331:1173.
46. Rogers MF, Thomas PA, Starcher ET, Noa MC, Bush TJ, Jaffe HW. Acquired immunodeficiency syndrome in children: report of the Centers for Disease Control National Surveillance, 1982 to 1985. Pediatrics 1987;79:1008.
47. Selik RM, Ward JW, Buehler JW. Trends in transfusion-associated acquired immune deficiency syndrome in the United States, 1982 through 1991. Transfusion 1993;33:890.
48. Busch MP, Eble BE, Khayam-Bashi H, et al. Evaluation of screened blood donations for human immunodeficiency virus type 1 infection by culture and DNA amplification of pooled cells. N Engl J Med 1991;325:1.
49. Bray GL. Recent advances in the preparation of plasma-derived and recombinant coagulation factor VIII. J Pediatr 1990;117:503.
50. Butler D. Making global blood safety a priority. Nature Med 1995;1:7.
51. Hersh BS, Popovici F, Apetrei RC, et al. Acquired immunodeficiency syndrome in Romania. Lancet 1991;338:645.
52. D'Angelo LJ, Bowler S, Sheon AR, D'Angelo LJ, Vermund SH. Adolescents and HIV infection: a clinician's perspective. Acta Paediatr Suppl 1994;400:88.
53. Centers for Disease Control and Prevention. Trends in sexual risk behavior among high school students—United States, 1990, 1991, and 1993. MMWR 1995;44:124.
54. Brunswick AF, Aidala A, Dobkin J, Howard J, Titus SP, Banaszak-Holl J. HIV-1 seroprevalence and risk behaviors in an urban African-American community cohort. Am J Public Health 1993;83:1390.
55. Hirschfeld S, Chanock SJ. Selected issues in human immunodeficiency virus infection in adolescents. Curr Opin Pediatr 1992;4:599.
56. Goodman E, Cohall AT. Acquired immunodeficiency syndrome and adolescents: knowledge, attitudes, beliefs, and behaviors in a New York City adolescent minority population. Pediatrics 1989;84:36.
57. Koopman C, Rotheram-Borus MJ, Henderson R, Bradley JS, Hunter J. Assessment of knowledge of AIDS and beliefs about AIDS prevention among adolescents. AIDS Educ Prev 1990;2:58.
58. Simonds RJ, Chanock S. Medical issues related to caring for human immunodeficiency virus-infected children in and out of the home. Pediatr Infect Dis J 1993;12:845.
59. Fitzgibbon JE, Gaur S, Frenkel LD, Laraque F, Edlin BR, Dubin DT. Transmission from one child to another of human immunodeficiency virus type 1 with a zidovudine-resistant mutation. N Engl J Med 1993;329:1835.
60. Centers for Disease Control and Prevention. Human immunodeficiency virus transmission in household settings-United States. MMWR 1994;43:347.
61. American Academy of Pediatrics Committee on Sports Medicine and Fitness. Human immunodeficiency virus (acquired immunodeficiency syndrome [AIDS] virus) in the athletic setting. Pediatrics 1991;88:640.
62. Palasanthiran P, Robertson P, Ziegler JB, Graham GG. Decay of transplacental human immunodeficiency virus type 1 antibodies in neonates and infants. J Infect Dis 1994;170:1593.
63. Consensus Workshop. Maternal factors involved in mother-to-child transmission of HIV-1. J Acquir Immune Defic Syndr 1992;5:1019.
64. Burgard M, Mayaux M-J, Blanche S, et al. The use of viral culture and p24 antigen testing to diagnose human immunodeficiency virus infection in neonates. N Engl J Med 1992;327:1192.
65. Simonds RJ, Lindegren ML, Thomas P, et al. Prophylaxis against Pneumocystis carinii pneumonia among children with perinatally acquired human immunodeficiency virus infection in the United States. N Engl J Med 1995;332:786.
66. Marion RW, Wiznia AA, Hutcheon RG, Rubinstein A. Human T-cell lymphotropic virus type III (HTLV-III) embryopathy. Am J Dis Child 1986;140:638.
67. Iosub S, Bamji M, Stone RK, Gromisch DS, Wasserman E. More on human immunodeficiency virus embryopathy. Pediatrics 1987;80:512.
68. Qazi QH, Sheikh TM, Fikrig S, Menikoff H. Lack of evidence for craniofacial dysmorphism in perinatal human immunodeficiency virus infection. J Pediatr 1988;112:7.
69. Embree JE, Braddick M, Datta P, et al. Lack of correlation of maternal human immunodeficiency virus infection with neonatal malformations. Pediatr Infect Dis J 1989;8:700.
70. Blanche S, Mayaux M-J, Rouzioux C, et al. Relation of the course of HIV infection in children to the severity of the disease in their mothers at delivery. N Engl J Med 1994;330:308.
71. Blanche S, Tardieu M, Duliege A-M, et al. Longitudinal study of 94 symptomatic infants with perinatally acquired human immunodeficiency virus infection. Am J Dis Child 1990;144:1210.
72. Duliege A-M, Messiah A, Blanche S, Tardieu M, Griscelli C, Spira A. Natural history of human immunodeficiency virus type 1 infection in children: prognostic value of laboratory tests on the bimodal progression of disease. Pediatr Infect Dis J 1992;11:630.
73. Scott GB, Hutto C, Makuch RW, et al. Survival in children with perinatally acquired human immunodeficiency virus type 1 infection. N Engl J Med 1989;321:1791.
74. The European Collaborative Study. Natural history of vertically acquired human immunodeficiency virus-1 infection. Pediatrics 1994;94:815.
75. Frederick T, Mascola L, Eller A, et al. Progression of human immunodeficiency virus disease among infants and children infected perinatally with human immunodeficiency virus or through neonatal blood transfusion. Pediatr Infect Dis J 1994;13:1091.
76. Tovo PA, De Martino M, Gabiano C, et al. Prognostic factors and survival in children with perinatal HIV-1 infection. Lancet 1992;339:1249.
77. Thomas P, Singh T, Williams R, Blum S. Trends in survival for children reported with maternally transmitted acquired immunodeficiency syndrome in New York City, 1982 to 1989. Pediatr Infect Dis J 1992;11:34.
78. Butler KM, Husson RN, Lewis LL, Mueller BU, Venzon D, Pizzo PA. CD4 status and p24 antigenemia. Are they useful predictors of survival in HIV-infected children receiving antiretroviral therapy? Am J Dis Child 1992;146:932.
79. Tudor-Williams G, Mueller BU, Stocker V, et al. Serum p24 antigen levels and disease progression in HIV-1 infected children. Abstract. Presented at the Keystone Symposium, Albuquerque, NM, 1993.
80. Pantaleo G, Graziosi C, Demarest JF, et al. HIV infection is active and progressive in lymphoid tissue during the clinically latent stage of disease. Nature 1993;362:355.
81. Frost SDW, McLean AR. Germinal center destruction as a major pathway of HIV pathogenesis. J Acquir Immune Defic Syndr 1994;7:236.
82. Sei S, Kleiner DE, Kopp JB, et al. Quantitative analysis of viral burden in tissues from adults and children with symptomatic human immunodeficiency virus type 1 infection assessed by polymerase chain reaction. J Infect Dis 1994;170:325.
83. Fox CH, Tenner-Racz K, Racz P, Firpo A, Pizzo PA, Fauci AS. Lymphoid germinal centers are reservoirs of human immunodeficiency virus type 1 RNA. J Infect Dis 1991;164:1051.
84. Saag MS, Crain MJ, Decker WD, et al. High-level viremia in adults and children infected with human immunodeficiency virus: relation to stage of disease and CD4+ lymphocyte levels. J Infect Dis 1991;164:72.
85. Erkeller-Yuksel FM, Deneys V, Hannet I, et al. Age-related changes in human blood lymphocyte subpopulations. J Pediatr 1992;120:216.
86. McKinney RE, Wilfert CM. Lymphocyte subsets in children younger than 2 years old: normal values in a population at risk for human immunodeficiency virus infection and diagnostic and prognostic application to infected children. Pediatr Infect Dis J 1992;11:639.
87. The European Collaborative Study. Age-related standards for T lymphocyte subsets based on uninfected children born to human immunodeficiency virus 1-infected mothers. Pediatr Infect Dis J 1992;11:1018.
88. Aldhous MC, Raab GM, Doherty KV, Mok JYQ, Bird AG, Froebel KS. Age-related ranges of memory, activation, and cytotoxic markers on CD4 and CD8 cells in children. J Clin Immunol 1994;14:289.
89. D'Arminio Monforte A, Novati R, Galli M, et al. T-cell subsets and serum immunoglobulin levels in infants born to HIV-seropositive mothers: a longitudinal evaluation. AIDS 1990;4:1141.
90. Centers for Disease Control. Guidelines for prophylaxis against Pneumocystis carinii pneumonia for children infected with human immunodeficiency virus. MMWR 1991;40:1.
91. Joshi VV, Oleske JM, Saad S, et al. Thymus biopsy in children with acquired immunodeficiency syndrome. Arch Pathol Med 1986;110:837.
92. Plaeger-Marshall S, Isacescu V, O'Rourke S, Bertolli J, Bryson YJ, Stiehm ER. T cell activation in pediatric AIDS pathogenesis: three-color immunophenotyping. Clin Immunol Immunopathol 1994;71:19.
93. Luzuriaga K, Koup RA, Pikora CA, Brettler DB, Sullivan JL. Deficient human immunodeficiency virus type 1-specific cytotoxic T cell responses in vertically infected children. J Pediatr 1991;119:230.
94. Vigano A, Principi N, Villa ML, et al. Immunologic characterization of children vertically infected with human immunodeficiency virus, with slow or rapid disease progression. J Pediatr 1995;126:368.

95. Clerici M, Roilides E, Butler KM, et al. Changes in T-helper cell function in human immunodeficiency virus-infected children during didanosine therapy as a measure of antiretroviral activity. Blood 1992;80:2196.

96. Buseyne F, Blanche S, Schmitt D, Griscelli C, Riviere Y. Detection of HIV-specific cell-mediated cytotoxicity in the peripheral blood from infected children. J Immunol 1993;8:3569.

97. Roilides E, Clerici M, DePalma L, Rubin M, Pizzo PA, Shearer GM. Helper T-cell responses in children infected with human immunodeficiency virus type 1. J Pediatr 1991;118:724.

98. Schnittman SM, Lane HC, Higgins SE, Folks T, Fauci AS. Direct polyclonal activation of human B lymphocytes by the AIDS virus. Science 1986;233:1084.

99. Roilides E, Black C, Reimer C, Rubin M, Venzon D, Pizzo PA. Serum immunoglobulin G subclasses in children infected with human immunodeficiency virus type 1. Pediatr Infect Dis J 1991;10:134.

100. Roilides E, Mertins S, Eddy J, Walsh TJ, Pizzo PA, Rubin M. Impairment of neutrophil chemotactic and bactericidal function in children infected with human immunodeficiency virus type 1 and partial reversal after in vitro exposure to granulocyte-macrophage colony-stimulating factor. J Pediatr 1990;117:531.

101. Roilides E, Venzon D, Pizzo PA, Rubin M. Effects of antiretroviral dideoxynucleosides on polymorphonuclear leukocyte function. Antimicrob Agents Chemother 1990;34:1672.

102. Roilides E, Holmes A, Blake C, Pizzo PA, Walsh TJ. Defective antifungal activity of monocyte-derived macrophages from human immunodeficiency virus-infected children against *Aspergillus fumigatus*. J Infect Dis 1993;168:1562.

103. Forte M, Maartens G, Campbell F, et al. T-lymphocyte responses to *Pneumocystis carinii* in healthy and HIV-positive individuals. J Acquir Immune Defic Syndr 1992;5:409.

104. Madhok R, Gracie JA, Forbes CD, Lowe GDO. B cell dysfunction in haemophilia in the absence and presence of HIV-1 infection. Thromb Haemost 1991;65:7.

105. Ellis M, Gupta S, Galant S, et al. Impaired neutrophil function in patients with AIDS or AIDS-related complex: a comprehensive evaluation. J Infect Dis 1988;158:1268.

106. Brettler DB, Forsberg A, Bolivar E, Brewster F, Sullivan J. Growth failure as a prognostic indicator for progression to acquired immunodeficiency syndrome in children with hemophilia. J Pediatr 1990;117:584.

107. McKinney RE, Robertson WR, Duke Pediatric AIDS Clinical Trials Unit. Effect of human immunodeficiency virus infection on the growth of young children. J Pediatr 1993;123:579.

108. Krentz AJ, Koster FT, Crist DM, et al. Anthropometric, metabolic, and immunological effects of recombinant human growth hormone in AIDS and AIDS-related complex. J Acquir Immune Defic Syndr 1993;6:245.

109. Laue L, Pizzo PA, Butler K, Cutler GB. Growth and neuroendocrine dysfunction in children with acquired immunodeficiency syndrome. J Pediatr 1990;117:541.

110. Fischer GD, Rinaldo CR, Gbadero D, et al. Seroprevalence of HIV-1 and HIV-2 infection among children diagnosed with protein-calorie malnutrition in Nigeria. Epidemiol Infect 1993;110:373.

111. Pizzo PA. Pediatric AIDS: problems within problems. J Infect Dis 1990;161:316.

112. Burr CK, Emery LJ. Speaking with children and families about HIV infection. In: Pizzo PA, Wilfert CM, eds. Pediatric AIDS. The challenge of HIV infection in infants, children, and adolescents. 2nd ed. Baltimore: Williams & Wilkins, 1994:923.

113. Wiener L, Theut S, Steinberg SM, Riekert KA, Pizzo PA. The HIV-infected child: parental responses and psychosocial implications. Am J Orthopsychiatry 1994;64:485.

114. Belman AL, Diamond G, Dickson D, et al. Pediatric acquired immunodeficiency syndrome. Neurologic symptoms. Am J Dis Child 1988;142:29.

115. Civitello LA. Neurologic complications of HIV infection in children. Pediatr Neurosurg 1991;17:104.

116. Dickson DW, Belman AL, Park YD, et al. Central nervous system pathology in pediatric AIDS: an autopsy study. APMIS Suppl 1989;8:40.

117. Schmitt B, Seeger J, Kreuz W, Enenkel S, Jacobi G. Central nervous system involvement of children with HIV infection. Dev Med Child Neurol 1991;33:535.

118. The European Collaborative Study. Neurologic signs in young children with human immunodeficiency virus infection. Pediatr Infect Dis J 1990;9:402.

119. DeCarli C, Civitello LA, Brouwers P, Pizzo PA. The prevalence of computed tomographic abnormalities of the cerebrum in 100 consecutive children symptomatic with the human immunodeficiency virus. Ann Neurol 1993;34:198.

120. Brouwers P, Belman A, Epstein L. Central nervous system involvement: manifestations, evaluation, and pathogenesis. In: Pizzo PA, Wilfert CA, eds. Pediatric AIDS. The challenge of HIV infection in infants, children, and adolescents. 2nd ed. Baltimore: Williams & Wilkins, 1994:318.

121. Wolters PL, Brouwers P, Moss HA, Pizzo PA. Adaptive behavior of children with symptomatic HIV infection before and after zidovudine therapy. J Pediatr Psychol 1994;19:47.

122. Lyman WD, Kress Y, Kure K, Rashbaum WK, Rubinstein A, Soeiro R. Detection of HIV in fetal central nervous system tissue. AIDS 1990;4:917.

123. Srugo I, Wittek AE, Israele V, Brunell PA. Meningoencephalitis in a neonate congenitally infected with human immunodeficiency virus type 1. J Pediatr 1992;120:93.

124. Kauffman WM, Sivit CJ, Fitz CR, Rakusan TA, Herzog K, Chandra RS. CT and MR evaluation of intracranial involvement in pediatric HIV infection: a clinical-imaging correlation. Am J Neuroradiol 1992;13:949.

125. Brouwers P, Heyes MP, Moss HA, et al. Quinolinic acid in the cerebrospinal fluid of children with symptomatic human immunodeficiency virus type 1 disease: relationships to clinical status and therapeutic response. J Infect Dis 1993;168:1380.

126. Gallo P, Laverda AM, De Rossi A, et al. Immunological markers in the cerebrospinal fluid of HIV-1 infected children. Acta Paediatr Scand 1991;80:659.

127. Surtees R, Hyland K, Smith I. Central-nervous-system methyl-group metabolism in children with neurological complications of HIV infection. Lancet 1990;335:619.

128. Lipton SA, Gendelman HE. Dementia associated with the acquired immunodeficiency syndrome. N Engl J Med 1995;332:934.

129. Geleziunas R, Schipper HM, Wainberg MA. Pathogenesis and therapy of HIV-1 infection of the central nervous system. AIDS 1992;6:1411.

130. Stiehm ER, Bryson YJ, Frenkel LM, et al. Prednisone improves human immunodeficiency virus encephalopathy in children. Pediatr Infect Dis J 1992;11:49.

131. Park YD, Belman AL, Kim T-S, et al. Stroke in pediatric acquired immunodeficiency syndrome. Ann Neurol 1990;28:303.

132. Husson RN, Saini R, Lewis LL, Butler KM, Patronas N, Pizzo PA. Cerebral artery aneurysms in children infected with human immunodeficiency virus. J Pediatr 1992;121:927.

133. Sharer LR, Dowling PC, Michaels J, et al. Spinal cord disease in children with HIV-1 infection: a combined molecular biological and neuropathological study. Neuropathol Appl Neurobiol 1990;16:317.

134. Pizzo PA, Butler K, Balis F, et al. Dideoxycytidine alone and in an alternating schedule with zidovudine in children with symptomatic human immunodeficiency virus infection. J Pediatr 1990;117:799.

135. Bottoni F, Gonnella P, Autelitano A, Orzalesi N. Diffuse necrotizing retinochoroiditis in a child with AIDS and toxoplasmic encephalitis. Graefes Arch Clin Exp Ophthalmol 1990;228:36.

136. Medlock MD, Tilleli JT, Pearl GS. Congenital cardiac toxoplasmosis in a newborn with acquired immunodeficiency syndrome. Pediatr Infect Dis J 1990;9:129.

137. Miller MJ, Remington JS. Toxoplasmosis in infants and children with HIV infection or AIDS. In: Pizzo PA, Wilfert CM, eds. Pediatric AIDS. The challenge of HIV infection in infants, children, and adolescents. Baltimore: Williams & Wilkins, 1991:299.

138. Walsh TJ. Fungal infections complicating pediatric HIV infection. In: Pizzo PA, Wilfert CM, eds. Pediatric AIDS. The challenge of HIV infection in infants, children, and adolescents. 2nd ed. Baltimore: Williams & Wilkins, 1994:321.

139. Frenkel LD, Gaur S, Tsolia M, Scudder R, Howell R, Kesarwala H. Cytomegalovirus infection in children with AIDS. Rev Infect Dis 1990;12:820.

140. Belec L, Tayot J, Tron P, Mikol J, Scaravilli F, Gray F. Cytomegalovirus encephalopathy in an infant with congenital acquired immuno-deficiency syndrome. Neuropediatrics 1990;21:124.

141. Epstein LG, DiCarlo FJ, Joshi VV, et al. Primary lymphoma of the central nervous system in children with acquired immunodeficiency syndrome. Pediatrics 1988;82:355.
142. Krasinski K, Borkowsky W, Bonk S, Lawrence R, Chandwani S. Bacterial infections in human immunodeficiency virus-infected children. Pediatr Infect Dis J 1988;7:323.
143. Roilides E, Marshall D, Venzon D, Butler K, Husson R, Pizzo PA. Bacterial infections in human immunodeficiency virus type 1-infected children: the impact of central venous catheters and antiretroviral agents. Pediatr Infect Dis J 1991;10:813.
144. Janoff EN, Breiman RF, Daley CL, Hopewell PC. Pneumococcal disease during HIV infection. Epidemiology, clinical, and immunologic perspectives. Ann Intern Med 1992;117:314.
145. Farley JJ, King JC, Nair P, Hines SE, Tressler RL, Vink PE. Invasive pneumococcal disease among infected and uninfected children of mothers with human immunodeficiency virus infection. J Pediatr 1994;124:853.
146. Andiman WA, Mezger J, Shapiro E. Invasive bacterial infections in children born to women infected with human immunodeficiency virus type 1. J Pediatr 1994;124:846.
147. Roilides E, Butler KM, Husson RN, Mueller BU, Lewis LL, Pizzo PA. *Pseudomonas* infections in children with human immunodeficiency virus infection. Pediatr Infect Dis J 1992;11:547.
148. Braun MM, Cauthen G. Relationship of the human immunodeficiency virus epidemic to pediatric tuberculosis and bacillus Calmette-Guerin immunization. Pediatr Infect Dis J 1992;11:220.
149. Dumois JA. Tuberculosis in children with HIV infection. Pediatr AIDS HIV Infect Fetus Adolesc 1992;3:177.
150. Moss WJ, Dedyo T, Suarez M, Nicholas SW, Abrams E. Tuberculosis in children infected with human immunodeficiency virus: a report of five cases. Pediatr Infect Dis J 1992;11:114.
151. Khoury YF, Mastrucci MT, Hutto C, Mitchell CD, Scott GB. *Mycobacterium tuberculosis* in children with human immunodeficiency virus type 1 infection. Pediatr Infect Dis J 1992;11:950.
152. Gutman LT, Moye J, Zimmer B, Tian C. Tuberculosis in human immunodeficiency virus-exposed or -infected United States children. Pediatr Infect Dis J 1994;13:963.
153. Starke JR, Jacobs RF, Jereb J. Resurgence of tuberculosis in children. J Pediatr 1992;120:839.
154. Abadco DL, Steiner P. Gastric lavage is better than bronchoalveolar lavage for isolation of *Mycobacterium tuberculosis* in childhood pulmonary tuberculosis. Pediatr Infect Dis J 1992;11:735.
155. Lewis LL, Butler KM, Husson RN, et al. Defining the population of human immunodeficiency virus-infected children at risk for *Mycobacterium avium-intracellulare* infection. J Pediatr 1992; 121:677.
156. Masur H, The Public Health Service Task Force on Prophylaxis and Therapy for *Mycobacterium avium* Complex. Recommendations on prophylaxis and therapy for disseminated *Mycobacterium avium* complex disease in patients infected with the human immunodeficiency virus. N Engl J Med 1993;329:898.
157. Husson RN, Ross LA, Sandelli S, et al. Orally administered clarithromycin for the treatment of systemic *Mycobacterium avium* complex infection in children with acquired immunodeficiency syndrome. J Pediatr 1994;124:807.
158. Nightingale SD, Cameron W, Gordin FM, et al. Two controlled trials of rifabutin prophylaxis against *Mycobacterium avium* complex infection in AIDS. N Engl J Med 1993;329:828.
159. Lewis L, Jacobsen F, Mueller B, et al. Phase I/II assessment of oral rifabutin suspension for the prophylaxis of *Mycobacterium avium* complex (MAC) bacteremia in HIV-infected children. First National Conference on Human Retroviruses and Related Infections. Washington, DC, 1993.
160. Kawimbe B, Bem C, Patil PS, Bharucha H. Cytomegalovirus ileitis presenting as massive rectal bleeding in infancy. Arch Dis Child 1991;66:883.
161. Mustafa MM. Cytomegalovirus infection and disease in the immunocompromised host. Pediatr Infect Dis J 1994;13:249.
162. Jura E, Chadwick EG, Josephs SH, et al. Varicella-zoster virus infections in children infected with human immunodeficiency virus. Pediatr Infect Dis 1989;8:586.
163. Srugo I, Israele V, Wittek AE, Courville T, Vimal VM, Brunell PA. Clinical manifestations of varicella-zoster virus infections in human immunodeficiency virus-infected children. Am J Dis Child 1993;147:742.
164. American Academy of Pediatrics. AIDS and HIV infections. In: Report of the committee on infectious diseases (red book). Elk Grove Village, IL: American Academy of Pediatrics, 1991:115.
165. Joshi VV, Kauffman S, Oleske JM, et al. Polyclonal polymorphic B-cell lymphoproliferative disorder with prominent pulmonary involvement in children with acquired immune deficiency syndrome. Cancer 1987;59:1455.
166. Katz BZ, Berkman AB, Shapiro ED. Serologic evidence of active Epstein-Barr virus infection in Epstein-Barr virus–associated lymphoproliferative disorders of children with acquired immunodeficiency syndrome. J Pediatr 1992;120:228.
167. Andiman WA, Martin K, Rubinstein A, et al. Opportunistic lymphoproliferations associated with Epstein-Barr viral DNA in infants and children with AIDS. Lancet 1985;2:1390.
168. Rohrlich P, Lescoeur B, Rahimy C, Vilmer E, Brousse N, Foulon E. Epstein-Barr virus associated B-cell lymphoproliferation in an infant treated for acute lymphoblastic leukemia. Blood 1993;81:264.
169. Kaplan LJ, Daum RS, Smaron M, McCarthy CA. Severe measles in immunocompromised patients. JAMA 1992;267:1237.
170. Nadel S, McGann K, Hodinka RL, Rutstein R, Chatten J. Measles giant cell pneumonia in a child with human immunodeficiency virus infection. Pediatr Infect Dis J 1991;10:542.
171. Markowitz LE, Chandler FW, Roldan EO, et al. Fatal measles pneumonia without rash in a child with AIDS. J Infect Dis 1988;158:480.
172. Krasinski K, Borkowsky W. Measles and measles immunity in children infected with human immunodeficiency virus. JAMA 1989;261:2512.
173. King JC, Burke AR, Clemens JD, et al. Respiratory syncytial virus illnesses in human immunodeficiency virus-and noninfected children. Pediatr Infect Dis J 1993;12:733.
174. Walsh TJ, Gonzales C, Roilides E, et al. Fungemia in children infected with the human immunodeficiency virus: new epidemiologic patterns, emerging pathogens, and improved outcome with antifungal therapy. Clin Infect Dis 1995;20:900.
175. Ting SF, Glader BE, Prober CG. Cryptococcus infection in a nine-year-old child with hemophilia and the acquired immunodeficiency syndrome. Pediatr Infect Dis J 1991;10:76.
176. Butcher JD, Krober MS. Cryptococcal meningitis in a child with acquired immunodeficiency syndrome. Pediatr AIDS HIV Infect Fetus Adolesc 1991;2:134.
177. Leggiadro RJ, Kline MW, Hughes WT. Extrapulmonary cryptococcosis in children with acquired immunodeficiency syndrome. Pediatr Infect Dis J 1991;10:658.
178. Byers M, Feldman S, Edwards J. Disseminated histoplasmosis as the acquired immunodeficiency syndrome-defining illness in an infant. Pediatr Infect Dis J 1992;11:127.
179. Mortier E, Pouchot J, Bossi P, Molinié V. Maternal-fetal transmission of *Pneumocystis carinii* in human immunodeficiency virus infection. N Engl J Med 1995;332:825.
180. Leibovitz E, Rigaud M, Pollack H, et al. *Pneumocystis carinii* pneumonia in infants infected with the human immunodeficiency virus with more than 450 CD4 T lymphocytes per cubic millimeter. N Engl J Med 1990;323:531.
181. Bernstein LJ, Bye MR, Rubinstein A. Prognostic factors and life expectancy in children with acquired immunodeficiency syndrome and *Pneumocystis carinii* pneumonia. Am J Dis Child 1989;143:775.
182. Kovacs A, Frederick T, Church J, Eller A, Oxtoby M, Mascola L. CD4 T-lymphocyte counts and *Pneumocystis carinii* pneumonia in pediatric HIV infection. JAMA 1991;265:1698.
183. Bye MR, Bernstein LJ, Glaser J, Kleid D. *Pneumocystis carinii* pneumonia in young children with AIDS. Pediatr Pulmonol 1990;9:251.
184. Connor E, Bagarazzi M, McSherry G, et al. Clinical and laboratory correlates of *Pneumocystis carinii* pneumonia in children infected with HIV. JAMA 1991;265:1693.
185. Gosey LL, Howard RM, Witebsky FG, et al. Advantages of a modified toluidine blue O stain and bronchoalveolar lavage for the diagnosis of *Pneumocystis carinii* pneumonia. J Clin Microbiol 1985;22:803.
186. Ognibene FP, Gill VJ, Pizzo PA, et al. Induced sputum to diagnose *Pneumocystis carinii* pneumonia in immunosuppressed pediatric patients. J Pediatr 1989;115:430.
187. Sleasman JW, Hemenway C, Klein AS, Barrett DJ. Corticosteroids improve survival of children with AIDS and *Pneumocystis carinii* pneumonia. AJDC 1993;147:30.

188. Rigaud M, Pollack H, Leibovitz E, et al. Efficacy of primary chemo-prophylaxis against *Pneumocystis carinii* pneumonia during the first year of life in infants infected with human immunodeficiency virus type 1. J Pediatr 1994;125:476.

189. Mueller BU, Pizzo PA, Steinberg S. Failure of intravenous pentamidine prophylaxis for *Pneumocystis carinii* pneumonia. (Reply to a letter). J Pediatr 1993;122:163.

190. Mueller BU, Butler KM, Husson RN, Pizzo PA. *Pneumocystis carinii* pneumonia despite prophylaxis in children with human immunodeficiency virus infection. J Pediatr 1991;119:992.

191. Nachman SA, Mueller BU, Mirochnik M, Pizzo PA. High failure rate of dapsone and pentamidine as *Pneumocystis carinii* pneumonia prophylaxis in human immunodeficiency virus-infected children. Pediatr Infect Dis J 1994;13:1004.

192. Curry A, Turner AJ, Lucas S. Opportunistic infections in human immunodeficiency virus disease: review highlighting diagnostic and therapeutic aspects. J Clin Pathol 1991;44:182.

193. Cordell RL, Addiss DG. Cryptosporidiosis in child care settings: a review of the literature and recommendations for prevention and control. Pediatr Infect Dis J 1994;13:310.

194. Marolda J, Bonforte RJ, Kotin NM, Rabinowitz J, Kattan M. Pulmonary manifestations of HIV infection in children. Pediatr Pulmonol 1991;10:231.

195. Moran CA, Suster S, Pavlova Z, Mullick FG, Koss MN. The spectrum of pathological changes in children with the acquired immunodeficiency syndrome: an autopsy study of 36 cases. Hum Pathol 1994;25:877.

196. Pitt J. Lymphocytic interstitial pneumonia. In: Edelson PJ, ed. Childhood AIDS. Philadelphia: WB Saunders, 1991:89.

197. Connor EM, Marquis J, Oleske JM. Lymphoid interstitial pneumonitis. In: Pizzo PA, Wilfert CM, eds. Pediatric AIDS. The challenge of HIV infection in infants, children, and adolescents. Baltimore: Williams & Wilkins, 1991:343.

198. Amorosa JK, Miller RW, Laraya-Cuasay L, et al. Bronchiectasis in children with lymphocytic interstitial pneumonia and acquired immune deficiency syndromes. Plain film and CT observations. Pediatr Radiol 1992;22:603.

199. Joshi VV, Oleske JM, Connor EM. Morphologic findings in children with acquired immune deficiency syndrome: pathogenesis and clinical implications. Pediatr Pathol 1990;10:155.

200. Joshi VV. Systemic lymphoproliferative lesions in children with AIDS. Pediatr AIDS HIV Infect Fetus Adolesc 1990;1:44.

201. Lipshultz SE, Chanock S, Sanders SP, Colan SD, Perez-Atayde A, McIntosh K. Cardiovascular manifestations of human immunodeficiency virus infection in infants and children. Am J Cardiol 1989;63:1489.

202. Luginbuhl LM, Orav EJ, McIntosh K, Lipshultz SE. Cardiac morbidity and related mortality in children with HIV infection. JAMA 1993;269:2869.

203. Steinherz LJ, Brochstein JA, Robins J. Cardiac involvement in congenital acquired immunodeficiency syndrome. Am J Dis Child 1986;140:1241.

204. Stewart JM, Kaul A, Gromisch DS, Reyes E, Woolf PK, Gowitz MH. Symptomatic cardiac dysfunction in children with human immunodeficiency virus infection. Am Heart J 1989;117:140.

205. Lipshultz SE, Orav EJ, Sanders SP, Hale AR, McIntosh K, Colan SD. Cardiac structure and function in children with human immunodeficiency virus infection treated with zidovudine. N Engl J Med 1992;327:1260.

206. Lipshultz SE, Fox CH, Perez-Atayde AR, et al. Identification of human immunodeficiency virus-1 RNA and DNA in the heart of a child with cardiovascular abnormalities and congenital acquired immune deficiency syndrome. Am J Cardiol 1990;66:246.

207. Joshi VV, Gadol C, Connor E, Oleske JM, Mendelson J, Marin-Garcia J. Dilated cardiomyopathy in children with acquired immunodeficiency syndrome: a pathologic study of five cases. Hum Pathol 1988;19:69.

208. Domanski MJ, Sloas MM, Follmann DA, et al. Effect of zidovudine and didanosine treatment on heart function in children infected with human immunodeficiency virus. J Pediatr 1995;127:137.

209. Joshi VV, Pawel B, Connor E, et al. Arteriopathy in children with acquired immune deficiency syndrome. Pediatr Pathol 1987;7:261.

210. Soberman N, Leonidas JC, Berdon WE, et al. Parotid enlargement in children seropositive for human immunodeficiency virus: imaging findings. Am J Radiol 1991;157:553.

211. Kotloff KL, Johnson JP, Nair P, et al. Diarrheal morbidity during the first 2 years of life among HIV-infected infants. JAMA 1994;271:448.

212. Nicholas SW. The opportunistic and bacterial infections associated with pediatric human immunodeficiency virus disease. Acta Paediatr Suppl 1994;400:46.

213. Oshitani H, Kasolo FC, Mpabalwani M, et al. Association of rotavirus and human immunodeficiency virus infection in children hospitalized with acute diarrhea, Lusaka, Zambia. J Infect Dis 1994;169:897.

214. Thea DM, St. Louis ME, Atido U, et al. A prospective study of diarrhea and HIV-1 infection among 429 Zairian infants. N Engl J Med 1993;329:1696.

215. Yolken RH, Li S, Perman J, Viscidi R. Persistent diarrhea and fecal shedding of retroviral nucleic acids in children infected with human immunodeficiency virus. J Infect Dis 1991;164:61.

216. Yolken RH, Hart W, Oung I, Shiff C, Greenson J, Perman JA. Gastrointestinal dysfunction and disaccharide intolerance in children infected with human immunodeficiency virus. J Pediatr 1991;118:359.

217. Miller TL, Orav EJ, Martin SR, Cooper ER, McIntosh K, Winter HS. Malnutrition and carbohydrate malabsorption in children with vertically transmitted human immunodeficiency virus 1 infection. Gastroenterology 1991;100:1296.

218. Persaud D, Bangaru B, Greco A, et al. Cholestatic hepatitis in children infected with the human immunodeficiency virus. Pediatr Infect Dis J 1993;12:492.

219. Leggiadro RJ, Lewis D, Whitington GL, Pendergrass LB, Langston C. Chronic hepatitis associated with perinatal HIV infection. AIDS Reader 1992;March/April:57.

220. de Martino M, Tovo P-A, Zuccotti GV, et al. Transferase values in infants at risk from human immunodeficiency virus type 1 perinatal infection. Pediatr Infect Dis J 1993;12:248.

221. Miller TL, Winter HS, Luginbuhl LM, Orav EJ, McIntosh K. Pancreatitis in pediatric human immunodeficiency virus infection. J Pediatr 1992;120:223.

222. Butler KM, Venzon D, Henry N, et al. Pancreatitis in human immunodeficiency virus-infected children receiving dideoxyinosine. Pediatrics 1993;91:747.

223. Hart CC. Aerosolized pentamidine and pancreatitis. Ann Intern Med 1989;111:691.

224. Kumar S, Schnadig VJ, MacGregor MG. Fatal acute pancreatitis associated with pentamidine therapy. Am J Gastroenterol 1989;451:451.

225. Cappell MS, Hassan T. Pancreatic disease in AIDS—a review. J Clin Gastroenterol 1993;17:254.

226. Cappell MS, Marks M. Acute pancreatitis in HIV-seropositive patients: a case control study of 44 patients. Am J Med 1995;98:243.

227. Strauss J, Abitol C, Zilleruelo G, et al. Renal disease in children with the acquired immunodeficiency syndrome. N Engl J Med 1989;321:625.

228. Ingulli E, Tejani A, Fikrig S, Nicastri A, Chen CK, Pomrantz A. Nephrotic syndrome associated with acquired immunodeficiency syndrome in children. J Pediatr 1991;119:710.

229. Schoeneman MJ, Ghali V, Lieberman K, Reisman L. IgA nephritis in a child with human immunodeficiency virus: a unique form of human immunodeficiency virus-associated nephropathy? Pediatr Nephrol 1992;6:46.

230. Kimmel PL, Phillips TM, Ferreira-Centeno A, Farkas-Szallasi T, Abraham AA, Garrett CT. Brief report: idiotypic IgA nephropathy in patients with human immunodeficiency virus infection. N Engl J Med 1992;327:702.

231. Scott GB, Buck BE, Leterman JG, Bloom FL, Parks WP. Acquired immunodeficiency syndrome in infants. N Engl J Med 1984;310:76.

232. McKinney RE, Pizzo PA, Scott GB, et al. Safety and tolerance of intermittent intravenous and oral zidovudine therapy in human immunodeficiency virus-infected pediatric patients. J Pediatr 1990; 116:640.

233. Ellaurie M, Burns ER, Rubinstein A. Hematologic manifestations in pediatric HIV infection: severe anemia as a prognostic factor. Am J Pediatr Hematol Oncol 1990;12:449.

234. Hilgartner M. Hematologic manifestations in HIV-infected children. J Pediatr 1991;119:S47.

235. Griffin TC, Squires JE, Timmons CF, Buchanan GR. Chronic human parvovirus B19-induced erythroid hypoplasia as the initial manifestation of human immunodeficiency virus infection. J Pediatr 1991;118:899.

236. Parmentier L, Boucary D, Salmon D. Pure red cell aplasia in an HIV-infected patient. AIDS 1992;6:234.

237. Frickhofen N, Abkowitz JL, Safford M, et al. Persistent B19 parvovirus infection in patients infected with human immunodeficiency virus type 1 (HIV-1): a treatable cause of anemia in AIDS. Ann Intern Med 1990;113:926.

238. Dalle JH, Dollfus C, Courpotin C, et al. Human immunodeficiency virus-associated hemophagocytic syndrome in children. Pediatr Infect Dis J 1994;13:1159.

239. Mueller BU, Jacobsen F, Jarosinski P, Lewis LL, Pizzo PA. Erythropoietin for zidovudine-associated anemia in children with HIV-infection. Pediatr AIDS HIV Infect Fetus Adolesc 1994;5:169.

240. Butler KM, Husson RN, Balis FM, et al. Dideoxyinosine in children with symptomatic human immunodeficiency virus infection. N Engl J Med 1991;324:137.

241. Pizzo PA, Eddy J, Falloon J, et al. Effect of continuous intravenous infusion of zidovudine (AZT) in children with symptomatic HIV infection. N Engl J Med 1988;319:889.

242. Mueller BU, Jacobsen F, Butler KM, Husson RN, Lewis LL, Pizzo PA. Combination treatment with azidothymidine and granulocyte colony-stimulating factor in children with human immunodeficiency virus infection. J Pediatr 1992;121:797.

243. Mueller BU. Hematological problems and their management in children with HIV infection. In: Pizzo PA, Wilfert CM, eds. Pediatric AIDS. The challenge of HIV infection in infants, children, and adolescents. 2nd ed. Baltimore: Williams & Wilkins, 1994:591.

244. Labrune P, Blanche S, Catherine N, Maier-Redelsperger M, Delfraissy JF, Tchernia G. Human immunodeficiency virus-associated thrombocytopenia in infants. Acta Paediatr Scan 1989;78:811.

245. Rigaud M, Leibovitz E, Sin Quee C, et al. Thrombocytopenia in children infected with human immunodeficiency virus: long term follow-up and therapeutic considerations. J Acquir Immune Defic Syndr 1992;5:450.

246. Bussel JB, Graziano JN, Kimberly RP, Pahwa S, Aledort LM. Intravenous anti-D treatment of immune thrombocytopenic purpura: analysis of efficacy, toxicity, and mechanism of effect. Blood 1991;77:1884.

247. Pollak AN, Janinis J, Green D. Successful intravenous immune globulin therapy for human immunodeficiency virus-associated thrombocytopenia. Arch Intern Med 1988;148:695.

248. Schwartz LJ, St Louis Y, Wu R, Wiznia A, Rubinstein A, Saenger P. Endocrine function in children with human immunodeficiency virus infection. Am J Dis Child 1991;145:330.

248a. Hirschfeld S. Laue L, Culter GB, Jr., Pizzo PA. Thyroid abnormalities in children infected with human immunodeficiency virus. J Pediatr 1996;128:70.

249. Blethen SL, Nachman S, Chasalow FI. Thyroid function in children with perinatally acquired antibodies to human immunodeficiency virus. J Pediatr Endocrinol 1994;7:1.

250. Grinspoon SK, Bilezikian JP. HIV disease and the endocrine system. N Engl J Med 1992;327:1360.

251. Butler KM, De Smet MD, Husson RN, et al. Treatment of aggressive cytomegalovirus retinitis with ganciclovir in combination with foscarnet in a child infected with human immunodeficiency virus. J Pediatr 1992;120:483.

252. Lopez JS, deSmet MD, Masur H, Mueller BU, Pizzo PA, Nussenblatt RB. Orally administered 566C80 for treatment of ocular toxoplasmosis in a patient with the acquired immunodeficiency syndrome. Am J Ophthalmol 1992;113:331.

253. De Smet MD, Nussenblatt RB. Ocular manifestations of HIV in pediatric populations. In: Pizzo PA, Wilfert CM, eds. Pediatric AIDS. The challenge of HIV infection in infants, children, and adolescents. 2nd ed. Baltimore: Williams & Wilkins, 1994:457.

254. Whitcup S, Butler K, Pizzo P, Nussenblatt R. Retinal lesions in children treated with dideoxyinosine. N Engl J Med 1992;326:1226.

255. Saran BR, Maguire AM, Nichols C, et al. Hypopyon uveitis in patients with acquired immunodeficiency syndrome treated for systemic *Mycobacterium avium* complex infection with rifabutin. Arch Ophthalmol 1994;112:1159.

256. Prose NS. Cutaneous manifestations of HIV infection in children. In: AIDS: a ten-year perspective. , 1991:543.

257. Nance K, V., Smith ML, Joshi VV. Cutaneous manifestations of acquired immunodeficiency syndrome in children. Int J Dermatol 1991; 30:531.

258. Prose NS. Mucocutaneous disease in pediatric human immunodeficiency virus infection. Pediatr Dermatol 1991;38:977.

259. Prose NS, von Knebel-Doeberitz C, Miller S, Milburn PB, Heilman E. Widespread flat warts associated with human papillomavirus type 5: a cutaneous manifestation of human immunodeficiency virus infection. J Am Acad Dermatol 1990;23:978.

260. Hughes WT, Parham DM. Molluscum contagiosum in children with cancer or acquired immunodeficiency syndrome. Pediatr Infect Dis J 1991;10:152.

261. Leibovitz E, Kaul A, Rigaud M, Bebenroth D, Krasinski K, Borkowsky W. Chronic varicella zoster in a child infected with human immunodeficiency virus: case report and review of the literature. Cutis 1992;49:27.

262. Cabanillas F, Armitage J, Pugh WC, Weisenburger D, Duvic M. Lymphomatous papulosis: a T-cell dyscrasia with a propensity to transform into malignant lymphoma. Ann Intern Med 1995; 122:210.

263. Mueller BU, Pizzo PA. Cancer in children with primary or secondary immunodeficiencies. J Pediatr 1995;126:1.

264. Arico M, Caselli D, D'Argenio P, et al. Malignancies in children with human immunodeficiency virus type 1 infection. Cancer 1991; 68:2473.

265. DiCarlo FJ, Joshi VV, Oleske JM, Connor EM. Neoplastic diseases in children with acquired immunodeficiency syndrome. Prog AIDS Pathol 1990;2:163.

266. Connor E, Boccon-Gibod L, Joshi V, et al. Cutaneous acquired immunodeficiency syndrome-associated Kaposi's sarcoma in pediatric patients. Arch Dermatol 1990;126:791.

267. Buck BE, Scott GB, Valdes-Dapena M, Parks WP. Kaposi sarcoma in two infants with acquired immune deficiency syndrome. J Pediatr 1983;103:911.

268. Gutierrez-Ortega P, Hierro-Orozco S, Sanchez-Cisneros R, Montana LF. Kaposi's sarcoma in a 6-day-old infant with human immunodeficiency virus. Arch Dermatol 1989;125:432.

269. Mueller BU, Butler KM, Feuerstein IM, et al. Smooth muscle tumors in children with human immunodeficiency virus infection. Pediatrics 1992;90:460.

270. McClain KL, Leach CT, Jenson HB, et al. Association of Epstein-Barr virus with leiomyosarcomas in young people with AIDS. N Engl J Med 1995;332:12.

271. Lee ES, Locker J, Nalesnik M, et al. The association of Epstein-Barr virus with smooth muscle tumors occurring after organ transplantation. N Engl J Med 1995;332:19.

272. Pizzo PA, Wilfert C. Antiretroviral therapy for infection due to human immunodeficiency virus in children. Clin Infect Dis 1994;19:177.

273. Balis FM, Pizzo PA, Eddy J, et al. Pharmacokinetics of zidovudine administered intravenously and orally in children with human immunodeficiency virus infection. J Pediatr 1989;114:880.

274. Balis FM, Pizzo PA, Murphy RF, et al. The pharmacokinetics of zidovudine administered by continuous infusion in children. Ann Intern Med 1989;110:279.

275. Balis FM, Poplack DG. Drug development and clinical pharmacology. In: Pizzo PA, Wilfert CA, eds. Pediatric AIDS. The challenge of HIV infection in infants, children, and adolescents. Baltimore: Williams & Wilkins, 1991:457.

276. Lyman WD, Tanaka KE, Kress Y, Rashbaum WK, Rubinstein A, Soeiro R. Zidovudine concentrations in human fetal tissue: implications for perinatal AIDS. Lancet 1990;335:1280.

277. Chavanet P, Diquet B, Waldner A. Perinatal pharmacokinetics of zidovudine. N Engl J Med 1989;321:1548.

278. Watts DH, Brown ZA, Tartaglione T, et al. Pharmacokinetic disposition of zidovudine during pregnancy. J Infect Dis 1991;163:226.

279. Boucher FD, Au DS, Martin DM, et al. Pharmacokinetics and safety of azidothymidine (AZT) in infants less than three months old, exposed at birth to HIV. Clin Res 1989;37:190A.

280. Boucher FD, Modlin JF, Weller S, et al. Phase I evaluation of zidovudine administered to infants exposed at birth to the human immunodeficiency virus. J Pediatr 1993;122:137.

281. Brouwers P, Moss H, Wolters P, et al. Effect of continuous-infusion zidovudine therapy on neuropsychologic functioning in children with symptomatic human immunodeficiency virus infection. J Pediatr 1990;117:980.

282. DeCarli C, Fugate L, Falloon J, et al. Brain growth and cognitive improvement in children with human immunodeficiency virus-induced encephalopathy after 6 months of continuous infusion zidovudine therapy. J Acquir Immune Defic Syndr 1991;4:585.

283. McKinney RE, Maha MA, Connor EM, et al. A multicenter trial of oral zidovudine in children with advanced human immunodeficiency virus disease. N Engl J Med 1991;324:1018.

284. Balis FM, Pizzo PA, Butler KM, et al. Clinical pharmacology of 2′,3′-dideoxyinosine in human immunodeficiency virus-infected children. J Infect Dis 1992;165:99.

285. Mueller BU, Butler KM, Stocker VL, et al. Clinical and pharmacokinetic evaluation of long-term therapy with didanosine in children with HIV infection. Pediatrics 1994;94:724.

286. Blanche S, Calvez T, Rouzioux C, et al. Randomized study of two doses of didanosine in children infected with human immunodeficiency virus. J Pediatr 1993;122:966.

287. Whitcup SM, Butler KM, Caruso R, et al. Retinal toxicity in human immunodeficiency virus-infected children treated with 2′,3′-dideoxyinosine. Am J Ophthalmol 1992;113:1.

287a. Kline MW, Dunkle LM, Church JA, et al. A phase I/II evaluation of stavudine (d4T) in children with human immunodeficiency virus infection. Pediatrics 1995;96:247.

288. Husson RN, Mueller BU, Farley M, et al. Zidovudine and didanosine combination therapy in children with human immunodeficiency virus infection. Pediatrics 1994;93:316.

289. Centers for Disease Control and Prevention. Recommendations of the Advisory Committee on Immunization Practices (ACIP): use of vaccines and immune globulins in persons with altered immunocompetence. MMWR 1993;42:1.

290. Adamson PC, Wu TC, Meade BD, Rubin M, Manclark CR, Pizzo PA. Pertussis in a previously immunized child with human immunodeficiency virus infection. J Pediatr 1989;115:598.

291. Mofenson LM, Moye J Jr, Bethel J, et al. Prophylactic intravenous immunoglobulin in HIV-infected children with CD4 counts of $0.02 \times 10^9/L$ or more. Effect on viral, opportunistic, and bacterial infections. JAMA 1992;268:483.

292. Yap PL. Does intravenous immune globulin have a role in HIV-infected patients? Clin Exp Immunol 1994;1:59.

293. The National Institute of Child Health and Human Development Intravenous Immunoglobulin Study Group. Intravenous immune globulin for the prevention of bacterial infections in children with symptomatic human immunodeficiency virus infection. N Engl J Med 1991;325:73.

294. Schiff RI. Transmission of viral infections through intravenous immune globulin. N Engl J Med 1994;331:1649.

PART V

Treatment of HIV Infection

AIDS: Biology, Diagnosis, Treatment and Prevention, fourth edition, edited by Vincent T. DeVita, Jr., Samuel Hellman, and Steven A. Rosenberg. Lippincott–Raven Publishers, © 1997

CHAPTER 21

Strategies and Progress in the Development of Antiretroviral Agents

Steven M. Schnittman and Carla B. Pettinelli

The development of effective antiviral therapies for the treatment of individuals infected with the human immunodeficiency virus (HIV) presents unique challenges. The integration of the virus into the host cell DNA, the dependence of the virus on host cell machinery, the high mutation rate of HIV reverse transcriptase, and the chronicity of viral replication represent formidable obstacles to the development of specific and effective antiretroviral therapies. HIV presents other challenges as well because of its progressive destruction of the cells critical for orchestrating the immune response against the virus and opportunistic diseases.

It is the goal of HIV therapeutics to attempt to cure HIV infection or, if that is not possible, to stop HIV disease progression while preserving a high quality of life for the afflicted. This may be achieved by effectively interfering with the viral life cycle and the pathogenic processes and by slowing or reversing the progressive immunologic dysfunction that leads to the complications of HIV infection. Considerable progress has been made in understanding the virus and HIV disease pathogenesis, which led to the discovery and development of a variety of agents that might have a role in treating HIV infection.

This chapter reviews the most important progress and strategies for HIV antiviral treatment research for adult HIV-infected patients. These priorities include discovery and development of new antiretroviral compounds and their application as monotherapies and in combination therapy

approaches; understanding the mechanisms of HIV resistance to antiretroviral agents and developing strategies for overcoming them; novel antiviral approaches, including gene therapy; the role of surrogate markers in clinical trials for speeding the development of promising therapies; and clinical research to expand our knowledge of the pathogenesis of HIV infection, especially primary HIV infection.

ANTIRETROVIRAL THERAPIES

Nucleoside Reverse Transcriptase Inhibitors

The only drugs approved for the treatment of HIV-1 infection are zidovudine (ZDV, AZT), didanosine (ddI), zalcitabine (ddC), and stavudine (d4T)).They belong to the class of nucleoside reverse transcriptase (RT) inhibitors (Fig. 21-1).

ZDV delays HIV progression and improves survival in HIV-1–infected patients with advanced disease.[1] The beneficial effect of ZDV, however, appears to diminish over time.[2] Early therapeutic interventions in asymptomatic individuals showed an initial clinical benefit that does not appear to be maintained for a prolonged period.[3-5] The drugs ddI and d4T have produced a beneficial effect in ZDV-treated patients.[6,7] The drug ddC appears to be at least as efficacious as ddI in delaying disease progression and death in patients who are intolerant of or are failing ZDV,[8] but it is not effective in ZDV-experienced patients.[9]

Overall, the clinical benefit provided by monotherapy with a nucleoside RT inhibitor is modest. Several factors may contribute to this finding: limited biologic activity with incomplete viral suppression, development of drug resistance, poor long-term tolerability, evolution of more virulent HIV strains, and possible development of "cellular resistance" to the nucleosides. In individuals with advanced HIV-1 infection, changes in CD4+ T-cell counts or in levels of HIV viremia as measured by plasma HIV RNA poly-

Steven M. Schnittman, Therapeutics Research Program, Division of AIDS, National Institutes of Allergy and Infectious Diseases, National Institutes of Health, Room 2C22, 6003 Executive Boulevard, Rockville, MD 20952.
Carla B. Pettinelli, Therapeutics Research Program, Division of AIDS, National Institutes of Allergy and Infectious Diseases, National Institutes of Health, Room 2C22, 6003 Executive Boulevard, Rockville, MD 20952.

Steps in Viral Replication
 1. Attachment

 2. Uncoating
 3. Reverse Transcription*

 4. RNAseH Degradation
 5. DNA Synthesis of Second Strand

 6. Migration to Nucleus
 7. Integration*

 8. Latency

 9. Activation of Virus*

 10. Transcription or RNA Processing*

 11. Protein Synthesis

 12. Protein Glycosylation*

 13. Assembly of Virus

 14. Release of Virus
 15. Maturation*

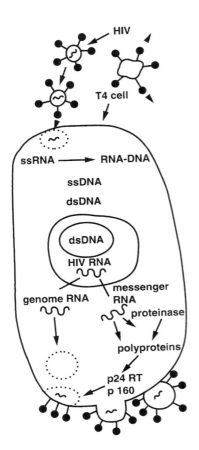

FIG. 21-1. The life cycle of HIV-1. (Adapted from Devita VT, Hellman S, Rosenberg SA (eds). AIDS: etiology, diagnosis, treatment and prevention, Philadelphia: JB Lippincott, 1992. *steps in viral replication for which therapeutic agents are described in the text.

merase chain reaction (PCR) methods predict clinical outcome.[10,11] In HIV-infected patients, nucleoside RT inhibitors are less potent with respect to their impact on such immunologic and virologic parameters than some of the protease and (at least initially) nonnucleoside RT inhibitors. Resistance to nucleosides has been observed in vitro and in vivo,[12] and data have shown that high-level resistance to ZDV predicted more rapid clinical progression and death of patients with advanced disease.[13] Despite the limited clinical benefit, the quest for more efficacious, less toxic, less resistance-inducing nucleoside RT inhibitors has continued, particularly with the goal of evaluating combination therapies.

Lamivudine (3TC) is a relatively new RT inhibitor with potent antiretroviral activity in vitro, good oral bioavailability, and less toxicity than ZDV. Resistance has been generated against 3TC in vitro and in vivo, caused by a unique single base change at position 184, which appears to fortuitously restore sensitivity to ZDV in vitro.[14] HIV-1 isolates with this mutation show less growth in vitro than the wild type.[15] A combination of 3TC with ZDV has produced profound and sustained immunologic and virologic responses[16,17] and is now in advanced clinical testing.

Some of the other nucleosides in early clinical testing include the Wellcome compounds 524W91, 1592U89, and 935U83 and U.S. BioScience's F-ddA. They are all potent inhibitors of RT in vitro with less toxicity than ZDV in pre-

clinical studies. These compounds are synergistic in vitro and generally non–cross-resistant with other RT inhibitors.

Because of incomplete viral suppression, the availability of nucleoside RT inhibitors with different toxicity profiles, the general lack of in vitro antagonism when tested in combination, the different activity in resting and proliferating cells, and the fact that some mutations induced in the RT may suppress ZDV resistance mutations, the evaluation of nucleoside RT inhibitors in combination has been a high clinical research priority. Concomitant combination therapy has produced sustained higher CD4+ T-cell counts and more profound viral suppression compared with monotherapy.[17–20] However, the limited clinical data available (ie, only in advanced patients with >6 months of therapy) are not encouraging.[9] No clinical efficacy data are available for antiretroviral-naive patients, who potentially may benefit the most from combination therapy. Completion of several clinical trials during the latter half of 1995 should provide a better understanding of the role of nucleoside RT inhibitors in the overall treatment of HIV infection.

Nonnucleoside Reverse Transcriptase Inhibitors

Nonnucleoside RT inhibitors (NNRTIs) are potent inhibitors of HIV-1 (but not of other retroviruses) RT. They target a nonsubstrate binding site of the RT enzyme and do not require activation through cellular metabolism. NNRTIs are synergistic in vitro with nucleoside RT inhibitors, and they inhibit ZDV-resistant isolates. Unfortunately, they induce the rapid development of resistance in vitro[21] and in vivo,[22–24] which appears to be temporally related to the loss of antiviral activity. Despite the emergence of resistance, certain patients still appear to benefit from NNRTIs.[24]

Establishing a role for NNRTIs in the management of HIV disease is a challenging task. Their development is being pursued, particularly in combination with nucleoside RT inhibitors. Such combinations could prevent the emergence of resistant isolates, or NNRTI-induced mutations may restore sensitivity to ZDV or other NNRTIs. However, combination with ZDV has not prevented the emergence of NNRTI resistance[25] even though a delayed development of NNRTI-resistant isolates has been observed.[26,27] A phase II clinical study comparing triple drug combination nevirapine (an NNRTI), ddI, and ZDV to the combination of ddI and ZDV showed that the triple combination had more potent immunologic and virologic effect.[28] Clinical efficacy trials are evaluating NNRTIs (ie, delavirdine plus nevirapine) in double or triple combination with RT inhibitors.

Protease or Proteinase Inhibitors

HIV-1 encodes a unique protease that enzymatically cleaves the Gag-Pol polyprotein to produce individual structural proteins and enzymes (see Fig. 21-1).[29] This proteolytic process is essential for the production of mature, infectious virions. HIV-1 protease belongs to the aspartyl protease class, and its function and three-dimensional structure have been known for several years.[30,31] HIV-1 protease is a dimer exhibiting twofold rotational (C2) symmetry on crystallography. Protease has been an important target for directed drug design,[32] and numerous pharmaceutical manufacturers have actively pursued discovery programs for inhibitors of this enzyme (Fig. 21-2).

Several protease inhibitors, such as Ro 31-8959, MK-639 (formerly L-735,524), and ABT-538, are being evaluated in phase II/III clinical testing of HIV-infected individuals. These compounds are peptidomimetic and share common properties, including potent in vitro inhibitory effect on HIV-1 replication in acutely and chronically infected cells; in vitro synergy with RT inhibitors in single or multiple combinations; complex synthetic process with consequent limited drug availability; and development of resistance in vitro or in vivo,[33–35] with preliminary evidence of cross-resistance.[35]

Preliminary data from phase I and II clinical trials have shown potent antiretroviral effect as measured by increases in CD4+ T-cell counts and declines in plasma HIV RNA. The antiretroviral activity, however, appears transient, with a peak in the first weeks of therapy followed by a slow return toward baseline by weeks 12 to 24.[36–38] This loss of antiretroviral effect in vivo appears to be temporally associated with resistance as has been shown for L-735,524.[39]

Protease inhibitors are synergistic with RT inhibitors, and consequently, multitarget combination studies are being conducted. A phase II study evaluating saquinavir with one or two nucleoside RT inhibitors has shown that the triple drug combination (ie, saquinavir [Ro 31-8959] plus ddC plus ZDV) has greater immunologic and virologic activity

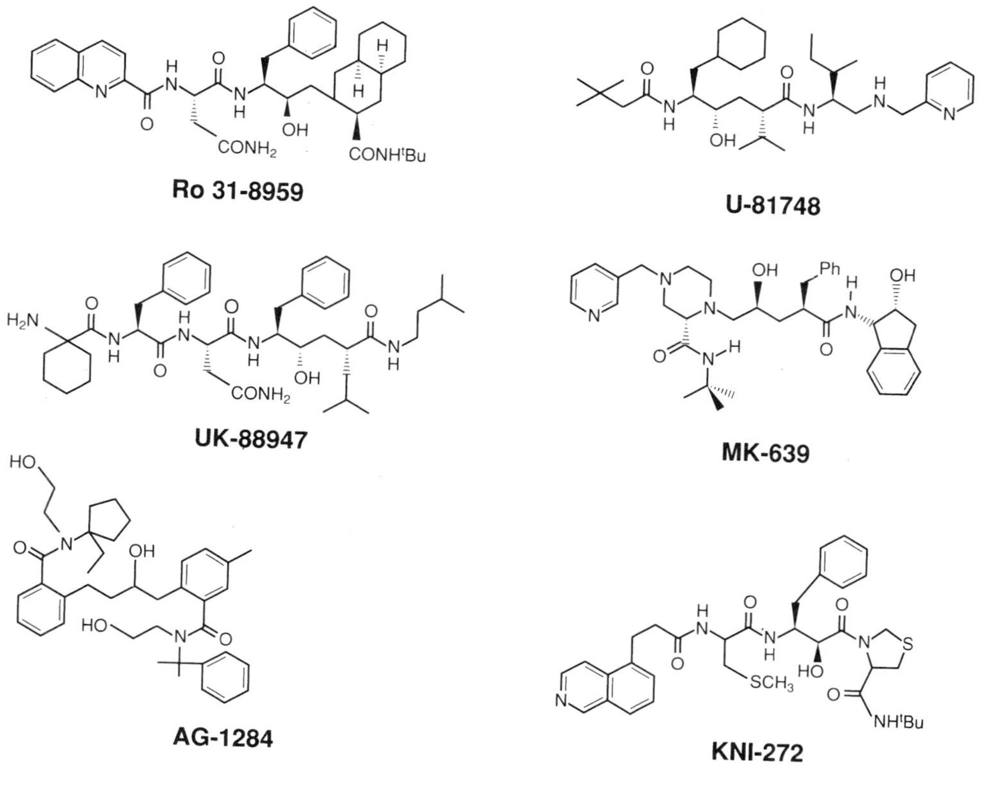

FIG. 21-2. Representative inhibitors of HIV-1 protease.

than the combination of saquinavir plus ZDV or ddC plus ZDV.[40] This triple combination is being evaluated for clinical efficacy in phase III studies. It is critical to assess how the biologic activity of protease inhibitors can predict their potential clinical efficacy.

Combination studies aimed at assessing the clinical efficacy of nucleoside RT inhibitors with other protease inhibitors, including MK-639 or ABT-538, are also underway. Considering their biologic potency, it will be important to evaluate protease inhibitors in combination, regardless of cross-resistance and possible pharmacologic interactions. Despite the challenges, including the observation that the binding of a protease inhibitor to the human serum α_1-acid glycoprotein leads to major decreases in cell uptake and subsequent decreased activity in vitro and in vivo,[41,42] several new proteinase inhibitors with novel structures, including KNI-272, AG-1343, and VTX-478[43-45] are being evaluated in early clinical trials, and several others are undergoing preclinical testing.

Integrase Inhibitors

Integration of HIV-1 DNA into the genome of the host cell is an essential step in the HIV-1 life cycle (see Fig. 21-1). Integrase, a unique HIV enzyme with no known analogous function in humans, catalyzes several steps (ie, cleavage, strand transfer, disintegration) of the integration process.[46] Until recently, the progress in identifying appropriate integrase inhibitors was hindered by the inability to determine its structure and by the lack of an adequate in vitro cellular screen. The poor solubility of HIV-1 integrase has made it difficult to crystallize, but Dyda and collaborators have been able to crystallize and identify the structure of the catalytically active core domain of the integrase after improving its solubility through the insertion of a single amino acid substitution (Fig. 21-3).[47]

The structure of the core domain consists of a central five-stranded beta sheet and six helices and is similar to ribonuclease H. This finding should facilitate the identification of suitable integrase inhibitors. In vitro acellular screening systems for integrase inhibitors have been optimized for high-output screening. Using such assays, several inhibitors have been identified, including topoisomerase inhibitors (ie, doxorubicin-like agents),[48] intercalators,[48] aurintricarboxylic acids,[49] and nucleotides. The normal metabolites of ZDV can inhibit HIV-1 integrase at concentrations achievable in vitro, suggesting the possibility that inhibition of viral integration may contribute to the in vivo potency of ZDV.[50] In general, most of the compounds identified in the screen are nonspecific and highly toxic in vitro. PCR-based assays that can detect the rate of viral integration in intact cellular systems have been developed and allow identification of compounds capable of blocking integrase specifically in vivo. Several pharmaceutical companies are actively pursuing this field, and integrase inhibitors may be soon in clinical trials.

Tat Inhibitors

The *tat* gene encodes an 86–amino acid protein that is a potent activator of HIV replication.[51,52] *Tat*-defective HIV-1 clones have been shown to be unable to replicate in most in vitro systems. However, tumor necrosis factor-α can replace the requirement for a functional Tat protein.[53] In 1991, a potent in vitro Tat antagonist (ie, Ro 5-3335) with activity in acutely

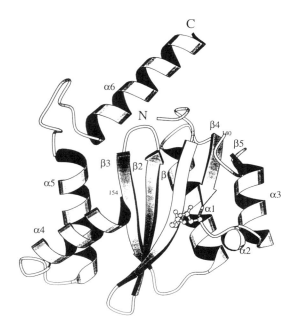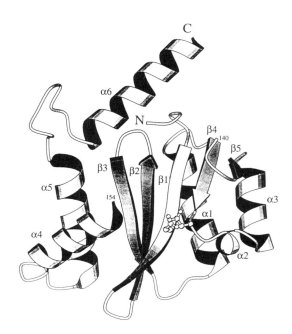

FIG. 21-3. Structure of HIV-1 integrase; stereoscopic image pair of the catalytically active core domain (Courtesy of Dr. Frederick Dyda, National Institutes of Health, Bethesda, MD).

and chronically infected cells was discovered.[54] An analog of this compound (Ro 24-7429) with similar potency was tested in a phase I/II study in HIV-1–infected individuals.[55] Unfortunately, Ro 24-7429 failed to show any evidence of biologic activity, even at doses that have produced plasma concentrations well above the in vitro 90% inhibitory concentration (IC_{90}). The reason for the lack of Ro 24-7429 antiretroviral activity is not fully understood, but several hypotheses have been suggested, including high protein binding and cell-dependent activity.[56] More research is needed to define the roles of Tat antagonists as antiretrovirals.

Other Inhibitors

Glycosidase Inhibitors

Compounds aimed at interfering with the glycosylation of gp120 have been identified and are in clinical testing (see Fig. 21-1). SC-48334 is an α-glucosidase I inhibitor that blocks HIV replication and syncytial formation in vitro and is synergistic with nucleoside RT inhibitors.[57,58] When tested in early clinical trials, SC-48334 was poorly tolerated; the most common side effect was severe diarrhea associated with weight loss.[59] A prodrug, SC-49483, appears to ameliorate this toxicity profile and is being evaluated in combination with ZDV in a phase II study. This study also is attempting to determine if the activity of SC-48334 is mainly directed toward syncytia-inducing HIV viruses. MDL-28,574 is another glucosidase I inhibitor being tested in a phase I study in early asymptomatic patients. Positive results from any of these trials could enhance the interest in this therapeutic approach.

Antisense Oligonucleotides

Sequence-specific antisense oligodeoxynucleotides that can potentially bind to viral RNA, viral mRNA, or integrated viral DNA have been under consideration as a possible tool for HIV-1 therapeutic intervention (see Fig. 21-1).[60] These nucleotides inhibit HIV replication in vivo, but specificity, cell delivery, and cellular degradation have been some of the obstacles in identifying antisense oligonucleotides appropriate for clinical evaluation. Phosphorothioate oligonucleotides appear to be good candidates; they are nuclease resistant, can hybridize with their mRNA target at physiologic temperature, and appear to be internalized in cells. Antisense oligonucleotides directed to the HIV-1 *rev-, tar-,* and *gag*-encoded mRNA have been evaluated in vitro.

Only one antisense oligonucleotide specifically directed against HIV-1, gene-expression modulator 91 (Gem 91), is in phase I/II clinical trials. Gem 91 is an investigational 25-nucleotide antisense oligodeoxynucleotide phosphorothioate complementary to the gag mRNA and therefore designed to inhibit the translation of the *gag*-encoded mRNA. In vitro, GEM 91 undergoes rapid uptake by lymphocytes and monocytes and is a potent inhibitor of laboratory and clini-

cal strains of HIV-1.[61] In animals, GEM 91 is widely distributed in tissues. Single dose escalating studies have shown the compound to be safe, and further evaluations aimed at establishing the safety and preliminary antiviral activity are ongoing.

Inhibitors of Accessory Proteins

HIV-1 encodes genes for at least five auxiliary proteins (ie, Vif, Vpr, Tat, Rev, Vpu, and Nef)[62,63] in addition to the Gag, Pol, and Env structural proteins. Although Tat or Rev are essential for viral replication in several in vitro systems, the others appear mainly to modulate viral replication. Vpr (viral protein R) is of particular interest because of a report in which Vpr appears to regulate HIV-1 transactivation and viral replication through the glucocorticoid receptor type II complex DNA target sequence.[64] Vpr augments viral production mainly in primary macrophages. Mifepristone, a specific inhibitor of the glucocorticoid pathway that has been studied in humans for other indications, is a potent inhibitor of virus replication and can inhibit the increase in virus production stimulated by Vpr or steroids in vitro.[64] This finding permits studies that can define the effect that a glucocorticoid receptor type II complex inhibitor has on virus production in vivo.

GENE THERAPY FOR HIV INFECTION

Progress in the development of conventional antiretroviral therapies that can arrest HIV viral replication, eradicate infected cell reservoirs, and restore a functional immune system has demonstrated the severe limitations in these efforts. Consequently, the development of novel treatment strategies such as gene therapy are receiving significant attention. In its broadest concept, gene therapy is an approach in which genes that can protect against HIV spread or permit reconstitution of an immune system that is resistant to HIV infection can be used to treat the infected host.[65]

Intracellular immunization is a term used to describe a process in which cells are genetically altered to become resistant to pathogens.[66] This process is achieved by stable introduction into cells of a DNA template (ie, a resistance gene) whose continuous expression inhibits the expression of an essential viral gene and hence inhibits viral replication. Because HIV infects hemopoietic cells, insertion of resistance genes into such cells could reduce the spread of virus in the body.

One such approach involves a novel inhibition strategy employing *trans*-acting–response (TAR) element decoys to block the function of the HIV *tat* gene.[67,68] Overexpression of RNA containing TAR is capable of acting as a decoy for Tat binding, preventing its binding to the TAR sequence in the viral RNA. This inhibited HIV viral replication with laboratory HIV isolates in established cell lines more completely than with clinical isolates, although virus breakthrough eventually occurred in all studies.

An extension of this inhibition strategy to the Rev system (ie, Rev-responsive element [RRE] decoys) appears to be much more potent than TAR decoys.[69] RRE decoys have been designed that are only 13 nucleotides long and are unable to bind host cell factors and are therefore less likely to cause cellular toxicity when expressed.[70] Expression of these RRE decoys in established and primary peripheral blood lymphocytes (PBLs) completely blocks HIV replication in vitro.

Another gene therapy approach involves the use of transdominant mutants of HIV-1 regulatory genes, such as *rev* and *tat,* which would be incapable of binding RRE and TAR, respectively, thereby blocking HIV replication.[71–75] Studies of a transdominant *rev* mutant (M10) in vitro have demonstrated complete inhibition of virus growth and protection of cells for as long as 30 days for laboratory strains and shorter for clinical isolates (Fig. 21-4).[76] A phase I clinical trial in HIV-infected individuals to assess the survival of M10-modified CD4 cells began in mid-1994.[76] Combinations of Tat/Rev fusion transdominant inhibitors are being studied and appear to be more effective in blocking HIV replication than either transdominant alone.

Ribozymes, or self-catalytic RNAs, represent another approach to inhibit the function of a critical portion of the viral genomic RNAs.[77] These nucleic acid enzymes have been successfully introduced into T-cell lines and PBLs from patients with HIV infection, as well as into progenitor hematopoietic cells, and protection against HIV infection was demonstrated in these cells.[78–82] In these studies, ribozymes were shown to be capable of destroying HIV RNA as it enters an uninfected cell in vitro, thereby diminishing the number of provirus copies in the host genome. Once fully developed, ribozymes may block the establishment of virus in target cells. In other studies, ribozymes were designed that co-localize with viral RNA, thereby destroying newly synthesized genome as it buds out of the infected cell. Ribozymes that include a combination of activities targeting different HIV RNAs are under development.[83] A phase I study involving the *ex vivo* modification of autologous PBL-derived CD4+ T cells with anti-HIV ribozyme and their reinfusion is planned.

Another intracellular antiviral approach involves single-chain intracellular antibodies.[84,85] This technology uses genes that are tailored to produce intracellular antibody (single-chain) fragments that bind HIV Env, Rev, Tat, or RT and that have the capacity to sequester the target protein in an inappropriate subcellular compartment. These single-chain antibody–HIV protein complexes are trapped in the subcellular compartment, blocking HIV replication or maturation.

Each of these approaches depends on the development of appropriate retroviral or other vectors or methods to deliver the gene of interest safely to the target cell and to ensure that appropriate levels of expression are maintained and controlled. Most experience has been with retrovirus vectors that express the transferred gene after integration but do not result in production of virions capable of a round of infection.[86] Retroviral vectors generally produce low titers of recombinant viruses and express low levels of the genes of interest in primary hemopoietic cells. These nonreplicating vectors require dividing cells to be expressed. Because of the deficiencies with retroviral vectors, other approaches are being developed. Progress is being made with adeno-associated virus vectors, which are nonpathogenic and can infect nonreplicating cells.[87,88] Progress is also being made with nonpathogenic HIV vectors designed for the specific use in HIV-infected patients; such vectors should target an antivi-

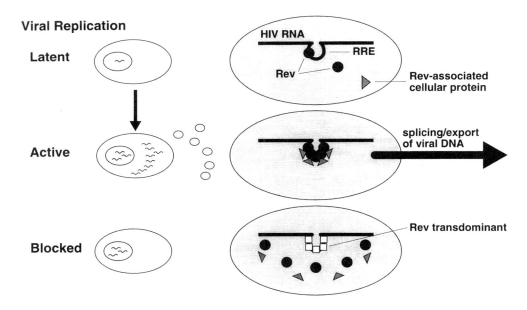

FIG. 21-4. Gene Therapy. Schematic of a M10 transdominant rev mutant (M10) that is incapable of binding the Rev Responsive Element (RRE), thereby blocking HIV replication (Courtesy of Dr. Gary Nabel, University of Michigan.)

ral gene to the same cells that are normally susceptible to HIV infection.[89,90] Much attention is being given to the development of nonviral delivery methods, such as liposomes and gene guns; these approaches obviate the risk of viral vectors to patients.

For the most part, gene therapies for HIV have used mature CD4+ T cells as targets because of the ease of availability from patient PBLs. However, PBLs have many limitations, including their limited in vivo growth and differentiation potential and their limited life span. Consequently, intense efforts are underway to develop approaches that employ pluripotent hematopoietic stem cells derived from one of several sources, including bone marrow, cord blood, and peripheral blood after mobilization from the bone marrow. Theoretically, such cells should be protected with an anti-HIV gene and could convey this protection to all of their hemopoietic progeny of various stages of differentiation and development. With the considerable progress that is being made in isolation and purification of human stem cells, there is hope that this approach will eventually be successful.

STRATEGIES AND PRIORITIES FOR SURROGATE END POINTS OF HIV INFECTION

HIV infection or AIDS is a chronic disease in which the clinical end points of time to opportunistic disease and death require considerable time and great expense in the context of clinical trials. However, it is the goal of researchers and their patients to assess the effectiveness of new drugs to treat HIV infection as rapidly as possible. The challenge to drug developers, study designers, and regulatory reviewers is one of balancing the need to accelerate decision making with the desire for a better understanding of how best to use any new drug or therapeutic intervention.

There are advantages to trial design, cost, and feasibility when a rare or distal end point is replaced by a more frequent or proximate end point. The true end point measurement may be unduly invasive, uncomfortable, or expensive, and the researcher therefore may accept a degree of measurement error regarding the timing or even the occurrence of a true end point. End point events close in time to the treatment or intervention under study may be more readily interpreted than more distal end points, such as study subject death, which may be confounded by secondary treatments or competing risks.

The median time from initial HIV infection to the development of symptomatic AIDS is about 11 years. The use of ZDV and other antiretroviral agents has extended survival to a median of 3 years after the diagnosis of AIDS.[91] Wide use of prophylactic therapies, such as those to prevent *Pneumocystis carinii* pneumonia, can delay the development of opportunistic complications until much further in the course of immunosuppression.

There have been many definitions of a surrogate end point, including the following:

An end point employed when the end point of interest is too difficult or expensive to measure routinely and when another, more readily measurable end point is sufficiently well correlated with the first[92]

An end point measured in lieu of another "true" end point[93]

An observed variable that relates in some way to the variable of primary interest, which we cannot conveniently observe directly[94]

A response for which a test of the null hypothesis of no relationship to the treatment groups under comparison is also valid of the corresponding null hypothesis based on the true end point (ie, Prentice criteria).[95]

A useful surrogate end point should have the potential to yield unambiguous information about differential treatment effects on the true end point. The surrogate variable should capture any relationship between the treatment and the true end point, a notion that can be operationalized by requiring the true end point rate at any follow-up time to be independent of treatment, given the preceding history of the surrogate variable.

An important distinction must be made between activity markers, prognostic markers, and surrogate end points. An activity marker is any measure of disease that may be affected by a therapeutic intervention but that may or may not translate into a clinical outcome benefit. A prognostic marker is a parameter of disease that can predict a clinical outcome or disease progression (Table 21-1). For HIV infection, typical activity and prognostic markers include immunologic parameters[96] such as CD4+ T-cell number, levels of β_2-microglobulin, or serum neopterin; proliferative responses to anti-CD3 monoclonal antibodies; and virologic markers such as HIV RNA viremia and HIV DNA and viral phenotypes.[97] Few activity or prognostic markers have been formally evaluated for their ability to serve as a surrogate marker, to demonstrate a change in response to a therapeutic intervention in a way that parallels or predicts the change in clinical outcome in response to such a therapy. A study is needed that has already demonstrated a differential clinical outcome before it is possible to test the strength of surrogacy–and these are rare in HIV or AIDS clinical trials.

CD4+ T-cell number has been studied in numerous antiretroviral clinical trials and has been found to be a partial

TABLE 21-1. *Markers correlated with HIV disease progression*

Immunologic Markers	Virologic Markers
CD4 cell number*, percent	p24 Antigen, ICD p24
β_2-microglobulin	Quantitative viral culture
Serum neopterin	HIV DNA
Lymphocyte proliferation	Quantitative HIV RNA*
Delayed-type hypersensitivity	Antiviral resistance
	Biologic phenotype (SI, NSI)

*Formally demonstrated to behave as partial surrogate markers for nucleoside antiretrovirals.

surrogate end point at best. In these evaluations, the effect of a treatment on the CD4+ T-cell number generally can explain no more than 30% of the effect of a nucleoside treatment on clinical outcome.[98] The failure of CD4+ T-cell number to serve as a surrogate marker for clinical outcomes is best highlighted by the Concorde trial, in which individuals were randomized to receive ZDV immediately or later with the onset of symptoms.[99] Despite an elevation in the CD4+ T-cell count of a mean of 30 cells/mm³, which persisted for the duration of the study, no difference in progression to AIDS-related complex, AIDS, or death was seen between the two arms. The incompleteness of CD4+ T-cell number as a surrogate marker for clinical end points may only reflect the low potency of the agents that have been studied. For therapies with a much greater impact on overall disease progression, it is entirely possible that changes in CD4 numbers may be a much better predictor of therapeutic response.

The investigation of virologic markers in HIV-infected individuals appears more promising. Changes in HIV viremia in response to an antiviral, as measured by semi-quantitative HIV RNA PCR-based analyses of plasma, have been able to explain a larger fraction of the effect of such a drug on the differential clinical outcome.[11,100]

Data from clinical studies, natural history studies, and studies of vertical transmission suggest that there may be a lower limit of viral burden below which disease progression is significantly diminished (ie, threshold effect).[97] These studies demonstrate an association of higher baseline HIV-1 plasma RNA copy number in patients with more rapid clinical progression than in patients with lower copy numbers. The trials also demonstrate that a decrease in HIV-1 plasma RNA copy number in response to a nucleoside is associated with a decreased relative risk of disease progression. Antiviral activity, as measured by short-term increases in CD4+ T-cell number and an early delay in progression of disease, is greatest in patients with higher viral loads.[100–103] Many of these surrogate variables are highly correlated with each other; lower CD4+ T-cell counts, the development of genotypic resistance to nucleosides, and the diagnosis of AIDS are all correlated with increases in viral copy number.

Those involved in the development of clinical trials of HIV therapies are all too aware of the inability to do prolonged trials that can reach meaningful clinical end points and of the great difficulty in being able to maintain patients on their assigned study drugs for very long. It is therefore one the highest priorities of clinical research that further evaluation of potential surrogate end points continues unabated.

PRIMARY HIV INFECTION

In an effort to more fully understand the pathogenesis of HIV-1 infection, there has been considerable investigation of the period immediately following the initial onset of infection with the virus. This period of new infection and the constellation of symptoms associated with it is referred to as primary or acute HIV-1 infection (PHI).

There are estimated to be at least 40,000 new cases of HIV-1 infection in the United States annually, most of whom will develop a spectrum of symptoms.[104,105] The clinical syndrome of PHI is typified by the acute onset of a febrile illness resembling acute mononucleosis, with symptoms that may include headache, myalgia, pharyngitis, lymphadenopathy, maculopapular rash, aphthous ulcers, weight loss, retroorbital pain, nausea, diarrhea, or meningeal signs.[106] Patients with symptomatic PHI usually present for medical attention about 2 to 6 weeks after exposure to HIV-1. The symptoms, which typically resolve within 1 to 2 weeks, occur in tandem with high-grade viremia, as measured by p24 serum antigen, plasma viremia (including RNA PCR), and high-titer HIV-1 cell co-cultures. The rapid development of HIV-specific antibodies[107–110] and HIV-1–specific cytotoxic T lymphocytes occurs with the prompt disappearance of the virologic parameters. This development of specific host immunity, which leads to a several-log decline in measurable HIV-1 plasma virus, strongly suggests the importance of the immune system in controlling HIV-1 replication in the earliest stages of infection.

What the prognostic implications of symptomatic and asymptomatic PHI are remains uncertain. There is evidence from retrospective analyses that individuals who develop symptomatic PHI are at risk for more rapid disease progression than those who are asymptomatic.[111] These observations appear to be confirmed by experience with patients enrolled in prospective clinical trials.[112,113]

The period of PHI is one marked by highly dynamic properties of virologic and immunologic parameters. The levels of p24 antigen, plasma viremia, and viral cell co-culture during PHI are extraordinarily high, commonly with 10^{10} to 10^{11} HIV viral particles per microliter of blood detected. These viral titers decrease substantially over the ensuing few weeks.[107–109] Studies in which the virus of patients taken from the period of PHI is cloned and sequenced reveals a remarkable homogeneity, typically with only one principal strain that is usually monocytotropic.[114] This is in distinct contrast to the considerable heterogeneity of virus that is seen in chronic HIV infection.

There is evidence of substantial immune activation, as measured by high levels of serum neopterin, β_2-microglobulin, interferon-α, and T_{H2}-type cytokines, as well as the number of circulating activated T cells during this period.[109,115] Serum antibodies rapidly appear against HIV, although it seems that specific neutralizing antibodies occur much later. The detection of cytotoxic T lymphocytes may precede the establishment of humoral responses to the virus, further underlining the critical importance of the cell-mediated immune response in the initial clearing of viremia.[116] Responses to other antigens and mitogens are also acutely impaired and begin to return to normal values over the next 6 to 12 months.[117,118]

The CD4+ T cells typically decrease to a mean of 349 cells/mm³[119] within 6 to 12 months after seroconversion, followed by the more gradual decline typical of chronic HIV-1 infection. This decline in CD4+ T cells is usually accompanied by an expansion of CD8+ T cells, leading to a reversal of the ratio of CD4 to CD8 cells. Preliminary evidence suggests that the pattern of T-cell receptor V-β usage, which recognizes HIV epitopes during early HIV infection, is associated with the rate of disease progression; monoclonal or oligoclonal T-cell receptor V-βs employed are associated with more rapid progression compared with polyclonal responses.[120]

The effects of antiviral therapies on acute retroviral replication have been described in numerous animal studies.[106] Interpretation of these studies must be tempered by the innumerable variables, including the retrovirus species and animal species employed, inoculum size, route of infection, timing of treatment and intervention, method of viral detection, and length of follow-up. In general, murine or feline oncogenic models evaluating postexposure therapies have been unsuccessful in preventing or eradicating retroviral infections. There is some evidence, however, for suppression or reduction of viral load, diminished clinical manifestations, and prolonged survival.[106]

Studies have also been performed with lentivirus models to evaluate possible benefits of prophylactic or postexposure antiretroviral therapy. Prophylactic ZDV can decrease acute viremia in the feline immunodeficiency virus cat model.[106] In the simian immunodeficiency virus (SIV) rhesus macaque infection model, prophylactic ZDV has been able to prevent development of SIV infection in only one study, while decreasing viral burden in other studies.[106]

The early experience with postexposure or early intervention treatment of PHI in humans includes a study of 11 subjects treated with ZDV (1g daily) for a median of 2 months.[121] Although the treatment was well tolerated, there did not appear to be any significant delay in the development of AIDS nor significant increases in CD4+ T-cell counts compared with historical controls. The small size of the study and the lack of a control group make interpretation of these observations problematic. The literature contains a handful of anecdotal cases in which postexposure ZDV therapy failed to prevent HIV infection after percutaneous inoculation with HIV-1.[106]

The opportunity to extend our understanding of the pathophysiologic mechanisms that interact during the initial dissemination of virus and immune response to HIV-1 infection, as well as the chance to slow disease progression by intervention, strongly supports the need for controlled therapeutic trials in humans. To this end, two major clinical trials to assess the efficacy of antiretroviral therapy begun at the time of PHI onset are underway,[122] one of which has produced some interesting preliminary data.

The European-Australian study that began in June 1991 was developed to assess the effect of ZDV initiated during PHI on clinical and laboratory parameters.[112] The 77 patients enrolled had one clinical criterion (ie, acute retroviral syndrome, exposure to HIV <3 months, or both) and one laboratory (ie, p24 antigenemia, negative or low-positive anti-HIV antibody screening test results, or both) criterion. Patients

were randomized to receive ZDV (250 mg twice daily) or ZDV placebo for 24 weeks. The end points included clinical symptoms (ie, duration of PHI, progression to CDC stage IV, or death) and laboratory parameters (eg, p24 antigen, CD4 cell count, viral replication). Ninety-one percent of enrolled patients had an acute retroviral syndrome. At an interim evaluation by a data and safety monitoring board,[112] it was determined that patients receiving ZDV had CD4+ T-cell counts that exceeded the counts of placebo patients by 120 cells/mm³ at 6 months and 80 cells/mm³ at 12 months after study entry; these differences were statistically significant. There were six minor opportunistic infections on the placebo arm (ie, thrush, oral hairy leukoplakia, herpes simplex virus) and only one on the ZDV arm.

Preliminary viral parameters suggests some small differences in viral load at the 6 and 12 month points (<0.5 log) between the treatment and control arms. As many as 15% of enrollees entered the study with virus already resistant to ZDV, a finding that may be a harbinger of a major problem to come. It remains to be seen how these early, promising surrogate end points will translate into a long-term clinical outcome for the patients on this study.

In the U.S. study, which began in January 1993, sponsored by the Division of AIDS Treatment Research Initiative, patients with symptomatic PHI are being randomized to ZDV (200 mg five times daily) or ZDV placebo for 24 weeks. Clinical, virologic, and immunologic parameters are closely monitored. In a follow-up to the studies previously described, a collaborative study of European, Australian, and U.S. investigators is in development; it will examine the ability of potent three- or four-drug antiretroviral combinations to influence the virologic and immunologic parameters of PHI.

ACKNOWLEDGMENTS

The authors offer special thanks to Dr. Pamela Clax and Mrs. Kathy Store for their expertise in preparing the manuscript and figures.

REFERENCES

1. McLeod G, Hammer S. Zidovudine: five years later. Ann Intern Med 1992;117:487.
2. Sande M, Carpenter C, Cobbs C, et al. Antiretroviral therapy for adult HIV infected patients: recommendations from a state-of-the-art conference. JAMA 1994;271:1830.
3. Volberding PA, Lagakos SW, Koch MA, et al. Zidovudine in asymptomatic human immunodeficiency virus infection: a controlled trial in persons with fewer than 500 CD4 positive cells per cubic millimeter. N Engl J Med 1990;322:941.
4. Volberding P, Lagakos S, Grimes J, et al. The duration of zidovudine benefit in person with asymptomatic HIV infection. JAMA 1994;272:437.
5. Concorde Coordinating Committee. Concorde: MRC/ANRS randomized double-blind controlled trial of immediate and deferred zidovudine in symptom-free HIV infection. Lancet 1994;343:871.
6. Kahn JO, Lagakos SW, Richman DD, et al. A controlled trial comparing continued zidovudine with didanosine in human immunodeficiency virus infection. N Engl J Med 1992;327:582.
7. Pazia A. Clinical response to stavudine therapy. Presented at the Sante Fe Antiviral Meeting, Sante Fe, NM, April 1995.

8. Abrams D, Goldman A, Launer C, et al. Comparative trial of didanosine and zalcitabine in patients with human immunodeficiency virus infection who are intolerant of or have failed zidovudine therapy. N Engl J Med 1994;330:657.

9. Fischl M, Stanley K, Collier A, et al. Combination and monotherapy with zidovudine and zalcitabine in patients with advanced HIV disease. Ann Intern Med 1995;122:24.

10. Welles S, Jackson J, Yen-Lieberman, et al. Prognostic capacity of plasma HIV-1 RNA copy number in ACTG 116-A. Abstract. Second National Conference on Human Retroviruses and Related Infections, Washington, DC, 1995.

11. O'Brien WA, Hartigan P, McCreedy B, Hamilton JD. Predictive value of plasma viral RNA and β_2-microglobulin in determining clinical outcome. Abstract 1208. The 34th Interscience Conference on Antimicrobial Agents and Chemotherapy, October 1994.

12. Johnson V. Nucleoside reverse transcriptase inhibitors and resistance of human immunodeficiency virus type 1. J Infect Dis 1995;17(Suppl 2):S140.

13. D'Aquila R, Johnson V, Welles S, et al. Zidovudine resistance and HIV-1 disease progression during antiretroviral therapy. Ann Intern Med 1995;122:401.

14. Tisdale M, Kemp S, Parry N, et al. Rapid in vitro selection of human immunodeficiency virus type 1 resistant to 3′-thiacytidine inhibitors due to a mutation in the YMMD region of reverse transcriptase. Proc Natl Acad Sci USA 1993;90:5653.

15. Wakefield J, Jablonski S, Morrow C. In vitro enzymatic activity of human immunodeficiency virus type 1 reverse transcriptase mutants in the highly conserved YMDD amino acid motif correlates with the infectious potential of the proviral genome. J Virol 1992;66:6806.

16. Eron J, Benoit S, Jemsek J, et al. A randomized double-blind multicenter trial of Lamivudine (3TC) monotherapy vs. zidovudine (ZDV) monotherapy in naive patients CD4 200–500 mm³. Abstract. Second National Conference on Human Retroviruses and Related Infections, Washington, DC, 1995.

17. Staszewski S, European Lamivudine HIV working group. Combination 3TC/ZDV vs ZDV monotherapy in ZDV experienced HIV-1 positive patients with a CD4 of 100–400 cells/mm³. Abstract. Second National Conference on Human Retroviruses and Related Infections, Washington, DC, 1995.

18. Collier AC, Coombs RW, Fischl MA, et al. Combination therapy with zidovudine and didanosine compared to zidovudine alone in human immunodeficiency virus type one infection. Ann Intern Med 1993;119:786.

19. Meng T, Fischl MA, Boota AM, et al. Combination therapy with zidovudine and dideoxycytidine in patients with advanced human immunodeficiency virus infection: a phase I/II study. Ann Intern Med 1992;116:13.

20. BW-34225-02. Physician's desk reference. Montvale, NJ: Medical Economics, 1993.

21. Nunberg JH, Scheif WA, Boots EJ, et al. Viral resistance to human immunodeficiency virus type 1-specific pyridinone reverse transcriptase inhibitors. J Virol 1991;65:4887.

22. Saag M, Emini E, Laskin O, et al. A short-term clinical evaluation of L-697,661, a non-nucleoside inhibitor of HIV-1 reverse transcriptase. N Engl J Med 1993;329:1065.

23. Wathen L, Freimuth W, Batts D, et al. Phenotypic and genotypic characterization of HIV-1 viral isolates from patients treated with combined AZT and delarvidine mesylate (DLV) therapy. Third International Workshop on HIV and Drug resistance, Kauai, Hawaii, 1994.

24. Havlir D, Cheeseman S, McLaughlin M, et al. High-dose nevirapine: safety, pharmacokinetics, and antiviral effect in patients with human immunodeficiency virus infection. J Infect Dis 1995;171:537.

25. Richman DD. Resistance of clinical isolates of human immunodeficiency virus to antiretroviral agents. Antimicrob Agents Chemother 1993;37:1207.

26. Campbell TB, Young RK, Eron JJ, D'Aquila RT, Tarpley WG, Kuritzkes DR. Inhibition of human immunodeficiency virus type 1 replication in vitro by the bisheteroarylpiperzine ateviridine (U-87201E) in combination with zidovudine or didanosine. J Infect Dis 1993;168:372.

27. Emini EA, Schleif WA, Sardana VV, et al. Combination therapy with AZT prevents selection of HIV variants that are highly resistant to non-nucleoside reverse transcriptase inhibitor L-697,661. Presented at the HIV Drug-Resistance Workshop, Noordwijk, The Netherlands, June 3–5, 1993.

28. D'Aquila R, Hughes M, Liou S for the NIAID AIDS clinical Trial Group (ACTG) Protocol 241 Team. A comparative study of a combination of zidovudine, didanosine, and double-blinded nevirapine versus a combination of zidovudine and didanosine. Abstract. Second National Conference on Human Retroviruses and Related Infections, Washington, DC, 1995.

29. Katz R, Skalka A. The retroviral enzymes. Annu Rev Biochem 1994;63:133.

30. Miller M, Jaskolski M, Rao JKM, Leis J, Wlodawer A. Crystal structure of a retroviral protease proves relationship to aspartic protease family. Nature 1989;337:576.

31. Navia MA, Fitzgerald PMD, McKeever BM, et al. Three-dimensional structure of aspartyl protease from human immunodeficiency virus HIV-1. Nature 1989;337:615.

32. Wlodawer A, Erickson JW. Structures based inhibitors of HIV-1 protease. Annu Rev Biochem 1993;62:543.

33. Jacobsen H, Yasargil K, Winslow DL, Craig JC, et al. Characterization of human immunodeficiency virus type 1 mutants with decreased sensitivity to proteinase inhibitor Ro 31-8959. Virology 1995;206:527.

34. Markowitz M, MO H, Kempf DJ, et al. Selection and analysis of human immunodeficiency virus type 1 variants with increased resistance to ABT-538, a novel protease inhibitor. Virology 1995;69:701.

35. Condra J, Schleif W, Blahy O, et al. Mutations in HIV Protease Conferring resistance to inhibitor L-735,524. Abstract. Second National Conference on Human Retroviruses and Related Infections, Washington, DC, 1995.

36. Markowitz M, Jalil L, Hurley A, et al. Evaluation of the antiviral activity of orally administered ABT-538, an inhibitor of HIV-1 Protease. Abstract. Second National Conference on Human Retroviruses and Related Infections, Washington, DC, 1995.

37. Mellors J, Steigbigel R, Gulick R, et al. A randomized, double blind study of the oral HIV protease Inhibitor, L-735,524 vs. zidovudine (ZDV) in p24 antigenic, HIV-1 infected patients with <500 CD4 cells/mm³. Abstract. Second National Conference on Human Retroviruses and Related Infections, Washington, DC, 1995.

38. Schapiro J, Winters M, Merigan T. First efficacy and safety results of the high dose Saquinavir monotherapy trial. Abstract. Second National Conference on Human Retroviruses and Related Infections, Washington, DC, 1995.

39. Condra JH, Schleif WA, Blahy OM, et al. In vivo emergence of HIV-1 variants resistant to multiple protease inhibitors. Nature 1995;374:569.

40. Collier A, Coombs R, Timpone J, et al. Comparative study of Ro 31-8959 and zidovudine (ZDV) and zalcitibine (ddC) vs. Ro 31-8959, ZDV and ddC. Abstract. Tenth International Conference on AIDS, Yokohama, Japan, 1994.

41. Sommadossi JP, Schinazi R, McMillan A, et al. A human serum glycoprotein profoundly affects antiviral activity of the protease inhibitor SC-52151 by decreasing its cellular uptake. Abstract. Second National Conference on Human Retroviruses and Related Infections, Washington, DC, 1995.

42. Fischl M, Richman D, Flexner C, et al. Phase I study of two formulations and dose schedules of SC-52151, a protease inhibitor. Abstract. Second National Conference on Human Retroviruses and Related Infections, Washington, DC, 1995.

43. Mimoto T, Imai J, Kisanuki S, et al. Kynostatin (KNI)-227 and 272, highly potent anti-HIV agents: conformationally constrained tripeptide inhibitors of HIV protease containing allophenylnostatine. Chem Pharm Bull (Tokyo) 1992;40:2251.

44. Quart B, Chapman S, Peterkin J, et al. Phase I safety, tolerance, pharmacokinetics and food effect studies of AG1343-A novel protease inhibitor. Abstract. Second National Conference on Human Retroviruses and Related Infections, Washington, DC, 1995.

45. Painter G, St. Clair M, Demiranda P, et al. An overview of the preclinical development of the HIV protease inhibitor VX-478(141W94). Abstract. Second National Conference on Human Retroviruses and Related Infections, Washington, DC, 1995.

46. Vink C, Plasterk R. The human immunodeficiency virus integrase protein. Trends Genet 1993;9:433.

47. Dyda F, Hickman AB, Jenkins TM, et al. Crystal structure of the catalytic domain of HIV-1 integrase: similarity to other polynucleotidyl transferase. Science 1994;266:1981.

48. Fesen N, Kohn K, Leteurtre F, et al. Inhibitors of human immunodeficiency virus integrase. Proc Natl Acad Sci USA 1993;90:2399.

49. Cushman M, Sherman P. Inhibition of HIV-1 integration by aurintricarboxylic acid monomers, monomer analogs and polymer fractions. Biochem Biophys Res Commun 1992;1:85,1992.

50. Mazumder A, Cooney D, Agbaria R, et al. Inhibition of human immunodeficiency virus type 1 integrase by 3′-azido-3′-deoxythymidylate. Proc Natl Acad Sci USA 1994;91:5771.

51. Felber BK, Pavlakis GN. Molecular Biology of HIV-1: positive and negative regulatory elements important for virus expression. AIDS 1993;7(Suppl 1):S51.

52. Lever A. Regulatory proteins of HIV. Med Virol 1991;3:155.

53. Luznik L, Kraus G, Guatelli J, et al. Tat-independent replication of human immunodeficiency viruses. J Clin Invest 1995;95:328.

54. Hsu MC, Schutt AD, Holly M, et al. Inhibition of HIV replication in acute and chronic infections in vitro by a Tat antagonist. Science 1991;254:1799.

55. Haubrich R and the ACTG 213 team. A randomized study of safety, tolerance, pharmacokinetics, and activity of oral Ro 24-7429. Abstract. Ninth International Conference on AIDS, Berlin, Germany, 1993.

56. Witvrouw M, Pauwels R, Vandamme AM, et al. Cell type-specific anti-human immunodeficiency virus type I activity of the transactivation inhibitor Ro 5,3335. Antimicrob Agents Chemother 1992;36:2628.

57. Ratner L. Mechanism of action of N-butyl-deoxynojirimycin in inhibiting HIV-1 infection and activity in combination with nucleoside analogs. AIDS Res Hum Retrovirus 1993;9:291.

58. Fischl M, Resnick L, Coombs R, et al. The efficacy and safety of combination N-butyl-deoxynojirimicin (SC-48334) and zidovudine in patients with HIV-1 infection and 200-500 CD4 cells/mm³. J Acquir Immune Defic Syndr 1994;7:139.

59. Tierney M, Pottage J, Kessler H, et al. The tolerability and pharmacokinetics of N Butyl Deoxynojirimicyn in patients with advanced HIV disease (ACTG 100). J Acquir Immune Defic Syndr 1995;10:549.

60. Agrawal S. In: Wickstrom E, ed. Prospects for antisense nucleic acid therapy for cancer and AIDS. New York: Liss, 1994:143.

61. Lisziewicz J, Sun D, Weichold F, et al. Antisense oligodeoxynucleotide phosphorothioate complementary to Gag mRNA blocks replication of human immunodeficiency virus type 1 in human peripheral blood cells. Proc Natl Acad Sci USA 1994;91:7942.

62. Cullen B. Mechanism of action of regulatory proteins encoded by complex retroviruses. Microbiol Rev 1992;56:375.

63. Subbramanian R, Cohen E. Molecular biology of the human immunodeficiency virus accessory Proteins. J Virol 1994;68:6831.

64. Refaeli Y, Levy DN, Weiner DB. The glucocorticoid receptor type II complex is a target of the HIV-1 vpr gene product. Proc Natl Acad Sci USA 1995;92:3621.

65. Bridges SH, Sarver N. Gene therapy and immune restoration for HIV disease. Lancet 1995;345:427.

66. Baltimore D. Intracellular immunization. Nature 335:395, 1988.

67. Sullenger BA, Gallardo HF, Ungers GE, et al. Overexpression of TAR sequences renders cells resistant to human immunodeficiency virus replication. Cell 1990;63:601.

68. Lisziewicz J, Sun D, Smythe J, et al. Inhibition of human immunodeficiency virus type 1 replication by regulated expression of a polymeric Tat activation response RNA decoy as a strategy for gene therapy in AIDS. Proc Natl Acad Sci USA 1993;90:8000.

69. Lee TC, Sullenger BA, Gallardo HF, Ungers GE, Gilboa E. Overexpression of RRE-derived sequences inhibits HIV-1 replication in CEM cells. New Biologist 1992;4:66.

70. Lee SW, Gallardo HF, Gilboa E, Smith E. Inhibition of human immunodeficiency virus type 1 in human T-cells by a potent Rev response element decoy consisting of the 13-nucleotide minimal Rev binding domain. J Virol 1994;68:8254.

71. Feinberg MB, Trono D. Intracellular immunization: trans-dominant mutants of HIV gene products as tools for the study and interruption of viral replication. AIDS Res Hum Retroviruses 1992;8:1013.

72. Green M, Ishino M, Loewenstein PM. Mutational analysis of HIV-1 Tat minimal domain peptides: identification of trans-dominant mutants that suppress HIV-LTR-driven gene expression. Cell 1989;58:215.

73. Pearson L, Garcia J, Wu F, et al. A transdominant tat mutant that inhibits Tat-induced gene expression from the human immunodeficiency virus long terminal repeat. Proc Natl Acad Sci USA 1990;87:5079.

74. Malim MH, Bohnlein S, Hauber J, Cullen BR. Functional dissection of the HIV-1 Rev trans-activator—derivation of a trans-dominant repressor of Rev function. Cell 1989;58:205.

75. Kubota S, Furuta R, Maki M, Hatanaka M. Inhibition of human immunodeficiency virus type 1 Rev function by a Rev mutant which interferes with nuclear/nucleolar localization of Rev. J Virol 1992;66:2510.

76. Nabel GJ, Fox BA, Post L, Thompson CB, Woffendin C. A molecular genetic intervention for AIDS—effects of transdominant negative form of Rev. Hum Gene Ther 1994;5:79.

77. Rossi JJ, Elkins D, Zaia JA, Sullivan S. Ribozymes as anti-HIV therapeutic agents: principles, applications, and problems. AIDS Res Hum Retroviruses 1992;8:183.

78. Sarver N, Cantin EM, Chang PS, et al. Ribozymes as potential anti-HIV therapeutic agents. Science 1990;247:1222.

79. Dropulic B, Lin NH, Martin MA, Jeang K. Functional characterization of a U5 ribozyme: intracellular suppression of human immunodeficiency virus type 1 expression. J Virol 1992;66:1432.

80. Weerasinghe M, Liem SE, Sabah S, Read SE, Joshi S. Resistance to human immunodeficiency virus type 1 (HIV-1) infection in human CD4+ lymphocyte-derived cell lines conferred by using retroviral vectors expressing an HIV-1 RNA-specific ribozyme. J Virol 1991;65:5531.

81. Ojwang JO, Hampel A, Looney DJ, Wong-Staal F, Rappaport J. Inhibition of human immunodeficiency virus type 1 expression by a hairpin ribozyme. Proc Natl Acad Sci USA 1992;89:10802.

82. Sioud M, Drlica K. Prevention of human immunodeficiency virus type 1 integrase expression in Escherichia coli by a ribozyme. Proc Natl Acad Sci USA 1991;88:7303.

83. Zhou C, Bahner IC, Larson GP, et al. Inhibition of HIV-1 in human T lymphocytes by retrovirally transduced anti-tat and rev hammerhead ribozymes. Gene 1994;4:149.

84. Duan L, Bagasra O, Laughlin MA, Oakes JW, Pomerantz RJ. Potent inhibition of human immunodeficiency virus type 1 replication by an intracellular anti-Rev single chain antibody. Proc Natl Acad Sci USA 1994;91:5075.

85. Chen S-Y, Khouri Y, Bagley J, Marasco WA. Combined intra- and extracellular immunization against human immunodeficiency virus type 1 infection with a human anti-gp120 antibody. Proc Natl Acad Sci USA 1994;91:5932.

86. Miller AD. Retrovirus packaging cells. Hum Gene Ther 1990;1:5.

87. Chatterjee S, Wong KK, Rose J, Johnson P. Transduction of intracellular resistance to HIV production by an adeno-associated virus-based antisense vector. In: Channock RM, Ginsberg H, Brown F, Lerner RA, eds. Vaccines 91: modern approaches to new vaccines, including the prevention of AIDS. Cold Spring Harbor, NY: Cold Spring Harbor Laboratory, 1991:85.

88. Kotin RM, Siniscalco M, Samulski RJ, et al. Site-specific integration by adeno-associated virus. Proc Natl Acad Sci USA 1990; 87:2211.

89. Poznansky M, Leveer A, Bergeron L, Haseltine W, Sodroski J. Gene transfer into human lymphocytes by a defective human immunodeficiency virus type 1 vector. J Virol 1991;65:532.

90. Buchschacher GL Jr, Panganiban AT. Human immunodeficiency virus vectors for inducible expression of foreign genes. J Virol 1992;66:2731.

91. Hirsch MS, D'Aquila RT. Therapy for human immunodeficiency virus infection. N Engl J Med 1993;328:1686.

92. Ellenberg SS, Hamilton JM. Surrogate endpoints in clinical trials: cancer. Stat Med 1989;8:405.

93. Wittes J, Lakatos E, Probstfield J. Surrogate endpoints in clinical trials: cardiovascular diseases. Stat Medicine 1989;8:415.

94. Hillis A, Siegel D. Surrogate endpoints in clinical trials: ophthalmologic disorders. Stat Med 1989;8:427.

95. Prentice RL. Surrogate endpoints in clinical trials: definition and operational criteria. Stat Med 1989;8:431.

96. Tsoukas CM, Bernard NF. Markers predicting progression of human immunodeficiency virus-related disease. Clin Microbiol Rev 1994;7:14.

97. Coombs RW, Reichelderfer PS. Viral burden, virulence and viral threshold in HIV-1 disease: implications for clinical trial design and studies on pathogenesis. J Cell Biochem (abstract) 1995;S21B:204.

98. Choi S, Lagakos SW, Schooley RT, Volberding PA. CD4+ T lymphocytes are an incomplete surrogate marker for clinical progression in persons with asymptomatic HIV infection taking zidovudine. Ann Intern Med 1993;118:674.

99. Aboulker JR, Swart AM. Preliminary analysis of the Concorde Trial. (Letter) Lancet 1993;341:889.

100. Coombs R, DeGruttola V, Reichelderfer PS, O'Brien WA, Jackson B. Clinical correlates of virological measurements; roundtable symposium. Abstract. Second National Conference on Human Retroviruses and Related Infections, session 12, Washington, DC, January 30, 1995.

101. Fiscus SA, DeGruttola V, Gupta P, et al. Human immunodeficiency virus type I quantitative microculture as a measure of antiviral efficacy in a multicenter clinical trial. J Infect Dis 1995;171:305.

102. Welles SL, Jackson JB, Yen-Lieberman B, et al. Prognostic capacity of plasma HIV-1 RNA copy number in ACTG 116A. Abstract 229. Second National Conference on Human Retroviruses and Related Infections, Washington, DC, January 31, 1995.
103. Collier AC, Coombs RW, Timpone J, et al. Comparative study of Ro 31-8959 and zidovudine (ZDV) vs ZDV and zalcitabine (ddC) vs Ro 31-8959, ZDV and ddC. Abstract 058B. Tenth International Conference on AIDS, Yokohama, Japan, August 1994.
104. Centers for Disease Control. Estimates of HIV prevalence and projected AIDS cases: summary of a workshop, October 31–November 1, 1989. MMWR 1990;49:110.
105. Cooper DA, Gold J, MaClean P, et al. Acute AIDS retrovirus infection. Lancet 1985;1:537.
106. Niu MT, Stein DS, Schnittman SM. Primary human immunodeficiency virus type-1 infection: review of pathogenesis and early treatment intervention in humans and animal retroviral infections. J Infect Dis 1993;168:1490.
107. Clark SJ, Saag MS, Decker WD, et al. High titers of cytopathic virus in plasma of patients with symptomatic primary HIV-1 infection. N Engl J Med 1991;324:954.
108. Daar ES, Moudgil T, Meyer RD, Ho DD. Transient high levels of viremia in patients with primary human immunodeficiency virus type 1 infection. N Engl J Med 1991;324:961.
109. Gaines H. Primary HIV infection. Scand J Infect Dis Suppl 1989;61:1.
110. Wall RA, Denning DW, Amos A. HIV antigenemia in acute HIV infection. Lancet 1987;1:566.
111. Pedersen C, Linhardt BO, Jensen BL, et al. Clinical course of primary HIV infection: consequences for subsequent course of infection. Br Med J 1989;299:154.
112. Hoen S, Hoen B, Cooper D, et al. Treatment of primary HIV infection with zidovudine. Abstract 002B. Tenth International Conference on AIDS, Yokohama, Japan, 1994.
113. DATRI 002 Study Team. Abstract. International Conference on AIDS and Associated Cancers, 35th Interscience Conference on Antimicrobial Agents and Chemotherapy. San Francisco, September, 1995.
114. Zhu T, Mo H, Ning W, et al. Genotypic and phenotypic characterization of HIV-1 in patients with primary infection. Science 1993;261:1179.
115. Gaines H, von Sydow MAE, von Stedingk LV, et al. Immunological changes in primary HIV-1 infection. AIDS 1990;4:995.
116. Safrit JT, Andrews CA, Zhu T, Ho DD, Koup RA. Characterization of human immunodeficiency virus type-1 specific cytotoxic T lymphocyte clones isolated during acute seroconversion: recognition of autologous virus sequences within a conserved immunodominant epitope. J Exp Med 1994;179:463.
117. Cooper DA, Tindall B, Wilson EJ, Imrie AA, Penny R. Characterization of T lymphocyte responses during primary infection with human immunodeficiency virus. J Infect Dis 157:889, 1988.
118. Pedersen C, Dickmeiss E, Gaub J, et al. T-cell subset alterations and lymphocyte responsiveness to mitogens and antigen during severe primary infection with HIV: a case series of seven consecutive HIV seroconverters. AIDS 1990;4:523.
119. Stein DS, Korvick JA, Vermund SH. CD4+ lymphocyte enumeration for prediction of clinical course of human immunodeficiency virus disease: a review. J Infect Dis 1992;165:352.
120. Pantaleo G, Demarest JF, Soudens H, et al. Major expansion of CD8+ T cells with a predominant VB usage during the primary immune response to HIV. Nature 1994;370:463.
121. Tindall B, Gaines H, Imrie A, et al. Zidovudine in the management of primary HIV-1 infection. AIDS 1991;167:291.
122. Niu MT, Jermano JA, Reichelderfer P, Schnittman SM. Summary of the National Institutes of Health Workshop on primary human immunodeficiency virus type-1 infection. AIDS Res Hum Retroviruses 1993;9:913.

AIDS: Biology, Diagnosis, Treatment and Prevention, fourth edition, edited by Vincent T. DeVita, Jr., Samuel Hellman, and Steven A. Rosenberg. Lippincott–Raven Publishers, © 1997

CHAPTER **22**

Pharmacology of Antiretroviral Agents

Charles Flexner and Craig Hendrix

The optimal clinical application of antiretroviral therapy is most likely to be achieved if clinicians thoroughly understand the pharmacology of the agents involved. The body's effect on the drug (ie, pharmacokinetics) and the drug's effect on the body (ie, pharmacodynamics) generally determine how useful a drug is and how it should be used. A quantitative understanding of these two terms often provides all the information needed for the rational use of approved drugs and the rational development of investigational drugs. Clinical pharmacology becomes especially critical in an era when standard antiretroviral regimens employ multiple drugs. These regimens are developed to exploit synergy and nonoverlapping drug toxicities, but they are complicated by potential pharmacokinetic and pharmacodynamic interactions.

Failure to define the clinical pharmacology of new antiretrovirals has led to some notable mistakes early in drug development. For example, the polysulfated polyanion dextran sulfate, a potent antiretroviral, was administered orally in a large clinical trial[1] before it was shown to have negligible oral bioavailability.[2] When this drug was administered as the maximally tolerated continuous intravenous infusion, it had no discernible activity against the human immunodeficiency virus (HIV) and was unacceptably toxic.[3] Zidovudine, the first approved antiretroviral, was administered in initial clinical trials at a dose associated with significant hematologic toxicity,[4] and this dosing regimen was chosen for clinical therapy. Subsequent trials demonstrated that this dose was too high and that lower doses of drug were associated with much less hematologic toxicity and equivalent clinical and virologic benefit.[5,6]

When pharmacodynamics are not understood, patients may be given drug doses or dosing regimens that are chosen with little scientific rationale and little chance of under-

standing a drug's potential benefit. For example, the relation between the dose of mismatched, double-stranded RNA (ie, ampligen or atvogen) and its limited biologic activity was defined only after the drug had been used in a variety of clinical trials employing a wide range of dosing regimens.[7]

Several pharmacologic factors must be taken into account when new drugs are introduced into clinical use. The four basic components of drug disposition—absorption, distribution, metabolism, and excretion—should be defined early in drug development, and individual factors contributing to pharmacokinetic variability should be anticipated as the drug is being used in a broader population. Additional pharmacologic factors, such as systemic bioavailability, protein binding effects, distribution into target cells and tissues, generation of active or toxic drug metabolites, and drug-drug interactions, may influence clinical drug utility and need to be considered. The quantitative human pharmacodynamics of a drug—the relation between drug exposure and drug effect (ie, beneficial activity and toxicity)—should be used to develop dosing regimens that are safe and cost effective.

Rapid advances in the discovery and clinical testing of antiretroviral drugs and the accelerated pace of antiretroviral drug approval have produced several challenges for clinicians and clinical investigators using these agents. With increasing pressure to bring new agents rapidly to the clinic, there is an increasing effort to understand their basic and clinical pharmacology to take full advantage of antiviral potency, minimize toxicity, and exploit unfilled therapeutic niches. We discuss several of these advances in this chapter.

BIOCHEMICAL PHARMACOLOGY OF NUCLEOSIDE ANALOGS

Understanding the molecular mechanisms of drug action and toxicity can improve clinical drug use by providing new ways to reduce toxicity and increase antiviral activity. The development of synergistic drug combinations, alternative dosing regimens, and modified compounds with greater

Charles Flexner, Division of Clinical Pharmacology, The Johns Hopkins University School of Medicine, Baltimore, MD 21287.

Craig Hendrix, Military Medical Consortium for Applied Retroviral Research, Rockville, MD 20307.

selective toxicity are often the result of insights provided by biochemical pharmacology.

The dideoxynucleosides (ddNs) inhibit HIV replication by blocking reverse transcription of the viral RNA genome, preventing formation of the double-stranded DNA that would serve as the template for future viral replication. These ddNs are prodrugs that must first enter the infected cell and then be phosphorylated to the active triphosphate moiety, similar to the natural deoxynucleosides whose functions they mimic (Fig. 22-1). Zidovudine (3'-azido-2',3'-dideoxythymidine [AZT]), stavudine (2',3'-didehydro-2',3'-dideoxythymidine [d4T]), and alovudine (3'-fluoro-2',3'-dideoxythymidine [FLT]) serve as analogs of deoxythymidine (dT); zalcitabine (2',3'dideoxycytidine [ddC]), and lamivudine (2'-deoxy-3'-thiacytidine [3TC]) are analogs of deoxycytidine (dC); didanosine (2',3'-dideoxyinosine [ddI]) and 9-(2-phosphonylmethoxyethyl) adenine (PMEA) are analogs of deoxyadenosine (dA).

As triphosphates, the ddNs act through inhibition of viral reverse transcriptase by means of substrate competition with natural deoxynucleosides and through chain termination of the nascent DNA being transcribed by the viral reverse transcriptase by means of incorporation of the dideoxynucleoside triphosphate (ddNTP) that lacks the 3'-hydroxyl group. The amount of intracellular triphosphate formation correlates most closely with reduction of HIV infectivity and cytopathic effects.[8] The differences in the mechanisms of phosphorylation (eg, anabolism), metabolism, and specificity for viral and cellular polymerases explain much of the variation in antiviral activity and clinical toxicity among these compounds.

Zidovudine

AZT uses the same cellular enzymes as dT to form the triphosphate AZTTP. The relatively high efficiency (V_{max}/K_m) of the initial phosphorylation step is roughly one half that of the natural dT substrate in H9 and peripheral blood mononuclear cells (PBMCs).[9] The efficiency of the thymidylate kinase in phosphorylating AZT monophosphate (AZTMP) to form AZT diphosphate (AZTDP), however, is very low because the maximum rate of AZTDP formation is only 0.3% of the dTMP rate of formation. Essentially, AZTMP blocks its own phosphorylation, as well as that of deoxythymidine monophosphate (dTMP) and other dideoxynucleoside monophosphates (dNMPs), acting as a substrate inhibitor of thymidylate kinase. As a result, AZTMP accumulates in lymphocytes with relatively little formation of AZTDP or AZTTP. Based on in vitro studies, increasing extracellular concentrations of AZT (ie, picomolar to micromolar range) result in proportionally increasing AZTMP concentrations but relatively small or no increases in AZTTP.[10,11] In cells taken from patients with acquired immunodeficiency syndrome (AIDS) after a 250-mg oral dose of AZT, the intracellular AZTMP to AZTTP ratio varies from 10- to 24-fold, depending on the time after dosing.[12] The absolute levels of all AZT phosphates vary widely,

even among clinically similar subjects. The intracellular phosphorylated AZT concentration in PBMCs from HIV-infected patients begins to decline, with a half-life of approximately 2.5 hours in the mono-, di-, and triphosphate moieties.[13,14] In clinical studies, in which clinical pharmacokinetics constitute an important additional variable, there seems to be relatively steady mean levels of the intracellular AZTTP concentration for up to 6 hours after dosing.

AZT anabolism also differs in different cell types. In monocyte-macrophage cells, which are important sources of HIV replication, AZT is monophosphorylated primarily by constitutively produced mitochondrial thymidine kinase (TK2) rather than the S-phase–specific cellular thymidine kinase (TK1), which is the predominant monophosphorylating enzyme in stimulated lymphocytes.[15,16] Although TK2 has a 15-fold lower specific activity than TK1, the larger cell volume of monocyte-macrophages results in a per cell TK activity only 77% lower in monocyte-macrophages than in activated lymphocytes. Because dT catabolism is more rapid in monocyte-macrophage cells, the level of AZTTP in essentially resting cells is sufficient to inhibit HIV.[17]

Other factors influence the intracellular concentrations of AZTTP. Phytohemagglutinin stimulation of PBMCs collected from HIV-infected and uninfected patients results in 60- to 150-fold and 10- to 17-fold increases, respectively, in the rate of intracellular AZT phosphorylation.[14,18] Consistent with this finding, cells taken from AIDS patients, presumably with high levels of lymphocyte activation, have phosphorylated AZT concentrations 10-fold higher than HIV-seronegative volunteers after the same 250-mg AZT dose.[12] Other studies report that AZT is actively pumped out of cells in a manner similar to, but independent of, the P-glycoprotein mechanism, which adds additional variation to intracellular concentrations and diminishes antiviral activity.[19]

The complicated intracellular pharmacology of AZT suggests that a wide range of AZTTP concentrations result within the lymphocyte, even among individuals taking the same dose of the drug with the same extracellular pharmacokinetic profile. Accordingly, AZT plasma concentrations should correlate poorly with clinical response to the drug, and total phosphorylated AZT concentrations in patients, reflecting mainly the inactive monophosphate moiety, should correlate only modestly with markers of HIV disease progression, as has been reported.[20] The heterogeneity of intracellular AZTTP concentrations despite uniform dosing in clinical trials may partially account for the modest clinical benefit of AZT despite its very high in vitro antiviral activity. Clinical studies have not correlated the concentration of the active drug moiety, AZTTP, with the antiviral or toxic effects. AZT is also a potent inhibitor of adenylate kinase ($K_i = 8$ μM) that takes part in the phosphorylation of adenosine analogs.[21]

Stavudine

Like AZT, the relative proportions of d4T mono-, di-, and triphosphate remain constant despite changes in the extra-

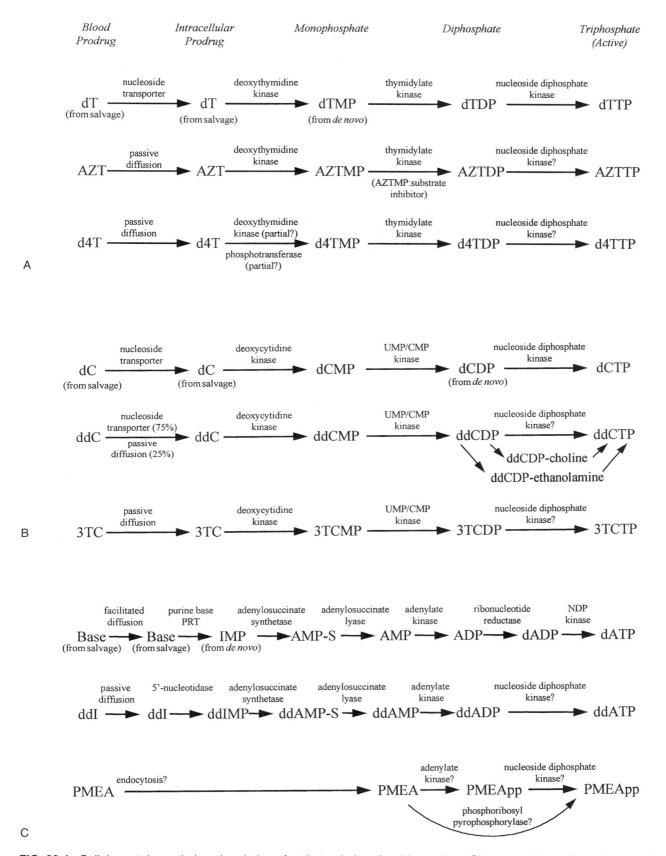

FIG. 22-1. Cellular uptake and phosphorylation of antiretroviral nucleoside analogs. Shown are the major pathways of cellular uptake and anabolism (phosphorylation) of (**A**) deoxythymidine (dT) and its analogs, zidovudine (AZT) and stavudine (d4T); (**B**) deoxycytidine (dC) and its analogs, zalcitabine (ddC) and lamivudine (3TC); (**C**) deoxyadenosine (purine base) and its analogs, didanosine (ddI) and 9-(2-phosphonylmethoxyethyl)-adenine (PMEA).

cellular concentration of the drug.[13,22] After incubation at clinically achievable 10 μM concentrations, intracellular d4TTP concentrations can be achieved that exceed the reverse transcriptase K_i by more than 10-fold.[23] At 10 μM, the triphosphate of d4T is more efficiently formed than AZTTP.[24] In lymphocyte cell lines, d4TTP has a 3.5-hour half-life after withdrawal of d4T from the culture medium, similar to AZTTP, in part because of resistance to hydrolysis by dT phosphorylase.[25]

At equimolar concentrations of d4T and AZT in CEM cells (ie, T-lymphoblastoid cell line), AZT monophosphorylation is unaffected, but d4T phosphorylation is reduced to 5% of its normal value, consistent with a much greater affinity of AZT for TK compared with d4T.[13] The potential clinical significance of this interaction is unclear. In TK-deficient Raji cells, in which AZT cannot be phosphorylated, d4T can be phosphorylated.[24] A phosphotransferase mechanism, by which phosphates are transferred from phenylphosphates or nucleoside monophosphates to pyrimidine nucleotides, has been suggested to account for such TK-independent phosphorylation. In resting cells that do not express TK1 activity, AZT can be phosphorylated, but d4T anabolites are not detectable.[23]

Zalcitabine

The mechanism of facilitated nucleoside diffusion accounts for much of ddC's penetration into lymphocytes, which is unique among the antiretroviral nucleosides.[26] In monocyte-macrophage cell cultures, dipyridamole inhibits dC salvage, but not ddC salvage, similar to the effects of dipyridamole on dT and AZT.[27,28] Unlike AZTMP, there is no substrate inhibition of the dCMP for the diphosphate kinase and therefore no accumulation of dCMP.[29] The ddC phosphorylation and antiviral activity is independent of the state of activation or infection of the cell. With a K_i/K_m ratio of 0.04, ddCTP is among the most potent of nucleoside analog reverse transcriptase inhibitors, having a much greater affinity for reverse transcriptase than the natural substrate, dC.[30,31] In combination studies, AZT and ddC do not alter each other's metabolism at clinically relevant concentrations.[29]

There is no evidence for any significant deamination of dC or its phosphates back to deoxyuridine moieties, nor is there evidence for the phosphorolysis of the dC phosphates back to dC.[26] Uniquely among nucleoside analogs, however, two liponucleotide metabolites of ddC, ddCDP-ethanolamine and ddCDP-choline exist.[26,29] Both of these metabolites have long half-lives and may, under some experimental conditions, exceed the concentration of ddCTP. It has been suggested that these metabolites may function as a long-acting storage form of ddC and may be related to the toxicity of this drug.

Lamivudine

Another dideoxy analog of cytidine, 3TC consists of a racemic mixture of β-D-(+)- and β-L-(−)-enantiomers that are equipotent in anti-HIV activity at nanomolar concentrations. The intracellular half-lives of the racemates differ (ie, 10.5 to 15.5 hours for the [−]-enantiomer and 3.5 to 7 hours for the [+]-enantiomer), but both are longer than the 3.5- to 4.5-hour half-lives of the thymidine analogs AZT, d4T, and FLT.[32] Resting and phytohemagglutinin-stimulated cells in culture phosphorylate 3TC to the triphosphate moiety to a similar extent. The active triphosphate form, 3TCTP, inhibits the viral reverse transcriptase enzyme with a K_i of 1 to 10 μM.[33] 3TC has activity against HIV laboratory strains in PBMCs, with a 50% inhibitory concentration (IC_{50}) of 2.5 to 90 nM, similar to that of AZT, but it is not active against HIV replication in chronically infected cell lines (eg, U937).[34] The (−)-racemate resists phosphorylase- and deaminase-mediated metabolism, but the (+)-racemate can be deaminated to 2′-deoxy-3′-thiauridine. 3TC does not alter the metabolism of other nucleotides.

Didanosine

The active form of ddI, ddATP, is a potent HIV reverse transcriptase inhibitor with a K_i/K_m ratio of 0.02, similar to ddCTP and AZTTP.[30] The antiviral drug ribavirin enhances the anti-HIV activity of ddI in culture by increasing the concentrations of ddIMP and, subsequently, of ddATP in PBMCs.[35] Hydroxyurea, at clinically achievable 0.1 mM concentrations, also potentiates the antiviral effects of ddI.[36] This has been attributed to selective inhibition of dATP synthesis by means of ribonucleotide reductase inhibition. The result is a favorable reduction in the dATP to ddATP ratio in ddI-treated cells, a principal determinant of ddI's antiviral activity. The 25- to 40-hour intracellular half-life of ddATP (from ddI) is the longest of the ddNTP analogs, especially compared with the pyrimidine triphosphate analogs half-lives of less than 4 hours.[37]

9-(2-Phosphonylmethoxyethyl) Adenine

The acyclic nucleotide analog PMEA inhibits HIV replication through PMEA diphosphate (PMEApp), the antivirally active moiety, which competitively inhibits reverse transcriptase and chain terminates virally encoded DNA at the same sites as dATP with a similar IC_{50} of less than 10 μM.[38] The lipophilic PMEA penetrates the cell through a slow, temperature-dependent, endocytosis-like mechanism, which is quite different from the nucleoside analogs discussed. Unlike the nucleoside analogs, the diphosphate form of PMEA is the antivirally active moiety, because PMEA already possesses a phosphate in a phosphonate configuration. Intracellular concentrations of PMEAp and PMEApp are proportional to extracellular PMEA concentrations in the 0.5 to 300 μM range, although they are typically 10- to 20-fold below the concentrations of the parent drug.[39] PMEA has no deaminated metabolites, and the rate of dephosphorylation by NDP kinase and ATPase is slow, resulting in a 16- to 18-hour intracellular half-life after removal of PMEA from the medium in tissue culture.

CLINICAL PHARMACOKINETICS OF NUCLEOSIDE ANALOGS

A variety of pharmacologic factors must be considered early in the clinical development of a new drug. This includes pharmaceutical factors such as formulation, route of administration, and intended dose and dosing regimen; pharmacokinetic factors such as oral and systemic bioavailability, distribution, and clearance; and pharmacodynamic factors such as target concentrations of drug needed to achieve antiviral effects or avoid toxicity (Table 22-1).

The clinical pharmacokinetics of the available antiretroviral nucleosides have been defined.[40] Summarized in the following paragraphs and Table 22-2 are the major pharmacokinetic features of these agents.

Bioavailability

Systemic bioavailability is generally high for the nucleoside analogs when administered orally, ranging from 60% to more than 90% for all but ddI, which is the single agent with low and variable absorption. ddI is acid labile, resulting in degradation at gastric acid pH, and it requires oral administration with a buffered carrier. Consequently, ddI should be administered in the fasted state, with food significantly decreasing absorption. The extent of absorption of the other nucleosides, as determined by the area under the curve (AUC), is not affected by food, although peak absorption (C_{max}) may be delayed. A high-fat[41] or high-protein meal[42] slows the rate of absorption of AZT, prolongs the time at which C_{max} occurs during a dosing interval, and reduces the mean C_{max}, but it does not significantly alter the AUC. This pattern of food effect is typical of all the nucleoside analogs except ddI.[40]

Clearance

Most of the nucleoside analogs are rapidly cleared from the plasma, with elimination half-lives averaging 1 hour. The half-lives of the active antiviral moieties, the intracellular

TABLE 22-1. Commonly used pharmacokinetic abbreviations

C_{max}	Maximum drug concentration during a dosing interval (peak)
C_{min}	Minimum drug concentration during a dosing interval (trough)
T_{max}	The time at which C_{max} occurs during a dosing interval
V_d	Volume of distribution; the apparent volume in which a drug is distributed, usually determined from plasma concentrations
CL	Clearance, expressed in volume per unit of time (eg, mL/min)
$t_{1/2}$	Elimination half-life; time required to eliminate 50% of remaining drug from a specified compartment, usually plasma
F	Bioavailability; fraction of drug absorbed systemically
AUC	Area under the concentration-time curve
CL/F	Oral clearance, often calculated as oral dose/AUC

NTPs, are considerably longer (see Table 22-2), accounting for the relatively long dosing intervals recommended for most of these agents. Clearance of these drugs, with the exception of AZT, is mainly achieved renally. Hepatic glucuronidation accounts for about 75% of AZT's elimination.

Protein Binding

Plasma protein binding is quite low for most of the nucleoside analogs (see Table 22-2) and appears to play no significant role in their disposition or in drug-drug interactions. This is in marked contrast to several other classes of antiretrovirals, for which high protein binding may be a more important factor in disposition.

Distribution and Central Nervous System Penetration

For the most part, the antiretroviral nucleosides are widely distributed in tissues and cells. Most nucleoside analogs

TABLE 22-2. Clinical pharmacokinetics of antiretroviral nucleoside analogs

Drug	Dose (mg)*	F (%)	C_{max} (µg/mL)	T_{max} (h)	$T_{1/2}$ (h)	Variability (%)†	Intr. $T_{1/2}$ (h)‡	Protein Binding (%)	V_d (L/kg)	CSF (%)	Clearance Route
Zidovudine	200	62–68§	0.9–1.2	0.5–1	0.9–1.4	30–40	2.5–3.5[13,14]	20	1.4–1.8	15–135	Hepatic (75%) Renal (15–20%)
Didanosine	375	21–54	1.95	1.0	0.6–1.7	26–50	25–40[37]	<5	0.9–4.9	21	Renal (60%)
Zalcitabine	5	86–100	0.08	1–2	1.1–1.8	38–50	NR	NR	0.5–0.6	9–37	Renal (75%)
Stavudine	200	82	4.1	0.5–1.0	1.0–1.6	16–30	3.5[25]	NR	0.5–1.1	11–160	Renal (34–41%)
Lamivudine	300	72–95	3.3	0.8–1.6	2.5	NR	10.5–15.5[32]	NR	1.0–1.6	NR	Renal (68–71%)

*Total single reference dose, normalized to a 70-kg subject if given in mg/kg.

†Percentage coefficient of variation for the area under the time-concentration curve during a dosing interval for an orally administered drug.

‡Intracellular half-life of the active triphosphate anabolite of the parent nucleoside.

§Ranges indicate published values from adult subjects without known hepatic or renal insufficiency. References for primary data are found in reference 40, except as indicated.

C_{max}, peak drug concentration during a dosing interval; CSF, percentage of drug in cerebrospinal fluid; $T_{1/2}$, time required to eliminate 50% of the remaining drug from a specified anatomic compartment; T_{max}, time at which C_{max} occurs during a dosing interval; V_d, apparent volume into which a drug is distributed, usually determined by plasma concentrations.

penetrate the central nervous system, with cerebrospinal fluid concentrations ranging from 10% to greater than 100% of simultaneous plasma levels (see Table 22-2). However, published studies suffer from limited sampling and an inadequate description of the cerebrospinal fluid concentration-time curve. The relation between central nervous system penetration and activity in HIV-associated encephalopathy has not been well characterized, although higher doses of AZT are associated with improved response in central nervous system disease.[43]

CLINICAL PHARMACOKINETICS OF OTHER REVERSE TRANSCRIPTASE INHIBITORS

Nucleotide Analogs

Because of its highly charged lipophilic nature, PMEA is poorly absorbed from the gastrointestinal tract. The prodrug, 9-[2-(bispivaloyloxymethyl) phosphonylmethoxyethyl] adenine (bis-POM PMEA), is an acylated ester of PMEA that masks the phosphonate moiety and significantly improves oral bioavailability to about 35% in humans.[44] The parent drug is renally cleared and has an elimination half-life of 1.1 to 2.0 hours.

Nonnucleoside Reverse Transcriptase Inhibitors

Several drugs, called nonnucleoside reverse transcriptase inhibitors (NNRTIs), are under development. These drugs are structurally unrelated, but they are similar in their potent inhibition of HIV-1 reverse transcriptase and are dissimilar to nucleoside analogs, which require phosphorylation intracellularly and have a narrower therapeutic index. Nevirapine (BI-RG-587) is a dipyridodiazepinone that potently inhibits reverse transcriptase (IC_{50} = 84 nM) and HIV-1 (IC_{50} = 40 nM).

Nevirapine is rapidly absorbed, with measurable drug detected within 15 minutes of administration and peak concentrations occurring at a mean of 2.2 hours. A concentration "plateau" at 80% of the C_{max} follows in many subjects and lasts 24 hours. Some patients have a secondary C_{max} at a mean of 14 hours possibly explained by enterohepatic recycling as observed in preclinical studies. The AUC and C_{max} are proportional at doses up to 100 mg but fall off slightly at the highest doses, where a 2-fold increase in dose results in a 1.2-fold increase in AUC and a 1.4-fold increase in C_{max}. The authors suggest enhanced clearance, as seen in preclinical studies, or saturated absorption to explain this diminished AUC and C_{max}.[45] The calculated half-life of nevirapine was 40 hours (range, 22 to 84 hours), with considerable variation not related to dose. The volume of distribution was 1.37 L/kg. Based on the results of this study, a 12.5 mg daily dose is predicted to achieve trough plasma concentrations at steady state from 13- to 36-fold of the in vitro IC_{50}.

CLINICAL PHARMACOKINETICS OF HIV PROTEASE INHIBITORS

The discovery of specific peptidomimetic inhibitors of the HIV-encoded protease produced one of the most rapid and widespread efforts to develop a new class of drugs in the history of the pharmaceutical industry. Within 4 years of the description of the first inhibitor, at least 22 clinical leads were developed, and 9 new agents were brought to clinical trials (see Chap. 23). These agents have a challenging pharmacology, related mainly to the fact that they are expensive and difficult to synthesize; often have poor oral bioavailability; are highly metabolized; and in several cases, are highly protein bound.

Saquinavir, the first of these agents to be studied clinically, was reported to have poor oral bioavailability (<5%), which was increased if the drug was taken with food. A 600-mg oral dose of saquinavir produced peak plasma concentrations (C_{max}) of 35 ng/mL, roughly threefold higher than the in vitro IC_{90}.[46] This agent is being studied in phase III trials in combination with AZT and ddC (see Chap. 23).

Unlike ddNs (but like the NNRTIs), protease inhibitors do not need to be "activated" inside cells before exerting their antiviral effect. Consequently, the relation between plasma concentrations and activity is likely to be less complex. This has generally proven true in clinical trials, where the most active regimens are those reported to achieve plasma trough concentrations near or above the IC_{90}. However, this association has been complicated in some cases by the high affinity binding of drug to plasma proteins.

Plasma protein binding has a significant impact on the activity of several investigational antiretrovirals in vitro, including polyanions,[47] an HIV Tat antagonist,[48] and certain peptidomimetic protease inhibitors.[49] As it pertains to clinical drug use, protein binding generally affects activity and toxicity equally, does not change the therapeutic index of a drug, and can be circumvented by increasing drug dose. However, protein binding may have an adverse impact on the clinical utility of a drug if drug substance is available in limited supply or is expensive to manufacture or if the drug's formulation is toxic or inconvenient to administer in greater mass.

Experience with the peptidomimetic protease inhibitor SC-52151 was especially instructive in this regard. In phase I pharmacokinetic studies, this agent had a pharmacokinetic profile similar to that of related drugs with significant antiretroviral efficacy in vivo (see Chap. 23). This included bioavailability of about 20% and a plasma elimination half-life of about 2 hours; the major route of clearance was through extensive hepatic metabolism.[50] This compound was poorly water soluble but was highly soluble in ethanol, necessitating administration in an elixir or emulsion with a high alcohol content.

SC-52151 was 90% to 95% bound by plasma protein in vitro and bound with high affinity to α_1-acid glycoprotein. As has been reported with related compounds,[49] addition of physiologic concentrations of α_1-acid glycoprotein greatly reduced the intracellular uptake of radiolabeled drug[51] and increased the in vitro IC_{95} by almost 20-fold.[50] In clinical trials, no significant antiretroviral activity was seen during 14 days' administration of this agent, despite achieving sustained plasma drug concentrations in excess of the IC_{95}. However, if plasma protein binding was considered and free drug concentrations estimated using known protein binding characteristics, plasma concentrations rarely reached the corrected IC_{95}.[50] Clinical failure of this compound likely resulted from the failure to take protein binding into account in determining target plasma drug concentrations. It is likely that higher concentrations of drug would have produced a measurable anti-HIV effect in vivo, but larger doses of drug could not be given because of concerns about long-term ethanol exposure from the formulation and the expense of manufacturing of drug substance.

TOXICITY OF NUCLEOSIDE ANALOGS

All licensed nucleoside analogs possess significant drug-specific dose-limiting toxicities, yielding a small therapeutic window between the minimally effective dose and the maximally tolerated dose. The more serious of these adverse effects includes bone marrow toxicity (eg, AZT, FLT), peripheral neuropathy (eg, ddC, ddI, d4T), pancreatitis (eg, ddI), myopathy (eg, AZT), and hepatic abnormalities (eg, AZT, ddI). Although mechanisms have been identified in vitro that are biologically plausible as the explanation of each of these clinical effects, only general correlations can be made without more precise data linking causes and effects. Perhaps more importantly, this information has not proven useful in managing the drugs clinically. When toxicity occurs, nucleoside doses are reduced or discontinued until symptoms become tolerable or resolve, prompting rechallenge or permanent discontinuation.

The principles for toxicity are similar to those for antiviral effect. The toxic nucleoside analog must enter the target cell, be anabolized or catabolized to the toxic moiety, enter the compartment of the cell wherein normal function is disordered, and achieve site-specific toxic concentrations for sufficient periods.

Much of the investigation of nucleoside analog toxicity has focused on the inhibition of cellular DNA polymerase α (ie, nuclear DNA synthesis), β (ie, endonuclease repair), γ (ie, mitochondrial DNA synthesis), δ (ie, exonuclease proof reading), and ε (ie, exonuclease repair), all of which use dNTP as substrates, as does the viral reverse transcriptase. Although ddN incorporation into cellular DNA correlates somewhat with cytotoxicity in vitro,[25,52] high concentrations of some ddNTPs in cell culture do not necessarily result in cytotoxicity.[30] Generally, the nuclear polymerases (ie, α and ε) are less sensitive to inhibitory effects than mitochondrial polymerase γ and repair polymerase β.[53] The net effect, however, is a far more complex picture than the inhibitory activity of any given nucleoside analog against a specific cellular polymerase.

Hematologic Toxicity

AZT-induced hematologic toxicity provides a useful example of the complex interactions of several factors that conspire to induce toxicity. Anemia secondary to AZT therapy occurs in fewer than 10% of patients with asymptomatic or mildly symptomatic disease,[5] but it occurs at several times that frequency in AIDS patients.[4] Other drugs for which there is substantive long-term clinical experience, such as ddC, ddI, and d4T, do not cause hematologic toxicity. Improvements in hemoglobin and white blood cell counts follow initiation of ddI.[54] The hematologic toxicities of AZT and FLT are reversible, dose or concentration dependent, occur within 1 month of starting either drug, and for AZT at least, the toxicity worsens with advanced stages of HIV disease.[4,55] One clinical study in which the concentration of AZT in the blood correlated with the occurrence of anemia, although not with the rate of clinical progression of disease, suggests that the determinants of AZT's clinical toxicity and clinical efficacy may be different.[56]

In vitro, hematologic toxicity is closely linked to extracellular AZT concentrations,[52] but this cytotoxicity can be reversed by addition of other nucleosides without a change in AZT's antiviral effect.[57] In Molt-4 and ATH-8 lymphoid cell lines, levels of AZTTP, the antivirally active moiety of AZT, do not correlate with cytostatic effects.[58] When intracellular AZTMP levels are reduced by two thirds (in a thymidine kinase–deficient mutant CEM cell line) with no effect on the level of AZTTP, cellular cytotoxicity is reduced 10-fold without altering the anti-HIV effect.[59] This suggests that AZT moieties other than the triphosphate form may play an important role in cellular growth inhibition.

AZTMP may play a significant part in the cellular toxicity of AZT. AZTMP inhibits cellular DNA polymerase δ's 3'- to 5'-exonuclease function, thereby reducing the excision of AZT incorporated into cellular DNA.[25,60,61] AZTMP inhibits production of dTTP and other nucleoside triphosphates through inhibition of thymidine kinase,[9,24] and AZTMP inhibits cellular protein glycosylation.[62] Mutant cells that accumulate less AZTMP experienced reduced cytotoxicity without affecting AZTTP concentrations or antiviral effects.[59] It has been demonstrated clinically that hematologic toxicity increases with HIV disease stage and that measured intracellular AZT phosphate levels and AZTMP, but not AZTTP, increased in patients with low CD4+ T-cell counts.[12] Although there is no demonstrated linkage between these findings, they are consistent with the in vitro findings, suggesting an important role for AZTMP in AZT hematologic toxicity.

With the equivalent of a 250-mg oral dose of AZT, an amino metabolite of AZT, 3'-amino-3'-deoxythymidine (AMT), achieves peak concentrations and an AUC that are one eighth and one fifth of the concentration of contemporaneous AZT.[63] In human bone marrow progenitor cell assays in vitro, AMT demonstrates toxicity to granulocyte-macrophage and erythroid progenitor cells at one fifth and one seventh, respectively, of the concentration of AZT.[64] These toxic effects appear to be independent of mitochondrial DNA inhibition.[65] Taken together, these findings suggest that AMT may be a contributing factor to the hematologic toxicity, especially erythroid, of AZT at clinically relevant doses.

Although it may be difficult to clarify which AZT moiety causes the toxic effects, several mechanisms of AZT hematologic toxicity have been proposed. AZT demonstrates dose-dependent inhibition of granulocyte-macrophage and erythroid progenitor cell proliferation and differentiation in bone marrow models in vitro.[65] Relative to concentrations of FLT or ddC, higher concentrations of AZT are required to inhibit the growth of the same cells. The amount of incorporation of AZT into DNA correlates closely with survival of bone marrow cells in culture.[52] Bone marrow progenitor cells may also be unresponsive to normal signals for erythroid differentiation, because micromolar concentrations of AZT reduce the intracellular mRNA levels coding for the erythropoietin receptor, resulting in reduced cell surface receptors for erythropoietin.[66] AZT and AMT, but not FLT, reduce globin production through decreased globin mRNA synthesis, although this may only occur at clinically irrelevant doses; bone marrow cytotoxicity can be partially reversed by the addition of hemin.[67,68] AZT also induces telomere shortening, with subsequently reduced cell viability,[69] which may have importance for rapidly dividing bone marrow cells, although AZT does not produce clinical toxicity in other rapidly dividing cell types.

The third thymidine analog, d4T, inhibits erythroid and granulocyte-macrophage lineage bone marrow progenitor cells at relatively late stages of development, similar to AZT and AMT, but at far higher concentrations than FLT or AZT.[65] Clinically relevant concentrations of d4T show no hematologic toxicity in vitro. Despite the fact that d4TTP concentrations accumulate in bone marrow, there is 10- to 50-fold less d4T incorporated into host DNA compared with AZT, possibly because of a much higher degree of exonuclease-mediated excision.[25] Unlike the situation in lymphocytes, bone marrow cells significantly catabolize d4TTP to d4TDP, which is not a substrate for incorporation into host DNA through the action of thymidine phosphorylase.[70] Unlike AZTMP, d4T does not affect intracellular nucleoside pools through thymidylate kinase inhibition.[24]

The dC analogs ddC and 3TC inhibit granulocyte-macrophage and erythroid cell lineages in vitro but not clinically. The ddC is equipotent against erythroid and granulocyte-macrophage lines in early stages of development and is even a more potent inhibitor of granulocyte-macrophage lineage cells than AZT, roughly equivalent to the potency of AMT.[65] However, because it is more potent against HIV reverse transcriptase and causes an etiologically different peripheral neuropathy at low doses, ddC does not achieve hematologically toxic concentrations in clinical use. The (+)-enantiomer of 3TC displays greater than 10-fold more hematologic toxicity than the (−)-enantiomer, with a CC_{50} around 2 μM, which is still far higher than the toxic concentrations of AZT or FLT.[71]

The purine analog ddI, which demonstrates no hematologic toxicity,[72] is restricted in its range of clinically usable doses because of nonhematologic dose-limiting toxicities, mainly neuropathy. PMEApp has a far lower K_i for nuclear polymerase α than d4TTP and AZTTP,[73] although no hematologic toxicity has been demonstrated in its limited clinical experience.

Neuropathy

A painful, peripheral sensorimotor neuropathy occurs in 15% to 20% of patients taking ddC, ddI, or d4T, and it is the dose-limiting toxicity for these medications.[74–76] A mild non–dose-limiting neuropathy has been observed in 20% of subjects in two FLT studies.[77] These neuropathies are insidious in onset, occur in or beyond the second month of treatment, and correlate with dose in time to onset and severity of symptoms. They characteristically begin as a tingling or burning sensation in a stocking and glove distribution, first noticed only while walking; with time, this pattern progresses to pain at rest. A "coasting" phenomenon occurs in which the symptoms may worsen for several weeks, even after discontinuation of the offending drug, but resolution is usually complete within a few weeks to months after discontinuation of the drugs.

Nerve conduction velocities in affected patients show absent or greatly diminished nerve action potentials consistent with axonal degeneration.[78] The ddC induces a primary myelinopathy with secondary distal and proximal axonopathy in rabbits that is accompanied by changes in mitochondrial morphology.[79,80] Schwann cells develop abnormally large, cup-shaped mitochondria with increased cristae. Molt-4 cells, in the presence of ddC, also develop abnormal mitochondrial ultrastructure with condensed cristae or vacuolization at 12 days.[81]

At the biochemical level, several ddNs inhibit purified, cell-free mitochondrial γ polymerase, and the degree of inhibition roughly correlates with Molt-4 cell mitochondrial DNA synthesis.[53] The magnitude of inhibition also roughly parallels the clinical occurrence of neuropathy; AZT and 3TC display far less inhibition of polymerase γ than ddC and d4T.[53] In proliferating CEM cells, the relative order of ddN-induced mitochondrial DNA (mtDNA) inhibition did not parallel the relative neurologic toxicity of these drugs, but when the ratio of cellular to mitochondrial toxicity was compared, the sequence more closely resembled this clinical picture: ddC > ddI > d4T > AZT.[82] In a resting neuronal cell model (ie, PC12 cells) that may approximate the target tissues of ddN-induced neuropathy, ddC demonstrated a dose-dependent reduction of mtDNA, and ddI induced mitochondrial toxicity.[82] AZT showed no effect on the cell to mtDNA ratio or cellular proliferation at concentrations up to 100 μM. Consistent with these findings, studies of bone marrow cells show that AZT does not alter the synthetic function of mitochondrial DNA polymerase γ or the nuclear DNA to mtDNA ratio at concentrations that inhibit 75% of granulocyte-macrophage or erythroid cell growth, unlike the effects of ddC, ddI, or d4T.[65] Although these in vitro studies demonstrate a consistent association of neuropathy-inducing drugs and mitochondrial toxicity, the exact mechanism awaits further clarification.

Myopathy

AZT has been associated with a reversible myopathy that is distinct pathologically from HIV-related myopathic changes, characterized by insidious onset of initially proximal muscle weakness and tenderness after an average of 1 year of AZT use.[83,84] Muscle biopsy shows areas of focal necrosis and "ragged red" fibers with mitochondria showing paracrystalline inclusions that correlate well with the clinical severity of the myopathy.[85,86] Studies of AZT-treated rats showed AZT to be a muscle mitochondrial toxin that interrupted oxidative phosphorylation coupling and respiratory chain activity.[87] However, the fact that AZT displays the least inhibition of polymerase γ or mtDNA among several ddN analogs,[82] none of which induce a similar myopathy, suggests a more complex process that may involve muscle cell—specific transport into and phosphorylation by mitochondria.

Pancreatitis

Pancreatitis, characterized by progressive abdominal pain, nausea, vomiting, and elevation of serum amylase, has been attributed to ddI in 5% of 7806 patients enrolled in the ddI expanded access program.[88] Although milder complications, such as abdominal pain, hyperamylasemia, or both, were reported in as many as 23% of patients. A few deaths (0.36%) have been attributed to ddI, largely as a consequence of pancreatitis. Although the pancreatitis is dose-related and reversible, rechallenge at lower doses frequently has not been successful.[89] A history of pancreatitis and concomitant alcohol use increase the risk for development of pancreatitis associated with ddI therapy. Pancreatitis has been reported only rarely with other nucleoside analogs (ie, ddC and cytosine arabinoside).[90,91] The biochemical mechanism of this complication is unknown.

Hepatic Steatosis With Lactic Acidosis

Severe hepatomegaly with macrovesicular steatosis occurred in 8 HIV-infected patients who had received at least 6 months of AZT; 6 of the 8 died of the disorder.[92] Metabolic acidosis was also seen in 5 of the 6 patients who died. Seven of the patients were women, and most were mildly to moderately obese. In another report, 7 patients developed unexplained lactic acidosis, 4 of whom died.[93] Two patients in this group were obese women who had extensive fatty liver at autopsy. Use of ddI has been associated with three cases of otherwise unexplained fulminant hepatic failure with lactic acidosis and microvesicular steatosis on biopsy.[94,95] An FLT

trial was terminated prematurely because of two unexplained cases of progressive hepatic failure.[77] These cases have roughly similar features: current or previous ddN exposure; hepatic abnormalities, including macrovesicular or microvesicular steatosis; and lactic acidosis. The mechanism of the syndrome remains unclear.

It has been postulated that the inhibition of mtDNA synthesis may play a role in the cases of hepatic steatosis and lactic acidosis. Lactic acid production results from dependence on glycolysis as a cellular energy source when mitochondrial oxidative phosphorylation is diminished and mitochondrially synthesized ATP is no longer available in quantities sufficient for the cell's energy needs. Many of the ddNs inhibit mitochondrial γ DNA polymerase, reduce mtDNA synthesis, and increase lactic acid production in a concentration-dependent fashion in cell culture.[53,82,96] However, the magnitude of change among these three parameters after exposure to ddNs does not correlate well, suggesting a more complex mechanism than simple γ DNA polymerase inhibition. In this context, it is intriguing that AZT inhibits adenylate kinase in vitro in the range of clinically achievable concentrations[21]; theoretically, AZT could also limit ATP availability by limiting the availability of ADP.

A clinical trial of the long-term effects of fialuridine (FIAU), an antiviral nucleoside analog with activity against hepatitis B virus, resulted in a frequently fatal syndrome with delayed onset of hepatic failure, severe refractory lactic acidosis, microvesicular fatty liver, and muscle, nerve, and pancreas involvement after several weeks of therapy.[97,98] In vitro investigations in U937 and Molt-4F cells indicated that FIAU-induced cytotoxicity was correlated with FIAU triphosphate concentrations and incorporation into DNA.[99] However, FIAU did not chain terminate DNA or increase lactate production. Another study using CEM cells and a hepatoblastoma cell line found that mtDNA replication was not inhibited, but lactic acid production was increased in a dose-dependent fashion.[98] This discordance between lactic acid production and mtDNA changes is also seen with antiretroviral ddNs.

SPECIAL TOPICS IN CLINICAL PHARMACOLOGY

Maternofetal Drug Transfer

The demonstration that perinatal administration of AZT substantially reduces the rate of vertical transmission of HIV[100] created increased interest in the transfer of antiretroviral drugs across the placenta during pregnancy. Unlike the central nervous system, the placenta generally is not a pharmacologically privileged compartment. Most drugs, especially those that are orally bioavailable, cross the placenta to some degree. This is particularly true for lipophilic agents and less so for compounds that are highly ionized in plasma. For example, nucleoside analogs such as AZT are uncharged in plasma and cross the placenta readily, but charged substances such as dextran sulfate or antisense oligonucleotides would be expected to cross the placenta poorly.

Most human and animal studies of placental transfer of antiretroviral drugs have involved nucleoside analogs. Plasma concentrations achieved in the fetus are proportional to those in maternal plasma.[40] Like many extrahepatic tissues, the placenta is capable of some drug metabolizing reactions, particularly glucuronidation, although this is probably an inconsequential means of clearance.

Like the placenta, mammary glands present no real barrier to drug distribution, and most orally available agents are expected to pass into breast milk to some extent. Lipophilic agents may be concentrated in breast milk and reach concentrations many times higher than those in maternal plasma. AZT concentrations in human breast milk are generally equal to or greater than simultaneous plasma concentrations, and the AUC of AZT in breast milk from lactating women is reported to be on average 50% higher than simultaneous plasma AUCs.[101] The possibility of nursing as an alternative way to deliver adequate oral AZT to neonates is being explored.

Pharmacokinetics in Special Populations

Possible differences in the efficacy and toxicity of AZT in women and ethnic minorities[102,103] prompted some attention to the comparative pharmacokinetics and pharmacodynamics of antiretroviral drugs in special subpopulations with HIV infection. Drug disposition in injection drug users, children and adolescents, and those with intercurrent opportunistic diseases and organ system failure have been considered as well.

A variety of inborn and exogenous factors can significantly alter drug clearance and drug response in an individual. As a general rule, broad genetic factors such as gender or race are less important determinants of individual variability in pharmacokinetics and pharmacodynamics than are more obvious conditions such as renal or hepatic failure or coadministration of drugs like probenecid or rifampin, which have a known propensity for inhibiting or accelerating the clearance of other agents. With few exceptions, most formal pharmacokinetic studies have found little or no significant effect of race or gender on drug disposition.[104] However, few studies have been published that specifically address this issue as it applies to antiretrovirals. The notable exceptions include neonates younger than 1 month of age, in whom some drug metabolizing pathways (eg, conjugation reactions) are not yet matured, and pregnant women in whom the volume of drug distribution may change significantly.[40,104] Neonates younger than 14 days of age, for example, have reduced clearance of AZT, most likely as a consequence of reduced glucuronidation.[105] However, AZT clearance in children and infants 14 days of age and older does not appear to be significantly different from that in adults.[106]

Drug Interactions

Clinically significant drug-drug interactions are a common complication of polypharmacy. More drug combinations are being developed to treat HIV infection and associated opportunistic diseases to exploit nonoverlapping toxicities and possible antimicrobial synergy. Unfortunately, this increases the probability of unanticipated pharmacokinetic interactions. Pharmacodynamic interactions are interactions in which the concentrations of coadministered drugs remain the same, but the effects of one or both agents are diminished or exaggerated. These interactions are recognized infrequently. An example of a pharmacodynamic interaction would be the unacceptable increase in hematologic toxicity seen when AZT and ganciclovir are coadministered.[107]

Any clinical regimen consisting of n different agents produces $n(n-1)/2$ possible two-drug combinations. A patient prescribed seven or eight pharmacologically active agents simultaneously—a common situation in late-stage disease, is exposed to almost 30 potential drug-drug interactions. Multidrug interactions (ie, those involving three or more agents) undoubtedly exist, but they are difficult to identify or evaluate.

The major mechanisms for pharmacokinetic drug-drug interactions include inhibition of absorption, renal clearance, or hepatic metabolism, and accelerated clearance. The latter is usually caused by inducers of hepatic drug metabolizing enzymes, such as rifampin or rifabutin. With antiretroviral regimens, the most worrisome pharmacokinetic interactions are those producing increased drug concentrations and increased toxicity or those producing decreased drug concentrations and a loss of beneficial clinical activity. The most likely scenarios are competition for renal clearance (ie, tubular secretion or glomerular filtration) or competition for phase I (eg, oxidation or reduction via cytochrome P450 isoforms) and phase II (eg, conjugation) drug metabolizing pathways in the liver. The former affects renally cleared drugs, such as ddI or d4T, and the latter affects drugs cleared predominately by phase I biotransformation, such as nevirapine or the peptidomimetic protease inhibitors, or by phase II conjugation, such as AZT. The list of agents known to significantly alter the pharmacokinetics of approved antiretroviral nucleosides is fortunately short (Table 22-3). However, for newer classes of antiretrovirals that are extensively metabolized, this may become a more important problem in clinical drug use.

As combination drug regimens proliferate, clinicians should be aware of potentially important pharmacokinetic interactions as soon as possible. An in vitro model system for predicting changes in the hepatic clearance of various drugs used in combination would be quite useful for those agents eliminated by the liver. Cultured human hepatocytes or human hepatic microsomes can be used to define metabolic pathways and estimate the effect of combining drugs on clearance. The predictive value of such systems has been examined in clinical trials, and results are mixed. In some

TABLE 22-3. *Pharmacokinetic drug-drug interactions affecting antiretroviral nucleoside analogs*

Drug	Increased AUC*	Decreased AUC*	No Effect
Zidovudine	Fluconazole Interferon-β Methadone[‡] Probenecid Valproic Acid[108]	Clarithromycin[125†] Rifampin	Acetaminophen Acyclovir Azithromycin Didanosine[126] Dipyridamole[116] Famciclovir[127] Foscarnet GM-CSF Ibuprofen Indomethacin Naproxen Oxazepam Pentoxifylline[128] Rifabutin[129] Trimethoprim/sulfa Zalcitabine[130]
Didanosine	Antacids[131§]		Forscarnet[132] Ganciclovir[131] Ranitidine[131,133] Stavudine[134] Zidovudine[126]
Zalcitabine			Zidovudine[130]
Stavudine			Didanosine[134]
Lamivudine			Zidovudine[135]

*Interactions listed are those that increase or decrease the AUC by a mean of ≥20%.

†Interaction can be avoided by separating administration by 2 hours or more. References for primary studies can be found in reference 40, except where indicated.

‡Conflicting data exist about whether a clinically significant pharmacokinetic interaction occurs.

§Already contained in commercially available formulations of drug.

AUC, area under the concentration-time curve; GM-CSF, granulocyte-macrophage colony-stimulating factor.

cases, such as AZT and valproic acid, a significant pharmacokinetic interaction was predicted in vitro and then confirmed in clinical studies.[108] In another case, significant interactions seen in vitro between AZT and nonsteroidal antiinflammatory drugs such as naproxen[109] were not seen in vivo when carefully tested in human subjects.[110] In the latter case, misleading results may have come from testing concentrations of naproxen in vitro that were much higher than those achievable in vivo.

Although drug-drug interactions are generally perceived as having a negative impact on therapeutics, some interactions may be beneficial. For example, the combination of AZT with probenecid[111] or valproic acid[108] in HIV-infected volunteers results in inhibition of AZT glucuronidation because these drugs compete for the same glucuronyl transferases in the liver. As a consequence, AZT's clearance is reduced, and plasma concentrations are increased, approximately doubling the AUC during a dosing interval. This strategy may allow a 50% reduction in the daily dose of AZT without sacrificing anti-HIV activity, saving substantially on the cost of drug therapy. However, the potential toxicities of the second agent in this combination, such as the rash associated with probenecid in HIV-infected sub-

jects[112] or the hepatotoxicity of valproic acid,[108] must be considered.

Other potentially beneficial pharmacokinetic interactions have been identified as being mediated through an effect on intracellular drug metabolism. The antiplatelet agent dipyridamole has synergistic anti-HIV activity with AZT and ddC in vitro, reducing by a factor of five the concentrations of AZT needed to suppress HIV replication.[28,113] This beneficial drug interaction is thought to be mediated by dipyridamole's effect on nucleoside transport. AZT enters the cell by passive diffusion, unlike native nucleosides that enter by means of a nucleoside transporter.[114] This transporter can be blocked by dipyridamole with no effect on intracellular concentrations of AZT, ultimately resulting in a favorable decrease in the dTTP to AZTTP ratio and an increase in the antiviral efficacy of AZT in vitro.[28,115] Inhibitory concentrations of dipyridamole have been achieved in clinical studies without clinical toxicity or interference with AZT pharmacokinetics.[116]

The antimetabolite hydroxyurea, an inhibitor of the enzyme ribonucleotide reductase, has been reported to enhance the anti-HIV activity of ddI through a similar mechanism. Hydroxyurea blocks a salvage pathway involved in the synthesis of deoxynucleosides, especially dATP.[36] Because ddI is converted to the active metabolite ddATP, hydroxyurea results in a decreased and therefore favorable intracellular ratio of dATP to ddATP, increasing the probability of incorporation of ddATP into the nascent viral RNA-DNA duplex.[36] Chronic low doses of hydroxyurea have been administered experimentally for the treatment of disorders like sickle cell anemia,[117] and studies are underway to evaluate the anti-HIV effects of concurrent hydroxyurea and ddI in HIV-infected subjects. Because hydroxyurea can suppress the bone marrow, caution must be exercised in the clinical use of this agent in HIV-infected patients, particularly those with advanced disease and poor bone marrow reserve.

Therapeutic Monitoring

Careful monitoring of drug exposure and drug effect are essential when dealing with agents that have a narrow therapeutic index. Often, therapeutic monitoring is as simple as ensuring compliance and assessing clinical improvement. However, for agents that have a high potential for toxicity, a well-defined threshold concentration for antiviral or toxic effects, or large interindividual pharmacokinetic variability, more intensive monitoring may be necessary. As is the case with anticonvulsants and antiarrhythmic drugs, therapeutic monitoring may require frequent dose adjustments to achieve a target physiologic effect or plasma concentration.

Many features of antiretroviral nucleoside analogs suggest a potential role for intensive therapeutic monitoring. This has not, however, been practical in most cases. A quantitative correlation between plasma drug concentrations and toxicity or anti-HIV activity has not been defined for most of these drugs, making dose adjustment an empiric exercise. Plasma concentrations of AZT are poorly correlated with anti-HIV activity or CD4 T-cell count changes.[20,118] This may be a function of the rapid elimination half-life of AZT from the plasma, making accurate assessment of cumulative drug exposure difficult in large clinical trials. Alternatively, this may reflect the fact that concentrations of the active metabolite, AZTTP, do not correlate well with extracellular or plasma concentrations of AZT.[10,11,119,120] Pharmacodynamics may be easier to define for newer antiretrovirals such as NNRTIs and protease inhibitors, which do not require intracellular activation.

In two cases, the quantitative pharmacodynamics of antiretroviral drugs have been defined as a function of plasma drug concentrations. The AZT analog FLT produces well-defined and predictable decreases in serum p24 antigen and quantitative PBMC microculture as a function of AUC and C_{min}.[77] A similar relation for p24 antigen effect has been reported as a function of foscarnet AUC.[121] In the case of FLT, this association was defined in concentration-controlled trials that required prospective dose individualization, and this drug has a plasma elimination half-life of 4.5

to 6 hours,[77] which is much longer than that of the other available nucleosides.

In vitro model systems have been developed to deliver drug concentrations to tissue culture cells grown in hollow fiber cartridges in a way that mimics human pharmacokinetics: first-order elimination of drugs.[122-124] This may prove useful in defining the pharmacodynamics of antiretroviral drugs early in development. Such pharmacokinetic-pharmacodynamic model systems could help produce more rational dosing regimens, and they may facilitate identification of appropriate target drug concentrations for treatment protocols.

Intensive therapeutic monitoring, especially dose adjustment based on plasma drug concentrations, seems unwarranted for antiretroviral nucleosides. This will probably remain true pending the identification of plasma drug concentrations that correlate with toxicity or antiviral efficacy. More rigorous therapeutic monitoring may become acceptable in the future as we learn more about the relation between plasma drug and intracellular anabolite concentrations and as new classes of antiretroviral drugs with different pharmacologic properties emerge.

REFERENCES

1. Abrams DI, Kuno S, Wong R, et al. Oral dextran sulfate (UA001) in the treatment of the acquired immunodeficiency syndrome (AIDS) and AIDS-related complex. Ann Intern Med 1989;110:183.
2. Lorentsen KJ, Hendrix CW, Collins JM, et al. Dextran sulfate is poorly absorbed after oral administration. Ann Intern Med 1989;111:561.
3. Flexner C, Barditch-Crovo PA, Kornhauser DM, et al. Pharmacokinetics, toxicity, and activity of intravenous dextran sulfate in human immunodeficiency virus infection. Antimicrob Agents Chemother 1991;35:2544.
4. Richman DD, Fischl MA, Grieco MH, et al. The toxicity of azidothymidine (AZT) in the treatment of patients with AIDS and AIDS-related complex. A double-blind, placebo-controlled trial. N Engl J Med 1987;317:192.
5. Volberding PA, Lagakos SW, Koch MA, et al. Zidovudine in asymptomatic human immunodeficiency virus infection. A controlled trial in persons with fewer than 500 CD4-positive cells per cubic millimeter. The AIDS Clinical Trials Group of the National Institute of Allergy and Infectious Diseases. N Engl J Med 1990;322:941.
6. Collier AC, Bozzette S, Coombs RW, et al. A pilot study of low-dose zidovudine in human immunodeficiency virus infection. N Engl J Med 1990;323:1015.
7. Hendrix CW, Margolick JB, Petty BG, et al. Biologic effects after a single dose of poly(I):poly(C12U) in healthy volunteers. Antimicrob Agents Chemother 1993;37:429.
8. Hao Z, Cooney DA, Hartman NR, et al. Factors determining the activity of 2',3'-dideoxynucleosides in suppressing human immunodeficiency virus in vitro. Mol Pharmacol 1988;34:431.
9. Furman PA, Fyfe JA, St Clair MH, et al. Phosphorylation of 3'-azido-3'-deoxythymidine and selective interaction of the 5'-triphosphate with human immunodeficiency virus reverse transcriptase. Proc Natl Acad Sci USA 1986;83:8333.
10. Balzarini J, Baba M, Pauwels R, Herdewijn P, De Clercq E. Anti-retrovirus activity of 3'-fluoro- and 3'-azido-substituted pyrimidine 2',3'-dideoxynucleoside analogues. Biochem Pharmacol 1988;37:2847.
11. Avramis VI, Markson W, Jackson RL, Gomperts E. Biochemical pharmacology of zidovudine in human T-lymphoblastoid cells (CEM). AIDS 1989;3:417.
12. Barry M, Howe JL, Ormesher S, et al. Pharmacokinetics of zidovudine and dideoxyinosine alone and in combination in patients with the acquired immunodeficiency syndrome. Br J Clin Pharmacol 1994;37:421.

13. Ho HT, Hitchcock MJ. Cellular pharmacology of 2′,3′-dideoxy-2′,3′-didehydrothymidine, a nucleoside analog active against human immunodeficiency virus. Antimicrob Agents Chemother 1989;33:844.

14. Tornevik Y, Jacobsson B, Britton S, Eriksson S. Intracellular metabolism of 3′-azidothymidine in isolated human peripheral blood mononuclear cells. AIDS Res Hum Retroviruses 1991;7:751.

15. Munch-Petersen B, Cloos L, Tyrsted G, Eriksson S. Diverging substrate specificity of pure human thymidine kinases 1 and 2 against antiviral dideoxynucleosides. J Biol Chem 1991;266:9032.

16. Arner ES, Eriksson S. Deoxycytidine and 2′,3′-dideoxycytidine metabolism in human monocyte-derived macrophages. A study of both anabolic and catabolic pathways. Biochem Biophys Res Commun 1993;197:1499.

17. Perno CF, Yarchoan R, Cooney DA, et al. Inhibition of human immunodeficiency virus (HIV-1/HTLV-IIIBa-L) replication in fresh and cultured human peripheral blood monocytes/macrophages by azidothymidine and related 2′,3′-dideoxynucleosides. J Exp Med 1988;168:1111.

18. Gao WY, Shirasaka T, Johns DG, Broder S, Mitsuya H. Differential phosphorylation of azidothymidine, dideoxycytidine, and dideoxyinosine in resting and activated peripheral blood mononuclear cells. J Clin Invest 1993;91:2326.

19. Dianzani F, Antonelli G, Turriziani O, et al. Zidovudine induces the expression of cellular resistance affecting its antiviral activity. AIDS Res Hum Retroviruses 1994;10:1471.

20. Stretcher BN, Pesce AJ, Frame PT, Stein DS. Pharmacokinetics of zidovudine phosphorylation in peripheral blood mononuclear cells from patients infected with human immunodeficiency virus. Antimicrob Agents Chemother 1994;38:1541.

21. Barile M, Valenti D, Hobbs GA, et al. Mechanisms of toxicity of 3′-azido-3′-deoxythymidine. Its interaction with adenylate kinase. Biochem Pharmacol 1994;48:1405.

22. August EM, Marongiu ME, Lin TS, Prusoff WH. Initial studies on the cellular pharmacology of 3′-deoxythymidin-2′-ene (d4T): a potent and selective inhibitor of human immunodeficiency virus. Biochem Pharmacol 1988;37:4419.

23. Zhu Z, Ho HT, Hitchcock MJ, Sommadossi JP. Cellular pharmacology of 2′,3′-didehydro-2′,3′-dideoxythymidine (D4T) in human peripheral blood mononuclear cells. Biochem Pharmacol 1990;39:R15.

24. Balzarini J, Herdewijn P, De Clercq E. Differential patterns of intracellular metabolism of 2′,3′-didehydro-2′,3′-dideoxythymidine and 3′-azido-2′,3′-dideoxythymidine, two potent anti–human immunodeficiency virus compounds. J Biol Chem 1989;264:6127.

25. Zhu Z, Hitchcock MJ, Sommadossi JP. Metabolism and DNA interaction of 2′,3′-didehydro-2′,3′-dideoxythymidine in human bone marrow cells. Mol Pharmacol 1991;40:838.

26. Cooney DA, Dalal M, Mitsuya H, et al. Initial studies on the cellular pharmacology of 2′,3-dideoxycytidine, an inhibitor of HTLV-III infectivity. Biochem Pharmacol 1986;35:2065.

27. Patel SS, Szebeni J, Wahl LM, Weinstein JN. Differential inhibition of 2′-deoxycytidine salvage as a possible mechanism for potentiation of the anti–human immunodeficiency virus activity of 2′,3′-dideoxycytidine by dipyridamole. Antimicrob Agents Chemother 1991;35:1250.

28. Szebeni J, Wahl SM, Betageri GV, et al. Inhibition of HIV-1 in monocyte/macrophage cultures by 2′,3′-dideoxycytidine-5′-triphosphate, free and in liposomes. AIDS Res Hum Retroviruses 1990;6:691.

29. Tornevik Y, Eriksson S. 2′,3′-Dideoxycytidine toxicity in cultured human CEM T lymphoblasts: effects of combination with 3′-azido-3′-deoxythymidine and thymidine. Mol Pharmacol 1990;38:237.

30. Hao Z, Cooney DA, Farquhar D, et al. Potent DNA chain termination activity and selective inhibition of human immunodeficiency virus reverse transcriptase by 2′,3′-dideoxyuridine-5′-triphosphate. Mol Pharmacol 1990;37:157.

31. Cheng YC, Dutschman GE, Bastow KF, Sarngadharan MG, Ting RY. Human immunodeficiency virus reverse transcriptase. General properties and its interactions with nucleoside triphosphate analogs. J Biol Chem 1987;262:2187.

32. Cammack N, Rouse P, Marr CL, et al. Cellular metabolism of (−) enantiomeric 2′-deoxy-3′-thiacytidine. Biochem Pharmacol 1992;43:2059.

33. Hart GJ, Orr DC, Penn CR, et al. Effects of (−)-2′-deoxy-3′-thiacytidine (3TC) 5′-triphosphate on human immunodeficiency virus reverse transcriptase and mammalian DNA polymerases alpha, beta, and gamma. Antimicrob Agents Chemother 1992;36:1688.

34. Coates JA, Cammack N, Jenkinson HJ, et al. (−)-2′-Deoxy-3′-thiacytidine is a potent, highly selective inhibitor of human immunodeficiency virus type 1 and type 2 replication in vitro. Antimicrob Agents Chemother 1992;36:733.

35. Balzarini J, Lee CK, Schols D, De Clercq E. 1-Beta-D-ribofuranosyl-1,2,4-triazole-3-carboxamide (ribavirin) and 5-ethynyl-1-beta-D-ribofuranosylimidazole-4-carboxamide (EICAR) markedly potentiate the inhibitory effect of 2′,3′-dideoxyinosine on human immunodeficiency virus in peripheral blood lymphocytes. Biochem Biophys Res Commun 1991;178:563.

36. Gao WY, Agbaria R, Driscoll JS, Mitsuya H. Divergent anti–human immunodeficiency virus activity and anabolic phosphorylation of 2′,3′-dideoxynucleoside analogs in resting and activated human cells. J Biol Chem 1994;269:12633.

37. Ahluwalia G, Cooney DA, Hartman NR, et al. Anomalous accumulation and decay of 2′,3′-dideoxyadenosine-5′-triphosphate in human T-cell cultures exposed to the anti-HIV drug 2′,3′-dideoxyinosine. Drug Metab Dispos 1993;21:369.

38. Balzarini J, Naesens L, Herdewijn P, et al. Marked in vivo antiretrovirus activity of 9-(2-phosphonylmethoxyethyl) adenine, a selective anti–human immunodeficiency virus agent. Proc Natl Acad Sci USA 1989;86:332.

39. Balzarini J, Hao Z, Herdewijn P, Johns DG, De Clercq E. Intracellular metabolism and mechanism of anti-retrovirus action of 9-(2-phosphonylmethoxyethyl) adenine, a potent anti–human immunodeficiency virus compound. Proc Natl Acad Sci USA 1991;88:1499.

40. Dudley MN. Clinical pharmacokinetics of nucleoside antiretroviral agents. J Infect Dis 1995;171(Suppl 2):S99.

41. Unadkat JD, Collier AC, Crosby SS, Cummings D, Opheim KE, Corey L. Pharmacokinetics of oral zidovudine (azidothymidine) in patients with AIDS when administered with and without a high-fat meal. AIDS 1990;4:229.

42. Sahai J, Gallicano K, Garber G, et al. The effect of a protein meal on zidovudine pharmacokinetics in HIV-infected patients. Br J Clin Pharmacol 1992;33:657.

43. Sidtis JJ, Gatsonis C, Price RW, et al. Zidovudine treatment of the AIDS dementia complex: results of a placebo-controlled trial. AIDS Clinical Trials Group. Ann Neurol 1993;33:343.

44. Barditch-Crovo PA, Toole J, Burgee H, et al. A randomized, double-blind, placebo-controlled phase I/II evaluation of 9-[-2-(bispivaloyloxymethyl) phosphonyl-methoxy] adenine (bis-POM PMEA), an orally bioavailable prodrug of the anti-HIV nucleotide, PMEA. (Abstract) Antiviral Res 1995;23:A229.

45. Cheeseman SH, Hattox SE, McLaughlin MM, et al. Pharmacokinetics of nevirapine: initial single-rising-dose study in humans. Antimicrob Agents Chemother 1993;37:178.

46. Vella S. HIV therapy advances: update on a protease inhibitor. AIDS 1994;8(Suppl 3):S25.

47. Hartman NR, Johns DG, Mitsuya H. Pharmacokinetic analysis of dextran sulfate in rats as pertains to its clinical usefulness for therapy of HIV infection. AIDS Res Human Retrovir 1990;6:805.

48. Georges DL, Hsu M-C, Connell E, Tam S, Lederman MM. The HIV-1 tat antagonist Ro 24-7429 is highly protein bound and relatively inactive at physiologic serum concentrations. Presented at the Second National Conference on Human Retroviruses and Related Infections, Washington, DC, February 1, 1995.

49. Kageyama S, Anderson BD, Hoesterey BL, et al. Protein binding of human immunodeficiency virus protease inhibitor KNI-272 and alteration of its in vitro antiretroviral activity in the presence of high concentrations of proteins. Antimicrob Agents Chemother 1994;38:1107.

50. Flexner C, Richman DD, Bryant M, et al. Effect of protein binding on the pharmacodynamics of an HIV protease inhibitor. (Abstract) Antiviral Res 1995;26:A282.

51. Sommadossi J-P, Schinazi RF, McMillan A, Xie M-Y, and Bryant M. A human serum glycoprotein profoundly affects antiviral activity of the protease inhibitor SC-52151 by decreasing its cellular uptake. Presented at the Second National Conference on Human Retroviruses and Related Infections, Washington, DC, January 30, 1995.

52. Sommadossi JP, Carlisle R, Zhou Z. Cellular pharmacology of 3′-azido-3′-deoxythymidine with evidence of incorporation into DNA of human bone marrow cells. Mol Pharmacol 1989;36:9.

53. Martin JL, Brown CE, Matthews-Davis N, Reardon JE. Effects of antiviral nucleoside analogs on human DNA polymerases and mitochondrial DNA synthesis. Antimicrob Agents Chemother 1994;38:2743.

54. Schacter LP, Rozencweig M, Beltangady M, et al. Effects of therapy with didanosine on hematologic parameters in patients with advanced human immunodeficiency virus disease. Blood 1992;80:2969.

55. Fischl MA, Richman DD, Causey DM, et al. Prolonged zidovudine therapy in patients with AIDS and advanced AIDS-related complex. AZT Collaborative Working Group. JAMA 1989;262:2405.

56. Mentre F, Escolano S, Diquet B, Golmard JL, Mallet A. Clinical pharmacokinetics of zidovudine: inter and intraindividual variability and relationship to long term efficacy and toxicity. Eur J Clin Pharmacol 1993;45:397.

57. Bhalla K, Birkhofer M, Li GR, et al. 2'-Deoxycytidine protects normal human bone marrow progenitor cells in vitro against the cytotoxicity of 3'-azido-3'-deoxythymidine with preservation of antiretroviral activity. Blood 1989;74:1923.

58. Balzarini J, Pauwels R, Baba M, et al. The in vitro and in vivo antiretrovirus activity, and intracellular metabolism of 3'-azido-2',3'-dideoxythymidine and 2',3'-dideoxycytidine are highly dependent on the cell species. Biochem Pharmacol 1988;37:897.

59. Tornevik Y, Ullman B, Balzarini J, Wahren B, Eriksson S. Cytotoxicity of 3'-azido-3'-deoxythymidine correlates with 3'-azidothymidine-5'-monophosphate (AZTMP) levels, whereas anti–human immunodeficiency virus (HIV) activity correlates with 3'-azidothymidine-5'-triphosphate (AZTTP) levels in cultured CEM T-lymphoblastoid cells. Biochem Pharmacol 1995;49:829.

60. Bridges EG, LeBoeuf RB, Weidner DA, Sommadossi JP. Influence of template primary structure on 3'-azido-3'-deoxythymidine triphosphate incorporation into DNA. Antiviral Res 1993;21:93.

61. Vazquez-Padua MA, Starnes MC, Cheng YC. Incorporation of 3'-azido-3'-deoxythymidine into cellular DNA and its removal in a human leukemic cell line. Cancer Commun 1990;2:55.

62. Hall ET, Yan JP, Melancon P, Kuchta RD. 3'-Azido-3'-deoxythymidine potently inhibits protein glycosylation. A novel mechanism for AZT cytotoxicity. J Biol Chem 1994;269:14355.

63. Stagg MP, Cretton EM, Kidd L, Diasio RB, Sommadossi JP. Clinical pharmacokinetics of 3'-azido-3'-deoxythymidine (zidovudine) and catabolites with formation of a toxic catabolite, 3'-amino-3'-deoxythymidine. Clin Pharmacol Ther 1992;51:668.

64. Cretton EM, Xie MY, Bevan RJ, Goudgaon NM, Schinazi RF, Sommadossi JP. Catabolism of 3'-azido-3'-deoxythymidine in hepatocytes and liver microsomes, with evidence of formation of 3'-amino-3'-deoxythymidine, a highly toxic catabolite for human bone marrow cells. Mol Pharmacol 1991;39:258.

65. Faraj A, Fowler DA, Bridges EG, Sommadossi JP. Effects of 2',3'-dideoxynucleosides on proliferation and differentiation of human pluripotent progenitors in liquid culture and their effects on mitochondrial DNA synthesis. Antimicrob Agents Chemother 1994;38:924.

66. Gogu SR, Malter JS, Agrawal KC. Zidovudine-induced blockade of the expression and function of the erythropoietin receptor. Biochem Pharmacol 1992;44:1009.

67. Weidner DA, Bridges EG, Cretton EM, Sommadossi JP. Comparative effects of 3'-azido-3'-deoxythymidine and its metabolite 3'-amino-3'-deoxythymidine on hemoglobin synthesis in K-562 human leukemia cells. Mol Pharmacol 1992;41:252.

68. Abraham NG, Bucher D, Niranjan U, et al. Microenvironmental toxicity of azidothymidine: partial sparing with hemin. Blood 1989;74:139.

69. Strahl C, Blackburn EH. The effects of nucleoside analogs on telomerase and telomeres in Tetrahymena. Nucleic Acids Res 1994;22:893.

70. Balzarini J, Kang GJ, Dalal M, et al. The anti-HTLV-III (anti-HIV) and cytotoxic activity of 2',3'-didehydro-2',3'-dideoxyribonucleosides: a comparison with their parental 2',3'-dideoxyribonucleosides. Mol Pharmacol 1987;32:162.

71. Sommadossi JP, Schinazi RF, Chu CK, Xie MY. Comparison of cytotoxicity of the (−)- and (+)-enantiomer of 2',3'-dideoxy-3'-thiacytidine in normal human bone marrow progenitor cells. Biochem Pharmacol 1992;44:1921.

72. Cooley TP, Kunches LM, Saunders CA, et al. Treatment of AIDS and AIDS-related complex with 2',3'-dideoxyinosine given once daily. Rev Infect Dis 1990;12(Suppl 5):S552.

73. Cherrington JM, Allen SJW, Bischofberger N, Chen MS. Kinetic interaction of the diphosphonates of 9-(2-phosphonylmethoxyethyl) adenine and other anti-HIV active purine congeners with HIV reverse transcriptase and human DNA polymerases alpha, beta, and gamma. Antiviral Chem Chemother 1995;6:217.

74. Friedland G. FDA approves d4T, an alternative to AZT, ddI, or ddC. AIDS Clin Care 1995;7:4.

75. Yarchoan R, Perno CF, Thomas RV, et al. Phase I studies of 2',3'-dideoxycytidine in severe human immunodeficiency virus infection as a single agent and alternating with zidovudine (AZT). Lancet 1988;1:76.

76. Lambert JS, Seidlin M, Valentine FT, Reichman RC, Dolin R. Didanosine: long-term follow-up of patients in a phase 1 study. Clin Infect Dis 1993;16(Suppl 1):S40.

77. Flexner C, van der Horst C, Jacobson MA, et al. Relationship between plasma concentrations of 3'-deoxy-3'-fluorothymidine (alovudine) and antiretroviral activity in two concentration-controlled trials. J Infect Dis 1994;170:1394.

78. Dubinsky RM, Yarchoan R, Dalakas M, Broder S. Reversible axonal neuropathy from the treatment of AIDS and related disorders with 2',3'-dideoxycytidine (ddC). Muscle Nerve 1989;12:856.

79. Feldman D, Brosnan C, Anderson TD. Ultrastructure of peripheral neuropathy induced in rabbits by 2',3'-dideoxycytidine. Lab Invest 1992;66:75.

80. Anderson TD, Davidovich A, Feldman D, et al. Mitochondrial schwannopathy and peripheral myelinopathy in a rabbit model of dideoxycytidine neurotoxicity. Lab Invest 1994;70:724.

81. Lewis W, Gonzalez B, Chomyn A, Papoian T. Zidovudine induces molecular, biochemical, and ultrastructural changes in rat skeletal muscle mitochondria. J Clin Invest 1992;89:1354.

82. Chen CH, Vazquez-Padua M, Cheng YC. Effect of anti–human immunodeficiency virus nucleoside analogs on mitochondrial DNA and its implication for delayed toxicity. Mol Pharmacol 1991;39:625.

83. Bessen LJ, Greene JB, Louie E, Seitzman P, Weinberg H. Severe polymyositis-like syndrome associated with zidovudine therapy of AIDS and ARC. (Letter) N Engl J Med 1988;318:708.

84. Helbert M, Fletcher T, Peddle B, Harris JR, Pinching AJ. Zidovudine-associated myopathy. (Letter) Lancet 1988;2:689.

85. Gorard DA, Henry K, Guiloff RJ. Necrotising myopathy and zidovudine. Lancet 1988;i:1050.

86. Dalakas MC, Illa I, Pezeshkpour GH, Laukaitis JP, Cohen B, Griffin JL. Mitochondrial myopathy caused by long-term zidovudine therapy. N Engl J Med 1990;322:1098.

87. Lamperth L, Dalakas MC, Dagani F, Anderson J, Ferrari R. Abnormal skeletal and cardiac muscle mitochondria induced by zidovudine (AZT) in human muscle in vitro and in an animal model. Lab Invest 1991;65:742.

88. Pike IM, Nicaise C. The didanosine expanded access program: safety analysis. Clin Infect Dis 1993;16(Suppl 1):S63.

89. Lambert JS, Seidlin M, Reichman RC, et al. 2',3'-Dideoxyinosine (ddI) in patients with the acquired immunodeficiency syndrome or AIDS-related complex. A phase I trial. N Engl J Med 1990; 322:1333.

90. Siemers RF, Friedenberg WR, Norfleet RG. High-dose cytosine arabinoside-associated pancreatitis. Cancer 1985;56:1940.

91. Aponte-Cipriani SL, Teplitz C, Yancovitz S. Pancreatitis possibly related to 2',3'-dideoxycytidine. Ann Intern Med 1993;119:539.

92. Freiman JP, Helfert KE, Hamrell MR, Stein DS. Hepatomegaly with severe steatosis in HIV-seropositive patients. AIDS 1993;7:379.

93. Chattha G, Arieff AI, Cummings C, Tierney LM, Jr. Lactic acidosis complicating the acquired immunodeficiency syndrome. Ann Intern Med 1993;118:37.

94. Lai KK, Gang DL, Zawacki JK, Cooley TP. Fulminant hepatic failure associated with 2',3'-dideoxyinosine (ddI). Ann Intern Med 1991; 115:283.

95. Bissuel F, Bruneel F, Habersetzer F, et al. Fulminant hepatitis with severe lactate acidosis in HIV-infected patients on didanosine therapy. J Intern Med 1994;235:367.

96. Tsai CH, Doong SL, Johns DG, Driscoll JS, Cheng YC. Effect of anti-HIV 2'-beta-fluoro-2',3'-dideoxynucleoside analogs on the cellular content of mitochondrial DNA and on lactate production. Biochem Pharmacol 1994;48:1477.

97. Marwick C. NIH panel report of "no flaws" in FIAU trial at variance with FDA report, new probe planned. JAMA 1994;272:9.

98. Colacino JM, Malcolm SK, Jaskunas SR. Effect of fialuridine on replication of mitochondrial DNA in CEM cells and in human hepatoblastoma cells in culture. Antimicrob Agents Chemother 1994; 38:1997.

99. Klecker RW, Katki AG, Collins JM. Toxicity, metabolism, DNA incorporation with lack of repair, and lactate production for 1-(2'-fluoro-2'-deoxy-beta-D-arabinofuranosyl)-5-iodouracil in U-937 and MOLT-4 cells. Mol Pharmacol 1994;46:1204.

100. Connor EM, Sperling RS, Gelber R, et al. Reduction of maternal-infant transmission of human immunodeficiency virus type 1 with zidovudine treatment. Pediatric AIDS Clinical Trials Group Protocol 076 Study Group. N Engl J Med 1994;331:1173.

101. Ruff A, Hamzeh F, Lietman P, et al. Excretion of zidovudine (ZDV) in human breast milk. Presented at the Thirty-Fourth Interscience Conference on Antimicrobial Agents and Chemotherapy, Orlando, FL, October 5, 1994.

102. Lagakos S, Fischl MA, Stein DS, Lim L, Volberding P. Effects of zidovudine therapy in minority and other subpopulations with early HIV infection. JAMA 1991;266:2709.

103. Easterbrook PJ, Keruly JC, Creagh-Kirk T, Richman DD, Chaisson RE, Moore RD. Racial and ethnic differences in outcome in zidovudine-treated patients with advanced HIV disease. Zidovudine Epidemiology Study Group. JAMA 1991;266:2713.

104. Fletcher CV, Acosta E, Strykowski JM. Gender differences in pharmacokinetics and pharmacodynamics. J Adolesc Health 1994;15:619.

105. Boucher FD, Modlin JF, Weller S, et al. Phase I evaluation of zidovudine administered to infants exposed at birth to the human immunodeficiency virus. J Pediatr 1993;122:137.

106. Mueller BU, Pizzo PA, Farley M, et al. Pharmacokinetic evaluation of the combination of zidovudine and didanosine in children with human immunodeficiency virus infection. J Pediatr 1994;125:142.

107. Hochster H, Dieterich D, Bozzette S, et al. Toxicity of combined ganciclovir and zidovudine for cytomegalovirus disease associated with AIDS. An AIDS Clinical Trials Group study. Ann Intern Med 1990; 113:111.

108. Lertora JJ, Rege AB, Greenspan DL, et al. Pharmacokinetic interaction between zidovudine and valproic acid in patients infected with human immunodeficiency virus. Clin Pharmacol Ther 1994;56:272.

109. Resetar A, Minick D, Spector T. Glucuronidation of 3'-azido-3'-deoxythymidine catalyzed by human liver UDP-glucuronosyltransferase. Significance of nucleoside hydrophobicity and inhibition by xenobiotics. Biochem Pharmacol 1991;42:559.

110. Barry M, Howe J, Back D, et al. The effects of indomethacin and naproxen on zidovudine pharmacokinetics. Br J Clin Pharmacol 1993;36:82.

111. Kornhauser DM, Petty BG, Hendrix CW, et al. Probenecid and zidovudine metabolism. Lancet 1989;2:473.

112. Petty BG, Kornhauser DM, Lietman PS. Zidovudine with probenecid: a warning. (Letter) Lancet 1990;335:1044.

113. Szebeni J, Wahl SM, Popovic M, et al. Dipyridamole potentiates the inhibition by 3'-azido-3'-deoxythymidine and other dideoxynucleosides of human immunodeficiency virus replication in monocyte-macrophages. Proc Natl Acad Sci USA 1989;86:3842; published erratum appears in Proc Natl Acad Sci USA 1989;86:5968.

114. Zimmerman TP, Prus KL, Mahony WB, Domin BA. 3'-Azido-3'-deoxythymidine and acyclovir: antiviral nucleoside analogues with unusual cell membrane permeation properties. Adv Exp Med Biol 1989;253B:399.

115. Betageri GV, Szebeni J, Hung K, et al. Effect of dipyridamole on transport and phosphorylation of thymidine and 3'-azido-3'-deoxythymidine in human monocyte/macrophages. Biochem Pharmacol 1990;40:867.

116. Hendrix CW, Flexner C, Szebeni J, et al. Effect of dipyridamole on zidovudine pharmacokinetics and short-term tolerance in asymptomatic human immunodeficiency virus-infected subjects. Antimicrob Agents Chemother 1994;38:1036.

117. Charache S, Terrin ML, Moore R, et al. Effect of hydroxyurea on the frequency of painful crises in sickle cell anemia. N Engl J Med 1995;332:1317.

118. Sale M, Sheiner LB, Volberding P, Blaschke TF. Zidovudine response relationships in early human immunodeficiency virus infection. Clin Pharmacol Ther 1993;54:556.

119. Slusher JT, Kuwahara SK, Hamzeh FM, Lewis LD, Kornhauser DM, Lietman PS. Intracellular zidovudine (ZDV) and ZDV phosphates as measured by a validated combined high-pressure liquid chromatography-radioimmunoassay procedure. Antimicrob Agents Chemother 1992;36:2473.

120. Robbins BL, Rodman J, McDonald C, Sriniva RV, Flynn PM, Fridland A. Enzymatic assay for measurement of zidovudine triphosphate in peripheral blood mononuclear cells. Antimicrob Agents Chemother 1994;38:115.

121. Fletcher CV, Collier AC, Rhame FS, et al. Foscarnet for suppression of human immunodeficiency virus replication. Antimicrob Agents Chemother 1994;38:604.

122. Bilello JA, Bauer G, Dudley MN, Cole GA, Drusano GL. Effect of 2',3'-didehydro-3'-deoxythymidine in an in vitro hollow-fiber pharmacodynamic model system correlates with results of dose-ranging clinical studies. Antimicrob Agents Chemother 1994;38:1386.

123. Moore MR, Hamzeh FM, Lee FE-H, Lietman PS. Activity of (S)-1-(3-hydroxy-2-phosphonylmethoxypropyl) cytosine against human cytomegalovirus when administered as single-bolus and continuous infusion in vitro cell culture perfusion system. Antimicrob Agents Chemother 1994;38:2404.

124. Hamzeh FM, Schaad HJ, Lietman PS. A pharmacokinetic/pharmacodynamic approach for the comparison of penciclovir and acyclovir: utilization on an in vitro model which simulates in vivo pharmacokinetics. (Abstract) Antiviral Res 1995;26:A338.

125. Petty B, Polis M, Haneiwich S, Dellerson M, Craft JC, Chaisson R. Pharmacokinetic assessment of clarithromycin plus zidovudine in HIV patients. Presented at the Thirty-Second Interscience Conference on Antimicrobial Agents and Chemotherapy, Anaheim, CA, October 11, 1992.

126. Barry M, Howe JL, Ormesher S, et al. Pharmacokinetics of zidovudine and dideoxyinosine alone and in combination in patients with the acquired immunodeficiency syndrome. Br J Clin Pharmacol 1994;37:421.

127. Siederer S, Scott S, Rousseau F, et al. Safe coadministration of famciclovir and zidovudine to HIV positive patients. (Abstract) Antiviral Res 1995;26:A287.

128. Dezube B, Lederman MM, Spritzler J, et al. High-dose pentoxifylline in patients with AIDS: inhibition of TNF production. J Infect Dis 1995;171:1628.

129. Gallicano K, Sahai J, Swick L, Pakuts A, Cameron W. The effect of rifabutin (R) on zidovudine pharmacokinetics. Presented at the Second National Conference on Human Retroviruses and Related Infections, Washington, DC, February 1, 1995.

130. Meng T-C, Fischl MA, Boota AM, et al. Combination therapy with zidovudine and dideoxycytidine in patients with advanced human immunodeficiency virus infection. Ann Intern Med 1992;116:13.

131. Hartman NR, Yarchoan R, Pluda JM, et al. Pharmacokinetics of 2',3'-dideoxyinosine in patients with severe human immunodeficiency infection. II. The effects of different oral formulations and the presence of other medications. Clin Pharmacol Ther 1991;50:278.

132. Aweeka FT, Mathur V, Dorsey R, et al. Concomitant foscarnet and didanosine: a pharmacokinetic (PK) evaluation in patients with HIV disease. Presented at the Second National Conference on Human Retroviruses and Related Infections, Washington, DC, February 1, 1995.

133. Knupp CA, Graziano FM, Dixon RM, Barbhaiya RH. Pharmacokinetic-interaction study of didanosine and ranitidine in patients seropositive for human immunodeficiency virus. Antimicrob Agents Chemother 1992;36:2075.

134. Seifert RD, Stewart MB, Sramek J, Conrad J, Kaul S, Cutler N. Pharmacokinetics of coadministered didanosine and stavudine in HIV-seropositive male patients. Br J Clin Pharmacol 1994;38:405.

135. Horton C, Yuen G, Mikolich D, et al. Pharmacokinetics of lamivudine administered alone and with zidovudine in asymptomatic patients with human immunodeficiency virus infection. (Abstract) Clin Pharmacol Ther 1994;55:198.

AIDS: Biology, Diagnosis, Treatment and
Prevention, fourth edition, edited by Vincent T.
DeVita, Jr., Samuel Hellman, and Steven A.
Rosenberg. Lippincott–Raven Publishers, © 1997

CHAPTER 23

Antiretroviral Therapy

Martin S. Hirsch, Richard T. D'Aquila, and Joan C. Kaplan

Although much is known about the replication of human immunodeficiency virus type 1 (HIV-1) and numerous agents have been developed that inhibit HIV-1 replication in vitro,[1] success in translating experimental studies into clinical practice has been meager. The major drawback in developing clinically useful antiretrovirals has been that available drugs provide only limited virus suppression for relatively short periods. It has become clear that HIV-1 burdens are substantial and high-level virus replication occurs at all stages of infection.[2-4] Even during asymptomatic and clinically quiescent periods, replication in lymphoid organs is extensive.[5,6] This high virus turnover drives the pathogenic process and the development of genetic variation. Under the selection pressure of drug therapy, viruses with resistance mutations accumulate, sometimes with complete replacement of wild-type virus by drug-resistant mutants in plasma after only 2 to 4 weeks of therapy.[2,3] Developing effective and sustained antiviral effects that allow reconstitution of the depleted immune system or prevent depletion altogether remains the major challenge for HIV-1 therapeutics.

This chapter reviews clinically available and promising agents and combinations, highlighting clinical trial results and resistance issues. The pharmacology and toxicity of individual compounds are reviewed in Chapter 22.

SITES FOR ATTACK

Within the HIV-1 replicative cycle are several potential targets for antiviral attack (Fig. 23-1). The initial steps in replication are attachment of the viral envelope glycoprotein to a specific receptor on the cell surface whose major component is CD4. After a membrane fusion event, HIV-1 is internalized and uncoated, and reverse transcription takes place in the cytoplasm within a preintegration complex of viral and possibly cellular proteins. This conversion of a single-stranded RNA genome to double-stranded DNA involves DNA polymerization and ribonuclease H (RNase H) enzymatic activities of HIV-1 RT and is the source of the extensive genetic heterogeneity of HIV-1. The DNA polymerization portion of this process is the target of most agents in clinical use and many of those under development.

While reverse transcription is occurring, cellular factors may specifically bind a nuclear localization signal site within the HIV-1 matrix protein to actively transport the viral preintegration complex into the nucleus.[7] Unlike other retroviruses, which do not integrate into DNA until nuclear membrane integrity is disrupted during mitosis, HIV-1 proviral DNA can be formed by the viral integrase that inserts viral genetic material into host chromosomal DNA of nondividing, terminally differentiated monocyte-macrophages and of CD4+ T lymphocytes arrested in G_2 and S phase.[7-9] Inhibition of any of the replication steps up to this point prevents the establishment of a productive infection.

Virus replication in cells that already contain integrated HIV-1 proviral DNA can only be inhibited by targeting steps late in the replication cycle. Integrated HIV-1 DNA is transcribed by host-cell RNA polymerase II, but the process is modulated by viral regulatory signals recognized by cellular transcription factors such as NF-kB[10] and virus-specific regulatory gene products. The mRNA and genomic RNA transcripts are spliced, capped, and polyadenylated and then transported to the cytoplasm, where they are translated into viral proteins. On some HIV-1 mRNAs, ribosomes shift reading frames to bypass a translational stop codon at the end of the Gag open reading frame; this frame shifting leads to an abundance of Gag precursor polypeptide and a smaller amount of the read-through Gag-Pol precursor polypeptide. Posttranslational processing includes myristylation and glycosylation; the glycosylation inhibitors cas-

Martin S. Hirsch, Infectious Disease Unit, Massachusetts General Hospital, Harvard Medical School, Boston, MA 02114.

Richard T. D'Aquila, Infectious Disease Unit, Massachusetts General Hospital, Harvard Medical School, Boston, MA 02114.

Joan C. Kaplan, Infectious Disease Unit, Massachusetts General Hospital, Harvard Medical School, Boston, MA 02114.

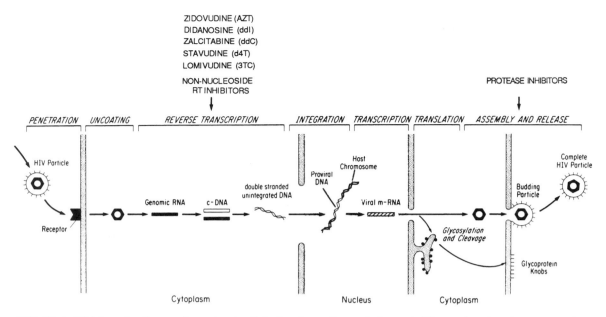

FIG. 23-1. HIV-1 replication cycle and potential sites for antiretroviral attack. The major sites for current therapeutic efforts are reverse transcriptase and protease.

tanospermine and deoxynojirimycin inhibit replication in vitro.[11,12]

HIV-1 regulatory gene products, including Tat, Rev, and Nef, modulate virus protein synthesis by acting at transcriptional or posttranscriptional levels. Inhibitors of Tat function have been identified by mechanism-based screening,[13] but they seem to act through cellular proteins and have been disappointing in clinical trials.[14] Viral structural proteins, replicative enzymes, and genomic RNA are assembled, associated with envelope glycoproteins, and released by budding from the plasma membrane where viral glycoproteins have congregated. Processing of HIV-1 proteins within budding virions includes specific cleavage of the Gag-Pol and Gag precursor polypeptides by the HIV-1 protease into mature forms, which are necessary to render the virion capable of reinitiating the infectious cycle when it encounters a susceptible host cell. At least three protease inhibitors have been approved in the United States, and other specific inhibitors of the HIV-1 protease are under investigation.

REVERSE TRANSCRIPTASE INHIBITORS

Zidovudine

Mechanism of Action

Zidovudine (azidothymidine, Retrovir, 3′-azido-3′-deoxythymidine [AZT]) is a synthetic pyrimidine analog that differs from thymidine in having an azido substituent instead of a hydroxyl group at the 3′ position of the deoxyribose ring. It was initially developed as an anticancer agent[15] and subsequently found to inhibit the reverse transcriptase (RT) of Friend leukemia virus.[16] Soon after the identification

of a human retrovirus as the etiologic agent of acquired immunodeficiency syndrome (AIDS), AZT was shown to have anti-HIV activity in vitro.[17]

The active form of zidovudine, AZT-triphosphate (AZT-TP), is a competitive inhibitor of RT. AZT-TP binds better to the HIV-1 RT than its natural substrate, thymidine triphosphate (TTP), and functions as an alternate substrate for the enzyme.[18,19] AZT-TP has a 100-fold greater affinity for RT than for cellular DNA polymerases alpha or beta.[20,21] The intracellular concentration of AZT-TP is greater than the K_i value for the HIV-1 RT but is less than K_i values for cellular polymerase alpha and beta.[21] AZT-TP is incorporated into growing DNA chains as AZT-monophosphate (AZT-MP), which leads to premature chain termination.[19] Because the incorporated AZT-MP does not provide a 3′-hydroxyl group to form a phosphodiester bond with the incoming nucleotide, chain elongation is terminated at thymidine residues.[19,21] Viral DNA synthesis is halted because the RT cannot excise the incorporated chain terminator.

AZT selectivity results from the preferential interaction of AZT-TP, rather than the physiologic TTP, with the RT.[19,21] Phosphorylation of AZT to its active form, AZT-TP, is accomplished by cellular enzymes.[17,21] AZT is an efficient substrate for the cellular thymidine kinase, which converts it to AZT-MP in infected and uninfected cells. AZT-MP accumulates in cells because of slow phosphorylation to AZT-diphosphate (AZT-DP) by host-cell thymidylate kinase, the rate-limiting step in AZT-TP formation. Some have suggested that high levels of AZT-MP may impair HIV-1 RT RNase H activity.[22] AZT-MP is a competitive inhibitor of thymidylate kinase and reduces the conversion of TMP to TDP, leading to decreased formation of TTP. Conversion of AZT-DP to AZT-TP is thought to be catalyzed by the cellular nucleoside diphosphate kinase.[20] Other metabolites of AZT may also be involved in its mechanism of action. Ribavirin antagonizes the in vitro anti-HIV-1 activity of AZT by inhibiting its phosphorylation.[23] Under certain experimental conditions, other agents, including ganciclovir[24] and stavudine,[25] may antagonize the anti-HIV-1 activity of AZT.

Resistance

Viruses resistant to AZT were first identified in isolates from patients treated with AZT for at least 6 months.[26] HIV-1 also develops resistance to AZT with in vitro serial passage in subinhibitory drug concentrations.[27] Specific substitutions in RT codons 41, 67, 70, 215, and 219 accumulate sequentially, resulting in increasing degrees of resistance.[28,29] The highest level of resistance, which is associated with four or five of these substitutions, results in a 100-fold increase in 50% inhibitory concentration (IC_{50}) of AZT. Clinical isolates from patients undergoing prolonged AZT therapy can have varied levels of resistance; many retain full susceptibility even after years of therapy. However, the likelihood of isolating an AZT-resistant virus increases with the duration of therapy and advancing disease.[30]

Resistant variants can be found at a low frequency (<1 in 10^3) in infected individuals before AZT exposure.[31] If antiretroviral therapy is terminated, AZT-resistant virus may be slowly replaced by more susceptible HIV-1, suggesting a selection advantage for wild-type virus in the absence of drug.[32]

The biochemical mechanisms by which the mutant RT confers AZT resistance to the virus require further definition. Substitutions at the base of the RT p66 "thumb" subdomain close to the polymerase active site (ie, codon 215[33] or codons 215 and 219[34]) decrease AZT-TP binding to purified RT enzyme in vitro. However, a mutant enzyme with mutations that confer high-level resistance to the virus can be inhibited just as effectively as wild-type enzyme by AZT-TP in vitro.[34,35] The structural model of the HIV-1 RT suggests that, in such highly resistant virus, not all residues altered by mutation cluster in a potential deoxynucleoside triphosphate binding site near the polymerase active site[36] but that some (ie, amino acids 41, 67, and 70 in the "fingers" subdomain) are physically distant and may affect RT function in other ways. Presumably, in vitro polymerase assays do not fully reflect RT enzyme function in the infected cell.

AZT-resistant virus is cross-resistant only to those HIV RT inhibitors that contain a 3'-azido substituent, such as 3'-azido-2',3'-dideoxyuridine.[26] Cloned mutant viruses that differ from the wild type only in that they possess specific AZT resistance mutations are not cross-resistant to didanosine (ddI), zalcitabine (ddC), or stavudine (d4T).[26] However, two clinical isolates with an AZT-resistant phenotype have been found to be cross-resistant to d4T.[37] Some investigators have observed a direct correlation between AZT IC_{50}s and ddI or ddC IC_{50}s of isolates from AZT-treated patients.[38] The genetic bases for these latter two phenomena remain to be elucidated.

AZT-resistant virus has been transmitted by documented[39] and presumed[40] parenteral exposure to HIV-1–infected blood. It has also been isolated from a patient with primary HIV-1 infection acquired by homosexual contact[41] and from apparent maternal-newborn transmission isolate pairs.[42] High-level AZT resistance has been associated with more rapid clinical progression during therapy than seen with AZT-susceptible isolates.[43–46] This association persists even when controlling for other factors that predict clinical deterioration.[43,44] However, therapeutic failure is complex and multifactorial, and patients can deteriorate while on AZT therapy, even if they harbor AZT-susceptible virus.

Clinical Trials

AZT was initially evaluated in a phase I trial studying 19 patients with AIDS or AIDS-related complex (ARC) at the National Cancer Institute (Bethesda, MD) and Duke University (Durham, NC).[47] There were suggestions of clinical and immunologic improvement and a possible virustatic effect in several patients; side effects were minimal in this 6-week clinical trial. Because of these results, large-scale, randomized, double-blind, placebo-controlled trials were instituted.

From February 1986 to the end of June 1986, 282 patients with advanced HIV infection were enrolled in a clinical trial at 12 different centers in the United States.[48,49] In this study, 145 patients received an oral dose of 250 mg of AZT every 4 hours, and 137 patients received placebo. By September 1986, it was apparent that differences in survival had emerged, and the study was terminated by an independent data safety monitoring board. Nineteen patients in the placebo group had died, compared with only one who received AZT. There was a significant difference in opportunistic infections (OI) in patients who received placebo (45 OI) compared with AZT recipients (24 OI). Patients who received AZT generally gained weight, but placebo recipients lost weight. Karnofsky scores of functional capability also improved for AZT recipients but did not improve for the placebo groups. Individuals who received AZT generally showed an increase in CD4 cells, although this effect was lost after 5 months in patients with AIDS.

Because of these results, AZT was approved in 1987 for patients with symptomatic HIV infections and fewer than 200 CD4+ lymphocytes/mm^3 of peripheral blood. The decreased mortality rates observed for patients receiving AZT were also seen during extended follow-up of the originally enrolled patients through 21 months of therapy.[50] Survival rates among those originally randomized to receive AZT were 84.5% and 57.6% at 12 and 21 months, respectively, after the initiation of therapy. In subsequent trials, lower doses of AZT (1200 mg daily for 1 month, followed by 600 mg daily) were equivalent in efficacy to high doses (1500 mg daily) in patients with advanced HIV infection and were associated with far less toxicity.[51]

Beginning AZT therapy before the onset of AIDS delays the progression of disease, as manifested by the delayed onset of opportunistic infections, neurologic disease, and tumors.[52,53] In two trials that together enrolled more than 2000 patients with early or no symptoms of HIV infection and CD4 cell counts less than 500/mm^3, AIDS developed earlier in the patients receiving placebo than in those treated with AZT. The rates of progression were similar in patients treated with 1500 mg daily and those treated with a lower dose (500 mg daily), although hematologic toxicity occurred more frequently in the former (11.8% and 2.95%, respectively). Additional studies of these subjects suggested that the duration of benefit was greatest for those with higher CD4 cell counts at entry and that survival differences were not evident over a mean follow-up of 2.6 years.[54]

Another study compared early and late AZT therapy (1500 mg daily) in 338 symptomatic patients with 200 to 500 CD4 cells/mm^3.[55] The patients in the late-treatment group received placebo until their CD4 counts fell below 200/mm^3 or until AIDS was diagnosed. During a mean follow-up of longer than 2 years, AIDS developed in 28 patients in the early-therapy group, compared with 48 in the late-therapy group ($P =.02$). However, the number of deaths was similar in the two groups (23 and 20 deaths, respectively), with a 3-year survival rate of approximately 80% in both.

The results of a large European trial, called Concorde,[56,57] indicated that survival of HIV-1–infected patients was equivalent whether AZT therapy was begun early or late in the course of infection. In this trial, 1749 patients with CD4 cell counts greater than 200/mm^3 were randomized to early or late AZT therapy; early was defined as entry into the study and late as when CD4 cell counts fell below 200/mm^3 or AIDS or ARC developed. The 3-year survival rates were equivalent in both groups.

No definitive recommendations can be made on the basis of these studies about the best time to institute AZT therapy. For many patients, however, prolonging the period of no or mild symptoms is preferable to extending the period between the diagnosis of AIDS and death. As discussed in subsequent sections, AZT monotherapy may no longer be the preferred initial therapy to use in adults. As of 1996, the U.S. recommendations are to begin AZT when CD4 cell counts drop below 500/mm^3 or to wait until symptoms appear in those with fewer than 500 CD4 cells/mm^3 or when CD4 counts fall even further (<200/mm^3).[58,59] One controlled trial suggested that even earlier treatment, when CD4 counts are between 400 and 800 CD4/mm^3, may offer clinical benefit,[60] but another suggested no additional benefit to starting AZT when CD4 cell counts were above 500/mm^3 compared with starting when CD4 cells fell below 500/mm^3.[61] A small but controlled pilot trial provided clinical and laboratory evidence that AZT administered during the primary HIV clinical syndrome may slow disease progression,[62] but long-term follow-up and further study are required to assess this approach.

In children with HIV infection, AZT therapy is associated with weight gain and improvements in cognitive function and virologic and immunologic markers.[63] Doses of 180 mg/m^2 of body surface area every 6 hours are recommended for children older than 3 months of age who have clinical or laboratory evidence of progressive HIV infection. However, AZT may be inferior to other alternatives (eg, ddI monotherapy, AZT plus ddI combination therapy) for initial therapy in children.[64] Anemia and leukopenia are the major side effects of AZT in children, as they are in adults.

AZT is well tolerated during pregnancy and does not cause fetal distress, malformation, or premature birth.[65] In a landmark study, investigators have shown that the transmission of HIV-1 from mother to newborn can also be reduced by AZT.[66] Women with CD4 counts greater than 200/mm^3 and minimal AZT experience were enrolled into a placebo-controlled trial of AZT between the 14th and 34th week of pregnancy. Within 24 hours of birth and for 6 weeks thereafter, newborns also received the same blinded medication as their mothers. Of 364 newborns tested, 53 had HIV infection, of whom 40 (25.5%) were placebo recipients and 13 (8.3%) were AZT recipients. On the basis of this study, it is now recommended that all pregnant women be offered HIV testing and that those who are HIV positive be given AZT. It is not clear, however, whether AZT would be efficacious for the prevention of mother-to-newborn transmission if given for shorter periods or to sicker women (CD4 cell counts <200/mm^3) with greater AZT experience. Retrospective studies of AZT-treated and untreated pregnant women support the results of the controlled trials.[67] Trials comparing AZT with other agents, such as ddI, have not been done in this setting.

AZT's role in prophylaxis among occupationally exposed health care workers is controversial, because several well-documented infections have occurred despite the administration of AZT soon after exposure.[58] However, retrospective case-control analysis of occupational exposures by the Centers for Disease Control suggests some benefit for early use of AZT prophylaxis.[68]

Didanosine, Zalcitabine, and Stavudine

Mechanism of Action

The drugs ddI (2′,3′-dideoxyinosine; didanosine [Videx]), ddC (2′,3′-dideoxycytidine; zalcitabine [Hivid]), and d4T (2′,3′-didehydro-3′-deoxythymdine; stavudine [Zerit]) compete with natural nucleoside triphosphate substrates when converted to their respective triphosphates and act as chain terminators if incorporation of the inhibitors occurs. Didanosine is converted to dideoxyadenosine (ddA) after absorption and before phosphorylation.

Resistance

Resistant viruses may emerge after months of ddI therapy. Substitutions in RT amino acids 74 (ie, Leu to Val),[34,69] 184 (ie, Met to Val),[70] and 65 (ie, Lys to Arg)[71] confer a minimal increase in IC$_{50}$ relative to viruses isolated from drug-naive individuals; substitution at codon 74 appears to be most common. The ddI-resistant mutations decrease inhibition of RT enzymatic activity by dideoxyadenosine triphosphate (ddATP), the active metabolite of ddI.[33,34,70,71] One report indicates that the codon 74 mutation in the "fingers" subdomain of the RT p66 subunit contacts the RNA template strand and reorients the terminus of the growing DNA chain downstream in the active site so that ddATP binding is decreased while binding of the natural substrate (dATP) is unimpaired.[72] These mutations confer cross-resistance between ddI and ddC. The clinical significance of ddI-resistant viruses has not yet been fully defined, although the results of one study suggest that appearance of the codon 74 mutation is associated with greater declines in CD4 cell counts and greater serum virus burdens during ddI monotherapy.[73]

Viruses resistant to ddC, another chain-terminating nucleoside analog, have not been extensively studied. Mutations in RT codons 69 (ie, Thr to Asp)[74] or 65 (ie, Lys to Arg)[71] are responsible for ddC resistance in cell culture. The codon 65 mutation also leads to resistance of the RT to inhibition by ddC triphosphate in vitro. Cross-resistance to ddI has been seen for RT codon 65 but not for codon 69 mutants.

The development of resistance to d4T was evaluated in patients treated for 18 to 22 months. Eleven pairs of pretreatment and posttreatment isolates were obtained, two of which showed moderately decreased sensitivity; no genetic basis was found for this resistance.[75] Resistance to d4T has been generated by passage of HIV-1 in vitro through increasing concentrations of drug; this resistance was associated with a Val-to-Thr substitution at RT residue 75.

Clinical Trials

The drug ddI was initially approved for use in patients with advanced HIV infection who were intolerant to AZT treatment or in whom such treatment had been unsuccessful. The approval was based on four small nonrandomized phase I trials involving 170 patients, a preliminary 12-week interim analysis of results in 412 patients enrolled in a randomized, double-blind study comparing AZT with ddI, and vast experience with toxicity accumulated in an expanded-access program involving several thousand patients.[58] In the phase I trials, there was improvement in weight, cutaneous hypersensitivity reactions, CD4 lymphocyte counts, and p24 antigenemia and, among children, improvement in IQ scores as well. Some of these trials have been extended for as long as 5 years.[76]

In subsequent trials, the safety and efficacy of AZT and ddI were compared in 913 adult patients who had received AZT previously for at least 16 weeks.[77] Two doses of ddI (500 mg and 750 mg) were compared with a 600-mg dose of AZT. The eligibility criteria included CD4 counts of less than 300/mm[3] in the case of patients with AIDS or ARC and less than 200/mm[3] in the case of asymptomatic patients. The patients who received the lower dose of ddI had significant delays in the onset of new AIDS-defining events compared with those who received AZT (P =.015). The benefit was not

associated with the duration of previous AZT therapy. The mortality rates in the three groups were similar. In another trial using patients with relatively advanced HIV-1 infection, the comparative effectiveness of ddI or AZT depended on the duration of previous AZT therapy.[78] AZT had greater efficacy in patients who had not received it previously, but ddI was more effective in those who had received AZT for 8 to 16 weeks before the randomized treatment began. These differences were evident with regard to the time to new AIDS-defining events and the time to death. In a third trial, 312 patients with CD4 cell counts of 300/mm[3] or less, greater than 6 months of AZT experience, and signs of clinical deterioration, switching to ddI was associated with fewer clinical end points than continuing AZT.[79] A fourth study reported similar results in patients with higher CD4 cell counts.[80] These results reinforce the concept that switching from AZT to ddI may be beneficial after a certain period of AZT therapy in patients with advanced disease, although the optimal time for a change in therapy is unclear.

Results from a large, randomized, blinded, and controlled clinical trial (AIDS Clinical Trials Group [ACTG] 175) again raised questions about what constitutes the optimal initial antiretroviral therapeutic regimen. In this study, 2467 eligible subjects with CD4 cell counts of 200 to 500/mm[3] were enrolled, 1067 of whom were antiretroviral-naive patients. The safety and efficacy of monotherapy with AZT or ddI were compared with those of combination regimens AZT plus ddC or AZT plus ddI. Aggregate end points included a 50% or greater decline in CD4 cell counts, an AIDS-defining end point, or death. The median duration of follow-up was 143 weeks.[81]

For the overall population, ddI monotherapy and the AZT plus ddC and AZT plus ddI combination regimens were significantly better than AZT monotherapy with respect to the aggregate end points (ddI monotherapy hazard ratio 0.61; confidence intervals 0.49, 0.76; P <.001). Similar differences were observed for AIDS and death (ddI monotherapy hazard ratio 0.69; confidence intervals 0.51, 0.94; P =.019) and death alone (ddI monotherapy hazard ratio 0.51; confidence intervals 0.32, 0.80; P =.011). These differences were seen in AZT-experienced and AZT-naive groups. The results differ from those described from ACTG 116A; however, in ACTG 116A, the population had more advanced disease, the numbers enrolled were smaller, progression rates were higher, end points occurred earlier, and follow-up was shorter. It appears that ddI may be preferable to AZT for initial therapy of adults with moderately advanced disease (ie, CD4 cell counts of 200 to 500/mm[3]).

Dose recommendations for ddI are related to weight for adults and to body surface area for children. In adults, 200 mg twice daily is recommended for those weighing more than 60kg; and 125 mg twice daily is recommended for those weighing less than 60 kg. In children, doses range from 25 mg twice daily to 100 mg twice daily.

The drug ddC has been studied as monotherapy and in combination with AZT. A 1-year interim analysis of a trial enrolling patients with baseline CD4 cell counts of less than

200/mm³ and less than 3 months of previous AZT therapy revealed poorer survival for the patients taking ddC than in those taking AZT. There were 59 deaths among 320 ddC-treated patients and 33 deaths among 315 AZT-treated patients (P =.007). No such differences were found in patients who entered comparative trials after prolonged AZT therapy.[82] In another trial, the efficacy of ddC was equivalent to that of ddI in patients in whom AZT therapy had been unsuccessful or who could no longer tolerate AZT.[83] Studies of ddI and ddC in combination with other agents are discussed in a subsequent section. The recommended doses for adults are 0.75 mg every eight hours.

Phase I trials of d4T have shown anti-HIV-1 activity (ie, decreased HIV-1 serum p24 antigen, increased or stable CD4 cell counts) at doses below those causing sensory peripheral neuropathy.[84] Controlled trials of d4T (40 mg twice daily) versus AZT (200 mg three times daily) were conducted using 822 patients with HIV infection (50 to 500 CD4 cells/mm³) and more than 6 months of AZT experience. Recipients of d4T had more consistent and pronounced improvement in CD4 cell counts, virus load, body weight, performance status, and clinical end points than those continued on AZT.[85] Other trials of d4T as monotherapy or in combination are in progress. Peripheral neuropathy is the major clinical toxic effect of d4T (15% to 21%) and is more common in those with previous neuropathy. Mild to moderate transaminase abnormalities may also occur. The recommended doses for adults are 40 mg twice daily for patients weighing more than 60 kg and 30 mg twice daily for patients weighing less than 60 kg.

Other Nucleoside Reverse Transcriptase Inhibitors

Lamivudine (2'-deoxy-3'-thiacytidine [3TC]) is a potent inhibitor of HIV-1 RT when converted intracellularly to its active triphosphate form. It is readily bioavailable and has a serum elimination half-life of 2.5 hours.[86] 3TC has activity against a wide spectrum of HIV-1 isolates, including those that are AZT resistant.[87] Rapid selection of resistant virus has been observed with 3TC in vitro[88–91] and in vivo.[92]

Early clinical trials of 3TC monotherapy indicate that it is generally well tolerated.[86,93] In a cohort of 3TC-treated individuals, a sharp decline (1 to 2 log) in viral load was seen within a week, followed by a slow rise in viral load toward but still below baseline.[86,92,93] 3TC resistance appears to be associated with changes at codon 184 of RT from methionine to valine or isoleucine.[88–91] The methionine to valine change, when introduced in a recombinant AZT-resistant virus, resulted in decreased resistance to AZT.[90] Although the rapid emergence of RT codon 184 mutant 3TC-resistant virus limits its use as a single agent, the same mutation at codon 184 suppresses AZT resistance, which suggests a potential mechanism for the sustained activity of the combination of AZT and 3TC.[94] Combinations of 3TC with AZT are discussed in a subsequent section. Several other nucleoside RT inhibitors are in various stages of clinical evaluation.

Nonnucleoside Reverse Transcriptase Inhibitors

Another class of agents directed specifically against the HIV-1 RT has been called the nonnucleoside RT inhibitors (NNRTIs), also known as HIV-1–specific RT inhibitors.[95] This class includes compounds with diverse chemical structures that are unrelated to nucleosides, such as nevirapine, TIBO compounds, atevirdine, and delavirdine, as well as a few agents such as TSAO and the HEPT compounds.

All of these inhibitors are uncompetitive with respect to substrates or primer template and potently inhibit HIV-1 RT in vitro with minimal cellular toxicity. They are extremely specific against HIV-1 RT, with no activity against the highly related HIV-2 RT. Structural modeling of the RT indicates that these compounds bind, with small differences, to a hydrophobic pocket of the p66 subunit near the active site.[36,96] They may indirectly affect residues in the polymerase active site or impair mobility of the "thumb" subdomain.[97] Resistant viruses emerge rapidly in vitro and can have one or more mutations that alter the RT-binding pocket. Clinical trials also demonstrate early emergence of resistant viruses often related to substitutions at specific residues (eg, 103–108, 179–190) parallel to those observed in vitro.[95] Emergence of resistant isolates are often accompanied by loss of clinical benefit, as evidenced by increasing virus loads and decreasing CD4 cell counts.[98–101]

In some patients, high doses of one NNRTI, nevirapine, resulted in sustained antiviral activity despite development of high-level resistance in vitro, perhaps because blood levels were achieved that exceeded the mean IC_{50} of resistant virus.[98,99] Resistance to one NNRTI may confer broad but not universal resistance to other NNRTIs.[102] In vitro, a delavirdine-selected mutation at RT residue 236 can resensitize virus having certain nevirapine-selected resistance mutations.[103] Alternating treatment with AZT and nevirapine does not prevent the development of nevirapine resistance.[104]

Although monotherapy with NNRTIs has only transient benefit, it is likely that combination therapy employing NNRTIs as one component will be more useful. This approach is discussed in greater detail in a subsequent section.

PROTEASE INHIBITORS

The HIV-1 protease is the best characterized of the virus's proteins, functionally and structurally.[105] It is an aspartyl protease similar in its catalytic mechanism to renin in humans. The posttranslational cleavage of Gag and Gag-Pol polypeptides by HIV-1 protease is essential for virion assembly and maturation within budding virions. If this function is blocked by an inactivating mutation or an inhibitor, immature, noninfectious virus particles bud from infected cell membranes.[106,107] Protease inhibitors appear capable of blocking late stages of the replicative cycle in vivo. They may also impair an early, preintegration event that depends on nucleocapsid protein cleavage within the virion.[108] The HIV-1 protease is a homodimer in which the two subunits are related by a twofold (C2) axis of symmetry, and a single peptide-binding active site is formed at the subunit interface. Its three-dimensional structure is known,[109] and its functional mechanism is similar to that of previously characterized aspartyl proteases.

Preclinical studies of protease inhibitors have been increasingly guided by structural data and have led to promising design principles and synthetic strategies. Crystallographic analyses of protease complexed with inhibitors have elucidated interactions between enzyme and inhibitor and have been used to identify lead compounds and improve the potency and specificity of lead compounds. The structures of many protease-inhibitor complexes have been described.[109] Most inhibitors are peptidomimetic, difficult to synthesize, and often have poor bioavailability, but smaller, nonpeptide compounds that are easier to synthesize are also under study. Although the active site of the enzyme is fairly symmetric, not all inhibitors are symmetric. The flexibility of the peptidomimetic inhibitor backbones appears to facilitate binding with the enzyme.

Several protease inhibitors are in clinical trials and three have been approved in the United States. The agent with the greatest clinical experience, as monotherapy and in combinations, is saquinavir. Monotherapy studies have been conducted using 49 AZT-naive asymptomatic, HIV-infected subjects with CD4 counts of 500/mm^3 of less.[110] Dose-response evaluations indicated favorable CD4 cell and virus load responses for up to 600 mg three times daily, and the drug was well tolerated. Although higher drug concentrations may be required for sustained effects, relatively poor oral bioavailability and difficult synthetic characteristics may limit the utility of saquinavir monotherapy. Newer oral formulations of saquinavir are under development. Combinations including saquinavir have been promising and are under extensive investigation.

Ritonavir is more orally bioavailable and, more active than saquinavir in its current formulation.[111] Substantial decreases in plasma viral RNA (1-2 logs) and increases in CD4 cell counts (100-200 cells/mm^3) have been seen in trials using ritonavir either as a single agent or in combination.[112-115] In advanced disease (CD4 cells <100/mm^3), addition of rotonavir to ongoing regimens has prolonged life and reduced clinical progression.[115] Toxicities are primarily gastrointestinal (nausea, vomiting, diarrhea) and neurologic (circumoral and peripheral paresthesias); elevated triglycerides and hepatic transaminases may also be observed. In addition, ritonavir is a potent inhibitor of cytochrome p450 3A activity and must be used with caution in combination with drugs that utilize this metabolic pathway. Resistance to ritonavir develops with prolonged use, related to the sequential accumulation of several protease gene mutations. Current recommended doses for adults are 600 mg twice daily.

Indinavir appears equivalent in antiviral potency to ritonavir, although the two protease inhibitors have not been directly compared. One to three log decreases in HIV plasma RNA together with increases in CD4 cell counts 100-200 cells/mm^3 have been observed when indinavir is used as monotherapy or in combination.[116] Toxicities include increases in indirect bilirubinemia and nephrolithiasis (2% to 3%). Resistance develops over time and is related to an accumulation of three or more mutations at various codons of the protease gene.[117] A characteristic ordered sequence of indinavir-associated mutations has not yet been defined; varied sets of mutations were noted in isolates from different patients.[117] Mutations induced by indinavir overlap with those induced by ritonavir. Thus, resistance to one of these agents may imply resistance to others. Prolonged indinavir use may result in broad cross-resistance among protease inhibitors;[117] this is also under study for other protease inhibitors. Optimal recommended indinavir doses appear to be 800 mg every 8 hours for adults.

Several other protease inhibitors are under development, as are strategies involving combinations of protease inhibitors with each other or with reverse transcriptase inhibitors (see below).

COMBINATION THERAPY

Combination therapy for controlling infection with HIV-1 provides several potential advantages over monotherapy. Two or more drugs may have additive or synergistic interactions that produce better efficacy than with either drug alone. Additive or synergistic combinations may also allow the use of drugs at lower doses than employed in monotherapy, possibly decreasing toxicity. Starting therapy with a combination regimen may also delay the emergence of resistant virus that can completely escape drug inhibition. If a virus resistant to one component is already present, broader coverage with combination therapy would also be useful. Combination therapy could target different cellular and tissue reservoirs of virus. One established mechanism for differential activity involves differences in nucleoside phosphorylation.[118,119]

Drug combinations may be administered in alternation, with a single drug given for a defined duration (eg, 1 week, 1 month) and then switched to a second drug for a defined period. Alternatively, they may be administered simultaneously, with two or more drugs administered during the entire period of treatment. The rationale for using alternating combination regimens is that they provide a period of washout, which may decrease toxicity. Two potential problems with this approach are decreased efficacy and no delay in the development of resistance. The concern with simultaneous combination therapy is that toxic effects may increase in frequency and severity.

When two or more drugs are combined, they may interact in several ways. In additive interactions, the activity of the drugs in the combination is equal to the sum of the activity of each drug used alone. In synergistic interactions, the activity of the drugs in the combination is greater than the sum of the activity of each drug used alone. In antagonistic interactions, the activity of the drugs in the combination is less than the sum of the activity of each drug used individually.

Several mathematical models have been used to study drug interactions, including the median-effect principle and the isobologram technique.[120] More complete discussions of mathematical methods and their advantages and disadvantages are described elsewhere.[121,122]

The goal of combination therapy is to find combinations of drugs that have additive or synergistic antiviral interactions without increased toxicity, although such interactions in vitro do not necessarily predict the effects in vivo. Nevertheless, evaluation of in vitro data is a logical way to select drug combinations that should also be tested individually for safety and toxicity in patients before combination studies are performed.

Clinical trials have been based on valuable information derived from a wide variety of in vitro studies, many of which have been reviewed elsewhere.[123] These in vitro studies have employed a variety of cell systems, looked at different multiplicities of virus input and stages of infection, and evaluated the degree of virus suppression and time of breakthrough virus replication. Several two- and three-drug regimens have been identified for further clinical study, and many of these preliminary trials have shown considerable promise.

Two-Drug Regimens

AZT and ddC

AZT and ddC have their own toxicities (see Chap. 22), but these are largely not overlapping. Because of synergistic in vitro antiviral activity[124] and nonoverlapping toxicities, these drugs have been widely used in combination regimens.

In a phase I/II, open-label study, a combination of AZT and ddC was studied in 56 previously untreated patients with advanced HIV-1 infection.[125] Patients were classified as having AIDS or advanced ARC, and all had CD4 cell counts of 200/mm³ or less. Six regimens of low dosages of AZT (150 to 600 mg/day) and ddC (0.015 or 0.03 mg/kg/day) were studied. No unexpected toxicity was associated with the combination therapy. The frequency of severe adverse events did not differ among patients who received one of the six regimens. All the regimens resulted in weight gain, increased CD4 cell counts, and decreased p24 antigen levels. The best responses were seen in patients treated with the combination of 600 mg of AZT and 0.03 mg of ddC/kg daily. On the basis of these results, large phase II/III trials of this combination were undertaken in patients who received previous therapy with AZT and in those who did not receive prior antiretroviral therapy.

Another trial of AZT and ddC studied alternating and intermittent regimens in 131 patients with AIDS or ARC and serum p24 antigenemia.[126] Most (96%) participants had not received AZT within 90 days of the study. Treatment regimens included weekly alternating doses of AZT and ddC, monthly alternating doses of AZT and ddC, intermittent doses of AZT, intermittent doses of ddC, and continuous doses of AZT. AZT was given at a dosage of 200 mg every 4 hours, and ddC was given as 0.01 mg/kg or 0.03 mg/kg every 4 hours.

There was a reduction in expected toxicities when AZT and ddC were given as alternating therapy. Patients receiving AZT in alternation with ddC had a significantly lower risk for hematologic toxic effects than did those who received AZT continuously (11% to 15% versus 33%, respectively). Rates of neuropathy among patients receiving three of the four alternating regimens (ie, weekly AZT and ddC [0.01 mg/kg] and monthly AZT and ddC [0.01 mg/kg and 0.03 mg/kg]) were similar to those among patients who did not receive ddC.[126] Two regimens, weekly alternating AZT (200 mg every 4 hours) and ddC (0.01 mg/kg every 4 hours) and monthly alternating AZT (200 mg every 4 hours) and ddC (0.03 mg/kg every 4 hours), provided the best responses with regard to weight gain, reductions in plasma levels of p24 antigen, and sustained increases in CD4 cell counts.[126]

This study suggested that alternating therapy with AZT and ddC reduces the toxicity associated with each drug alone while maintaining strong antiretroviral activity. However, neither alternating nor concomitant administration of the two antiretroviral agents has yet to demonstrate the ability to prevent the emergence of in vitro resistance to AZT.

The results of one large study evaluating combinations of AZT plus ddC (ACTG 155) have been reported.[127] This study enrolled 1001 patients with symptomatic HIV disease and CD4 cell counts of 300/mm³ or less or those with asymptomatic HIV disease and CD4 cell counts of 200/mm³ or less. All patients had received prior therapy with AZT for more than 6 months, and many had received the drug for more than 1 year. Participants were randomly assigned to receive AZT (600 mg/day), ddC (2.25 mg/day), or AZT (600 mg/day) plus ddC (2.25 mg/day).

The conclusion of this study using an intention-to-treat analysis was that there was no difference among the three treatment groups with respect to time until the occurrence of an AIDS-defining event or death for patients who had received previous prolonged therapy with AZT.[127] However, if the patients were grouped by pretreatment CD4 cell counts (<50, 50 to 150, and ≥150/mm³) in an exploratory analysis, there was a difference in time to disease progression or death. For patients with pretreatment CD4 cell counts of 150/mm³ or greater, those receiving combination therapy were significantly less likely to develop progressive disease or die than were those receiving AZT (relative risk, 0.51; 95% confidence interval, 0.28-0.93; P =.029). No differences between the groups receiving monotherapy with ddC and AZT were observed. For patients with CD4 cell counts of less than 150/mm³, there were no differences in disease progression or death among the three treatment groups.[127]

The incidence of severe toxic effects was also inversely correlated with the pretreatment CD4 cell count. Patients with CD4 cell counts of 150/mm³ or more tolerated therapy, with no apparent difference in the rates of severe toxic effects among the three treatment groups. Moderate or worsening peripheral neuropathy occurred more often in the group receiving ddC monotherapy (23%) and in the group receiving combination therapy (22%) than in the group receiving AZT monotherapy

(13%). However, the rate of severe peripheral neuropathy was not different among the three treatment groups. For patients with pretreatment CD4 cell counts of 50/mm³ or less, severe neutropenia (<750 cells/mm³) was more common in the group receiving AZT monotherapy (41%) and in the group receiving combination therapy (35%) than in the group receiving ddC monotherapy (18%).[127]

ACTG 175 also compared AZT and ddC in combination with AZT monotherapy in patients with CD4 lymphocyte counts between 200 and 500/mm³.[81] Using an aggregate end point of a CD4 cell decline of 50% or less, an AIDS-defining end point, or death, the combination was superior to AZT monotherapy (hazard ratio of 0.54; confidence intervals 0.43, 0.68; P <.001) in AZT-naive and AZT-experienced patients. A significant reduction in AIDS and death (51%) was also seen in the antiretroviral-naive group, favoring the combination of AZT and ddC; in the AZT-experienced population, the end points of AIDS and death were similar in the AZT plus ddC and the AZT monotherapy groups.

AZT and ddI

The effectiveness of monotherapy with AZT or ddI in treating HIV-1 infection, the drug's different toxicities, and their in vitro synergy against HIV-1 led to studies of combination therapy with AZT plus ddI. A clinical trial of combination therapy with AZT and ddI compared the use of AZT alone with the use of five combinations of AZT and ddI (ie, 150 mg of AZT/day and 90 mg of ddI/day; 300 mg of AZT/day and 334 mg of ddI/day; 600 mg of AZT/day and 334 mg of ddI/day; 300 mg of AZT/day and 500 mg of ddI/day; and 600 mg of AZT/day and 500 mg of ddI/day) in 55 patients with CD4 cell counts of less than 400/mm³.[128] There was no increased toxicity seen with the combinations compared with AZT monotherapy. There were similar increases in CD4 cell counts in the five groups receiving combination therapy, and these increases were greater than those in the group receiving AZT monotherapy. This increase in CD4 cell count persisted even after an adjustment for initial CD4 cell count and previous therapy with AZT. Titers of HIV-1 RNA in plasma decreased in 15 (83%) of 18 patients receiving combination therapy compared with 2 (29%) of 7 patients receiving AZT alone.[128]

A phase I/II, open-label, randomized trial compared ddI alone with three combinations of AZT and ddI in 116 asymptomatic HIV-positive patients.[129] Patients were randomized to one of four treatment arms: ddI alone (500 mg/day); a low-dose combination (150 mg of AZT/day and 134 mg of ddI/day); a moderate-dose combination (300 mg of AZT/day and 334 mg of ddI/day); and a high-dose combination (600 mg of AZT/day and 500 mg of ddI/day). All patients had CD4 cell counts between 200 and 500/mm³. The combinations of drugs were well tolerated; there was, however, an increase in hepatotoxic effects in hemophiliacs receiving AZT-containing regimens. Preliminary results showed an increase in CD4 cell counts in patients in all four treatment arms of the study, and

the serial quantitative viral cultures showed a decrease in titers of virus in patients in all treatment arms. Culture results for 10 (42%) of 24 patients receiving combination therapy with AZT and ddI for 12 months were negative. In contrast, culture results were negative for only 2 of 26 patients who received 12 months of monotherapy with AZT before enrolling in the study. Although combination therapy with AZT and ddI suppressed the load of virus, it did not prevent the development of AZT resistance.[130]

Results are also available from a pilot study comparing alternating and simultaneous regimens of AZT and ddI in 41 patients with AIDS or symptomatic HIV infection and CD4 cell counts of less than 350/mm³.[131] The simultaneous-treatment group received 100 mg of AZT every 8 hours and 250 mg of ddI every 24 hours. The alternating-treatment group received 100 mg of AZT every 4 hours and 250 mg of ddI every 12 hours at 3-week intervals. Patients who received simultaneous therapy had greater and more sustained increases in their CD4 cell counts than did patients receiving alternating therapy. There was also a trend toward decreased levels of HIV p24 antigen and fewer opportunistic infections in the patients receiving the simultaneous regimen than in those receiving the alternating regimen. The toxic effects of the two regimens were comparable, although one patient in the simultaneous treatment arm died of fulminant pancreatitis. Whether there is any difference in the development of drug resistance in the two groups remains to be investigated.[131]

ACTG 175 also compared the combination of AZT plus ddI with the effects of monotherapy using either agent alone in patients with CD4 lymphocyte counts between 200 and 500/mm³.[81] The combination proved superior to AZT monotherapy with respect to the aggregate primary study end points of a 50% or greater CD4 cell count decline, development of an AIDS-defining event, or death, as well as the solely clinical end points of AIDS and death or of death alone in the overall population. This was reflected by reductions of 50%, 35%, and 45% of these end points, respectively. Similar patterns were seen in AZT-experienced and AZT-naive groups.

In contrast to comparisons with AZT monotherapy, AZT plus ddI appeared comparable to ddI monotherapy or to AZT plus ddC combination therapy in ACTG 175, using an intent-to-treat analysis. Further evaluation of ACTG 175 is underway. Overall, the results of ACTG 175 for adults and ACTG 152 for children signal a reconsideration of initiating therapy with AZT alone. These results suggest the benefit of beginning treatment with ddI alone or with combinations of AZT and ddI or ddC (or possibly 3TC, which was not included in this study). Patient and physician preference, potential toxicities, and cost are factors that should enter into this judgment.

AZT and 3TC

Another promising combination studied is AZT combined with 3TC. These agents are strongly synergistic against

AZT-sensitive and AZT-resistant isolates of HIV-1 in vitro.[25] Moreover, the commonly observed 3TC-induced mutation at codon 184 in RT induces a phenotypic reversion to AZT sensitivity in AZT-resistant isolates.[94] Preliminary data suggest that 3TC may be useful in combination with AZT in previously antiretroviral-naive patients by impeding the emergence of AZT-resistant variants, although other mechanisms are also possible.[94]

Several small, randomized clinical trials have evaluated AZT and 3TC in combination in AZT-experienced and AZT-naive patients. In a randomized, open-label trial, 129 AZT-naive patients with CD4 cell counts between 100 and 400/mm^3 were treated with AZT alone or AZT plus 3TC for 24 weeks, at which time all subjects were offered open-label treatment with the combination for an additional 24 weeks.[132] Although AZT recipients had early rises in CD4 cell counts (mean rise, 34 cells/mm^3 at 4 weeks), by week 24, CD4 cell counts were below baseline (mean fall, 7/mm^3). In contrast, AZT plus 3TC recipients had mean CD4 cell counts that rose to 80/mm^3 above baseline at 8 weeks and were sustained for 24 weeks. Declines in plasma HIV-1 RNA, p24 antigen, cellular viremia, β_2-microglobulin, and neopterin were also greater and more sustained in the combination-therapy group.

In a parallel trial using AZT-experienced patients with CD4 cell counts of 100 to 400/mm^3, similar results were seen.[133] In the study, 223 patients were randomized to receive AZT alone or in combination with 300 mg or 600 mg of 3TC daily. After 24 weeks, all patients were offered open-label combination therapy. Mean CD4 cell counts fell to 21 cells/mm^3 below baseline in the AZT monotherapy group at 24 weeks, but the mean count rose to 47 cells/mm^3 above baseline in the combination groups; no significant differences were seen between the two doses of 3TC.

A third trial compared 3TC monotherapy, AZT monotherapy, and AZT plus 3TC combination therapy in 366 AZT-naive patients with CD4 cell counts between 200 and 500/mm^3; low-dose and high-dose 3TC regimens were employed.[134] Combination regimens were associated with greater increases in CD4$^+$ cells and more profound decreases in plasma HIV-1 RNA levels, without increases in adverse events. These differences were maintained for at least 52 weeks.

These trials were not designed or powered to look for clinical end point differences, and such studies have not yet been reported. Nevertheless, the lack of toxicity and sustained CD4 cell count and virologic results support the concept that AZT and 3TC may prove to be a useful combination in the years ahead.

Other Nucleoside Combinations

Based on in vitro observations of additive to synergistic anti-HIV effects, a number of pilot clinical trials with other combinations (ie, AZT plus d4T; d4T plus 3TC; d4T plus ddI) are in progress. The combination of AZT plus d4T shows positive interactions against some HIV-1 isolates but is antagonistic against others in vitro.[25]

Nucleoside and Nonnucleoside Reverse Transcriptase Inhibitors

Combinations of nevirapine (12.5, 50, 200, and 400 mg/day) and AZT (200 mg every 8 hours) have been studied in a small trial of 32 HIV-positive patients.[98] Several patients receiving 400 mg of nevirapine had dose-limiting rashes, but the combination was otherwise well tolerated. AZT plus nevirapine caused a greater and more sustained decrease in levels of p24 antigen than did nevirapine alone. Development of nevirapine resistance was neither prevented nor slowed by combining nevirapine with AZT.[99] However, the patterns of genotypic resistance observed with the combination were different from those seen with nevirapine monotherapy.[100]

L697,661 is a pyridinone compound; it is a nonnucleoside inhibitor of HIV-1 RT.[135] As with nevirapine, high-level resistance develops quickly in patients receiving monotherapy with L697,661.[101] As a result, studies were begun using this pyridinone in combination regimens. In a small number of patients, combination therapy with L697,661 and AZT seemed to delay the emergence of resistance to the pyridinone.[136]

In a larger trial involving 120 patients who had not received AZT previously and who had CD4 cell counts of 200 to 500/mm^3, patients received AZT (300 mg/day) alone, L697,661 (600 mg/day) alone, or AZT (300 mg/day) plus L697,661 (300 or 600 mg/day). Virus with high-level resistance to pyridinone was found only in the group receiving L697,661 monotherapy. In patients receiving AZT plus pyridinone, only strains of virus with low-level resistance to pyridinone could be isolated.[137] However in a trial involving patients with CD4 cell counts of less than 250/mm^3, the combination had only transient beneficial effects on levels of serum p24 antigen and viral RNA, and resistance to L697,661 developed rapidly in all patients, with some patients developing high-level pyridinone resistance. On the basis of this information, further clinical development of L697,661 was suspended (Massari F: personal communication).

Several other combinations of nucleosides and nonnucleosides are under investigation, including ddI plus delavirdine and AZT plus delavirdine.

Protease Inhibitors and Reverse Transcriptase Inhibitors

In vitro studies have shown additive and synergistic anti-HIV interactions between protease inhibitors and nucleoside and nonnucleoside RT inhibitors.[138,139] Preliminary clinical trials also suggest beneficial interactions between RT inhibitors and several different protease inhibitors.[140] On the basis of these preliminary data, saquinavir, ritonavir, and indinavir have been approved for combination therapy in the United States.

AIDS: *Biology, Diagnosis, Treatment and Prevention, fourth edition,* edited by Vincent T. DeVita, Jr., Samuel Hellman, and Steven A. Rosenberg. Lippincott–Raven Publishers, © 1997

Antiretroviral Therapy Update

Since completion of this chapter in early 1996, several new developments have occurred. These include a better understanding of the rapid rate of virus and CD4 cell turnover in peripheral blood, several studies indicating the importance of measuring plasma viral RNA in monitoring the effectiveness of therapy, and promising preliminary results of several three drug antiretroviral combination regimens. These developments have led to more aggressive recommendations for therapy in a wide variety of clinical situations.

Soon after starting therapy with potent antiretroviral regimens, plasma HIV-1 RNA levels drop approximately 100-fold as a result of clearance of free virions, the rapid loss of productively infected cells, and the prevention of new cell infection. This is followed by a slower second phase decrease in plasma virus, probably related to loss of latently-infected or long-lived cells. Mathematical models have been developed to estimate the length of treatment that might be required to eradicate virus from these pools.[1] It has been estimated that 1.5 to 3.0 years of potent therapy might be required to achieve this goal, and trials are being undertaken to evaluate this possibility. However, there are still many unknowns in HIV pathogenesis which may require revision of these estimates, including still other compartments with even slower cell and virus turnover rates.

One of the major advances in recent AIDS research has been the advent and implementation of techniques to accurately measure HIV-1 RNA in plasma. Assays employing either polymerase chain reaction (PCR) or branched chain DNA (bDNA) technology are now routinely used to monitor both disease progression and the effects of therapy.[2-5] The risk of disease progression (AIDS or death) appears directly related to levels of plasma HIV-1 RNA, referred to as plasma viral load, and this marker is a better predictor of outcome than numbers of peripheral blood CD4 cells. Moreover, changes in plasma viral load in response to effective therapies are rapid, and a rebound in viral replication predicts subsequent failure of treatment. Thus, although clinical endpoints remain the ultimate markers of successful therapy, clinical management of patients will depend more and more on monitoring levels of plasma viral RNA. Several recommendations have recently been made on how to use this marker in initiating or changing therapy.[5,6] Plasma HIV-1 RNA levels above 5,000 to 10,000 copies/mL should suggest initiation of therapy, regardless of clinical status or CD4 cell count, and the target of therapy should be to lower the levels below the limits of detection of the assay being employed. The minimum decrease indicative of antiviral activity is >0.5 log. A return to within 0.3 to 0.5 log of pre-treatment value suggests treatment failure, although any significant increase (>0.3log) from an achieved nadir might suggest reduction in drug effect. It is suggested that two baseline measurements be made 2 to 4 weeks apart, approximately 4 weeks after initiating or changing treatment, and then every 3 to 4 months thereafter.

Several recent clinical trials have shown remarkable sustained reductions of plasma viral RNA, often below the limits of assay detection for prolonged periods. These studies have generally employed three drug regimens with two nucleoside reverse transcriptase inhibitors plus another drug, either a potent protease inhibitor or a nonnucleoside reverse transcriptase inhibitor. One study employed indinavir, zidovudine, and lamivudine in zidovudine-experienced patients with over 20,000 copies/mL of HIV-1 RNA and 50 to 400 CD4 cells/mm^3 prior to starting therapy. After 24 to 44 weeks of follow-up, 83% to 92% of 3-drug recipients had plasma viral RNA levels below the limit of detection of the PCR assay detection (<500 copies/mL), compared with less than 36% of patients receiving one or two of these drugs.[7] Trials of ritonavir, zidovudine, and lamivudine in acutely infected individuals have also shown significant reductions of plasma virus below detectable levels, although numbers were small and follow-up periods were brief.[8] Preliminary trials of zidovudine, didanosine, and nevirapine (the latter recently approved for use in the USA) also show similar reductions in virus load below the detection limit in a large proportion of patients with relatively early stages of disease and limited prior drug treatment.[9] This contrasts with a lesser effect on plasma RNAQ levels in patients with greater prior antiretroviral experience.[10] The potent antiviral effects produced by these different three drug regimens appear to greatly reduce the emergence of drug resistant variants which are dependent on some viral replication for their selection, although many years of observation will be required before the duration of benefit can be established. In addition, the long term toxicity of each potent three drug regimen remains to be established.

Four Phase II trials of a two drug regimen, zidovudine plus lamivudine, have now been completed, using both drug-naive and experienced patients.[11-14] These studies showed dramatic reductions in plasma HIV1 RNA and increases in CD4 cell counts that were sustained for over a year. Moreover, a meta-analysis of all four trials involving 972 patients indicates that this combination also delays the clinical progression of disease when compared with control treatment regimens.[15]

On the basis of these and other studies, an international panel organized by the International AIDS Society-USA has recently published guidelines for therapy in a variety of clinical situations.[6] In addition, the US Public Health Service has promulgated provisional recommendations for the use of combination regimens in the occupational post-exposure prophylaxis setting.[16] Both groups emphasize that combination regimens using two reverse transcriptase inhibitors, plus or minus a potent protease inhibitor, are the optimal approaches for initiation of therapy. Both initiation and changes of treatment should be guided by clinical status, plasma virus RNA, and CD4 cell count, as well as available drug options, underlying conditions and concomitant medications. Recommendations and options in mid-1996 are summarized in Tables 23-1 through 23-3. It is clear that these guidelines will change as new data emerge, and that frequent updates and revisions will be generated. Nevertheless, the progress in the area of antiretroviral therapy in HIV-1 infection has been enormous, giving rise to considerable optimism for the future.

TABLE 23-1. Provisional Public Health Service recommendations for chemoprophylaxis after occupational exposure to HIV, by type of exposure and source material —1996

Type of exposure	Source material*	Antiretroviral prophylaxis†	Antiretroviral regimen‡
Percutaneous	Blood§		
	Highest risk	Recommend	ZDV plus 3TC plus IDV
	Increased risk	Recommend	ZDV plus 3TC, ± IDV‖
	No increased risk	Offer	ZDV plus 3TC
	Fluid containing visible blood, other potentially infectious fluid#, or tissue	Offer	ZDV plus 3TC
	Other body fluid (eg, urine)	Not offer	
Mucous membrane	Blood	Offer	ZDV plus 3TC, ± IDV**
	Fluid containing visible blood, other potentially infectious fluid#, or tissue	Offer	ZDV, + 3TC
	Other body fluid (eg, urine)	Not offer	
Skin, increased risk**	Blood	Offer	ZDV plus 3TC, ± IDV**
	Fluid containing visible blood, other potentially infectious fluid#, or tissue	Offer	ZDV, ± 3TC
	Other body fluid (eg, urine)	Not offer	

*Any exposure to concentrated HIV (eg, in a research laboratory or production facility) is treated as percutaneous exposure to blood with highest risk.

†*Recommend,* Postexposure prophylaxis (PEP) should be recommended to the exposed worker with counseling; *Offer,* PEP should be offered to the exposed worker with counseling; *Not offer,* PEP should not be offered because these are not occupational exposures to HIV-1.

‡Regimens: zidovudine (ZDV), 200 mg three times a day; lamivudine (3TC), 150 mg two times a day; indinavir (IDV), 800 mg three times a day (if IDV is not available, saquinavir may be used, 600 mg three times a day). Prophylaxis is given for 4 weeks. For full prescribing information, see package inserts.

§*Highest risk,* both larger volume of blood (eg, deep injury with large diameter hollow needle previously in source patient's vein or artery, especially involving an injection of source-patient's blood) and blood containing a high titer of HIV (eg, source with acute retroviral illness or end-stage AIDS; viral load measurement may be considered, but its use in relation to PEP has not be evaluated); *Increased risk,* either exposure to larger volume of blood or blood with a high titer of HIV; *No increased risk,* neither exposure to a larger volume of blood nor blood with a high titer of HIV (eg, solid suture needle injury from source patient with asymptomatic HIV infection).

‖Possible toxicity of additional drug may not be warranted.

#Includes semen, vaginal secretions, cerebrospinal, synovial, pleural, peritoneal, pericardial, and amniotic fluids.

**For skin, risk is increased for exposures involving a high titer of HIV, prolonged contact, an extensive area, or an area in which skin integrity is visibly compromised. For skin exposures without increased risk, the risk for drug toxicity outweighs the benefit of PEP.

(CDC Update: provisional recommendations for chemoprophylaxis after occupational exposure to human immunodeficiency virus. MMWR 1996;45:468)

Table 23-2. Recommendations for when to initiate treatment

Status	Recommendation
Symptomatic HIV disease*	Therapy recommended for all patients
Asymptomatic, CD4+ cell count <0.500 x 10^5/L	Therapy recommended†
Asymptomatic, CD4+ cell count >0.500 x 10^9/L	Therapy recommended for patients with >30,000-50,000 HIV RNA copies/mL or rapidly declining CD4- cell counts. Therapy should be considered for patients with >5,000-10,000 HIV RNA copies/mL

*Symptomatic human immunodeficiency virus (HIV) disease includes symptoms such as recurrent mucosal candidiasis, oral hairy leukoplakia, and chronic and unexplained fever, night sweats, and weight loss.

†Some would defer therapy in a subset of patients with stable CD4+ cell counts between 0.350 and 0.500 x 10^9/L and plasma HIV RNA levels consistently below 5,000–10,000 copies/mL.

(Carpenter CCJ, Fischl MA, Hammer SM for the International AIDS Society - USA. Antiretroviral therapy for HIV infection in 1996. Recommendations of an international panel. JAMA 1996;276:146)

Table 23-3. Recommendations for initial therapy regimens

Zidovudine/didanosine, or zidovudine/zalcitabine, or zidovudine/lamivudine, or didanosine monotherapy*	If a protease inhibitor is added to a nucleoside analogue-containing regimen, the choice of protease inhibitor should be based primarily on antiretroviral potency and secondarily on other considerations as described in the text.†

*Didanosine monotherapy may be less effective as initial therapy in patients with more advanced human immunodeficiency virus (HIV) disease. Other possible non-zidovudine-containing regimens include didanosine/stavudine, stavudine/lamivudine, and stavudine monotherapy, although these regimens are less well studied.

†Antiretroviral potency refers to plasma HIV RNA and CD4+ cell count responses associated with these drugs at approved doses and with currently available formulations.

(Carpenter CCJ, Fishl MA, Hammer SM for the International AIDS Society - USA. Antiretroviral therapy for HIV infection in 1996. Recommendations of an international panel. JAMA 1996;276:146)

REFERENCES

1. Perelson AS, Neumann AU, Markowitz M, Leonard JM, Ho DD. HIV-1 dynamics in vivo: virion clearance rate, infected cell life-span, and viral generation time. Science 1996;271:1582.
2. Mellors JW, Rinaldo CR Jr, Gupta P, White RM, Todd JA, Kingsly LA. Prognosis in HIV-1 infection predicted by the quantity of virus in plasma. Science 1996;272:1167.
3. O'Brien WA, Hatigan PM, Martin D, et al. Changes in plasma HIV-1 RNA and CD4+ lymphocyte count relative to treatment and progression to AIDS. N Engl J Med 1996;334:426.
4. Katzenstein DA, Hammer SM, Hughes MD, et al. Virologic and immunologic markers and clinical outcomes after nucleoside therapy of adults with 200 to 500 CD4 cells per cubic millimeter. N Engl J Med 1996;in press.
5. Saag MS, Holodniy M, Kuritzkes DR, et al. HIV viral load markers in clinical practice. Nature Medicine 1996;2:625.
6. Carpenter CCJ, Fischl MA, Hammer SM for the International AIDS Society - USA. Antiretroviral therapy for HIV infection in 1996. Recommendations of an international panel. JAMA 1996;276:146.
7. Gulick RM, Mellors J, Havlir D, et al. Potent and sustained antiretroviral activity of indinavir (IDV), zidovudine (ZDV) and lamivudine (3TC). Abstr ThB931. XI Internat Conf on AIDS. Vancouver, July 7-12, 1996.
8. Markowitz M, Cao Y, Hurley A, et al. Triple therapy with AZT, 3TC, and ritonavir in 12 subjects newly infected with HIV-1. Abstr. ThB933. XI Internat Conf on AIDS. Vancouver, July 7-12, 1996.
9. Myers MW, Montaner J for the Incas Study Group. A randomized, double-blinded comparative trial of the effects of zidovudine, didanosine and nevirapine combinations in antiviral naive, AIDS-free, HIV-infected patients with CD4 counts 200-600/mm³. Abstract MoB294. XI Internat Conf on AIDS. Vancouver, July 7-12, 1996.
10. D'Aquila RT, Hughes MD, Johnson VA, et al. Nevirapine, zidovudine, and didanosine compared with zidovudine and didanosine in patients with HIV-1 infection. A randomized, double-blind, placebo-controlled trial. Ann Intern Med 1996;124:1019.
11. Eron JJ, Benoit SL, Jemsek J, et al. Treatment with lamivudine, zidovudine, or both in HIV-positive patients with 200 to 500 CD4+ cells per cubic millimeter. N Engl J Med 1995;333:1662.
12. Staszewski S, Loveday C, Picazo JJ, et al. Safety and efficacy of lamivudine-zidovudine combination therapy in zidovudine-experienced patients. A randomized controlled comparison with zidovudine monotherapy. JAMA 1996;276:111.
13. Katlama C, Ingrand D, Loveday C, et al. Safety and efficacy of lamivudine-zidovudine combination therapy in antiretroviral-naive patients. A randomized controlled comparison with zidovudine monotherapy. JAMA 1996;276:118.
14. Bartlett JA, Benoit SL, Johnson VA, et al. Lamivudine plus zidovudine compared with zalcitabine plus zidovudine in patients with HIV infection. A randomized, double-blind, placebo-controlled trial. Ann Intern Med 1996;125:161.
15. Staszewski S, Bartlett J, Eron JJ, et al. Reductions in HIV-1 disease progression for AZT/3TC relative to control treatments: a meta analysis. Abstr ThB948. XI Internat Conf on AIDS. Vancouver, July 7-12, 1996.
16. CDC Update: Provisional recommendations for chemoprophylaxis after occupational exposure to human immunodeficiency virus. MMWR 1996;45:468.

Multidrug Combinations

Combinations of three or more antiretroviral agents are being employed in clinical trials, based in part on in vitro studies demonstrating greater and more sustained antiviral effects as the number of agents in simultaneous combination was increased.[139] This pattern was observed when the combinations contained agents acting at the same or at different target sites.

Two clinical trials have compared three- and two-drug regimens in HIV-1 infected individuals. In ACTG 241, 398 patients with 350 or fewer CD4 lymphocytes/mm^3 and more than 6 months prior nucleoside therapy were randomized to receive AZT and ddI in conventional doses with or without additional nevirapine (200 mg/day for 2 weeks, then 400 mg/day). After 48 weeks of therapy, patients assigned to the three-drug regimen had an 18% higher CD4 cell count (P =.001), 0.32 $\log_{10}$ lower mean infectious HIV-1 titer in peripheral blood mononuclear cells (P =.023), and 0.25 $\log_{10}$ lower mean plasma HIV-1 RNA level (P =.028) compared with those assigned the two-drug regimen.[141] There was no difference in disease progression, although the study had only moderate power to detect a major difference; severe rashes were more common in the three-drug recipients (9% versus 2%, P =.002).

A second trial, ACTG 229, compared the three-drug regimen of saquinavir, ddC, and AZT to the two-drug regimens of AZT plus ddC or AZT plus saquinavir.[140] The 302 patients enrolled had CD4 cell counts between 50 and 300/mm^3 and had received prior AZT for 4 months or longer. Patients were treated for 24 weeks; conventional doses of AZT and ddC were employed, and the saquinavir dose was 600 mg, administered three times daily. The rate of increase of CD4 cell counts was greater and viral load was lower in recipients of the three-drug combination, and there were no significant differences in toxicities. The study was not powered to detect clinical outcome differences.

Both of these studies support further exploration of three or more drug combinations in HIV-1 infections. Additional trials of these and other three-drug combinations are underway in patients with earlier disease and less antiretroviral experience, as are trials with sufficient size to detect significant clinical end point differences.

Other Combinations

Several studies comparing AZT with the combination of AZT plus acyclovir have had mixed results.[142] Although acyclovir itself has little or no antiretroviral activity, there is controversy about whether it can potentiate AZT activity in vitro. One European-Australian collaborative study reported improvement in survival when acyclovir was added to AZT in patients with AIDS (1 year rates of 0.54 versus 0.73; P =.014) and those with ARC (1-year rates of 0.81 versus 0.97, P =.045).[143] A second study reported similar results in treating 302 patients with advanced disease with CD4 cell counts of 150/mm^3 or less.[144] One retrospective analysis of a large HIV-1 infected cohort further supported this possibility,[145] but another did not.[146] The ACTG 063 study, involving 334 patients with AIDS randomly assigned to monotherapy or combination therapy including acyclovir (1000 mg/day), showed no differences in survival, opportunistic infections, or neoplasms.[147] No firm conclusions can be drawn on the value of acyclovir supplementation to antiretroviral regimens at this time.

Another interesting combination being tested in clinical trials is ddI plus hydroxyurea. Although hydroxyurea has little antiretroviral activity by itself, it does potentiate ddI activity in vitro, presumably by depleting deoxynucleoside triphosphate pools.[148] Because hydroxyurea has been used clinically for decades in the treatment of neoplastic disorders, it will be of interest to see whether it will be a useful adjunct to ddI in treating HIV disease as well.

REFERENCES

1. Hirsch MS, Kaplan JC, D'Aquila RT. Antiviral agents. In: Fields BN, Knipe DM, Howley PM, eds. Fields Virology. 3rd ed. New York: Raven Press 1996:431.
2. Ho DD, Neumann AU, Perelson AS, Chen W, Leonard JM, Markowitz M. Rapid turnover of plasma virions and CD4 lymphocytes in HIV-1 infection. Nature (London) 1995;373:123.
3. Wei X, Ghosh SK, Taylor ME, et al. Viral dynamics in human immunodeficiency virus type 1 infection. Nature (London) 1995;373:117.
4. Coffin JM. HIV population dynamics in vivo: implications for genetic variation, pathogenesis, and therapy. Science 1995;267:483.
5. Embretson J, Zupanic M, Ribas JL, et al. Massive covert infection of helper T lymphocytes and macrophages by HIV during the incubation period of AIDS. Nature (London) 1993;362:359.
6. Pantaleo G, Graziosi C, Demarest JF, et al. HIV infection is active and progressive in lymphoid tissue during clinically latent stage of disease. Nature (London) 1993;362:355.
7. Bukrinsky MI, Haggerty S, Dempsey MP, et al. A nuclear localization signal within HIV-1 matrix protein that governs infection of non-dividing cells. Nature (London) 1993;365:666.
8. Lewis P, Hensel M, Emerman M. Human immunodeficiency virus infection of cells arrested in the cell cycle. EMBO J 1992;11:3053.
9. Weinberg JB, Mathews TJ, Cullen BR, Malim MH. Productive human immunodeficiency virus type 1 (HIV-1) infection of nonproliferating human monocytes. J Exp Med 1991;174:1477.
10. Nabel G, Baltimore D. An inducible transcription factor activates expression of human immunodeficiency virus in T cells. Nature (London) 1987;326:711.
11. Gruters RA, Neefjes JJ, Tersmette M, et al. Interference with HIV-induced syncytium formation and viral infectivity by inhibitors of trimming glucosidase. Nature (London) 1987;330:74.
12. Walker BD, Kowalski M, Goh WC, et al. Inhibition of human immunodeficiency virus syncytium formation and virus replication by castanospermine. Nature (London) 1987;84:8120.
13. Hsu M-C, Schutt AD, Holly M, et al. Inhibition of HIV replication in acute and chronic infections in vitro by a tat antagonist. Science 1991;254:1799.
14. Haubrich RH, Flexner C, Lederman M, et al. Tat antagonist for HIV infection. A randomized trial of the activity and safety of Ro24-7429 (tat antagonist) versus nucleoside for HIV infection. J Infect Dis 1995;172:1246.
15. Horwitz JP, Chua J, Noel M. The mononesylates of 1-(2'-deoxy-beta-D-lyxofuranosyl) thymidine. J Organ Chem 1964;29:2076.
16. Ostertag W, Roesler G, Krieg CJ, et al. Induction of endogenous virus and of thymidine kinase by bromodeoxyuridine in cell cultures transformed by Friend virus. Proc Natl Acad Sci USA 1974;71:4980.
17. Mitsuya H, Weinhold KJ, Furman PA, et al. 3'-Azido-3'-deoxythymidine (BWA509U): an antiviral agent that inhibits the infectivity and cytopathic effect of human T-lymphotropic virus type 111/lymphadenopathy-associated virus in vitro. Proc Natl Acad Sci USA 1985;82:7096.
18. Cheng Y-C, Dutschman GE, Bastow KW, Sarngadharan MG, Ting RYC. Human immunodeficiency virus reverse transcriptase. General properties and its interactions with nucleoside triphosphate analogs. J Biol Chem 1987;262:2187.

19. St. Clair MH, Richards CA, Spector T, et al. 3′-Azido-3′-deoxythymidine triphosphate as an inhibitor and substrate of purified human immunodeficiency virus reverse transcriptase. Antimicrob Agents Chemother 1987;31:1972.

20. Furman PA, Barry DW. Spectrum of antiviral activity and mechanism of action of zidovudine. Am J Med 1988;85(Suppl 2A):176.

21. Furman PA, Fyfe JA, St. Clair MH, et al. Phosphorylation of 3′-azido-3′-deoxythymidine and selective interaction of the 5′-triphosphate with HIV reverse transcriptase. Proc Natl Acad Sci USA 1986; 83:8333.

22. Tan CK, Cival R, Mian AM, So AG, Downey KM. Inhibition of the RNase H activity of HIV reverse transcriptase by azidothymidylate. Biochemistry 1991;30:4831.

23. Vogt MW, Hartshorn KL, Furman PA, et al. Ribavirin antagonizes the effect of azidothymidine on HIV replication. Science 1987;235:1376.

24. Medina DJ, Hsiung GD, Mellors JW. Ganciclovir antagonizes the anti-human immunodeficiency virus type 1 activity of zidovudine and didanosine in vitro. Antimicrob Agents Chemother 1992;36:1127.

25. Merrill DP, Moonis M, Chou T-C, Hirsch MS. Lamivudine (3TC) or stavudine (d4T) in two- and three-drug combinations against HIV-1 replication in vitro. J Infect Dis 1996;173:355.

26. Larder BA, Darby G, Richman DD. HIV with reduced sensitivity to zidovudine (AZT) isolated during prolonged therapy. Science 1989;243:1731.

27. Larder BA, Coates KE, Kemp SD. Zidovudine-resistant human immunodeficiency virus selected by passage in cell culture. J Virol 1991;65:5232.

28. Kellam P, Boucher CAB, Larder BA. Fifth mutation in human immunodeficiency virus type 1 reverse transcriptase contributes to the development of high-level resistance to zidovudine. Proc Natl Acad Sci USA 1992;89:1934.

29. Larder BA, Kemp SD. Multiple mutations in HIV-1 reverse transcriptase confer high-level resistance to zidovudine (AZT). Science 1989;246:1155.

30. Richman DD, Grimes JM, Lagakos SW. Effect of stage of disease and drug dose on zidovudine susceptibilities of isolates of human immunodeficiency virus. J Acquire Immune Defic Syndr 1990;3:743.

31. Najera I, Holguin A, Quinones-Mateu ME, et al. *Pol* gene quasispecies of human immunodeficiency virus: mutations associated with drug resistance in virus: mutations associated with drug resistance in virus from patients undergoing no drug therapy. J Virol 1995;69:23.

32. Land S, McGavin K, Birch C, Lucas R. Reversion from zidovudine resistance to sensitivity on cessation of treatment. Lancet 1991;338:830.

33. Martin JL, Wilson JE, Haynes RL, Furman PA. Mechanism of resistance of human immunodeficiency virus type 1 to 2′,3′-dideoxyinosine. Proc Natl Acad Sci USA 1993;90:6135.

34. Eron JJ, Chow Y-K, Caliendo AM, et al. *Pol* mutations conferring zidovudine and didanosine resistance with different effects in vitro yield multiply resistant human immunodeficiency virus type 1 isolates in vivo. Antimicrob Agents Chemother 1993;37:1480.

35. Lacey SF, Reardon JE, Furfine ES, et al. Biochemical studies of the reverse transcriptase and RNase H activities from human immunodeficiency virus strains resistant to 3′-azido-3′-deoxythymidine. J Biol Chem 1992;267:15789.

36. Kohlstaedt LA, Wang J, Friedman JM, Rice PA, Steitz TA. Crystal structure at 3.5 A resolution of HIV-1 reverse transcriptase complexed with an inhibitor. Science 1992;256:1783.

37. Rooke R, Parniak MA, Tremblay M, et al. Biological comparison of wild-type and zidovudine-resistant isolates of human immunodeficiency virus type 1 from the same subjects: susceptibility and resistance to other drugs. Antimicrob Agents Chemother 1991;35:988.

38. Mayers D, Wagner KF, Chung RCY, et al. Drug susceptibilities of HIV isolates from patients receiving serial dideoxynucleoside therapy with ZDV, ddI and ddC. Abstract. Second International HIV Drug Resistance Workshop. Noordwijk, The Netherlands, 1993:47.

39. Anonymous. Clinical Practice: HIV seroconversion after occupational exposure despite early prophylactic zidovudine therapy. Lancet 1993;341:1077.

40. Fitzgibbon JE, Gaur S, Frenkel LD, Laraque F, Edlin BR, Dubin DT. Transmission from one child to another of human immunodeficiency virus type 1 with a zidovudine-resistance mutation. N Engl J Med 1993;329:1835.

41. Erice A, Mayers DL, Strike DG, et al. Brief report: primary infection with zidovudine-resistant human immunodeficiency virus type 1. N Engl J Med 1993;328:1163.

42. Frenkel LM, Wagner II LE, Demeter LM, et al. Effects of zidovudine use during pregnancy on resistance and vertical transmission of human immunodeficiency virus type 1. Clin Infect Dis 1995;20:1321.

43. D'Aquila RT, Johnson VA, Welles SL, et al. Zidovudine resistance and HIV-1 disease progression during antiretroviral therapy. Ann Intern Med 1995;122:401.

44. Montaner JSG, Singer J, Schecter MT, et al. Clinical correlates of in vitro HIV-1 resistance to zidovudine. Results of the Multicentre Canadian AZT Trial. AIDS 1993;7:189.

45. Ogino MT, Dankner WM, Spector SA. Development and significance of zidovudine resistance in children infected with human immunodeficiency virus. J Pediatr 1993;123:1.

46. Tudor-Williams G, St. Clair M, McKinney RE, et al. HIV-1 sensitivity to zidovudine and clinical outcome in children. Lancet 1992;339:15.

47. Yarchoan R, Klecker RW, Weinhold KJ, et al. Administration of 3′-azido-3′-deoxythymidine, an inhibitor of HTLV111/LAV replication, to patients with AIDS or AIDS-related complex. Lancet 1986;1:575.

48. Fischl MA, Richman GG, Grieco MH, et al. The efficacy of azidothymidine (AZT) in the treatment of subjects with AIDS and AIDS-related complex—a double-blind placebo-controlled trial. N Engl J Med 1987;317:185.

49. Richman DD, Fischl MA, Grieco MH, et al. The toxicity of azidothymidine (AZT) in the treatment of patients with AIDS and AIDS-related complex—a double-blind, placebo-controlled trial. N Engl J Med 1987;317:192.

50. Hirsch MS. AIDS commentary—azidothymidine. J Infect Dis 1988;157:427.

51. Fischl MA, Parker CB, Pettinelli C, et al. A randomized controlled trial of a reduced daily dose of zidovudine in patients with the acquired immunodeficiency syndrome. N Engl J Med 1990;323:1009.

52. Fischl MA, Richman DD, Hansen N, et al. The safety and efficacy of zidovudine (AZT) in the treatment of subjects with mildly symptomatic human immunodeficiency virus type 1 (HIV) infection. Ann Intern Med 1990;112:727.

53. Volberding PA, Lagakos SW, Koch MA, et al. Zidovudine in asymptomatic human immunodeficiency virus infection. A controlled trial in persons with fewer than 500 CD4-positive cells per cubic millimeter. N Engl J Med 1990;322:941.

54. Volberding PA, Lagakos SW, Grimes JM, et al. The duration of zidovudine benefit in persons with asymptomatic HIV infection: prolonged evaluation of protocol 019 of the AIDS Clinical Trials Group. JAMA 1994;272:437.

55. Hamilton JD, Hartigan PM, Simberkoff MS, et al. A controlled trial of early versus late treatment with zidovudine in symptomatic human immunodeficiency virus infection. N Engl J Med 1992;326:437.

56. Aboulker JP, Swart AM. Preliminary analysis of the Concorde trial. Lancet 1993;341:889.

57. Concorde Coordinating Committee. Concorde: MRC/ANRS randomised double-blind controlled trial of immediate and deferred zidovudine in symptom-free HIV infection. Lancet 1994;343:871.

58. Hirsch MS, D'Aquila RT. Therapy for human immunodeficiency virus infection. N Engl J Med 1993;325:1686.

59. Sande M, Carpenter CCJ, Cobbs GC, et al. Antiretroviral therapy for adult HIV-infected patients-recommendations from a state-of-the-art conference. JAMA 1993;270:2583.

60. Cooper DA, Gatell J, Kroon S, et al. Zidovudine in persons with asymptomatic HIV infection and CD4+ cell counts greater than 400 per cubic millimeter. N Engl J Med 1993;329:297.

61. Volberding PA, Lagakos SW, Grimes JM, et al. A comparison of immediate with deferred zidovudine therapy for asymptomatic HIV-infected adults with CD4 cell counts of 500 or more per cubic millimeter. N Engl J Med 1995;333:401.

62. Kinloch-DeLoes S, Hirschel BJ, Hoen B, et al. A controlled trial of zidovudine in primary human immunodeficiency virus infection. N Engl J Med 1995;333:408.

63. McKinney REJ, Maha MA, Conner EM, et al. A multicenter trial of oral zidovudine in children with advanced immunodeficiency virus disease. N Engl J Med 1991;324:1018.

64. Baker C, for the ACTG 152 Protocol Team. Executive summary, 1995.

65. Sperling RS, Stratton P, O'Sullivan M, et al. A survey of zidovudine use in pregnant women with human immunodeficiency virus infection. N Engl J Med 1992;326:857.

66. Connor, EM, Sperling, RS, Gelber, R, et al. Reduction of maternal-infant transmission of human immunodeficiency virus type 1 with zi-

dovudine therapy. Pediatric AIDS Clinical Trials Group Protocol 076 Study Group. N Engl J Med 1994;331:1173.

67. Matheson PB, Abrams EJ, Thomas PA, et al. Efficacy of antenatal zidovudine in reducing perinatal transmission of human immunodeficiency virus type 1. J Infect Dis 1995;172:353.

68. Cardo D, Srivastava P, Ciesielski R, et al. Case-control study of HIV seroconversion in health care workers (HCWs) after percutaneous exposure to HIV-infected blood. Abstract. Fifth Annual Meeting of the Society for Healthcare Epidemiology of America. San Diego, April 2–4. 1995.

69. St. Clair MH, Martin JL, Tudor-Williams G, et al. Resistance to ddI and sensitivity to AZT induced by a mutation in HIV-1 reverse transcriptase. Science 1991;253:1557.

70. Gu Z, Gao Q, Li X, Parniak MA, Wainberg MA. Novel mutation in the human immunodeficiency virus type 1 reverse transcriptase gene that encodes cross-resistance to 2′,3′-dideoxyinosine and 2′,3′-dideoxycytidine. J Virol 1992;66:7128.

71. Zhang D, Caliendo AM, Eron JJ, et al. Resistance to 2′,3′-dideoxycytidine conferred by a mutation in codon 65 of the human immunodeficiency virus type 1 reverse transcriptase. Antimicrob Agents Chemother 1994;38:282.

72. Boyer PL, Tantillo C, Jacobo-Molina A, et al. The sensitivity of wild-type human immunodeficiency virus reverse transcriptase to dideoxynucleosides depends on template length; the sensitivity of drug-resistant mutants does not. Proc Natl Acad Sci USA 1994;91:4882.

73. Kozal MJ, Kroodsma K, Winters MA, et al. Didanosine resistance in HIV-infected patients switched from zidovudine to didanosine monotherapy. Ann Intern Med 1994;121:263.

74. Fitzgibbon JE, Howell RE, Haberzettl CA, Sperber SJ, Gocke DJ, Dubin DT. Human immunodeficiency virus type 1 pol gene mutations which cause decreased susceptibility to 2′,3′-dideoxycytidine. Antimicrob Agents Chemother 1992;36:153.

75. Lin P, Samanta H, Rose RE, et al. Genotypic and phenotypic analysis of human immunodeficiency virus type-1 isolates from patients on prolonged stavudine therapy. J Infect Dis 1994;170:1157.

76. Nguyen B-Y, Yarchoan R, Wyvill KM, et al. Five-year follow-up of a phase I study of didanosine in patients with advanced immunodeficiency virus infection. J Infect Dis 1995;171:1180.

77. Kahn JO, Lagakos SW, Richman DD, et al. A controlled trial comparing continued zidovudine with didanosine in human immunodeficiency virus infection. N Engl J Med 1992;327:581.

78. Dolin R, Amato DA, Fischl MA, et al. Zidovudine compared to didanosine in patients with advanced HIV-1 infection and little or no previous experience with zidovudine. Arch Intern Med 1995;155:961.

79. Spruance SL, Pavia AT, Peterson D, et al. Didanosine compared with continuation of zidovudine in HIV-infected patients with signs of clinical deterioration while receiving zidovudine. A randomized, double-blind clinical trial. Ann Intern Med 1994;120:360.

80. Montaner JSG, Schecter MT, Rachlis A, et al and the Canadian HIV Trials Network Protocol 002 Study Group. Didanosine compared with continued zidovudine therapy for HIV-infected patients with 200 to 500 CD4 cells/mm³. A double blind randomized controlled trial. Ann Intern Med 1995;123:561.

81. Hammer SM, for ACTG 175 protocol team. Executive summary, September, 1995.

82. Fischl MA, Olsen RM, Follansbee SE, et al. Zalcitabine compared with zidovudine in patients with advanced HIV-1 infection who received previous zidovudine therapy. Ann Intern Med 1993;118:762.

83. Abrams D, Goldman A, Launer C, et al. A comparative trial of didanosine or zalcitabine in patients with human immunodeficiency virus infection. N Engl J Med 1994;330:657.

84. Browne MJ, Mayer KH, Chafee SBD, et al. 2′,3′-Didehydro-3′-deoxythymidine (d4T) in patients with AIDS or AIDS-related complex: a phase I trial. J Infect Dis 1993;167:21.

85. Pavia AT, Gathe J, et al and BMS-019 Study Group Investigators. Clinical efficacy of stavudine (d4T, Zerit) compared to zidovudine (ZDV, Retrovir) in ZDV-pretreated HIV positive patients. Abstract. Thirty-fifth International Conference on AIDS and Associated Cancers, San Francisco. September 17–20, 1995.

86. Van Leeuwen R, Katlama C, Kitchen V, et al. Evaluation of safety and efficacy of 3TC (lamivudine) in patients with asymptomatic or mildly symptomatic human immunodeficiency virus infection a phase I/II study. J Infect Dis 1995;171:1166.

87. Soudeyns H, Yao XJ, Gao Q, et al. Anti-human immunodeficiency virus type 1 activity and in vitro toxicity of 2′-deoxy-3′-thiacytidine (BCH-189), a novel heterocyclic nucleoside analog. Antimicrob Agents Chemother 1991;35:1386.

88. Gao Q, Gu Z, Hiscott J, Dionne G, Wainberg MA. Generation of drug-resistant variants of human immunodeficiency virus type 1 by in vitro passage in increasing concentrations of 2′,3′-dideoxycytidine and 2′,3′-dideoxy-3′-thiacytidine. Antimicrob Agents Chemother 1993;37:130.

89. Schinazi RF, LLoyd RM, Nguyen M-H, et al. Characterization of human immunodeficiency viruses resistant to oxathiolane-cytosine nucleosides. Antimicrob Agents Chemother 1993;37:875.

90. Tisdale M, Kemp SD, Parry NR, Larder BA. Rapid in vitro selection of human immunodeficiency virus type 1 resistant to 3′-thiacytidine inhibitors due to a mutation in the YMDD region of reverse transcriptase. Proc Natl Acad Sci USA. 1993;90:5653.

91. Boucher CAB, Cammack N, Schipper P, et al. High-level resistance to (−)enantiomeric 2′-deoxy-3′-thiacytidine in vitro is due to one amino acid substitution in the catalytic site of human immunodeficiency virus type 1 reverse transcriptase. Antimicrob Agents Chemother 1993;37:2231.

92. Schuurman R, Nijhuis M, van Leeuwen R, et al. Rapid changes in human immunodeficiency virus type 1 RNA load and appearance of drug-resistant virus populations in persons treated with lamivudine (3TC). J Infect Dis 1995;171:1411.

93. Pluda JM, Cooley TP, Montaner JSG, et al. A phase I/II study of 2′-deoxy-3′-thiacytidine (Lamivudine) in patients with advanced human immunodeficiency virus infection. J Infect Dis 1995;171:1438.

94. Larder BA, Kemp SD, Harrigan PR. Potential mechanism for sustained antiretroviral efficacy of AZT-3TC combination therapy. Science 1995;269:696.

95. De Clercq E. Antiviral Therapy for human immunodeficiency virus infections. Clin Microbiol Rev 1995;8:200.

96. Smerdon SJ, Jager J, Wang J, et al. Structure of the binding site for nonnucleoside inhibitors of the reverse transcriptase of human immunodeficiency virus type 1. Proc Natl Acad Sci USA 1994;91:3911.

97. Rogers DW, Gamblin SJ, Harris BA, et al. The structure of unliganded reverse transcriptase from the human immunodeficiency virus type 1. Proc Natl Acad Sci USA 1995;92:1222.

98. Cheeseman SH, Havlir D, McLaughlin MM, et al. Phase I/II evaluation of nevirapine alone and in combination with zidovudine for infection with human immunodeficiency virus. J Acquir Immune Defic Syndr 1995;8:141.

99. Havlir D, Cheeseman SH, Mclaughlin M, et al. High-dose nevirapine: safety, pharmacokinetics, and antiviral effect in patients with human immunodeficiency virus infection. J Infect Dis 1995;171:537.

100. Richman DD, Havlir D, Corbeil J, et al. Nevirapine resistance mutations of HIV-1 selected during therapy. J Virol 1994;68:1660.

101. Saag MS, Emini EA, Laskin OL, et al. A short-term clinical evaluation of L-697,661, a non-nucleoside inhibitor of HIV-1 reverse transcriptase. N Engl J Med 1993;329:1065.

102. Balzarini J, Velazquez S, San Felix A, et al. Human immunodeficiency virus type 1-specific [2′,5′-bis-O-(tert-butyldimethylsilyl)-beta-D-ribofuranosyl]-3′-spiro-5″-(4″-amino-1″-oxathiole-2″,2″-dioxide)-purine analogues show a resistance spectrum that is different from that of the human immunodeficiency virus type 1-specific non-nucleoside analogues. Mol Pharmacol 1993;43:109.

103. Duewecke TJ, Pushkarskaya TJ, Poppe SM, et al. A novel mutation in bisheteroaryl-piperazine-resistant HIV-1 reverse transcriptase confers increased sensitivity to other nonnucleoside inhibitors. Proc Natl Acad Sci USA 1993;90:4713.

104. deJong MD, Loewenthal M, Boucher CAB, et al. Alternating nevirapine and zidovudine treatment of human immunodeficiency virus type 1–infected persons does not prolong nevirapine activity. J Infect Dis 1994;169:1346.

105. Winslow DL, Otto MJ. HIV protease inhibitors. AIDS 1995;9(Suppl A):S183.

106. Kohl NE, Emini EA, Schleif WA, et al. Active human immunodeficiency virus protease is required for viral infectivity. Proc Natl Acad Sci USA 1988;85:4686.

107. McQuade TJ, Tomasselli AG, Liu L, et al. A synthetic HIV-1 protease inhibitor with antiviral activity arrests HIV-like particle maturation. Science 1990;247:454.

108. Nagy K, Young M, Baboonian C, Merson J, Whittle P, Oroszlan S. Antiviral activity of human immunodeficiency virus type 1 protease in-

hibitors in a single cycle of infection: evidence for a role of protease in the early phase. J Virol 1994;68:757.

109. Wlodawer A, Erickson JW. Structure-based inhibitors of HIV-1 protease. Ann Rev Biochem 1993;62:543.

110. Kitchen VS, Skinner CA, Lane EA, et al. Safety and activity of saquinavir in HIV infection. Lancet 1995;345:952.

111. Kempf DJ, Harsh KC, Denisson JF, et al. ABT-538 is a potent inhibitor of human immunodeficiency virus protease and had high oral bioavailability in humans. Proc Natl Acad Sci USA 1995;92:2484.

112. Danner SA, Carr A, Leonard JM, et al. A short-term study of the safety, pharmacokinetics, and efficacy of ritonavir, an inhibitor of HIV-1 protease. M Engl J Med 1995;333:1528.

113. Markowitz M, Saag M, Powderly WG, et al. A preliminary study of ritonavir, an inhibitor of HIV-1 protease, to treat HIV-1 infection. N Engl J Med 1995;333:1534.

114. Mathez D, deTruchis P, Gorin I, et al. Ritonavir, AZT, ddC as triple combination in AIDS patients. Abstr. 3rd Conference on Retroviruses and Opportunistic Infections, Washington. Jan 28-Feb 1, 1996.

115. Cameron B, Heath Chiozzi M, Kravick S, et al. Prolongation of life and prevention of AIDS in advanced HIV immunodeficiency with ritonavir. Abstr. 3rd Conference on Retroviruses and Opportunistic Infections, Washington. Jan 28-Feb 1, 1996.

116. Gulick R, Mellors J, Havlir D, et al. Potent and sustained antiretroviral activity of indinavir (IDV) in combination with zidovudine (ZDV) and lamivudine (3TC). Abstr. 3rd Conference on Retroviruses and Opportunistic Infections, Washington. Jan 28-Feb 1, 1996.

117. Condra JH, Schleif WA, Blahy OM, et al. In vivo emergence of HIV-1 variants resistant to multiple protease inhibitors. Nature (London) 1995;374:569.

118. Watson AJ, Wilburn LM. Inhibition of HIV infection of resting peripheral blood lymphocytes by nucleosides. AIDS Res Hum Retroviruses 1992;8:1221.

119. Gao W-Y, Shirasaka T, Johns DG, Broder S, Mitsuya H. Differential phosphorylation of azidothymidine, dideoxycytidine, and dideoxyinosine in resting and activated peripheral blood mononuclear cells. J Clin Invest 1993;91:2326.

120. Chou T-C, Talalay P. Quantitative analysis of dose-effect relationships: the combined effects of multiple drugs or enzyme inhibitors. Adv Enzyme Regul 1984;22:27.

121. Chou J, Chou T-C. Dose-effect analysis with microcomputers: quantitation of ED50, LD50, synergism, antagonism, low-dose risk, receptor-ligand binding and enzyme kinetics. A computer software for IBM-PC and manual. Cambridge, UK: Elsevier-Biosoft, 1987.

122. Chou T-C. The median-effect principle and the combination index for quantitation of synergism and antagonism. In: Chou T-C, Rideout DC, eds. Synergism and antagonism in chemotherapy. New York: Academic Press, 1991:61.

123. Wilson CC, Hirsch MS. Combination antiretroviral therapy for the treatment of human immunodeficiency virus type-1 infection. Proc Assoc Am Physician 1995;107:19.

124. Eron JJ Jr, Johnson VA, Merrill DP, Chou T-C, Hirsch MS. Synergistic inhibition of replication of human immunodeficiency virus type 1, including that of a zidovudine-resistant isolate, by zidovudine and 2',3'-dideoxycytidine in vitro. Antimicrob Agents Chemother 1992;36:1559.

125. Meng TC, Fischl MA, Boota AM, et al. Combination therapy with zidovudine and dideoxycytidine in patients with advanced human immunodeficiency virus infection. A phase I/II study. Ann Intern Med 1992;116:13.

126. Skowron G, Bozzette SA, Lim L, et al. Alternating and intermittent regimens of zidovudine and dideoxycytidine in patients with AIDS or AIDS-related complex. Ann Intern Med 1993;118:321.

127. Fischl MA, Stanley K, Collier AC, et al. Combination and monotherapy with zidovudine and zalcitabine in patients with advanced HIV disease. The NIAID AIDS Clinical Trials Group. Ann Intern Med 1995;122:24.

128. Collier AC, Coombs RW, Fischl MA, et al. Combination therapy with zidovudine and didanosine compared with zidovudine alone in HIV-1 infection. Ann Intern Med 1993;119:786.

129. Ragni MV, Amato DA, LoFaro ML, et al. Randomized study of didanosine monotherapy and combination therapy with zidovudine in hemophilic and non-hemophilic subjects with asymptomatic human immunodeficiency virus-1 infection. AIDS Clinical Trials Group. Blood 1995;85:2337.

130. Shafer RW, Iversen AKN, Winters MA, et al. Drug resistance and heterogeneous long-term virologic responses of human immunodeficiency virus type 1–infected subjects to zidovudine and didanosine combination therapy. J Infect Dis 1995;172:70.

131. Yarchoan R, Lietzau J, Nguyen B-Y, et al. A randomized pilot of alternating or simultaneous zidovudine (AZT) and didanosine (ddI) in patients with symptomatic human immunodeficiency virus infection. J Infect Dis 1994;169:9.

132. Katlama C. Combination 3TC/ZDV vs ZDV monotherapy in ZDV naive HIV positive patients with a CD4 of 100-400 cells/mm³. Abstract LB 31. Program and abstracts of the 2nd National Conference on Human Retroviruses and Related Infections. Washington, DC: American Society for Microbiology, 1995:173.

133. Staszewski S. Combination 3TC/ZDV vs ZDV monotherapy in ZDV experienced HIV-1 positive patients with a CD4 of 100-500 cells/mm³. Abstract LB 32. Program and abstracts of the 2nd National Conference on Human retroviruses and Related Infections. Washington, DC: American Society for Microbiology, 1995:173.

134. Eron JJ, Benoit SL, Jemsek J, et al. Treatment with lamivudine, zidovudine or both in HIV-positive patients with 200–500 CD4⁺ cells per cubic millimeter. N Engl J Med 1995;333:1662.

135. Goldman ME, Nunberg JH, O'Brien JA, et al. Pyridinone derivatives: specific human immunodeficiency virus type 1 reverse transcriptase inhibitors with antiviral activity. Proc Natl Acad Sci USA 1991;88:6863.

136. Kuritzkes D, Curtis M, Rosandich M, Stein D, Schooley R, Team AS. Delayed emergence of resistance to L-697,661, in patients receiving concomitant zidovudine. Abstract PO-B26-1994. Ninth International AIDS Conference, Berlin, 1993.

137. Staszewski S, Emini E, Massari F, et al. A double-blind randomized trial for safety, clinical efficacy, biological activity and susceptibility testing in 120 HIV positive patients treated with L-697,661, AZT and combinations of both drugs. Abstract WS-B26-4. Ninth International Conference on AIDS, Berlin, 1993.

138. Johnson VA, Merrill DP, Chou TC, Hirsch MS. Human immunodeficiency virus type 1 (HIV-1) inhibitory interactions between protease inhibitor Ro 31-8959 and zidovudine, 2',3'-dideoxycytidine, or recombinant interferon-α against zidovudine-sensitive or -resistant HIV-1 in vitro. J Infect Dis 1992;166:1143.

139. Mazzulli T, Rusconi S, Merrill DP, et al. Alternating versus continuous drug regimens in combination chemotherapy of human immunodeficiency virus type 1 infection in vitro. Antimicrob Agents Chemother 1994;38:656.

140. Collier AC, Coombs RW, Schoenfeld DA, et al. Combination therapy with saquinavir, zidovudine and zalcitabine. N Engl J Med 1996; in press.

141. Executive summary of results of ACTG protocol 241, November, 1994 and D'Aquila RT, Hughes M, Liou S-H, for the ACTG protocol 241 team. A comparative study of a combination of zidovudine, didanosine and double blinded nevirapine versus a combination of zidovudine and didanosine, Abstract. Second National Conference on Human Retroviruses, Washington, DC, January, 1995.

142. Caliendo AM, Hirsch MS. Combination therapy for infection due to human immunodeficiency virus type I. Clin Infect Dis 1994;18:516.

143. Cooper DA, Pehrson PO, Pedersen C, et al. The efficacy and safety of zidovudine alone or as cotherapy with acyclovir for the treatment of patients with AIDS and AIDS-related complex: a double-blind randomized trial. AIDS 1993;7:197.

144. Youle MS, Gazzard BG, Johnson MA, et al. Effects of high-dose oral acyclovir on herpes virus disease and survival in patients with advanced HIV disease: a double-blind, placebo-controlled study. AIDS 1994;8:641.

145. Stein DS, Graham NMH, Park LP, et al. The effect of the interactions of acyclovir with zidovudine on progression to AIDS and survival in the Multicenter Cohort Study. Ann Intern Med 1994;121:100.

146. Gallant JE, Moore RD, Keruly J, Richman DD, Chaisson RE. Lack of association between acyclovir use and survival in patients with advanced human immunodeficiency virus disease treated with zidovudine. J Infect Dis 1995;172:346.

147. Collier A, for the ACTG 063 protocol team. Executive summary, 1995.

148. Lori F, Malykha A, Cara A, et al. Hydroxyurea as an inhibitor of human immunodeficiency virus-type 1 replication. Science 1994;266:801.

AIDS: Biology, Diagnosis, Treatment and Prevention, fourth edition, edited by Vincent T. DeVita, Jr., Samuel Hellman, and Steven A. Rosenberg. Lippincott–Raven Publishers, © 1997

CHAPTER 24

Immunologic Approaches to the Treatment of Human Immunodeficiency Virus Infection

Michael C. Sneller and Clifford Lane

A unique feature differentiates human immunodeficiency virus (HIV) infection from other persistent viral diseases. By causing progressive dysfunction and depletion of CD4 T cells, HIV subverts the ability of the host to mount an adequate antiviral response. Over time, this HIV-induced depletion of CD4 T cells leads to collapse of the immune response and life-threatening immunodeficiency. A crucial element in the successful treatment of HIV infection is the restoration and preservation of immune competence.

Current therapy for HIV infection involves the administration nucleoside analogues that have antiretroviral activity. Although these drugs have improved survival times, they do not halt the progressive destruction of the immune system that characterizes HIV infection. Any design of a comprehensive therapeutic strategy for HIV disease must focus on blocking viral replication and on restoring immunocompetence. This chapter reviews the status of immune-based therapies for HIV infection.

PASSIVE IMMUNOTHERAPY

The passive transfer of immunoglobulins as a therapy for infectious diseases began in the late 19th century. This form of immunotherapy is based on the premise that correction of deficient humoral immunity through the administration of exogenous antibodies will result in clinical benefit.

The role of the humoral immune response in controlling HIV infection is unclear. Sera from most patients with HIV infection contain antibodies that can neutralize various laboratory strains of HIV.[1] The progression of HIV infection to clinical acquired immunodeficiency syndrome (AIDS) is often associated with a loss of neutralizing antibodies.[2,3] The generation of escape mutants is a frequently observed phenomenon in HIV infection; sera from HIV-infected patients neutralize laboratory strains of HIV but show little or no neutralizing activity when tested against the patient's own viral isolates.[4] It is not clear whether the generation of escape mutants and the loss of neutralizing antibody play a causative role in the progression of HIV infection or are merely a secondary phenomena. Nonetheless, it is possible that the administration of HIV-specific immunoglobulins to patients with advanced HIV infection may provide high titers of neutralizing antibodies that could help control viral replication and slow the progression of disease.

Another potential role for passive immunotherapy with anti-HIV immunoglobulins is in the prevention of mother-to-fetus transmission of HIV. Many cases of neonatal HIV infection occur during vaginal delivery.[5] Administration of HIV-neutralizing antibodies during labor possibly may reduce the frequency of maternal-fetal transmission during delivery. Similarly, administration of neutralizing antibodies to HIV-infected pregnant women throughout gestation may reduce the incidence of in utero transmission of HIV. The utility of this latter approach may be limited by logistical problems and the generation of epitope escape mutants during therapy.

Pooled HIV—Immune Plasma

Several controlled studies have investigated the clinical, immunologic, and virologic effects of passive immunotherapy with HIV–immune plasma preparations.[6–8] In these studies, purified γ-globulin fractions were obtained from HIV-infected donors with high titers of neutralizing anti-

Michael C. Sneller, Laboratory of Immunoregulation, National Institute of Allergy and Infectious Diseases, National Institutes of Health, Building 10, Room 11B-13, 9000 Rockville Pike, Bethesda, MD 20892.

Clifford Lane, Laboratory of Immunoregulation, National Institute of Allergy and Infectious Diseases, National Institutes of Health, 9000 Rockville Pike, Bethesda, MD 20892.

bodies. The HIV–immune plasma was then administered intravenously to patients with advanced HIV disease. Treatment with HIV immune plasma was consistently associated with a decline in serum p24 antigen levels. However, no significant decrease in plasma viremia, as measured by quantitative culture, was demonstrated.[6] The observed decline in p24 levels most likely represented binding of p24 antigen to infused p24 antibody rather than an effect on viral replication. In one study, treatment with 300 mL of immune plasma given every 2 weeks was associated with a statistically significant reduction in the cumulative incidence of AIDS-defining opportunistic infections and neoplasms.[7] Significant clinical benefits were not seen in the other studies, and none of the studies could show a beneficial effect of passive immunotherapy on survival.

Passive immunotherapy with HIV immune plasma is associated with several potential problems, including high cost and the requirement for a large pool of donors. It remains to be demonstrated whether this form of therapy has a role in clinical practice.

Monoclonal Antibodies

Another approach to passive immunotherapy involves the use of monoclonal antibodies that can neutralize a wide range of HIV isolates. Most of the neutralizing antibodies generated in response to HIV infection react with determinants on the surface glycoprotein gp120 and, to a lesser extent, the transmembrane protein gp41. For gp120, the V3 region and the discontinuous epitope forming the CD4 binding region seem to be especially important for antibody-mediated viral neutralization.[9–11] Monoclonal antibodies directed against these epitopes have been designed and, in some cases, can neutralize a diverse array of primary HIV isolates.[12–14] However, the heterogenicities of HIV strains and the ability of the virus to generate mutations in critical neutralizing epitopes represent major obstacles in the development of these agents for passive immunotherapy. It remains to be determined whether the use of combinations of monoclonal antibodies can overcome these problems. Clinical trials have been initiated in an attempt to answer these questions.

Pooled γ-Globulin From Normal Donors

Infection with HIV is associated with severe dysfunction in cellular and humoral immunity. In adults, the most common manifestation of immune deficiency is infection with opportunistic fungal, viral, and protozoan pathogens. HIV-infected children frequently develop severe and recurrent infections with encapsulated bacteria.

Several studies have shown that treatment of HIV-infected children with pooled γ-globulin (from healthy, non-infected donors) decreases the incidence of serious bacterial infections.[15–17] In a large, randomized, placebo-controlled trial, HIV-infected children who were treated with pooled γ-globulin experienced a significant reduction in bacterial infections compared with children receiving placebo.[18] The reduction in bacterial infections was most pronounced in the subgroup of children with CD4 counts of 200/mm^3 or more and was not associated with improved survival. Because this trial was conducted before therapy with zidovudine had become standard practice, a second trial was carried out. In this study, HIV-infected children were randomized to receive zidovudine plus pooled γ-globulin or zidovudine plus placebo.[19] The γ-globulin treatment reduced the occurrence of bacterial infections only in patients who were not receiving trimethoprim-sulfamethoxazole for *Pneumocystis carinii* prophylaxis. The results of this study suggest that prophylaxis with an oral antibiotic that has activity against gram-positive bacteria may be as effective as pooled γ-globulin in reducing the occurrence of bacterial infections in HIV-infected children. The results of multiple small trials suggest that pooled γ-globulin is not effective in preventing bacterial or opportunistic infections in HIV-infected adults.[20]

CYTOKINE THERAPY

Interferons

Interferons are a group of protein molecules with antiviral, antiproliferative, and immunomodulatory properties.[21] Interferons can be grouped into two distinct types based on their cell receptors and biologic effects. Type I interferons include interferon-α and interferon-β, which share a common cellular receptor and are produced by multiple cell types (eg, leukocytes, fibroblasts, epithelial cells). Type II interferon or interferon-γ is produced by activated T lymphocytes and natural killer (NK) cells and has a cellular receptor distinct from the type I interferons. There are at least 20 different interferon-α genes that encode at least 16 distinct protein products. In contrast, there is only one interferon-β and one interferon-γ gene.

Interferon-α

Even before the AIDS epidemic, interferon-α was known to exhibit antiretroviral activity. Studies of mice infected with murine leukemia virus indicated that interferon-α can inhibit viral replication in vitro by impeding the assembly and maturation of murine leukemia virus.[22] With the identification of HIV as the cause of AIDS, several laboratories began to examine the effects of interferon-α on HIV replication. It was initially shown that concentrations of interferon-α in the range of 100U/mL could suppress HIV replication in tissue culture.[23] This effect was most pronounced when interferon-α was continually present in the culture media and comparable in magnitude to the level of suppression seen with zidovudine. Subsequent work demonstrated that inhibition of HIV replication was more pronounced by class I interferons than by interferon-γ.[24] In T lymphocytes, interferon-α appears to suppress HIV replication by interfering with the assembly and release of progeny virus.[23,25] In contrast, nucleoside analogs, such as zidovudine, act early in the HIV life cycle by inhibiting reverse transcriptase.

The first therapeutic trials of interferon-α in HIV disease focused on the treatment of Kaposi's sarcoma. In these studies, interferon-α in doses of approximately 30 to 35 million units/day showed significant antitumor effect, with response rates of 20% to 67%.[26–31] An important finding of these studies was the strong correlation between clinical response and the level of immune competence, as measured by CD4 percentage or absolute CD4 T-cell number. For example, in one study, 5 of 5 patients with CD4 counts greater than 400 cells/mm^3 exhibited a partial or complete response of their Kaposi's sarcoma lesions, but none of 7 patients with CD4 counts less than 150 cells/mm^3 responded.[27] These results suggest that, rather than having a direct antiproliferative or antiviral effect, interferon-α is acting as a biologic response modifier to mediate its antitumor effect.

Based on these studies, interferon-α was licensed as therapy for patients with HIV-associated Kaposi's sarcoma. Although the package insert describes doses in the range of 35 million units/day, few patients can tolerate this dose because of flu-like symptoms, neutropenia, and elevations of hepatic transaminases. Most clinicians start with lower doses (1 to 5 million units) and escalate as tolerated on schedules ranging from daily to 3 times each week.

Besides the antitumor effect, these studies provided evidence that interferon-α also had an antiretroviral effect. Like the antitumor effect, this anti-HIV effect was strongly correlated with the level of immune competence, again suggesting that interferon-α was acting to enhance the immune response rather than having direct antiviral activity.

To better assess the antiretroviral activity of interferon-α, a randomized, placebo-controlled trial enrolling asymptomatic HIV-infected individuals with CD4 counts greater than 400 cells/mm^3 and positive cultures for HIV was carried out.[32] Of the 17 patients randomized to interferon-α treatment, 7 (41%) developed persistently negative cultures for HIV, and only 2 of 17 patients randomized to placebo became culture negative. During the treatment period, CD4 percentages remained stable or increased in patients receiving interferon-α and declined slightly in patients receiving placebo. Toxicity associated with interferon-α treatment was substantial, as indicated by the fact that 35% of patients randomized to interferon-α withdrew from the study because of toxic effects. The most prominent toxicities were flu-like symptoms, neutropenia, and elevations of hepatic transaminases.[32] The results of this trial suggest that, although it is associated with considerable toxicity, interferon-α may exhibit some antiretroviral activity in patients with more than 400 CD4 cells/mm^3.

Interferon-α and zidovudine inhibit HIV replication by different mechanisms, and the combination of zidovudine and interferon-α can act synergistically to inhibit HIV replication in vitro.[33] These considerations, combined with the limited ability of interferon-α to control HIV replication in vivo, led to several phase I/II trials of combination therapy with interferon-α and zidovudine.[34–37] These trials demonstrated that concurrent therapy with interferon-α and zidovudine is associated with a high frequency of certain toxicities (eg, neutropenia, thrombocytopenia, transaminase elevations) that are dose limiting. The maximum tolerated dose of interferon-α in these studies were between 4 and 10 million units/day, depending on the zidovudine dose. At these doses of interferon-α, the antitumor effect seen with combination therapy was equivalent to that observed with higher-dose interferon-α monotherapy. The combination of zidovudine and interferon-α also appeared to have significant anti-HIV activity in patients with higher CD4 counts, but it is not clear whether this effect is superior to that of zidovudine alone.[38]

Interferon-α is an important cytokine being evaluated for the therapy of HIV infection. Its well-documented efficacy in the treatment of HIV-associated Kaposi's sarcoma has made it approved therapy for this condition. The antitumor and antiviral effects of interferon-α critically depend on the level of immune competence, and treatment with this agent is unlikely to be effective in HIV-infected individuals with CD4 counts less than 150 cells/mm^3. Interferon-α can be used in combination with zidovudine, but significant toxicity, especially neutropenia, can result. Trials are underway comparing the long-term efficacy of interferon-α monotherapy, zidovudine monotherapy, and combination zidovudine plus interferon-α in the treatment of HIV-infected patients with CD4 counts greater than 500 cells/mm^3.

Interferon-β and Interferon-γ

Interferon-β is similar to interferon-α in its immunomodulatory effect and in vitro activity against HIV.[39] Results of a single trial in patients with HIV-associated Kaposi's sarcoma suggest that the antiretroviral and anti–Kaposi's sarcoma effect of interferon-β are similar or slightly less than that of interferon-α.[40]

The in vitro activity of interferon-γ against HIV is variable and depends on the tissue culture system that is used. Administration of interferon-γ to patients with HIV-associated Kaposi's sarcoma has shown no apparent clinical benefit.[41] Interferon-γ is a potent macrophage activator and may have a role as adjunctive therapy in the treatment of certain opportunistic infections.

Interleukins

Interleukin-2

Interleukin-2 (IL-2) is a glycoprotein produced by activated T lymphocytes that enhances the proliferation and differentiation of NK cells, T lymphocytes, and B lymphocytes. The rational for the use of IL-2 in the treatment of HIV infection comes from in vitro observations that IL-2 can enhance proliferation of peripheral blood T cells from HIV-infected individuals.[42-45] NK activity, which is depressed by HIV infection, can be restored by the incubation of peripheral blood mononuclear cells with IL-2.[46] These in vitro studies suggested that it might be possible to restore some degree of immune competence in vivo by treatment of HIV-infected patients with IL-2.

Early trials of IL-2 therapy in AIDS and AIDS-related complex patients met with little success.[47-49] Because of marked variations in the doses, length of treatment, and route of administration, it is difficult to compare the results of these trials. Nevertheless, no clinical benefits could be shown in these studies, and only transient changes in lymphocyte counts were observed.

The minimal immunologic changes seen with IL-2 monotherapy, along with concerns that IL-2–induced T-lymphocyte activation could lead to increased HIV replication and dissemination, prompted to several trials of IL-2 combined with zidovudine (Table 24-1). Continuous intravenous infusion of IL-2 at doses between 1.5 to 12×10^6 IU/m^2/day resulted in transient changes in CD4 counts and NK activity in patients with CD4 counts of 400/mm^3 or greater.[50] In a follow-up study,[51] 19 HIV-infected patients were treated with zidovudine combined with polyethylene glycol–conjugated IL-2 (PEG-IL-2). PEG-IL-2 has a prolonged half-life and was administered intravenously once each week. Acute dose-related increases in CD4 counts, HIV-specific cytotoxicity, and NK activity was seen. No increases in p24 antigenemia or HIV DNA (as detected by polymerase chain reaction) were seen.[51] The maximum tolerated dose of IL-2 in this study was 3×10^6 IU/m^2, with adverse reactions of hypotension, neutropenia, and neurotoxicity. Similar results

were obtained when IL-2 (0.2 to 2×10^6 IU/ m^2/day) or PEG -IL-2 (up to 1×10^6 IU/week) was administered by subcutaneous injection.[52,53] Administration of zidovudine combined with low doses of PEG-IL-2 (36,000 IU/week) given by subcutaneous injection to patients with CD4 counts greater than 100/mm^3 resulted in insignificant changes in CD4 counts and quantitative HIV cultures. Small but statistically significant increases in NK activity were detected.[54,55] Taken together, these studies indicate that administration of IL-2 combined with zidovudine results in transient immunologic changes and is associated with significant, dose-limiting toxicities.

Sustained rises in CD4 counts have been reported in HIV-infected patients treated with antiretrovirals combined with intermittent IL-2 therapy.[56] IL-2 was given at doses of 12 to 18 million units/day for 5 days every 8 weeks. In 6 of 10 patients with baseline CD4 counts higher than 200 cells/μL, intermittent IL-2 therapy was associated with at least a 50% increase in the number of CD4 cells. A decline in the percentage of CD8 cells that expressed HLA-DR was also seen. Four patients had transient but consistent rises in plasma HIV RNA at the end of each IL-2 infusion. In patients with baseline CD4 counts of less than 200 cells/μL, IL-2 therapy was associated with increased viral activation, few immunologic improvements, and substantial toxicity. The results of this study suggest that intermittent courses of IL-2 can improve some immunologic abnormalities associated with HIV infection in patients with CD4 counts higher than 200 cells/μL. The immunologic and clinical significance of these sustained increases in CD4 counts is unknown. Larger, controlled trials are underway to evaluate the role of intermittent IL-2 therapy in HIV infection.

TABLE 24-1. *Summary of interleukin-2 plus antiviral trials*

Study	Number of Patients	CD4 Count	Dose (IU)	Immunologic Effects	Effect on Viral Load
Schwartz[50]	10	>400	IV; 1.5–12 × 10^6/M^2 5 d/wk for 3 wk	Increase in CD4 count, increase in NK function	No increase in p24
Wood[51]	19	>400 200–400 <200	IV; PEG 1–5 × 10^6 weekly × 25 wk	Acute increase in CD4 count, increase in NK function	No increase in p24 or HIV by DNA PCR
McMahon[52]	16	AIDS/ARC	SC; 0.2–2.0 × 10^6 daily × 5 d	Increase in CD4 count, increase in NK function	No increase in p24
Waites[53]	25 25	>200 <200	SC; PEG 0.05–1 × 10^6 2 of 4 wk × 28 wk	Transient increase in CD4 count only in >200 group	No increase in p24
Teppler[54,55]	16	>100	ID; PEG 3.6 × 10^4/wk × 4 mo	Increased NK function, increased DTH recall	No increase in quantitative viral cultures
Kovacs[56]	25	>200 <200	IV; 6–18 × 10^6/d for 5 d every 8 wk	Sustained increases in CD4 counts only in >200 group	Transient increases in bDNA in >200; sustained increases in bDNA in <200

IV, intravenous; ID, intradermal; SC, subcutaneous; PEG, polyethylene glycol conjugated; interleukin-2; 400 IU = 1 μg of IL-2; 70 kg human = 1.8 M^2

Interleukin-12

Although IL-12 came late in the chronology of discovery, it is one of the earliest acting cytokines in the immune response to infection.[57] Macrophages begin to produce IL-12 shortly after they encounter pathogens. IL-12 then activates NK cells and T cells, resulting in enhancement of cytotoxic activity and interferon-γ production by both cell types. IL-12 also pushes uncommitted T cells to differentiate into T_{H1} cells, which produce interferon-γ and other cytokines associated with cell-mediated immunity. IL-4 is another cytokine that is important in shaping the immune response. Early in the immune response, IL-4 production, by yet unidentified cells, pushes uncommitted T cells to become T_{H2} effector cells that secrete cytokines associated with humoral immunity (ie, IL-4, IL-5, and IL-10).

Some in vitro studies have suggested that there is a progressive imbalance in the T-cell response to antigen in HIV-infected individuals, with a selective defect in T_{H1} type responses and predominance of T_{H2} responses.[45] Based on these studies, it has been proposed that a switch from a T_{H1} to a T_{H2} cytokine phenotype occurs early in the course of HIV infection and is a critical step in the progression of HIV disease.[58] However, later studies failed to find evidence for a T_{H1} to T_{H2} switch during the progression of HIV infection.[59,60] Although it is clear that defects in T_{H1}-type responses are present in HIV infection, it is not clear whether these defects results from a quantitative deficiency in T_{H1} cells that results from HIV-induced CD4 cell depletion or a qualitative switch from a T_{H1} to a T_{H2} response that then leads to accelerated CD4 cell loss and immunodeficiency.

Regardless of whether there is T_{H1} to T_{H2} shift in HIV infection, several in vitro observations suggest that IL-12 may have a role in the treatment of HIV infection. Peripheral blood mononuclear cells from HIV-infected patients produce 5-fold to 10-fold less IL-12 than normal controls, and addition of IL-12 to cell cultures from HIV-infected patients restores defective NK function.[61,62] IL-12 has also been reported to increase proliferation and interferon-γ production by peripheral blood mononuclear cells from HIV-infected patients.[63]

In animal models, exogenous IL-12 administration can have beneficial and detrimental effects on the outcome of infectious diseases. When administered at the initiation of infection, IL-12 in doses greater than or equal to 100 ng/day has been shown to limit infection and improve survival in certain strains of mice infected with intracellular parasites and bacteria.[64–66] This beneficial effect is related to the ability of the exogenously administered IL-12 to induce a protective T_{H1} response in mice genetically predisposed to mount a T_{H2} response to infection with intracellular pathogens. No beneficial effect is seen when IL-12 is administered later in the course of experimental infection, suggesting exogenous IL-12 administration cannot reverse an established T_{H2} response.

In mice infected with lymphocytic choriomeningitis virus, administration of IL-12 at doses greater than or equal to 100 ng/day results in a profound inhibition of virus-specific cytotoxic T-lymphocyte responses and increases viral replication.[67] These detrimental effects of IL-12 depended on endogenous tumor necrosis factor (TNF) production.[68] The results of these animal studies emphasize that administration of IL-12 may be beneficial or detrimental, depending on the type of infection and the particular endogenous immune responses. What role IL-12 may have in the treatment of HIV infection remains to be defined.

Tumor Necrosis Factor-α

Tumor necrosis factor-α (TNF-α) is a cytokine produced by many different cell types and plays an important role in host defense against a variety of pathogens.[69] Infection with HIV is associated with increased production of TNF-α. In tissue culture, B lymphocytes from HIV-infected patients spontaneously secrete high levels of TNF-α, and patients with advanced HIV disease frequently have increased serum levels of this cytokine.[70–72] It has been hypothesized that high TNF-α production may contribute to the wasting syndrome seen in some HIV-infected patients. TNF-α can also increase HIV expression in chronically infected T-lymphocyte and macrophage cell lines.[73] The overproduction of TNF-α in the HIV-infected patient may contribute to cachexia and wasting and may increase HIV replication and dissemination.

These observations raise the possibility that selectively blocking TNF-α production or action may reduce HIV replication in vivo and have a beneficial effect on the course of HIV disease. Thalidomide selectively inhibits TNF-α production in vitro and has been shown to reduce serum TNF-α levels in leprosy patients with erythema nodosum leprosum.[74] Pentoxifylline is a methylxanthene derivative used to treat peripheral vascular disease. In vitro, pentoxifylline can inhibit TNF-α production and decrease HIV replication.[75] Although clinical trials with pentoxifylline in HIV-infected patients are ongoing, it is unlikely that oral administration can produce levels of pentoxifylline that are sufficient to inhibit TNF-α production in vivo. Anti–TNF-α monoclonal antibody and recombinant soluble TNF-α receptor have been shown to inhibit TNF-α–induced HIV replication in vitro,[73,76] and phase I clinical trials with both agents have been conducted. When considering anti–TNF-α therapy, it must be emphasized that TNF-α plays an important role in host defense. Blocking TNF-α production or action may increase the HIV-infected patient's susceptibility to certain fungal, bacterial, and mycobacterial infections.

IMMUNOSUPPRESSIVE THERAPY

HIV infection is associated with a chronic state of immune activation. This chronic state of immune activation is manifested by polyclonal B-cell activation with hypergammaglobulinemia, increased production of certain cytokines (eg, TNF-α), increased expression of activation markers on peripheral blood T lymphocytes, increased circulating levels of β₂-microglobulin, reactive lymphoid hyperplasia, and autoimmune phenomenon. This chronic state of immune activation is seen throughout the course of HIV infection and is most likely a response to the persistence of virus and ongoing viral replication. Although activation of various components of the immune system is critical to generating a protective immune response, the chronic state of immune activation seen with HIV infection my have a detrimental effect on the course of disease. Abundant in vitro evidence indicates that HIV replication is more efficient in activated cells than in resting cells, and cell activation induces replication of HIV in latently infected cells.[77,78] The chronic state of immune activation may serve to enhance HIV replication and dissemination.

Besides the effects on viral replication, this chronic state of immune activation may be deleterious to the immune system itself by inducing programmed cell death (ie, apoptosis) of T cells. Apoptosis is an active form of cell death that requires protein and RNA synthesis and is characterized by the induction of endogenous endonucleases that cleave chromatin into nucleosomal fragments.[79] The hypothesis that HIV-induced apoptosis may contribute to CD4 cell depletion is based on several in vitro observations. It has been shown that CD4 T cells from asymptomatic HIV-infected individuals die by apoptosis when stimulated in vitro with mitogens or antigens.[80] Cell death was seen only in the CD4 population and could be prevented by pretreatment of the cells with cyclosporin A or antibody to CD28.[80] Additional studies have shown that crosslinking of CD4-bound gp120 (with anti-gp120 antibodies) on human T cells, followed by T-cell-receptor–mediated activation results in cell death by apoptosis.[81] Taken together, these results led to the hypothesis that the chronic state of immune activation, the gp120-mediated crosslinking of CD4, or both actions prime CD4 T cells from HIV-infected individuals to undergo apoptosis when activated through their antigen receptor.[82] This mechanism of CD4 cell depletion would not require that the cell be infected with HIV, because uninfected CD4 T cells that had bound circulating or cell-associated gp120 would undergo apoptosis on activation by microbial antigens or superantigens.

These considerations raise the possibility that selectively blocking immune activation in a HIV-infected individual may have beneficial effects on the progression of disease. Cyclosporin A is a potent immunosuppressive agent that inhibits T-cell functions by disrupting formation of a transcriptional activating factor (ie, NF-AT) that is required for normal T-cell activation.[83] Mixed results have been obtained when cyclosporin A was administered to HIV-infected patients in an attempt to downregulate the harmful effects of chronic immune activation. One study showed an apparent short-term benefit from cyclosporin A therapy,[84] and a second study showed clinical and immunologic deterioration.[85] It

was later shown that the cyclosporin A binding protein, cyclophilin A, binds the HIV-1 Gag protein and that this interaction is necessary for the formation of infectious HIV virions.[86,87] In vitro, cyclosporin A can inhibit the interaction between cyclophilin A and Gag and reduce virion infectivity.[86] Cyclosporin A can reduce HIV production by a mechanism independent of its immunosuppressive effect. Nonimmunosuppressive analogs of cyclosporin A that inhibit the cyclophilin A–Gag interaction have been developed and may prove useful in the treatment of HIV infection.

Glucocorticosteroids have a wide range of antiinflamatory and immunoregulatory properties and have been investigated as agents that could downregulate the immune system in HIV infection. In a recent uncontrolled study, 44 HIV-infected patients were treated with 0.3 to 0.5 mg/kg of prednisone for 1 year.[88] Prednisone treatment was associated with a significant decrease in serum immunoglobulins, β₂-microglobulin, and the percentage of CD4 cells expressing activation markers. Serum levels of HIV RNA remained stable after 1 year of prednisone, and CD4 counts increased by median of 119 cells/μL.[88]

It is not clear what role immunosuppressive therapy has in the treatment of HIV disease. This approach may be useful early in the course of HIV infection, before the development of significant immunodeficiency. However, immunosuppressive therapy also has the potential to adversely affect the immune response to HIV and accelerate the progression of immunologic deterioration.

ADOPTIVE IMMUNOTHERAPY

Attempts at Immunologic Reconstruction

Another approach to restoring immune competence in HIV-infected individuals involves the use of adoptive transfer of peripheral blood lymphocytes and bone marrow. Immunologic reconstitution by bone marrow transplantation has been shown to correct the immunologic defects in various forms of primary immunodeficiency, most notably severe combined immune deficiency.[89] Early attempts at achieving immunologic reconstitution in patients with AIDS using allogeneic bone marrow transplantation were unsuccessful, with patients usually dying from complications of the conditioning regimens.

After the development of zidovudine as antiretroviral therapy for HIV, work began on syngeneic bone marrow transplantation (ie, using identical twin pairs) in combination with zidovudine therapy as a means of achieving immunologic reconstitution. In the largest of these studies, a total of 16 HIV-infected patients were studied.[90] Patients were stratified according to CD4 counts and treated with zidovudine for 12 weeks combined with infusions of peripheral blood lymphocytes (at week 10) and bone marrow (week 12) from their HIV-negative, identical twin brothers. After transplantation, the patients were randomized to treatment with zidovudine or placebo. After bone marrow transplantation and adoptive transfer of lymphocytes, a small increase in the CD4 count was observed in most cases. The transfer of functional immunity was documented in that 8 of 9 patients had no skin test reactivity to keyhole-limpet hemocyanin before transplantation but developed delayed-type hypersensitivity reactions to this antigen after transplantation.[90] These immunologic changes were not associated with any significant clinical improvement and were transient, with CD4 counts declining to baseline after several months and keyhole-limpet hemocyanin skin test reactivity eventually disappearing.[90] Compared with the placebo group, there were no differences in the rate of decline in CD4 counts or keyhole-limpet hemocyanin immunity in patients randomized to receive zidovudine after transplantation.

Based on the results of this trial and the availability of candidate HIV vaccines, we initiated a trial of syngeneic bone marrow transplantation and adoptive lymphocyte transfer using HIV-negative, identical twin donors who were immunized with a recombinant gp160 vaccine. In this study, the HIV-infected patients were treated with an aggressive antiviral regimen consisting of zidovudine, interferon-γ, and a soluble recombinant CD4-Ig molecule. The uninfected twin donors were immunized with gp160, and lymphocytes were transferred at weeks 10 and 12, with bone marrow transplantation at week 12. In these studies, the increases in CD4 counts were transient, as in previous trials. Work continues in this area, most recently employing the in vitro expansion and activation of donor lymphocytes using anti-CD3 and IL-2.

Adoptive Transfer of CD8 Cells

Infection with HIV induces a cellular immune response that includes CD8, major histocompatibility complex (MHC)–restricted cytotoxic T lymphocytes (CTLs), and CD16+ cells, which mediate antibody-dependent cytotoxicity.[91] MHC class I–restricted CTLs are detectable at a high frequency in the peripheral blood of infected individuals and can inhibit viral replication in vitro.[92–94] During the acute phase of HIV infection, a vigorous polyclonal CD8 CTL response is seen.[95,96] The appearance of these HIV-specific CTLs is temporally correlated with a dramatic fall in plasma viremia.[96] In contrast to other persistent viral infections, such as Epstein-Barr virus and cytomegalovirus infections, the CTL response to HIV is only able to transiently control the infection. During the course of infection, there is a gradual loss of HIV-specific CTL activity that correlates with disease progression and the development of immunodeficiency.[91,97] However, individuals who are able maintain a HIV-specific CTL response may experience a more prolonged asymptomatic period and a more gradual loss of CD4 cells.[98] These observations suggest that HIV-specific CTLs play an important role in the immune response to HIV, but they are ultimately ineffective in preventing the spread of infection and eventual progression to AIDS.

It is unclear why the CTL response to HIV is unable to control the infection. Although the initial immune response to HIV infection can clear virus from the peripheral blood, studies indicate that a substantial viral burden persists in the peripheral lymphoid tissue.[99] It may be that the CTL response is not of sufficient magnitude to control a large HIV burden at this anatomic site. Another likely possibility is that the rapid rate of viral replication and error-prone nature of the reverse transcription process results in the generation of mutant virus that is continuously able to escape the CTL response. This process may continue until the immune system is so compromised that it is unable to generate a response to new viral mutants. Support for this hypothesis comes from the identification of variants of HIV that have mutated to escape a defined CTL response in HIV-infected patients.[100] If either of these hypotheses is correct, attempts to quantitatively and qualitatively improve the effector response through adoptive immunotherapy with in vitro expanded CTLs may be beneficial in treatment of HIV infection.

The principles and efficacy of adoptive transfer of in vitro expanded lymphocytes in the treatment of viral infections have been established in animal models.[101–103] Investigations of the adoptive transfer of in vitro expanded lymphocytes in the treatment human diseases have shown that this approach is technically feasible, and in vivo biologic effects of the transferred cells have been documented.[104–106]

In theory, it should be possible to augment the antiviral response in HIV-infected individuals with adoptive immunotherapy. Small phase I trials using in vitro expansion and adoptive transfer of uncloned populations of CD8 lymphocytes from HIV-infected individuals have been performed.[107–109] These studies show that CD8 lymphocytes can be purified from the peripheral blood of HIV-infected individuals, expanded in vitro to obtain large numbers of cells with enhanced anti-HIV activity, and safely infused into patients. However, the natural progression of HIV infection despite the development of virus-specific CTLs, perhaps because of the generation of CTL escape mutants, suggests that significant obstacles will be encountered in applying this form of adoptive immunotherapy to HIV infection.

In recognition of the general failure of the native immune system to maintain long-term effective host defense against HIV infection, several groups have developed strategies that involve genetic modification of CTLs to enhance their anti-HIV activity. In one approach, CTLs that can recognize antigen without the need for cognate recognition of the target cell have been created by transducing peripheral blood CD8 T lymphocytes with chimeric receptors containing immunoglobulin-like antigen-binding domains linked to the ζ-chain of the CD3 complex.[110] Another approach involves the introduction into CD8 T lymphocytes of hybrid genes that promote autocrine growth after stimulation through the T-cell receptor.[111] These strategies could potentially increase the efficacy and survival of adoptively transferred CD8 cells.

CONCLUSIONS

With a better understanding of the immunopathogenesis of HIV infection, our approaches to immunotherapy for this disease have evolved. Initial attempts using immune-based treatments have had mixed results. Although definite biologic effects have been seen, clinical benefits have been modest. Efforts are focused on restoring immune competence and improving the immune response to HIV through the use of cytokines, cytokine antagonists, and adoptive immunotherapy.

REFERENCES

1. Katzenstein DA, Vujcic LK, Latif A, et al. Human immunodeficiency virus neutralizing antibodies in sera from North Americans and Africans. J Acquir Immune Defic Syndr 1990;3:810.
2. Robert GM, Brown M, Gallo RC. HTLV-III-neutralizing antibodies in patients with AIDS and AIDS-related complex. Nature 1985;316:72.
3. Weber JN, Clapham PR, Weiss RA, et al. Human immunodeficiency virus infection in two cohorts of homosexual men: neutralising sera and association of anti-gag antibody with prognosis. Lancet 1987;1:119.
4. Arendrup M, Sonnerborg A, Svennerholm B, et al. Neutralizing antibody response during human immunodeficiency virus type 1 infection: type and group specificity and viral escape. J Gen Virol 1993;74:855.
5. European Collaborative Study. Children born to women with HIV-1 infection: natural history and risk of transmission. Lancet 1991;337:253.
6. Jacobson JM, Colman N, Ostrow NA, et al. Passive immunotherapy in the treatment of advanced human immunodeficiency virus infection. J Infect Dis 1993;168:298.
7. Vittecoq D, Chevret S, Morand JL, et al. Passive immunotherapy in AIDS: a double-blind randomized study based on transfusions of plasma rich in anti-human immunodeficiency virus 1 antibodies vs. transfusions of seronegative plasma. Proc Natl Acad Sci U S A 1995;92:1195.
8. Levy J, Youvan T, Lee ML. Passive hyperimmune plasma therapy in the treatment of acquired immunodeficiency syndrome: results of a 12-month multicenter double-blind controlled trial. The Passive Hyperimmune Therapy Study Group. Blood 1994;84:2130.
9. Javaherian K, Langlois AJ, McDanal C, et al. Principal neutralizing domain of the human immunodeficiency virus type 1 envelope protein. Proc Natl Acad Sci U S A 1989;86:6768.
10. Thali M, Olshevsky U, Furman C, et al. Characterization of a discontinuous human immunodeficiency virus type 1 gp120 epitope recognized by a broadly reactive neutralizing human monoclonal antibody. J Virol 1991;65:6188.
11. Lasky LA, Nakamura G, Smith DH, et al. Delineation of a region of the human immunodeficiency virus type 1 gp120 glycoprotein critical for interaction with the CD4 receptor. Cell 1987;50:975.
12. Burton DR, Pyati J, Koduri R, et al. Efficient neutralization of primary isolates of HIV-1 by a recombinant human monoclonal antibody. Science 1994;266:1024.
13. Ohno T, Terada M, Yoneda Y, et al. A broadly neutralizing monoclonal antibody that recognizes the V3 region of human immunodeficiency virus type 1 glycoprotein gp120. Proc Natl Acad Sci U S A 1991;88:10726.
14. Javaherian K, Langlois AJ, LaRosa GJ, et al. Broadly neutralizing antibodies elicited by the hypervariable neutralizing determinant of HIV-1. Science 1990;250:1590.
15. Hague RA, Yap PL, Mok JY, et al. Intravenous immunoglobulin in HIV infection: evidence for the efficacy of treatment. Arch Dis Child 1989;64:1146.
16. Wood CC, McNamara JG, Schwarz DF, et al. Prevention of pneumococcal bacteremia in a child with acquired immunodeficiency syndrome-related complex. Pediatr Infect Dis J 1987;6:564.
17. Calvelli TA, Rubinstein A. Intravenous gamma-globulin in infant acquired immunodeficiency syndrome. Pediatr Infect Dis 1986;5:s207.
18. The National Institute of Child Health and Human Developments Intravenous Immunoglobulin Study Group. Intravenous immune globulin for the prevention of bacterial infections in children with symptomatic human immunodeficiency virus infection. N Engl J Med 1991;325:73.
19. Spector SA, Gelber RD, McGrath N, et al. A controlled trial of intravenous immune globulin for the prevention of serious bacterial infections in children receiving zidovudine for advanced human immunodeficiency virus infection. Pediatric AIDS Clinical Trials Group. N Engl J Med 1994;331:1181.
20. De Simone C, Antonaci S, Chirigos M, et al. Report of the symposium on the use of intravenous gammaglobulin in adults infected with the human immunodeficiency virus. J Clin Lab Anal 1990;4:313.
21. Baron S, Tyring SK, Fleischmann WJ, et al. The interferons. Mechanisms of action and clinical applications. JAMA 1991;266:1375.
22. Pitha PM, Wivel NA, Fernie BF, et al. Effect of interferon and murine leukaemia virus infection. IV. Foramtion of non-infectious virus in chronically infected cells. J Gen Virol 1979;42:467.
23. Ho DD, Hartshorn KL, Rota TR, et al. Recombinant human interferon alfa-A suppresses HTLV-III replication in vitro. Lancet 1985;1:602.
24. Poli G, Orenstein JM, Kinter A, et al. Interferon-alpha but not AZT suppresses HIV expression in chronically infected cell lines. Science 1989;244:575.
25. Francis ML, Meltzer MS, Gendelman HE. Interferons in the persistence, pathogenesis, and treatment of HIV infection. AIDS Res Hum Retroviruses 1992;8:199.
26. deWit R, Schattenkerk JK, Boucher CA, et al. Clinical and virological effects of high-dose recombinant interferon-alpha in disseminated AIDS-related Kaposi's sarcoma. Lancet 1988;2:1218.
27. Lane HC, Kovacs JA, Feinberg J, et al. Anti-retroviral effects of interferon-alpha in AIDS-associated Kaposi's sarcoma. Lancet 1988;2:1218.
28. Volberding PA, Mitsuyasu R. Recombinant interferon-alpha in the treatment of acquired immune deficiency syndrome related KS. Semin Oncol 1985;12:2.
29. Gelmann EP, Preble OT, Steis R, et al. Human lymphoblastoid interferon treatment of Kaposi's sarcoma in the acquired immune deficiency syndrome. Clinical response and prognostic parameters. Am J Med 1985;78:737.
30. Groopman JE, Gottlieb MS, Goodman J, et al. Recombinant alpha-2 interferon therapy for Kaposi's sarcoma associated with the acquired immunodeficiency syndrome. Ann Intern Med 1984;100:671.
31. Real FX, Oettgen HF, Krown SE. Kaposi's sarcoma and the acquired immunodeficiency syndrome: treatment with high and low doses of recombinant leukocyte A interferon. J Clin Oncol 1986;4:544.
32. Lane HC, Davey V, Kovacs JA, et al. Interferon-alpha in patients with asymptomatic human immunodeficiency virus (HIV) infection. A randomized, placebo-controlled trial. Ann Intern Med 1990;112:805.
33. Jonhson VA, Barlow MA, Merrill DP, et al. Three-drug syngergistic inhibition of HIV-1 replication in vitro by zidovudine, recombinant soluble CD4, and recombinant interferon-gamma. J Infect Dis 1990;161:1059.
34. Kovacs JA, Deyton L, Davey R, et al. Combined zidovudine and interferon-gamma therapy in patients with Kaposi's sarcoma and the acquired immunodeficiency syndrome (AIDS). Ann Intern Med 1989;111:280.
35. Edlin BR, Weinstein RA, Whaling SM, et al. Zidovudine-interferon-alpha combination therapy in patients with advanced human immunodeficiency virus type 1 infection: biphasic response of p24 antigen and quantitative polymerase chain reaction. J Infect Dis 1992;165:793.
36. Fischl MA, Uttamchandani RB, Resnick L, et al. A phase I study of recombinant human interferon-alpha 2a or human lymphoblastoid interferon-alpha n1 and concomitant zidovudine in patients with AIDS-related Kaposi's sarcoma. J Acquir Immune Defic Syndr 1991;4:1.
37. Krown SE, Gold JW, Niedzwiecki D, et al. Interferon-alpha with zidovudine: safety, tolerance, and clinical and virologic effects in patients with Kaposi sarcoma associated with the acquired immunodeficiency syndrome (AIDS). Ann Intern Med 1990;112:812.
38. Berglund O, Engman K, Ehrnst A, et al. Combined treatment of symptomatic human immunodeficiency virus type 1 infection with native interferon-alpha and zidovudine. J Infect Dis 1991;163:710.
39. Hartshorn K, Neumeyer D, Vogt M, et al. Activity of interferons alpha, beta, and gamma against human immunodeficiency virus replication in vitro. AIDS Res Hum Retroviruses 1987;112:582.

40. Miles SA, Wang HJ, Cortes E, et al. Beta-interferon therapy in patients with poor-prognosis Kaposi sarcoma related to the acquired immunodeficiency syndrome (AIDS). A phase II trial with preliminary evidence of antiviral activity and low incidence of opportunistic infection. Ann Intern Med 1990;112:582.

41. Lane HC, Davey RT, Sherwin SA, et al. Phase I trial of recombinant interferon-gamma in patients with Kaposi's sarcoma and the acquired immunodeficiency syndrome (AIDS). J Clin Immunol 1989;9:351.

42. Murray HW, Welte K, Jacobs JL, et al. Production of and in vitro response to interleukin 2 in the acquired immunodeficiency syndrome. J Clin Invest 1985;76:1959.

43. Ciobanu N, Kruger G, Welte K. Defective T cell response to PHA and mitogenic monoclonal antibodies in male homosexuals with acquired immunodeficiency syndrome and its in vitro correction by interleukin-2. J Clin Immunol 1983;3:332.

44. Gupta S. Study of activated T cells in man: interleukin-2 receptor and transferrin receptor expression on T cells and production of interleukin-2 in patients with acquired immune deficiency syndrome. Clin Immunol Immunopathol 1986;38:93.

45. Clerici M, Hakim FT, Venzon DJ, et al. Changes in interleukin-2 and interleukin-4 production in asymptomatic, human immunodeficiency virus-seropositive individuals. J Clin Invest 1993;91:759.

46. Rook AH, Hooks JJ, Quinnan GV, et al. Interleukin-2 enhances the natural killer cell activity of acquired immunodeficiency syndrome patients through a gamma-interferon-independent mechanism. J. Immunol. 1985;134:1503.

47. Ernst M, Kern P, Flad HD, et al. Effects of systemic in vivo interleukin-2 (IL-2) reconstitution in patients with acquired immune deficiency syndrome (AIDS) and AIDS-related complex (ARC) on phenotypes and functions of peripheral blood mononuclear cells (PBMC). J Clin Immunol 1986;6:170.

48. Kern P, Toy J, Dietrich M. Preliminary clinical observations with recombinant interleukin-2 in patients with AIDS or LAS. Blut 1985;50:1.

49. Lane HC, Siegel JP, Rook AH, et al. Use of interleukin-2 in patients with acquired immunodeficiency syndrome. J Biol Response Modif 1984;3:512.

50. Schwartz DH, Skowron G, Merigan TC. Safety and effects of interleukin-2 plus zidovudine in asymptomatic individuals infected with human immunodeficiency virus. J Acquir Immune Defic Syndr 1991;4:11.

51. Wood R, Montoya JG, Kundu SK, et al. Safety and efficacy of polyethylene glycol-modified interleukin-2 and zidovudine in human immunodeficiency virus type 1 infection: a phase I/II study. J Infect Dis 1993;167:519.

52. McMahon DK, Armstrong JA, Huang XL, et al. A phase I study of subcutaneous recombinant interleukin-2 in patients with advanced HIV disease while on zidovudine. AIDS 1994;8:59.

53. Waites L, Fyfe G, Senechek D, et al. Polyethylene glycol modified interleukin-2 (PEG IL-2) therapy in HIV seropositive individuals. Abstract PuB 7580. Program and abstracts of the Eighth International Conference on AIDS (Amsterdam). Amsterdam: Congrex, Holland BV, 1992.

54. Teppler H, Kaplan G, Smith K, et al. Efficacy of low doses of the polyethylene glycol derivative of interleukin-2 in modulating the immune response of patients with human immunodeficiency virus type 1 infection. J Infect Dis 1993;167:291.

55. Teppler H, Kaplan G, Smith KA, et al. Prolonged immunostimulatory effect of low-dose polyethylene glycol interleukin 2 in patients with human immunodeficiency virus type 1 infection. J Exp Med 1993;177:483.

56. Kovacs JA, Baseler M, Dewar RJ, et al. Increases in CD4 T lymphocytes with intermittent courses of interleukin-2 in patients with human immunodeficiency virus infection. A preliminary study. N Engl J Med 1995;332:567.

57. Paul W, Seder R. Lymphocyte responses and cytokines. Cell 1994;76:241.

58. Clerici M, Shearer G. A T_{H1}-T_{H2} switch is a critical step in the etiology of HIV infection. Imunol Today 1993;14:107.

59. Maggi E, Mazzetti M, Ravina A, et al. Ability of HIV to promote a T_{H1} to T_{H0} shift and to replicate preferentially in T_{H2} and T_{H0} cells. Science 1994;265:244.

60. Graziosi C, Pantaleo G, Gantt KR, et al. Lack of evidence for the dichotomy of T_{H1} and T_{H2} predominance in HIV-infected individuals. Science 1994;265:248.

61. Chehimi J, Starr SE, Frank I, et al. Impaired interleukin 12 production in human immunodeficiency virus-infected patients. J Exp Med 1994;179:1361.

62. Chehimi J, Starr SE, Frank I, et al. Natural killer (NK) cell stimulatory factor increases the cytotoxic activity of NK cells from both healthy donors and human immunodeficiency virus-infected patients. J Exp Med 1992;175:789.

63. Clerici M, Lucey DR, Berzofsky JA, et al. Restoration of HIV-specific cell-mediated immune responses by interleukin-12 in vitro. Science 1993;262:1721.

64. Gladue RP, Laquerre AM, Magna HA, et al. In vivo augmentation of IFN-gamma with a rIL-12 human/mouse chimera: pleiotropic effects against infectious agents in mice and rats. Cytokine 1994;6:318.

65. Heinzel FP, Schoenhaut DS, Rerko RM, et al. Recombinant interleukin 12 cures mice infected with Leishmania major. J Exp Med 1993;177:1505.

66. Sypek JP, Chung CL, Mayor SE, et al. Resolution of cutaneous leishmaniasis: interleukin 12 initiates a protective T helper type 1 immune response. J Exp Med 1993;177:1797.

67. Orange JS, Wolf SF, Biron CA. Effects of IL-12 on the response and susceptibility to experimental viral infections. J Immunol 1994;152:1253.

68. Orange JS, Salazar MT, Opal SM, et al. Mechanism of interleukin 12-mediated toxicities during experimental viral infections: role of tumor necrosis factor and glucocorticoids. J Exp Med 1995;181:901.

69. Beutler B, Cerami A. The biology of cachectin/TNF-a primary mediator of the host response. Annu Rev Immunol 1989;7:625.

70. Rieckmann P, Poli G, Fox CH, et al. Recombinant gp120 specifically enhances tumor necrosis factor-alpha production and Ig secretion in B lymphocytes from HIV-infected individuals but not from seronegative donors. J Immunol 1991;147:2922.

71. Rieckmann P, Poli G, Kehrl JH, et al. Activated B lymphocytes from human immunodeficiency virus-infected individuals induce virus expression in infected T cells and a promonocytic cell line, U1. J Exp Med 1991;173:1.

72. Dezube BJ, Pardee AB, Beckett LA, et al. Cytokine dysregulation in AIDS: in vivo overexpression of mRNA of tumor necrosis factor-alpha and its correlation with that of the inflammatory cytokine GRO. J Acquir Immune Defic Syndr 1992;5:1099.

73. Poli G, Kinter A, Justement J, et al. Tumor necrosis factor alpha functions in an autocrine manner in the induction of human immunodeficiency virus expression. Proc Natl Acad Sci USA 1990;87:782.

74. Sampaio EP, Moreira AL, Sarno EN, et al. Prolonged treatment with recombinant interferon gamma induces erythema nodosum leprosum in lepromatous leprosy patients. J Exp Med 1992;175:1729.

75. Fazely F, Dezube BJ, Allen RJ, et al. Pentoxifylline (Trental) decreases the replication of the human immunodeficiency virus type 1 in human peripheral blood mononuclear cells and in cultured T cells. Blood 1991;77:1653.

76. Howard OM, Clouse KA, Smith C, et al. Soluble tumor necrosis factor receptor: inhibition of human immunodeficiency virus activation. Proc Natl Acad Sci U S A 1993;90:2335.

77. Rosenberg Z, Fauci A. Induction of expression of HIV in latently or chronically infected cells. AIDS Res Hum Retroviruses 1989;5:1.

78. Zack JA, Arrigo SJ, Weitsman SR, et al. HIV-1 entry into quiescent primary lymphocytes: molecular analysis reveals a labile, latent viral structure. Cell 1990;61:213.

79. Cohen J, Duke R, Fadok V, et al. Apoptosis and programmed cell death in immunity. Ann Rev Immunol 1992;10:267.

80. Groux H, Torpier G, Monte D, et al. Activation-induced death by apoptosis in CD4+ T cells from human immunodeficiency virus-infected individuals. J Exp Med 1992;75:331.

81. Banda NK, Bernier J, Kurahara DK, et al. Crosslinking CD4 by human immunodeficiency virus gp120 primes T cells for activation-induced apoptosis. J Exp Med 1992;176:1099.

82. Ameisen JC. The programmed cell death theory of AIDS pathogenesis: implications, testable predictions, and confrontation with experimental findings. Immunodefic Rev 1992;3:237.

83. Flanagan WM, Corthesy B, Bram RJ, et al. Nuclear association of a T-cell transcription factor blocked by FK-506 and cyclosporin A. Nature 1991;352:803.

84. Andrieu J, Even P, Venet A. Effects of cyclosporin on T-cell subsets in human immunodeficiency virus disease. Clin Immunol Immunopathol 1988;46:181.

85. Phillips A, Wainberg MA, Coates R, et al. Cyclosporine-induced deterioration in patients with AIDS. Can Med Assoc J 1989;140:1456.
86. Thali M, Bukovsky A, Kondo E, et al. Functional association of cyclophilin A with HIV-1 virions. Nature 1994;372:363.
87. Franke EK, Yuan HE, Luban J. Specific incorporation of cyclophilin A into HIV-1 virions. Nature 1994;372:359.
88. Andrieu JM, Lu W, Levy R. Sustained increases in CD4 cell counts in asymptomatic human immunodeficiency virus type 1-seropositive patients treated with prednisolone for 1 year. J Infect Dis 1995;171:523.
89. Vossen J. Bone marrow transplantation in the treatment of primary immunodeficiencies. Ann Clin Res 1987;19:285.
90. Lane HC, Zunich KM, Wilson W, et al. Syngenic bone marrow transplanations and adoptive transfer of peripheral blood lymphocytes combined with zidovudine in human immunodeficiency virus (HIV) infection. Ann Intern Med 1990;113:512.
91. Fauci AS, Schnittman SM, Poli G, et al. NIH conference. Immunopathogenic mechanisms in human immunodeficiency virus (HIV) infection. Ann Intern Med 1991;114:678.
92. Tsubota H, Lord C, Watkins D, et al. A cytotoxic T lymphocyte inhibits acquired immunodeficiency syndrome virus replication in peripheral blood lymphocytes. J Exp Med 1989;169:1421.
93. Walker B, Moody J, Sites D, et al. CD8+ T lymphocyte control of HIV replication in cultured CD4+ cells varies among infected individuals. Cell Immunol 1989;119:470.
94. Hoffenbach A, Langlade-Demoyen P, Dadaglio G, et al. Unusually high frequencies of HIV-specific cytotoxic T lymphocytes in humans. J Immunol 1989;142:452.
95. Pantaleo G, Demarest JF, Soudeyns H, et al. Major expansion of CD8+ T cells with a predominant V beta usage during the primary immune response to HIV. Nature 1994;370:463.
96. Koup RA, Safrit JT, Cao Y, et al. Temporal association of cellular immune responses with the initial control of viremia in primary human immunodeficiency virus type 1 syndrome. J Virol 1994;68:4650.
97. Carmichael A, Jin X, Sissons P, et al. Quantitative analysis of the human immunodeficiency virus type 1 (HIV-1)-specific cytotoxic T lymphocyte (CTL) response at different stages of HIV-1 infection: differential CTL responses to HIV-1 and Epstein-Barr virus in late disease. J Exp Med 1993;177:249.
98. Cao Y, Qin L, Zhang L, et al. Virologic and immunologic characterization of long term survivors of human immunodeficiency virus type 1 infection. N Engl J Med 1995;332:201.
99. Pantaleo G, Graziosi C, Demarest JF, et al. HIV infection is active and progressive in lymphoid tissue during the clinically latent stage of disease. Nature 1993;362:355.
100. Couillin I, Culmann PB, Gomard E, et al. Impaired cytotoxic T lymphocyte recognition due to genetic variations in the main immunogenic region of the human immunodeficiency virus 1 NEF protein. J Exp Med 1994;180:1129.
101. Byrne JA, Oldstone MB. Biology of cloned cytotoxic T lymphocytes specific for lymphocytic choriomeningitis virus: clearance of virus in vivo. J Virol 1984;51:682.
102. Larsen HS, Feng MF, Horohov DW, et al. Role of T-lymphocyte subsets in recovery from herpes simplex virus infection. J Virol 1984;50:56.
103. Lukacher AE, Braciale VL, Braciale TJ. In vivo effector function of influenza virus-specific cytotoxic T lymphocyte clones is highly specific. J Exp Med 1984;160:814.
104. Rosenberg S, Packard B, Read E, et al. Use of tumor infiltrating lymphocytes and IL-2 in the immunotherapy of patients with metastatic melanoma: a preliminary report. N Engl J Med 1988;319:1676.
105. Rosenberg S, Lotze M, Muul L, et al. Observation on the systemic administration of autologous lymphokine-activated killer cells and recombinant interleukin 2 to patients with metastatic cancer. N Engl J Med 1985;313:1485.
106. Riddell SR, Watanabe KS, Goodrich JM, et al. Restoration of viral immunity in immunodeficient humans by the adoptive transfer of T cell clones. Science 1992;257:238.
107. Whiteside TL, Elder EM, Moody D, et al. Generation and characterization of ex vivo propagated autologous CD8+ cells used for adoptive immunotherapy of patients infected with human immunodeficiency virus. Blood 1993;81:2085.
108. Torpey D, Huang XL, Armstrong J, et al. Effects of adoptive immunotherapy with autologous CD8+ T lymphocytes on immunologic parameters: lymphocyte subsets and cytotoxic activity. Clin Immunol Immunopathol 1993;68:263.
109. Ho M, Armstrong J, McMahon D, et al. A phase 1 study of adoptive transfer of autologous CD8+ T lymphocytes in patients with acquired immunodeficiency syndrome (AIDS)-related complex or AIDS. Blood 1993;81:2093.
110. Roberts MR, Qin L, Zhang D, et al. Targeting of human immunodeficiency virus-infected cells by CD8+ T lymphocytes armed with universal T-cell receptors. Blood 1994;84:2878.
111. Riddell SR, Gilbert MJ, Greenberg PD. CD8+ cytotoxic T cell therapy of cytomegalovirus and HIV infection. Curr Opin Immunol 1993;5:484.

AIDS: Biology, Diagnosis, Treatment and
Prevention, fourth edition, edited by Vincent T.
DeVita, Jr., Samuel Hellman, and Steven A.
Rosenberg. Lippincott–Raven Publishers, © 1997

CHAPTER 25

Gene Therapy

Thierry VandenDriessche, Marinee K.L. Chuah, and Richard A. Morgan

An estimated 5 to 10 million people worldwide are now infected with the human immunodeficiency virus type 1 (HIV-1), and approximately 1 million new cases of acquired immunodeficiency syndrome (AIDS) will occur over the next 5 years. Among hemophiliacs and users of illicit drugs, AIDS is now the leading cause of death. AIDS is a uniformly fatal viral infection for which no curative therapy exists. Therapeutic strategies for AIDS include anti–HIV-1 retroviral drug therapy, immunomodulator therapy, and immune restoration by bone marrow or lymphocyte transfer. Strategies are being developed for intervening in the secondary effects of HIV-1 infection, such as treatment and prophylaxis of opportunistic infections and antitumor therapy (eg, Kaposi 's sarcoma).

 The anti-HIV retroviral drugs approved by the U.S. Food and Drug Administration (FDA) for AIDS include reverse transcriptase inhibitors such as the nucleoside analogs zidovudine (AZT), dideoxyinosine (ddI), dideoxycytosine (ddC), stavudine (d4T), and lamivudine (3TC). Although survival times are lengthened and frequency of opportunistic infections are reduced in patients taking reverse transcriptase inhibitors, complete and sustained improvement of immune status had not been achieved.[1] An important drawback of reverse transcriptase inhibitors is that they have no effect on already integrated HIV-1 proviruses and HIV-1 gene expression. The toxic effects associated with these antiretroviral drugs and the emergence of drug-resistant HIV-1 strains also may limit their usefulness for the treatment of AIDS. Despite the advances in treating HIV disease,

more efficacious and less toxic therapies with novel mechanisms of action are needed.

Because the primary problem in AIDS is induced immunodeficiency associated with quantitative loss of functional T cells, immunologic reconstitution (with or without AZT treatment) has been attempted. Various methods of immune reconstitution have been tested, including syngeneic or allogeneic bone marrow transplantation, peripheral blood lymphocyte infusions, and lymphokine-based (eg, interleukin-2, interferon-α) immunotherapy.[3–9] These studies confirmed the safety of adoptive transfer of peripheral blood lymphocyte or bone marrow cells in AIDS patients, but only a transient improvement in immune function and no sustained clinical benefit was seen. Other clinical trials involving adoptive transfer of HIV-1 specific cytotoxic T lymphocytes (CTLs) have also been initiated in an attempt to restore immune function (Lieberman J and colleagues, Walker R and coworkers: personal communications).

Because no effective strategy is available to treat AIDS, it is important to explore and develop new modalities for the treatment of this deadly disease. Gene therapy, defined as the introduction of new genetic material into cells of an individual with resulting therapeutic benefit, may be an effective treatment for a variety of disorders.[10] Because HIV-1 integrates itself into the host's genome, AIDS can be considered an "acquired genetic disease" and is therefore potentially amenable to treatment using gene therapy. Gene therapy for HIV-1 requires the introduction of anti–HIV-1 genes into cells to prevent or inhibit HIV-1 viral gene expression or function and consequently to limit HIV-1 replication and AIDS pathogenesis. Anti–HIV-1 gene therapy offers new opportunities for the intervention of HIV-1 replication at the molecular level, such as the possibility to target conserved cis-acting regulatory sequences or essential HIV-1 proteins. Another potential advantage of gene therapy is that it can downregulate HIV-1 gene expression, in contrast to conventional drug therapies such as reverse transcriptase inhibitors. This is important in view of the findings

Thierry VandenDriessche, Clinical Gene Therapy Branch, National Center for Human Genome Research, National Institutes of Health, 49 Convent Drive, Bethesda, MD 20892.

Marinee K.L. Chuah, Genetic Therapy Inc., 19 Firstfield Road, Gaithersburg, MD 20878.

Richard A. Morgan, Gene Transfer Technology Section, Clinical Gene Therapy Branch, National Center for Human Genome Research, National Institutes of Health, 10 Center Drive, Building 10, Room 10C103, Bethesda, MD 20892.

that certain HIV-1 gene products may be associated with virus-independent pathology.[11-17] Gene therapy may permit constitutive expression of anti-HIV gene products in HIV-1–infected individuals, potentially leading to a prolonged improvement of the patient's immune status.

Various anti–HIV-1 gene therapy strategies have been developed and shown to inhibit HIV-1 replication or expression in vitro. The introduction of anti-HIV genes into cells allows for the intracellular inhibition of HIV-1. In addition to this intracellular intervention, gene therapy may also be used to intervene with HIV-1 viral spread at the extracellular level. This could be achieved in vivo by sustained expression of a secreted anti–HIV-1 protein at high local concentrations or by stimulation of an anti–HIV-1 immune response.

The anti–HIV-1 gene therapy strategies that have been developed include approaches based on proteins (eg, *trans*-dominant mutant HIV-1 proteins, cellular proteins, gene vaccines, toxic "suicide" proteins), RNA (eg, antisense RNA decoys, ribozymes), or DNA (eg, antisense oligonucleotides).[18-21] Alternatively, a combination of different anti–HIV-1 genes can be simultaneously introduced into cells to target multiple stages in the viral life cycle. We published a detailed description of each of the different anti-HIV gene therapy strategies,[19] and only selected strategies are presented here. In this chapter, we describe the anti-HIV clinical gene therapy protocols that have been approved by the Recombinant DNA Advisory Committee (RAC) and the FDA. The preclinical studies and the experimental design of each of the clinical trials are the main focus of this review.

ANTI-HIV GENE THERAPY CLINICAL TRIALS

Eight anti-HIV gene therapy clinical protocols were reviewed and approved by the RAC as of April 1995. These protocols can be divided into three different categories: gene-marker studies, intracellular inhibition, and immune stimulation. There are two gene-marking studies, one involving the transfer of neomycin resistance gene (*neo^R*)-marked syngeneic peripheral T cells in HIV-1–discordant identical twins[22] and a second analyzing the transfer of autologous anti-HIV CTLs engineered with a marker or suicide gene, the hygromycin resistance–thymidine kinase (*hy-tk*) fusion gene.[23] There are three gene therapy strategies aimed at inhibiting HIV-1 intracellularly. These strategies include the use of a *trans*-dominant mutant version of the HIV-1 Rev protein, by itself[24] or in combination with antisense-TAR (ie, *trans*-acting response element)[25] or a ribozyme specific for the HIV-1 leader sequence.[26] Three gene therapy strategies are aimed at stimulating an anti–HIV-1 immune response by expression of a chimeric CD4-ζ chain universal receptor on CTLs[27] or by intracellular expression of HIV-1 IIIB Env.[28,29] Expression of HIV-1 IIIB Env is achieved by ex vivo engineering of autologous fibroblasts[28] or by direct intramuscular injection of HIV-IIIB Env retroviral vectors.[29]

Marking of Syngeneic T Cells

A gene-marker study on the safety and survival of the adoptive transfer of genetically marked syngeneic lymphocytes in HIV-discordant identical twins has been initiated by Walker and colleagues.[22] The objective of this phase I/II pilot project is to evaluate the distribution and survival, tolerance, safety, and efficacy of infusions of activated, gene-marked syngeneic T lymphocytes obtained from HIV-seronegative identical twins on the functional immune status of HIV-infected twin recipients.

This protocol represents the initial step in a sequence of studies designed to evaluate the potential value of genetically modified T lymphocytes (CD4+ and CD8+) in an attempt to prevent or control HIV infection. This study will provide the initial baseline data needed to prospectively evaluate the fate of activated CD4+ and CD8+ cells after reinfusion in HIV-infected individuals. In association with other protocols in development that are using adoptive transfer of ex vivo expanded and activated cells without gene marking, this study will allow differentiation of the effects of gene modification of the cells from those effects of activated T-cell infusions alone. By monitoring functional immune status, measure of viral burden, and physiologic markers, it may be possible to determine whether this approach is feasible and safe. The knowledge gained from a careful analysis of gene-marked CD4+ and CD8+ T-cell survival, when correlated with quantitative assays of HIV viremia and immune status, may serve as an important method for monitoring disease progression. The availability of healthy T cells from the uninfected donor permits rigorous expansion under conditions that may be difficult with T cells from infected patients.

The experimental design for this protocol is outlined in Figure 25-1A. Lymphocytes from each seronegative twin are obtained by apheresis, and polyclonal T-cell proliferation is induced with anti-CD3 antibodies and recombinant interleukin-2 (rIL-2) stimulation. After the cells begin dividing, they are engineered with a *neo^R* gene-containing retroviral vector, and the cell numbers are expanded 10- to 1000-fold during approximately 2 weeks in culture. These marked T cells are then infused into the seropositive twins. Efficacy evaluation includes assessment of the survival of the uniquely marked T-cell populations by semiquantitative determination of the *neo^R* gene in peripheral blood lymphocytes by vector-specific polymerase chain reaction (PCR) serial determinations of CD4+ and CD8+ counts and percentages, T-cell proliferative responses and cytotoxicity, serial p24 antigen levels, and serial quantitative determinations of HIV viremia.

Six twin pairs have undergone the protocol. At the time of entry into the study, three patients had CD4 counts above 200/mm³, and three had counts below 200/mm³. Preliminary results indicate that gene-marked T cells (CD4+ and CD8+) could be detected in the circulation from all six infused patients (Walker R: personal communication). The first

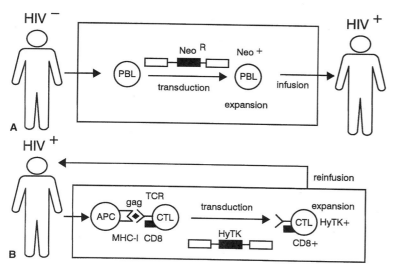

FIG. 25-1. Adoptive transfer of gene-marked T cells (**A**) in identical twins disordant for HIV-1 infection and (**B**) in an HIV-1-infected person. Peripheral blood T lymphocytes (PBL) from each seronegative twin are induced to polyclonal proliferation with anti-CD3 and rIL-2 stimulation, transduced with a Neo^R retroviral vector and expanded. These marked T-cell fractions are then infused into the seropositive twins, followed by safety and efficacy evaluations. Adoptive transfer of autologous cytotoxic T lymphocytes (CTL) involves ex vivo expansion of major histocompatibility complex class-I (MHC-I) restricted CD8+ CTL clones specific for the HIV-1 Gag protein. These clones are obtained by confronting CD8+ T cells with autologous antigen-presenting cells (APC) that present HIV-1 Gag-derived peptides in association with MHC-I to the T-cell receptor (TCR) of the CD8+ T cells. These CTL clones are marked with a HyTK vector that serves as a marker and as a built-in safety feature. Transduced cells are expanded and reinfused into the HIV-1 seropositive individual, followed by safety and efficacy evaluation.

patient remained vector positive out to 20 weeks after infusion of the *neo*^{R} gene-marked T cells. All patients have tolerated the therapy well, and no side effects related to the gene transfer procedure have been observed. Data is still being accrued from this protocol.

Marking of Cytotoxic T Cells

A second gene-marking study involves adoptive immunotherapy using genetically modified HIV-specific CD8+ T cells for HIV seropositive patients.[23] The objectives of this trial are to evaluate the safety and toxicity of administering increasing doses of autologous CD8+ class I major histocompatibility complex (MHC)–restricted HIV-specific cytotoxic T-cell clones transduced by retrovirus-mediated gene transfer to express a marker-suicide gene; to determine the survival of adoptively transferred HIV-specific T-cell clones; and to evaluate markers of HIV disease activity in these recipients.

The importance of MHC class I–restricted CD8+ CTL in controlling infection has not been as well documented for HIV as for other viruses for which small animal models exist, but it is supported by correlative data from HIV-1–infected patients. Before developing AIDS, HIV-seropositive patients commonly have MHC class I–restricted CD8+ CTLs that are detectable in high concentrations in peripheral blood and specific for numerous HIV proteins, including Env, Gag, Pol, Vif, and Nef.[30–36] The rationale for using HIV-specific T-cell clones to limit HIV-1 infection is based on the observations that CD8+ T cells inhibit replication of HIV-1 in human lymphocytes in vitro.[37] Circumstantial evidence also suggests that maintenance of HIV-specific CTLs may retard the development of AIDS.[38–42] Adoptive immunotherapy using in vitro expanded cytomegalovirus (CMV)-specific clones has proven effective for reconstituting CMV-specific T-cell responses after bone marrow transplantation.[43] Adoptive immunotherapy with in vitro expanded HIV-specific CD8+ CTLs therefore may have a beneficial antiviral effect.

The initial HIV-1–infected patients enrolled in this clinical trial were infused with ex vivo expanded CD8+ CTL clones specific for the HIV-1 Gag protein, concurrent with AZT administration (Fig. 25-1*B*). These CTL clones were marked with a retroviral vector that expressed a bifunctional hybrid fusion protein (*hy-tk*) of the hygromycin resistance gene (*hyg*^{R}) and the herpes simplex virus thymidine kinase (HSV-*tk*) gene.[44] The rationale of using this *hy-tk* fusion construct is that it serves as a marker to follow the persistence of the infused CTL clones and as a built-in safety feature. HSV-*tk* is a conditionally lethal (suicide) gene, and engineered cells can therefore be ablated in vivo by administration of ganciclovir to the CTL recipient if unexpected CTL growth or an unexpectedly vigorous CTL response is observed. Alteration of *hy-tk*–engineered cells in vivo has been demonstrated in animal models.

Assessment of the clinical data includes determination of survival of the infused CTL clones by PCR or Southern blot analysis, characterization of HIV-specific CTL generation, and HIV-1 status, such as quantitation of serum p24 antigen levels. Analysis of the in vivo data is still in progress, but preliminary results indicate that the CTL clones may persist for a few weeks. This strategy and other approaches employing CD8+ cells (see the universal chimeric T-cell receptor protocol described later) may be affected by the decline in CD4+ cell function during AIDS progression, because CD4+ T-cell help is needed to sustain an effective CTL response. In contrast to other viruses, such as CMV and Epstein-Barr virus (EBV), for which virus-specific CD8+ CTL responses persist throughout life, HIV-infected patients gradually lose detectable HIV-specific CTLs, and this decline in CTL responses correlates with increases in plasma viremia, reductions in CD4+ T-cell counts, and the development of clinical AIDS.[36–38] It may be possible to overcome these limitations by the development of helper-independent CTL clones, potentially by engineering the CD8+ cells to secrete IL-2 in an autocrine fashion.

Trans-dominant Rev

Preclinical Studies

The HIV-1 *rev* gene encodes an essential regulatory protein that mediates transactivation of HIV-1 gene expression by binding onto the HIV-1 mRNA Rev-responsive element (RRE) sequence. The Rev-RRE interaction strongly transactivates HIV-1 by facilitating the extranuclear transport of unspliced and singly spliced mRNAs that encode HIV-1 structural proteins.[45-48] Inhibition of Rev function may therefore preclude HIV-1 replication and inhibit structural gene expression. This may be important because the HIV-1 envelope protein (gp120) may be associated with virus-independent pathologic manifestations. These virus-independent, gp120-related pathologies include effects on uncontrolled lymphocyte proliferation, activation-induced apoptosis, and potential neuronal damage.[14-17] Because expression of gp120/gp41 depends on *rev* expression, gene therapy aimed at inhibiting the function of *rev* may specifically downregulate *env* gene expression and potentially diminish its pathologic effects.

The Rev protein is composed of three distinct domains; an N-terminal arginine-rich tract that binds to the RRE and is required for nuclear localization, followed by a motif that is involved in oligomerization, and a C-terminal domain that contains a conserved leucine-rich region and is thought to mediate interaction with a host cell factors.[45-51] Mutations in the first two domains generally inactivate Rev, but mutations in the C-terminal activation domain can confer a dominant-negative (ie, *trans*-dominant) phenotype. By definition, such mutants lack intrinsic wild-type activity and inhibit the function of their cognate wild-type protein in *trans*. Inhibition may occur because the mutant competes for an essential substrate or cofactor that is available in limiting amounts, or for proteins that form multimeric complexes, such as Rev, the mutant may associate with wild-type monomers to form an inactive mixed multimer.[52]

A *trans*-dominant negative mutant form of the HIV-1 Rev protein, designated as M10, contains two adjacent point mutations in the activator domain (ie, Leu^{78} to Asp^{78} and Glu^{79} to Leu^{79}). This mutant inhibits wild-type Rev by forming nonfunctional complexes with the wild-type Rev protein but resembles its wild-type counterpart in its ability to localize in the nucleus and in its capacity to bind to the RRE.[49,52] Preclinical studies revealed that expression of M10 inhibited HIV-1 replication when co-transfected with a proviral DNA molecular clone or in stably transduced T-cell lines.[49,53,54] More importantly, replication of HIV-1 laboratory strains and clinical HIV-1 isolates was inhibited in primary CD4+ T lymphocytes transduced with a retroviral vector expressing M10.[55] Inhibition of HIV-1 was also observed when the *M10* gene was transfected into the CD4+ T lymphocytes by gold particle–mediated gene transfer.[55] Expression of Rev M10 did not appear to interfere with normal cellular functions, because mitogen-induction of IL-2 secretion or NF-kB induction of HIV in T-cell lines was unaffected.[53]

Clinical Protocol

Based on the encouraging preclinical data obtained with the Rev mutant M10, a clinical protocol was proposed by Nabel and colleagues in which CD4+ T lymphocytes from an HIV-1–infected individual will be engineered with Rev M10 expression vectors.[24] In this study, the efficacy of intracellular inhibition of HIV-1 infection by the M10 *trans*-dominant mutant Rev protein will be evaluated. The aim of this proposal is to determine whether expression of M10 can prolong the survival of peripheral blood lymphocytes in AIDS patients, conferring protection against HIV-1 infection. CD4+ T lymphocytes will be genetically modified in patients using particle-mediated gene transfer (Fig. 25-2*Ai*) or retrovirus-mediated gene transfer (Fig. 25-2*Aii*). In each case, a control vector identical to the Rev M10, but with a frameshift that inactivates gene expression, will be used to transduce a parallel population of CD4+ cells. Retroviral transductions and particle-mediated transfections will be performed after stimulation of CD4+-enriched cells with IL-2 and anti-CD3 or anti-CD28 antibodies. Activation of endogenous HIV-1 will be inhibited by addition of reverse transcriptase inhibitors plus an HIV-specific toxin (ie, fusion protein between soluble CD4 and *Pseudomonas* enterotoxin CD4-PE40). The engineered and expanded cells will be returned to the patient, and the survival of the cells in each group will be compared by limiting-dilution PCR. The effect of Rev M10 on HIV-1 status and immunologic parameters will also be evaluated. Preliminary data using gold particle–mediated gene transfer shows a small percentage of vector-engineered cells in the circulation of four patients treated.

Trans-dominant Rev in Combination With Antisense-TAR

Preclinical Studies

Activation of the HIV-1 provirus initiates the transcription of multiply spliced RNAs early in the HIV-1 life cycle, and these produce the two key HIV-1 regulatory proteins Tat and Rev.[45] The HIV-1 Tat and Rev proteins are essential, conserved regulatory proteins that are powerful transactivators of HIV-1 viral gene expression. Inhibition of Tat or Rev function may preclude HIV-1 gene expression and replication. We therefore developed anti-HIV gene therapy strategies aimed at specifically inhibiting the function of Tat and Rev by *trans*-dominant mutant Rev protein and antisense-TAR, respectively.

To specifically inhibit the function of Rev, we generated a *trans*-dominant Rev mutant (Rev^{TD}), based on the previously described Rev M10 mutant, and showed that the presence of just one point mutation in the activator domain (Leu^{78} to Asp^{78}) was sufficient to confer a dominant-negative phenotype.[56] This mutant inhibited expression of a Rev-dependent chloramphenicol acetyltransferase reporter gene in transient transfection assays and greatly reduced syncytia

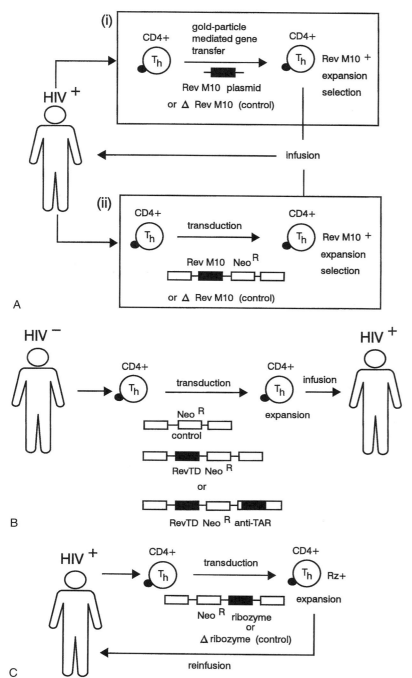

FIG. 25-2. Gene therapy protocols aimed at inhibiting HIV-1 intracellularly. These strategies include the use of (**A**) a *trans*-dominant mutant version of the HIV-1 Rev protein, (**B**) a *trans*-dominant mutant version of the HIV-1 Rev protein in combination with antisense-TAR, or (**C**) a ribozyme specific for the HIV-1 leader sequence. CD4+ T cells are obtained from HIV-1–infected patients and subjected (**Ai**) to gold-particle–mediated gene transfection ("gene gun") of an expression vector encoding the Rev M10 *trans*-dominant protein (or a control vector that contains a deletion preventing Rev M10 expression—Δ Rev M10) or (**Aii**) to transduction with a retroviral vector expressing the Rev M10 (or a control—ΔRev M10). Transfected or transduced cells can be expanded (and selected if necessary), reinfused into the HIV-1 infected person, and further analyzed for efficacy and safety. (**B**) CD4+ T cells from each seronegative twin are transduced with distinctive Neo[R] control retroviral vectors (LNL6 or G1Na) and a vector expressing a *trans*-dominant mutant version of Rev (Rev[TD]), with or without antisense-TAR. These marked T-cell fractions are then infused into the seropositive twins after combining the individual CD4+ fractions, followed by safety and efficacy evaluations. (**C**) In the ribozyme protocol, CD4+ T lymphocytes from an HIV-1 seropositive patient are subjected to retroviral transduction with a vector expressing the leader ribozyme or a control vector. After expansion and autologous transfer into the HIV-1-infected patient, safety and efficacy are monitored.

formation by preventing *env* gene expression in HeLa T4 cells. Preclinical studies further demonstrated that expression of the Rev[TD] protein inhibited production of HIV-1 laboratory strains in stably transduced T-cell lines and protected the cells from viral lysis. No virus escape mutants were observed in vitro, because viruses that emerged late in infection from Rev[TD]-engineered cultures remained sensitive to Rev-mediated inhibition. In situ hybridization and Northern analysis revealed that Rev[TD] acts by inhibiting unspliced and singly spliced mRNA accumulation, possibly by preventing their extranuclear transport.

To inhibit Tat function, we developed an antisense strategy targeted at the HIV-1 transactivation response (TAR) element. The TAR element corresponds to an RNA stem-loop structure within the untranslated leader sequence of all HIV-1 transcripts, including the RNA genome, and it is required for HIV-1 Tat function.[57] The interaction between Tat and TAR can lead to potent transactivation (increasing expression by 20- to 100-fold) by inducing transcriptional initiation, elongation, or both actions.[45,58–61] We constructed a retroviral vector that uses an RNA polymerase III promoter to express a chimeric tRNA$_i^{Met}$ antisense-TAR fusion transcript complementary to the HIV-1 TAR region.[62] Using transient and stable transfection assays, we showed that anti-sense-TAR inhibited Tat-mediated transactivation of the HIV-1 long terminal repeat–chloramphenicol acetyltransferase gene in a dose-dependent fashion. Decreased HIV-1 viral production was observed in a SupT1 T-cell line that was transduced with the antisense-TAR retroviral vector. The exact mechanism involved in this inhibition is not fully understood but may involve inhibition of Tat binding on the TAR element or RNase degradation of the RNA duplex between the antisense TAR and its complementary target sequence. This RNA duplex may also inhibit ribosome binding and consequently inhibit translation.

To evaluate the efficacy of Rev[TD] and antisense-TAR in conditions relevant for clinical anti-HIV gene therapy, primary patient HIV-1 isolates, including AZT-resistant strains, were used to challenge CD4+ T lymphocytes that were transduced with retroviral vectors expressing Rev[TD], antisense-TAR, or a combination of both elements in the same vector. We demonstrated effective protection against the primary patient isolates with all the vectors tested, but greater inhibition of HIV-1 was observed with Rev[TD] than with antisense-TAR.[56,63] Expression of Rev[TD] or antisense-TAR did not appear to interfere with normal cellular functions, because expression of T-cell activation or differentiation antigens (eg, CD2, CD3, CD4, CD8, IL-2R, MHC-I, MHC-II) and lymphokine secretion patterns (eg, IL-3, IL-4, IL-6, granulocyte-macrophage colony-stimulating factor, interferon-γ) in transduced primary T cells was unaffected (unpublished observations). These preclinical efficacy and safety data support the use of Rev[TD] and antisense-TAR as a gene therapy strategy for inhibiting HIV-1 in infected persons.

Clinical Protocol

We have proposed a clinical protocol for AIDS gene therapy using retrovirus-mediated gene transfer to deliver antisense-TAR and Rev[TD] genes to syngeneic lymphocytes in identical twins discordant for HIV-1 infection (Fig. 25-2B). This phase I/II pilot study is based on the preclinical data obtained with the antisense-TAR and Rev[TD] retroviral vectors and on the adoptive transfer of neo[R]-marked syngeneic CD4+ T cells in HIV-1 discordant identical twins.[22] The trial will evaluate the safety, survival, and potential efficacy of the adoptive transfer of genetically engineered syngeneic lymphocytes obtained from HIV-seronegative identical twins on the functional immune status of HIV-infected twin recipients.[25]

The experimental design for this protocol is outlined in Figure 25-2B and is similar in design to the twin marker study.[22] A unique feature of this design is the availability of healthy T cells from the uninfected donor that permits rigorous expansion that does not require culture conditions that inhibit the spread of endogenous HIV-1 during the transduction process. T cells from each seronegative twin will be obtained by periodic apheresis, enriched for CD4+ T cells by immunomagnetic depletion of CD8+ T cells and induced

to polyclonal proliferation with anti-CD3 antibodies and rIL-2 stimulation. The CD4+ T-cell cultures will be divided into aliquots, which will be transduced with a control neo[R] retroviral vectors (LNL6 or G1Na) and up to two additional retroviral vectors containing the potentially therapeutic antisense-TAR or rev[TD] genes (or both). These engineered T-cell populations will be expanded 10- to 1000-fold during approximately 2 weeks in culture before infusion into the seropositive twin. The relative survival of the uniquely engineered T-cell populations will be analyzed by vector-specific PCR, and the recipient's immune condition and HIV-1 status will be monitored.

Anti-HIV Ribozyme

Preclinical Studies

Ribozymes are catalytic RNA molecules that hybridize specifically to a complementary RNA target, analogous to conventional antisense molecules but also functionally inactivating it by cleaving the phosphodiester backbone at a specified location. The cleavage reaction is catalytic in that more than one substrate molecule is processed per ribozyme molecule.

Wong-Staal and colleagues designed an HIV-1–specific hairpin ribozyme.[64–66] This ribozyme was derived from the minimum catalytic center of the negative strand of the tobacco ringspot viroid and cleaves HIV-1 RNA in the untranslated leader sequence (at nucleotides +111/+112 relative to the transcription initiation site). This target is conserved among most of the known HIV-1 isolates and is present in early and late viral gene products, including the viral genome. The leader sequence is essential for reverse transcription, transactivation, 5'-capping, and translation.[45] Unlike hammerhead ribozymes, hairpin-based ribozymes may be particularly advantageous because the conditions required for optimal function of hairpin ribozymes are almost physiologic.[65] Cleavage of the target RNA occurs at a GUC sequence and involves hydrolysis of a 3',5'-phosphodiester bond.[64–66] In vitro analysis of this ribozyme revealed a specific and highly efficient cleavage activity.

To evaluate its antiviral activity, a plasmid expressing the ribozyme from the human β-actin promoter was co-transfected with HIV-1 proviral DNA into HeLa cells.[66] HIV-1 expression was inhibited, as measured by p24 antigen levels and reduced Tat activity. The inhibition primarily resulted from the ribozyme catalytic activity rather than merely acting as conventional antisense, because a three-base mutation of the catalytic center significantly reduced its inhibitory potential. By cleaving at this site, the ribozyme renders the RNA capless and presumably exposed to degradation. The uncapped mRNAs are most likely poorly translated. This ribozyme was also cloned into a retroviral vector, using RNA polymerase III (tRNA[Val], adenovirus VA1) or polymerase II (MoMLV) promoters and shown to effectively inhibit diverse strains of HIV-1 in transduced Molt-4 T-cell lines or HeLa cells co-transfected with proviral DNA.[67,68]

This ribozyme was shown to act by cleaving afferent HIV-1 genomes and efferent viral mRNA and therefore target HIV-1 at multiple stages in the viral life cycle, even at the preintegration stage.[68] Although the presence of one nucleotide substitution in the leader sequence of the HIV-1$_{SF}$ strain was sufficient to significantly reduce the effectiveness of the ribozyme, ribozyme-sensitive HIV-1 strains did not convert to a resistant phenotype in vitro when confronted with ribozyme-expressing T-cell lines. However, it cannot be excluded that ribozyme-resistant HIV-1 escape mutants may readily emerge in vivo by virtue of the error-prone reverse transcriptase activity combined with the inherently rapid HIV-1 replication rate in AIDS patients.[69]

To evaluate the efficacy of the ribozyme in conditions that more closely mimic clinical anti-HIV gene therapy, CD4+ T lymphocytes were transduced with the ribozyme vector and challenged with primary patient HIV-1 isolates.[70] HIV-1 production was significantly inhibited in the transduced primary cells without affecting their viability or proliferation kinetics.

Retroviral vectors carrying the ribozyme gene were used to transduce purified CD34+ stem or progenitor cells from human fetal cord blood, prestimulated with stem cell factor, IL-3, and IL-6.[71] Transduction and ribozyme expression had no apparent adverse effect on cell differentiation or proliferation. Macrophage-like cells differentiated from the stem or progenitor cells in vitro when granulocyte-macrophage colony-stimulating factor was added to the cultures. The cells expressed the ribozyme gene and resisted infection by the macrophagetropic HIV-1$_{Bal}$ strain. These results suggest the feasibility of stem cell gene therapy in HIV-1–infected patients.

Clinical Protocol

A clinical protocol for AIDS gene therapy using the HIV-1 leader-specific hairpin ribozyme has been proposed by Wong-Staal and coworkers. In this phase I clinical trial, the safety and efficacy of ribozyme gene therapy will be evaluated in HIV-1–infected patients (CD4 counts between 250 and 500/mm^3) by reinfusing autologous CD4+ T cells that have been transduced ex vivo with a retroviral vector that expresses the HIV-1 leader sequence ribozyme (Fig. 25-2C).

Transduction of HIV-1–infected cells in vitro will require culture conditions that inhibit the spread of endogenous HIV-1 (eg, using nevirapine and CD4-PE40). The in vivo kinetics and survival of ribozyme-transduced cells will be compared by limiting-dilution PCR with those of a separate aliquot of cells transduced with a control vector that is identical except for the ribozyme cassette. The level and persistence of ribozyme expression will also be assessed. The results will determine whether this ribozyme can protect CD4+ T cells in patients with HIV-1 infection and will aid the design of future trials of hematopoietic stem cell gene therapy for AIDS.

Universal Chimeric T-Cell Receptor

Preclinical Studies

As outlined earlier in the section on the gene-marker studies, adoptive transfer of HIV-specific MHC class I–restricted CD8+ CTLs may have potential as an immunotherapy for HIV-infected individuals. Investigators at Cell Genesys, Inc., have designed a universal, MHC class I–unrestricted, chimeric T-cell receptor that can redirect the antigenic specificity of peripheral blood mononuclear cell–derived CD8+ T-cell populations to recognize the HIV-1 envelope protein gp120 on the surface of the infected cells.[27] This anti-HIV chimeric universal receptor (UR) is composed of the extracellular domain of the human CD4 receptor that recognizes the gp120 moiety of the HIV-1 Env, fused to the cytoplasmic domain of the ζ chain, which is responsible for signal transduction in T cells. On binding to gp120, these CD4-ζ URs initiate T-cell activation, resulting in induction of effector functions, including cytolysis of the virus-infected cell. Using retrovirus-mediated transduction with replication-defective retroviral vectors, T-cell populations expressing high levels of HIV-specific URs could routinely be obtained. Preclinical studies further demonstrated that the UR+CD8+ T-cell population exhibits highly efficient cytolytic activity against T cells infected with HIV-1 in vitro, including low-passage lymphocytotropic strains. This strategy using CTLs engineered to express gp120-specific CD4-ζ URs could have potentially therapeutic benefit in HIV-1–infected individuals.

Clinical Protocol

This protocol is similar in design to the identical twin marker study[22] (see Fig. 25-1A), but in this case, CD8+ CTLs will be transduced with a retroviral vector encoding the universal, MHC class I–unrestricted, chimeric CD4-ζ receptor (Fig. 25-3A). A phase I/II pilot study has been approved by RAC and the FDA to assess the safety and tolerance of the adoptive transfer of syngeneic gene-modified CTLs in HIV-infected identical twins.[27] The objective of this project is to evaluate the distribution and survival, tolerance, safety, and efficacy of infusions of CTLs obtained from HIV-seronegative identical twins that will be transduced with a gene encoding a universal, chimeric CD4-ζ anti-HIV receptor on the functional immune status of HIV-infected twin recipients. The proposed study is an open-label, comparative, sequentially randomized treatment with genetically modified or unmodified ex vivo expanded T lymphocytes.

This study is divided into two treatment periods. In the initial period, single doses of genetically unmodified T lymphocytes or single, escalating doses of genetically modified T lymphocytes will be administered. In the second period, multiple doses of the maximum tolerated cell dose will be administered. The feasibility and safety of this approach will be assessed by monitoring functional immune status, viral burden, clinical symptoms, organ function, and persistence of circulating gene-modified T lymphocytes.

Gene Vaccines

Preclinical Studies

Conventional immunization procedures involve the administration of soluble antigens, such as inactivated viruses or recombinant viral proteins, to enhance antibody production that clears viral infection.[72] Although most HIV-1–infected persons develop antibodies, some of which possess neutralizing activity in vitro, such antibodies appear to be unable to clear HIV-1 infection. Most HIV-1 vaccines and immunotherapeutics have generated HIV-1–reactive antibodies, but they fail to prevent disease progression.

Circumstantial evidence suggests that the CTL response may play an important role in controlling HIV-1 infection.[37–42] The development of a vaccine that would augment CTL activity instead of antibody production may induce a beneficial clinical effect in HIV-1–infected patients. Although soluble proteins have been shown to induce CTL activity, efficient activation of MHC class I–restricted CD8+ CTLs generally occurs by intracellular synthesis of foreign proteins and subsequent antigen processing and presentation through the endogenous MHC class I presentation pathway. Retroviral vector-mediated immunization or "genetic vaccination" for HIV-1 provides a means of introducing HIV-1 genes into the genome of the host cells and of delivering intracellular HIV-1–derived antigenic peptides to the endogenous MHC class I antigen-presentation pathway, leading to CTL activation.

Preclinical studies showed that a nonreplicating MoMLV-based vector encoding the HIV-1 IIIB Env and Rev proteins (N2 IIIBenv) can provide endogenous production of these HIV-1 proteins for MHC class I antigen presentation in murine and nonhuman primate cells.[73–75] Induction of antigen-specific class I MHC–restricted CD8+ CTL responses in mice and rhesus monkeys was observed after injection of ex vivo N2 IIIBenv vector-transduced autologous fibroblasts. Most importantly, murine CTLs induced by vector-transduced cells also exhibited cross-reactivity by lysing cells infected with different HIV-1 prototypic strains and clinical HIV-1 isolates.

Because direct in vivo administration of the vector provides a more feasible approach for retroviral vector-mediated immunization compared with ex vivo transduced cells, vector immunization was also examined by direct intramuscular injection of the N2 IIIBenv vector.[76] Vector-immunized mice, macaques, and baboons generated long-lived (4 to 6 months) HIV-1–specific CD8+ MHC class I–restricted CTLs, and in mice and baboons, an HIV-1 Env-specific antibody response was also detectable. These preclinical observations underscore the potential of gene transfer for the generation of an HIV-1–specific CTL response in HIV-1–infected individuals that may provide heterologous protection against different polymorphic HIV-1 isolates.

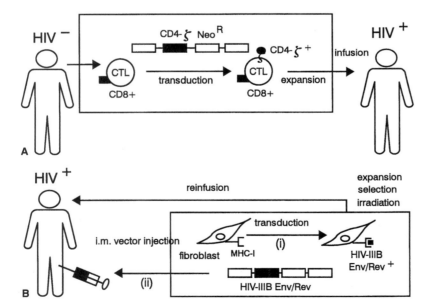

FIG. 25-3. Gene therapy strategies aimed at stimulating an anti-HIV-1 immune response (**A**) by expression of a chimeric CD4-ξ chain universal receptor on cytotoxic T lymphocytes (CTL) or (**B**) by intracellular expression of HIV-1 IIIB Env/Rev. Expression of HIV-IIIB Env is achieved (**Bi**) by ex vivo engineering of autologous fibroblasts or (**Bii**) by direct intramuscular injection of HIV-IIIB Env retroviral vectors. (**A**) The universal receptor protocol is similar in design to the identical twin marker study (see Fig. 25-1A), but in this case, CD8+ CTL obtained from HIV-seronegative identical twins are transduced with a retroviral vector encoding the universal, MHC class I–unrestricted chimeric CD4-ξ receptor that is specific for HIV-1 Env. On binding to gp120, these CD4-ξ universal receptors initiate T-cell activation, resulting in induction of effector functions, including cytolysis of the virally infected cell. Transduced cells are infused into the HIV-1-seropositive twin after expansion, and safety and efficacy parameters are then determined. (**B**) For the gene vaccine studies, HIV-1–infected patients have their fibroblasts removed for ex vivo transduction with a potentially immunotherapeutic MoMLV-based retroviral vector encoding the HIV-1 Env/Rev proteins (designated as HIV-IT). These fibroblasts are obtained from a skin biopsy and subsequently transduced with the HIV-IT vector, selected, irradiated, quality control tested, and returned to the donor. Several injections or doses are given, and then safety and efficacy are analyzed. The direct in vivo injection protocol involves the administration of the HIV-IT vector or a diluent control to HIV-infected, seropositive, asymptomatic individuals. Direct vector treatment consists of a series of three monthly intramuscular injections using a two-tier dosing schedule, and safety and efficacy are monitored.

Clinical Protocol

Two related clinical protocols have been approved by the RAC and FDA to test the safety and potential efficacy of genetic vaccination in HIV-1–infected individuals. In one protocol,[28] HIV-1–infected patients will have their fibroblasts removed for ex vivo transduction (Fig. 25-3Bi) with a potentially immunotherapeutic MoMLV-based retroviral vector (designated as HIV-IT) encoding the HIV-1 Env and Rev proteins, and in the other protocol,[29] HIV-IT will be injected intramuscularly into the HIV-1–infected patient to achieve in situ transductions (Fig. 25-3Bii).

The ex vivo genetic vaccination phase I clinical protocol involves three successive doses (and a booster set of three successive doses) of HIV-IT transduced autologous fibroblasts. These fibroblasts will be obtained from a skin biopsy and subsequently transduced with the HIV-IT vector, selected, irradiated, quality control tested, and returned to the donor. The direct in vivo injection protocol is a phase I placebo-controlled clinical trial involving the administration of the HIV-IT vector or a diluent control to HIV-infected, seropositive, asymptomatic individuals not currently receiving antiretroviral treatment. Direct vector treatment consists of a series of three monthly intramuscular injections (using a two-tier dosing schedule). Treated individuals will be evaluated for acute toxicity and for normal clinical parameters, CD4+ T-cell levels, HIV-specific T-cell responses, and viral load before, during, and after treatment.

Preliminary clinical data suggest that HIV-infected patients treated with vector-transduced autologous fibroblasts show augmented HIV-1 IIIB Env specific CD8+ CTL responses. It is hoped that the retroviral vector-mediated immunization will result in a balanced in vivo immune attack by HIV-specific CTLs and antibody responses that may eliminate HIV-infected cells and clear cell-free virus from an HIV-1–infected individual.

CONCLUSIONS

A large variety of anti–HIV-1 gene therapy strategies have been developed that effectively inhibit HIV-1 in vitro.[19] Significant progress has been made in demonstrating that primary CD4+ T lymphocytes can be protected from infection with HIV-1, including primary patient isolates, using gene therapy approaches based on trans-dominant mutant HIV-1 proteins, antisense elements, and ribozymes.[55,63,70] The data obtained by vector-mediated immunization are also encouraging, because long-term persistence of CTLs and cross-protection against heterologous polymorphic HIV-1 strains have been demonstrated in animal models.[73–76] Based on these preclinical findings, several anti-HIV gene therapy strategies have received RAC and FDA approval for testing in HIV-1–infected individuals.

These clinical trials will be able to address the question of whether rendering a cell resistant to HIV-1 infection by gene therapy will have a therapeutic benefit to the patient, particularly late in the course of infection. Although inhibition of HIV-1 was demonstrated in vitro, it is still not clear which in vitro HIV-1 challenge dose mimics the true in vivo condition, which depends on the clinical stage and anatomic location.[77,78] Expression of the anti-HIV genes may be sufficiently high to protect engineered cells from HIV-1 infection in vivo when exposed to the typically low levels of HIV-1 viral particles in the circulation. In contrast, because HIV-1 infection is active and progressive in the lymph nodes during the clinically latent stage of the disease, it is likely that the engineered cells, when administered in vivo, would be confronted with a large number of HIV-1–infected cells in the lymphoid tissues. However, this does not necessarily imply that the engineered cells would be exposed to a high viral dose of replication-competent HIV-1 particles, because the high rate of errors in retroviral replication could result in many defective HIV-1 quasispecies.[79,80] A large proportion of the cells in the germinal centers of the lymph nodes are latently infected with HIV-1 and do not express any HIV-1 RNA.[77]

These proposed protocols should also help in the design of future trials to test whether resistance to HIV-1 can ultimately be transferred to the entire lymphohematopoietic system by gene transfer into hematopoietic precursor or stem cells. The demonstration that CD34+-enriched hematopoietic stem or progenitor cells can be engineered with anti-HIV vectors and confer HIV-1 resistance to the macrophage lineage is encouraging.[67] Some gene transfer and gene therapy protocols should also elucidate the mechanisms of immunopathogenesis leading to AIDS. The gene vaccine protocols and the adoptive transfer of gene-marked CTLs should help to evaluate the potential importance of CTLs in limiting HIV-1 infection. Ultimately, if these techniques prove beneficial, it will be necessary to develop alternative gene-delivery systems to minimize ex vivo manipulation of a patient's cells and to make gene therapy accessible on a wider scale.

ACKNOWLEDGMENTS

We would like to thank Theresa Lumsden for her secretarial assistance

REFERENCES

1. Concorde Coordinating Committee. Concorde: MRC/ANRS randomized double-blind controlled trial of immediate and deferred zidovudine in symptom-free HIV infection. Lancet 1994;343:871.
2. Rook AH, Masur H, Lane HC, et al. Interleukin-2 enhances the depressed natural killer and cytomegalovirus-specific cytotoxic activities of lymphocytes from patients with the acquired immunodeficiency syndrome. J Clin Invest 1987;72:398.
3. Walker R. A study of the safety and survival of the adoptive transfer of genetically marked syngeneic lymphocytes in HIV-infected identical twins. Hum Gene Ther 1993;4:659.
4. Vilmer E, Rhodes-Feuillette A, Rabian C, et al. Clinical and immunological restoration in patients with AIDS after marrow transplantation, using lymphocyte transfusions from the marrow donor. Transplantation 1987;44:25.
5. Lane HC, Masur H, Longo D, et al. Partial immune reconstitution in a patient with the acquired immunodeficiency syndrome. N Engl J Med 1984;311:1099.

6. Lane HC, Kovacs JA, Feinberg J. Anti-retroviral effects of interferon-alpha in AIDS-associated Kaposi's sarcoma. Lancet 1988;2:1218.

7. Verdonck LF, de Gast GC, Lange JM, et al. Syngeneic leukocytes together with suramin failed to improve immunodeficiency in a case of transfusion-associated AIDS after syngeneic bone marrow transplantation. Blood 1988;71:666.

8. Lane HC, Zunich KM, Wilson W, et al. Syngeneic bone marrow transplantation and adoptive transfer of peripheral blood lymphocytes combined with zidovudine in human immunodeficiency virus (HIV) infection. Ann Intern Med 1990;113:512.

9. Kovacs JA, Baseler M, Dewar RJ, et al. Increases in CD4 T lymphocytes with intermittent courses of interleukin-2 in patients with human immunodeficiency virus infection. N Engl J Med 1995;332:567.

10. Anderson WF. Prospects toward human gene therapy. Science 1984;226:401.

11. Ensoli B, Barillari G, Salahuddin SZ, Gallo RC, Wong-Staal F. Tat protein of HIV-1 stimulates growth of cells derived from Kaposi's sarcoma lesions of AIDS patients. Nature 1990;344:84.

12. Laurence J, Astrin SM. Human immunodeficiency virus induction of malignant transformation in human B lymphocytes. Proc Natl Acad Sci USA 1991;88:7635.

13. Sabatier J-M, Vives E, Mabrouk K, et al. Evidence for neurotoxic activity of tat from human immunodeficiency virus type 1. J Virol 1991;65:961.

14. Banda NK, Bernier J, Kurahara DK, et al. Crosslinking CD4 by human immunodeficiency virus gp120 primes T cells for activation-induced apoptosis. J Exp Med 1992;176:1099.

15. Miller SB, Tse H, Rosenspire AJ, King SR. CD4-independent inhibition of lymphocyte proliferation mediated by HIV-1 envelope glycoproteins. Virol 1992;191:973.

16. Hill JM, Mervis RF, Avidor R, Moody TW, Brenneman DE. HIV envelope protein-induced neuronal damage and retardation of behavioral development in rat neonates. Brain Res 1993;603:222.

17. Lu Y-Y, Koga Y, Tanaka K, et al. Apoptosis induced in CD4+ cells expressing gp160 of human immunodeficiency virus type 1. J Virol 1994;68:390.

18. Morgan RA, Anderson WF. Gene therapy for AIDS. In: Kumar A, ed. Advances in molecular biology and targeted treatments for AIDS. New York: Plenum Press, 1991:301.

19. VandenDriessche T, Chuah MKL, Morgan RA. Gene therapy for acquired immune deficiency syndrome. AIDS Updates 1994;7:1.

20. Yu M, Poeschla E, Wong-Staal F. Progress towards gene therapy for HIV infection. Gene Ther 1994;1:13.

21. Gilboa E, Smith C. Gene therapy for infectious diseases: the AIDS model. Trends Genet 1994;10:139.

22. Walker R, et al. Clinical protocol: a study of the safety and survival of the adoptive transfer of genetically marked syngeneic lymphocytes in HIV infected identical twins. 1993;.

23. Ridell SR, et al. Phase I study of cellular adoptive immunotherapy using genetically modified CD8+ HIV-specific T cells for HIV seropositive patients undergoing allogeneic bone marrow transplant. Hum Gene Ther 1992;3:319.

24. Nabel G, Fox BA, Post L, Thompson CB, Woffendin C. A molecular genetic intervention for AIDS—effects of a transdominant negative form of Rev. Hum Gene Ther 1994;5:79.

25. Morgan RA, et al. Clinical protocol: gene therapy for AIDS using retroviral mediated gene transfer to deliver HIV-1 antisense TAR and transdominant REV protein genes to syngeneic lymphocytes in HIV infected identical twins. NIH Review. Hum Gene Ther 1995;12:1644.

26. Wong-Staal F, et al. Clinical protocol: a phase I clinical trial to evaluate the safety and effects in HIV-1 infected humans of autologous lymphocytes transduced with a ribozyme that cleaves HIV-1 RNA. NIH Review. Hum Gene Ther 1994;5:655.

27. Walker RE. Clinical protocol: a phase I/II pilot study of the safety of the adoptive transfer of syngeneic gene-modified cytotoxic T-lymphocytes in HIV-infected identical twins. Hum Gene Ther 1996;7:367.

28. Galpin JE, et al. Clinical protocol: a phase I clinical trial to evaluate the safety and biological activity of HIV-IT (TAF) (HIV-1IIIBenv-transduced, autologous fibroblasts) in asymptomatic HIV-1 infected cells. Hum Gene Ther 1994;5:997.

29. Haubrich R, McCutchan JA, Holdredge R, et al. An open label, phase I/II clinical trial to evaluate the safety and biological activity of HIV-IT(V) (HIV-III Benv-rev retroviral vector) in HIV-1 infected subjects. Hum Gene Ther 1995;6:941.

30. Walker BD, Chakrabarti S, Moss B, et al. HIV-specific cytotoxic T lymphocytes in seropositive individuals. Nature 1987;328:345.

31. Langlade-Demoyen P, Michel F, Hoffenbach A, et al. Immune recognition of AIDS virus antigens by human and murine cytotoxic T lymphocytes. J Immunol 1988;141:1949.

32. Walker BD, Flexner C, Paradis TJ, et al. HIV-1 reverse transcriptase is a target for cytotoxic T lymphocytes in infected individuals. Science 1988;240:64.

33. Riviere Y, Tanneau-Slavadori F, Regnault A, et al. Human immunodeficiency virus-specific cytotoxic T lymphocytes in infected individuals: distinct types of effector cells mediate killing of targets expressing gag and env proteins. J Virol 1989;63:2270.

34. Culmann B, Gomard E, Kieny M-P, et al. An antigen peptide of the HIV-1 NEF protein recognized by cytotoxic T lymphocytes of seropositive individuals in association with different HLA-B molecules. Eur J Immunol 1989;19:2383.

35. Hosmalin A, Clerici M, Houghten R, et al. An epitope in human immunodeficiency virus 1 reverse transcriptase recognized by both mouse and human cytotoxic T lymphocytes. Proc Natl Acad Sci USA 1990;87:2344.

36. McChesney M, Tanneau F, Regnault A, et al. Detection of primary cytotoxic T lymphocytes specific for the envelope glycoprotein of HIV-1 by deletion of env amino-terminal signal sequence. Eur J Immunol 1990;20:215.

37. Tsubota H, Lord CI, Watkins DI, Morimoto C, Letvin NL. A cytotoxic T lymphocyte inhibits acquired immunodeficiency syndrome virus replication in peripheral blood lymphocytes. J Exp Med 1989;169:142.

38. Pantaleo G, Koenig S, Baseler M, et al. Defective clonogenic potential of CD8+ lymphocytes in patients with AIDS: expansion in vivo of a nonclonogenic CD3+ CD8+ DR+ CD25- T cell population. J Immunol 1990;144:1696.

39. Walker BD, Plata F. Cytotoxic T lymphocytes against HIV. AIDS 1990;4:177.

40. Fauci AS, Schnittman SM, Poli G, et al. Immunopathogenic mechanisms in human immunodeficiency virus (HIV) infection. Ann Intern Med 1991;114:678.

41. Kundu SK, Merigan TC. 1991. Inverse relationship of CD8+CD11+ suppressor T cells with human immunodeficiency virus (HIV)-specific cellular cytotoxicity and natural killer cell activity in HIV-infection. Immunology 1991;74:567.

42. Carmichael A, Jin X, Sissons P, Borysiewicz L. Quantitative analysis of the human immunodeficiency virus type 1 (HIV-1)-specific cytotoxic T lymphocyte (CTL) response at different stages of HIV-1 infection: differential CTL responses to HIV-1 and Epstein-Barr virus in late disease. J Exp Med 1993;177:249.

43. Reusser P, Riddell SR, Meyers JD, Greenberg PD. Cytotoxic T-lymphocyte response to cytomegalovirus after human allogeneic bone marrow transplantation: pattern of recovery and correlation with cytomegalovirus infection and disease. Blood 1991;78:1373.

44. Lupton SD, Brunton LL, Kalkerg VA, et al. Dominant positive and negative selection using a hygromycin phosphotransferase-thymidine kinase fusion gene. Mol Cell Biol 1991;11:3374.

45. Vaishnav YN, Wong-Staal F. The biochemistry of AIDS. Annu Rev Biochem 1991;60:577.

46. Malim MH, Cullen B. Rev and the fate of pre-mRNA in the nucleus: implications for the regulation of RNA processing in eukaryotes. Mol Cell Biol 1993;13:6180.

47. Fischer U, Meyer S, Teufel M, et al. Evidence that HIV-1 Rev directly promotes the nuclear export of unspliced RNA. EMBO J 1994;13:4105.

48. Kalland KH, Szilvay AM, Brokstad KA, Saetrevik W, Haukenes G. The human immunodeficiency virus type 1 Rev protein shuttles between the cytoplasm and nuclear compartments. Mol Cell Biol 1994;14:7436.

49. Malim MH, Bohnlein S, Hauber J, Cullen BR. Functional dissection of the HIV-1 Rev trans-activator: derivation of a trans-dominant repressor of rev function. Cell 1989;58:205.

50. Mermer B, Felber BK, Campbell M, Pavlakis GN. Identification of transdominant HIV-1 rev protein mutants by direct transfer of bacterially produced proteins into human cells. Nucleic Acids Res 1990;18:2037.

51. Venkatesh LK, Chinnadurai G. Mutants in a conserved region near the carboxy-terminus of HIV-1 Rev identify functionally important residues and exhibit a dominant negative phenotype. Virology 1990;178:327.

52. Hope TJ, Klein NP, Elder ME, Parslow TG. Trans-dominant inhibition of human immunodeficiency virus type 1 rev occurs through formation of inactive protein complexes. J Virol 1992;66:1849.

53. Malim MH, Freimuth WW, Liu J, et al. Stable expression of transdominant rev protein in human T cells inhibits human immunodeficiency virus replication. J Exp Med 1992;176:1197.

54. Bahner I, Zhou C, Yu XJ, Guatelli JC, Kohn DB. Comparison of transdominant inhibitory mutant human immunodeficiency virus type 1 genes expressed by retroviral vectors in human T lymphocytes. J Virol 1993;67:3199.

55. Woffendin C, Yang, Z-Y, Udaykumar, et al. Nonviral and viral delivery of a human immunodeficiency virus protective gene into primary human T cells. Proc Natl Acad Sci USA 1994;91:11581.

56. Ragheb JA, Bressler P, Daucher M, et al. Analysis of transdominant mutants of the HIV-1 rev protein for their ability to inhibit Rev function, HIV-1 replication, and their use as anti-HIV gene therapeutics. AIDS Res Hum Retroviruses 1995;11:1343.

57. Frankel AD. Activation of HIV transcription by Tat. Curr Opin Genet Dev 1992;2:293.

58. Muesing MA, Smith DH, Capon DJ. Regulation of mRNA accumulation by a human immunodeficiency virus trans-activator protein. Cell 1987;48:691.

59. Laspia MF, Rice AP, Mathews MB. HIV-1 tat protein increases transcriptional initiation and stabilizes elongation. Cell 1989;59:283.

60. Berkhout B, Silverman RH, Jeang KT. Tat trans-activates the human immunodeficiency virus through a nascent RNA target. Cell 1989;59:273.

61. Cullen BR. Does HIV-1 Tat induce a change in viral initiation rights? Cell 1993;73:417.

62. Chuah MKL, VandenDriessche T, Chang H, Ensoli B, Morgan RA. Inhibition of human immunodeficiency virus type-1 by retroviral vectors expressing antisense TAR. Hum Gene Therapy 1995;5:1467.

63. VandenDriessche T, Chuah MKL, Chiang L, et al. In press. Inhibition of clinical HIV-1 isolates in primary CD4+ T lymphocytes by retroviral vectors expressing anti-HIV genes. J Virol 1995;69:4045.

64. Hampel A, Tritz R, Hicks M, Cruz P. Hairpin catalytic RNA model: evidence for helices and sequence requirement for substrate RNA. Nucleic Acids Res 1990;18:299.

65. Hampel A, Tritz R, Hicks M, Cruz P. . Nucleic Acids Res 1990;18:299.

66. Ojwang JO, Hampel A, Looney DJ, Wong-Staal F, Rappaport J. Inhibition of human immunodeficiency virus type 1 expression by a hairpin ribozyme. Proc Natl Acad Sci USA 1992;89:10802.

67. Yu M, Ojwang J, Yamada O, et al. A hairpin ribozyme inhibits expression of diverse strains of human immunodeficiency virus type 1. Proc Natl Acad Sci USA 1993;90:6340.

68. Yamada O, Yu M, Yee JK, et al. Intracellular immunization of human T cells with a hairpin ribozyme against human immunodeficiency virus type 1. Gene Ther 1994;1:38.

69. Coffin J. HIV population dynamics in vivo: implications for generic variation, pathogenesis, and therapy. Science 1995;267:483.

70. Leavitt MC, Yu M, Yamada O, et al. Transfer of an anti–HIV-1 ribozyme gene into primary human lymphocytes. Hum Gene Ther 1994; 5:1115.

71. Yu M, Leavitt MC, Maruyama M, et al. Intracellular immunization of human fetal cord blood stem/progenitor cells with a ribozyme against human immunodeficiency virus type 1. Proc Natl Acad Sci USA 1995;92:699.

72. Fast P, Walker MC, Wescott SL, Schultz AM. Phase I/II trials of candidate HIV-1 vaccines. AIDS Res Hum Retroviruses 1994;10:S114.

73. Warner JF, Anderson C-G, Laube L, et al. Induction of HIV-specific CTL and antibody responses in mice using retroviral vector-transduced cells. AIDS Res Hum Retroviruses 1991;7:645.

74. Chada S, DeJesus CE, Townsend K, et al. Cross-reactive lysis of human targets infected with prototypic and clinical human immunodeficiency virus type 1 (HIV-1) strains by murine anti–HIV-1 IIIB env-specific cytotoxic T lymphocytes. J Virol 1993;67:3409.

75. Laube LS, Burrascano M, De Jesus CE, et al. Cytotoxic T lymphocytes (CTL) and antibody responses generated in rhesus monkeys immunized with retroviral vector transduced fibroblasts expressing HIV-1 IIIB env/rev proteins. Hum Gene Ther 1994;5:583.

76. Irwin MJ, Laube LS, Lee V, et al. Direct injection of recombinant retroviral vector induces human immunodeficiency virus-sepcific immune responses in mice and nonhuman primates. J Virol 1994; 68:5036.

77. Embretson J, Zupancic M, Ribas JL, et al. Massive covert infection of helper T lymphocytes and macrophages by HIV during the incubation period of AIDS. Nature 1993;362:359.

78. Pantaleo G, Graziosi C, Demarest JF, et al. HIV infection is active and progressive in lymphoid tissue during the clinically latent stage of disease. Nature 1993;362:355.

79. Li Y, Kappes J, Conway JA, et al. Molecular characterization of human immunodeficiency virus type 1 cloned directly from uncultured human brain tissue: identification of replication-competent and -defective viral genomes. J Virol 1991;65:3973.

80. Temin HM, Bolognesi DP. Where has HIV been hiding? Nature 1993;362:292.

PART VI

Psychosocial Aspects

AIDS: Biology, Diagnosis, Treatment and
Prevention, fourth edition, edited by Vincent T.
DeVita, Jr., Samuel Hellman, and Steven A.
Rosenberg. Lippincott–Raven Publishers, © 1997

CHAPTER 26

Counseling Persons Seropositive for Human Immunodeficiency Virus Infection and Their Families

Lynda S. Doll and Beth A. Dillon

Through June 1994, 401,749 persons with AIDS had been reported to the Centers for Disease Control and Prevention.[1] More than 600,000 additional persons are thought to be infected with HIV in the United States,[2] although as many as 50% may not have been tested and notified of their infection status.[3] As the number of persons with HIV infection and AIDS increases, so too does the need for high-quality counseling to address the social, psychologic, and medical needs of infected persons and their families.

To date, the published literature on HIV-related counseling has focused largely on counseling issues and techniques surrounding the initial notification of test results.[4] This chapter expands on this literature by reviewing available data on issues and concerns of adult persons with HIV infection and their families, not only at initial notification but throughout the chronic infection phase of the disease. Because there are excellent references describing counseling techniques,[5,6] we focus here on an overview of selected counseling themes that may be particularly salient across the disease course. These are specific issues that may be amenable to short-term, focused counseling intervention by a range of health professionals working with HIV-infected persons and their families. These individuals may also require in-depth psychotherapy from trained mental health professionals for concerns such as depression and severe anxiety.

The research literature on the experiences of infected persons and their families is at this point quite small and qualita-

tive in nature. The extant quantitative literature focuses largely on gay men and may not be representative of other populations.

THE HIV DISEASE COURSE

Medical and counseling professionals must be knowledgeable about the HIV disease course to understand the experiences and concerns of infected persons and their families. The HIV infection course is usually divided into three phases: (1) an acute infection phase, characterized by flu-like symptoms, which is experienced by 50% to 70% of infected persons[7]; (2) a much longer, chronic infection phase, characterized by initial symptom-free periods and then gradual impairment of the immune system and the occurrence of a spectrum of medical conditions that can lower quality of life[8]; and (3) a final crisis phase, characterized by collapse of the immune system and the presence of AIDS-defining illnesses. Progression through these phases varies among individuals, both in length of time and in severity of HIV-related manifestations. Median time from HIV infection to AIDS diagnosis is estimated to be approximately 10 years among adults.[9] Median survival time from severe immunosuppression or AIDS diagnosis is estimated to be 18 to 24 months (Debra Hanson, personal communication, CDC, March 1995).

HIV DISEASE AND THE FAMILY

Research and clinical reports have emphasized the importance of the family in the emotional, physical, and financial support of infected persons. This same literature has also highlighted the complex emotional burdens and caregiving responsibilities challenging families and the difficulties they experience in

Lynda S. Doll and Beth A. Dillon: National Center for HIV, STD, and TB Prevention, Centers for Disease Control and Prevention, US Public Health Service, Department of Health and Human Services, 1600 Clifton Road, Mailstop D21, Atlanta, GA 30333, phone 404-639-0935, fax 404-639-0910.

performing these tasks.[10,11] In working with HIV-infected persons, health professionals must broaden their definition of family to encompass both biologic and functional families, including sex partners and close social networks among homosexual men.[12] Health professionals must also be aware of the broader context of the lives of many families with HIV-infected members, which may include homelessness, single parenthood, unsafe physical environments, and substance abuse. It may be impossible to address HIV-related issues without also addressing some of these larger concerns.

Partners or other family members may ask to be present during contacts with the health professional, including initial notification of test results. Some clinicians have suggested that the family, and not the individual alone, should be the basic unit of care for purposes of counseling.[12] The preference of the seropositive patient must be the deciding factor in decisions related to family involvement in counseling. However, other important factors may include the duration of the relationship, whether there has been mutual disclosure between partners or family members about risk behaviors, and the supportive quality of the relationship.

COUNSELING ISSUES ACROSS THE DISEASE PHASES

The individual variability that occurs in length and severity of the disease course also occurs in the range of emotional and social responses of both patients and family members to the HIV infection. The characteristic coping strategies, social support structure, previous interpersonal experience with HIV, and the health status of each individual at the time of engagement with the health professional all influence the response to HIV infection and predict the counseling techniques and resources required. Assessment of each of these factors is critical to providing appropriate and beneficial counseling throughout the disease course.

IMMEDIATE POSTNOTIFICATION PHASE

The immediate tasks of the health professional after notifying an individual of a seropositive test result are to provide emotional support, to give accurate, up-to-date information about HIV infection, to encourage the identification of social support, and to provide referral for medical care, social services, and risk reduction interventions, including drug treatment. The health professional must also assist in the development of a short-term plan of action.[13,14]

Individual reactions to receipt of a seropositive test result range from intense emotion to resignation or shock.[15-17] Research suggests that these reactions depend on a number of factors, including test result expectations, whether the initial notification occurred simultaneously with an AIDS diagnosis or with the experiencing of significant AIDS-related symptoms, and whether the individual is part of a social network that includes persons with similar AIDS-related concerns.[4] In some cases, the anxiety associated with having an HIV test may have been so severe that the impact of positive results is softened by the resolution of uncertainty.

Health professionals should be cautioned to avoid preconceived expectations about a patient's response to result notification and corresponding needs for counseling, support, and referral.[15] One person may require intensive counseling although the immediate medical situation requires only routine follow-up. Another person may encounter a critical medical situation yet have good social and emotional support and require little counseling.

Stress management workshops before or after HIV testing may be helpful for some. Research has suggested that such interventions may buffer the psychologic impact of receiving positive test results. For example, a prenotification, cognitive-behavioral stress management intervention significantly decreased the level of depression among gay men receiving positive results.[18] Similarly, in a study of seropositive, asymptomatic adults, psychologic distress significantly decreased among individuals who received postnotification stress prevention training, compared with persons who received standard counseling.[19]

Health professionals should also be cautioned against attempting to address the continuum of informational, support, and clinical care issues in the same counseling session in which notification occurs. The individual's emotional reaction and capacity to absorb information should determine the content, duration, and intensity of the session.[15] Several sessions may be required to complete an adequate assessment of the patient's support needs.

CHRONIC INFECTION PHASE

After the immediate postnotification period, HIV-infected individuals and their families face a number of tasks and issues that may impact long-term quality of life and access to health care. Among these are (1) disclosing their serostatus to significant others; (2) seeking meaning in living with an HIV diagnosis; (3) making critical decisions about safer sexual behavior and drug use, reproductive choices, and custody planning for children; (4) adopting healthy coping strategies; (5) seeking social support; (6) managing social distancing in relationships; and (7) coping with the uncertainty of the disease course.

Disclosure

A critical task of health care providers in the immediate postnotification period is to counsel infected individuals and their families on when and to whom to disclose their serostatus. Disclosure permits the infected person to access much-needed physical and social support, to openly seek health care, and to follow medical regimens. It may also facilitate discussions about safer sex with partners and custody planning for children. Disclosure to close family members may be particularly important to facilitate family cohesion and provide opportunities for anticipatory grieving.

Data on actual disclosure patterns show that HIV-infected persons selectively inform significant others. Furthermore, at least among gay men, the amount of disclosure increases with the stage of illness and overt physical symptoms.[20,21] Disclosure rates among gay men vary but have generally been found to be highest for sex partners, somewhat lower for mothers, siblings, coworkers, and friends, and lowest for fathers, employers, landlords, and religious leaders.[20,21] Disclosure to family members and colleagues may not occur until HIV symptoms appear. Fisher and associates[22] found the percentage of family members informed by gay men of their status to range from 50% among seropositive patients to 81% among men diagnosed with AIDS.

Studies of infected women have shown high rates of disclosure to at least one person (95%) and relatively high rates to five or more persons (60%).[23] High rates of disclosure to primary male partners (81% to 85%) have also been found, with most of this disclosure (86%) occurring within a few weeks of notification.[24] No published quantitative data are available on the frequency of disclosure by families members to others.

Concerns that may impact disclosure decisions include anticipated AIDS-related stigma or discrimination; expectations of rejection or relationship disruption, including violent behavior; and desire to protect significant others, particularly children.

Concerns About Stigma or Discrimination

Specific instances of discrimination against persons with HIV or their families have been described in the published literature.[25–28] The actual frequency of experiences of AIDS-related stigma or discrimination is unknown but may be less common than anticipated by infected persons. For example, although 75% of 54 HIV-infected injecting drug users expected seronegative persons to avoid touching infected persons, only 15% had experienced such occurrences. Nonetheless, both expectations and experiences with stigma were associated with depression and anxiety in this sample.[29] Such concerns may significantly affect disclosure decisions.

Concerns About Rejection

Data on expected versus actual experiences of rejection or relationship disruption after disclosure follow a similar pattern. In a qualitative study of 50 infected women, Gielen and colleagues[23] found that although two thirds expected negative responses such as rejection and violence from their primary male partner, more than three fourths reported acceptance, support, and understanding after disclosure. Similarly, Clark and colleagues[24] found that infected women who had not disclosed their serostatus to their main partner (19% of 122 women) feared psychologic rejection, relationship disruption, anger, or physical violence if they did so, but among those who had disclosed, 95% reported feeling very or moderately accepted by their main partner.

Studies of gay men have also shown concerns about anticipated negative reactions.[20,21] Fisher and colleagues[22] found that the least favorable reactions were from male family members, landlords, and sex partners. However, overall in the two studies that have examined this issue in gay men, disclosure was well received within the social networks of the participants,[30] and the majority of men reported that their primary relationships remained strong 6 months after notification.[31]

Concerns About Violence

Concerns about violence toward infected persons have surfaced not only in the context of disclosure but more generally as well. Approximately 7% of women interviewed by Gilien and colleagues[23] had experienced some violence as a result of disclosure. Most of these violent episodes were verbal fights or threats. In a national convenience sample of HIV-infected persons,[27] 17% of women and 12% of men reported experiencing violence in the home, and 21% of both groups reported experiencing violence in the community because of their seropositive status. Moore and associates[32] found that approximately 10% of 510 women studied had been physically attacked or raped within the past 12 months, with the rates equally high for infected and uninfected women. Neither study associated the violent episodes temporally with disclosure of HIV serostatus.[27,32] Research on the frequency and social context of violence targeted toward infected persons is limited and yet essential in order to understand the daily stressors experienced by these patients. Health professionals should routinely screen for the potential for violence and be prepared to provide appropriate social service referrals.

There are few quantitative data available on perceived concerns and consequences of families related to disclosure. Qualitative research has suggested that disclosure by family members to their extended social networks may be avoided because of the association between HIV and homosexuality, illicit drug use, and perceived sexual infidelity.[12] Although the data are limited, HIV-infected parents report that disclosure to their children is the most difficult decision they face.[33] Mothers report not wanting to burden their children, in order to allow them to "just be children." Mothers also report concern about whether younger children will broadly disclose their parent's illness to others and potentially face AIDS-related stigma themselves.

In discussing disclosure decisions, the health professional should encourage individuals to weigh the likelihood of both positive and negative responses from others. In addition, the individual should be encouraged to consider the pros and cons of when to disclose, including the emotional distress of maintaining secrecy until later in the disease course.[20,33,34] Learning about other persons' positive experiences with disclosure (eg, through support groups) may be helpful in dispelling fears about potential stigma, relationship disruption, and violence. Ultimately, however, decisions about when and whom to inform must be made by the

HIV-infected person and his or her family members, and the health professional must guard against encouraging premature disclosure.

Sense of Meaning

A second critical task of health professionals, and one that has received less research attention, is helping infected persons and their families assimilate the HIV diagnosis and set new life goals. Clinical reports and qualitative research results have suggested that HIV disease can lead to major disorganization in the lives of infected persons and their families. Alternatively, it can result in refocusing with new and purposeful life goals.[16,35,36] Linn and associates[37] found that persons who rated themselves as having achieved a sense of meaning and purpose in their lives reported higher self-esteem and less anxiety.

Health professionals may help infected persons gain a sense of meaning by helping them mentally process and reframe the illness as an opportunity for personal growth and challenge.[38] The process of life review can be used to help individuals evaluate their past goals and accomplishments and establish directions and priorities for the future.[16] It is important also to give patients both a sense of optimism and realistic information about what to expect. Depending on the stage of illness, the counselor may need to help the infected person to plan for living with a chronic, progressively debilitating disease, or, for those approaching death, to work through their grief related to the many losses they are experiencing.

Critical Decisions

A third critical task of health professionals is to assist infected persons and their family members in a series of critical decisions related to risk reduction behaviors, reproductive choices, and, if necessary, custody planning for children.

Risk Reduction Behaviors

The effectiveness of single-session, face-to-face counseling in promoting safer sexual behaviors and drug use has primarily been examined in conjunction with HIV counseling and testing. These data suggest limited success with long-term behavior change after a single counseling session, although research has shown greater behavior change among seropositive than among seronegative individuals.[4] Reviews of the behavior change literature suggest that risk reduction counseling should occur repeatedly over time to assist the individual to initiate and maintain behavior change.[39] To be effective, counseling should also (1) review information on how to avoid transmission, (2) encourage development of skills to implement the behavior changes (eg, purchasing condoms, negotiating with partners), (3) ensure that the needed devices are available (eg, condoms, clean needles and syringes, bleach), (4) identify strategies and social support for behavior change, and (5) motivate behavior change by addressing the social and psychologic context within which risk behaviors occurs.[39] Because continued risk behaviors frequently occur within primary relationships,[40,41] counseling of couples may be particularly beneficial. Similarly, given the frequency of sexual risk behaviors in the context of drug and alcohol use,[42] the health professional should initiate discussions about substance use and advocate for treatment.

Reproductive Choices

Approximately 7000 HIV-infected women give birth each year.[43] Some of these women chose to conceive or to deliver despite knowledge of their seropositive status. Others learn their serostatus when they give birth. The reasons infected women choose to give birth are complex and may include wishing to experience motherhood for its personal or social meanings, to replace a child lost through death, or to leave behind a "living legacy."[44] The reasons infected women choose not to conceive or to abort a pregnancy are equally complex, ranging from fears of perinatal transmission, to concerns about leaving the child behind when they die, to the impact of the pregnancy on their own disease progression.[33] The role of health professionals in reproductive decisionmaking is to provide sound medical information and a supportive, nonjudgmental environment in which the woman can explore the choices available to her. Health professionals should help patients explore their own personal values related to motherhood as well as the social pressures that they may be encountering.

Custody Planning

Health professionals may also need to assist parents in making choices about custody plans for their children. It has been estimated that by the year 2000 there will be as many as 125,000 children in the United States who have lost their mothers to HIV,[45] and many of these mothers will have provided the only consistent parenting that these children have known. Mothers differ in their ability to become involved in custody planning. Some actively seeking placement through a relative, friend, or social service agency; others fail to make any plans. If available, social service programs such as New York City's Early Permanency Planning Program[46] are excellent referral sources. These programs attempt to ease the child's transition into alternative care by assisting the mother in disclosing her illness to family members and in selecting a custody placement. They also try to ensure that social service entitlements continue to be available for the child in the new home.

Coping Strategies

A fourth critical issue health professionals may need to address is the coping strategies that patients and their families use to manage living with HIV infection. These include

(1) problem-focused strategies, such as planning a course of action, negotiating, and maintaining health-promoting behaviors such as proper diet, exercise, and sleep; (2) emotion-focused strategies, such as maintaining a positive attitude; using mental distraction, and seeking social support; and (3) escape or avoidance strategies, such as avoiding social contact, drug or alcohol abuse, excessive sleeping, and denial of serostatus or the presence of symptoms.

In studies of gay men[38,47] and of men with hemophilia (Rex Forehand, PhD, Institute for Behavioral Research, University of Georgia, personal communication, March 1995), problem-focused strategies have been associated with less psychologic distress, higher self-esteem, and fewer self-reported physical symptoms than have avoidance strategies. Emotion-focused strategies have been found to be common responses to HIV infection among gay men and injecting drug users, perhaps because they are strategies aimed at managing the emotional consequences of the uncontrollable aspects of the disease.[48,49] In a study of a large, diverse sample of persons with AIDS, Fleishman and Fogel[47] found that avoidance strategies were used more frequently by persons of color. Moreover, such strategies increased with length of time since notification, symptom intensity, and use of injection drugs. Avoidance strategies are particularly problematic, in part because they may prevent individuals from receiving social support. No quantitative data are available on coping strategies used by family members of persons with HIV infection.

In counseling infected persons and their families, health professionals should build on individual and family strengths, including previously successful methods of coping.[11] Problem- and emotion-focused coping strategies should be encouraged, especially strategies that are associated with higher levels of social support.[16] Emotion-focused coping may be particularly helpful if the stressful event or condition cannot be changed.[48] Group-based interventions have also been successfully tested that include instruction in these strategies.[50] Finally, screening and referral for increased drug or alcohol use may be necessary.[34]

Social Support

A fifth critical task of health professionals is to assist the patient in identifying sources of social support. Social support is defined as the comfort, information, and assistance provided by family, friends, and institutional representatives such as health care providers.[51] Adequate availability and perceived satisfaction from social support have been shown to be associated with lower psychologic distress and the use of healthy coping strategies among persons with HIV.[38,51–53] Additional studies have suggested an inverse relation between social support and self-reported physical health.[52,54]

During counseling, health professionals must assess the infected person's existing support networks and encourage the identification of new sources. Support groups, volunteer buddies, and health professionals are sources of formal support and may become increasingly important later in the dis-

ease course.[16,55] Research has suggested that peers, rather than family members, are the most common and most effective sources of support among gay men.[51] African American gay men[38] and injecting drug users[47] have been shown to seek social support less frequently than white gay men.

There are few data on the availability of social support for HIV-infected heterosexual men and women or for families of infected persons. Qualitative research suggests that health professionals may need to counter the perception that HIV-related support systems, such as those found in gay communities, are not available to heterosexual men and women.[12] This literature also suggests that the caregiving provided by women to children and other infected family members may complicate their own ability to access social support[16] and that families with an infected member frequently choose to maintain secrecy and thus are often isolated from extended support networks.[56] Because of this isolation, health professionals may play a particularly important support role for families with infected members.

Social Distancing

A sixth phenomenon experienced in varying forms by infected persons and their families is social distancing. This distancing can occur in close personal relationships and within more formal relationships, including those with health care providers and employers. Social distancing may occur because of attitudes toward behaviors or medical conditions associated with HIV (eg, homosexual behavior, severe hemophilia)[52] or toward the terminal prognosis of the disease.[54] Fears of contagion can motivate physical distancing and constrain sexual and affectional intimacy between sex partners and family members.[57] Anxiety related to transmission may also hamper the physical caregiving provided by family members to infected persons. Despite widespread knowledge about routes of HIV transmission among the American public, counseling of infected persons and their families regarding the likelihood of transmission through casual contact continues to be an important role of health professionals.

To counterbalance negative experiences related to social distancing, the health professional should help infected individuals and their families identify sources of formal or informal support early in the disease course, rather than seeking support only during severe distress.[47] As the disease progresses, infected individuals may find themselves increasingly weakened and isolated because of debilitating illnesses and thus unable to seek new support.[54]

Uncertainty About Disease Course

Anxieties about the uncertainty of the HIV disease course have been well documented in the qualitative nursing literature.[35,36] Reactions to this uncertainty may begin with initial notification and intensify over time. For example, infected persons report monitoring of visual signs and symptoms such as weight loss, skin problems, oral thrush, and T-cell counts to assess disease progression.[16,34]

Symptomatic persons have been shown to need extensive information from their health care providers about their treatment options, health insurance and prognosis, as well as how their experiences compare with those of others. In a sample of symptomatic gay men, degree of satisfaction with informational support was critical in buffering stress associated with physical symptoms.[51] In contrast, research suggests that asymptomatic gay men may have fewer informational needs and in fact may avoid AIDS-related information. By understanding the psychologic impact of uncertainty and helping the individual gather information on physical symptoms and the disease course, the health professional may contribute to the individual's sense of control and predictability over the disease course.[51]

INTERVENTION MODELS

The social and medical issues associated with HIV infection complicate the already difficult task of providing counseling to patients and families dealing with a chronic and terminal illness. The evolving needs of HIV-infected persons and their families require multiple counseling approaches and extensive referral sources.[5,16,58] As we have noted, counseling may be required for numerous concerns including disclosure, intimacy, sexuality, substance abuse, family planning, and death and dying. Approaches may include brief counseling interventions, crisis intervention, long-term psychotherapy, support and recovery groups, and family counseling. Each of these areas of focus and models of counseling requires specific expertise and skill.

Ideally, a multidisciplinary team should collaborate to meet the needs of the patient and the family. At any given time, a physician, nurse, nutritionist, social worker, psychologist, AIDS service provider, "buddy," or chaplin may be needed to address complex counseling and support needs. The interplay between medical and psychosocial issues in managing HIV infection strongly argue for an integrated approach to clinical care and counseling support.[59] This integrated and multidisciplinary approach provides a model for ensuring that the HIV-infected person and his or her family receive the counseling and support services responsive to their evolving needs.

CONCLUSION

Although our knowledge about responses to HIV has increased over time, additional research is needed to guide our counseling efforts. We must better understand at what age and point in the disease course parents should disclose their serostatus to a child, how individuals cope with social distancing or instances of discrimination, and which counseling models are most effective with different concerns and at different points along the disease course. We also need to better understand the influence of provider characteristics on counseling effectiveness. Most importantly, we must understand how to encourage the large and diverse group of professionals who work with HIV-infected persons and their families to develop and utilize effective counseling skills to help improve the quality of life among those living with HIV infection.

REFERENCES

1. Centers for Disease Control and Prevention. HIV/AIDS surveillance report, midyear edition, vol 6. Atlanta: Centers for Disease Control and Prevention, 1994.
2. Centers for Disease Control. Estimates of HIV prevalence and projected AIDS cases: summary of a workshop, October 31–November 1, 1989. MMWR 1989;39:110.
3. Anderson JE, Fichtner R, Campbell CH. How many HIV positive persons in the U.S. have been tested for HIV antibodies? Presented at the Ninth International AIDS Conference, Berlin, 1993.
4. Doll LS, Kennedy MB. HIV counselling and testing: what is it and how well does it work? In: Schochetman G, George JR, eds. AIDS testing, 2nd ed. New York: Springer-Verlag, 1994:302.
5. Bor R, Miller R, Goldman E. Theory and practice of HIV counselling. London: Cassell, 1992.
6. Davis H, Fallowfield L. Counselling and communication in health care. Chichester, England: John Wiley & Sons, 1991.
7. Smith D, Moore J. Epidemiology, manifestations, and treatment of HIV infection in women. In: O'Leary A, Jemmott L, eds. Women and AIDS: the emerging epidemic. New York: Plenum (in press).
8. Stulberg I, Buckingham SL. Parallel issues for AIDS patients, families, and others. Social Casework 1988;69:355.
9. Rutherford GW, Lifson AR, Hessol NA, et al. Course of HIV-1 infection in a cohort of homosexual and bisexual men: an 11-year follow-up study. BMJ 1990;301:1183.
10. Williams RJ, Stafford WB. Silent casualties: partners, families, and spouses of persons with AIDS. Journal of Counselling & Development 1991;69:423.
11. Lippmann SB, James WA, Frierson RL. AIDS and the family: implications for counselling. AIDS Care 1993;5:71.
12. Tiblier KB, Walker G, Rolland JS. Therapeutic issues when working with families of persons with AIDS. Marriage and Family Review 1989;13:81.
13. Centers for Disease Control and Prevention. HIV counselling, testing and referral standards & guidelines. Atlanta: Centers for Disease Control and Prevention, 1994.
14. World Health Organization. Guidelines for counselling about HIV infection and disease. WHO AIDS Series 8. Geneva: World Health Organization, 1990.
15. Bor R, Miller R, Goldman E, Scher I. The meaning of bad news in HIV disease: counselling about dreaded issues revisited. Counseling Psychology Quarterly 1993;6:69.
16. Hoffman MA. Counseling the HIV-infected client: a psychosocial model for assessment and intervention. Counsel Psychol 1991;19:467.
17. Roncone R, Core L, Casacchia M. Counselling and psychoeducational interventions in HIV infection. New Trends in Experimental and Clinical Psychiatry 1993;9:137.
18. Antoni MH, Baggett L, Ironson G, et al. Cognitive-behavioral stress management intervention buffers distress responses and immunologic changes following notification of HIV-1 seropositivity. J Consult Clin Psychol 1991;59:906.
19. Perry S, Fishman B, Jacobsberg L, Young J, Frances A. Effectiveness of psychoeducational interventions in reducing emotional distress after human immunodeficiency virus antibody testing. Arch Gen Psychiatry 1991;48:143.
20. Hays RB, McKusick L, Pollack L, Hilliard R, Hoff C, Coates TJ. Disclosing HIV seropositivity to significant others. AIDS 1993;7:425.
21. Marks G, Bundek NI, Richardson JL, Ruiz MS, Maldonado N, Mason HRC. Self-disclosure of HIV infection: preliminary results from a sample of Hispanic men. Health Psychol 1992;11:300.
22. Fisher L, Goldschmidt RH, Hays RB, Catania JA. Families of homosexual men: their knowledge and support regarding sexual orientation and HIV disease. J Am Board Fam Pract 1993;6:25.

23. Gielen AC, O'Campo P, Faden RR, Eke A. Women with HIV: disclosure concerns and experiences. Presented at the HIV Infection in Women Conference, Washington DC, 1995.

24. Clark LF, Solomon L, Schoenbaum E, Schuman P, Boland B. HIV positive women's disclosure of HIV status to primary partners. Presented at the annual meetings of the American Psychological Association, Los Angeles, 1994.

25. Pryor JB, Reeder GD. Collective and individual representations of HIV/AIDS stigma. In: Pryor JB, Reeder GD, eds. The social psychology of HIV infection. Hillsdale, NJ: Lawrence Erlbaum Associates, 1993:263.

26. Herek GM, Glunt EK. Public attitudes toward AIDS-related issues in the United States. In: Pryor JB, Reeder GD, eds. The social psychology of HIV infection. Hillsdale, NJ: Lawrence Erlbaum Associates, 1993:229.

27. National Association of People With AIDS. HIV in America: a profile of the challenges facing Americans living with HIV. Washington DC: National Association of People With AIDS, 1992.

28. Powell-Cope GM, Brown MA. Going public as an AIDS family caregiver. Soc Sci Med 1992;34:571.

29. Demas PA, Wills TA. HIV-related stigma and psychosocial adjustment in the injecting drug user population. Presented at the annual meeting of the Society for Behavioral Medicine, 1995.

30. Stempel R, Moulton J, Moss AR. Disclosure of HIV-antibody test results, reactions, and reasons for non-disclosure. Presented at the International AIDS Conference, Berlin, 1990.

31. Schnell DJ, Higgins DL, Wilson RM, Goldbaum G, Cohn DL, Wolitski RJ. Men's disclosure of HIV test results to male primary sex partners. Am J Public Health 1992;82:1675.

32. Moore J, Solomon L, Schoenbaum E, et al. Factors associated with stressful events and depressive symptoms among HIV infected and uninfected women. Presented at the HIV Infection in Women Conference, Washington DC, 1995.

33. Armistead L, Forehand R. For whom the bell tolls: parenting decisions and challenges faced by mothers who are HIV seropositive. Clin Psychol: Science and Practice (in press).

34. Demas P, Schoenbaum EE, Wills TA, Doll LS, Klein RS. Stress, coping and attitudes toward treatment in injecting drug users: a qualitative study. AIDS Educ Prev 1995;7:429.

35. Brown MA, Powell-Cope GM. AIDS family caregiving: transitions through uncertainty. Nurs Res 1991;40:338.

36. McCain NL, Gramling LF. Living With dying: coping with HIV disease. Issues Ment Health Nurs 1992;13:271.

37. Linn JG, Lewis FM, Cain VA, Kimbrough GA. HIV-illness, social support, sense of coherence, and psychosocial well-being in a sample of help-seeking adults. AIDS Educ Prev 1993;5:254.

38. Leserman L, Perkins DO, Evans DL. Coping with the threat of AIDS: the role of social support. Am J Psychiatry 1992;149:11.

39. Choi KH, Coates TJ. Prevention of HIV infection. AIDS 1994;8:1371.

40. Doll LS, Byers RH, Bolan G, et al. Homosexual men who engage in high-risk sexual behavior: a multicenter comparison. Sex Transm Dis 1991;18:170.

41. Padian NS, O'Brien TR, Chang Y, Glass S, Francis DP. Prevention of heterosexual transmission of human immunodeficiency virus through couple counseling. J Acquir Immune Defic Syndr 1993;6:1043.

42. Coates TJ, Faigle, M, Koijane J, Stall RD. Does HIV prevention work for men who have sex with men? Washington DC: Office of Technology Assessment, 1995.

43. Centers for Disease Control. Update: AIDS among women—United States, 1994. MMWR 1995;44:84.

44. Wander N, Downing M, Fogarty L, Lockaby T, Milstein B, CDC Prevention of HIV in Women and Infants Demonstration Project Investigators. The many meanings of motherhood for women affected by HIV. Presented at the meeting of the American Psychological Association on Psychological and Behavioral Factors in Women's Health. Washington DC, 1994.

45. Levine C, Stein GL. Orphans of the HIV epidemic: unmet needs in six U.S. cities. New York: The Orphan Project, 1994.

46. Prince RJ. The child welfare administration's early permanency planning project. In: Levine C, ed. Orphans of the HIV epidemic. New York: United Hospital Fund of New York, 1993.

47. Fleishman JA, Fogel B. Coping and depressive symptoms among people with AIDS. Health Psychol 1994;13:156.

48. Taylor SE, Kemeny ME, Schneider SG, Aspinwall LG. Coping with the threat of AIDS. In: Pryor JB, Reeder GD, eds. The social psychology of HIV infection. Hillsdale, NJ: Lawrence Erlbaum Associates, 1993:305.

49. Namir S, Wolcott DL, Fawzy FI, Alumbaugh MJ. Coping with AIDS: psychological and health implications. J Appl Soc Psychol 1987;17:309.

50. Chesney MA, Folkman S. Psychological impact of HIV disease and implications for intervention. Psychiatr Clin North Am 1994;17:163.

51. Hays RB, Turner H, Coates TJ. Social support, AIDS-related symptoms, and depression among gay men. J Consult Clin Psychol 1992;60:463.

52. Green G. Editorial review: social support and HIV. AIDS Care 1993;5:87.

53. Kelly JA, Murphy DA, Bahr GR, et al. Factors associated with severity of depression and high-risk sexual behavior among persons diagnosed with human immunodeficiency virus (HIV) infection. Health Psychol 1993;12:215.

54. Namir S, Alumbaugh MJ, Fawzy FI, Wolcott DL. The relationship of social support to physical and psychological aspects of AIDS. Psychol Health 1989;3:77.

55. Catania JA, Turner HA, Choi KH, Coates TJ. Coping with death anxiety: help-seeking and social support among gay men with various HIV diagnoses. AIDS 1992;6:999.

56. Cates JA, Graham LL, Boeglin D, Tielker S. The effect of AIDS on the family system. Families in Society 1990;71:195.

57. Moneyham L, Seals B, Demi A, Sowell R, Cohen L, Guillory J. Perceptions of stigma in women infected with HIV. Presented at HIV Infection in Women Conference, Washington DC, 1995.

58. Martelli LJ, Peltz FD, Messina W. When someone you know has AIDS. New York: Crown Publishers, 1987.

59. Feingold A, Slammon WR. A model integrating mental and primary care services for families with HIV. Gen Hosp Psychiatry 1993;15:290.

AIDS: Biology, Diagnosis, Treatment and Prevention, fourth edition, edited by Vincent T. DeVita, Jr., Samuel Hellman, and Steven A. Rosenberg. Lippincott–Raven Publishers, © 1997

CHAPTER 27

Psychiatric Considerations in Human Immunodeficiency Virus Disease

David G. Ostrow

The increasingly chronic nature of infection with human immunodeficiency virus-1 (HIV-1) and risk of transmission of this still incurable infection creates a natural history of mental health functioning and coping that parallels the physiologic effects of HIV-1. This natural history ranges from preoccupations about risk of becoming infected (ie, the "worried well"), to initial infection, through asymptomatic and symptomatic infection, to acquired immunodeficiency syndrome (AIDS), to terminal illness.

This chapter describes the psychologic challenges and adaptation of persons living with HIV-1 infection (PWHIVs). Attention has been focussed on the 10% to 20% of PWHIVs, also referred to as nonprogressors, whose illness does not appear to progress to AIDS over 10 or more years of infection and on persons with AIDS, also referred to as long-term survivors, who have survived 5 or more years since the AIDS diagnosis. In terms of the neuropsychiatric natural history of HIV-1 infection, it has similarly been observed that most PWHIVs do not experience major dysfunctional episodes, prompting more attention on the factors that confer psychologic resilience among most PWHIVs. I also discuss the vulnerabilities and resources that each individual brings to the experience of living with this virus and the roles that psychiatrists and other mental health professionals can play in recognizing these individual coping factors and working with each patient to minimize the negative impact while maximizing the positive impact that HIV-1 infection can have on their life course (Table 27-1).

The mental health natural history of HIV-1 infection may also be divided into sequential phases (see Table 27-1).[1] In the first phase, the at-risk person is engaging in sexual or drug use behaviors, placing them at significant risk for acquiring primary HIV-1 infection. The second phase encompasses the period between primary infection or exposure and the emergence of antibodies to HIV-1 seroconversion. This period may range from a few weeks to months, but seroconversion usually usually occurs within 6 months of exposure. The third phase is known as the asymptomatic phase; it is that period between seroconversion and the development of serious symptoms. This period is highly variable, lasting from months to many years, although averaging 9 to 10 years for gay, white men.[2] Although an individual may not experience severe or life-threatening disease during this phase, he may experience intermittent symptoms such as night sweats, rashes, or diarrhea. Some persons may experience more serious physiologic symptoms, such as fatigue and weight loss, which can be incapacitating at times. The fourth phase begins with symptoms of severe immunosuppression or the diagnosis of significant neurologic impairment, a life-threatening opportunistic infection, a secondary neoplasm, a debilitating wasting syndrome, or a CD4 lymphocyte count below 200/µL. At this point, a person is diagnosed as having AIDS according to specific criteria developed by the Centers for Disease Control (CDC).[3]

During each of these stages, an individual may experience a variety of mental health problems. Specific problems that are more likely to occur at a particular stage of HIV-1 infection are indicated in Table 27-1.

A biopsychosocial conceptualization of HIV-1 disease means that mental health, well-being, and cognitive functioning become the ultimate determinants of the quality of life. Many of the proponents of holistic health would argue that mental health influences physical health, measured in terms of length of survival (ie, long-term survival), rate of immunologic deterioration (ie, psychoimmunology), and neurologic functioning (ie, psychoneuroimmunology). If mental disorders are properly detected and treated among HIV-1–infected

David G. Ostrow, Medical College of Wisconsin, Department of Psychiatry and Behavioral Medicine, 1201 N. Prospect Avenue, Milwaukee, WI 53202.

TABLE 27-1. *Overview of individual and family psychosocial issues in relation to stage of HIV infection*

Stage of HIV-1 Infection	Time	Developing Psychosocial Issues	
		Infected Individual	Family
Exposure	0 Years	High-risk behaviors, denial, fear	High-risk behaviors: denial, secrecy, Stage of HIV-1 Infection concern, fear
I. Testing HIV positive		Crisis reaction: shock, denial, depression, suicide thoughts, guilt, withdrawal, anger, relief Disclosure: fear	Crisis reaction: shock, denial, depression, uncertainty Disclosure: fear
II. Symptom-free period		Reestablish equilibrium: search for meaning, restore self-esteem, try to gain control, uncertainty Changes in lifestyle	Reestablish equilibrium: search for meaning, uncertainty Possible changes in lifestyles
III. Signs and symptoms		Loss of control and independence: guilt, anger, depression, suicide thoughts, support reciprocity, disfigurement, treatment decisions, bargaining	Caregiving: support reciprocality, treatment decisions, bargaining
IV. AIDS		Grief, possible relief at diagnosis, depression	Anticipatory grief, depression
Terminal stage		Preparation for death: depression, acceptance, treatment decisions, assisted suicide	Preparation for death: caregiver burnout, final treatment decisions, depression, acceptance, requests for assistance
Death	2 to 10+ years		Bereavement recovery

Adapted from Adelman M. Social support and AIDS. AIDS Public Policy J 1989;4 New York:31.
Kubler-Ross E. AIDS: the ultimate challenge. New York:Macmillan, 1987.
Wadland WC, Gleeson CJ. A model for psychosocial issues in HIV disease. Fam Pract 1991;33:82.

individuals, the quality of life would improve, as quite possibly would immune functioning and the length of survival. Although this is still an area of considerable debate and controversy, several studies of gay and bisexual cohorts have suggested that, at least among men in the earlier stages of HIV-1 infection, depression and social isolation are associated with faster rates of immunologic decline.[4,5] These results were not supported, however, by studies of stress[6,7] or depression[8,9] effects on immune competency in the same or similar longitudinal cohorts. Although strong arguments can be made for reducing stress and for diagnosing and treating depression to improve the quality of life of persons with HIV infection, the argument that such interventions will alter disease progression remains unproven.

As has been found for most persons with chronic illnesses, correlations exist between levels of stress and levels of mental health functioning among PWHIVs, but the resulting levels of distress and psychopathology vary widely among persons suffering equivalent levels of stress.[10,11] Coping styles and social support can mediate the relation between stress and distress, with the ability to positively or negatively affect outcomes. Several studies have indicated that familial or prior history of mental illness are additional strong predictors of mental dysfunction among gay or bisexual men,[12–15] intravenous drug users (IDUs), and hemophiliacs[16] with HIV-1 or AIDS. Premorbid substance abuse or dependence can also seriously compromise mental health and behavioral functioning at any stage of the HIV-1 spectrum (see Chap. 30).

Sources of distress for PWHIVs include the knowledge that they carry a lethal infectious virus; have a highly stigmatized disease that the larger society associates with an equally stigmatized lifestyle; may be socially ostracized, with significant risk of loss of job, income, housing, family, and other support; and may eventually suffer from a disfiguring, painful, and terminal illness (Table 27-2). Bisexual men, closeted gay men, and IDUs may be at even greater risk of suffering depression and isolation than self-identified gay men,[17] perhaps because self-identified gay men are more connected to supportive networks in their community, while bisexual men and IDUs fear rejection from their social networks and may not readily identify with a supportive community.[18]

Several studies have demonstrated that specific coping mechanisms, such as active appraisal and adaptation and supportive social interactions can contribute to well-being and improved quality of life for PWHIVs (see Table 27-2).[10,19–21] Denial or passive fatalism; the use of alcohol, recreational drugs, or casual sex as distraction coping responses; and conflict with a person's social network are maladaptive coping strategies that can contribute negatively to well-being and significantly impact the quality of life. Gay men, bisexual men, and IDUs experience social conflict as a result of others' responses to their infection and because of societal reactions to their homosexuality or drug abuse.[22,23] This social conflict may be compounded by fear of eviction from their housing, termination from their place of employ-

TABLE 27-2. *Resources and vulnerabilities determining HIV mental health outcomes*

RESOURCES

Positive or active coping styles
Adequate and perceived helpful social support networks of family and friends
Trusted confidants
Strong partnership with health care providers
Maintenance of mobility and sense of good health
Lack of prior significant mental health history
Adequate health insurance coverage and financial independence
Integration into community
Lack of current substance abuse
Ability to work or find alternative productive activities
Good self-esteem and maintenance of hope for future

VULNERABILITIES

Distraction, denial, or fatalistic coping styles
Inadequate or perceived unavailable social support networks
Lack of trusted confidants
Weak or distrustful relationship with health care providers
Declining mobility or overall health
Prior history of major psychiatric or suicidal history
Inadequate or no health insurance coverage; economic dependence
Social isolation and lack of community integration
Low self-esteem and lack of hope for future
Current substance abuse
Inability to work or find alternative productive activities

ment, and loss of their health insurance in reaction to the diagnosis.[24] Social conflict has been found to increase the symptoms of depression among men at risk for AIDS.[25] Not surprisingly, social support groups have proven to be effective in ameliorating distress and isolation experienced by PWHIVs.[26] The earliest community support programs, such as Shanti and Gay Mens' Health Crisis, were based on such a social support and coping model.

INTERVENTION ISSUES FOR THE AT-RISK PERSON

Psychologic reactions to the threat of HIV-1 or AIDS itself are quite varied, but according to our experience, they can be divided into three types. The first are those that are exacerbations or recurrences of preexisting psychopathology under the stress of HIV or AIDS but that have little to do with the infectious process other than its acting as a source of distress. Second are the types of problems are focussed on in the remainder of this chapter: disorders related directly to the stresses involved in having a diagnosis of HIV or AIDS. Third are the neuropsychiatric illnesses that result directly from HIV infection of the central nervous system (CNS), which are briefly reviewed at the conclusion of this chapter. A continuing case study is used to illustrate some of the more salient psychiatric issues at each stage of HIV-1 infection.

Before seroconversion, at-risk persons may begin to manifest psychologic symptoms from the stress of potentially becoming HIV-1 infected.[27] Such persons have been described as the "worried well."[28–30] Their psychologic distress may take the form of generalized or AIDS-specific anxieties, panic attacks, hypochondriasis, or obsessive-compulsive disorders.[28] Persons at risk for HIV-1 illness, especially gay or bisexual men who are well integrated into the community, may be experiencing the illness or death of friends and lovers, which may cause depression directly and through the loss of their significant social supports or the threat of their own premature mortality.[22,23] While observing these reactions, it is important for clinicians to account for preexisting psychiatric disorders, including substance abuse or dependency, that may become exacerbated by the threat of HIV-1 illness.

HIV-1 Antibody Testing Issues

Counseling related to HIV antibody testing is often the first contact that HIV-infected persons have with mental health caregivers. According to the CDC,[3] ". . . successful HIV prevention counseling involves four essential components: personalized risk assessment to facilitate a realistic self perception of risk; identification and discussion of barriers to behavior change and reinforcement of behavior change already initiated by the client; negotiation between the counselor and the client of a realistic and incremental risk reduction plan; and establishment of a specific plan to receive test results and after test counseling."

Prevention also requires the need for the strictest confidentiality to develop trust and protect clients from possible discrimination. Of paramount importance is the evaluation of all patients for possible adverse behavioral or mental health consequences of testing and provision of psychologic therapies aimed at ameliorating those responses. Often, this means referring a patient to one or more community-based AIDS service organizations that provide HIV-1 psychosocial and case management services (see Chap. 26). The following ongoing case example illustrates the various psychiatric concerns that can arise at each stage of treatment of a bisexual male with HIV-1 infection.

CASE STUDY

Steve is a 28-year-old white, bisexual man who comes to see you with the complaint of increasing anxiety, insomnia, fatigue, and poor appetite, with 10-pound weight loss over the past month. The precipitant appears to be his recent breakup with a male lover of 5 years and the ex-lover's informing Steve that he had tested positive for HIV-1 antibodies. Steve reports frequent nightmares and daytime anxiety attacks, all focusing on fears that he has AIDS and will soon die, alone and disfigured. At times, suicidal thoughts occupy his thinking, and he is unable to concentrate on his work or household chores. He has withdrawn from friends and his female lover, Sarah, for fear that they will notice his illness and react negatively. He was referred to you for psychiatric evaluation by his internist, who found mildly swollen axillary lymph glands on examination of this otherwise healthy-appearing but extremely anxious patient.

During Steve's first visit, you listen to his concerns and provide reassurance and factual information regarding the natural history of HIV-1 infection, the signs and symptoms of AIDS, and the practical aspects of HIV-1 antibody testing. After discussing his anxiety attacks, you decide to prescribe an anxiolytic medication. You then take a detailed sexual behavior history, noting Steve's significant potential exposure history and his continuing sexual activities with Sarah. After discussing the pros and cons of HIV-1 antibody testing, you and Steve agree that a test is indicated, and blood is drawn for the ELISA and confirmatory Western blot analyses. You schedule a follow-up appointment for 1 week later, at which time you will evaluate Steve's response to anxiolytic therapy and discuss the result of his HIV-1 antibody test. You provide him with some written materials about HIV-1 testing and encourage him to call you if he experiences any anxiety attacks or problems with the medication. On leaving your office, Steve informs you that he feels relieved about finally being tested and discussing his fears with you.

A realistic personalized plan for behavior modification based on the client's own risk behavior history needs to be developed during the pretest counseling session. It is important that both counselor and client agree on the feasibility of this plan and that possible barriers to the suggested changes are discussed and reactions to them anticipated. Although behavioral risk assessment and planning for behavioral change are essential, it is also important that the therapist take into account the psychologic needs and state of the person seeking the test. For at-risk persons requesting testing, there are a number of highly emotionally charged issues: feelings that they may have put themselves or partners at risk for HIV-1 and may soon learn that they are HIV-1 seropositive; thoughts about the possible consequences of a positive test and fears of having to disclose the result (and related indiscretions) to loved ones; and the associated fears of abandonment. For women, HIV testing often occurs as part of prenatal screening, raising issues of reproductive health, decision making, and the potential loss of the ability to care for their existing or future children.

In anticipation of these fears, the therapist should walk the client through different scenarios, explaining possible emotional reactions and asking what the client will do if he or she is HIV-1 positive or negative. A counselor or therapist can and should be as helpful as possible in pointing out behavioral, emotional, societal, legal, and psychologic consequences of both scenarios. Sufficient time should be spent discussing the test procedures, the meaning and limitations of the laboratory findings, and the recommended follow-up procedures for each individual.

There are many ethical and legal issues that complicate the patient-therapist relationship when HIV-1 testing or treatment is involved.[31] Many states have passed legislation or public health regulations that define the therapist's obligations and the conditions under which patient privacy may be breached for public health considerations. Psychiatrists

need to be familiar with their local laws and regulations related to patient confidentiality and HIV-1 testing and discuss their implications with all new at-risk patients.

Seroconversion and Disclosure Issues

Varied and conflicting reports have been made about the impact of testing and disclosure of serostatus for those who are at risk for HIV-1. Possible impacts include depression, suicidal ideation or suicidal attempts, anxiety and somatic preoccupations, an increased sense of isolation, anger, substance abuse or other forms of distraction coping, symptoms of adjustment disorder, and mild transient patterns of psychologic distress[22,32-36] Some researchers have reported a sharp rise in anxiety and depression for some individuals at the time of diagnosis of HIV-1 infection but found that these states dissipated with time.[37] However, specific concerns about AIDS and the long-term impact of being HIV-1 seropositive significantly increase after learning about being infected; dealing with these "AIDS worries" is often a major goal of therapy for HIV-1–seropositive persons. Substance abuse and other forms of maladaptive coping may increase or recur, and issues of informing spouses, sexual partners, and other significant persons are frequently central to therapy in the period after disclosure.

CASE STUDY

Steve returns for his posttest counseling appointment, at which time he reports a significant decrease in his anxiety, with no incapacitating attacks or suicidal ideation during the past week. However, he reports significant increased anxiety this morning, focusing on his reaction to an expected positive test result. He appears somewhat relieved when you tell him that his test was positive but that he is in the earliest stage of infection. Steve's anxiety returns when the issue of informing his girlfriend, Sarah, about his HIV-1 seropositivity is raised. Although she has always been aware of his bisexuality and Steve expects her to be supportive of him, he feels extreme embarrassment and guilt over the thought that he might have infected her. You reassure Steve and counsel him about the importance of HIV-1 testing for Sarah and any other unprotected sexual contacts he might have had in the past year. You and Steve agree on the need to continue the anxiolytic therapy and weekly psychotherapy with you, focusing on his anxiety and AIDS-specific worries. Because Steve expresses a preference for seeing a gay physician specializing in HIV and AIDS care, you refer him to the infectious disease practitioner you work closest with and provide him with a list of local AIDS service organizations.

Social Support Issues and Interventions for Recently Seropositive Persons

In addition to the psychologic impact of HIV-1 infection, there are also positive and negative social effects. Researchers have speculated on the occurrence of depression and suicidal ideation at the time of HIV-1 antibody testing and again at the time of an AIDS diagnosis. Most clinicians believe that recently diagnosed HIV-1–positive persons need to be watched closely for suicidality. Although Marzuk and colleagues[38] reported the relative risk for suicide by men between the ages of 20 and 59 years to be 36 times greater for those with AIDS than for men without the diagnosis, Perry[36] found that the increased risk for suicide dissipated 2 months after diagnosis. Less reassuring, Perry found that suicidal ideation persisted after notification for 15% of seropositive and seronegative gay men.

Regardless of the initial psychologic reaction at the time of a seropositive test notification, it is important to perform a suicide potential assessment[39] and begin appropriate intervention if indicated. The usual risk factors for serious suicide potential apply to the recently diagnosed HIV-1–seropositive patient: preexisting affective illness, prior suicidality, substance abuse, social isolation and conflict, extreme hopelessness, and impulsivity. These issues may be difficult to assess during the immediate posttest counseling period, because the patient may be in a state of acute shock.[37] After immediate attention has been paid to the acute psychologic reaction, a follow-up session should be arranged, at which time further assessment and initiation of appropriate treatment can take place. Often, individual psychotherapy and social support group interventions are sufficient to reduce suicidal ideation. However, if serious suicidality persists, it may be necessary to consider more intense intervention, including possible inpatient treatment.

ISSUES FOR SEROPOSITIVE PERSONS

During stages II and III (see Table 27-1), patients may experience a wide range of intermittent physiologic symptoms, such as thrush, diarrhea, or night sweats. These symptoms vary in both magnitude and frequency among all HIV-1-seropositive individuals, but will generally not be serious or meet the criteria for AIDS until several to ten or more years after the initial infection. For those who experience minor symptoms, they serve as frequent reminders that they are ill; and for those who do not experience symptoms or are unaware that their symptoms are HIV-1 related, the lack of symptoms may add to the denial that they are infected. Psychologic reactions, such as depression, may take the form of sadness, hopelessness, or anticipatory grief. Some authors have reported difficulty differentiating between depression as a reaction to HIV-1 infection, demoralization, and hopelessness, and as symptoms of HIV-1 infection, which may be similar to depression, such as difficulty sleeping, poor concentration, and fatigue.[40,41] Multiple AIDS-related bereavements are related to increased levels of hopelessness, depression, and HIV-1-related symptoms.[6,42,43,44]

Depression: Prevalence, Diagnosis and Treatment Issues

This case illustrates a common difficulty in the management of depressive symptoms in an otherwise asymptomatic person with more than 500 CD4 cells:

CASE STUDY

Steve returns quarterly after the resolution of his initial anxiety attacks at the time of his HIV-1 diagnosis. He has done well for the past 4 years in terms of physical and mental health. He has continued working as a massage therapist, stayed active in his support group, and not needed any antiretroviral or prophylactic medications. His helper T lymphocyte (CD4) cell counts have fluctuated between 1000 and 600 cells/mm^3, but more recently, they have been in the 500 to 650 range. When you see him on the fifth anniversary of his initial positive antibody test, he complains of feeling depressed, frequently tired and unable to get out of bed, poor appetite, loss of interest in social activities, and occasionally being tearful. He reports first noticing these symptoms after Tim, one of the long-term members of his support group and Steve's "buddy" when he first joined the group, died of an opportunistic infection. Aside from fatigue, he denies difficulties in his work as a massage therapist, but he does complain of occasional forgetfulness, which is unusual for him.

You and Steve decide that even if his depressive symptoms are in reaction to Tim's death, a trial of an antidepressant that may restore his energy, concentration, and mood is warranted because of the degree of discomfort he is suffering. You start him on a low dose of an activating antidepressant, and he reports an immediate improvement in sleep, appetite, and energy levels. Over the next several weeks, you gradually increase his dosage as his mood returns to normal. You keep him on a maintenance dose of the antidepressant for 6 months, while continuing psychotherapy that focuses on the issues of loss and coping with his physical deterioration and that of close friends. Steve eventually volunteers to be a buddy for someone else in the group, and he volunteers one evening per week in the HIV clinic of the local medical center.

Although the likelihood that the symptoms are organic in origin is exceedingly small, it may be extremely difficult to differentiate symptoms that are reactive to HIV-related losses from "pseudo-depression" resulting directly from HIV-1 infection of the brain. The situation is made even more difficult if typical vegetative signs and symptoms are not present but the person appears to be significantly impaired in work or social performance. The field is still divided over whether to be aggressive in the treatment of what may be reactive or subsyndromal depression in such patients. Although prospective cohort studies of largely asymptomatic gay men have indicated low rates of major depression,[7,45,46] clinicians frequently see various levels of depression in HIV-1–infected patient populations. Many have also described the effects on PWHIVs of living with a chronic disease.[22,28] Several of the symptoms of depression seen with HIV-1 infection are similar to those seen with other chronic diseases, such as cancer, heart disease, or Alzheimer's disease. Although PWHIVs may share some of the same concerns—such as the prospect of debilitating disease, loss of financial resources, or early death—HIV-1–related conditions additionally elicit fear and stigma from the community at large.[33]

African Americans with HIV-1 infection may be at even greater risk of depression and suicide than their white counterparts. Cochran and Mays[47] found that one third to almost

TABLE 27-3. *Traditional and nontraditional antidepressants used for HIV patients*

Antidepressant	Product Name	Type	Response*	Stage Recommend	Side-Effect Profile
Imipramine		TCA	Medium	Early stages	Anticholinergic, sedative, weight gain, constipation
Desipramine		TCA	Medium	Early stages	Anticholinergic, activating, weight loss
Fluoxetine	Prozac	Serotonin reuptake	Medium	All	Sexual dysfunction, insomnia, nausea blocker
Sertraline	Zoloft	Serotonin reuptake blocker	Fast	All	Sexual dysfunction, insomnia, nausea
Venlafaxine	Effexor	Combined NE and serotonin reuptake blocker	Medium	Not known, presumably all	Activating, hypertension, , nausea weight loss
Bupropion	Welbutron	Dopamine and NE stimulation	Medium	All, but particularly useful in anergic/ fatigue patients	Lowers seizure threshold, activating
Dextroamphetamine or methylpenidate	Ritalin	Psychostimulant	Fast	Late, especially if fatigue and/or concentration problems	Activating, "nervousness," insomnia, psychosis (rare)
Testosterone		Androgen hormone	Medium	Late, especially if accompanied by hypogonadism or weight loss	Hair loss, irritability

NE, norepinephrine; TCA, tricyclic antidepressant.
*Fast, significant response within 2 weeks; medium, significant response within 2 to 6 weeks; slow, response may be delayed beyond 2 months.

one half of HIV-1–positive African-American gay or bisexual men reported elevated levels of depression symptoms, compared with 10% to 20% of white gay or bisexual men in most studies.[45,46] Given the theorized contributions of social stigma and isolation to distress related to HIV-1 infection, it is likely that racial or ethnic minority PWHIVs in general are at increased risk of depression. This problem will become even more evident as the distribution of new infections and disease continues to increasingly predominate in minority populations (Table 27-3).

Depression occurring in PWHIVs can be treated with an increasingly wide spectrum of antidepressants, regardless of the underlying cause, as long as the medications are matched carefully in terms of the patient's symptoms and the medications' side-effect profiles (see Table 27-3) and are given in judicious doses.[46,48,49,50] There appear to be no untoward immunologic effects of acute antidepressant treatment of patients with HIV-1 infection.[49,50] One study of HIV-infected gay and bisexual men suggested that depressed individuals suffer more accelerated deterioration of their immune systems than nondepressed individuals,[4] although this finding remains controversial,[6,9,51] and the converse—that treatment of depression may lead to slower progression of immunodeficiency in HIV-1—has not been demonstrated. The emphasis should be on maximizing the quality of life, and aggressive treatment of depression in PWHIVs has been shown to markedly improve their quality of life and preference for life-sustaining treatments.[52]

Anxiety: Differential Diagnosis and Treatment

Most persons with adverse reactions to their initial HIV-1 diagnosis experience a decrease in anxiety symptoms on acceptance into psychosocial treatment; some, as in the case study, respond well to a combination of acceptance, reassurance, and brief anxiolytic therapy. However, a careful evaluation of anxiety symptoms is necessary before beginning treatment to determine the underlying causes and type of disorder.

The differential diagnosis of anxiety in HIV-infected patients is similar to that for any person facing a life-threatening chronic illness—complicated by concerns about loss of social support due to the stigmatization of AIDS and HIV-transmitting lifestyles. Assessment of possible underlying medical disorders (eg, hyperthyroidism), excess caffeine consumption, stimulant drug usage or withdrawal, and medications used in the treatment of HIV or AIDS that can also have anxiety-producing side effects is necessary. Evaluation of any patient presenting with excess anxiety should also include consideration of possible depression or panic disorder, both of which may present with prominent anxiety symptoms. Because of the relatively high degree of overlap between anxiety, depression, and somatic symptoms frequently observed in PWHIVs, diagnoses of "subsyndromal" anxiety or "mixed anxiety-depression" may be relatively common.[53]

Supportive or cognitive psychotherapy is the first-line treatment for anxiety, and often includes referral to AIDS social organizations offering support group services. Counseling of a patient's partners, close friends, and family members can often help to relieve social conflict or fears of abandonment. Anxiolytic treatment should be considered if the anxiety is severe and disabling or is accompanied by panic attacks or if a diagnosis of generalized anxiety disorder or posttraumatic stress disorder is made. There is an increasing spectrum of anxiolytic medications available, and nonbenzodiazepine medications should be considered for all patients not previously treated chronically with a benzodiazepine compound, as well as those who can be successfully tapered off of benzodiazepines.

Neuropsychology

Anxiety and depression can be accompanied by mild cognitive deficits, such as poor concentration or short-term memory. For the person with HIV-1 infection, these symptoms can themselves be stressful, because they may be experienced as indicators of early HIV-1 brain involvement. If the cognitive symptoms are mild and in keeping with the degree of affective dysfunction, the patient should be counseled that the symptoms will probably disappear after the anxiety or depression is adequately treated. However, if the cognitive symptoms appear out of proportion to the degree of affective involvement or they do not respond to adequate antidepressant or anxiolytic treatment, a neuropsychologic evaluation is indicated, even for patients with more than 500 CD4 cells/mm^3.

In terms of HIV-1 and mental functioning, it is not clear if significant CNS involvement precedes the development of full-blown AIDS.[54–56] In part, this controversy reflects our lack of knowledge about the highly variable natural history of HIV-1 infection of the CNS and the etiopathogenesis of HIV-1–related cognitive and motor disease. Further complicating the picture are the myriad factors that may influence neuropsychologic functioning of PWHIVs: prescribed drug and recreational drug side effects, the stresses of living with HIV and its manifest social consequences, nutritional deficiencies, CNS opportunistic infections and neoplasms, and altered affective states. Careful assessment, which may include formal neuropsychologic testing, and treatment of any underlying conditions that may be contributing to cognitive dysfunction are essential before a diagnosis of HIV-1–associated cognitive or motor syndrome is made. A list of the most common signs and symptoms of HIV CNS infection at the various stages of development of HIV-related cognitive-motor dysfunction is given in Table 27-4.S Psychostimulant treatment has been shown to be particularly useful in ameliorating mixed affective and cognitive symptoms in persons with later stage HIV-1 illness.[57]

SYMPTOMATIC INFECTION, AIDS, AND TERMINAL ILLNESS

Grief over receiving a diagnosis of AIDS may begin with an acute response of shock and denial, which may than be followed by guilt, anger, or sadness. This is frequently fol-

TABLE 27-4. *Signs and symptoms of HIV-related central nervous system infection*

EARLY COGNITIVE IMPAIRMENTS

Short-term memory deficits; "forgetfulness" rather than amnesia
Decreased concentration and attention
Confusion and disorientation
Difficulty following other speakers, especially when multiple sensory inputs exist
Overall intellectual ability generally well preserved until late
Visuospatial perception deficits (rare)

CHANGES IN PERSONALITY AND BEHAVIOR

Apathy, decreased interest
Impaired judgment
Erratic or hypomanic behavior
Social withdrawal
Rigidity of thinking
Later: speech impairment, slowing, dysarthria, hypophonia

PSYCHOTIC SYMPTOMS

Hallucinations
Suspiciousness and delusions
Agitation and inappropriate behavior
Full mania, particularly in AIDS, and possibly exacerbated by antivirals

MOTOR SYMPTOMS

Ataxia
Loss of coordination
Weakness, especially in distal extremities
Tremors

GENERALIZED SYSTEMIC SYMPTOMS

Fatigue, sleep changes including hypersomnia
Anorexia, weight loss
Enuresis
Hypersensitivity to medications, alcohol and substances of abuse

COGNITIVE SYMPTOMS ASSOCIATED WITH ADVANCED DEMENTIA

Global cognitive impairment
Rudimentary social functgioning
Disorientation
Psychomotor retardation, decreased spontaneity
Agitation, "sundowning" (eg, nighttime delusions, agitation)
Mutism, vacant stare
Coma

MOTOR SYMPTOMS ASSOCIATED WITH ADVANCED DEMENTIA

Ataxia
Spastic weakness
Paraplegia, quadraparesis
Hyperreflexia, myclonus
Seizures
Bladder and bowel incontinence

lowed by a transitional state during which individuals may alternate between anger, guilt, self-pity, anxiety, and denial.[23] These feelings can be particularly distressing and confusing, with changes in self-esteem, identity, and considerations of suicide. New symptoms or events may precipitate new crises for the individual. This has caused some to describe the uncertainty of HIV-1 illness as an "emotional roller coaster."[23]

Many will find reinforcement for their denial through recurring reports in the press and popular media about the "myth of HIV-1" being the cause of AIDS, and others are forced to acknowledge the life-threatening nature of AIDS when hearing media accounts of disappointments in antiviral drug development. Inevitably, issues of loss reemerge at the time of an AIDS diagnosis and complicate the management of end-of-life issues.

CASE STUDY

After almost 10 years of living and working with HIV-1 infection, Steve learns that his CD4 cell count has gone below 200 cells/mm^3, qualifying him for the diagnosis of AIDS according to current criteria.[58] Through his work with you and the support group, he has prepared himself for this eventuality. This has included writing a living will and formally designating his long-term female partner as the person responsible for medical and financial decisions if he becomes incapacitated. When you next see him, he is somewhat sad, having just retired from work and applied for SSI disability and Medicaid coverage. You discuss the plans he has made for this, the fourth and final stage of his HIV-1 natural history. In response to your questions about suicidal ideation, Steve tells you that he has decided to end his life if and when he becomes mentally incapacitated. You suggest a group counseling session with Steve, Sarah, the support buddy, and other members of his immediate support network. That session is very emotional, but it provides an opportunity for Steve to make his terminal care preferences known to his support network and for them to reaffirm their support for him.

Psychologic treatment must usually be refocussed on helping clients adapt to changes in their levels of mental and physical functioning and associated fears of debilitation and dependency on others, management of pain, maximizing quality of life, and terminal care preferences. It may be particularly difficult for psychotherapists who have worked with patients across multiple stages of HIV-1 infection to discuss those patients' fears and wishes about terminal care, especially plans for assisted suicide. The involvement of spiritual and palliative care can be extremely important for improving the quality of life of the terminal patient and preventing depression and burnout among mental health caregivers.

CONCLUSIONS

Consideration in this chapter of the complex interrelations among the various goals in treating PWHIVs—physical health, immunocompetence, mental health, social and functional well-being, and overall quality of life—and the accompanying case study have emphasized the importance of an integrated biopsychosocial treatment approach. Given the central role of quality of life issues in the treatment of any person living with HIV, the coordinating role of the mental health care provider has been emphasized. An integrated holistic or biopsychosocial treatment approach works best when it is applied to the full range of problems experienced by HIV-infected persons and includes all the diverse elements of health care required. For this reason, many communities have established central HIV and AIDS care coordinating organizations, which provide or contract for comprehensive HIV case management services. Because of the complexity and multidisciplinary nature of coordinated biopsychosocial HIV-1 care, frequently involving, in addition to medical and mental health services, a host of education and support services for patients and their families, it is extremely important that a case management model of care be used whenever possible.

The establishment of interdisciplinary care teams, AIDS task forces, and HIV case management systems does not automatically solve the major problems inherent in the delivery of such care for PWHIVs. For example, programs that provide comprehensive long-term care need to minimize actions that will isolate patients from mainstream society, while maximizing the availability of specialized services. The intense stigma and discrimination to which HIV-infected patients are still subject requires extraordinary attention to the confidentiality of medical records, while ensuring adequate communication among the diverse care team members.

The prevalence of dual or triply diagnosed patients—most usually a combination of a functional mental health disorder, a substance use disorder, and organic illness—means that already limited treatment facilities for such patients are often unavailable, and specific efforts have to be made to create appropriate treatment options. The occurrence of cognitive deficits in late-stage HIV-1 illness means that patients may have difficulty with the complicated diagnostic and treatment regimens made necessary by the nature of their illness. The close involvement of AIDS service organizations able to provide in-home assistance, support buddies, and transportation can frequently make outpatient treatment possible across the full spectrum of HIV-1 infection.

The daily stresses of working in the HIV and AIDS health care arena, combined with the experience of seeing relatively young patients deteriorate and die despite the physician's best efforts is a formula for burnout.[59,60,61] Any viable AIDS and HIV treatment program must provide adequate education, emotional support, and counseling for the patients and for those who care for them. In achieving this goal, mental health caregivers can contribute enormously to the compassionate care of all persons living with HIV-1 infection, improving the quality of life of their patients while setting a leadership example for the practice of holistic health care.

REFERENCES

1. Ostrow DG, Wren PA. Mental health aspects of HIV/AIDS. Ann Arbor: University of Michigan, 1993.
2. Bacchetti P, Moss AR. Incubation period of AIDS in San Francisco. Nature 1989;338:251.
3. Centers for Disease Control. Technical guidance on HIV counseling. MMWR 1993;42:11.

4. Burack JH, Barrett RD, Stall MA, Chesney MA, Ekstrand ML, Coates TJ. Depressive symptoms and CD4 lymphocyte decline among HIV-infected men. JAMA 1993;270:2568.
5. Caumartin S, Joseph JG, Chmiel J. Premorbid psychosical factors associated with differentiated survival time in AIDS patients. Paper presented at VII International AIDS Conference, Florence, Italy, June, 1991.
6. Kessler RC, Foster C, Joseph J, et al. Stressful life events and symptom onset in HIV infection. Am J Psychiatry 1991;148:733.
7. Williams JBW, Rabkin JG, Remien RH, et al. Multidisciplinary baseline assessment of homosexual men with and without human immunodeficiency virus infection. Arch Gen Psychiatry 1991;48:124.
8. Perry S, Fishman B, Jacobsberg L, Francis A. Relationships over 1 year between lymphocyte subsets and psychosocial variables among adults with infection by human immunodeficiency virus. Arch Gen Psychiatry 1992;49:396.
9. Lyketsos CG, Hoover DR, Guccione M, Senterfitt W, Morgenstern H. Depressive symptoms as predictors of medical outcomes in HIV infection. JAMA 1993;270:2563.
10. Folkman S, Chesney MA, Pollack L, Coates T. Stress, control, coping and depressive mood in human immunodeficiency virus-positive and -negative gay men in San Francisco. J Nerv Ment Dis 1993;181:409.
11. Lackner JB, Joseph JG, Ostrow DG, et al. A longitudinal study of psychological distress in a cohort of gay men: effects of social support and coping strategies. J Nerv Ment Dis 1993;181:4.
12. Atkinson JH, Grant I, Kennedy CJ, Richman DD, Spector SA, McCutchan JA. Prevalence of psychiatric disorders among men infected with human immunodeficiency virus. Arch Gen Psychiatry 1988;45:859.
13. O'Dowd MA, Biderman DJ, McKegney FP. Incidence of suicidality in AIDS and HIV-positive patients attending a psychiatry outpatient program. Psychosomatics 1993;34:33.
14. Perry S, Jacobsberg L, Card CA, Ashman T, Frances A, Fishman B. Severity of psychiatric symptoms after HIV testing. Am J Psychiatry 1993;150:775.
15. Perkins DO, Stern RA, Golden RN, Murphy C, Naftolowitz D, Evans DL. Mood disorders in HIV infection: prevalence and risk factors in a nonepicenter of the AIDS epidemic. Am J Psychiatry 1994;151:233.
16. Wickland BM, Jackson MA. Coping with AIDS in hemophilia. In: Ahmed PI, ed. Living and dying with AIDS. New York: Plenum Press, 1992:255.
17. Ostrow DG, Monjan A, Joseph J, et al. HIV-related symptoms and psychological functioning in a cohort of homosexual men. Am J Psychiatry 1989;146:737.
18. Dew MA, Ragni MV, Nimorwica P. Infection with human immunodeficiency virus and vulnerability to psychiatric distress. Arch Gen Psychiatry 1990;47:737.
19. Hays RB, Turner H, Coates TJ. Social support, AIDS-related symptoms and depression among gay men. J Consult Clin Psychol 1992;60:463.
20. Halman LJ, Ostrow DG, Eshleman S, Caumartin S, Joseph J. Structure of coping in a gay cohort at risk for AIDS. Presented at AIDS' Impact: 2nd International Conference on Biopsychosocial Aspects of HIV Infection, Brighton, England, July, 1994.
21. Wolf TM, Galson PM, Morse EV, et al. Relationship of coping style to affective state and perceived social support in asymptomatic and symptomatic HIV-infected persons: implications for clinical management. J Clin Psychiatry 1991;52:171.
22. Holland JC, Tross S. The psychosocial and neuropsychiatric sequelae of the acquired immunodeficiency syndrome and related disorders. Ann Intern Med 1985;103:760.
23. Nichols SE. Psychosocial reactions of persons with the acquired immunodeficiency syndrome. Ann Intern Med 1985;103:765.
24. Cassens BJ. Social consequences of the acquired immunodeficiency syndrome. Ann Intern Med 1985;103:768.
25. O'Brien K, Wortman CB, Kessler RC, Joseph JG. Social relationships of men at risk for AIDS. Soc Sci Med 1993;36:1161.
26. Kelly JA, Murphy DA, Bahr GR, Kalichman SC, Bernstein BM. Outcome of cognitive-behavioral and support group brief therapies for depressed, HIV-infected persons. Am J Psychiatry 1993;150:1671.
27. Joseph J, Caumartin S, Tal M, et al. Psychological functioning in a cohort of gay men at risk for AIDS. J Nerv Ment Dis 1990;178:607.
28. Faulstich ME. Psychiatric aspects of AIDS. Am J Psychiatry 1987;144:551.
29. Jenike M, Pato C, Disabling fear of AIDS responsive to imipramine. Psychosomatics 1986;27:143.
30. Morin SF, Charles KA, Mayon AK. The psychological impact of AIDS on gay men. Am Psychologist 1984;39:1288.
31. Wren PW. Legal and ethical issues. In: Ostrow DG, Wren PA, eds. Mental health aspects of HIV/AIDS. Ann Arbor: University of Michigan, 1993:227.
32. Jacobsen PB, Perry SW, Hirsch DA. Responses to HIV antibody testing: behavioral and psychological responses to HIV antibody testing. J Consult Clin Psychol 1987;58:31.
33. Kelly JA, Murphy DA, Bahr GR, et al. Factors associated with severity of depression and high-risk behavior among persons diagnosed with immunodeficiency virus (HIV) infection. Health Psychol 1993;12:215.
34. Kelly JA, St. Lawrence JS. The AIDS health crisis: psychological and social interventions. New York: Plenum Press, 1988.
35. Ostrow DG, Joseph JG, Kessler R, et al. Disclosure of HIV antibody status: behavioral and mental health correlates. AIDS Prev Educ 1988;1:1.
36. Perry S, Jacobsberg L, Fishman B. Suicidal ideation and HIV testing. JAMA 1990;263:679.
37. Ostrow DG, Leite MC, Lackner J, Eshleman S. Time course, mental health, and social support changes after learning HIV serostatus in the Chicago MACS/CCS cohort. Presented at the Neuroscience of HIV Satellite Meeting, Amsterdam, June 1992.
38. Marzuk PM, Tierney H, Tardiff K, et al. Increased risk of suicide in persons with AIDS. JAMA 1988;259:1333.
39. Beckett A, Shenson D. Suicide risk in patients with human immunodeficiency virus infection and acquired immunodeficiency syndrome. Harvard Rev Psychiatry 1993;1:27.
40. Ostrow D, Grant I, Atkinson H. Assessment and management of AIDS patients with neuropsychiatric disturbances. J Clin Psychiatry 1991;49:14.
41. Kalichman SC, Sikkema KJ, Somlai A. Assessing persons with Human Immunodeficiency virus (HIV) infection using the Beck depression inventory: disease processes and other potential confounds. J Pers Assess 1995;64:86.
42. Martin JL. Psychological consequences of AIDS-related bereavement among gay men. J Consult Clin Psychol 1988;56:856.
43. Neugebauer R, Rabkin J, Williams J, Remien R, Goetz R, Gorman J. Bereavement reactions among homosexual men experiencing multiple losses in the AIDS epidemic. Am J Psychiatry 1992;149:1374.
44. Rabkin JG, Williams JB, Neugebauer R, Remien R, Goetz R. Maintenance of hope in HIV-spectrum homosexual men. Am J Psychiatry 1990;147:1322.
45. Kalichman SC, Sikkema KJ. Psychological sequelae of HIV infection and AIDS: Review of empirical findings. Clin Psychol Rev 1994;14:611.
46. Markowitz JC, Rabkin JG, Perry SW. Treating depression in HIV-positive patients. AIDS 1994;8:403.
47. Cochran S, Mays V. Depressive distress among homosexually active African-American men and women. Am J Psychiatry 1994;151:524.
48. Fernandez F. Anxiety and the neuropsychiatry of AIDS. J Clin Psychiatry 1989;50(Suppl):9.
49. Rabkin JG, Rabkin R, Harrison W, Wagner G. Imipramine effects on mood and enumerative measures of immune status in depressed patients with HIV illness. Am J Psychiatry 1994;151:516.
50. Rabkin JG, Rabkin R, Wagner G. Fluoxetine effects on mood and immune status in depressed patients with HIV illness. J Clin Psychiatry 1994;55:92.
51. Perry S, Fishman B. Depression and HIV: how does one affect the other? JAMA 1993;270:2609.
52. Fogel BS, Mor V. Depressed mood and care preferences in patients with AIDS. Gen Hosp Psychiatry 1993;15:203.
53. Hintz S, Kuck J, Peterkin JJ, Volk DM, Zisook S. Depression in the context of human immunodeficiency virus infection: implications for treatment. J Clin Psychiatry 1990;51:497.
54. Grant I, Atkinson JH, Hesselink JR, et al. Evidence for early central nervous system involvement in the acquired immunodeficiency virus (HIV) infections. Ann Intern Med 1987;107:823.
55. Levy RM, Bredesen DE. Central nervous system dysfunction in acquired immunodeficiency syndrome. J Acquir Immune Defic Syndr 1988;1:13.

56. Ostrow DG. Psychiatric aspects of human immunodeficiency virus infection. Kalamazoo: Scope Publications, 1990.

57. Fernandez F, Adams F, Levy JK. Cognitive impairment due to AIDS-related complex and its response to psychostimulants. Psychosomatics 1988;29:38.

58. Centers for Disease Control. 1993 Revised classification system for HIV infection and expanded surveillance case definition for AIDS among adolescents and adults. MMWR 1992;41:1.

59. Ostrow DG, Gayle TC. Psychosocial and ethical issues of AIDS health care programs. Qual Rev Bull 1986;12:284.

60. Fawzi FI, Fawzy NW, Pasnau RO. Bereavement in AIDS. Psychiatr Med 1994; 12.

61. McDaniel S, Farber EW, Summerville MB. Mental health care providers working with HIV: avoiding stress and burnout. In: Homosexuality and mental health: a comprehensive review. Washington, DC: American Psychiatric Press.

AIDS: Biology, Diagnosis, Treatment and Prevention, fourth edition, edited by Vincent T. DeVita, Jr., Samuel Hellman, and Steven A. Rosenberg. Lippincott–Raven Publishers, © 1997

CHAPTER 28

The Community-Based Response to Acquired Immunodeficiency Syndrome

Derek Hodel

Since it was first reported among groups of homosexual males in 1981,[1] acquired immunodeficiency syndrome (AIDS) has escalated to become the leading cause of death among adults between the ages of 25 and 44 in the United States in 1994.[2] More than 440,000 AIDS cases have been reported to the Centers for Disease Control and Prevention (CDC), and more than 270,870 Americans have died, contributing to the most profound mortality trends since the flu pandemic of 1918.[3] AIDS cases have been reported in all 50 states, eight territories, the District of Columbia, and the Commonwealth of Puerto Rico. In San Francisco alone, AIDS has claimed more than 20,750 lives, a number equivalent to nearly 3% of that city's total population.[4] In New York City, there are more than 23,500 persons living with AIDS.[5] According to the Surgeon General's estimates, 40,000 to 80,000 new infections occur annually in the United States.[6]

Although no racial or socioeconomic group has remained untouched, the epidemic has decimated the ranks of certain population groups, including injection drug users and gay men. Among these same groups, the seroprevalence rates in certain urban centers exceed 50%, a level viewed by some researchers as a potential saturation point.[7] AIDS disproportionately affects the poor, predominantly persons of color, and women and young gay men constitute the fastest growing demographic groups.[8,9]

In its short course, AIDS has disturbed America's complacency toward infectious diseases and pierced an unwillingness among members of the public to talk frankly about homosexuality, sexuality in general, and to a lesser degree, drug use. It has called into question certain fundamental tenets of public health, perhaps most notably the medical model employed against sexually transmitted diseases that emphasizes compulsory treatment, contact tracing, and partner notification.[10] More than any time since the Tuskegee Syphilis Experiment exposé prompted a presidential commission to issue new guidelines for the protection of human research subjects almost 20 years ago,[11] AIDS has prompted the scientific research community to rethink central paradigms in clinical research methodology and has empowered patients to participate in decision making to a heretofore unheard of degree.[12] Perhaps to a greater extent than any time since Congress passed the Kefauver amendment to the Food, Drug, and Cosmetic Act in 1960 in response to the thalidomide crisis in Europe, AIDS has sparked a reevaluation and revamping of the federal system of drug regulation.[13]

The demands placed by AIDS on urban health care systems, especially those caring for large numbers of the poor, have called into question the nation's ability to cope with health care emergencies and have surely influenced the public drive for health care reform.[14] Continuous legal challenges posed by discrimination against persons with AIDS contributed to the landmark passage of the Americans With Disabilities Act (ADA) in the 101st Congress.[10,15] AIDS is a defining event of the 1980s and is likely so to define the 1990s and perhaps many years into the next millennium.

DEFINITIONS

For the purposes of this chapter, I employ the term *community resources* to describe opportunities or services provided by nongovernmental organizations, referred to broadly in the United States as *community-based organizations* (CBOs), for persons with or affected by human immunodeficiency virus (HIV) disease. The term CBO suggests a measure of self-help and operational involvement on the part of the affected com

Derek Hodel, Director of Public Policy, Gay Men's Health Crisis, Inc., 129 West 20th Street, New York, NY 10011.

munity.[15] Early in the AIDS epidemic, this involvement did not necessarily include individuals with AIDS, a tension that would become a significant source of division within the community and that would provide the ideologic framework for the self-empowerment movement.[16]

In defining community resources, the distinction from government resources is key. The birth of most CBOs was prompted by dissatisfaction with the government services available to them.[17] With AIDS, this dynamic has proved particularly keen, sometimes even volatile. Many attribute the breadth, robustness, and durability of the community response directly to government neglect.[18]

The challenges inherent in defining community resources pale in comparison with the difficulties posed by defining *community* itself. With AIDS, disputes within and among the various communities affected by the epidemic have punctuated the history of community definition, generally calling into question any given community's ability to serve or represent another.[15] Although this phenomenon is not unique to AIDS, it is more pronounced than with other diseases; ironically, this may be a direct result of the AIDS communities' successes in attaching greater significance to the voices of their affected members.

Significantly, the public defines many AIDS communities in other, often powerful ways, a fact that may work to the advantage and to the detriment of the community in question. For example, although the spread of many infectious diseases and the designation of a community may understandably parallel socioeconomic, geographic, or lifestyle communities, nowhere is this more the case than with AIDS.[19] AIDS has disproportionately affected groups identified primarily through behavior for which they are otherwise characteristically and powerfully stigmatized (eg, homosexual sex, drug use). As a result, with respect to the organizational and political development of communities, AIDS has effectively collapsed the distinction between disease and identity politics. This is particularly, but not exclusively, true in the gay community.[20] Insofar as a thoroughgoing discussion of the definition of community would entail a sociologic treatise and because my primary concern in this chapter is to avail the reader of practical information for persons living with HIV or AIDS or their caregivers, I will not struggle further to define the term more precisely.

A COMMUNITY RESPONDS

Historical Background

That the decade preceding the AIDS epidemic saw the explosive growth of a previously embryonic gay civil rights movement was fortunate, at least insofar as it contributed to the development of a community infrastructure capable of rapidly responding to a crisis. The existing CBOs were capable of mobilizing or at least contacting their members. A sense of community identity, although perhaps not mature,

had evolved, and the community had the beginnings of a political identity.[23] Perhaps key, a young but vibrant press existed that was capable of disseminating critical information early, before the government saw fit to educate the public about the dangers of what was first called "gay cancer," the "gay plague," or GRID (gay-related immune deficiency). A homophobic response provoked by the early identification of AIDS as a gay disease, combined with the pressures of intractable poverty, may have short-circuited an otherwise natural tendency to organize in other strong communities that exist among other groups, in particular African-American and Latino populations.

In contrast, incipient organizing among communities with high numbers of drug users or among users themselves was confined primarily to Europe, where drug users were not so demonized as they are in the United States.[22] Gay men of color also faced significant barriers posed by dual discrimination from the broader communities of color, who were loath to acknowledge homosexuality, and from their more privileged white counterparts, who initially made little effort to transcend discrimination based on race or class.[21] To the American public, the early epidemic was signified by middle-class, white, gay men, while casualties among other groups went ignored.

The association of AIDS with groups that were otherwise strongly politically identified and stigmatized contributed to its conceptualization as a sociopolitical as much as a medical problem. Elected officials, ever mindful of offending conservative constituencies, were reluctant to confront the burgeoning epidemic early, particularly in the critical areas of research, education, and prevention.[23] For example, the provision of sexually explicit educational material and sterile injection equipment, both of which public health experts agreed were likely to reduce the transmission of HIV, was essentially prohibited for most of the decade after the epidemic was first reported.

In response, at a more rapid pace than at any other time in modern U.S. medical history, community-based groups organized themselves to serve the growing legions of those affected by the disease. By 1982, about 45 such organizations existed, mostly within the gay community. By the end of the decade, more than 600 such groups were in existence.[12] By 1992, the number of groups surged to an estimated 16,000.[15]

Community-based providers supply comprehensive medical care, perform confidential counseling and HIV antibody testing, administer psychosocial counseling, secure stable assisted housing, and deliver hot meals to the homebound. Volunteer attorneys write wills, defend victims of discrimination, and advocate for the civil rights of persons with AIDS. Agencies founded by white, middle-class, gay men now deliver child care, family counseling, and support for individuals with addiction problems.

Spearheaded by persons with AIDS, groups such as the People With AIDS (PWA) Coalition in New York City maintain treatment hotlines, offer support groups and peer counseling, and sponsor tea dances for persons who are HIV positive to provide an environment where the disclosure of HIV status becomes moot. Often in defiance of local laws and conservative prohibition, radical volunteers, many themselves ex-junkies, distribute sterile needles to addicts on street corners in an effort to prevent the further spread of HIV in already devastated communities. Their courage and the "medical necessity" of their actions has been upheld in a court of law,[24] and their method has been copied by nonprofit providers and even by some public health departments.

AIDS activists organized to protest the lack of research focused on finding a cure. One such protest was held in Washington, D.C., outside the White House in June of 1987 (Fig. 28-1). In that same year, a demonstration on Wall Street, sponsored by a nascent, renegade group of street activists calling themselves by the mnemonic acronym Act Up (AIDS Coalition to Unleash Power), sparked a worldwide social movement that grew to capture the attention of world governments, the powerful pharmaceutical industry, Hollywood, and the upper echelons of the Catholic church.[12] Their pressure within the scientific research community produced fundamental shifts in the relationship between doctor and patient, between researcher and subject.[25]

Artists with AIDS and an art community devastated by AIDS have produced works that speak to the struggles posed by a modern day epidemic,[26] and the entertainment industry has rallied with glittering, star-studded benefits. In a moving affront to the rigidly conservative notion of family values, many gay men, lesbians, and others have adopted the children left orphaned by young parents who succumbed to AIDS; many of these children are themselves infected.

In 1983, a caucus of AIDS "victims" at an early National AIDS Forum captured the spirit of all these myriad, community-based responses to the AIDS crisis best when they declared, "We condemn attempts to label us as 'victims,' a term which implies defeat, and we are only occasionally 'patients,' a term which implies passivity, helplessness, and dependence on the care of others. We are 'People With AIDS.'"[16]

Those groups most sharply affected by the epidemic, most notably the gay community, have been transformed by their own brief history, by the devastation wrought by the epidemic, and through their experiences in responding to it.[21] For all its carnage, AIDS has supplied the gay community in particular with a sense of cohesion lacking in earlier decades of the movement and has helped to unify men and women with markedly different perspectives, agendas, and lives.[27,28]

Long traditions of social activism and volunteerism predate AIDS, from organizations such as the American Social Hygiene Association at the turn of the century to the modern private, voluntary health agencies, such as the Red Cross or the March of Dimes. Self-help, patient advocacy, and even so-called empowerment organizations also predate AIDS: Alcoholics Anonymous, Heart-to-Heart, Added Care, and others.[37] With AIDS, the concept of self-empowerment has reached its zenith, enhancing the license and resolve of sufferers of other diseases, most notably breast cancer activists.[38] CBOs provide the foundation for such community organizing and development. AIDS has provided a powerful example that community development can lead to a greater capacity for effective advocacy, which can lead to enhanced government services.[28,30]

Although adversarial at its outset, the relationship between public (government) and private (community) AIDS service providers has evolved to become symbiotic

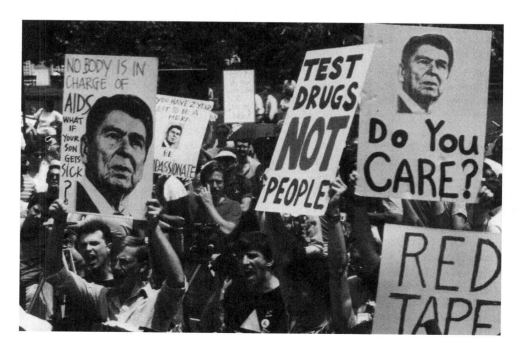

FIG. 28-1. AIDS activists protest government inaction at the White House in June 1987. (Photograph courtesy of Jane Rosett.)

and interdependent, if not any less mutually suspicious.[20] In perhaps the most striking example, the United States Congress passed the Ryan White Comprehensive AIDS Resources Emergency (CARE) Act, which disburses nearly $1 billion to state and local jurisdictions, who contract with CBOs to provide services for persons with AIDS. Initially as an outgrowth of many great society programs and later as a key strategy to privatize the federal bureaucracy, CBOs are now the recipients of large numbers of government grants or contracts specifically for health care services at a local level. With AIDS, the extent to which such relationships characterize the United States' overall response to a health care emergency has escalated dramatically.

A Selective History: Case Histories of the Community Responses to AIDS

Provided in the following sections are case histories of some of the many CBOs formed in response to the AIDS epidemic, many of which inspired other groups like them around the country and around the world. The organizations described are not intended to constitute an exhaustive or even a representative history, but they are offered as examples of the many innovative, often courageous, always moving responses to AIDS.

1981—Birth of the AIDS Community: The Gay Men's Health Crisis

In 1981, a small report buried in the New York Times was headlined, "Rare Cancer [Kaposi's Sarcoma] Seen in 41 Homosexuals."[31] Within a small group of gay men in New York City, the emergence of a deadly disease of unknown etiology provoked panic. A hastily called meeting at the home of playwright Larry Kramer resulted in the formation of the Gay Men's Health Crisis (GMHC), a volunteer group dedicated to raising money for research and to helping victims of the disease. That night, $6635 was raised by passing the hat.[23,32]

As the first AIDS organization, the newly formed GMHC was besieged first by requests for information and then by volunteers offering their help. The group formed the first volunteer AIDS hotline, initially set up on an answering machine, and received more than 100 calls the first night. To quell growing fears in the community, they wrote and distributed a 34-page health newsletter. Open community forums were presented to capacity crowds, and more than 250,000 flyers were distributed to the city's many gay bars. By the end of 1982, GMHC had developed a Patients Services Program. Crisis intervention counselors, all trained volunteers, helped patients at times of crisis, whether medical, legal, spiritual, or emotional. A corps of volunteer buddies was inaugurated to help with daily chores, such as laundry, errands, and cooking. To provide emotional support for frightened patients and caregivers, GMHC established support therapy groups. GMHC board officers met with city and state health officials and traveled to the CDC to urge

greater action. After a series of fundraisers, the GMHC donated almost $50,000 to local academic research centers. The AIDS community was born.[33]

In addition to early volunteer, education, development, and patient programs, GMHC instituted financial advocacy, legal advocacy, public policy programs, and an Ombudsman's office. Later, Child Life, Medical Information, Treatment Education and Advocacy, a Lesbian AIDS project, TB Education and Treatment Support, and Substance Use Education and Counseling were added. As early as 1982, similar organizations, many originating in the gay community and modeled on GMHC, existed in Atlanta, Baltimore, Boston, Chicago, Denver, Los Angeles, Chicago, Houston, Philadelphia, San Francisco, and Washington, D.C.[34] Like GMHC, which now employs more than 270 professional staff members and raises $27 million annually, many of these organizations have matured to become full-spectrum social service agencies, and they provide the foundation in their local community for a network of other organizations dedicated to serving persons living with AIDS.

1982—Community-Based AIDS Research: The American Medical Foundation

Joseph Sonnabend, a New York physician who worked in the gay community in the late 1970s, had been trained as a research scientist. After seeing a case of *Pneumocystis carinii* pneumonia (PCP) in his practice and then reading about similar cases in the *Morbidity and Mortality Weekly Report,* Sonnabend knew that an epidemic was at hand. With his colleague Dr. Mathilde Krim, a respected interferon researcher and the wife of Hollywood magnate Arthur Krim, the two began experiments in Krim's laboratory at Memorial Sloan-Kettering. Sonnabend also conducted experiments with the assistance of volunteers from his practice. In one of the earliest clinical AIDS experiments in the country, Sonnabend managed to have T4 cells measured among patients stratified by sexual history, thereby establishing a clear link between sexually transmitted diseases and immune suppression.[35]

In early 1982, Sonnabend published his first warning to gay men in the *New York Native,* urging them to abandon sexual promiscuity because of his findings. Although vilified in the community, Sonnabend's research caught the attention of a publisher who was interested in starting a journal to cover this new disease. With Sonnabend at the helm, *AIDS Research,* the first journal of its kind, began publication in 1983.[32]

Largely in an effort to fund Sonnabend's research, Krim founded the American Medical Foundation (AMF) in 1982. Although neither Sonnabend nor Krim had previous experience in financing research, the AMF established an institutional review board (IRB), solicited proposals, and ultimately funded the first clinical trial of an anti-HIV treatment (ie, isoprinosine) in the world. Raising money proved difficult even for Krim, a reflection of the stigmatism associated with AIDS. Although their first fundraiser at Manhattan's chic Studio 54 raised $100,000, Krim's requests for help were politely rebuffed at Ford, Rockefeller, and other traditional philanthropic foundations. The AMF would later merge with the nascent National AIDS Research Foundation, formed by Dr. Michael Gottlieb and Elizabeth Taylor with a bequest from the estate of Rock Hudson, to form the American Foundation for AIDS Research, now the world's largest AIDS research foundation.

1983—Community Health and Gay and Lesbian Clinics: The Whitman Walker Clinic

Originally founded in 1973 as the Gay Men's VD Clinic, Whitman Walker Clinic was one of several community-based clinics targeting gay men and lesbians in cities around the country, including the Howard Brown Clinic in Chicago, the St. Mark's Community Health Project in New York, the Gay and Lesbian Community Services Center in Los Angeles, the Fenway Clinic in Boston, and others. Modeled largely on the women's health movement, these groups offered culturally sensitive, nonjudgmental care to gay men and lesbians, many of whom were uncomfortable discussing issues related to their health and especially their sexuality with mainstream providers. As with other gay community organizations, these health clinics proved to be well positioned, if not prepared or equipped, to care for the many persons with AIDS that they began to see in the early 1980s.[19]

By early 1983, when 22 cases of AIDS had been reported in the District of Columbia, Whitman Walker recognized that it would have a key role to play in the community's response. That year, following the first AIDS fundraiser in the District, Whitman Walker sponsored a community forum attended by 1200 gay men, distributed its first AIDS education pamphlet, received the first city AIDS contract for the operation of an "AIDS Infoline," sponsored the first Education Forum targeting persons of color, and awarded the organization's first grant to a person with AIDS.

With a staff of 200, Whitman Walker is now the largest gay and lesbian organization in the United States. In locations throughout the District and Northern Virginia, Whitman Walker offers anonymous HIV testing, outpatient medical and dental care, gynecologic care, an on-site pharmacy, a food bank, and supported housing for persons with AIDS. The clinic also manages a research unit affiliated with the National Institute of Allergy and Infectious Diseases' (NIAID) AIDS Clinical Trials Group, operates a speakers' bureau, sponsors countless public education forums, distributes educational literature, and aggressively advocates on public policy issues associated with HIV and AIDS.[36]

1983—Self-Empowerment Movement: The People With AIDS Coalition

In 1982 in San Francisco, self-proclaimed "KS Poster Boy" Bobbi Campbell, usually sporting a button that proclaimed

"SURVIVE," began an influential column in the San Francisco Sentinel, a local gay paper, describing his experiences and offering advice. Later, in collaboration with Dan Turner, Campbell held a meeting from which the first AIDS self-empowerment organization would emerge. Coining a moniker that would come to signify a movement, Campbell called his organization People With AIDS (PWA) San Francisco. Shortly thereafter, the KS/AIDS Foundation (later the San Francisco AIDS Foundation), which had grown out of an early AIDS hotline started by Dr. Marcus Conant and activist Cleve Jones, invited PWA San Francisco to submit recommendations for its board of directors. The notion that the sick should participate in the operation of the organizations that served them was new and controversial; GMHC did not add an openly HIV-positive member to its board until 1987. Campbell was also instrumental in producing San Francisco's first safe-sex brochure, Can We Talk? In May 1983, many members of PWA San Francisco organized the first candlelight march and vigil, marching behind a banner that proclaimed "Fighting For Our Lives."[16]

Meanwhile, in New York, gay community activists Michael Callen and Richard Berkowitz published a controversial article in the New York Native urging gay men to reduce their number of sexual partners.[37] In November 1983, they formed a group called Gay Men With AIDS to provide peer support for men with AIDS and sexual addiction problems.[32] Callen and Berkowitz later took their message one step further by publishing and widely distributing a 40-page pamphlet, How to Have Sex in an Epidemic.[38] Although it foreshadowed safe-sex education campaigns that would become the standard fare of AIDS service organizations worldwide, the pamphlet was revolutionary in New York, where AIDS community leaders, mainly constituted at GMHC, initially were disinclined to issue any instructions regarding matters of sexuality.[39]

Callen and Berkowitz also attended the AIDS Network, a group formed by lesbian activist Virginia Apuzzo and others. Kramer, who had become increasingly disaffected with GMHC, which he perceived to be too conservative, also attended. The Network had taken its cue from the women's health movement and was discussing demonstrations at a time that GMHC was talking about negotiations. In a seminal article, "1,112 and Counting," Kramer called for 3000 volunteers for acts of civil disobedience.[40] On May 10, 1983, the AIDS Network held its first small picket in torrential rain outside Lenox Hill Hospital, where Mayor Koch was to address a historic AIDS conference.[39] The group's feminist ideology taught Callen (and perhaps even Kramer) much about political organizing and power. Ultimately, this growing awareness was to fuel Callen's own drive for self-empowerment.[32]

The idea that AIDS organizations should sponsor AIDS patients to attend the Second National AIDS Forum, which was to be convened in Denver in 1983, originated in San Francisco but quickly swept across the country. In New York, GMHC provided tepid resistance to the idea.[41] However, in Denver, Callen, Berkowitz, Campbell, Turner, and others caucused in a hospitality suite hastily provided for them to air their concerns. Out of their discussions came a vision for the National Association of People With AIDS and a series of statements later dubbed "The Denver Principles" (Table 28-1).[16]

TABLE 28-1. *The Denver principles*

RECOMMENDATIONS FOR HEALTH CARE PROFESSIONALS

1. Come out, especially to their patients who have AIDS
2. Always clearly identify and discuss the theory they favor about the cause of AIDS, because this bias affects the treatments and advice they give
3. Get in touch with their feelings (eg, fears, anxieties, hopes) about AIDS and not simply deal with AIDS intellectually
4. Take a thorough personal inventory and identify and examine their own agendas around AIDS
5. Treat people with AIDS as whole people, and address psychosocial issues as well as biophysical ones
6. Address the question of sexuality in people with AIDS specifically, sensitively and with information about gay male sexuality in general, and the sexuality of people with AIDS in particular

RECOMMENDATIONS FOR ALL PEOPLE

1. Support us in our struggle against those who would fire us from our jobs, evict us from our homes, refuse to touch us or separate us from our loved ones, our community or our peers, because available evidence does not support the view that AIDS can be spread by casual, social contact
2. Not scapegoat people with AIDS, blame us for the epidemic or generalize about our lifestyles

RECOMMENDATIONS FOR PEOPLE WITH AIDS

1. Form caucuses to choose their own representatives, to deal with the media, to choose their own agenda and to plan their own strategies
2. Be involved at every level of decision making and specifically serve on the boards of directors of provider organizations
3. Be included in all AIDS forums with equal credibility as other participants, to share their own experiences and knowledge
4. Substitute low-risk sexual behaviors for those which could endanger themselves or their partners; we feel that people with AIDS have an ethical responsibility to inform their potential sexual partners of their health status

RIGHTS OF PEOPLE WITH AIDS

1. To as full and satisfying sexual and emotional lives as anyone else
2. To quality medical treatment and quality social service provision without discrimination of any form including sexual orientation, gender, diagnosis, economic status or race
3. To full explanations of all medical procedures and risks, to choose or refuse their treatment modalities, to refuse to participate in research without jeopardizing their treatment and to make informed decisions about their lives
4. To privacy, to confidentiality of medical records, to human respect and to choose who their significant others are
5. To die—and to LIVE—in dignity

Today, the PWA Coalition New York is a thriving, self-help organization that maintains an information hotline staffed by persons with AIDS, provides social and emotional support services to these persons and their loved ones, and publishes the *PWA Newsline*, a newsletter read by many thousands of persons with AIDS each month. Organizations like it in many cities and towns across the country are represented in Washington by the National Association of People With AIDS.

1983—A National Presence and the De-Gaying of AIDS: The Federation of AIDS-Related Organizations

At the Second National AIDS Forum, activists called for a national organization to coordinate the efforts of the many AIDS groups scattered across the country. Of particular importance, many attendees described a desire to dissociate the new organization with the gay rights movement, a step thought necessary to secure needed credibility and money. The Federation of AIDS-Related Organizations, which ironically included only one nongay member organization at its inception, quickly set up a national clearinghouse and hired a Washington lobbyist. Its efforts to raise its projected budget failed, however, and the organization was reconstituted in 1984 as the AIDS Action Council (AAC), a group dedicated solely to lobbying.[19] That year also saw the first targeted federal funds made available to CBOs.

AAC met several times with Surgeon General Koop as he prepared his report on the epidemic. In 1985, AAC convened its first conference of CBOs. At this meeting, the group formed the National AIDS Network, a now-defunct organization dedicated to providing technical assistance to member groups. In 1987, AAC inaugurated the National Organizations Responding to AIDS, a coalition of mainstream public health organizations that strongly influenced the passage of the Ryan White CARE Act. AAC is now the leading national AIDS advocacy organization, representing more than 1000 community-based groups nationwide.

1983—Housing for People With AIDS: The AIDS Resource Center and Bailey-Holt House

In April 1983, a group of community activists and artists, led by Rev. Lee Hancock of the Judson Memorial Baptist Church, became concerned with the increasing number of persons with AIDS who lost their homes as a result of the disease. Because virtually no options existed for these homeless persons, the group formed the AIDS Resource Center (ARC), which started the first housing program for persons with AIDS in New York City, with a single room in a board member's apartment. The group sought to create a space that was neither a nursing home nor a leper colony, but a place where persons with AIDS could live safely, comfortably, and independently. The next year, ARC rented its first apartment with private monies, although it was not until 1987 that the City of New York would contract with ARC to provide 20 scattered-site apartments.

In 1985, recognizing that secure housing enhanced survival and was a prerequisite for other services and benefits, ARC successfully lobbied New York Mayor Ed Koch's administration to purchase a six-story hotel in Greenwich Village and lease it to ARC. Over the opposition of local businesses, the former River Hotel was transformed into a 44-room facility offering each resident a private room and bath, telephone, and three meals each day. Although Bailey House experienced early difficulties (eg, it took a lawsuit to get the building wired for cable, garbage men refused to carry the trash, the copier went without service because repairmen refused to enter the building), it quickly became a model for supportive housing programs worldwide. Named in honor of ARC founder Mead Bailey and later renamed in memory of Fritz Holt, the partner of ARC board member Barry Brown, Bailey-Holt House now offers a wide range of support services, including substance abuse and bereavement counseling, bilingual case management, and psychiatric and recreational therapy.

1984—Grassroots Political Action: Mobilization Against AIDS

In 1984, meeting in an apartment in San Francisco's Castro neighborhood, 10 concerned activists formed Mobilization Against AIDS (MAA), a nonpartisan, gay organization. The group declared its intention to emulate the tactics of Vietnam War protestors, and in an early brochure, declared: "We exist to push the Federal government into giving meaningful support and funding to the other AIDS organizations." In January 1985, MAA targeted its first demonstration at California elected officials, including Senator Alan Cranston, Representative John Burton, and the San Francisco Board of Supervisors. In rapid succession, the renegade group targeted regents of the University of California at San Francisco, the U.S. Department of Health and Human Services (in San Francisco), and the California State Legislature.

In August 1985, MAA member Patty Rose completed a 130-mile walk across Death Valley in a pointed challenge to President Reagan to say the word AIDS in public. At a September press conference, Reagan finally said the word after being asked whether he would support a moon-shot effort to defeat AIDS, an idea originated by MAA.

In May 1985, MAA organized the AIDS Candlelight Memorial in more than 40 cities on four continents, the largest simultaneous AIDS action to date. Later, at an MAA demonstration targeting a fundraiser for Senator Pete Wilson, then Vice President Bush told the press, "I just hope that persons don't think a lack of statements is equated with a lack of concern" (written communication, Mobilization Against AIDS, April 28, 1995). The following year, MAA produced San Francisco's first AIDS Dance-a-thon. In June 1990, MAA helped organized the "HIV/AIDS March: A United Call to Action" at the closing of the Sixth International Conference on AIDS. In a symbolic show of collaboration and respect, 20,000 demonstrators, including many of the world's leading AIDS scientists chanted, "300,000 dead from AIDS. Where is George [Bush]?"[42]

1985—Community-Based AIDS Research: The San Francisco County Community Consortium

The idea that AIDS drugs could be tested in physicians' offices occurred to Donald Abrams and Paul Volberding, both doctors at San Francisco General. Initially begun as a series of meetings to discuss communication between community and academic physicians (Abrams was the former, Volberding the latter), the San Francisco County Community Consortium (CCC) was inaugurated in March of 1985. The group's intention was to conduct rigorous clinical trials out of physicians' offices, a strategy pursued with some success in cancer research.[25]

Two years later, at a 1987 meeting organized by Timothy Westmoreland, aide to Representative Henry Waxman, a group of activists including Callan, Kramer, and GMHC's Dr. Barry Gingell and Nathan Kolodner, faced off with NIAID Director Anthony Fauci. Callen pleaded with Fauci to issue guidelines for using pentamidine, a drug then suspected to prevent PCP, the leading killer of persons with AIDS. Fauci argued that he could neither produce such guidelines nor convene a conference without scientific data. Callen was incensed, because PCP prophylaxis was standard-of-care in many community physicians' offices. He decided then that the community, not the million-dollar Federal bureaucracy, would have to take the responsibility for testing pentamidine. Callen, Sonnabend, and Hannan would later form New York's Community Research Initiative (CRI) to do just that.[32]

For its first efforts, CCC elected to study pentamidine. Although pentamidine was in use in the community, no studies had been conducted to evaluate efficacy. In a departure from clinical research practice, the principal investigator's pentamidine trial elected to eschew a placebo control, instead conducting a dose study. (An earlier Bactrim study had infuriated activists, who viewed the use of a placebo when Bactrim had established efficacy in preventing PCP in an immunocompromised host to be unethical.) Although NIAID declined to fund the study, although the institute had rated pentamidine a high-priority drug, CCC eventually secured funding from the University of California and the drug's manufacturer, Lyphomed. On May 1, 1989, an Food and Drug Administration (FDA) advisory committee voted unanimously to approve pentamidine, based principally on data submitted by San Francisco's CCC and New York City's CRI.[25]

Following a recommendation from the Presidential Commission on the HIV Epidemic,[43] NIAID ultimately funded its own consortium of community-based research centers (which ironically did not include New York's CRI), the Community Program for Clinical Research on AIDS. The American Foundation for AIDS Research, headed by Krim, managed to raise $1 million at a concert at Carnegie Hall, which it quickly parlayed into a network of 16 community-based research centers, the Community Based Clinical Trials program.[32]

1985—Treatment Education and Advocacy: Project Inform

In the mid-1980s, before the licensure of a single drug to treat HIV infection, enterprising gay men traveled to Mexico to purchase ribavirin and isoprinosine, two supposed AIDS treatments. Although little scientific data supported their beliefs that the drugs would be helpful, they were undaunted. Martin Delaney, then a communications consultant in San Francisco, was among those making repeated smuggling runs to Tijuana. Delaney built a reputation for resourcefulness and tenacity. In an early public speaking role, he took on a representative from the FDA at a public forum sponsored by MAA. After many such trips, Delaney proposed evaluating the drugs in a clinical trial of sorts, run in the community and monitored by community physicians. Although ridiculed by the establishment, the organization he formed to oversee the trial, Project Inform, grew to be the first AIDS treatment information and advocacy organization.[44]

From the outset, Project Inform advocated aggressive treatment, arguing that treatment was preferable to no treatment, even if scientific data were inconclusive. While trying to organize his trial, Delaney, a charismatic speaker, perfected a town meeting format, in which he would offer the latest treatment information and opine on treatment strategies. The town meetings had the tenor of revival meetings and quickly developed an enthusiastic following; Delaney later toured around the country.

The most controversial of Project Inform's endeavors was the conduct of a multisite, underground clinical trial of the purported AIDS drug, Compound Q. The drug was one in a long series of putative AIDS cures that in the mid-1980s blew through the community like wildfire. In several ways, however, it was different. It was administered intravenously, it was available only in China, and it was known to have side effects, some very serious. Project Inform's underground study enrolled patients in four cities and was by all accounts a serious effort to conduct a by-the-books clinical trial. The trial was harshly criticized, however, by the FDA, by the mainstream medical establishment, and by the community. More than one patient died during the Q trial, and ethicists later argued that the clandestine nature of so-called underground trials compromised ethical standards for medical research.[45]

Delaney was not to be dismissed, however. Even after his Compound Q trial was halted, he was invited to present data to the FDA, who later permitted a more rigorously monitored trial to continue. Although Delaney later suggested that this vindicated him of any breach in medical research standards, he continued to be roundly criticized and interest in Compound Q eventually faded.[42]

Also of note, Project Inform would later convene a series of scientific meetings called Project Immune Restoration. At these "think-tank" style gatherings, leading AIDS researchers were encouraged to brainstorm together, an all too rare opportunity in science. Today, Project Inform runs a national experimental treatment hotline, and is an influential advocate for more efficient drug development and clinical trials.[32]

1985—Advocacy for Drug Users: The Association for Drug Abuse Prevention and Treatment

By 1983, the Association for Drug Abuse, Prevention and Treatment (ADAPT) was moribund. Founded some years earlier by professionals (many were ex-users) concerned about drug abuse to pressure for additional drug treatment slots, the organization's members had drifted apart. Several former ADAPT members began to notice the impact of the AIDS epidemic among drug users in New York, and they urged that the organization be resuscitated. Yolanda Serrano became the newly reinvigorated organization's executive director.

Although New York was home for the highest concentration of drug users in the United States, it also had among the nation's strictest syringe possession laws. As a result, sterile "works" (ie, injection equipment) were scarce, forcing addicts to share. HIV seroprevalence among New York City injection drug users soared to a level exceeding 50%.[46] ADAPT soon became legendary for its outreach efforts in New York City's infamous "shooting galleries," where addicts could rent works long enough for them to inject, after which they would be rented to others. With access to drug treatment a fantasy for most of New York's 200,000 users, ADAPT strongly advocated the use of bleach to clean injection equipment and distributed thousands of kits for that purpose.

Although the Health Commissioner David Sencer had proposed the idea of distributing sterile syringes to addicts in 1985, no proposal had yet been approved as of 1988. The idea met with strong resistance from New York's African-American and Latino leaders, some of whom likened needle exchange to genocide.[47] ADAPT, in a risky move, announced to the media that if the city failed to move forward, they would commence providing clean needles on their own. Although the threat had serious consequences (ie, New York City froze ADAPTs funding and closed its offices for 2 days), a limited needle exchange program was approved by the State Health Commissioner, although numerous other obstacles would have to be cleared before it finally got underway.[47]

1986—The AIDS Treatment Newsletter: AIDS Treatment News

In May 1986, John James turned what had been his biweekly column in the *San Francisco Sentinel* into a biweekly newsletter called *AIDS Treatment News*. The first issue focused on AL721, a reputed AIDS therapy concocted from egg lipids. James, although not a scientist, provided a bibliography of scientific references and presented information so as to be understandable to his lay readers. In an approach that would later characterize the AIDS treatment activist movement, James refused to accept the mysticism that often surrounded medicine.[32] *AIDS Treatment News*'s spare format and even, objective prose lent it a considerable following among persons with AIDS, physicians, policy makers, and caregivers. Still edited by James out of a Victorian row house on San Francisco's Church Street, *AIDS Treatment News* has a circulation of more than 5000.[12] Similar, all-purpose newsletters are printed with various degrees of regularity by Project Inform (*PI Perspectives*), GMHC (*Treatment Issues*), the San Francisco AIDS Foundation (*BETA*), and *Critical Path* (Table 28-2). Myriad sources of information are available through local groups, national clearinghouses, and hotlines (Table 28-3).

1987—AIDS Defines a Social Movement: Act Up!

On March 10, 1987, after Nora Ephron canceled as the featured speaker at the New York Lesbian and Gay Community Services Center's speakers series, Larry Kramer was asked to fill in. His angry speech was a call to action, another plea for social protest and civil disobedience.[39] Two days later, 300 men and women met again at the Center and founded Act Up, "a diverse nonpartisan group united in anger and committed to direct action to end the global AIDS epidemic." The group's first action was a demonstration on Wall Street to protest, among other things, the $10,000 annual price tag of zidovudine (AZT). Hundreds of demonstrators choked Wall Street in the first major act of civil disobedience related to the AIDS epidemic.[32] That year, AIDS activists protested at New York City's Main Post Office on April 15, at the White House on June 1, at New York's Federal Plaza on June 30, at New York's Memorial Sloane-Kettering Hospital for 4 days beginning on July 21, at Northwest Airlines on August 4, at the first meeting of the President's Commission on the HIV epidemic on September 9, and at the Supreme Court on October 13.[48]

Several later demonstrations would solidify the image of Act Up (and AIDS activism generally) in the minds of the American public. In September 1988, a huge demonstration was held at the headquarters of the FDA, in Rockville, Maryland. In 1989, Act Up demonstrated on the Golden Gate Bridge, snarling rush hour traffic for hours and delaying the opening of the San Francisco Opera season. In November 1989, infuriated that New York's Cardinal O'Con-

TABLE 28-2. *Newsletters that discuss AIDS*

Community Newsletters	Cost	Address/Phone
AIDS Treatment News (biweekly)	$100/individuals, $115/nonprofit organ., $230/businesses	AIDS Treatment News P.O. Box 411256 San Francisco, CA 94110 1-800-TREAT-1-2
Bulletin of Experimental Treatments for AIDS (quarterly)	Free	San Francisco AIDS Foundation 25 Van Ness St San Francisco, CA 94110
GMHC Treatment Issues (10 times/year)	$35/individuals, $70/businesses and int. sliding scale for PWA	Gay Men's Health Crisis 129 West 20th St New York, NY 10011
Notes From the Underground (bimonthly)	$35/year or sliding scale for PWA/low income	PWA Health Group 150 W 26th St, Rm 201 New York, NY 10001
PWA Coalition Newsline & SIDAAhora (monthly)	$35/year, PWAs free	PWA Coalition 50 W 17th Street, 8th Floor New York, NY 10011
Body Positive (monthly)	Free but $35 donation suggested	Body Positive 19 Fulton Street, Suite 308B New York, NY 10038 1-800-566-6599
Critical Path (quarterly)	$50/year, PWAs free	Critical Path AIDS Project 2062 Lombard Street Philadelphia, PA 19146 215-545-2212
Positively Aware (bimonthly)	Free but donation suggested	Test Positive Aware 1258 West Belmont Street Chicago, IL 60657
PI Perspectives Newsletter (quarterly)	Free but donation suggested	Project Inform 1965 Market St, Ste 220 San Francisco, CA 94103 1-800-822-7422

TABLE 28-3. *AIDS hotlines*

Hotlines	Phone Number	Type of Information Provided
CDC HIV/AIDS Information Line	1-800-342-AIDS	General information, referrals to local agencies or community-based organizations
AIDS Clinical Trials Information Service (ACTIS)	1-800-874-2572	Current information on federally and privately sponsored clinical trials for HIV infected individuals, and on the drugs being investigated in these trials
Body Positive Helpline	1-800-566-6599	Support and counseling, referrals, for HIV-positive individuals
HIV/AIDS Treatment Information Service (ATIS)	1-800-448-0440	Information about federally approved treatments for HIV and AIDS
Project Inform Treatment Hotline	1-800-822-7422	Information on experimental drug treatments for HIV and AIDS
National Association of People With AIDS (NAPWA)	202-898-0414	Information on HIV and AIDS issues; referrals

ner would reject the National Conference of Catholic Bishops' call for limited tolerance of condom use as a protection against a deadly disease, Act Up heckled the Cardinal while he celebrated mass in St. Patrick's Cathedral, in a demonstration dubbed "Stop the Church."[49] The protest was decried by Governor Mario Cuomo and President George Bush.

It was Act Up's Treatment and Data Committee (T+D) that proved to have the greatest influence on AIDS research. T+D members proved themselves adept at understanding the science behind AIDS research and drug regulation, taught themselves the intricacies of bureaucratic regulation, and demanded reform.[15] By mastering scientific concept and jargon while testifying at the influential Lasagna Committee, T+D members Mark Harrington, Jim Eigo, and Iris Long almost singlehandedly legitimized Act Up in the scientific world with their careful analysis of drug regulation. In an insightful criticism of the AIDS clinical trials system, Harrington called for participation of the AIDS community in research design; a comprehensive plan for drug development and testing; equal attention to antiretrovirals and antiinfectives; the inclusion of women, drug users, and persons of color in clinical trials; the elimination of restrictions on concomitant medications; and fairly priced drugs. Harrington's analysis suggested that more humanely designed clinical trials would prove to be more efficient. In the years to come, many of his suggestions would come to pass.[32]

T+D's zenith was the result of a characteristic double-pronged strategy to target the venerable National Institutes of Health (NIH). While Harrington scuffled with Fauci for permission to attend the scientific meetings of the AIDS Clinical Trials Group (ACTG), T+D planned the next in a series of spectacular demonstrations, "Storm the NIH." At first, T+D members attended ACTG meetings uninvited, but they were discouraged to be treated like interlopers, sometimes being physically removed from certain closed-door meetings. They demanded participant status. The ACTG leadership relented by creating the Community Constituent Group (CCG), which at first the activists regarded as mere tokenism. Despite Fauci's assurances that he was doing everything possible, the activists were still barred from key committees.

The action at NIH saw 1000 activists marching with placards among colored smoke bombs through the otherwise bucolic campus of the NIH. Police arrested 82 activists, who chanted "Ten years later, one billion dollars, one drug, big deal." By November 1990, NIAID announced that community representatives would sit on every committee of the ACTG.[25] Although Act Up's T+D committee is still active, the most influential of its members later split from the organization to form the Treatment Action Group (TAG).

1987—Mourning Community Loss: The Names Project AIDS Memorial Quilt

In 1985, as San Francisco activist Cleve Jones helped prepare the annual candlelight march in honor of Harvey Milk, the openly gay Supervisor who was assassinated in 1978, he realized that the number of San Franciscans who had died of AIDS had reached the 1000 mark. Jones asked his fellow marchers to write the names of deceased friends and loved ones on placards, and above a sea of candlelight, he and others taped those placards to the walls of the San Francisco Federal Building. The image reminded him of a patchwork quilt. A little over a year later, Jones created the first panel for a larger memorial, the NAMES Project AIDS Memorial Quilt, in memory of his friend Marvin Feldman, to whom the quilt is dedicated. In June 1987, Jones and others organized the NAMES Project Foundation. At a workshop in a San Francisco storefront, while a group of friends prepared panels to memorialize loved ones, panels from New York, Los Angeles, San Francisco, and other cities began to arrive daily.

In October 1987, the NAMES Project displayed the quilt for the first time on Capitol Mall in Washington, D.C., at the National March on Washington for Lesbian and Gay Rights. It was made of 1920 panels, covered a space larger than a football field, and was visited by 500,000 persons. On display in Washington, D.C., in 1992, the number of panels had risen to 20,064 (Fig. 28-2). Today, there are 38 NAMES Project Chapters and 29 independent quilt initiatives around the world. More than 5,000,000 persons have visited the quilt at thousands of displays. The quilt includes more than 30,000 individually made panels. The quilt is the largest example of a community art project in the world and was

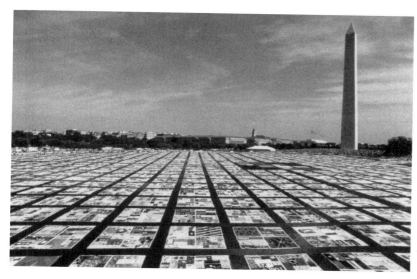

FIG. 28-2. The NAMES Project AIDS Memorial Quilt, comprising 20,064 panels, on display in Washington, DC in October 1992. (Photograph courtesy of Jane Rosett.)

nominated for a Nobel Peace Prize in 1989. The film *Common Threads: Stories From the Quilt* won the Academy Award for best feature-length documentary in 1989.

1987—The AIDS Underground: People With AIDS Health Group

In the mid-1980s, although ribavirin and isoprinosine had caught the attention of persons with AIDS and inspired a certain amount of smuggling, nothing proved more intriguing to activists than AL-721, a mixture created from egg lipids and described by Dr. Robert Gallo in a brief letter to the *New England Journal of Medicine* as "promising." Besides its purported therapeutic benefits, AL-721 had the allure of being natural, an important consideration for many individuals. However, like many so-called natural products, AL-721 was anything but—although made up of egg lipids, its extraction required acetone and other solvents. Some persons with AIDS traveled to Israel, where the substance was under study, and others attempted to produce it at home. When the level of interest became clear, Callen and Hannan arranged with a pharmaceutical contractor to manufacture a batch of AL-721. The two speculated that if they could demonstrate a market for AL-721, a manufacturer would seize the initiative. That turned out to be a mistake; nothing of the sort happened, and Callen and Hannan found themselves in business.

Taking orders from persons with AIDS from around the city, the two formed a business partnership to handle the transactions, and immediately sold out their first lot. Mindful of FDA regulations, Callen declared that AL-721 was a food and therefore did not qualify for regulation as a drug. Nevertheless, the group took elaborate precautions, going so far as to require detailed release forms, picture identification, and certified checks. To discourage imaginary gun-toting FDA agents, they distributed goods from the sanctuary of a church basement. In a matter of weeks, Callen and Han-

nan were overwhelmed by orders, egg lipids, and cash flow. In 1987, the two established People With AIDS Working For Health, Inc., the first of the so-called buyers' clubs in the country. By the time the Health Group hired their first employee in September 1988, the group had logged more than $2 million in transactions.

Contrary to the Health Group's stated intention to "put themselves out of business," the PWA Health Group soon offered a range of medications, including many pharmaceutical products that were available in markets overseas. In response to pressure from activists, in 1988, FDA Commissioner Frank Young had relaxed FDA regulations to permit "personal use" importations of such drugs. The Health Group interpreted the commissioner's move to apply to drugs received through the mail and set about offering mail-order service to its several thousand clients. In 1988, dextran sulfate was the drug of choice. In 1989, the PWA Health Group made headlines by importing fluconazole. England had approved the drug more than a year before the United States; for those lucky enough to afford it, fluconazole as maintenance therapy for cryptococcal meningitis presented an alternative to amphotericin B, which had been dubbed "amphoterrible" or "shake-and-bake" by patients. Later, the PWA Health Group helped members in importing clarithromycin, azithromycin, roxithromycin, albendazole, and other drugs, all before their U.S. marketing approval. In 1990, the PWA Health Group caught the attention of the United States Congress by importing vials of pentamidine at a cost to patients of $40, nearly $100 less than the price in the United States. The PWA Health Group's activities were designed to provoke the FDA and in some measure contributed to FDA reforms of compassionate use and early access protocols.

AIDS SERVICE ORGANIZATIONS

National, regional, and local hotlines (see Table 28-3) can provide referrals to local community-based AIDS organizations. Listings of such organizations and the services they provide also can be found in published directories (Table 28-4). The types of services provided by CBOs vary widely, depending on resources, the magnitude of the local epidemic, the demographics of the local community, and federal and state funding. Although terminology varies among providers, the following paragraphs outline the range of services available through community-based providers.

Coping with daily activities can prove challenging for those with HIV disease. Buddies are individuals, usually volunteers, who will perform certain daily chores, such as laundry, cooking, cleaning, or errands. Typically, a buddy visits a client once or more a week, for an hour or more at a time. Although a buddy is not a replacement for home care and most are not trained to provide sophisticated services, buddies can assist persons with AIDS in retaining their independence, and often provide welcome companionship.

Occasionally, the problems posed by HIV disease can mount to the point where employment, housing, or medical stability is threatened. Such problems are frequently cumulative and interdependent (eg, the loss of housing can portend a loss of employment and a deterioration in health) and can mount quickly. Crisis intervention workers are volunteers who have received additional training to resolve more difficult or complex problems. Although buddies are generally assigned long term, crisis intervention workers typically are available until problems are resolved. For particularly intractable problems, some agencies employ an ombudsman (ie, client advocate) to advocate on the client's behalf.

For women with HIV, the demands of child care and homemaking can preclude seeking medical care. Accordingly, some agencies provide child care to relieve women of the need to watch their children while they receive treatment or to help in caring for children with AIDS.

Finding appropriate medical care can be difficult for persons with HIV disease, particularly outside urban centers. Many general practitioners are unfamiliar with the myriad manifestations of HIV disease, and unfamiliar providers are sometimes insensitive and can be reluctant, or even unwilling to provide care. In the United States, refusing to provide medical care because a person has HIV or AIDS is against federal law.

Outpatient medical care is provided by some groups in a supportive, AIDS-sensitive setting. Many such groups provide exclusively HIV-related services, often on a sliding scale. Such clinics are often equipped to provide routine medical care, including x-ray films, diagnostic testing, and other laboratory work, as well as dental, obstetric-gyneco-

logic, and ophthalmologic care. On-site pharmacies are sometimes available. Some clinics maintain affiliations with major hospitals and can refer clients for inpatient care.

HIV testing is available from many CBOs in anonymous (where no identification is required) or confidential settings. Community-based HIV test sites frequently provide superior referrals for early intervention or other medical care and are more culturally sensitive than government-operated sites.

In some cities, day treatment programs offer more sophisticated medical care and can serve as an alternative to inpatient or home care. By its nature, the treatment of HIV disease evolves rapidly. Keeping up with the standard of care can be challenging for primary care providers, let alone their patients. Beyond the many medical journals and other sources for clinical information, treatment information for a lay audience is available concerning the entire range of options available to persons with HIV disease, from opportunistic infections through end-stage disease. Although much information is written for those with a relatively sophisticated understanding of science and biomedical research, brochures, pamphlets, multimedia materials, and hotlines are widely available for many different reading and education levels. Lay literature is available on the natural history of HIV disease and on the range of AIDS-related opportunistic infections; on treatments for HIV and HIV-related infections, experimental and fully approved; on general health promotion and maintenance; on medical decision making and the doctor-patient relationship; on the interpretation of laboratory markers; on alternative and holistic treatments; and on matters of public policy concerning treatment and research. Many organizations offer public forums, discussion groups, electronic bulletin boards, or specialized training in this area (Table 28-5).

The emotional burden of coping with HIV disease or with providing care to someone living with HIV can be debilitating by itself. Consequently, many groups offer a range of options, including peer support groups, individual and group therapy, or referrals to qualified psychotherapists. Providers design such specialized support to acknowledge the difficulties associated with serious illnesses and to recognize the stigma or discrimination faced by many persons with AIDS. Because many individuals have experienced multiple losses due to AIDS, bereavement groups focus on issues relating to loss, grief, and depression, and help is available to persons with and persons affected by HIV/AIDS. Psychological support is also available for families struggling with one or more members with HIV or

TABLE 28-4. *Community-based organizations*

Directories of Community Based AIDS Organizations	Publisher	Order Number
National Organizations Providing HIV/AIDS Services	CDC National AIDS Clearinghouse	1-800-458-5231
The AIDS Directory ($250.00)	LRP Publications	1-800-341-7874, ext 274
Local AIDS Services: The National Directory ($15.00)	U.S. Conference of Mayors	202-293-7330

TABLE 28-45. *Bulletin boards discussing AIDS*

Selected AIDS-related Bulletin Boards	Address and Phone or Homepage address	Type of Information
National AIDS Clearinghouse	http://cdcnac.aspensys.com:86	AIDS news and research courtesy of the CDC.
The Body Homepage	http://thebody.com	A multimedia AIDS and HIV information Resource. Links to AIDS organization.
HIV Info Web	http://www.jri.org/infoweb	Guide to online AIDS resources
Project Inform	http://www.projinf.org	Updates on experimental AIDS treatments
Gay Men's Health Crisis	http://www.gmhc.org	Tips on living with AIDS and HIV; the basics on HIV testing.
Critical Path	2062 Lombard St. Philadelphia, PA 19146 p:215-545-2212	Extensive series of forums, treatment information
HandsNet (Registration fee and monthly fees)	20195 Stevens Creek Blvd., Suite 120 Cupertino, CA 95014 p:408-257-4500	Prevention, policy, and funding
NIH Information Center	Dennis Rodrigues p:301-496-6610	Press releases, articles, and document summaries
CDC Wonder/PC	1600 Clifton Road, NE, Atlanta, GA 30333 p:404-332-4569	CDC epidemiologic data, public health reports, and guidelines.

AIDS, for children of HIV-infected parents, and for parents of HIV-infected children.

In part because of the episodic nature of HIV disease and in some cases because of discrimination, many persons with AIDS are vulnerable to the loss of housing, particularly after losing employment. Recognizing that stable and secure housing is a prerequisite for good health, many AIDS organizations provide housing services specifically targeted to persons with AIDS. Scattered-site apartments are subsidized units specifically equipped for persons with AIDS who have low-threshold medical needs. Supportive housing programs, often in a group-home setting, are equipped to provide a more substantial range of medical and social support services and can serve as a bridge between independent living and inpatient or nursing home care. In some cities, rent vouchers are available to persons with AIDS to cover part of their housing expenses.

In San Francisco, 30% of persons with AIDS are eligible for Medicaid at time of death, emblematic of the pauperization commonly associated with AIDS—in New York City, the proportion is closer to 80%. It is not uncommon for those with HIV disease to experience considerable difficulty in meeting daily living expenses at some point during their illness. In response, many organizations maintain food banks or offer hot meal programs. Eligible clients can receive staples or nonperishable food items or can join others for nutritious, hot meals. Meals-on-Wheels or similar programs delivers hot, balanced meals to the homebound in many cities. Often, the food provided is enough for an additional meal. Most such organizations rigorously monitor the nutritional balance of their meals and are equipped to follow special dietary restrictions if necessary.

Since the outset of the epidemic, persons with HIV disease have experienced particular difficulties with the Social Security Administration and other government bureaucra-

cies. Early in the epidemic, the time required to complete benefit applications could exceed a patient's life span, and many patients died before receiving benefits. In other cases, support and disability compensation programs were ill equipped to deal with the episodic nature of HIV disease; individuals may suffer bouts of serious illness alternating with periods of relative stability. Financial advocates or entitlement counselors can assist in negotiating complex government bureaucracies to obtain benefits. Typically, counselors offer information, instructions, and assistance in applying for Medicaid, MediCare, social security disability, social security supplemental income, rent assistance, unemployment, and other benefits. Sometimes, counselors are available to advocate on behalf of clients who experience particular difficulties.

Legal services and advocacy are offered by some organizations. Beyond helping clients to write wills, lawyers (usually volunteer) assist with AIDS-related discrimination, immigration problems, landlord-tenant disputes, health care access problems, or difficulties with the criminal justice system. Although certain specialized groups, such as the American Civil Liberties Union or the Lambda Legal Defense and Education Fund, limit their services to impact litigation designed to influence public policy, others provide more routine services, usually free of charge.

For individuals who use illicit injection drugs, obtaining drug treatment can present significant challenges. To make matters worse, many states prohibit the possession or sale of syringes, and it can be almost impossible to obtain sterile injection equipment. Although still controversial, some organizations run needle exchange programs in convenient locations (sometimes mobile). These programs dispense or exchange clean "works," refer users to drug treatment programs or medical care, provide safe-sex counseling, offer encouragement, and supply users with condoms, bleach, alcohol swabs (to prevent endocarditis), and clean cotton. Such programs operate based on a harm reduction philosophy, which acknowledges that many individuals cannot or will not stop taking drugs, and seeks to help them in reducing the risks associated with drug taking. The harm reduction model is nonjudgmental, accepts whatever steps the individual is prepared to make in reducing drug associated risks in their lives, and is non-coercive. Some of these same groups also conduct narcotics anonymous groups and operate drug treatment facilities.

Among the early AIDS service organizations, the provision of personal services was offered to clients, many of whom had been refused services elsewhere. Many continue to offer haircuts, massages, exercise, or yoga instruction. PWA Coalitions and other AIDS groups also provide recreation activities for clients who may otherwise become isolated. Often by soliciting donations, many groups offer free or reduced-price tickets to theater, movies, or special events and provide other social activities. Some groups, such as Body Positive, offer a range of activities aimed specifically at HIV-positive singles.

AIDS has become a defining political event of the time. Consequently, a range of opportunities is available for the politically motivated. Political protest groups such as Act Up have formed in cities all over the country, offering members the opportunity to contribute to a range of activities. Increasingly, mainstream AIDS service providers and advocacy groups also rely on community organizing and grassroots mobilization. For persons with AIDS seeking to advocate on their own behalf, there are opportunities to write letters, make phone calls, or participate in legislative lobbying visits.

Most CBOs rely on volunteers, many of whom are themselves living with AIDS. Volunteers frequently attribute an enhanced sense of well-being to their volunteer work and find helping others to be a source of strength. Typically, volunteers participate in almost every aspect of running the organization, from stuffing envelopes and answering phones to provide technical, medical or legal services. In some instances, AIDS agencies rely on volunteers for up to 75% of their total labor hours. Most CBOs use persons with AIDS and their caregivers as members of their board of directors.

Other spiritual and self-empowerment activities abound. There are numerous 12-step programs for persons with AIDS, offering group support for recovery and other abuse issues; church and other religious services; healing circles and spiritual groups such as the Course in Miracles and Northern Lights Alternatives. Many such groups focus on holistic treatment; some offer physical activities such as yoga.

Largely because of the pressure brought to bear by treatment activists, many clinical research centers now use community advisory boards to help them in research protocol planning, recruitment, and oversight. These community advisory boards review protocols, offer guidance concerning recruitment materials and serve as ombudsmen for research volunteers. The many community-based research sites use volunteers for a variety of administrative and other functions.

CONCLUSIONS

By its nature, the community-based response to the AIDS epidemic is in flux, as the epidemic and the communities affected by it evolve and as those who fight the disease are themselves transformed by their experiences. Ultimately, as the many AIDS communities' perimeters expand and overlap, the scope of the disease will obviate the need for such distinctions. Integral to that process is the realization that AIDS is not rightfully characterized as a problem of the "other" but is instead a challenge and a responsibility for society as a whole. Until that time, the community-based individuals and organizations dedicated to fighting AIDS will continue to shape and reshape their relationships with mainstream health providers, planners, and researchers and to collectively confront the most serious domestic epidemic of our time.

REFERENCES

1. Centers for Disease Control and Prevention. *Pneumocystis* pneumonia—Los Angeles. MMWR 1981;30.
2. National Center for Health Statistics. Annual Summary of Births, Marriages, Deaths, and Divorces: United States, 1993. Hyattsville, MD: United States Department of Health and Human Services, Public Health Service, Centers for Disease Control and Prevention, 1994.
3. Brandt A. No magic bullet: a social history of venereal disease in the United States since 1880. New York: Oxford University Press, 1987.
4. Centers for Disease Control and Prevention. HIV/AIDS surveillance report. 1994;6.
5. New York City Department of Health, Office of AIDS Surveillance. AIDS surveillance update, third quarter, 1994.
6. Centers for Disease Control and Prevention, Health Resources and Services Administration, National Institutes of Health. Surgeon General's report to the American public on HIV infection and AIDS. Washington, DC, (no date).
7. Des Jarlais DC, Friedman SR, Sotheran JL. The first city: HIV among intravenous drug users in New York City. In: Fee E, Fox DM, eds. AIDS: the making of a chronic disease. Los Angeles: University of California Press, 1992.
8. Centers for Disease Control and Prevention. Update: AIDS among women-United States. MMWR 1995;44.
9. Osmond D, Page K, Wiley J, et al. HIV infection in homosexual men 18 to 29 years of age: the San Francisco young men's health study. Am J Public Health 1994;84.
10. Bayer R, Kirp DL. The United States: at the center of the storm. In: Bayer R, Kirp DL, eds. AIDS in the industrialized democracies: passions, politics, and policies. New Brunswick, NJ: Rutgers University Press, 1992.
11. National commission for the Protection of Human Subjects of Biomedical and Behavioral Research. Belmont report. Ethical principles and guidelines for the protection of human subjects of research. Washinton, DC: U.S. Government Printing Office, 1979.
12. National Research Council. The social impact of AIDS in the United States. Washinton, DC: National Academy Press, 1993.
13. Edgar H and Rothman DJ. New rules for new drugs: the challenge of AIDS to the regulatory process. Milbank Q 1990;68 (Suppl 1).
14. Bartlett L. Financing health care for persons with AIDS:balancing public and private responsibilities. In: Gostin L, ed. AIDS and the health care system. New Haven, CT: Yale University Press, 1990.
15. Altman D. Power and community: organizational and cultural responses to AIDS. Bristol, PA: Taylor & Francis, 1994.

16. Callen M, Turner D. A history of the PWA self-empowerment movement. In: Callen M, ed. Surviving and thriving with AIDS: collected wisdom. New York: People With AIDS Coalition, 1988.
17. Stoddard T. Paradox and paralysis: an overview of the American response to AIDS. In: Carter E, Watney S, eds. Taking liberties: AIDS and cultural politics. London: Serpent's Tail, 1989.
18. Chambre SM. The volunteer response to the AIDS epidemic in New York City: implications for research on voluntarism. Nonprofit Voluntar Sector Q 1991;20(Suppl 3).
19. Altman D. AIDS in the mind of America. New York: Anchor Books, 1987.
20. Altman D. Legitimation through disaster: AIDS and the gay movement. In: Fee E, Fox DM, eds. AIDS: the burdens of history. Los Angeles: University of California Press, 1988.
21. Padgug RA, Oppenheimer GM. Riding the tiger: AIDS and the gay community. In: Fee E, Fox DM, eds. AIDS: the making of a chronic disease. Los Angeles: University of California Press, 1992.
22. Hunter N, Rubenstein W, eds. AIDS agenda. New York: The New Press, 1992.
23. Shilts R. And the band played on. New York: The Penguin Group, 1987.
24. State of New York v. Gregg Bordowitz, et al. (NYC criminal court. Dockets 90NO28423–26, 90NO28440–1, 90NO28453–4.) June 25, 1991.
25. Arno PS, Feiden KL. Against the odds: the story of AIDS drug development, politics & profits. New York: HarperCollins, 1992.
26. Crimp D. AIDS: cultural analysis/cultural activism. October, 1987 (winter); 43.
27. Goldstein R. AIDS and the social contract. In: Carter E, Watney S, eds. Taking liberties: AIDS and cultural politics. London: Serpent's Tail, 1989.
28. Patton C. Sex and germs: the politics of AIDS. Boston: South End Press, 1985.
29. Ellis SJ, Noyes KH. By the people: a history of America as volunteers. San Francisco: Jossey-Bass, 1990.
30. Kayal P. Bearing witness: Gay men's health crisis and the politics of AIDS. Boulder, CO: Westview Press, 1993.
31. Altman L. Rare cancer seen in 41 homosexuals. New York Times. July 3, 1981.
32. Nussbaum B. Good intentions. New York: The Atlantic Monthly Press, 1990.
33. Gay Men's Health Crisis. The history of Gay Men's Health Crisis, Inc. In: The biggest gay event of all time (benefit program). November 30, 1983.
34. Gay Men's Health Crisis, Inc. AIDS newsletter (pamphlet). 1983.
35. Garrett L. The coming plague: newly emerging diseases in a world out of balance. New York: Farrar, Straus, & Giroux, 1994.
36. Whitman Walker Clinic. 1992 Annual report. Washington, DC: Whitman Walker Clinic, 1992.
37. Callen M, Berkowitz R. We know who we are: two gay men declare war on promiscuity. New York Native November 8–21, 1982.
38. Callen M, Berkowitz R. How to have sex in an epidemic (pamphlet). New York: News from the Front, 1982.
39. Kramer L. Reports from the holocaust: the making of an AIDS activist. New York: St. Martin's Press, 1989.
40. Kramer L. 1,112 and counting. New York Native 1983;59.
41. Callen M. Surviving AIDS. New York: HarperCollins, 1990.
42. Wachter RM. The fragile coalition: scientists, activists, and AIDS. New York: St. Martin's Press, 1991.
43. Presidential Commission on the Human Immunodeficiency Virus Epidemic. Report of the Presidential Commission on the human immunodeficiency virus epidemic. Document 0-214-701:QL 3. Washington, DC: U.S. Government Printing Office, 1988.
44. Kwitny J. Acceptable risks. New York: Poseidon Press, 1992.
45. Levine C, Dubler NN, Levine RJ. Building a new consensus: ethical principles and policies for clinical research on HIV/AIDS. IRB: a review of human subjects research. 1991;13).
46. National Commission on AIDS. Report: the twin epidemics of substance use and HIV. Washington, DC: U.S. Government Printing Office, 1991.
47. Perrow C, Guillen MF. The AIDS disaster: the failure of organizations in New York and the nation. New Haven, CT: Yale University Press, 1990.
48. Bordowitz G. Picture a coalition. October, 1987 (Winter); 43.
49. Crimp D, Rolston A. AIDS demographics. Seattle: Bay Press, 1990.

PART VII

Prevention and Public Health

AIDS: Biology, Diagnosis, Treatment and Prevention, fourth edition, edited by Vincent T. DeVita, Jr., Samuel Hellman, and Steven A. Rosenberg. Lippincott–Raven Publishers, © 1997

CHAPTER 29 Risk Factors for Sexual Transmission

29.1 Risk Factors for Sexual Transmission of Human Immunodeficiency Virus

Scott D. Holmberg

Although most HIV transmission in the world occurs through sexual contact, transmission by this route is relatively inefficient. In one review, only 15% of more than 1600 female sex partners exposed by vaginal sex with HIV-infected men—on average, 100 or more times—were themselves HIV-infected.[1] This percentage may overestimate the actual probability of heterosexual transmission of the virus, because some persons in developed countries whose infections are attributed to sexual intercourse may, like their partners, be injection drug users and also exposed by that route.

The per contact probability of an uninfected woman acquiring HIV infection from vaginal sex with an infected man is probably less than 0.2%.[1] For an uninfected man having sex with an infected woman, this probability is even lower because male-to-female spread of HIV generally seems to be less than female-to-male spread (Table 29.1-1). Among homosexual men, the likelihood of HIV infection from anal sexual intercourse is higher than for heterosexual partners having vaginal sex, but it is still low. In one study,[8] the likelihood of an uninfected man's acquiring HIV from anal sex with an HIV-infected male partner was calculated to be 0.5% to 3% per contact. These rates may be contrasted with a man's likelihood of acquiring gonorrhea from a single exposure with an infected prostitute, which is estimated to be about 25%.[9,10]

However, the statistically low probability of heterosexual or homosexual transmission of HIV per individual sexual act obscures great variability of actual likelihood of acquiring HIV from sexual contact. Some sex partners of HIV-infected persons remain HIV seronegative despite hundreds or thousands of sexual contacts.[7] Conversely, there are

apparent "super-spreaders" or "disseminators" who infect most or all of their contacts after only one or a few sexual contacts.[6,11] The hypothesis that has gained progressively more credence over the past decade is that the number of different sex partners—not the number of sex contacts with any given HIV-infected partner—determines one's risk of HIV infection from sexual contact.[12,13] In almost all studies that compare the number of lifetime sex partners of HIV-infected with uninfected persons of the same HIV risk group, homosexual men and heterosexual men and women who have had the greatest number of different sex partners are most likely to be HIV infected.[14–16] The implication is that, on a population basis, the rate at which sexually active persons acquire new partners determines the spread of HIV within the population, as progressively more susceptible persons are exposed to HIV-infected spreaders. Risk factors or cofactors in the transmitter and the host and the type of virus involved putatively play a critical role in the sexual transmission of HIV.

BEHAVIORAL FACTORS

Although comparisons of the specific risk of sexual transmission from vaginal, oral, and anal sex are complicated by unavoidable problems in defining the actual risk of each of them, broad outlines are evident.[17] Anal sex has been consistently found to be the most "risky" sex act in a host of studies of heterosexual[4,18–21] and homosexual[16,22] partner pairs. For the heterosexual or homosexual receptive partner, the deposition of HIV-infected semen in the easily abraded rectum carries the highest risk of HIV transmission.[17] Other behavioral cofactors may augment this risk. For example, the use of inhaled nitrites (ie, "poppers") may dilate rectal veins, make them more friable, and facilitate homosexual transmission of HIV.[23]

Scott D. Holmberg, Special Studies Section, Division of HIV/AIDS, MS E-45, Centers for Disease Control and Prevention, Atlanta, GA 30333.

TABLE 29.1-1. *Relative efficiency* of male-to-female compared with female-to-male sexual transmission of HIV in several studies*

	No. HIV-infected/No. Susceptibles		Relative Efficiency*
	(% infected)		
Study Location	Men	Women	
Italy[2]	20/206 (10%)	126/524 (24%)	2.3
Thailand[3]	77/1,115 (7%)		
Europe[4]	19/159 (12%)	82/404 (20%)	1.7
USA[5]	1/72 (1%)	61/307 (20%)	14.3
England[6]	1/8 (12%)	15/78 (19%)	1.5
USA[7]	2/25 (8%)	10/55 (18%)	2.3

*Relative efficiency refers to the calculated ratio of male-to-female compared with female-to-male transmission.

Vaginal sex is usually considered less risky than anal (or rectal) sex but much more risky than oral sex.[17] The degree of trauma during sex has also been considered in studies of the likelihood of male-to-female or male-to-male transmission of HIV. Although it is impossible to determine this effect precisely, such trauma has been quantitated on the basis of "bleeding" during or after sex. Heterosexual women who report bleeding during or after sex are more likely to be HIV seropositive.[21]

In this hierarchy of risk from types of sexual contact, the risk of HIV infection from receptive oral sex is of more than academic interest, because many homosexual and some heterosexual partner pairs have adopted this sex contact as presumably "safe." Unfortunately, this route of HIV transmission is the most difficult to demonstrate or refute, because it is confounded by the various other sex acts almost always practiced between partners. Some anecdotal evidence suggests that the deposition of HIV-infected semen in the buccal mucosa, particularly when this mucosa is abraded, fosters the transmission of HIV.[24] However, these anecdotal reports must be weighed against the very low risk of transmission of HIV by vaginal sex and the consideration that HIV transmission by oral sex must be even lower. In one study, "crack" cocaine-using young women who had had oral blisters, fissures, and other lesions from hot crack pipes were at an minimally increased risk of HIV infection from receptive oral intercourse, when all other major risk factors for HIV transmission were controlled for (Faruque S: unpublished observations). Salivary factors also may decrease the infectivity of HIV in the oral cavity.[25,26]

The protective effect of condom use is unequivocal.[27] Latex condoms, appropriately used, apparently decrease the low risk of transmission by sexual routes at least one or two orders of magnitude for exposed heterosexual women and men[19,28,29] and homosexual men.[16] Of all sexual behavior interventions other than complete abstinence, condom use is widely accepted as the most efficacious.

The effectiveness of using other chemical and mechanical contraceptive devices in reducing the risk of HIV transmission is much less clear. Vaginal spermicides, notably nonoxynol-9,, may inhibit or kill HIV in vitro, but they have untested effectiveness in actual sexual situations.[30] Oral contraceptive pills have been reported as increasing[31,32] or decreasing[29] the risk of HIV infection by vaginal intercourse. A major problem in interpreting any research in this area is that oral contraceptive use diminishes the rationale for using other contraceptives that may provide an effective mechanical barrier, such as condoms. Cervical ectopy may be increased or decreased by oral contraceptive use,[1] and the role of cervical ectopy in facilitating HIV transmission to susceptible women is unknown.[33]

One of the most important behavioral determinants of sexual transmission of HIV is the use of substances that alter mental status and decision-making during times of potential sexual contact. For example, approximately 17% of women and 29% of men who had AIDS reportedly from heterosexual contact were categorized as "potentially alcoholic."[15] An inebriated homosexual man at a gay bar may be more likely to initiate unprotected sex contact.[34] A young, female crack cocaine smoker may have unprotected sex to obtain money or drugs.[35,36] In such situations, the decision to have "safe" sex or no sex may be affected by the substance being used. One critical effect of preventing drug and alcohol abuse will be to diminish unprotected sexual contacts during times of impaired thinking and impulse control.

The disquieting conclusion is that a susceptible partner can be infected by an infectious partner during almost any sexual contact in which biologic fluids are exchanged. Eventually, given enough different and unprotected sexual contacts, the infectiousness of the transmitter, the susceptibility of the exposed partner, the infectivity of the viral strain, or some combination of these factors will lead to the sexual transmission of HIV. For example, in several studies, one half or more of repeatedly exposed African prostitutes are found to be HIV-infected.[32] These considerations segue to the research concerning the biologic factors that may enhance or inhibit such transmission.

BIOLOGIC FACTORS

The probability of HIV transmission between an HIV-infected person and his or her uninfected partner—regardless of the type of contact—relies on the infectiousness of the transmitting partner, the strain of the virus presented to the uninfected partner, and the susceptibility of that uninfected partner. The last factor has been most studied.

Factors Determining the Susceptibility of an Uninfected Partner

Considerable information has now accumulated to support the theory that any factor that disrupts the vaginal or rectal mucosal integrity of an HIV-uninfected, susceptible person increases that person's chance of acquiring HIV from an infected sex partner. Although there is some evidence that HIV can penetrate intact epithelium,[37] it is intuitively appealing to consider mechanical breaks in the mucosa as portals of entry for HIV.[38] Most research regarding cofactors in HIV sexual transmission has focused on agents that disrupt this barrier.

Genital ulcerative diseases (GUDs), notably herpes simplex virus type 2 (HSV-2), syphilis, and chancroid, expose the vaginal or rectal mucosa and bloodstream to HIV from an infected partner. Such GUDs in the susceptible partner have been thought to be important to the heterosexual transmission of HIV from man to woman,[15,28,31] from woman to man,[15,28,39,40] and from man to man.[16,41] Less appreciated, GUDs may even increase the infectiousness of a receptive HIV-infected female partner for her insertive uninfected male partner.[42] The importance of genital ulcerative diseases in disrupting the mucosal integrity and exposing uninfected persons to additional HIV transmission risk has been reported from populations as diverse as white homosexual men in San Francisco and female prostitutes in Nairobi, Kenya, and in study designs that are retrospective, cross-sectional, or prospective.

Because the methods of acquisition of GUDs and HIV are the same, analysis of one in relation to the other is easily confounded; highly sexually active persons who have just acquired HIV are at increased risk of having had GUDs at some time before their HIV infection. However, when researchers have tried to control for the number of sex partners or other variables denoting sexual activity or have performed prospective studies, they have still found that the acquisition of HIV is independently associated with antecedent GUD. The preponderance of evidence and the attitude of most experts is that GUDs in susceptible heterosexual men and women and homosexual men facilitate HIV transmission.

Several mechanical factors that may abrade or disrupt the vaginal or rectal mucosa have been proposed as risk factors for HIV infection. One study indicated that tampon users may have an increased HIV susceptibility, presumably because of desiccation and abrasion of the vagina.[43] The use of vaginal desiccants by African women[44] to promote "hot, dry" and thereby more pleasurable sex for the male partner may also put them at increased risk of HIV infection. For postmenopausal women,[7] senile atrophic vaginitis and a resultant propensity to bleed during vaginal sex may likewise increase the risks of HIV transmission. For homosexual men, activities that cause anorectal injury, such as rectal douching, perianal bleeding, receipt of objects in ano, or receptive fisting, may increase the likelihood of HIV transmission.[16] The unifying mechanism for these risk factors is mechanical abrasion of the vagina or rectum and putative exposure of the bloodstream to HIV.

For heterosexual and homosexual men who are insertive sex partners, lack of penile circumcision may also be a risk factor for HIV infection.[45,46] The mechanism is again thought to be trauma and abrasion of the thin epithelium of the prepuce during intercourse, balanitis, longer contact of HIV trapped under the intact foreskin, easier maceration of the penis, or some combination of all these factors. However, this association is controversial, because it may be confounded by many factors.

The role of nonulcerative sexually transmitted organisms, such as those causing gonorrhea, syphilis, or chlamydial infections, in fostering the susceptibility of HIV-uninfected persons to HIV acquisition from an infected partner is unclear. Although some researchers have discerned a role for these in increasing the susceptibility of an uninfected sex partner,[47] others have not been able to confirm such infections as risk factors.[48]

Viral Infectivity and Virulence

Strains of HIV may differ considerably in their ability to infect a new host. This ability could be the result of two properties of the virus. *Infectivity* describes the ability of the virus to breach host defenses and gain entry to the target cell, tissue, or organ; *virulence* is its ability to replicate and cause damage in host cells. Both are essential for the virus to spread successfully.

This is probably the most difficult-to-evaluate biologic risk factor for sexual transmission of HIV,[49] because it is rarely possible to identify which virus has been transmitted from one person to another. HIV manifests a high degree of variability in vivo and in vitro, and genetically different strains can be recovered from the same HIV-infected person at different times or even the same time.[50-53] Which of these recovered strains represents "infective" virus? How does the clinician compare infectivity of different isolates recovered from the same or different persons?

One approach has been to evaluate the tropism or propensity of viral stains to infect various cell lines in vitro.[54,55] The same cell types from different persons may have markedly different susceptibility to infection; for example, there appears to be differential susceptibility of CD4+ T lymphocytes from different persons to infection with the same HIV strains.[56] However, most virologic research has been directed toward determinants of infectivity of the virus rather than the susceptibility of target cells.

A single-point mutation in the HIV genome may confer markedly different phenotypic properties.[57] Many mutations, particularly those in the *gag, pol, tat,* or *rev* regions, lead to HIV variants incapable of replication. Other mutations, such as in the *sor* (*vif*), *nef,* or *vpu* genes, can lead to mutations that are replicative but may have decreased HIV infectivity in vivo.[58] Because the viral envelope attaches to the CD4 receptor of target monocytic cells and so is considered critical to HIV infectivity,[59-61] much research has been directed toward finding *env* variants, specifically in their gp120 envelope proteins,[62-66] associated with more or less infective HIV strains. Single genotypic mutations in *env* apparently confer markedly different phenotypic ability to infect target cells in vitro,[67-69] but it is unknown how important such changes detected in vitro are to viral infectivity during actual sexual transmission of HIV.

HIV isolates from patients with advanced clinical disease appear to grow more rapidly or to be more "virulent," as determined by reverse transcriptase production, than isolates from asymptomatic HIV-infected persons.[70] HIV strains recovered late in HIV disease are capable of inducing syncytia in vitro,[71,72] a property thought to correlate with cell-to-cell infectivity. These syncytium-inducing (SI) viral strains, compared with non–syncytium-inducing (NSI) strains, have received much attention because of the increased recovery of SI strains later in disease, usually at the time a patient has AIDS. Do SI strains that have higher replicative capacity also have greater infectivity? The hypothesis is appealing because some researchers have indicated that patients who are late in their disease course and have symptomatic AIDS, when they are more likely to have SI strains recovered, are also more likely to transmit HIV to susceptible partners. However, contrary to this expectation, analysis of strains recovered from persons recently infected with HIV show these to be not SI but NSI.[66,73,74] Sequences of transmitted viruses actually correlate better with "minor," usually NSI, virus variants recovered from the transmitting partner.

Transmission may occur very early[75] or late in the course of HIV infection of the transmitting sex partner. The several weeks immediately after HIV infection and the period late in the course of HIV (AIDS) share low CD4+ T-lymphocyte counts, HIV antigen recoverability, and high viremia as quantified by polymerase chain reaction or viral culture.[76] The increased viral burden may be a critical biologic factor in determining HIV transmission, may obscure the relative contribution of HIV genotype or phenotype in HIV infectivity, or both. To further complicate the problems in discerning factors determining viral infectivity as a risk factor for HIV transmission, it is possible that viruses of low virulence may disappear from the population as the epidemic progresses.

Host Infectiousness

Some persons are apparently highly *infectious* (eg, a property of the human host, as distinct from *infective,* a property of the virus). These effective disseminators[11,77,78] are thought to be important to the spread of HIV within populations and probably explain why the number of different sex partners, not the number of contacts with a single partner, best predicts actual risk of infection.[12–14] Conversely, it is also known that the wives of some HIV-infected men may remain uninfected despite hundreds of unprotected vaginal sexual contacts with their infected spouses.[7,28] Presumably, some of the nontransmitting men in these studies are relatively or completely noninfectious.

However, little research has been directed toward risk factors for transmission from the HIV-infected partner, because these persons traditionally have been very hard to identify. Most homosexually and heterosexually infected persons have had multiple partners, many of whom are HIV-infected or of unknown HIV infection status, usually making definite identification of the source of the transmitted virus impossible.

Many epidemiologic date indicate that HIV transmission is most likely to occur late in the course of the infection, when symptoms of AIDS are evident.[20,21,28,78–84] Limited data also suggest that the likelihood of HIV transmission from an infectious partner may be increased very early in the course of HIV infection[75]—immediately after (ie, "primary") infection of the infectious partner.[85] These early and late periods in the course of HIV infection are times when T-lymphocyte (CD4+ cell) counts are low[76] and antigenemia[86] is more readily detected. These are the periods when HIV is more easily recovered or quantitatively greater in the infected person's blood,[76] semen,[87–89] or cervicovaginal secretions.[90,91] Variations in viral load in these clinical specimens are thought to indicate potential infectiousness of a sex partner,[92] representing an important biologic risk factor for the sexual transmission of HIV.

In addition to the level of viremia or its indices (eg, low CD4+ cell count, high antigenemia), genital tract inflammation in men and women leads to greater numbers of host cells harboring HIV and increases the infectiousness of the individual. Genital tract inflammation in men[93,94] and women[90,91,95] has been associated with increased recovery of infectious virions or actual transmission of HIV.

The role of zidovudine and probably other antiretroviral therapies in decreasing infectiousness of HIV-infected men is unclear. Some researchers have not found an association between zidovudine use and decreased shedding of HIV in semen;[96] but others[87] have found that there is decreased seminal recovery in the period after zidovudine is first administered. However, from a public health and preventive viewpoint, this may be of more academic interest than tangible impact, because HIV can apparently be transmitted from persons taking zidovudine.[97]

Because most women do not normally secrete from the cervix monocytic cells that can host HIV except during menses,[98] vaginal sex during menstruation has been posited as a risk factor for HIV transmission to susceptible male sex partners. The evidence has been limited, but the latest data from European studies of heterosexual partner pairs[19] suggest that sex during menses may be a risk factor for female-to-male transmission.

In addition to the recruitment of leukocytes to the inflamed genital tract, it has been suggested that GUDs may facilitate sexual spread of HIV from the HIV-infected sores of the infecting partner.[95]

CONCLUSIONS

The likelihood of sexual transmission of HIV is apparently determined by myriad behavioral and biologic risk factors. Some susceptible persons become infected after one or only a few contacts, but others remain uninfected despite hundreds or even thousands of unprotected exposures to an HIV-infected partner. The risk of contracting HIV infection from sexual contact is low but unpredictable. This risk seems to be determined more by the number of different sex partners than the number of acts with a specific sex partner. Some of the risk factors for sexual transmission seem rather clear and are agreed on by experts, but these factors are apparently many, complicated, and of unclear relative importance.

Rectal sex is thought to be more risky than vaginal sex, which is considered more risky than oral sex. Risk is substantially reduced by the use of condoms, but it is increased when decisions are made under the influence of alcohol or drugs.

GUDs and other factors that mechanically disrupt the vaginal or rectal mucosa increase an uninfected person's susceptibility. Greater excretion of virus, as measured by plasma viremia or by viral recovery from semen or cervicovaginal samples, correlates with increased infectiousness of the HIV-infected sex partner. HIV infectivity may be influenced by genotypic and phenotypic factors of the virus, particularly those relating to the viral envelope; these changes apparently determine cell tropism in vitro and may influence infectivity in vivo.

REFERENCES

1. Holmberg SD, Horsburgh CR Jr, Ward JW, Jaffe HW. Biologic factors in the sexual transmission of human immunodeficiency virus. J Infect Dis 1989;160:116.
2. Nicolosi A, Musicco M, Saracco A, Lazzarin A, Italian Study Group on HIV Heterosexual Transmission. Risk factors for woman-to-man sexual transmission of the human immunodeficiency virus. J Acquir Immune Defic Syndr 1994;7:296.
3. Mastro TD, Satten GA, Nopkesorn T, Sangkharomya S, Longini IM Jr. Probability of female-to-male transmission of HIV-1 in Thailand. Lancet 1994;343:204.
4. European Study Group. Risk factors for male to female transmission of HIV. Br Med J 1989;298:411.
5. Padian NS, Shiboski SC, Jewell NP. Female-to-male transmission of human immunodeficiency virus. JAMA 1991;266:1664.
6. Johnson AM, Petherick A, Davidson SJ, et al. Transmission of HIV to heterosexual partners of infected men and women. AIDS 1989;3:367.
7. Peterman TA, Stoneburner RL, Allen JR, Jaffe HW, Curran JW. Risk of human immunodeficiency virus transmission from heterosexual adults with transfusion-associated infections. JAMA 1988;259:55.
8. DeGruttola V, Seage III GR, Mayer KH, Horsburgh CR Jr. Infectiousness of HIV between male homosexual partners. J Clin Epidemiol 1989;42:849.
9. Holmes KK, Johnson DW, Trostle HJ. An estimate of the risk of men acquiring gonorrhea by sexual contact with infected females. Am J Epidemiol 1970;91:170.
10. Hooper RR, Reynolds GH, Jones OG, et al. Cohort study of venereal disease. I. The risk of gonorrhea transmission from infected women to men. J Infect Dis 1978;108:136.
11. Clumeck N, Taelman H, Hermans P, Piot P, Schoumacher M, De Wit S. A cluster of HIV infection among heterosexual people without apparent risk factors. N Engl J Med 1989;321:1460.
12. Blower SM, Boe C. Sex acts, sex partners, and sex budgets: implications for risk factor analysis and estimation of HIV transmission probabilities. J Acquir Immune Defic Syndr 1993;6:1347.
13. Padian NS, Shiboski SC, Jewell NP. The effect of number of exposures on the risk of heterosexual HIV transmission. J Infect Dis 1990;161:883.
14. Centers for Disease Control. Number of sex partners and potential risk of sexual exposure to human immunodeficiency virus. MMWR 1986;37:565.
15. Diaz T, Chu SY, Conti L, et al. Risk behaviors of persons with heterosexually acquired HIV infection in the United States: results of a multistate surveillance project. J Acquir Immune Defic Syndr 1994;7:958.
16. Caceres CF, van Griensven GJP. Male homosexual transmission of HIV-1. AIDS 1994;8:1051.
17. AIDS Institute, New York State Department of Health. Expert Panel on Sexual Transmission of HIV. Summary of the proceedings of the meeting of June 18, 1993.
18. Lazzarin A, Saracco A, Musicco M, Nicolosi A, Italian Study Group on HIV Heterosexual Transmission. Man-to-woman sexual transmission of the human immunodeficiency virus. Risk factors related to sexual behavior, man's infectiousness, and woman's susceptibility. Arch Intern Med 1991;151:2411.
19. European Study Group on Heterosexual Transmission of HIV. Comparison of female to male and male to female transmission of HIV in 563 stable couples. Br Med J 1992;304:809.
20. Giesecke J, Ramstedt K, Granath F, Ripa T, Rådö G, Westrell M. Partner notification as a tool for research in HIV epidemiology: behavior change, transmission risk and incidence trends. AIDS 1992;6:101.
21. Seidlin M, Vogler M, Lee E, Lee YS, Dubin N. Heterosexual transmission of HIV in a cohort of couples in New York City. AIDS 1993;7:1247.
22. Samuel MC, Hessol N, Shiboski S, Engel RR, Speed TP, Winkelstein W Jr. Factors associated with human immunodeficiency virus seroconversion in homosexual men in three San Francisco cohorts. J Acquir Immune Defic Syndr 1993;6:303.
23. Seage GR, Mayer KH, Horsburgh CR Jr, Holmberg SD, Moon MW, Lamb GA. The relation between nitrite inhalants, unprotected receptive anal intercourse, and the risk of human immunodeficiency virus infection. Am J Epidemiol 1992;135:1.
24. Lifson AR, O'Malley PM, Hessol NA, Buchbinder SP, Cannon L, Rutherford GW. HIV seroconversion in two homosexual men after receptive oral intercourse with ejaculation: implications for counseling concerning safe sexual practices. Am J Public Health 1990;80:1509.
25. Fultz P. Components of saliva inactivate human immunodeficiency virus. (Letter) Lancet 1986;2:1215.
26. Levy JA, Greenspan D. HIV in saliva. (Letter) Lancet 1988;2:1248.
27. Feldblum PJ. Results from prospective studies of HIV-discordant couples. (Letter) AIDS 1991;5:1265.
28. de Vincenzi I, European Study Group on Heterosexual Transmission of HIV. A longitudinal study of human immunodeficiency virus transmission by heterosexual partners. N Engl J Med 1994;331:341.
29. Saracco A, Musicco M, Nicolosi A, et al. Man-to-woman sexual transmission of HIV: longitudinal study of 343 steady partners of infected men. J Acquir Immune Defic Syndr 1993;6:497.
30. Stone KM, Peterson HB. Spermicides, HIV, and the vaginal sponge. (Editorial) JAMA 1992;268:521.
31. Plummer FA, Simonsen JN, Cameron DW, et al. Cofactors in male-female sexual transmission of human immunodeficiency virus type 1. J Infect Dis 1991;163:233.
32. Simonsen JN, Plummer FA, Ngugi EN, et al. HIV infection among lower socioeconomic strata prostitutes in Nairobi. AIDS 1990;4:139.
33. Moss GB, Clemetson D, D'Costa L, et al. Association of cervical ectopy with heterosexual transmission of human immunodeficiency virus: results of a study of couples in Nairobi, Kenya. J Infect Dis 1991;164:588.
34. McCusker J, Westenhouse J, Stoddard AM, Zapka JG, Zorn MW, Mayer KH. Use of drugs and alcohol by sexually active men in relation to sexual practices. J Acquir Immune Defic Syndr 1990;3:729.
35. Edlin BR, Irwin KL, Faruque S, et al. Intersecting epidemics—crack cocaine use and HIV infection among inner-city young adults. N Engl J Med 1994;331:1422.
36. Ellerbrock TV, Lieb S, Harrington PE, et al. Heterosexually transmitted human immunodeficiency virus infection among pregnant women in a rural Florida community. N Engl J Med 1992;327:1704.
37. Phillips DM, Zacharopoulos VR, Tan X, Pearce-Pratt R. Mechanisms of sexual transmission of HIV: does HIV infect intact epithelia? Trends Microbiol 1994;2:454.
38. Miller CJ, Alexander NJ, Sutjipto S, et al. Genital mucosal transmission of simian immunodeficiency virus: animal model for heterosexual transmission of human immunodeficiency virus. J Virol 1989;63:4277.
39. Telzak EE, Chaisson MA, Bevier PJ, Stoneburner RL, Castro KG, Jaffe HW. HIV-1 seroconversion in patients with and without genital ulcer disease. Ann Intern Med 1993;119:1181.
40. Ryder RW, Ndilu M, Hassig SE, et al. Heterosexual transmission of HIV-1 among employees and their spouses at two large businesses in Zaire. AIDS 1990;4:725.
41. Holmberg SD, Stewart JA, Gerber AR, et al. Prior herpes simplex virus type 2 infection as a risk factor for HIV infection. JAMA 1988;259:1048.
42. Kreiss JK, Coombs R, Plummer F, et al. Isolation of human immunodeficiency virus from genital ulcers in Nairobi prostitutes. J Infect Dis 1989; 160:380.
43. Goedert JJ, Eyster ME, Ragni MV, Biggar RJ, Gail MH. Rate of heterosexual HIV transmission and associated risk with HIV antigen [ab-

stract 4019]. In: Program and abstracts of the Fourth International Conference on AIDS, book 1. Stockholm: Swedish Ministry of Health and Social Affairs, 1988:264.

44. Irwin K, Mibandumba N, Mbuyi K, Ryder R, Sequeira D. More on vaginal inflammation in Africa. (Letter) N Engl J Med 1993; 328:888.

45. Simonsen JN, Cameron W, Gakinya MN, et al. Human immunodeficiency virus infection among men with sexually transmitted diseases. Experience from a cohort study. Ann Epidemiol 1990;1:117.

46. Cameron DW, D'Costa LJ, Maitha GM, et al. Female to male transmission of human immunodeficiency virus type 1: risk factors for seroconversion in men. Lancet 1989;2:403.

47. Laga M, Manoka A, Kivuvu M, et al. Non-ulcerative sexually transmitted diseases as risk factors for HIV-1 transmission in women: results from a cohort study. AIDS 1993;7:95.

48. Weir SS, Feldblum PJ, Roddy RE, Zekeng L. Gonorrhea as a risk factor for HIV acquisition. AIDS 1994;8:1605.

49. Kim MY, Lagakos SW. Estimating the infectivity of HIV from partner studies. Ann Epidemiol 1990;1:117.

50. Fisher AG, Ensoli B, Looney D, et al. Biologically diverse molecular variants within a single HIV-1 isolate. Nature 1988;334:444.

51. McNeary T, Hornickova Z, Klostner B, et al. Evolution of sequence divergence among human immunodeficiency virus type 1 isolates derived from a blood donor and a recipient. Pediatr Res 1993;33:36.

52. Saag MS, Hahn BH, Gibbons J, et al. Extensive variation of human immunodeficiency virus in vivo. Nature 1988;334:440.

53. Wolfs TFW, Zwart G, Bakker M, Goudsmit J. HIV-1 genomic RNA diversification following sexual and parenteral virus transmission. Virology 1992;189:103.

54. Sakai K, Dewhurst S, Ma X, Volsky D. Differences in cytopathogenicity and host cell range among infectious molecular clones of human immunodeficiency virus type 1 simultaneously isolated from an individual. J Virol 1988;62:4078.

55. Schuitemaker H, Kootstra N, Groenick M, de Goede REY, Miedema F, Tersmette M. Differential tropism of clinical HIV-1 isolates for primary monocytes and promonocytic cell lines. AIDS Res Hum Retroviruses 1992;9:1679.

56. Williams LM, Cloyd MW. Polymorphic human gene(s) determines differential susceptibility of CD4 lymphocytes to infection by certain HIV-1 isolates. Virology 1991;184:723.

57. Reitz MS, Wilson C, Naugle C, Gallo RC, Robert-Guroff M. Generation of a neutralization-resistant variant of HIV-1 is due to selection for a point mutation in the envelope gene. Cell 1988;54:57.

58. Fisher AG, Ensoli B, Ivanoff, et al. The sor gene of HIV-1 is required for efficient virus transmission in vitro. Science 1987;237:888.

59. Ivanoff LA, Dubay JW, Morris JF, et al. V3 loop region of the HIV-1 gp120 envelope protein is essential for virus infectivity. Virology 1992;187:423.

60. Chesebro B, Wehrly K, Nishio J, Perryman S. Macrophage-tropic human immunodeficiency virus isolates from different patients exhibit unusual V3 envelope sequence homogeneity in comparison with T-cell–tropic isolates: definition of critical amino acids involved in cell tropism. J Virol 1992;66:6547.

61. Goudsmit J, Wolfs TFW, Kuiken CL. Biological significance of human immunodeficiency virus envelope variability. In: Koff WC, Wong-Staal F, Kennedy RC, eds. AIDS research reviews, vol 1. New York: Marcel Dekker, 1991:35.

62. Hansen BD, Nara PL, Maheshwari RK, et al. Loss of infectivity by progeny virus from alpha interferon-treated human immunodeficiency virus type 1-infected T cells is associated with defective assembly of envelope gp120. J Virol 1992;66:7543.

63. Ho DD, Kaplan JC, Rackauskas IE, Gurney ME. Second conserved domain of gp120 is important for HIV infectivity and antibody neutralization. Science 1988;239:1021.

64. Stamatatos L, Cheng-Mayer C. Evidence that the structural conformation of envelope gp120 affects human immunodeficiency virus type 1 infectivity, host range, and syncytium-forming ability. J Virol 1993;67:5635.

65. Zhang LQ, MacKenzie P, Cleland A, Holmes EC, Leigh Brown AJL, Simmonds P. Selection for specific sequences in the external envelope protein of human immunodeficiency virus type 1 upon primary infection. J Virol 1993;67:3345.

66. Zhu T, Mo H, Wang N, et al. Genotypic and phenotypic characterization of HIV-1 in patients with primary infection. Science 1993;261:1179.

67. Schulz TF, Reeves JD, Hoad JG, et al. Effects of mutations in the V3 loop of HIV-1 gp120 on infectivity and susceptibility to proteolytic cleavage. AIDS Res Hum Retroviruses 1993;9:159.

68. Shioda T, Levy JA, Cheng-Mayer C. Small amino acid changes in the V3 hypervariable region of gp120 can affect the T-cell line and macrophage tropism of human immunodeficiency virus type 1. Proc Natl Acad Sci USA 1992;89:9434.

69. Willey RL, Smith DH, Lasky LA, et al. In vitro mutagenesis identifies a region within the envelope gene of the human immunodeficiency virus that is critical for infectivity. J Virol 1988;62:139.

70. Cheng-Mayer C, Seto D, Tateno M, Levy JA. Biologic features of HIV-1 that correlate with virulence in the host. Science 1988;240:80.

71. Tersmette M. de Goede REY, Al BJM, et al. Differential syncytium-inducing capacity of human immunodeficiency virus isolates: frequent detection of syncytium-inducing isolates in patients with acquired immunodeficiency syndrome (AIDS) and AIDS-related complex. J Virol 1988;62:2026.

72. Richman DD, Bozzette SA. The impact of the syncytium-inducing phenotype of human immunodeficiency virus on disease progression. J Infect Dis 1994;169:968.

73. Roos MTL, Lange JPA, de Goede REY, et al. Viral phenotype and immune response in primary human immunodeficiency virus type 1 infection. J Infect Dis 1992;165:427.

74. Wolinsky SM, Wike CM, Korber BTM, et al. Selective transmission of human immunodeficiency virus type-1 variants from mothers to infants. Science 1992;255:1134.

75. O'Brien TR, Busch MP, Donegan E, et al. Heterosexual transmission of human immunodeficiency virus type 1 from transfusion recipients to their sex partners. J Acquir Immune Defic Syndr 1994;7:705.

76. Pantaleo G, Graziosi C, Fauci As. The immunopathogenesis of human immunodeficiency virus. N Engl J Med 1993;328:327.

77. Padian N, Marquis L, Francis DP, et al. Male-to-female transmission of human immunodeficiency virus. JAMA 1987;258:788.

78. Staszewski S, Shieck E, Rehmet S, Helm EB, Stille W. HIV transmission from male after only two sexual contacts. (Letter) Lancet 1987;2:628.

79. Laga M, Taelman H, Van der Stuyft P, Bonneux L, Vercauteren G, Piot P. Advanced immunodeficiency as a risk factor for heterosexual transmission of HIV. AIDS 1989;3:361.

80. Goedert JJ, Eyster ME, Biggar RJ, Blattner WA. Heterosexual transmission of human immunodeficiency virus: association with severe depletion of T-helper lymphocytes in men with hemophilia. AIDS Res Hum Retroviruses 1987;3:355.

81. Eyster ME, Goedert JJ. Apparent heterosexual transmission of HIV infection from an asymptomatic haemophiliac to his wife three or more years after seroconversion. (Letter) AIDS 1987;1:131.

82. Osmond D, Bacchetti P, Chaisson RE, et al. Time of exposure and risk of HIV infection in homosexual partners of men with AIDS. Am J Public Health 1988;78:944.

83. Nicolosi A, Corrêa Leite ML, Musicco M, Arici C, Gavazzeni G, Lazzarin A. The efficiency of male-to-female and female-to-male transmission of the human immunodeficiency virus: a study of 730 stable couples. Epidemiology 1994;5:570.

84. Hira SK, Nkowane BM, Kamanga J, et al. Epidemiology of human immunodeficiency virus in families in Lusaka, Zambia. J Acquir Immune Defic Syndr 1990;3:83.

85. Jacquez JA, Koopman JS, Simon CP, Longini IM Jr. Role of primary infection in epidemics of HIV infection in gay cohorts. J Acquir Immune Defic Syndr 1994;7:1169.

86. Laurian Y, Peynet J, Verroust F. HIV infection in sexual partners of HIV seropositive patients with hemophilia. (Letter) N Engl J Med 1989;320:183.

87. Anderson DJ, O'Brien TR, Politch JA, et al. Effects of disease stage and zidovudine therapy on the detection of human immunodeficiency virus type 1 in semen. JAMA 1992;267:2769.

88. Tindall B, Evans L, Cunningham P, et al. Identification of HIV-1 in semen following primary HIV-1 infection. AIDS 1992;6:949.

89. Hamed KA, Winters MA, Holodniy M, Katzenstein DA, Merigan TC. Detection of human immunodeficiency virus type 1 in semen: effects of disease stage and nucleoside therapy. J Infect Dis 1993;167:798.

90. Clemetson DBA, Moss GB, Willerford DM, et al. Detection of HIV DNA in cervical and vaginal secretions: prevalence and correlates among women in Nairobi, Kenya. JAMA 1993;269:2860.

91. Zorr B, Schäfer APA, Dilger I, Habermehl K-O, Kosh M. HIV-1 detection in endocervical swabs and mode of HIV-1 infection. (Letter) Lancet 1994;343:852.

92. Simmonds P. Variation in HIV virus load of individuals at different stages in infection: possible relationship with risk of transmission. AIDS 1990;4(Suppl):S77.

93. Wolff H, Anderson DJ. Potential human immunodeficiency virus-host cells in human semen. (Letter) AIDS Res Hum Retroviruses 1988;4:1.

94. Wolff H, Anderson DJ. Male genital tract inflammation associated with increased numbers of potential human immunodeficiency virus host cells in semen. Andrologia 1988;20:404.

95. Kreiss J, Willerford DM, Hensel M, et al. Association between cervical inflammation and cervical shedding of human immunodeficiency virus DNA. J Infect Dis 1994;170:1597.

96. Krieger JN, Coombs RW, Collier AC, et al. Recovery of human immunodeficiency virus type 1 from semen: minimal impact of stage of infection and current antiviral therapy. J Infect Dis 1991;163:386.

97. Routy JP, Blanc AP, Allegre T, Chardon H, Arriodare C. HIV-1 transmission by a heterosexual man treated with zidovudine. (Letter) J Acquir Immune Defic Syndr 1991;4:1166.

98. Hill JA, Anderson DJ. Quantitation of human vaginal leukocytes and effects of vaginal secretions on mechanisms of HIV transmission. Abstract 2551. In: Program and abstracts of the Fourth International Conference on AIDS, book 2. Stockholm: Swedish Ministry of Health and Social Affairs, 1988:113.

AIDS: Biology, Diagnosis, Treatment and Prevention, fourth edition, edited by Vincent T. DeVita, Jr., Samuel Hellman, and Steven A. Rosenberg. Lippincott–Raven Publishers, © 1997

29.2

Effectiveness of Behavioral Interventions to Prevent Sexual Transmission of Human Immunodeficiency Virus Infection

David R. Holtgrave

BACKGROUND

"What works?" is one of the most frequently asked questions in HIV prevention. This question is important, but it is frustrating. The question is general, and it possesses a troubling hidden aspect. Underlying the "what works" inquiry is the criterion that the questioner uses to gauge the success of HIV prevention programs. Any of the following could be used to judge whether prevention programs work:

Does the program successfully change high-risk sexual behaviors?
Does the intervention significantly modify risky drug using behaviors?
Can my service organization afford to provide the intervention?
Does this program save society money?
Is it cost effective?

Other criteria can be articulated, and in this chapter, we acknowledge the importance of all of these yardsticks, but we focus on the first standard. The literature contains helpful review papers that address the other four questions.[1-4]

In 1994, there were 80,691 new AIDS case diagnoses.[5] The reported HIV-exposure categories for these cases indicate that a substantial portion of HIV transmissions are by means of sexual behavior. Of the 80,691 cases, 34,974 were through male homosexual or bisexual contact, and 8300 were through heterosexual contact. Using just these two

exposure categories probably underestimates the number of sexual transmissions because some AIDS cases classified into the exposure categories of "history of injecting-drug use" and "no reported risk" could have involved sexual transmission. Similar conclusions about the importance of sexual transmission are reached by examining 1993 data on HIV infection from states with confidential reporting systems.[6] Of 15,047 reported HIV infections that year among male and female adults and adolescents, 6781 were classified into homosexual or heterosexual exposure categories, which is likely to be an underestimate of infections due to sexual transmission.

OVERVIEW

High-risk sexual behaviors can be modified through behavioral interventions. This is the conclusion of multiple, detailed reviews of a substantial and scientifically sound literature consisting of several dozen studies on the effectiveness of HIV prevention interventions.[7-9] At least two dozen of these studies are randomized trials.[7,9] Most intervention studies have demonstrated a favorable impact on HIV-related sexual risk behaviors.[7-9]

A variety of behavioral interventions have been tested. These interventions can be grouped into a few general types. In the following sections, we provide a description and discussion of the four major kinds of behavioral interventions for the prevention of sexually transmitted HIV infection: individual, small-group, community, and societal actions. Each type is defined and described, key citations are provided, and important strengths and weakness of the intervention type are presented. We also describe some important limitations in this literature and suggest a few key areas of needed research. The

David R. Holtgrave, Center for AIDS Intervention Research, Department of Psychiatry and Behavioral Medicine, Medical College of Wisconsin, 1201 North Prospect Avenue, Milwaukee, WI 53202.

literature cited here is not exhaustive; readers interested in a complete listing of studies in this area should consult previously conducted reviews,[7-9] as well as the most recent behavioral, social, and biomedical science databases.

INDIVIDUAL INTERVENTIONS

Definition and Examples

Individual-level interventions provide risk reduction services to one client at a time. Usually, only one service provider is involved. The prototypic individual level intervention is HIV counseling and testing; however, there is no reason that individual counseling necessarily must be linked to HIV antibody testing.[9]

The Centers for Disease Control and Prevention (CDC) have articulated important components of HIV counseling and testing services.[10] Pretest counseling should include the following behavioral components: risk assessment, assessment of and augmenting knowledge about modes of HIV transmission, identification of behavioral risk reduction goals, and negotiation and development of an initial plan for taking first steps toward those risk reduction goals. Posttest counseling for persons engaged in high-risk behavior (regardless of HIV serostatus) should include follow-up on initial risk reduction progress, setting subsequent risk reduction goals, practice of safer sex skills, and referral to other behavior-change, prevention services, as needed.[10]

Strengths and Weaknesses of Individual Interventions

Studies have shown that HIV counseling and testing services, which are one manifestation of individual-level intervention, can have an impact on risky sexual behaviors.[11] However, this result varies by HIV serostatus and by population.[9,11] Most studies show that persons testing HIV seronegative do not subsequently modify risky sexual behaviors,[11-14] others show some evidence of increased risky behavior,[11,15,16] and one evidences risk reduction.[17]

The findings are different for persons testing HIV seropositive.[9,11] For heterosexual couples in which one person is seronegative and the other positive, HIV counseling and testing services have led to greatly increased condom use.[11] Studies on the behavioral effects of HIV counseling and testing services for injection drug users shows little if any behavioral effect; the same is true for research focusing on HIV seropositive women and subsequent reproductive decision making.[11] The literature on the effects of counseling and testing for men who have sex with men is mixed, with some studies showing a positive behavioral effect but some showing no impact.[11]

A primary limitation to studies of the impact of HIV counseling and testing on risky sexual behaviors is a definitional one. Most researchers refer to their intervention as counseling without clearly specifying the components of the counseling. To compare studies and adequately summarize the literature, such articulation of intervention components is crucial. This definitional problem is the primary obstacle to the completion of quantitative metanalyses on the behavioral effects of HIV counseling and testing.

Another difficulty is the translation of counseling interventions from the research setting to less well supported field settings. An expert panel reviewed the CDC's publicly funded counseling and testing program and found that although the CDC's counseling guidance was basically sound, the field implementation was inadequate.[18]

A third problem with individual-level interventions is their limited reach to multiple clients. However, some service providers are considering the benefits of using group pretest counseling for some clients. This limited reach of counseling services must be balanced with the ability of individual interventions to be especially intensive and highly tuned to the needs of individual clients. Unfortunately, most counseling interventions do not take advantage of this potential for tailoring and follow-up; many counseling sessions are rapidly delivered, often lasting only a few minutes. This suggests a real need to strengthen the intensity, duration, and quality of counseling that accompanies HIV antibody testing.[18]

SMALL-GROUP INTERVENTIONS

Definition and Examples

Small-group interventions involve several clients, often 6 to 10, jointly engaging in activities designed to increase HIV prevention knowledge, modify inappropriate beliefs about HIV prevention issues, increase risk reduction skills, and follow-up on attempts to reduce high-risk behaviors. The leader or facilitator of the group may be a group member, a peer, or a professional service provider. Small-group interventions may last from one to tens of sessions. Most of these group interventions seize the opportunity to use the group setting to role play (practice) safer sex negotiation skills and to reinforce the social norms that safer sex is highly valued and reinforced by other members of, at least, the small group. Small-group interventions to reduce high-risk sexual practices have been developed and evaluated for youth in high-risk situations, men who have sex with men, and women in urban settings.[7-9,19-24]

In an example of this kind of small-group intervention, a program was developed for gay men who reported recent histories of high-risk sexual behavior.[22] Participants in the intervention attended a series of 12 weekly 90-minute sessions in groups of 8 to 15 men with two facilitators. The group program addressed four major areas: risk and risk reduction education, along with correcting misconceptions about HIV; sexual assertiveness training to resist coercion to engage in risky sex, communicate health concerns, and negotiate safer sex understanding; self-management skills training to help participants identify and develop different ways to handle "triggers," including drinking, loneliness, and other factors that may potentiate vulnerability and high-risk behaviors; and strategies to develop relationships characterized by low-risk behaviors, plan and reinforce risk reduction steps, and accept responsibility for protecting oneself and others. Similar topics were addressed and exercises used in an intervention for women at elevated risk for HIV infection.[24]

Strengths and Weaknesses of Small-Group Interventions

Much sexual behavior is social in nature. The small-group setting allows for role play that in at least some respects approximates this social aspect of actual sexual situations. The perceived social norms are an extremely important factor in human behavior,[25] and small-group members who work together on safer sex exercises, almost by definition, articulate and reinforce a norm that safer sex is valued and important. This perceived norm can be key if a group member has a sex partner who is unwilling to adopt safer practices. Stated another way, small-group interventions that possess the characteristics described previously address several important determinants of human behavior[26] and emphasize social norms that are a crucial behavioral determinant.[9,25,26] Small-group interventions with these characteristics rest on a firm foundation of behavioral and social science theories of behavior change.

Another strength is that many small-group interventions are multisession. Having this additional work time in the group allows a number of behavioral determinants to be addressed (e.g., knowledge, attitudes, beliefs, skills, self-efficacy, intentions, social norms). It is difficult to address all of these factors in brief interventions. The extra work time also allows the group to positively reinforce its members for successive approximations to safer sexual behaviors. This allows each person's behavior change to emerge over time. Behaviors generally do not change suddenly and permanently. They are modified, perhaps evolving through a number of stages, over time.[9,27] One-time interventions do not possess this important feature. However, if only a single session is feasible, it is important to attempt to inform clients about consciously reinforcing their own behavior when they make strides toward behavior change, even if imperfect steps are taken.

Besides the conceptual and theoretical strength of small-group interventions, their empiric basis also is strong. Randomized trials have been done to assess small-group interventions for women in high-risk situations, gay men, and adolescents.[19,20,22–24] All found statistically significant changes in high-risk sexual behaviors. For instance, the small-group intervention for gay men (described previously) led to statistically significant changes in condom use behaviors over an 8-month follow-up period. In the intervention condition, condom use, increased from 23% before intervention to 77% at the 8-month follow-up. No increase was seen in the control group.

Small groups do have limitations. A primary difficulty is arranging the group sessions. Participants have to be motivated to modify their schedules to meet with the group at a particular time. They must be committed enough to return to group sessions—perhaps several times. Participants also have to be willing to discuss highly sensitive sexual matters in a group setting. Groups cannot be individually tailored to the needs of individuals clients as can individual-level interventions.

COMMUNITY-LEVEL INTERVENTIONS

Definition and Examples

Community-level interventions seek to modify individual behavior, but they also aim to directly influence the social norms of a community. This goes beyond using perceived social norms to help change individual behavior and involves attempting to modify a community's social norms. After this community-level change is accomplished, individual-level change should follow. The changed social norms should help to sustain the behavior changes over time.

Community-level interventions use the concept of diffusion of innovations to achieve this change in social norms and individual behavior.[28] This is best described by an example. In a set of studies focused on populations of gay men in small cities, researchers tested community-level interventions that began by identifying persons well liked, popular, and well trusted within their circle of friends and social networks.[29–31] These opinion leaders were then approached and invited to attend a series of group session that taught the popular persons ways to effectively recommend and endorse the importance of behavior changes to their friends and acquaintances. After extensive practice and role play training, the cadre of opinion leaders were then encouraged to initiate such conversations with friends in bars, everyday meeting places, and other settings. This approach is considered a diffusion of innovations model because it engages a small group of influential and popular persons to initially endorse and recommend an innovative behavior change—in this case, risk avoidance and safer sex—with the expectation that sustained conversations with friends will cause the change to gradually diffuse, be adopted by others, and cause a shift in social norms that makes risk reduction behavior changes more accepted.

Another family of community-level interventions is the AIDS Community Demonstration Projects funded and administered by the Centers for Disease Control and Prevention.[32] These interventions were implemented in five U. S. cities. They address several different populations who received the intervention: young persons in high-risk situations, men who have sex with men but do not self-identify as gay, women who have sex with injection drug users, and female commercial sex workers. All interventions had several characteristics in common. First, they were based on actual success stories of behavior change by community

members. These success stories were translated into suc-
cinct "role model stories" and printed on various "small
media" (e.g., baseball card–sized handouts, pamphlets,
booklets). Small-media role model stories were prepared for
persons at several different stages of behavior change. The
small media were delivered in street settings by members of
the community who volunteered and received some special
training in HIV prevention issues.

Strengths and Weaknesses of
Community-Level Interventions

Social norms play a key role in modifying human behavior.
Community-level interventions can modify these norms
directly and at a broad level. Community norms supportive
of safer sexual behaviors are important determinants of individual behavior. They can help to sustain behavior change in
community long after an HIV prevention intervention is
over. Hence, there is a sound theoretical rationale supporting
community-level interventions.

   Although few, careful empiric studies have shown that
community-level intervention can lead to real changes in risk
behaviors. In the example described earlier in which popular
opinion leaders were identified in the gay communities of
small cities and engaged to diffuse behavior change endorsement message to their friends,[29–31] large-scale anonymous surveys were administered to men entering gay bars in each city
before and after the community intervention program. Before
intervention, over one third of men surveyed in each city
reported engaging in high-risk sexual behavior during the past
2 months. After the intervention, declines were found in the
proportion of men who reported risky practices, and survey
data indicated a strengthening in perceived peer norms supporting safer sex as an expected way to behave. In most of the
cities in the trial, there was about a 30% reduction from initial
levels in the number of men who reported unsafe sex.[29–31] The
empiric literature suggests that community-level interventions are promising behavioral interventions for preventing
the sexual transmission of HIV infection.

   There are limitations to community-level interventions.
First, they require greater start-up effort than do small-group
interventions and therefore may be beyond the capacity of
some service provider organizations to develop and provide.
Second, they are more difficult to coordinate and staff than
individual or small-group interventions. Third, because the
intervention is implemented at the community level, randomized trials of intervention effectiveness pose several
methodologic challenges: sufficient matching of communities on nonintervention variables, identification of sufficient
numbers of communities to make meaningful statistical
comparisons, and difficulty in controlling historical trends
in several communities that may differently impact citizens'
behavior during the study period. It can be difficult to define
the "community" to target for the intervention. The intervention developer must ask whether the community is to be
defined geographically, demographically, or behaviorally.

SOCIETAL INTERVENTIONS

Definition and Examples

In general, society-level interventions use broad scale
changes in laws, policies, governmental procedures, and
mass communications to achieve some fundamental change
in society that, if successful, will lead eventually to reductions in HIV transmission. Examples of society-level interventions include the following:

Changes in a state's needle and syringe purchase laws
A school board's decision to distribute condoms in school-
   based health facilities
Modifications in a federal agency's requirements that its
   grantees receive community input when planning prevention programs
Decisions to allow distribution of safer information in correctional facilities.

   Some policy changes can directly reduce barriers that
would otherwise stifle persons attempting to change HIV-
related sexual risk behaviors (e.g., allowing greater information about and access to condoms).

   Mass communication efforts can have many different
types of goals at several different levels.[33] Some earlier HIV-
related mass media campaigns in the United States (e.g.,
"American Responds to AIDS")[34] sought, among other
goals, to educate the general public about modes of HIV
transmission and basic methods of self-protection. A later
U.S. campaign, the CDC's Prevention Marketing Initiative,
sought to increase the correct and consistent use of latex
condoms among young persons.[35]

Strengths and Weakness of Societal Interventions

Societal interventions are so heterogeneous that general statements of their strengths are weaknesses are difficult to make.
Some advantages of societal interventions are they sweeping
in scope and able to affect many persons at once. Some society-level interventions carry the weight of law, although
human behavior cannot always be legislated. Societal interventions are the least tailored of all types of interventions.
Although they may move society as a whole, they may not
meet the exact intervention needs of any one citizen.

   These types of interventions may be the most difficult of
all to evaluate. Control groups often do not exist, and sometimes even baseline measures are unavailable. For further
discussion of these evaluative complexities, we recommend
a recent review of the HIV-related mass media campaigns.[33]

OVERALL LIMITATIONS OF THE LITERATURE

HIV prevention research is applied research by its very
nature. Applied research aims to fill important knowledge
gaps of practical significance. The information needs of persons who make decisions about HIV prevention programs

must be addressed. These persons include governmental policy makers at the local, state and federal levels; HIV-prevention community planning groups; and managers and staff of nongovernmental organizations, including community-based organizations. They must make choices about which types of interventions to adopt in their programs, which to stop funding, and how to mix the various levels of interventions for optimal effectiveness.

Although it is important to use the sizable literature on behavioral intervention effectiveness, it is fair to say that these important information needs race well ahead of the available literature. There exist no studies on the mixture of multicomponent HIV-prevention programs. Not all types of interventions have been studied across all populations. Rigorous empiric studies on the effects of societal interventions are difficult to find. External validity challenges abound, as in, for example, how to take the research literature and apply it to a particular field setting. These challenges suggest that behavioral intervention research in the future will take on many of the characteristics of phase IV studies, health services research, and research translation efforts. We need research on what works best for whom, in what settings, for how long, in what combinations, and at what cost.[36] Several of the criteria that may be used to judge the success of HIV prevention programs should be used and addressed in future research.

CONCLUSIONS

Although there are limitations to this literature, the intervention studies provide us with a great deal of powerful information. Research has demonstrated that high-risk sexual behaviors can be modified. This is most readily demonstrated for small-group and community-level interventions.

Even when we do not have specific studies of particular interventions in certain populations, important information is available about other interventions for a given population or the effects in other populations for a given intervention. This is an important starting place. This empiric information, combined with practical behavioral and social science theory gives us an informed starting point for HIV-prevention intervention program development, regardless of the novelty of the situation at hand. We must build HIV-prevention programs on this solid base of behavioral information.

ACKNOWLEDGMENTS

The author is grateful to Jeffrey A. Kelly, Ph.D., for his insightful review of an earlier version of this chapter. Preparation of this chapter was supported in part by grant P30-MH52776 from the National Institute of Mental Health.

REFERENCES

1. Des Jarlais DC, Friedman SR. AIDS and the use of injected drugs. Sci Am 1994;270:82.
2. Stephens RC, Simpson DD, Coyle SL, McCoy CB, and the National AIDS Research Consortium. Comparative effectiveness of NADR interventions. In: Brown BS, Beschner GM, eds. Handbook on risk of AIDS: injection drug users and sexual partners. Westport, CT: Greenwood Press, 1993:519.
3. Holtgrave DR, Valdiserri RO, West GA. Quantitative economic evaluations of HIV-related prevention and treatment services: a review. Risk 1994;5:29.
4. Holtgrave DR, Qualls NL. Threshold analysis and programs for HIV prevention. Med Decis Making 1995;15:311.
5. Centers for Disease Control and Prevention. Update: acquired immune deficiency syndrome—United States, 1994. MMWR 1995;44:64.
6. Centers for Disease Control and Prevention. HIV/AIDS surveillance report. 1994;5:1.
7. Choi KH, Coates TJ. Prevention of HIV infection. AIDS 1994;8:1371.
8. Kelly JA, Murphy DA, Sikkema KJ, Kalichman SC. Psychological interventions to prevent HIV infection are urgently needed: new priorities for behavioral research in the second decade of AIDS. Am Psychol 1993;48:1023.
9. Holtgrave DR, Qualls NL, Curran JW, Valdiserri RO, Guinan ME, Parra WC. An overview of the effectiveness and efficiency of HIV prevention programs. Public Health Rep 1995;110:134.
10. Centers for Disease Control and Prevention. Recommendations for HIV testing services for inpatients and outpatients in acute-care hospital settings and technical guidance on HIV counseling. MMWR 1993;42(RR-2):8.
11. Higgins DL, Galavotti C, O'Reilly KR, et al. Evidence for the effects of HIV antibody counseling and testing on risk behaviors. JAMA 1991;266:2419.
12. Doll LS, O'Malley P, Pershing A, Darrow WW, Hessol N, Lifson A. High-risk sexual behavior and knowledge of HIV-antibody status in the San Francisco city clinic cohort. Health Psychol 1990;9:253.
13. McCusker J, Stoddard AM, Mayer KH, Zapka J, Morrison C, Saltzman SP. Effects of HIV antibody test knowledge on subsequent sexual behaviors in a cohort of homosexually active men. Am J Public Health 1988;78:462.
14. Wenger NS, Greenberg JM, Hilborne LH, Kusseling F, Mangotich M, Shapiro MF. Effect of HIV antibody testing and AIDS education on communication about HIV risk and sexual behavior: a randomized, controlled trial in college students. Ann Intern Med 1992;117:905.
15. Fox R, Odaka NJ, Brookmeyer R, Polk BF. Effect of HIV antibody disclosure on subsequent sexual activity in homosexual men. AIDS 1987;1:241.
16. Otten MW, Zaida AA, Wroten JE, Witte JJ, Peterman TA. Changes in sexually transmitted disease rates after HIV testing and posttest counseling, Miami, 1988 to 1989. Am J Public Health 1993;83:529.
17. Wenger NS, Linn LS, Epstein M, Shapiro MF. Reduction of high-risk sexual behavior among heterosexuals undergoing HIV antibody testing: a randomized clinical trial. Am J Public Health 1991;81:1580.
18. CDC Advisory Committee on the Prevention of HIV Infection. External review of CDC's HIV prevention strategies. Atlanta, GA: Centers for Disease Control and Prevention, 1994:1.
19. Hobfoll SE, Jackson AP, Lavin J, Britton PJ, Shepherd JB. Reducing inner-city women's AIDS risk activities: a study of single, pregnant women. Health Psychol 1994;13:397.
20. Jemmott JB, Jemmott LS, Fong GT. Reductions in HIV risk-associated sexual behaviors among black male adolescents: effects of an AIDS prevention intervention. Am J Public Health 1992;82:372.
21. Rotheram-Borus MJ, Koopman C, Haignere C, Davies M. Reducing HIV sexual risk behaviors among runaway adolescents. JAMA 1991;266:1237.
22. Kelly JA, St. Lawrence JS, Hood HV, Brasfield TL. Behavioral intervention to reduce AIDS risk activities. J Consult Clin Psychol 1989;57:60.
23. Valdiserri RO, Lyter DW, Leviton LC, Callahan CM, Kingsley LA, Rinaldo CR. AIDS prevention in homosexual and bisexual men: results of a randomized trial evaluating two risk reduction interventions. AIDS 1989;3:21.
24. Kelly JA, Murphy DA, Washington CD, et al. The effects of HIV/AIDS intervention groups for high-risk women in urban clinics. Am J Public Health 1994;84:1918.
25. Fishbein M, Middlestadt SE, Hitchcock PJ. Using information to change sexually transmitted disease-related behaviors: an analysis based on the theory of reasoned action. In: DiClemente RJ, Peterson JL, eds. Preventing AIDS: theories and methods of behavioral intervention. New York: Plenum Press, 1994:61.

26. National Commission on AIDS. Behavioral and social sciences and the HIV/AIDS epidemic. Washington, DC: National Commission on AIDS, 1993:1.

27. Prochaska JO, DiClemente CC, Norcross JC, Steiger JH. In search of how people change: applications to addictive behaviors. Am Psychol 1992;47:1102.

28. Dearing JW, Meyer G, Rogers EM. Diffusion theory and HIV risk behavior change. In: DiClemente RJ, Peterson JL, eds. Preventing AIDS: theories and methods of behavioral intervention. New York: Plenum Press, 1994:79.

29. Kelly JA, St. Lawrence JS, Diaz YE, et al. HIV risk behavior reduction following intervention with key opinion leaders of a population: an experimental community-level analysis. Am J Public Health 1991;81:168–171.

30. Kelly JA, St. Lawrence JS, Stvenson LY, et al. Community AIDS/HIV risk reduction: the effects of endorsement by popular people in three cities. Am J Public Health 1992;82:1483.

31. Kelly JA, Winett RA, Roffman RA, et al. Social diffusion models can produce population-level HIV risk behavior reduction: field trial results and mechanisms underlying change. Abstract PO-C23-3167. Ninth International Conference on AIDS, Berlin, June 6–11, 1993.

32. O'Reilly KR, Higgins DL. AIDS Community Demonstration Projects for HIV prevention among hard-to-reach groups. Public Health Rep 1991;106:714.

33. Flora JA, Maibach EW, Holtgrave DR. Communication campaigns for HIV prevention: using mass media in the next decade. Background Report for the Institute of Medicine, National Academy of Science, 1995 [available from DR Holtgrave].

34. Woods DR, Davis D, Westover BJ. America Responds to AIDS: its content, development process, and outcome. Public Health Rep 1991;106:616.

35. Centers for Disease Control and Prevention. 1994 Fact Book. (Document HIV/OAD/7-94-046) Atlanta, GA: Centers for Disease Control and Prevention, 1994.

36. Holtgrave DR, Qualls NL. HIV prevention programs. Science 1994;266:16.

AIDS: Biology, Diagnosis, Treatment and Prevention, fourth edition, edited by Vincent T. DeVita, Jr., Samuel Hellman, and Steven A. Rosenberg. Lippincott–Raven Publishers, © 1997

CHAPTER **30**

Acquired Immunodeficiency Syndrome and the Injection of Illicit Psychoactive Drugs

Don C. Des Jarlais

Injection of illicit psychoactive drugs has been reported from 118 different countries, and human immunodeficiency virus (HIV) infection among injecting drug users (IDUs) has been reported in 80 different countries.[1] The injection of illicit psychoactive drugs does not by itself transmit HIV. When someone injects drugs intravenously, he or she typically draws blood into the syringe to be certain that a vein has been located. If the same needle and syringe are then used by a second person without effective disinfection, the resulting microtransfusion is a relatively effective method for transmitting blood-borne pathogens.

In many areas, HIV has spread extremely rapidly among IDUs, with the HIV seroprevalence rate (ie, percentage of IDUs infected with HIV) increasing from less than 10% to 40% or greater within a period of 1 to 2 years.[2] Two factors have been associated with extremely rapid transmission of HIV among IDUs: the lack of awareness about HIV infection and acquired immunodeficiency syndrome (AIDS) as a local threat and the mechanisms for rapid, efficient mixing or sharing of injection equipment within the local IDU population. Without an awareness of AIDS as a local threat, IDUs are likely to use each other's equipment frequently. Before an awareness of HIV and AIDS, providing previously used equipment to another IDU was probably considered an act of solidarity among IDUs or as a service for which a person could legitimately charge a small fee.

Shooting galleries (ie, places where IDUs can rent injection equipment, which is then returned to the gallery owner for rental to other IDUs) and dealer's works (ie, injection equipment kept by a drug seller, which can be lent to successive drug purchasers) are examples of situations that provide rapid, efficient mixing within an IDU population. The sharing of injection equipment is rapid because many IDUs may use the gallery or the dealer's

injection equipment within very short periods. The infectiousness of HIV may be many times greater in the period immediately after initial infection compared with the long period between initial infection and the development of severe immunosuppression. Rapid mixing can lead to highly infectious IDUs transmitting HIV to very large numbers of other drug injectors.

Efficient mixing refers to the sharing of drug injection equipment with few restrictions on who shares with whom. Efficient mixing spreads HIV across potential social boundaries, such as friendship groups, which otherwise might have served to limit transmission. Shooting galleries and dealer's works situations tend to arise where there are legal restrictions on sale and possession of drug injection equipment. These restrictions can make it difficult to purchase sterile injection equipment and make it difficult for IDUs to carry their own equipment with them for fear of being arrested.[3]

In some European countries, such as Spain and Italy, injecting drug use has long been the most common risk factor for HIV infection and AIDS. In the United States, injecting drug use has been associated with approximately one third of the cumulative cases of AIDS.[4] More than one half of the U.S. heterosexual transmission cases have involved transmission from an IDU, and more than one half of the perinatal transmission cases have occurred in women who injected drugs themselves or were the sexual partners of IDUs. In the United States, approximately one half of all new infections in the country are occurring among IDUs.[5]

OUTCOMES OF HIV INFECTION AMONG INJECTING DRUG USERS

In sharp contrast to the situation with HIV infection among homosexual and bisexual men, HIV infection among IDUs leads to a wider variety of illnesses than the original oppor-

Don C. Des Jarlais, Director of Research, Chemical Dependency Institute, Beth Israel Medical Center, New York, NY.

TABLE 30.1. *Infections associated with HIV immunosuppression among injecting drug users*

Disease	Comments	Investigation
Bacterial pneumonia	Higher incidence, higher morbidity, more severe course	Selwyn et al.,[60] Stoneburner et al.,[6] Nelson et al.[61]
Endocarditis	Higher incidence, higher morbidity, more severe course	Stoneburner et al.,[6] Nelson et al.[61]
Tuberculosis	Higher incidence, higher morbidity, and reactivation of pre-existing infection, multi-drug resistant	Stoneburner et al.,[6] 1988; Nelson et al.[61]
Pelvic inflammatory disease	Possible more severe course	Minkoff & DeHovitz[62]
Cervical cancer	Interaction with human papillomavirus (HPV) infection	Vermund et al.[63]

tunistic infections that were used to define AIDS. Table 30-1 presents some of the infections for which concurrent HIV infection may increase morbidity, severity, and mortality among IDUs. The 1987 and 1993 revisions of the Centers for Disease Control surveillance definition for AIDS were based in part on the studies showing this wider spectrum of HIV-related illnesses among IDUs. Before these revisions, many IDUs were dying of HIV-related illnesses without ever being classified as having AIDS.[6]

The mechanisms through which HIV infection leads to this wider spectrum of illnesses have not been identified. Tuberculosis infection is controlled primarily through cell-mediated immunity, and HIV infection could be expected to lead to increased reactivation of latent tuberculosis infection and increased susceptibility to tuberculosis infection. HIV infection can also affect humoral immune functioning,[7] and resistance to many infectious agents may be compromised. The lifestyle of many IDUs may put them at greater risk for exposure to a wide variety of pathogens and reduce immune functioning through mechanisms such as poor nutrition.

Whether continued use of psychoactive drugs influences the course of HIV infection has been an important question since AIDS was first noticed among IDUs. A wide variety of psychoactive substances have at least some in vitro effects on components of the immune system, but epidemiologic studies have not yet shown any consistent deleterious effects of continued drug use on the course of HIV infection. Immune system activation, however, may increase replication of HIV,[8] so that very high frequencies of unsterile injections or the development of other infections such as bacterial pneumonias may increase progression of HIV infection. A high-frequency drug-use lifestyle may also interfere with adherence to medical treatment regimens, including antiviral medications for HIV infection and treatments for opportunistic infections.

Some psychoactive drugs may also interact with medications needed by HIV-infected persons. The interaction between methadone and rifampin is the best known. IDUs on methadone maintenance treatment who must take rifampin may need to have their methadone dosage adjusted upward to provide proper methadone medication.

There is no vaccine to prevent HIV infection and no cure for HIV infection. Public health efforts to reduce morbidity and mortality related to HIV among IDUs must focus on reducing the HIV risk behavior of IDUs. The remainder of this chapter therefore focuses on current knowledge of HIV prevention programs for IDUs. Although there are still important issues to be addressed, much has been learned during the last 15 years, and it is possible to assess many prevention activities in terms of their effects on HIV transmission.

THEORIES OF HIV PREVENTION PROGRAMMING

As with other initial AIDS prevention programs, the first programs for IDUs focused on simply providing factual information about AIDS. The first evidence that IDUs would change their risk behavior in response to information about AIDS came from several studies in New York City[9,10] which actually were conducted before the implementation of any formal HIV prevention programs for IDUs in the city. In both of these studies, most drug users reported that they knew about AIDS, that they knew that it was transmitted through the sharing of needles and syringes, and that they had already made at least some changes in their injection behavior (eg, reduced sharing of injection equipment).

IDUs in New York had learned about AIDS through the mass media and through their own oral communication networks. Because of the relatively large number of cases of AIDS among IDUs in New York City even in the early 1980s, there had been a considerable amount of mass-media coverage. The relatively large number of cases of AIDS among IDUs in New York also meant that a substantial number of them knew someone firsthand who had developed AIDS or knew someone who knew someone who had developed AIDS. Another potentially important factor in this early behavior change and risk reduction was the expansion of the illicit market in sterile injection equipment.[11]

The importance of basic factual information about HIV and AIDS—or the lack of such basic information—can also be seen in the very rapid spread of HIV in many areas of south Asia.[12-15] In all of these countries, the rapid spread of HIV among IDUs occurred before any education about AIDS.

Although the early studies indicated that IDUs would learn about AIDS from the mass media and through oral communication networks, it became clear by the mid-1980s that there would be many additional advantages to providing face-to-face AIDS education for IDUs. Face-to-face education would permit transmitting more detailed information; use of culturally appropriate terminology that might not have been possible in mass media; answering questions that the drug users might have; and adopting an tone attuned to the emotional state of individual IDUs participating in the immediate communication.

Drug abuse treatment programs were one logical site for providing such face-to-face AIDS education for IDUs. Many programs did implement such efforts. There were several difficulties, however, in using drug abuse treatment programs for AIDS education.[16] First, it was necessary to provide extensive AIDS education for the staff of the treatment programs before it was possible to work with the drug users in treatment. The education for the staff needed to include strong reassurances that AIDS was not transmitted through the types of casual contact that occurred in the treatment programs. Second, education about how AIDS was transmitted (eg, through sharing drug injection equipment) carried an implication that the person in treatment was likely to inject drugs again. Many drug treatment staff believed that such education would undermine the effectiveness of their programs because it would weaken the drug user's treatment-based expectation that he or she was going to successfully avoid all future use of illicit drugs.

The most important problem was that relatively few IDUs were in treatment at any one time. In the United States, only an estimated 15% to 20% of persons with drug abuse problems are in treatment at any given time, and perhaps as many as one half have never received drug abuse treatment. To reach large numbers of IDUs at risk for AIDS, it was necessary to develop "street outreach" programs to reach IDUs who were not in treatment. Street outreach programs were implemented in New Jersey, New York, Chicago, and San Francisco in the mid-1980s. These programs often employed ex-addicts as peer educators.

Using Psychologic Theories of Health-Related Behavior

Although early studies did show some effect from providing general education about AIDS in reducing HIV risk behavior among IDUs, it also became clear that information-only prevention programs were not likely to be very successful in producing long-term behavior change. Knowledge of possible long-term adverse consequences is rarely sufficient to change behavior in the health field. Various theories of health-related behavior, including the Health Belief model,[17] social learning theory,[18] and the theory of reasoned action,[19] have been used in HIV prevention programs. Although there are differences among these theories, there are also more important similarities. All include elements of expectancy-value decision-making analyses. These theories tend to emphasize perceived probabilities (eg, of getting or avoiding AIDS, of being able to success-

fully perform new behaviors) and subjective valuations of different outcomes (eg, the perceived seriousness of developing AIDS, perceived costs of performing new behaviors if one's injecting or sexual partners were resistant). With some variation, these theories also consider social factors (eg, role models, perceived social norms) and various barriers to changing HIV risk behaviors.

Using these psychologic theories of health behavior required more than the one-way communication possible in mass-media approaches and more than the usually brief conversations that occur between outreach program workers and IDUs encountered in the streets. The National AIDS Demonstration Research and AIDS Targeted Outreach Model (NADR/ATOM) program was begun in the United States in 1987, and it eventually included 41 projects in almost 50 cities.[20] (In all of the cities, the NADR/ATOM project involved street outreach to IDUs not in treatment programs. The eligibility requirements for subjects to be enrolled in the research component of the NADR/ATOM projects required that the person must have injected illicit drugs in the previous 6 months and must not have been in drug abuse treatment in the preceding 1 month. Approximately 40% of the more than 30,000 subjects enrolled in the NADR/ATOM projects reported that they had never been in treatment for drug abuse.

Many of the NADR/ATOM projects used experimental designs to test psychologic theories of health-behavior change. All subjects were provided with a "standard" intervention to reduce HIV risk behavior, which included information about HIV and AIDS, a baseline risk assessment, and the option of HIV counseling and testing. Some of these subjects were then randomly assigned to an "enhanced" condition, which typically involved several additional hours of counseling, education, and skill-training and which incorporated components of the psychologic theories of health behavior. Subjects were followed at 6-month intervals to assess changes in HIV risk behaviors and the incidence of new HIV infections.

The NADR/ATOM projects provided a wealth of data about HIV risk behaviors among IDUs not in drug treatment programs. With respect to changes in HIV risk behaviors, there were two strong and consistent findings. First, almost all of the NADR/ATOM projects showed substantial reductions in injection risk behavior from the baseline assessment to the follow-up interviews, with the percentage of IDUs reporting that they did not "always use a sterile needle" declining from 64% to 41% and those reporting ever sharing needles declined from 54% to 23%.[21]

The second salient finding was that few of the various projects showed significant differences in risk reduction between the standard intervention and the enhanced program. The general lack of differences between the standard and the enhanced interventions should not be interpreted as meaning that the psychologic theories of health behavior are not useful for HIV risk reduction among IDUs. These results instead suggest two other possible explanations.

First, after the provision of basic information about AIDS (as in the standard intervention), 2 to 6 hours of additional education and counseling does little to further strengthen anti-AIDS attitudes, perceptions, and intentions. A second explanation is that risk reduction among IDUs after basic HIV and AIDS education is primarily a function of social processes among IDUs rather than of the characteristics of individual IDUs.

Social-Change Theories of HIV Risk Reduction Among Injecting Drug Users

There is increasing evidence that social-change processes, particularly peer influences, are particularly important in HIV risk reduction among IDUs.[22,23] Almost all injection risk behaviors (eg, sharing of injection equipment) and all sexual risk behaviors occur within social settings. Successful risk reduction may require social changes in addition to such individual changes as learning about AIDS and developing intentions to practice new behaviors. Initiating and maintaining safer injection practices and safer sexual behaviors may require changes in the social relationship among IDUs and their sexual partners.

In an analysis of factors associated with risk reduction among IDUs in four of the cities (ie, Bangkok, Glasgow, Rio de Janeiro and New York City) participating in the World Health Organization's Multi-Centre Study of AIDS and Drug Injection, "talking with drug-using friends" was significantly associated with risk reduction in all four cities.[24] Despite the substantial variation in the drugs injected in these cities (ie, heroin in Bangkok, heroin and buprenorphine in Glasgow, cocaine in Rio de Janeiro, and heroin and cocaine in New York) and the obvious cultural differences among IDUs in these cities, peer influence appeared to be an important component of risk reduction in all four cities.

The use of current drug users as change agents for HIV prevention was initiated in Amsterdam. In 1984, the "Junkie Bond," an organization of drug users and concerned nonusers, worked with the municipal health department to establish a syringe exchange program.[25] A pharmacy in the center of the city had ended its previous policy of selling needles and syringes to drug users, and the users and the health department were concerned at that time about possible increases in hepatitis among the users. (The HIV antibody test had not yet been developed, and no one was yet concerned about AIDS among drug injectors in Amsterdam.) The Junkie Bond and the health department worked together to establish the first syringe exchange program in the city. When the HIV antibody test was developed during the next year, testing of drug users showed that about 30% were already infected with HIV. The Amsterdam syringe exchange program was then greatly expanded, and health department officials worked with the Junkie Bonds in other Dutch cities to establish syringe exchanges and other HIV prevention activities.

Australia was the second country to work with drug user groups to implement syringe exchanges and other HIV prevention efforts. As in the Netherlands, the Australian user groups received modest amounts of government funding, often directly operated the syringe exchange programs, and produced brochures, pamphlets, and newsletters for AIDS prevention.[25]

Several of the NADR/ATOM models also explicitly focused on peer influence and social-change processes. The Chicago project[26] had its origins in the long tradition of ethnography, community research and outreach to drug users by researchers at the University of Chicago. In this particular project, ex-addicts, under the supervision of trained ethnographers, conducted outreach to IDUs not in treatment. Specific efforts were made to enroll influential persons (ie, indigenous leaders) within drug-use networks into the project and to have them use their influence on other IDUs to practice safer injection. This project used the naturally occurring social structure among IDUs to change HIV risk behaviors. A cohort research design was used, with subjects followed for 5 years. The subjects reported dramatic reductions in injection risk behavior. At the start of the project, 95% of subjects reported engaging in injection risk behavior, and this declined to only 15% of the subjects reporting injection risk behavior by the fifth year of the study.

One of the New York City NADR projects involved "self-organization" among IDUs.[25,27,28] The Dutch "Junkie Bonds"—one of which had initiated the first syringe-exchange program in Holland—served as a model for how IDUs can act together to further their own health interests. In the New York City project, outreach workers recruited IDUs and assisted them in developing self-help groups to address HIV transmission and other issues of importance to them. In particular, the subgroup of commercial sex workers among IDUs had a number of common interests. Regular group meetings were held to discuss how the participants could change peer norms about injection and sexual risk behaviors. Attending the meetings was strongly associated with the subjects' own risk reduction and with their efforts to change the behavior of other IDUs.[28]

Social-change theories do not necessarily replace "AIDS education" and psychologic theories of health-related behavior. Knowledge of HIV infection and AIDS and of how to practice safer sex and safer injection are still important, as are perceptions of risk and a sense of efficacy in practicing safer behaviors. Social-change theories do, however, offer important additional tools for reducing HIV risk behaviors. Influencing others to adopt new behaviors can also serve to strengthen the intentions of prevention program participants to change their own risk behaviors. If social norms about injection and sexual behavior can be changed, it becomes possible to change the behavior of IDUs who do not directly participate in the prevention program. The peer approval that comes with following the new norms can itself serve to reinforce safer injection and safer sex practices among IDUs.

PROVIDING THE MEANS FOR BEHAVIOR CHANGE

Reducing HIV risk behavior often requires providing or facilitating access to the actual means for behavior change. Reducing sexual risk behaviors requires access to condoms, reducing drug injection often requires access to drug abuse treatment, and reducing unsafe injection-related HIV risk behaviors requires access to sterile injection equipment or at least to the means for disinfecting HIV-contaminated injection equipment. In many developed countries, increasing legal access to sterile injection equipment was an important aspect of initial efforts to reduce HIV transmission among IDUs. For example, in 1985, the city of Amsterdam rapidly expanded existing syringe-exchange services that were previously implemented to reduce hepatitis B transmission. In 1987, the United Kingdom implemented a nationwide system of syringe-exchange programs.[29] In 1987, France repealed its laws requiring prescriptions for the sale of sterile injection equipment and set up a program that encouraged pharmacists to sell injection equipment to IDUs.[30,31] Australia repealed its prescription requirement laws in 1984 and established a system of syringe-exchange programs.

In many European countries, such as Italy, Germany, and Spain, there had been no legal restrictions on the sale and possession of injection equipment before awareness of HIV infection among IDUs, and education programs were implemented to educate and encourage IDUs to inject with sterile equipment. Many of these countries have since established syringe-exchange programs as a means for providing face-to-face outreach efforts to IDUs and safe disposal of the exchanged (potentially HIV-contaminated) injection equipment.[32] Providing legal access to sterile injection equipment, whether through expanded pharmacy sales, syringe exchange, or both, is now a standard aspect of HIV prevention in almost all industrialized countries.

In the United States, there was some early consideration of providing legal access to sterile injection equipment as a method for reducing HIV transmission among IDUs.[33] Early exchanges were implemented by activists in the Northeast and by community-based organizations in the Northwest.[32] There were many impediments to providing legal access to sterile injection equipment for IDUs in the U.S.[3,32,34] The states with the largest numbers of IDUs (ie, New York, California, and Illinois) had laws requiring prescriptions for the sale of injection equipment, and almost all states had previously enacted laws criminalizing the possession of equipment for injecting illicit drugs.

Efforts to increase access by IDUs to sterile injection equipment—whether through changing laws or by implementing "underground" syringe exchanges in defiance of existing statues—often generated intense controversy about whether it would increase illicit drug use or represent official condoning of illicit drug use.[32] In some areas, racial and ethnic group antagonisms compounded the controversies.[35]

In 1989, federal legislation was enacted that prohibited the use of any federal funds to support syringe exchanges or other distribution of sterile injection equipment to persons who inject illicit drugs. This prohibition remains in effect.

Given these legal, political, and funding difficulties in providing legal access to sterile injection equipment, there was an obvious need to find some other means to assist IDUs in practicing safer injection. Based on ethnographic interviews with IDUs, the Mid-City Consortium in San Francisco[36] identified criteria for possible disinfection of HIV-contaminated drug injection: the disinfectant should be strong and readily available; the disinfection procedure should be quick; it should not harm the injection equipment; and it should not harm the injector in the event that small amounts of disinfectant were injected. Of the various possible disinfectants, household bleach appeared to be the closest to meeting these criteria. Outreach workers began distributing small bottles of bleach with instructions on how to use the bleach as a disinfectant: two rinses of the needle and syringe with bleach, followed by two rinses with clean water. The use of bleach was readily accepted by most IDUs in San Francisco. Within 1 year after the bleach distribution program was started, more than one half of the IDUs in the city reported using bleach as a disinfectant.[37]

After the initial success in getting IDUs in San Francisco to use bleach as a disinfectant, many other outreach programs adopted bleach distribution. Most NADR/ATOM programs included bleach distribution.

Although the controversy surrounding syringe-exchange programs was much greater, there still was some controversy about whether the distribution of bleach would encourage drug use. Outreach workers employed by the State of New Jersey and by Los Angeles County were forbidden to distribute bleach. The initial authorization for funding of these programs by the U.S. Department of Health and Human Services in 1988 contained a provision that would have forbidden use of federal funds for bleach distribution. This bill was eventually vetoed for reasons not related to bleach distribution, and the prohibition on bleach distribution was removed from the final bill.

Effects of Providing Means for Safer Injection

Because of the controversy about whether syringe-exchange programs might lead to increased illicit drug use, this question has been explicitly addressed in a number of syringe-exchange studies. The cumulative research on syringe exchange has been quite clear in the lack of evidence that syringe-exchange programs lead to any detectable increase in illicit drug injection. The U.S. Government Accounting Office (GAO) review[38] included five study projects that addressed this question and met the GAO criteria for "strong evidence." Four of these study projects showed no increase in illicit drug injection, and one even showed a decrease concurrent with the implementation of a local syringe exchange.

A report by Lurie and colleagues[32] also reviewed the existing literature and included focus-group interviews with current drug injectors on this topic. The report concluded that "there is no evidence of a change in injecting or non-injecting drug use associated with the opening or operation" of any syringe exchange (p. 359). Lurie's group also examined various indicators of illicit drug use, such as the Drug Abuse Warning Network and the Drug Use Forecasting system, to see if there were any indications of increased illicit drug use in communities that had implemented syringe-exchange programs. They were not able to detect any effect of a local syringe-exchange program on rates of illicit drug use.

If syringe-exchange programs led to an increased number of IDUs, investigators could expect to see relatively large numbers of young, newer injectors at the syringe-exchange programs or at least in the cities in which they are located. This has not happened. The best available data may be from Amsterdam, where—despite the massive expansion of the syringe-exchange program from 100,000 needles and syringes exchanged in 1985 to more than 6,000,000 exchanged in 1995—the number of IDUs in the city has remained stable at an estimated 3000, and the average age of the IDU population has increased from 26.8 years in 1983 to 30.8 years in 1990.[39]

Later data also support the conclusion that syringe-exchange programs do not lead to any detectable increase in illicit drug injection. A San Francisco study[40] also found an increase in the mean age of IDUs in the city during the years of operation of the syringe-exchange programs. In a New York study,[41] a large shift from injection to intranasal use of heroin occurred in the city during the same time as the implementation and operation of the "underground" syringe-exchange programs. This increase in intranasal use is itself in the opposite direction from a prediction that access to syringe exchanges would lead to an increase in injecting drug use.

Although identifying the factors that lead some persons to start injecting illicit drugs despite knowing about the risk of AIDS remains an important question for future research, the presence of a syringe-exchange program in these cities does not appear to have caused any increase in illicit drug injection.

There has also been some controversy about whether bleach-distribution programs would lead to an increase in illicit drug use. Studies of outreach bleach-distribution programs have not focused on this question of increased drug injection to the same extent that syringe-exchange studies have, but the available data are consistent with the findings of the syringe-exchange studies. Participants in outreach bleach-distribution programs also tend to have very long histories of injecting drug use.[20] Few of these participants are recent initiates into injection drug use. There is no evidence to support the hypothesis that the opportunity to obtain bleach from an outreach program lures people into initiating injection drug use.

HIV Incidence in Outreach Projects

Almost all evaluations of HIV prevention programs have shown self-reported risk reduction among participating IDUs. In most of the research on the effects of the prevention programs on risk behaviors, however, important differences in research designs have precluded comparisons across studies. Different questions about risk behavior were used, different follow-up intervals were used, and different methods of recruiting comparison groups were used, and the initial levels of risk behavior differed among the groups participating in the prevention programs. It has not been possible to compare the reductions in risk behavior resulting from the different prevention programs.

The major exception to this lack of comparability has been the NADR/ATOM projects, in which similar research methods were used across different interventions in the same city and across interventions in different cities. The most common finding from the NADR/ATOM studies, however, was that the standard intervention led to as much risk reduction as the enhanced intervention in almost all cities. (Inclusion of a no-intervention control group would have been unethical in research with persons at high risk for infection with a fatal virus.) Overall, the data from these projects do indicate substantial risk reduction among the participants, but the NADR/ATOM projects do not provide a firm basis for attempting to identify more effective or less effective interventions.

There has been sufficient research that examined the rate of new HIV infections among participants in outreach programs that it is possible to assess the potential impact of prevention programs on the rate of new HIV infections. Table 30-2 presents data on new HIV infections among participants in the NADR/ATOM projects for which HIV incidence data are available.[42] The cities are not identified individually, because researchers in those cities are preparing individual research reports.

There are two clear findings from the NADR/ATOM HIV incidence studies. First, the new infection rates are substantially lower in the cities where the initial (background) HIV seroprevalence rates were low. Second, background HIV seroprevalence and the new infection rates are generally much lower in areas that permit over-the-counter sales of sterile injection equipment (ie, areas that do not have prescription requirements for equipment).

The higher new infection rates in areas with higher HIV seroprevalence are easily understood in epidemiologic terms. An uninfected person who engages in risk behavior (eg, sharing of drug injection equipment, unprotected sexual intercourse) is more likely to encounter an HIV-infected risk partner in a high-prevalence area.

The overall incidence was also much lower in areas with legal over-the-counter sales of injection equipment (0.79 per 100 person-years at risk) than in areas that had prescription requirements for sale of injection equipment (1.99 per 100 person-years at risk).[4]

TABLE 30-2. *HIV seroprevalence and HIV seroconversions per 100 person-years at risk among injecting drug users in fourteen localities* according to legal status of over-the-counter syringe sales*

No. HIV Negative	No. HIV Positive	Percent HIV Positive	Seroconversions	Person-Years at Risk†	Seroconversions per 100 Person-Years at Risk
LOCALITIES WHERE OVER-THE-COUNTER SALES ARE ILLEGAL					
288	311	51.9%	4	49.3	8.11
1088	908	45.5%	6	146.1	4.10
855	589	40.8%	3	81.9	3.66
669	194	22.5%	17	262.8	6.47
1222	76	5.9%	2	956.1	0.21
787	14	1.7%	0	109.0	0.00
LOCALITIES WHERE OVER-THE-COUNTER SALES ARE LEGAL					
1760	138	7.3%	7	184.0	3.80
652	43	6.2%	5	187.0	2.67
1968	61	3.0%	8	732.5	1.09
651	17	2.5%	0	225.3	0.00
2099	31	1.5%	2	765.1	0.26
891	13	1.4%	3	983.4	0.31
372	4	1.1%	0	18.0	0.00
514	5	1.0%	0	53.7	0.00

*The principal investigators of specific sites are preparing detailed analyses of their data on seroconversion rates. Data are publicly available (with locality identifiers removed) through Nova Research Company, Bethesda, Maryland.

†Numbers presented for person-years at risk by locality do not add up to those for the summary table because of a rounding error.

Because of the difficulties in establishing the factors that account for current HIV seroprevalence in U.S. cities where over-the-counter sales of injection equipment are legal, researchers must be cautious in drawing conclusions about causal relationships between such sales and lower rates of HIV incidence. The data in Table 30-2, however, strongly suggest that legal over-the-counter sales may be one factor in facilitating safer injection among IDUs. Studies from France,[30,31] Glasgow, Scotland,[43] and Connecticut,[44] where the prescription requirement was recently repealed, all show HIV risk reduction associated with over-the-counter sales, supporting the interpretation of a causal role for over-the-counter sales in reducing HIV transmission among IDUs.

In the high HIV seroprevalence areas, the outreach bleach-distribution programs also appear to have led to substantial risk reduction among IDUs, but the rates of new HIV infections ($\geq$3/100 person-years at risk) must still be considered unacceptable from a public health standpoint. In these areas, more prevention efforts are needed. These may include better access to sterile injection equipment, better access to drug abuse treatment, and programs to reduce the numbers of persons starting to inject illicit drugs.

Effectiveness of Bleach as a Disinfectant for Drug Injection Equipment

Although the outreach programs have led to substantial risk reduction among IDUs and to low rates of new HIV infections in low-seroprevalence areas, questions have arisen about the actual effectiveness of using bleach as a disinfec-

tant for injection equipment. Recent studies from Baltimore[45] and New York City[46] have failed to show any relation between self-reported use of bleach to disinfect injection equipment and protection from infection with HIV. There are numerous difficulties in attempting to find such an association. Reports on the frequency and circumstances of using bleach may not be very accurate. Drug users may not now how to properly use bleach to disinfect injection equipment (the current recommendation is for 30 seconds of contact time of undiluted bleach in the needle and syringe). Even if the drug injectors know how to properly use bleach, they may not be using it properly under field conditions.[47]

The apparent effectiveness of the outreach bleach-distribution programs in lowering rates of new HIV infections among IDUs may be a result of participants obtaining more sterile injection equipment from pharmacies or on the illicit market, rather than a result of the actual use of bleach to disinfect used injection equipment.

HIV Incidence and Syringe Exchange

Determining whether syringe-exchange programs have led to reductions in the rate of new HIV infections involves complex methodologic problems. Many of these methodologic problems also hold for assessing outreach bleach programs, but the problems have been examined in much more detail for syringe-exchange programs. There have been no random-assignment clinical trials of syringe-exchange programs, and because of the logistical and ethical problems in conducting such a study, there may never be. Moreover, syringe exchanges may indirectly protect IDUs who do not actually attend the exchange. If HIV-infected IDUs return their used injection equipment to an exchange without passing it on to others, the other IDUs may be protected against HIV, even though they do not use the exchange themselves. For these and other methodologic reasons, most reviews have generally not drawn conclusions about the direct effectiveness of syringe-exchange programs in reducing transmission of blood-borne viruses among IDUs.

One way of studying the potential effectiveness of syringe-exchange programs on HIV transmission is to examine HIV seroincidence among IDUs participating in syringe-exchange programs. Table 30-3 presents such HIV incidence data.[48] First, as with the outreach bleach-distribution programs, HIV incidence is quite low in areas with low background HIV prevalence. HIV incidence is, among other factors, related to the probability of a seronegative IDU sharing equipment with a seropositive IDU. Because of this, it may be that any modestly effective HIV prevention program will be associated with low HIV incidence in a low-seroprevalence area. Conversely, the presence of syringe-exchange programs or other good access to sterile injection equipment may itself be an important reason why HIV seroprevalence and HIV incidence has remained low in many populations of IDUs.

IDUs from the Montreal exchange, however, have an HIV incidence rate notably above that of the other cities in Table 30-3. The Montreal program appears to attract a subgroup of IDUs with extremely high initial risk levels,[49,50] including high rates of cocaine injection and high levels of unprotected commercial sex work. However, additional data are needed to fully explain the Montreal incidence, and new studies are being initiated in Montreal.[51]

The HIV incidence data from the three high-seroprevalence U.S. cities (ie, New Haven, Chicago, and New York) with syringe-exchange programs are based on relatively small sample sizes of person-years at risk. Nevertheless, these results must be considered extremely encouraging with respect to reducing HIV transmission in high-seroprevalence areas. These data are also consistent with the previously developed mathematical model to assess the effectiveness of the New Haven syringe-exchange program.[51]

A case-control study of incident hepatitis B and hepatitis C infection among IDUs in Tacoma, Washington, may contain the strongest evidence for the effectiveness of syringe-exchange programs in reducing transmission of blood-borne viruses.[52,53] Pierce County (Tacoma) is one of the four counties in the U.S. Centers for Disease Control Hepatitis Surveillance System, and it has among the best data on hepatitis incidence in the United States. Cases of hepatitis B and hepatitis C among IDUs were identified through the surveillance reporting system. Controls were identified among IDUs attending the drug treatment and HIV counseling clinics in Pierce County. Sera is collected at both clinics and could be tested to identify IDUs who were seronegative for hepatitis. Demographic data, drug-injection history data, and whether the subject had ever used the local syringe-exchange program were abstracted from the clinics' records.

Multiple logistic regression analyses were used to identify statistically independent factors differentiating the inci-

TABLE 30-3. *HIV seroconversion rates among injecting drug users participating in syringe exchange*

City or Country	HIV Prevalence*	Measured HIV Seroconversions†	Estimated HIV Seroconversions†	Investigation
Lund	Low	0		Ljungberg et al.[64]
Glasgow	Low		0–1 (2)	WHO Multi-Centre[65]
Sydney	Low		0–1 (2)	WHO Multi-Centre[65]
Toronto	Low		1–2 (2)	WHO Multi-Centre[65]
England and Wales (except London)	Low		0–1 (1)	Stimson (personal communication, 1994)
Kathmandu	Low	0		Maharjan et al.[66]
Tacoma, WA	Low	<1		Hagan et al.[67]
Portland, OR	Low	<1		Oliver et al.[68]
Montreal	Moderate	13		Hankins et al.[50]
London	Moderate		1–2 (3)	Stimson (personal communication, 1994)
Amsterdam	High	4		Van den Hoek, personal communication, 1994)
Chicago, IL	High	0		O'Brien et al.[69]
New York, NY	Very high	2		Paone et al.[70]
New Haven, CT	Very high		0 (4)	Kaplan and Heimer[71]

*Low, 0 to 5%; moderate, 6% to 20%; high, 21% to 40%; very high, 41+%.

†Cohort study or repeated testing of participants in per 100 person-years at risk, estimated from (1) stable, very low <2% seroprevalence in area, (2) self-reports of previous seronegative test and a current HIV blood or saliva test, (3) stable or declining seroprevalence, (4) from HIV testing of syringes collected at exchange per 100 person-years at risk.

dent IDU hepatitis cases from the controls. Failure to use the local syringe exchange (versus any use) was strongly associated with incident hepatitis B and incident hepatitis C. The adjusted odds ratios for not using the exchange were both greater than 5 for incident hepatitis B and hepatitis C infections.

A panel of the U.S. National Academy of Sciences reviewed the accumulated evidence on syringe-exchange programs.[54] Going beyond the conclusions of previous reviews, this group concluded that syringe-exchange programs do reduce the transmission of HIV among IDUs. Although there has not yet been (and for ethical reasons probably never will be) a randomized clinical trial of syringe-exchange programs, several lines of evidence were used to reach this conclusion. First, there is the highly consistent evidence that participation in syringe exchanges does lead to reductions in injection risk behavior. The HIV incidence data (see Table 30-3) is also almost perfectly consistent in showing low rates of new HIV infections among syringe-exchange participants. The combined data from the evaluations of the New Haven and Tacoma exchanges were particularly important in the conclusions of the National Academy of Sciences panel. The behavior change and hepatitis data from Tacoma and the mathematical modeling based on the syringe-tracking system from New Haven provide some of the strongest evidence that participation in syringe-exchange programs is causally associated with low rates of infection with blood-borne viruses.

CURRENT STATE OF PREVENTION RESEARCH

Prevention programs for IDUs in low-seroprevalence areas appear to be capable of achieving control over HIV transmission.[52] These programs cannot prevent all new HIV infections, but it does appear that they can maintain low seroprevalence indefinitely. In these low-seroprevalence areas, almost all of the remaining risk behavior among IDUs occurs among persons who are HIV-seronegative and occurs without transmission of the virus. In high-seroprevalence areas, even moderate levels of injection risk behavior are likely to involve persons of different HIV serostatus and may lead to transmission of the virus. Analyses conducted by Holmberg[5] of the CDC suggest that transmission of HIV among IDUs in high-seroprevalence areas may represent the plurality of new HIV infections in the United States.

A new generation of HIV prevention programs may be needed for IDUs in high-seroprevalence areas. In addition to more intensive programs focusing on safer injection, there is a need for programs to reduce the numbers of persons injecting illicit drugs in high-seroprevalence areas. Massive expansion of drug abuse treatment could lead to large reductions in the numbers of persons who are injecting illicit drugs. Programs to reduce initiation into drug injection would also be very useful for high-seroprevalence areas, because these would also lead to a reduction over time in the numbers of IDUs.[55]

HARM REDUCTION

The worldwide epidemic of HIV infection among IDUs has led to important conceptual developments on injecting drug use as a health problem. HIV and AIDS have dramatically increased the adverse health consequences of injecting drug use and have led to seeing psychoactive drug use as a health problem and not just a criminal justice problem. HIV infection can be prevented without requiring the cessation of injecting drug use, and this potential separation of a severe adverse potential consequence of drug use from the drug use itself has encouraged analysis of other areas in which adverse consequences of drug use might be reduced without necessarily requiring cessation of drug use.

The ability of many IDUs to modify their behavior to reduce the chances of HIV infection has also led to consideration of drug addicts as concerned about their health and as capable of acting on that concern without denying the compulsive nature of drug dependence. These ideas have formed much of the basis for what has been called the "harm reduction" perspective on psychoactive drug use.[56–59] Harm reduction is a rapidly developing perspective on the use and misuse psychoactive drugs, without a single set of uniform precepts accepted by all persons who consider themselves to be advocates of harm reduction. Space limitations prohibit a full explication of harm reduction here, but it is important to understand some of the basic tenets of the perspective.

Harm reduction is conceptually distinct from the old drug legalization versus drug prohibition debate. Within harm reduction theory, criminal and civil laws are powerful and important tools to reduce the harms associated with psychoactive drug use, and permitting unrestricted marketing of all psychoactive drugs would undoubtedly greatly increase the total harm to society from drug use. Nicotine (in tobacco products) is perhaps the most compelling example of the enormous harm that can occur from unrestricted marketing of a powerful psychoactive drug.

The conceptual power of harm reduction is in its ability to reject the extremes of the legalization versus prohibition debate and to encourage public health officials and policy makers to think about methods for reducing drug-related harms that do not require legalization or prohibition. Syringe-exchange programs are a prototypical harm-reduction activity. They do not lead to increased illicit drug injection, they certainly do not require legalization of the drugs that are injected, and syringe-exchange programs can reduce the transmission of HIV among IDUs, their sexual partners, and their children.[54] Other examples of harm-reduction activities include designated-driver and call-a-taxicab programs to reduce drunken driving and the potential banning of cigarette vending machines, because minors can easily and illegally obtain cigarettes from such machines. Neither designated-driver nor call-a-taxicab programs require prohibition of alcohol, and banning cigarette vending machines would not require prohibition of nicotine.

The harm-reduction perspective emphasizes the pragmatic need to reduce harmful consequences of psychoactive drug use while acknowledging that eliminating psychoactive drug use or drug misuse is not likely to be feasible for the foreseeable future. One of the major strengths of the perspective is its applicability to licit and illicit psychoactive drug use.

ACKNOWLEDGMENTS

Sections of this chapter were originally prepared as reports to the United Kingdom Department of Health and for the United States Congressional Office of Technology Assessment.

REFERENCES

1. Stimson GV. The health and social costs of drug injecting: the challenge to developing countries. Sixth International Conference on the Reduction of Drug-Related Harm. Florence, Italy, 1995:26.
2. Des Jarlais DC, Friedman SR, Choopanya K, Vanichseni S, Ward TP. International epidemiology of HIV and AIDS among injecting drug users. AIDS 1992;6:1053.
3. Des Jarlais DC, Friedman SR. The AIDS epidemic and legal access to sterile equipment for injecting illicit drugs. Annals of the American Academy of Political and Social Science, 1992;521:42.
4. Centers for Disease Control and Prevention. HIV/AIDS surveillance report. Atlanta, GA: Centers for Disease Control, 1994.
5. Holmberg SD. Emerging epidemiological patterns in the USA. 6th Annual Meeting of the National Cooperative Vaccine Development Group for AIDS. Alexandria, VA, 1993.
6. Stoneburner RL, Des Jarlais DC, Benezra D, et al. A larger spectrum of severe HIV-1-related disease in intravenous drug users in New York City. Science 1988;242:916.
7. Zolla-Pazner S, Des Jarlais DC, Friedman SR, et al. Nonrandom development of immunologic abnormalities after infection with human immunodeficiency virus: implications for immunologic classification of the disease. Proceedings of the National Academy of Sciences 1987;84:5404.
8. Zagury D, Bernard J, Leonard R, et al. Long-term cultures of HTLV-III-infected T cells: a model of cytopathology of T-cell depletion in AIDS. Science 1986;231:850.
9. Friedman SR, Des Jarlais DC, Sotheran JL, Garber J, Cohen H, Smith D. AIDS and self-organization among intravenous drug users. International Journal of the Addictions 1987;22:201.
10. Selwyn PA, Feiner C, Cox CP, Lipshutz C, Cohen R. Knowledge about AIDS and high-risk behavior among intravenous drug abusers in New York City. AIDS 1987;1:247.
11. Des Jarlais DC, Friedman SR, Hopkins W. Risk reduction for the acquired immunodeficiency syndrome among intravenous drug users. Annals of Internal Medicine 1985;103:755.
12. Goa Q-L. HIV among drug injectors in China. Oral presentation at the III International Conference on the Reduction of Drug Related Harm. Melbourne, Australia, 1992.
13. Naik TN, Sarkar S, Singh HL. Intravenous drug users—a new high-risk group for HIV infection in India. AIDS 1991;5:117.
14. Poshyachinda V. Drug injection and HIV infection among the population of drug abusers in Asia. Bulletin on Narcotics 1993;45:77.
15. Stimson GV. Reconstruction of sub-regional diffusion of HIV infection among injecting drug users in South-East Asia: implications for early intervention. AIDS 1994;8:1630.
16. Des Jarlais DC, Friedman SR, Sotheran JL. The first city: the spread of HIV among intravenous drug users and the treatment program response in New York City. In: Fox DM, Fee E, eds. AIDS: The Making of a Chronic Disease. Berkeley: University of California Press, 1992:279.
17. Becker MH, Joseph JK. AIDS and behavioral change to reduce risk: a review. American Journal of Public Health 1988;78:394.
18. Bandura A. Social learning theory. Engelwood, NJ: Prentice-Hall, 1977.
19. Fishbein M, Ajzen I. Belief, attitude intention, and behavior: an introduction to theory and research. Reading MA: Addison-Wesley, 1975.
20. Brown BS, Beschner GM. Introduction: at risk for AIDS—injection drug users and their sexual partners. In: Brown BS, Beschner GM, eds. Handbook on risk of AIDS. Westport, CT: Greenwood Press, 1993.
21. Stephens RC, Simpson DD, Coyle SL, McCoy CB, and the National AIDS Research Consortium. Comparative effectiveness of NADR interventions. In: Brown BS, Beschner GM, eds. Handbook on risk of AIDS. Westport CT: Greenwood Press, 1993:519.
22. Friedman SR, Des Jarlais DC, Ward TP. Social models for changing health-relevant behavior. In: DiClemente R, Peterson J, eds. Preventing AIDS: theories & methods of behavioral interventions. New York: Plenum Press, 1994;95.
23. Neaigus A, Friedman SR, Curtis R, et al. The relevance of drug injectors' social networks and risk networks for understanding and preventing HIV infection. Social Science and Medicine 1994;38:67.
24. Des Jarlais DC, Friedman SR, Friedmann P, et al. HIV/AIDS-related behavior change among injecting drug users in different national settings. AIDS 1995;9(6):611.
25. Friedman SR, de Jong W, Wodak A. Community development as a response to HIV among drug injectors. AIDS 92/93 1993;7(suppl. 1): S263-S269.
26. Wiebel W, Jimenez A, Johnson W, Ouellet L, Murray J, O'Brien M. Positive effect on HIV seroconversion of street outreach intervention with IDU in Chicago, 1988-1992. Presented at the Ninth International Conference on AIDS, Berlin, 1993.
27. Friedman SR, Sufian M, Curtis R, Neaigus A, Des Jarlais DC. Organizing drug users against AIDS. In: Huber J, Schneider BE, eds. The social context of AIDS. Newbury, CA: Sage, 1992:115.
28. Friedman SR, Wiebel W, Jose B, Levin L. Changing the culture of risk. In: Brown BS, Beschner GM, eds. Handbook on risk of AIDS. Westport, CT: Greenwood Press, 1993:499.
29. Stimson GV, Alldritt LJ, Dolan KA, Donoghoe MS, Lart RA. Injecting equipment exchange schemes: final report. London: Monitoring Research Group, Goldsmith's College, 1988.
30. Espinoza P, Bouchard I, Ballian P, Polo DeVoto J. Has the open sale of syringes modified the syringe exchanging habits of drug addicts? Presented at the Fourth International Conference on AIDS, Stockholm, Sweden, 1988.
31. Ingold FR, Ingold S. The effects of the liberalization of syringe sales on the behavior of intravenous drug users in France. Bulletin on Narcotics, 1989;41:67.
32. Lurie P, Reingold AL, Bowser B, eds. The public health impact of needle-exchange programs in the United States and abroad, volume 1. Atlanta, GA: Centers for Disease Control and Prevention, 1993.
33. Des Jarlais DC, Hopkins W. "Free" needles for intravenous drug users at risk for AIDS: current developments in New York City (letter). N Engl J Med 1985;313:1476.
34. Gostin L. The interconnected epidemics of drug dependency and AIDS. Harvard Civil Liberties-Civil Rights Law Review 1991;26:114.
35. Anderson W. The New York needle trial: the politics of public health in the age of AIDS. American Journal of Public Health 1991;81:1506.
36. Newmeyer JA. Why bleach? Development of a strategy to combat HIV contagion among San Francisco intravenous drug users. In: Battjes RJ, Pickens RW, eds. Needle sharing among intravenous drug users: national and international perspectives Washington, DC: U.S. Government Printing Office, 1988:151.
37. Chaisson RE, Osmond D, Moss AR, Feldman HW, Biernacki P. HIV, bleach and needle sharing (letter). Lancet 1987:1430.
38. U.S. General Accounting Office. Needle exchange programs: research suggests promise as an AIDS prevention strategy. Report to the Chairman, Select Committee on Narcotics Abuse and Control, House of Representatives. Washington, DC: U.S. House of Representatives, 1993.
39. Buning EC. Effects of the Amsterdam needle and syringe exchange. International Journal of the Addictions 1991;26:1303.
40. Watters JK, Estilo MJ, Clark GL, Lorvick J. Syringe and needle exchange as HIV/AIDS prevention for injection drug users. Journal of the American Medical Association. 1994;271:115.
41. Des Jarlais DC, Friedman SR, Sotheran JL, et al. Continuity and change within an HIV epidemic: injecting drug users in New York City, 1984 through 1992. JAMA. 1994;271:121.
42. Friedman SR, Jose B, Deren S, Des Jarlais DC, Neaigus A, National AIDS Research Consortium. Risk factors for HIV seroconversion among out-of-treatment drug injectors in high- and low- seroprevalence cities. American Journal of Epidemiology 1995;142(8):864.

43. Goldberg D, Watson H, Stuart F, Miller M, Gruer L, Follett E. Pharmacy supply of needles and syringes—the effect on spread of HIV in intravenous drug misusers. Presented at the Fourth International Conference on AIDS, Stockholm, Sweden, 1988.

44. Valleroy L, Groseclose S. Legislative changes: the Connecticut experience. Presentation given at the National Academy of Sciences Workshop on Needle Exchange and Bleach Distribution Programs, Baltimore, MD, 1993.

45. Vlahov D, Astemborski J, Solomon L, Nelson KE. Field effectiveness of needle disinfection among injecting drug users. Journal of Acquired Immune Deficiency Syndromes 1994;7:760.

46. Titus S, Marmor M, Des Jarlais DC, Kim M, Wolfe H, Beatrice S. Bleach use and HIV seroconversion among New York City injection drug users. Journal of Acquired Immune Deficiency Syndromes 1994;7:700.

47. Gleghorn AA, Doherty MC, Vlahov D, Celentano DD, Jones TS. Inadequate bleach contact times during syringe cleaning among injection drug users. Journal of Acquired Immune Deficiency Syndromes 1994;7:767.

48. Des Jarlais DC, Friedmann P, Friedman SR. The protective effect of self-reported AIDS risk reduction among injecting drug users: a cross-national study. (submitted).

49. Bruneau J, Lamothe F, Lachance N, Soto J, Vincelette J. HIV prevalence and incidence in a cohort of IDUs in Montreal, according to their needle exchange attendance. Presented at the Tenth International Conference on AIDS, Yokohama, Japan, 1994.

50. Hankins C, Gendron S, Tran T. Montreal needle exchange attenders versus non-attenders: what's the difference? Presented at the Tenth International Conference on AIDS, Yokohama, Japan, 1994.

51. O'Keefe E, Kaplan E, Khoshnood K. Preliminary report: city of New Haven needle exchange program. New Haven, CT: New Haven Health Department, 1991.

52. Des Jarlais DC, Hagan H, Friedman SR, et al. Maintaining low HIV seroprevalence in populations of injecting drug users. JAMA 1995;274(15):1226.

53. Hagan H, Des Jarlais DC, Friedman SR, Purchase D, Alter MJ. Reduced risk of hepatitis B and hepatitis C among injecting drug users participating in the Tacoma syringe-exchange program. American Journal of Public Health 1995;85(11):1531.

54. Normand J, Vlahov D, Moses L, eds. Preventing HIV transmission: the role of sterile needles and bleach. Washington, DC: National Academy Press, 1995.

55. Des Jarlais DC, Casriel C, Friedman SR, Rosenblum A. AIDS and the transition to illicit drug injection: results of a randomized trial prevention program. British Journal of Addiction 1992;87:493.

56. Brettle RP. HIV and harm reduction in injection drug users. AIDS 1991;5:125.

57. Des Jarlais DC. Harm reduction—a framework for incorporating science into drug policy (editorial). American Journal of Public Health 1995;85(1):10.

58. Des Jarlais DC, Friedman SR, Ward TP. Harm reduction: a public health response to the AIDS epidemic among injecting drug users. Annual Review of Public health 1993;14:413.

59. Heather N, Wodak A, Nadelmann E, O'Hare P, eds. Psychoactive drugs and harm reduction: from faith to science. London: Whurr Publishers, 1993.

60. Selwyn PA, Feingold AR, Hartel D, et at. Increased risk of bacterial pneumonia in HIV-infected intravenous drug users without AIDS. AIDS 1988;2:267.

61. Nelson KE, Vlahov D, Cohn S, Lindsay A, Solomon L, Anthony JC. Diabetes is protective against HIV infections in IV drug users. Paper presented at the Sixth International Conference on AIDS, San Francisco, CA, 1990.

62. Minkoff HL, DeHovitz JA. Care of women infected with the human immunodeficiency virus. JAMA 1991;266:2253.

63. Vermund SH, Kelley KF, Klein RS, et al. High risk of human papillomavirus infection and cervical squamous intraepithelial lesions among women with symptomatic human immunodeficiency virus infection. Am J Obstet Gynecol 1991;165(2):392.

64. Ljungbery B, Christensson B, Tunving K, et al. HIV prevention among injecting drug users: three years of experience from a syringe exchange program in Sweden. Journal of Acquired Immune Deficiency Syndromes 1991;4:890.

65. World Health Organization, Program on Substance Abuse. Multi-centre study on drug injecting and risk of HIV infection. A report prepared on behalf of the International Collaborative Group. Geneva: World Health Organization, 1993.

66. Maharjan SH, Peak A, Rana S, Crofts N. Declining risk for HIV among IDUs in Kathmandu: impact of a harm reduction programme. Paper presented at the Tenth International conference on AIDS. Yokohama, Japan, 1994.

67. Hagan H, Des Jarlais DC, Friedman SR, Purchase D. Risk for human immunodeficiency virus and Hepatitis B virus in users of the Tacoma syringe change program. In: Proceedings: workshop on needle exchange and bleach distribution programs. Washington, DC: National Academy Press, 1994:24.

68. Oliver K, Maynard H, Friedman SR, Des Jarlais DC. Behavioral and community impact of the Portland syringe exchange program. In: Proceedings of the workshop on needle exchange and bleach distribution programs. Washington, DC: National Academy Press, 1994:35.

69. O'Brien M, Murray JR, Rahemian A, Wiebel W. Three topics from the Chicago needle exchange cohort study: seroconversion, the behavior of HIV-positive NX users, and the need for additional prevention around non-needle injection risks. Paper presented at the Annual North American Syringe Exchange Conference, Santa Cruz, CA, 1994.

70. Paone D, Des Jarlais DC, Caloir S, Friedmann PB, Ness I, Friedman SR. New York City syringe exchange: an overview. In: Proceedings: workshop on needle exchange and bleach distribution programs. Washington, DC: National Academy Press, 1994:47.

71. Kaplan E, Heimer R. What happened to HIV transmission among HIV drug injectors in New Haven? Chance: New Directions for Statistics and Computing 1993;6:9.

AIDS: Biology, Diagnosis, Treatment and Prevention, fourth edition, edited by Vincent T. DeVita, Jr., Samuel Hellman, and Steven A. Rosenberg. Lippincott–Raven Publishers, © 1997

CHAPTER 31

Human Immunodeficiency Virus Transmission Through Blood, Blood Products, and Tissue and Organ Donations

Cladd E. Stevens

Patients given blood or blood components or treated with certain blood products were at risk of infection with the human immunodeficiency virus (HIV) in the late 1970s through early 1985, before antibody tests to screen donors were available. An estimated 12,000 to 15,000 transfusion recipients were infected, as were most hemophiliacs who received clotting factor concentrates during this period. Recipients of blood and components that cannot be sterilized or patients exposed to blood through other donated tissue or organs remain at some risk, albeit quite small. Although the overall residual risk now is extremely low, blood and tissue banks, scientists, and public health authorities must seek to reduce or eliminate that risk and must remain alert to changes in the epidemic that could again increase the risk. This chapter reviews data on the epidemic of transfusion-transmitted HIV infection in the United States, the current risk of infection through transfusion, and efforts to improve further the safety of the blood supply.

TRANSFUSION-ASSOCIATED AIDS

Hemophiliacs

The first acquired immunodeficiency syndrome (AIDS) cases associated with blood or blood products were reported in 1982 among hemophiliacs.[1] It is estimated that 75% to 85% of the cohort of hemophiliacs in the United States treated in the early 1980s with clotting factor concentrates were infected.[1–10] At that time, each lot of clotting factor concentrate was made from the pooled plasma of several thou-

Cladd E. Stevens, Laboratory of Epidemiology, The New York Blood Center, 310 East 67th Street, New York, NY 10021.

sand donors, and the products were not inactivated for viral infection. The incidence of HIV type 1 (HIV-1) infection among hemophiliacs in the United States and Western Europe is estimated to have peaked in 1982 at 22 per 100 person-years.[10] Patients who received cryoprecipitate, a product made from much smaller donor pools, were at substantially lower risk.[4–6] Since 1984, when clotting factor concentrates began to undergo heat or chemical inactivation, transmission to hemophiliacs through blood products has been negligible.[10–15]

By the end of 1994, 3863 AIDS cases among hemophiliacs had been reported to the U.S. Centers for Disease Control and Prevention (CDC), according to the 1994 AIDS Public Information Data Set (these numbers are somewhat low because of delayed reporting). Despite the current lack of risk of acquiring HIV, AIDS cases and deaths due to AIDS continue to be observed among hemophiliacs, a reflection of the long incubation period between infection and the onset of clinical disease. In the United States, the annual number of hemophiliac AIDS cases seemed to have stabilized in the late 1980s, although the number increased again after the 1993 revision of the AIDS surveillance case definition to include severe cellular immunodeficiency (Fig. 31-1). In a study of HIV-infected hemophiliacs in Great Britain, however, the mortality rate continued to rise after 1984, reaching a peak of 81 cases per 1000 patients in 1991 and 1992.[16] This continuing increase in mortality may reflect the effect of treatments for specific AIDS diseases and the consequent prolongation of life.

The number of new cases will diminish eventually, because hemophiliacs are no longer being infected through blood products. Given an average interval between the onset of infection and clinical AIDS of 9 to 10 years and a peak incidence of HIV

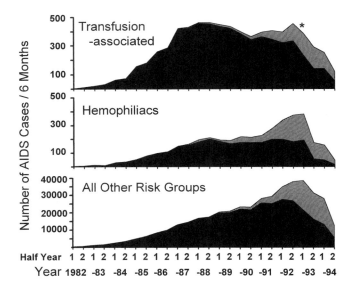

FIG. 31-1. Number of AIDS cases reported to the US Centers for Disease Control and Prevention (CDC). Number of cases reported (six month intervals): *solid black,* cases meeting the 1993 clinical AIDS diagnostic criteria; *hatched,* cases with number of CD4+ T-lymphocytes < 200 per mm³, but no specific clinical diagnosis; *, the CD4 criteria were added to the case definition. Number of cases reported for the first and second half of 1994 are expected not to be accurate because of delays in reporting.

infection in 1982, a decline in the number of AIDS cases is expected after 1992 or 1993, a pattern that should become clearer as the statistics are compared during the next few years.

Blood and Blood Component Recipients

The first case of AIDS associated with single-donor component transfusion was reported in 1982 in a child who had been given red blood cells and platelets as a newborn.[17] Follow-up of the donors to this child implicated one platelet donor, a homosexual man who developed AIDS and died 17 months after his blood donation. Additional infected persons who had no other known risks accrued throughout 1983, and as with the child, follow-up of the donors to these cases identified one or more donor in each case who was an AIDS-risk group member, providing firm evidence that AIDS was caused by a transfusion-transmissible agent.[18-22]

By the end of 1994, 7223 AIDS cases (ie, 6866 adults and 357 children younger than 13 years) had been reported in the United States among recipients who had no other risks for AIDS, constituting as many as 4% of cases reported annually to the CDC, according to the 1994 AIDS Public Information Data Set. The number of transfusion-associated AIDS cases is still lower than, but approaching, the number of patients projected in early studies to have been infected through blood transfusion between 1978 and early 1985 and surviving the immediate posttransfusion period, estimated at 12,000 to 15,000 cases among survivors 13 to 65 years of age.[23,24]

A study from the Irwin Memorial Blood Center in San Francisco, a high-risk area for AIDS, estimated that as many as 1.9% of surviving blood and component recipients were infected with blood from their center during this period (assuming an average of four units per recipient), with a peak risk of 1.1% per unit in 1982, before any efforts to eliminate donations from high-risk donors were in place.[25] The researchers projected more than 2000 cases from their center alone, an estimate that now seems rather high (Busch MP: personal communication). Retrospective testing of stored sera from a 1984 through 1985 survey (ie, after implementation of donor exclusion or surrogate testing but before antibody screening) of blood donors in four U.S. cities with the highest AIDS risk at the time, including San Francisco, detected HIV-specific antibody (anti-HIV) in only 0.16%.[26] Even these data probably exaggerate the risk at the time, because the survey focused on the highest-risk areas within their respective regions. These data, moreover, did not reflect the transfusion risk at that time in the United States as a whole.

As for hemophiliacs, the annual number of transfusion-associated cases peaked around 1988 and has declined steadily since (see Fig. 31-1). Some of the apparent decline in transfusion-associated AIDS cases is an artifact of "missing" cases among older HIV-infected transfusion recipients who may be more likely than younger recipients to die of their underlying diseases in the immediate posttransfusion period or to die later of other, non–AIDS-related causes before they develop a clinical AIDS disease (Fig. 31-2).[23-28]

When reported transfusion-associated AIDS cases are analyzed by their year of transfusion, the annual incidence of AIDS drops precipitously for cases transfused after donor anti-HIV screening was instituted March 1985 (Fig. 31-3).[27] After intensive investigation of the AIDS cases that were initially reported as "transfusion associated" in the era after antibody screening, Selik and colleagues identified other risk

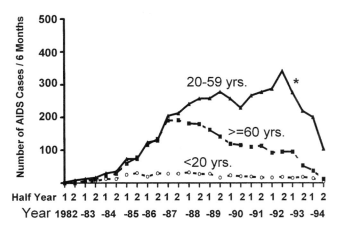

FIG. 31-2. Number of transfusion-associated AIDS cases reported to the CDC in six-month intervals among adults and children by age at diagnosis.*, the surveillance case definition changed to include low CD4 T-lymphocyte number.

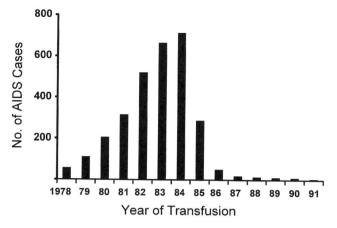

FIG. 31-3. Number of transfusion-associated AIDS cases reported to the CDC by year of transfusion. These data include only cases meeting the 1987 surveillance case definition reported through June 1992 (adapted from Selik RM, Ward JW, Buehler JW. Trends in transfusion-associated acquired immune deficiency syndrome in the United States, 1982 through 1991. Transfusion 33:890–893, 1993.)

factors in nearly 75% of cases, reducing the annual numbers of cases with no other risk to about 5 cases per year.[27] This number undoubtedly underestimates the total number of transfusion-acquired infections after antibody testing, because the full incubation period to the expression of disease had not been realized, and some individuals were expected to die of other causes before they developed clinical AIDS.

BLOOD DONOR SCREENING

After the association of AIDS with blood transfusions was recognized, a variety of measures were implemented to reduce the risk of HIV transmission through blood, nonsterile blood products, and donated tissues and organs. Before the virus itself was identified, blood centers attempted to reduce the risk that blood would be collected from a member of a recognized AIDS-risk group.[29–33] In addition to advising risk-group members not to donate, individuals who thought they might be at risk were asked to inform the center that their blood should not be used for transfusion. Some centers tested for possible surrogate markers of at-risk behavior, such as the antibody to the core protein of hepatitis B virus (anti-HBc), or they tested for the immunologic consequences of AIDS, such as low numbers of helper T lymphocytes (CD4-positive T cells), the primary target cells of HIV infection, although such testing was not implemented universally.

The effectiveness of any of these measures has been difficult to assess. The timeliness and adequacy of the efforts undertaken before the availability of specific tests for antibody to HIV has been criticized, as has the lack of an overall, coordinated, rigorous public health approach for dealing with the epidemic to protect the blood supply.[34] After HIV

was identified, specific antibody assays rapidly followed and have been improved in sensitivity since then.[35] In September 1995, the U.S. Food and Drug Administration (FDA) announced its recommendation to add HIV p24 antigen, a soluble core protein, screening to the test battery. HIV p24 antigen is thought to be detectable several days before antibody appears, shortening the period between HIV infection and its serologic detectability.[36,37] Licensure and implementation occurred in March 1996.

Anti-HIV Testing

In March 1985, the FDA licensed the first antibody tests to screen donors for infection with HIV-1.[35] Simultaneously, local public health services offered free, anonymous anti-HIV testing, in part to further protect the blood supply by making testing readily available outside of the blood bank setting and thereby minimizing the possibility that people at high risk would donate blood to be tested.[38] A second-generation assay with improved sensitivity was adopted in 1987, and a further improved third-generation assay covering HIV-1 and HIV-2 was implemented universally in June 1992.[36,37] Comparison of assays indicates that the window period between the onset of infection or infectivity and antibody seroconversion was reduced from an average of 55 days to about 42 days (90% <141 days) with second-generation assays and by another 20 days (95% confidence interval [CI] of 8 to 32 days) with third-generation assays.[37,39]

Current tests for screening blood donors detect antibodies to HIV-1 and HIV-2, even though very few HIV-2 infections have been reported in the United States. Although most HIV-2 infections have been found among immigrants from West Africa, the virus has been detected in three U.S. blood donors, one in 1986 and two later identified with the HIV-1/HIV-2 assays.[40–44] A variant of HIV-1 (ie, subtype O), first found in France among immigrants from West-Central Africa, has been reported predominantly in Cameroon, Gabon, and the Central African Republic.[45–51] Some of these variants are not detected by current screening tests, especially some of the more sensitive tests based on recombinant or synthetic peptides.[50] One identified variant showed no reactivity to any of the HIV-1 V3 loop peptides tested.[50] Assay systems licensed in the United States have not been modified yet to cover this variant. Such modifications, however, need to ensure retention of sensitivity for antibody to HIV-1 and HIV-2, which remain the greatest risk for blood donations in North America and Western Europe.

P24 Antigen Testing

HIV p24 antigen testing was added to the battery of routine donor screening tests in early 1996, after assays were licensed for donor screening by the FDA. Several attempts have been made to estimate the number of infections that could be prevented by screening donated blood for p24 antigen using models of the number of blood donors who might donate while in the window period before antibody becomes detectable and using estimates of the duration of p24 antigen positivity before antibody seroconversion. HIV p24 antigen testing is estimated to further reduce the window period by an average of 5 to 10 days.[37,39,52-57]

Based on the screening procedures in place in 1988, Mendelson estimated that p24 antigen testing would identify approximately one infected component in 4.9 million not otherwise detected or about four HIV-infected components per year.[54] Le Pont and colleagues estimated that three to five infected donations might have been positive for p24 antigen alone in 1992 in the United States.[58] This estimate, however, assumed only 10 million donations per year, no donations split into components, and the same prevalence of window-period donations in first-time as in repeat blood donors. Busch, on the other hand, estimates 0.7 antigen positives will be detected per 1 million anti-HIV–negative donations in the United States, based on an assumed incidence of new HIV infections among donors of 50 per 1 million donor-years.[56,57] From this estimate, about 8 to 10 donations or about 13 infected components (among the 19 million transfused each year) would be found positive only by p24 antigen testing. Although p24 antigen testing should identify additional HIV antibody–negative infections, some infectious donations will still be missed.[37,39,53,56-59] Estimates of the period of infectivity, for example, leave a residual window period of approximately 3 weeks, on average, of infectivity before HIV p24 antigen is positive.[37,39,53,56-59]

Despite the desirability of eliminating additional infected donations, the decision to test donors for p24 antigen has been controversial.[58,60-63] Some questioned whether it is worth the added expense (estimated at up to $80 million per year) for such a small increment of theoretical benefit. A more important question, however, is whether p24 antigen testing will make the blood supply safer. Any potential benefit could be completely eliminated, or the overall risk even increased, if some individuals who fear that they have been recently exposed to HIV choose to donate blood as a means of being tested for this early marker of infection. In one survey of gay and bisexual men in Portland, Oregon, and Tucson, Arizona, higher risk was a predictor of repeat testing.[64] Blood donation by such high-risk individuals could replace the few HIV p24 antigen-positive donations eliminated by screening with other undetected infectious donations, a possibility easily attainable because of the small number of donations expected to be positive for p24 antigen alone. Making p24 antigen testing available as part of all routine HIV testing would help reduce the incentive to donate blood just to be tested for the p24 antigen.

Surrogate Markers

When AIDS was first recognized as a blood-transmissible disease, nonspecific blood tests were proposed by some as possible surrogate markers to identify donors with a risk of HIV infection by detecting the immunologic consequences of infection, such as low CD4-positive T-lymphocyte numbers and elevated β_2-microglobulin levels, or a possible indicator of a high-risk lifestyle, such as anti-HBc, a marker of infection with hepatitis B virus (HBV), an agent that is also transmissible by sexual contact or blood. The potential value of surrogate marker testing was controversial, in part because volunteer donors had to be "healthy" at the time of donation and because those with certain venereal diseases or a history of hepatitis were automatically excluded. The applicability of data from AIDS cases or high-risk group members to volunteer blood donors was not clear, especially after strategies to exclude risk group members were adopted. Testing for surrogate markers was neither implemented uniformly nor officially recommended by public health authorities.

Although anti-HBc testing was not universally adopted as a surrogate marker for AIDS risk, it was added to donor screening in most of the United States in 1986 and 1987 (except for areas with a high background prevalence) as a surrogate for the risk of non-A, non-B hepatitis.[65,66] Even though the primary etiologic agent of non-A, non-B hepatitis, the hepatitis C virus (HCV), was identified in 1988 and specific serologic tests became available in 1990, anti-HBc has remained part of the donor screening battery, initially because of evidence that first-generation anti-HCV assays did not detect all HCV infections or that other transfusion-transmissible hepatitis agents might exist and because of evidence that some donors who were positive only for anti-HBc were infectious for HBV.[67]

In view of current donor-screening practices, the potential efficacy of anti-HBc as a surrogate marker for HIV risk in blood donors is limited to those who give blood during the infectious window period before antibody or antigen seroconversion. In one study of repeat blood donors who seroconverted between 1987 and 1990, anti-HBc was detected in only 18% of their previous negative donations and only 9% of those known to have seroconverted within a 6-month interval or less (ie, those most likely in the infectious window period), rates that are substantially less than those observed among early AIDS cases (≥80%) or during the first years of blood donor anti-HIV testing (30% to 50%).[57,68-70] The relatively poor association between anti-HBc and incident HIV infections in the donor population may reflect the effects of donor selection and changes in the epidemic that may diminish the epidemiologic parallels between HIV and HBV. Although donor anti-HBc screening now contributes negligibly or not at all to preventing HIV transmission, it undoubtedly prevents some residual HBV infections among transfusion recipients, providing enough rationale for its continued use, as recommended by a National Institutes of Health Consensus Conference.[67,71]

Confidential Unit Exclusion and Direct Donor Deferral

After the link between AIDS and blood transfusion became apparent, blood centers developed several formal strategies to exclude people at high risk from donating blood, including confidential unit exclusion (CUE) at the time of donation and "call-back" for at-risk donors.[29–33] These strategies allowed candidate donors to give blood, but instructed those who thought they were at risk of HIV infection to indicate at the time of donation that their blood should not be used for transfusion or to call the blood center later with this information. These strategies recognized the social pressures to donate blood under many circumstances. High-risk donors could continue to donate, but selection of CUE or call-back options would remove their blood from the transfusion pool. Subsequently, direct oral queries about the risks of HIV exposure was added to donor-screening procedures and was shown to increase donor deferral but not to have any apparent impact on the safety of the blood supply as measured by HIV antibody seroprevalence.[72]

Although CUE had some efficacy in the first few years of application, its apparent utility declined rapidly after antibody testing was implemented. For example, only 3% to 5% of donors at 40 U.S. blood centers who seroconverted between 1985 and December 1990 had self-excluded at the time of their last anti-HIV–negative donation (ie, the potential infectious window period donation).[73–75] All of the seroconverting donors who used the CUE option were at one of two blood centers, where CUE efficacy reached 12% to 13%. Moreover, when queried at follow-up, most of the anti-HIV–positive donors were found to have a known risk.[73] As a consequence of the lack of efficacy for CUE, in April 1992, the FDA made the use of CUE an option rather than a requirement for U.S. blood centers.

TRANSPLANT DONOR SCREENING

Organ and tissue transplants differ from blood transfusion in several important aspects that affect some of the procedures for screening donors and assessing their potential risk for HIV and other infectious disease transmission. Blood donation poses little risk or sacrifice on the part of the donor. Moreover, finding a suitable unit of blood under most circumstances depends only on ABO blood group and Rh compatibility, is relatively easy to accomplish, and does not depend on any one individual's donation. Transplants, however, may require matching for human leukocyte antigens (HLA), an especially critical consideration for bone marrow transplants, because HLA-mismatched transplants usually result in severe, often fatal graft-versus-host disease. An HLA-compatible organ or tissue donation may represent the only chance of survival for a transplant candidate, and the choice often must be made on a now-or-never basis.

Although organ and tissue donor-screening procedures follow the same general guidelines used for blood donors, important exceptions are made, depending on the circumstances. Cadaver donors, for example, cannot be queried about their risks, making serologic testing the central mechanism for preventing HIV transmission with these donations, along with accurate tracking of any tissues banked for future transplantation. In one instance, for example, several trans-

plant recipients of organs and tissues from a single anti-HIV–negative cadaver donor were later found to have developed AIDS.[76] Retrospective testing of stored residual tissue and blood specimens confirmed the antibody negativity but detected HIV-1 by culture and polymerase chain reaction (PCR) methods. The records of all harvested tissues had not been kept in this case, and all tissues could not be accounted for. If tissues are to be banked long term for future use, accurate record keeping, including linkage to tissues distributed elsewhere, is essential to ensure that banked materials from donors later found to be infectious can be traced and are not transplanted to additional patients in the future.

Bone marrow transplants are further complicated by the need to prepare patients well in advance, including a period for marrow ablation before the transplant. Donor screening is allowed to take place up to 30 days before the donation, and the patient is committed to the transplant regardless of interim changes in the donor's risk or serostatus. Placental or umbilical cord blood harvested after birth is a rich source of hematopoietic stem cells and is being used as an alternative to bone marrow for sibling and unrelated transplants.[77–79] This stem cell source has an advantage over bone marrow in that the donated tissue itself can be tested. Placental blood has a potential disadvantage, however, because the infectious disease risks are derived from the "donor's" mother for those agents capable of crossing the placenta in utero or of leaking into the fetal circulation during labor and delivery.[78] The mother of the infant donor and her risks need to be assessed when placental blood is the hematopoietic stem cell source.

CALCULATING AND REDUCING THE RISK OF HIV INFECTION BY TRANSFUSION

After the application of sensitive serologic tests, the risk of HIV infection through transfusion or transplantation became limited to circumstances in which the donor had been infected recently with HIV but had not yet developed any serologic marker; to infections with variants that are not detected by the current assays, such as some of the HIV-1 subtype 0 variants identified among North Africans living in Europe; and to human error.[45–51,80–86] A rare possibility can occur in the transplant setting if a patient makes a decision knowingly to receive tissue from an HIV-infected donor for an otherwise fatal disease when no other compatible donor source is available. At least one such case has occurred with a bone marrow donation from a sibling (Adamson J: personal communication).

The risk of HIV infection through the transfusion of blood and blood components can be estimated by a variety of approaches: monitoring reported AIDS cases, prospective evaluation of transfusion recipients for incident infections, detection of HIV in blood from antibody-negative donors, and projections based on the rate of new HIV infections among blood donors. The number of infections occurring annually must take into account the number of units of blood and components transfused each year, the number of units given per patient, and the expected survival of transfusion recipients.

In the United States, 12 to 14 million units of blood are collected and a small proportion imported from Europe each year from volunteer donors, 80% to 85% of which are eventually transfused.[87-92] The overall number of whole blood units collected has been declining gradually since the mid-1980s, but the proportion of patients donating blood for themselves (ie, autologous transfusion) has increased steadily, reaching 8% of total collections in 1992.[87-96]

Approximately 90% of donations are split into components to create packed red blood cells, platelet concentrates, cryoprecipitate, and fresh-frozen plasma. Random donor platelet concentrates are being replaced by single-donor platelet concentrates collected by apheresis, allowing greater use of platelets taken from smaller numbers of donors.[92] Some donations are split into three to four small-volume packs for transfusion of newborn infants. As a consequence of splitting whole blood into components, many donations go to more than one patient recipient. A total of approximately 19 million units of whole blood, packed red blood cells, pooled platelet or white blood cell concentrates, single-donor apheresis platelet units, cryoprecipitate, or fresh-frozen plasma units are transfused annually, with the recipient patients exposed to an average of three to four donors.[87-92] Although some types of patients are still treated with cryoprecipitate, most hemophiliacs are treated with clotting factor concentrates that are virus inactivated when made from pools of donated blood or are manufactured by recombinant technology from a nondonor source.[11,97,98] In addition to exposure to donated blood and components, several thousand patients are exposed to human blood each year through tissue and organ transplantation.

The number of reported AIDS cases attributable only to transfusion given after donor anti-HIV screening averaged about five per year of transfusion for 1986 through 1991.[27] However, this figure underestimates the transfusion risk, because 55% to 65% of infected patients die of other causes before developing AIDS, and given an average incubation period of 9 to 10 years, other cases will not have developed yet. This figure probably represented no more than one fifth to one fourth of the transfusion-transmitted HIV infections occurring each year during this period. If these assumptions are valid, these data suggest a total of 20 to 30 infections per year for 1986 to 1991, because only 45% survive long enough to develop AIDS, and only one third to one half of the potential cases would have developed by the time of the report. Assuming about 19 million transfusions were given, these data suggest a risk during the era of first- and second-generation testing of about 1 to 2 cases per 1 million units transfused.

In a prospective study of cardiovascular surgery patients carried out in Baltimore, Maryland, and Houston, Texas, from 1985 through 1991 (when testing was by first- and second-generation antibody assays), Nelson and his colleagues detected two new HIV infections among the recipients of 120,312 units of anti-HIV–negative blood or single-donor blood components.[81,84] Follow-up identified a donor who seroconverted in each case. The observed risk of transfusion-associated HIV infection from this study was 17 per 1 million units, with an upper bound (95% CI) of 53, comparable to an earlier estimate by Ward and coworkers of 26 per 1 million units.[80] If representative of the risk throughout the United States, these data suggest a total of about 300 to 400 transfusion-associated HIV infections each year in the United States (upper bound of 1007), a figure that is quite discordant with the estimate based on reported AIDS cases.

Accurately assessing the prevalence of HIV infection in anti-HIV–negative blood donors by testing donated blood with assays to detect the virus or HIV p24 antigen is an enormous task because of the expected low prevalence. In two studies involving almost 500,000 donations, no units positive only for p24 antigen were found.[61,62] A smaller study of blood donations in Western Europe also detected no p24 antigen–positive donors who were not also anti-HIV positive.[60] However, HIV p24 antigen testing is not expected to detect a substantial proportion of antibody-negative, infectious donations.[39] Using a strategy to reduce the number of tests, Busch and colleagues pooled specimens from more than 70,000 blood donations (50 donations per pool) given in San Francisco in 1987 to 1989 and sought evidence of HIV infection by culture, PCR, or both methods of assaying peripheral blood mononuclear cells.[99] One HIV infection was found. Given some loss of sensitivity due to pooling, these researchers estimated an HIV infection rate of 16 per 1 million donations (with an upper 95% CI of 94). Assuming that these data were representative of the United States, a total of about 300 infections per year would be expected for this period (upper bound of 1786).

Data on the incidence of HIV infection in donors and estimates of the duration of the infectious window period provide a somewhat more conservative estimate of the risk.[23,24,39,52,57] The Retrovirus Epidemiology Donor Study of repeat donors in 1991 and 1992 found an HIV incidence of 2.6 cases per 100,000 person-years.[57] Assuming an average infectious window period of 42 days before detection of antibody (with second-generation assays) and 19 million components transfused each year gives an estimate of about 60 transfusion-transmitted infections per year (26 per 1 million person-years × 42/365 × 19 million transfusions) or 3 per 1 million units, a rate closer to that projected from the transfusion-associated AIDS cases reported.[23,24,57] This estimate assumes, however, that the risk is the same for donations from first-time as for repeat donors, a potential source for underestimating the risk.[26]

The preceding estimates of the risk of HIV and AIDS from transfusions are quite discordant. Estimates derived from reported AIDS cases gave the lowest projected risk. Although the effect from reporting delays and the effect of the prolonged incubation period were taken into account, the assumptions used still may have underestimated the risk. It seems unlikely, however, that there is significant underreporting of transfusion-associated AIDS cases, considering the concerns about the safety of the blood supply. Estimates from studies of recipients and donors gave the highest estimates. However, these studies detected very few infections and therefore have rather unstable risk estimates with broad confidence limits. Moreover, some of the participating cities have had a high incidence of AIDS cases, and risk estimates from these sites may not be representative of the United States as a whole. Estimates based on incident infections in repeat donors were more compatible with those from reported AIDS cases and suggested a risk of about 3 cases per 1 million units for patients given blood screened by second-generation assays.

Third-generation antibody tests are projected to reduce the infectious window period by about 20 days and should reduce the risk of transfusion-associated HIV infection by about one half to 1.5 cases per 1 million units.[39,56,57] Whether p24 antigen testing will provide any additional benefit depends on whether the availability of testing through blood donation motivates high-risk men and women to give blood.

Reducing Patient Exposure to Blood

One way to reduce the individual patient's risk of acquiring HIV through blood transfusion is to reduce the number of units of blood transfused. This can be accomplished by improving surgical procedures to minimize blood loss or, when possible, using the patient's own blood through transfusion of predeposited units or by intraoperative blood salvage.

Autologous Blood Transfusion

Donating blood for oneself has long been an option for persons with rare blood types who can elect to cryopreserve their own red blood cells for future use. With the AIDS epidemic, donation in advance, also called predeposit, to avoid the risk of exposure to infection from other donors has become an option for individuals scheduled to undergo elective surgery.[87-96] Fresh whole blood can be stored for 35 to 42 days before reinfusion, depending on the anticoagulant and preservatives used, and during this time, patients can donate as many as 3 to 5 units of packed red blood cells. Toy and her colleagues estimate that up to 72% of transfusions required for elective surgery could be covered by autologous blood.[93] Although autologous donation is still vastly underused, data suggest that rates are improving as physicians and patients become more informed about the procedure.[88-92,95]

The newborn infant presents a special opportunity for possible autologous transfusion that deserves exploration. Intensive monitoring and blood testing of premature infants often produces an iatrogenic anemia in the first few weeks of life, requiring repeated blood transfusion, usually in small volumes (10 to 25 mL each) and often from multiple donors. The blood remaining in the placenta and umbilical cord blood after delivery of the infant can be easily harvested from the umbilical vein during the third stage of labor.[78] An estimated one third of the blood volume in the fetal circulation is con-

tained in the cord and placenta, and the volume of blood that can be collected therefore varies directly with the size of the infant and its gestational age. Nevertheless, 40 to 80 mL of blood should be salvageable for most premature infants, which is in the range of their transfusion requirements.

Blood Salvage and Improved Surgical Procedures

Procedures have been developed to collect blood lost into the operative site during surgery and return this blood to the patient, a procedure that has proven most effective in certain thoracic, abdominal, and orthopedic surgeries, which account for most intraoperative transfusions.[100] Intraoperative blood salvage, however, reduces the number of units transfused by only a modest amount, estimated on average at about one unit. Improved surgical techniques, with better control of blood loss, continue to reduce transfusion requirements and probably have had a greater overall impact.[89,91,92]

Viral Inactivation of Plasma Products

Clotting factors are required to treat certain inherited deficiencies such as hemophilia A, factor IX deficiency, and von Willebrand disease. In the 1960s and into the 1970s, most patients were treated with cryoprecipitate after sustaining significant trauma or in preparation for elective surgical procedures.[101] This crises approach to treatment was dictated by the only treatment then available, cryoprecipitate, and did not prevent all of the lifestyle restrictions or debilitating orthopedic and neurologic sequelae these patients suffered. The clotting factor concentrates introduced during the 1970s had a relatively long shelf life and could be stored and administered at home, greatly improving the life of hemophiliacs through rapid, early treatment of bleeding episodes and prophylaxis.[101] The concentrates, however, were made from pools of several thousand blood donations, virtually ensuring inclusion of hepatitis viruses and, later, HIV in many lots of the final product.

Beginning in the early 1980s, initially in response to the recognized risk of viral hepatitis, clotting factor manufacturers explored methods to inactivate factor concentrates.[11,101] Factor VIII and factor IX complex are labile, however, necessitating rather gentle treatment. Inactivation methods included dry or wet heat at various temperatures and durations; solvent-detergent (SD) treatment, designed to dissolve the lipoprotein coat of enveloped viruses, with or without ultraviolet light; and immune-affinity purification.[11,101-104] Spiking experiments documented clearance of several logs of HIV, as well as HBV and HCV. Surveillance by the CDC, however, detected a residual risk of HIV infection in recipients of concentrates made by short-duration, low-temperature, dry-heat inactivation.[11] Evidence of transmission of non-A, non-B hepatitis resulted in withdrawal of all dry-heat–inactivated products. Although SD treatment is not expected to inactivate nonenveloped virus, there has been some indication of possible failures of this procedure for enveloped viruses as well. Outbreaks of hepatitis A have occurred in hemophiliacs receiving SD-treated concentrates from at least one European manufacturer.[105,106] These events may reflect breakdowns in production procedures, and some manufacturers now apply SD and heat inactivation. Several clotting factors produced by recombinant technology are available and have proven efficacious and safe.[98,107,108]

As a consequence of donor screening, viral inactivation, and the use of recombinant clotting factors, most clotting factor recipients have not been at risk of HIV infection since 1984 or 1985. The cohort of hemophiliacs born in the last decade has been spared. An exception may be a few patients with severe von Willebrand disease or other bleeding disorders who may still require treatment with cryoprecipitate. Many of these patients have been treated successfully with a vasopressin analog that releases factor VIII and von Willebrand factor from the tissues or with virus-inactivated concentrates or recombinant von Willebrand factor, depending on the specific disease variant.[101,109,110]

CONCLUSIONS AND TRENDS

The dramatic reduction in the risk of HIV infection from transfused blood and blood components or plasma products has been one of the major successes in the AIDS epidemic, with current estimates of the risk in the range of 1 HIV infection per 300,000 to 700,000 units transfused and no risk for most hemophiliacs. The challenge for the future will be to reduce the risk from blood and component transfusions further or eliminate it altogether. The community must remain alert to the possibility of variants that elude detection by current assays and modify the tests as needed.

In addition to ongoing efforts to reduce exposure to blood, one potential strategy to reduce the risk of transfusion-transmitted HIV infection is development of new tests to detect HIV during the residual infectious window period. Assays to detect the virus, such as PCR, have not yet been standardized nor formatted to make them practical for the large-scale testing required for screening fresh blood and components, although progress is being made in this direction. Another strategy would be inactivation of virus in fresh-frozen plasma and cellular components. Fresh-frozen plasma is indicated for a limited number of bleeding disorders for which no specific component is yet available. Most fresh plasma is used, however, during surgical procedures, especially as a means of replacing presumed "lost clotting factors" or for volume expansion after massive blood loss. A large number of patients are exposed to fresh-frozen plasma as a consequence, many for dubious indications.[111]

A virus-inactivated plasma is being developed.[112] For practical reasons, however, inactivation requires some pooling, thereby increasing the potential risk of viral infection in the pooled starting material or increasing the risk of infection with nonenveloped viruses in the final product unless other inactivation steps are included. Nevertheless, the relative benefit of eliminating all risk of HIV infection probably outweighs any risk of infection from other agents.

A greater challenge has been the effort to inactivate cellular blood components for viral agents (some of which may be cell associated) without simultaneously damaging the cells. Several reports have shown encouraging results with photoreactive dyes that inactivate cell-free virus while apparently leaving red blood cells intact.[113–117] However, these approaches are not expected to inactivate intracellular virus, a challenge that persists.[118]

REFERENCES

1. Anonymous. Pneumocystis carinii pneumonia among persons with hemophilia A. MMWR 1982;31:365.
2. Johnson RE, Lawrence DL, Evatt BL, et al. Acquired immunodeficiency syndrome among patients attending hemophilia treatment centers and mortality experience of hemophiliacs in the United States. Am J Epidemiol 1985;121:797.
3. Evatt BL, Gomperts ED, McDougal JS, Ramsey RB. Coincidental appearance of LAV/HTLV-III antibodies in hemophiliacs and the onset of the AIDS epidemic. N Engl J Med 1985;312:483.
4. Ragni MV, Tegtmeier GE, Levy JA, et al. AIDS retrovirus antibodies in hemophiliacs treated with factor VIII or factor IX concentrates, cryoprecipitate, or fresh frozen plasma: prevalence, seroconversion rate, and clinical correlations. Blood 1986;67:592.
5. Eyster ME, Gail MH, Ballard JO, Al-Mondhiry H, Goedert JJ. Natural history of human immunodeficiency virus infections in hemophiliacs: effects of T-cell subsets, platelet counts, and age. Ann Intern Med 1987;107:1.
6. Ragni MV, Winkelstein A, Kingsley L, Spero JA, Lewis JH. 1986 Update of HIV seroprevalence, seroconversion, AIDS incidence, and immunologic correlates of HIV infection in patients with hemophilia A and B. Blood 1987;70:786.
7. Curran JW, Jaffe HW, Hardy AM, Morgan WM, Selik RM, Dondero TJ. Epidemiology of HIV infection and AIDS in the United States. Science 1988;239:610.
8. Jason J, Lui K-J, Ragni MV, Hessol NA, Darrow WW. Risk of developing AIDS in HIV-infected cohorts of hemophilic and homosexual men. JAMA 1989;261:725.
9. Goedert JJ, Kessler CM, Aledort LM, et al. A prospective study of human immunodeficiency virus type 1 infection and the development of AIDS in subjects with hemophilia. N Engl J Med 1989;321:1141.
10. Kroner BL, Rosenberg PS, Aledort LM, Alvord WG, Goedert JJ. for the Multicenter Hemophilia Cohort Study. HIV-1 infection incidence among persons with hemophilia in the United States and Western Europe, 1978. J Acquir Immune Defic Syndr 1994;7:279.
11. Epstein JS, Fricke WA. Current safety of clotting factor concentrates. Arch Pathol Lab Med 1990;114:335.
12. Dietrich SL, Mosley JW, Lusher JM, et al, and The Transfusion Safety Study Group. Transmission of human immunodeficiency virus type 1 by dry-heated clotting factor concentrates. Vox Sang 1990;59:129.
13. Gjerset GF, Mosley JW. Safety of factor VIII. Ann Intern Med 1991;114:171.
14. Mannucci PM, Schimpf K, Abe T, et al, and the International Investigator Group. Low risk of viral infection after administration of vapor-heated factor VIII concentrate. Transfusion 1992;32:134.
15. Shapiro A, Abe T, Aledort LM, et al, and the International Factor Safety Study Group. Low risk of viral infection after administration of vapor-heated factor VII concentrate or factor IX complex in first-time recipients of blood components. Transfusion 1995;35:203.
16. Darby SC, Ewart DW, Giangrande PLF, et al on behalf of the UK Haemophilia Centre Directors' Organisation. Mortality before and after HIV infection in the complete UK population of haemophiliacs. Nature 1995;377:79.
17. Ammann AJ, Cowan MJ, Wara DW, Weintrub P, Dritz S, Goldman H, Perkins HA. Acquired immunodeficiency in an infant: possible transmission by means of blood products. Lancet 1983;1:956.
18. Curran JW, Lawrence DN, Jaffe H, et al. Acquired immunodeficiency syndrome (AIDS) associated with transfusions. N Engl J Med 1984;310:69.
19. Curran JW, Morgan WM, Hardy AM, Jaffe HW, Darrow WW, Dowdle WR. The epidemiology of AIDS: current status and future prospects. Science 1985;229:1352.

20. Jaffe HW, Sarngadharan MG, DeVico AL, et al. Infection with HTLV-III/LAV and transfusion-associated acquired immunodeficiency syndrome. Serologic evidence of an association. JAMA 1985;254:770.
21. Peterman TA, Jaffe HW, Feorino PM, et al. Transfusion-associated acquired immunodeficiency syndrome in the United States. JAMA 1985;254:2913.
22. Leparc GF. Case 46-1984: AIDS associated with transfusion of blood products. N Engl J Med 1985;312:648.
23. Peterman TA, Liu K-J, Lawrence DN, Allen JR. Estimating the risks of transfusion-associated acquired immune deficiency syndrome and human immunodeficiency virus infection. Transfusion 1987;27:371.
24. Kalbfleisch JD, Lawless JF. Estimating the incubation time distribution and expected number of cases of transfusion-associated acquired immune deficiency syndrome. Transfusion 1989;29:672.
25. Busch MP, Young MJ, Samson SM, et al, and Transfusion Safety Study Group. Risk of human immunodeficiency virus (HIV) transmission by blood transfusions before the implementation of HIV-1 antibody screening. Transfusion 1991;31:4.
26. Kleinman SH, Niland JC, Azen SP, et al, and the Transfusion Safety Study Group. Prevalence of antibodies to human immunodeficiency virus type 1 among blood donors prior to screening. Transfusion 1989;29:572.
27. Selik RM, Ward JW, Buehler JW. Trends in transfusion-associated acquired immune deficiency syndrome in the United States, 1982 through 1991. Transfusion 1993;33:890.
28. Donegan E, Perkins H, Vyas G, and The Transfusion Safety Study Group. Mortality in the recipients of blood in the Transfusion Safety Study. Blood 1986;68:296a.
29. Anonymous. Joint statement on acquired immune deficiency syndrome (AIDS) related to transfusion. Transfusion 1983;23:87.
30. Recommendations to decrease the risk of transmitting acquired immune deficiency syndrome (AIDS) from blood donors. Memorandum to blood establishments. Bethesda, MD: Food and Drug Administration, Public Health Service, US Department of Health and Human Services, March 1983.
31. Revised recommendations to decrease the risk of transmitting acquired immune deficiency syndrome (AIDS) from blood donors. Memorandum to blood establishments. Bethesda, MD: Food and Drug Administration, Public Health Service, US Department of Health and Human Services, December 1984.
32. Pindyck J, Waldman A, Zang E, Oleszko W, Lowy M, Bianco, C. Measures to decrease the risk of acquired immunodeficiency syndrome transmission by blood transfusion. Transfusion 1985;25:3.
33. Revised recommendations to decrease the risk of transmitting acquired immune deficiency syndrome (AIDS) from blood donors. Memorandum to blood establishments. Bethesda, MD: Food and Drug Administration, Public Health Service, US Department of Health and Human Services, 1990.
34. Leveton LB, Sox HC Jr, Stoto MA, eds, for the Institute of Medicine. HIV and the blood supply. An analysis of crisis decision making. Washington, DC: National Academy Press, 1995.
35. Petricciani JC. Licensed tests for antibody to human T-lymphotropic virus type III: sensitivity and specificity. Ann Intern Med 1985;103:726.
36. Zaaijer HL, Exel-Oehlers PV, Kraaijeveld T, Altena E, Lelie PN. Early detection of antibodies to HIV-1 by third generation assays. Lancet 1992;340:770.
37. Busch MP, Lee LLL, Satten GA, et al. Time course of detection of viral and serologic markers preceding human immunodeficiency virus type 1 seroconversion: implications for screening of blood and tissue donors. Transfusion 1995;35:91.
38. Snyder AJ, Vergeront JM. Safeguarding the blood supply by providing opportunities for anonymous HIV testing. N Engl J Med 1988;319:374.
39. Busch MP. HIV and blood transfusion: focus on seroconversion. Vox Sang 1994;67(Suppl 3):13.
40. O'Brien TR, Polon C, Schable CA, et al. HIV-2 in an American. AIDS 1991;5:85.
41. Anonymous. Update: HIV-2 infection among blood and plasma donors—United States, June 1992–June 1995. MMWR 1995;44:603.
42. Couroucé A. HIV-2 in blood donors and in different risk groups in France. Lancet 1987;1:1151.
43. George JR, Rayfield MA, Phillips S, et al. Efficacies of U.S. Food and Drug Administration-licensed HIV-1 screening enzyme immunoassays for detecting antibodies to HIV. AIDS 1990;4:321.
44. O'Brien TR, George JR, Holmberg SD. Human immunodeficiency virus type 2 infection in the United States. Epidemiology, diagnosis and public health importance. JAMA 1992;267:2775.
45. De Leys R, Vanderborght B, Haesevelde MV, et al. Isolation and partial characterization of an unusual human immunodeficiency retrovirus from two persons of West-Central African origin. J Virol 1990;64:1207.
46. Gürtler LG, Hauser PH, Eberle J, et al. A new subtype of human immunodeficiency virus type 1 (MVP-5180) from Cameroon. J Virol 1994;68:1581.
47. Haesevelde MV, Decourt J-L, De Leys RJ, et al. Genomic cloning and complete sequence analysis of a highly divergent African human immunodeficiency virus isolate. J Virol 1994;68:1586.
48. Loussert-Ajaka I, Ly TD, Chaix ML, et al HIV-1/HIV-2 seronegativity in HIV-1 subtype O infected patients. Lancet 1994;343:1393.
49. Dondero TJ, Hu DJ, George JR. HIV-1 variants: yet another challenge to public health. Lancet 1994;343:1376.
50. Schable C, Zekeng L, Pau C-P, et al. Sensitivity of United States HIV antibody tests for detection of HIV-1 group O infections. Lancet 1994;344:1333.
51. Simon F, Ly TD, Bailou-Beaufils A, et al. Sensitivity of screening kits for anti-HIV-1 subtype O antibodies. AIDS 1994;8:1628.
52. Petersen LR, Satten GA, Dodd R, et al, and The HIV Seroconversion Study Group. Duration of time from onset of human immunodeficiency virus type 1 infectiousness to development of detectable antibody. Transfusion 1994;34:283.
53. Stramer SL, Heller JS, Coombs RW, Parry JV, Ho DD, Allain J-P. Markers of HIV prior to IgG antibody seropositivity. JAMA 1989;262:64.
54. Mendelson DN, Sandler SG. A model for estimating incremental benefits and costs of testing donated blood for human immunodeficiency virus antigen (HIV-Ag). Transfusion 1990;30:73.
55. Gallarda JL, Henrard DR, Liu D, et al. Early detection of antibody to human immunodeficiency virus type 1 by using an antigen conjugate immunoassay correlates with the presence of IgM antibody. J Clin Microbiol 1992;30:2379.
56. Busch MP, Mosley JW, Alter HJ, Epstein JS. Case of HIV-1 transmission by antigen-positive, antibody-negative blood. N Engl J Med 1991;325:1174.
57. Schreiber GB, Busch MP, Gilcher RO, et al, for the NHLBI Retrovirus Epidemiology Donor Study (REDS). Incidence rates of infectious disease makers in repeat blood donors. Transfusion 1994;34(Suppl):74S.
58. Le Pont F, Costagliola D, Rouzioux C, Valleron AJ. How much would the safety of blood transfusion be improved by including p24 antigen in the battery of tests? Transfusion 1995;35:542.
59. de Saussure P, Yerly S, Tullen E, Perrin LH. Human immunodeficiency virus type 1 nucleic acids detected before p24 antigenemia in a blood donor. Transfusion 1993;33:164.
60. Bäcker U, Weinauer W, Gathof G, Eberle J. HIV antigen screening in blood donors. Lancet 1987;2:1213.
61. Alter HJ, Epstein JS, Swenson SG, et al, and the HIV-Antigen Study Group. Prevalence of human immunodeficiency virus type 1 p24 antigen in U.S. blood donors—an assessment of the efficacy of testing in donor screening. N Engl J Med 1990;323:1312.
62. Busch MP, Taylor PE, Lenes BA, et al, and the Transfusion Safety Study Group. Screening of selected male blood donors for p24 antigen of human immunodeficiency virus type 1. N Engl J Med 1990;323:1308.
63. Busch MP, Alter HJ. Will human immunodeficiency virus p24 antigen screening increase the safety of the blood supply and, if so, at what cost? Transfusion 1995;35:536.
64. Phillips KA, Paul J, Kegeles S, Stall R, Hoff C, Coates TJ. Predictors of repeat HIV testing among gay and bisexual men. AIDS 1995;9:769.
65. Stevens CE, Aach RD, Hollinger FB, et al. Hepatitis B virus antibody in blood donors and the occurrence of non-A, non-B hepatitis in transfusion recipients. Ann Intern Med 1984;101:733.
66. Koziol DE, Holland PV, Alling DW, et al. Antibody to hepatitis B core antigen as a paradoxical maker for non-A, non-B hepatitis agents in donated blood. Ann Intern Med 1986;104:488.
67. Mosley JW, Stevens CE, Aach RD, et al. Donor screening for antibody to hepatitis B core antigen and hepatitis B virus infection in transfusion recipients. Transfusion 1995;35:5.
68. Korelitz JJ, Busch MP, Kleinman SH, et al, and the NHLBI Retrovirus Epidemiology Donor Study (REDS). Ability of anti-HBc to detect retrovirus seropositive blood donors. Transfusion 1994;34:37S.

69. Busch MP, Dodd RY, Petersen LR, and the CDC HIV-1 Seroconverting Donor Study. Value of anti-HBc as a surrogate marker for window phase HIV-1 infection. Transfusion 1994;34(Suppl):64S.
70. Petersen LR, Doll LS, and the HIV Blood Donor Study Group. Human immunodeficiency virus type 1-infected blood donors: epidemiologic, laboratory, and donation characteristics. Transfusion 1991;31:698.
71. Consensus Conference. Surrogate marker screening of blood donors. Bethesda, MD: National Institutes of Health, January 1995.
72. Johnson ES, Doll LS, Satten GA, et al. Direct oral questions to blood donors: the impact on screening for human immunodeficiency virus. Transfusion 1994;34:769.
73. Doll LS, Petersen LR, White CR, Ward JW, and the HIV Blood Donor Study Group. Human immunodeficiency virus type 1-infected blood donors: behavioral characteristics and reasons for donation. Transfusion 1991;31:704.
74. Petersen LR, Lackritz E, Lewis WF, et al The effectiveness of the confidential unit exclusion option. Transfusion 1994;34:865.
75. Korelitz JJ, Williams AE, Busch MP, et al. Demographic characteristics and prevalence of serologic markers among donors who use the confidential unit exclusion process: the Retrovirus Epidemiology Donor Study. Transfusion 1994;34:870.
76. Simonds RJ, Holmberg SD, Hurwitz RL, et al. Transmission of human immunodeficiency virus type 1 from a seronegative organ and tissue donor. N Engl J Med 1992;326:726.
77. Gluckman E, Broxmeyer HE, Auerbach AD, et al. Hematopoietic reconstitution in a patient with Fanconi anemia by means of umbilical-cord blood from an HLA-identical sibling. N Engl J Med 1989;321:1174.
78. Rubinstein P, Rosenfield RE, Adamson JW, Stevens CE. Stored placental blood for unrelated bone marrow transplantation. Blood 1993;81:1679.
79. Kurtzberg J, Graham M, Casey J, Olson J, Stevens C, Rubinstein P. The use of umbilical cord blood in mismatched related and unrelated hemopoietic stem cell transplantation. Blood Cells 1994;20:275.
80. Ward JW, Holmberg SD, Allen JR, et al. Transmission of human immunodeficiency virus (HIV) by blood transfusions screened as negative for HIV antibody. N Engl J Med 1988;318:473.
81. Cohen ND, Muñoz A, Reits BA, et al. Transmission of retroviruses by transfusion of screened blood in patients undergoing cardiac surgery. N Engl J Med 1989;320:1172.
82. Cumming PD, Wallace EL, Schorr JB, Dodd RY. Exposure of patients to human immunodeficiency virus through the transfusion of blood components that test antibody-negative. N Engl J Med 1989;321:941.
83. Donahue JG, Nelson KE, Muñoz A, et al. Transmission of HIV by transfusion of screened blood. N Engl J Med 1990;323:1709.
84. Nelson KE, Donahue JG, Muñoz A, et al. Transmission of retroviruses from seronegative donors by transfusion during cardiac surgery. A multicenter study of HIV-1 and HTLV-I/II infections Ann Intern Med 1992;117:554.
85. Linden JV, Paul B, Dressler KP. A report of 104 transfusion errors in New York State. Transfusion 1992;32:601.
86. Linden JV, Kaplan HS. Transfusion Errors: causes and effects. Transfus Med Rev 1994;8:169.
87. Surgenor DM, Wallace EL, Hao SHS, Chapman RH. Collection and transfusion of blood in the United States, 1982. N Engl J Med 1990;322:1646.
88. Wallace EL, Surgenor DM, Hao SHS, An J, Chapman RH, Churchill WH. Collection and transfusion of blood and blood components in the United States. Transfusion 1993;33:139.
89. McCullough J. The nation's changing blood supply system. JAMA 1993;269:2239.
90. Forbes JM, Laurie ML. Blood collections by community blood centers, 1988 through 1992. Transfusion 1994;34:392.
91. Heaton WAL. Changing patterns of blood use. Transfusion 1994;34:365.
92. Wallace EL, Churchill WH, Surgenor DM, et al. Collection and transfusion of blood and blood components in the United States. Transfusion 1995;35:802.
93. Toy PTCY, Strauss RG, Stehling LC, et al. Predeposited autologous blood for elective surgery. N Engl J Med 1987;316:517.
94. Surgenor DM. The patient's blood is the safest blood. N Engl J Med 1987;316:542.
95. Toy PTCY, McVay PA, Strauss RG, Stehling LC, Ahn DK. Improvement in appropriate autologous donations with local education: 1987 to 1989. Transfusion 1992;32:562.
96. Toy PTCY, Kaplan EB, McVay PA, et al, and The Preoperative Autologous Blood Donation Study Group. Blood loss and replacement in total hip arthroplasty: a multicenter study. Transfusion 1992;32:63.
97. Anonymous. Safety of therapeutic products used for hemophilia patients. MMWR 1988;37:441.
98. Schwartz RS, Abildgaard CF, Aledort LM, et al, and The Recombinant Factor VIII Study Group. Human recombinant DNA-derived antihemophilic factor (Factor VIII) in the treatment of hemophilia A. N Engl J Med 1990;323:1800.
99. Busch MP, Eble BE, Khayam-Bashi H, et al. Evaluation of screened blood donations for human immunodeficiency virus type 1 infection by culture and DNA amplification of pooled cells. N Engl J Med 1991;325:1.
100. Consensus Conference. Perioperative red blood cell transfusion. JAMA 1988;260:2700.
101. Kasper CK, Lusher JM, and the Transfusion Practices Committee. Recent evolution of clotting factor concentrates for hemophilia A and B. Transfusion 1993;33:422.
102. Horowitz B, Wiebe ME, Lippin A, Stryker MH. Inactivation of viruses in labile blood derivatives. Transfusion 1985;25:516.
103. Gomperts ED. Procedures for the inactivation of viruses in clotting factor concentrates. Am J Hematol 1986;23:295.
104. Prince AM, Horowitz B, Brotman B. Sterilisation of hepatitis and HTLV-III viruses by exposure to tri(n-butyl) phosphate and sodium cholate. Lancet 1986;1:706.
105. Mannucci PM. Outbreak of hepatitis A among Italian patients with hemophilia. Lancet 1992;339:819.
106. Gerritzen A, Schneweis KE, Brackmann HH, et al. Acute hepatitis A in haemophiliacs. Lancet 1992;340:1231.
107. Lusher JM, Arkin S, Abildgaard CF, Schwartz RS, and the Kogenate Previously Untreated Patient Study Group. Recombinant factor VIII for the treatment of previously untreated patients with hemophilia A. Safety, efficacy and development of inhibitors. N Engl J Med 1993;328:453.
108. Bray GL, Gomperts ED, Courter S, et al, and the Recombinant Study Group. A multicenter study of recombinant factor VIII (Recombinate): safety, efficacy, and inhibitor risk in previously untreated patients with hemophilia A. Blood 1994;83:2428.
109. Mannucci PM. Desmopressin (DDAVP) for treatment of disorders of hemostasis. Prog Hemostas Thrombos 1986;8:19.
110. Lusher JM. Response to 1-deamino-8-D-arginine vasopressin in von Willebrand disease. Haemostasis 1994;24:276.
111. Consensus Conference. Fresh frozen plasma. JAMA 1985;253:551.
112. Horowitz B, Bonomo R, Prince AM, Chin SN, Brotman B, Shulman RW. Solvent/detergent-treated plasma: a virus-inactivated substitute for fresh plasma. Blood 1992;79:826.
113. Horowitz B, Williams B, Rywkin S, et al. Inactivation of viruses in blood with aluminum phthalocyanine derivatives. Transfusion 1991;31:102.
114. Lavie G, Mazur Y, Lavie D, et al. Hypericin as an inactivator of infectious viruses in blood components. Transfusion 1995;35:392.
115. Ben-Hur E, Rywkin S, Rosenthal I, Geacintov NE, Horowitz B. Virus inactivation in red cell concentrates by photosensitization with phthalocyanines: protection of red cells but not of vesicular stomatitis virus with a water-soluble analogue of vitamin E. Transfusion 1995;35:401.
116. Wagner SJ, Cifone MA, Murli H, Dodd RY, Myhr B. Mammalian genotoxicity assessment of methylene blue in plasma: implications for virus inactivation. Transfusion 1995;35:407.
117. Rywkin S, Ben-Hur E, Reid ME, Oyen R, Ralph H, Horowitz B. Selective protection against IgG binding to red cells treated with phthalocyanines and red light for virus inactivation. Transfusion 1995;35:414.
118. Vyas GN. Inactivation and removal of blood-borne viruses. Transfusion 1995;35:367.

AIDS: Biology, Diagnosis, Treatment and Prevention, fourth edition, edited by Vincent T. DeVita, Jr., Samuel Hellman, and Steven A. Rosenberg. Lippincott–Raven Publishers, © 1997

CHAPTER 32 AIDS Vaccines

32.1 Acquired Immunodeficiency Disease Vaccines: Design and Development

Tun-Hou Lee

Human immunodeficiency virus (HIV) is projected to infect 40 million persons by the turn of this century.[1,2] Historically, the most effective public health intervention for infectious diseases has been vaccination of the at-risk population.[3] Although developing a cost-effective vaccine for HIV remains a formidable task, it is hoped that the availability of such a vaccine will slow the spread of HIV and diminish the cases of acquired immunodeficiency syndrome (AIDS). This chapter highlights the previous decade's efforts of HIV vaccine development and discusses the challenges to future HIV vaccine design and development. Because most vaccine development efforts are focused on HIV type 1, the term HIV is used for brevity.

THE FIRST DECADE OF HIV VACCINE DEVELOPMENT

T-Cell-Line–Adapted HIV

The discovery that HIV could be propagated in continuous T-cell lines[4-7] has had a significant impact on HIV prevention. The ability to grow large quantities of HIV led to the development of serologic assays for HIV, which helped to limit its spread through contaminated blood and blood products. This discovery also facilitated the subsequent molecular cloning and characterization of HIV. However, as was learned much later, the convenience of growing HIV in continuous T-cell lines resulted in a disproportionate focus on T-cell-line--adapted HIV.

Among the most often cited and better characterized T-cell-line–adapted strains of HIV are HIVLAI (previously designated IIIB or LAV) and HIVSF2 (previously desig-

nated ARV). Molecular clones of HIVLAI and HIVSF2 were generated by several laboratories, and complete nucleotide sequences of these strains were determined.[8-11] Many open reading frames with the potential to encode HIV proteins were identified before the discovery of the actual proteins. Undoubtedly, the pace of technologic advancement was faster than the pace at which AIDS pathogenesis was deciphered during this period. The skewed focus on T-cell-line–adapted HIV in the first decade of vaccine development can be attributed to the convenience of culturing HIV in T cells and the availability of molecular clones and DNA sequence information. As discussed later, most candidate vaccine antigens in clinical trials are subunit derivatives of T-cell-line–adapted HIV.[12-14]

Hypervariable Region V3

The HIV envelope gene encodes a precursor protein (gp160),[15] which is further processed into two mature subunits, surface glycoprotein gp120[15] and transmembrane glycoprotein gp41.[5,7] The identification of these envelope proteins and the determination of their N-terminal amino acid sequences for the HIVLAI strain allowed the precise deduction of envelope protein sequences for other strains of T-cell-line–adapted HIV.[15,16]

Alignment of envelope protein sequences of a few strains of T-cell-line–adapted HIV soon revealed that gp120 contains five hypervariable regions, designated V1 to V5.[17,18] These hypervariable regions are interspersed between five constant regions, C1 to C5, which contain amino acid residues shared by different strains of T-cell-line–adapted HIV. A large number of envelope DNA sequences have been compiled and are updated every year by the Los Alamos National Laboratory.[19] The original observation of hypervariable and constant regions of gp120 remains valid for all HIV strains analyzed.

Tun-Hou Lee, Department of Cancer Biology, Harvard School of Public Health, 665 Huntington Avenue, Boston, MA 02115.

The V3 region of gp120 has been referred to as the principal neutralizing domain (PND) and has been a major focus of the first decade of HIV vaccine development. Recombinant proteins corresponding to different regions of the HIVLAI envelope were expressed in bacteria, and antibodies were raised against them.[20] One hyperimmune serum raised against these recombinant proteins was shown to block infection of target T cells by HIVLAI. Subsequent analyses using synthetic peptides corresponding to the V3 region demonstrated that the neutralizing activity in the hyperimmune serum could be mapped to V3. These original observations were later confirmed by experiments using antisera raised against V3 peptides of T-cell-line–adapted HIV.[21] Similarly, many V3-specific monoclonal antibodies were shown to neutralize T-cell-line–adapted HIV in vitro. In one experiment, seroconversion was prevented in a chimpanzee inoculated with HIVLAI after it had been preincubated with a V3-specific monoclonal antibody.[22]

A common theme that emerged from these and many other related studies is that the V3 region of T-cell-line–adapted HIV is a target of neutralizing antibodies. The V3 epitopes involved comprise mainly continuous amino acid residues. Under most circumstances, neutralizing monoclonal antibodies targeting a given V3 sequence do not cross-neutralize HIV strains lacking the same V3 sequence.

The recognition that V3 could be an important target for candidate vaccines led to large-scale genotyping of HIV strains circulating in North America. The intent was to determine the degree of V3 divergence.[23] It was found that most of the HIV surveyed had not been adapted to continuous T-cell lines and that their V3 sequences were representative of HIV strains now commonly referred to as primary isolates.

The total number of amino acid residues in V3 is relatively constant because insertions or deletions in this region are rare, a feature not shared by other hypervariable regions. The tendency for certain amino acid residues to appear in particular positions in V3 was also noticed, and based on this survey, a consensus V3 sequence was derived. As was later learned, sequence divergence in V3 appears to be under some structural constraint, because covariation of certain residues at particular positions can be observed.[24]

Another T-cell-line–adapted strain of HIV that has undergone much study is HIVMN. The subunit derivatives of HIVMN are candidate vaccines in clinical trials. Although a synthetic peptide corresponding to the HIVLAI V3 sequence reacted with only 14% of sera tested, a similar peptide corresponding to the V3 region of HIVMN reacted with 66% of sera from 57 HIV-seropositive individuals (Table 32.1-1). This relatively high percentage of serologic reactivity was used as a rationale to choose HIVMN over other HIV strains for vaccine development. The V3 sequence of HIVMN was found to differ from the consensus sequence at six positions, including the arginine residue preceding the GPGR amino acid motif and the asparagine residue near the C-terminal end of V3. These two residues are determinants of the syncytium-inducing genotype.[25,26] Viruses with such a genotype are less frequently found in early HIV infection,[27–29] raising the question of whether other primary isolates without the syncytium-inducing genotype would have been a better choice than HIVMN.

CD4 Receptor Binding Site

Interaction between the CD4 receptor and HIV gp120 is an important event in the early stages of HIV infection. The initial CD4 receptor binding site on gp120 was initially characterized using a monoclonal antibody that blocked interaction between gp120 and CD4 in vitro.[30] This monoclonal antibody recognized a proteolytic fragment of gp120 that mapped to the C4 region. The residues in C4 that were thought to be critical for CD4 receptor binding were further mapped using a series of gp120 mutants. Using linker insertion mutants of gp120, it was determined that residues in C3, C4, and C5 were involved in CD4 receptor binding.[31] Subsequent studies showed that substitution of some residues in C2[32] and deletion of some residues in C1[33] can affect CD4 binding. These findings are in agreement with another study that reported that 62 N-terminal and 20 C-terminal residues along with the V1, V2, and V3 regions of gp120 were not involved in CD4 receptor binding.[34] Whether the residues identified in these studies are directly or indirectly involved in CD4 receptor binding cannot be resolved until the three-dimensional structure of gp120 becomes available. However, the consensus seems to be that the CD4 receptor binding site of gp120 probably involves discontinuous amino acid residues in the constant regions.

TABLE 32.1-1. *Frequency of PND peptide reactivity with 86 randomly selected sera*

Isolate	V3 Sequence	Number of HIV Sera Reacting With PND Peptides (%)
Consensus	C T R P N N N T R K S I H I . . G P G R A F Y T T G E I I G D I R Q A H C	
HIVSC/41	– – – – – – – – T R – – – – . . – – – – – – – A – – D – – – – – – – – –	56 (65)
HIVMN/51	– – – – – Y K – – R – – – . . – – – – – – – – – K N – – – T – – – – – –	57 (66)
HIVWMJ-2/122	– – – – Y – – V – R – L S – . . – – – – – – – . R – R – – – – I – – – – –	61 (71)
HIVLAI/167	– – – – – – – – – – – R – Q R – – – – – – V – I – K – . – N M R – – – –	12 (14)
HIVRF/194	– – – – – – – – – – – T K . . – – – – V I – – T – Q – – – – – – K – – –	19 (22)

Modified from LaRosa GJ, Davide JP, Weinhold K, et al. Conserved sequence and structural elements in the HIV-1 principal neutralizing determinant. Science 1993;249:932.

Several human monoclonal gp120 antibodies neutralize more than one T-cell-line–adapted HIV strain, although these strains have different V3 sequences.[35,36] These monoclonal antibodies also block binding of gp120 to CD4 in vitro. CD4 receptor blocking activity appears to account for the broad neutralizing activity of these monoclonal antibodies. The amino acid residues of gp120 involved in the binding of broadly neutralizing human monoclonal antibodies were subsequently probed, and the residues were mapped to several constant regions of gp120, based on binding of the antibodies to various gp120 mutants.[37] Not surprisingly, most regions previously identified as important for CD4 binding overlap with those regions important for the binding of broadly neutralizing human monoclonal antibodies.[38] These studies have helped to identify amino acid residues or domains of gp120 that should be considered if epitopes recognized by broadly neutralizing human monoclonal antibodies are to be preserved in a candidate vaccine.

The importance of discontinuous gp120 residues for broadly neutralizing activity is compatible with the observation that broadly neutralizing human monoclonal antibodies are sensitive to conformational changes of gp120.[35,36] Eighteen highly conserved cysteine residues are present in HIV gp120.[19] The nine disulfide bonds formed by these cysteine residues probably play a role in bringing these discontinuous residues close to each other in a fully folded gp120.[39] This conjecture is supported by the observation that the reduced form of gp120 is unreactive with broadly neutralizing human monoclonal antibodies.[35] The recognition that the CD4 receptor binding site represents a more universal target of neutralizing antibodies than V3 and that the integrity of gp120 conformation is more critical for broadly neutralizing antibodies than those targeting V3 led to the suggestion that recombinant envelope subunit vaccines with a native gp120 conformation would be more desirable than those without.

Candidate Vaccines in Clinical Trials

All candidate HIV vaccines in clinical trials for preventive purposes are subunit vaccines. Envelope gene-encoded products have been the composition of choice for most candidate vaccines.[12] Three other candidate vaccines use *gag* gene-encoded products, *pol* gene-encoded products, or both.[12] An inactivated "whole" virus preparation that does not contain the envelope protein has been tested in HIV-infected persons for therapeutic purposes,[40] but it is not covered in this chapter.

The envelope protein was chosen for vaccine development largely because the outermost coat of HIV is a target of neutralizing antibodies and because it plays a critical role in HIV entry. The peptide p17 was chosen because antisera to p17 can neutralize HIV,[41] p24 was targeted because a decrease in p24 antibody titer has been linked to AIDS progression.[42] The *gag*- and *pol*-encoded proteins are less variable than *env*-encoded proteins, and cytotoxic T cells (CTLs) have been detected against these proteins.

Candidate vaccines can be grouped into four major categories according to the method of production: synthetic peptide, recombinant subunit, live recombinant vector, and a combination of live recombinant vector and recombinant subunit. Synthetic envelope peptides are monovalent or polyvalent synthetic peptides, which correspond to the V3 sequences of different T-cell-line–adapted HIV strains.[43–47] Polyvalent V3 synthetic peptides are presented in the more traditional monomeric form or in an octameric form.[48,49] One Gag synthetic peptide being tested as a candidate vaccine corresponds to a segment of p17 that bears a relatively weak sequence homology with α_1-thymosin.[50,51]

Recombinant envelope subunits are produced by different expression vectors in insect, yeast, or mammalian cells. Recombinant envelope proteins are gp160 and gp120. The recombinant Gag subunit protein, p24, is produced in yeast as a virus-like particle.[52] The live recombinant vectors used to produce gp160 are vaccinia virus and canarypox virus. In one candidate vaccine preparation, vaccinia virus was used to produce pseudovirions containing *gag*-, *pol*-, and *env*-encoded products.[53] Combination approaches have adopted the strategy of priming the vaccine recipient with recombinant gp160 expressed by live vaccinia virus and boosting them with recombinant envelope subunits, gp160 or gp120, expressed in insect or mammalian cells.[54–56]

Candidate vaccines can also be categorized based on the anticipated immune response. Recombinant proteins that are expressed endogenously by live vectors, such as vaccinia virus or canarypox virus, are expected to elicit a CTL response. Synthetic peptides and recombinant subunit proteins that are exogenously presented to the immune system are expected to elicit a humoral response. Priming with an endogenously presented antigen and boosting with an exogenously presented subunit recombinant protein is expected to elicit humoral and CTL responses.

The method used to produce candidate HIV vaccines can have a significant impact on how closely the recombinant subunit vaccine resembles the native HIV protein. For instance, one recombinant gp160 vaccine expressed by baculovirus in insect cells retains the V3 epitope, but it lacks several broadly neutralizing epitopes found in the native HIV envelope protein. The basis of this dissimilarity is unknown. However, significant defects in this expression system appear unlikely, because the baculovirus expression system has been used to produce many other biologically functional proteins. It is generally assumed that the procedure used to isolate and purify the relatively insoluble recombinant gp160 from insect cells contributes to the alteration of antigenicity. What contributes to the insolubility of gp160 is unknown, but the possibility that the baculovirus expression system is not ideally suited to express highly glycosylated proteins, such as gp160 and gp120, should be considered.

In another method of vaccine production, a recombinant gp120 expressed in yeast is unglycosylated. This recombinant protein retains the continuous V3 epitope, but it lacks broadly neutralizing epitopes found in native gp120. Most of the recombinant gp160 and gp120 expressed in mammalian cells by mammalian expression vectors or by live recombinant vectors are known to retain CD4 receptor–binding ability and the broadly neutralizing epitopes found in the native HIV envelope protein. This accounts for the predominance of candidate vaccines that use envelope proteins expressed in mammalian cells.

During the first decade of HIV vaccine development, there was an enthusiastic pursuit of new adjuvants. The number of adjuvants that have been brought to clinical trials during this relatively short period is unprecedented. In addition to alum, new adjuvants have been tried with some recombinant subunit vaccines.[12,57,58] There are indications that the CTL response can be elicited by exogenously presented recombinant subunit vaccines when some of these adjuvants are used. The precise mechanism by which the adjuvants influence the immune system is not well understood, but it is likely that the observed effect is mediated by cytokines that regulate different arms of the immune response.

The results of the phase I and phase II clinical trials of HIV candidate vaccines are covered in another chapter of this book and therefore are not discussed in detail here. It is generally recognized that candidate HIV vaccines that have been tested in clinical trials do not elicit long-lasting antibodies or CTL responses. The information gleaned from the past decade of vaccine development nevertheless helped to dispel safety concerns about certain potentially deleterious effects that were predicted by laboratory observations. A decade of vaccine development efforts has also increased the possibility that some of the new adjuvants, which are likely to be immunologically more potent than alum, will be fully developed for human vaccines.

OBSTACLES TO HIV VACCINE DEVELOPMENT

It was decided that phase III clinical trials would not be conducted in the United States to assess the efficacy of certain candidate HIV vaccines that have completed phase I and phase II clinical trials.[59] This pause in HIV vaccine development efforts has been regarded by some as a setback, but others have applauded the decision. Such diametrically opposing views reflect the inability of the scientific community to reach a consensus on the likelihood of success of any candidate HIV vaccine. Several obstacles to HIV vaccine development efforts are discussed here. This may also serve to elucidate why it has been difficult to reach a consensus.

Indicators of Protection

The sharpest contrast between viral infections for which effective vaccines have been produced and HIV infection is that natural immunity does not appear to have a strong impact on the final outcome of HIV infection. For instance, approximately 90% of the persons infected with hepatitis B virus (HBV) develop antibodies to the surface antigen and do not become chronic carriers. This observation and other clinical experimentation, some of which would have difficulty receiving human subject approval today, indicate that a strong humoral response to the surface antigen of HBV is correlated with protection. The application of recombinant technology to produce a molecular replica of the surface antigen of HBV would not by itself produce an efficacious HBV vaccine if an effective humoral response to the surface antigen did not clear HBV in most infected individuals.

The question of whether natural immunity in HIV infection is protective is not well understood. The high mortality rate associated with HIV infection tends to support the argument that natural immunity is not sufficient in most HIV-infected individuals to prevent progression to AIDS.

In most infected individuals, broadly neutralizing antibodies to T-cell-line–adapted HIV are detectable. However, the in vivo significance of such neutralizing antibodies remains unknown. Recently, emphasis has been placed on neutralization assays using primary HIV isolates and primary cultures of peripheral blood mononuclear cells. Based on such an assay, it was reported that broadly neutralizing antibodies to primary HIV isolates were only detectable in long-term slow progressors but not in progressor controls.[60,61] These findings suggest the possibility that neutralizing antibodies to primary HIV isolates may account for slow clinical progression. If this interpretation is correct, understanding why such antibodies do not appear to be present in most HIV-infected persons who follow a more usual course of clinical progression could be as important as discovering how these antibodies were elicited in long-term slow progressors.

Longitudinal studies of persons at a very early stage of HIV infection demonstrated that the CTL response preceded a sharp reduction of plasma virus RNA.[62] The CTL response in these early seroconverters was often detected before the circulating neutralizing antibodies were detected in the blood. These memory CTLs were directed at *gag-*, *pol-*, or *env-* encoded products, and no absolute correlation was observed between any of the CTL responses and the reduction of plasma RNA. The relative contribution of CTL response to virus clearance in early HIV infection was often compared with that of neutralizing antibodies. Although it is tempting to conclude that the CTL response plays a more significant role than neutralizing antibodies, in some cases, the contribution of neutralizing antibodies cannot be ruled out.[62] Moreover, the level of plasma RNA reduction does not always correlate with the increase in CTLs over time.

Another line of study suggested that the CTL response may be correlated with disease protection. Comparisons of CTL precursor frequency between a group of long-term slow progressors and their progressor controls revealed that higher levels of CTL activity correlated with slower disease progression.[63]

Findings from these studies and other related studies are not sufficient for a definitive identification of immune correlates of protection in HIV infection. The average time between the onset of HIV infection and progression to AIDS is 10 to 12 years.[64] Because HIV was discovered only about 12 years ago and most natural history cohort studies have not followed HIV-infected persons long enough to allow for comprehensive studies of immune correlates of protection, future studies with more subjects will be needed to elucidate the indicators of protection in HIV infection.

Genetic Variability

HIV is a large family of related viruses. This genetic diversity poses serious challenges to HIV vaccine design and development. Genotypically, HIV is classified into M (major) and O (outlier) groups.[19] The M group comprises clades or subtypes A through I. These 9 subtypes are genetically equidistant. The O group is genetically distinct from the M group and comprises viruses first isolated from Cameroon citizens. These strains of HIV are not uniformly distributed throughout the world.[65] For instance, the predominant subtype in North America and Western Europe is the B subtype. In Thailand, subtypes B and E have been isolated, although the predominant subtype, E, is more closely linked to the heterosexual epidemic. Epidemiologically, heterosexual transmission accounts for most HIV epidemics outside of North America and Western Europe. The unique restriction of the B subtype in North America and Western Europe, where HIV has spread primarily through homosexual contact or through the use of contaminated needles by intravenous drug users, raises the possibility that the B subtype has been counterselected for heterosexual transmission.[66,135]

Besides the variability found in HIV from individuals in different regions, HIV sequences have also been known to vary, albeit to a lesser extent, within infected individuals. The term *quasispecies* has been coined to describe this intrasubject divergence.[67–71] Based on a relatively high ratio of nonsynonymous to synonymous changes (ie, nucleotide acid changes that induce amino acid changes versus those that do not), it is thought that HIV variability is influenced by selection pressure, which may include the immune response.[72–77] Another factor likely to have significant impact on HIV variability, at least in later stages of HIV infection, is the rapid turnover of HIV observed in infected persons with fewer than 500 CD4-positive cells/mm^3.[78,79]

Genetic variability of HIV can be expected to result in phenotypic changes. Phenotypic studies have categorized HIV into syncytium-inducing (SI) and non–syncytium-inducing (NSI) classes.[80–82] SI viruses are found in about one half of all AIDS patients, and a switch from the NSI to the SI phenotype precedes progression to AIDS.[83,84] Subtle genetic changes in V3 were found to be linked to the phenotypic switch.[25,26] Phenotypically, HIV has also been classified as monocyte-macrophage tropic or T-cell-line tropic.[85,86] Studies conducted to identify genetic sequences responsible for the monocyte-macrophage tropism also reported that V3 was the key determinant.[87–90] Most SI viruses do not replicate

in monocyte-macrophages, and some studies have suggested that SI virus less efficiently transmitted than NSI.[28] Similarly, genetic variability can have a significant impact on the antigenicity of HIV proteins. Sequence variation in V3 has been known to account for strain-specific neutralization of T-cell-line–adapted HIV. Studies of a neutralization escape mutant demonstrated that genetic changes outside of V3 could confer antigenic changes in V3.[91]

Animal Models

The lack of an adequate animal model has hampered progress in HIV vaccine development. Experiments conducted in nonhuman primate species using HIV and various simian immunodeficiency viruses (SIV) are covered in another chapter of this book and therefore are not discussed in detail here. The only nonhuman primate species that can be reproducibly infected by HIV is the chimpanzee. Besides the issue of availability of chimpanzees, HIV does not replicate persistently in chimpanzees, nor does HIV consistently cause AIDS in this species. Initial enthusiasm about using pig-tailed macaques for HIV infection has waned,[92] and efforts to develop a model based on an SIV/HIV hybrid (ie, SHIV) are ongoing.[93] The pathogenesis of SIV in rhesus macaques mirrors that observed with HIV. However, SIV-encoded proteins differ in antigenicity and immunogenicity from HIV, raising the question of immediate applicability of any successful SIV vaccine design.

A commonly held view is that a candidate HIV vaccine should not proceed to a phase III clinical trial until some efficacy can be demonstrated by the candidate vaccine or by an equivalent SIV preparation in some animal models. There is no doubt that any protection achieved in an animal model may offer the opportunity to understand the nature of immunity that is correlated with protection in that animal model. However, there is no convincing basis to conclude that protection observed in any of the animal models is suitable to predict vaccine efficacy in humans. It may also be argued that the lack of protection in any of the animal models does not rule out the possibility that the candidate vaccine may still be efficacious in humans.

Lack of Incentives

Because a sufficiently high risk-benefit ratio has become a critical criteria for testing candidate HIV vaccines in phase III trials, developing countries that have a high HIV seroincidence appear to be the logical places to conduct such trials. A general consensus at this time is that candidate vaccines matching the subtype prevalent in the target population should be used in such trials, because this may increase the likelihood of success. For instance, subunit derivatives of HIV subtype E should be considered key components of any candidate vaccine to be tested in Thailand.

However, most candidate HIV vaccines that have completed phase I and phase II clinical trials are subunit derivatives of T-cell-line–adapted HIV of the B subtype. Vaccine manufacturers are not likely to receive market approval for these candidate vaccines from the regulatory agency in the near future, because phase III clinical trials have been halted in the United States. At this juncture, business considerations apparently have precluded a firm commitment from vaccine manufacturers to develop candidate vaccines based on HIV subtypes prevalent in developing countries. At the same time, expertise and technology needed for HIV vaccine development are not yet available in the developing countries where most new HIV infection occurs. Innovative profit- and risk-sharing arrangements are needed to move HIV vaccine development forward.

FUTURE HIV VACCINE DESIGN AND DEVELOPMENT

Future efforts to develop an HIV vaccine probably will move beyond current approaches, which have been influenced by available technology rather than by an appreciation of AIDS pathogenesis. The knowledge base for HIV and AIDS has increased substantially since the discovery of the virus. However, without an adequate animal model or firmly established indicators of protection, the validity of any new concept regarding HIV vaccine design can only be determined through clinical trials.

Composition of a Candidate HIV Vaccine

There are two fundamental approaches to address the issue of what components should be included in a candidate HIV vaccine. The "build-down" approach seeks to include the entire virus; the "build-up" approach includes only certain subunits of HIV. The former approach does not have a bias regarding which component of the virus will confer protection. By including multiple components of the virus, this approach may help to limit the possible effects of immune escape. The fully assembled virus includes native HIV antigens, such as oligomeric envelope proteins, which can be difficult to reproduce on a meaningful scale. The drawbacks associated with the build-down approach include the possible ramifications of incomplete inactivation. The potential difficulty of identifying the protective components of such vaccine preparations may also make further improvement to vaccine design more difficult. An additional complexity may involve the ability to differentiate vaccinees from HIV-infected persons. Vaccinees of a whole virus preparation are more likely to develop an antibody profile, however transient it may be, similar to that of HIV-infected persons.

A whole-virus vaccine for HIV probably will be delivered as a killed vaccine preparation. Pseudovirions containing most of the virion components are a possible alternative. However, subtle yet potentially critical differences that exist between pseudovirions and native virus may not be easily identified. The prospect of testing a live attenuated HIV vaccine in humans is extremely remote. It is likely that only a

noninfectious and nonreplicating HIV, which does not integrate into the host genome, will totally alleviate safety concerns. The formidable, if not insurmountable, challenge facing the development of a live attenuated HIV vaccine is to create an HIV strain that is sufficiently attenuated to alleviate safety concerns but that retains its infectivity and its ability to replicate in vivo.

Modification of HIV Antigens

Candidate vaccines containing native HIV antigens are likely to elicit immune responses that largely mimic natural immunity. A critical question is whether a conventional vaccine design that elicits an immune response mimicking natural immunity will be efficacious for HIV prevention. The relatively rapid emergence of drug-resistant mutants suggests that natural immunity is not sufficiently effective in blocking new rounds of HIV replication in vivo.[78,79] Similarly, natural immunity has not been sufficient to reduce the high mortality rate associated with HIV infection.

One of the alternatives to the conventional approach is to modify native HIV antigens for the purpose of improving antigenicity and immunogenicity. An example of such an approach involves modifying antigenicity through deletion of N-linked glycosylation sites on the HIV envelope protein.

In natural infection, the humoral response to gp120 is largely directed to conformational epitopes that are highly dependent on the integrity of disulfide bonds.[94-96] Reduction of gp120 was reported to destroy conformational epitopes of gp120, and most sera from HIV-infected persons were not found to react with the reduced form of gp120 by Western blot assays.[94,95] This finding demonstrates the conformational constraints of the naturally immunogenic gp120 epitopes.

Preserving the native conformation of the envelope protein has been regarded by some as extremely critical for candidate HIV vaccines containing such a component. In addition to disulfide bonds, modification by glycosylation plays an important role in folding of the HIV envelope protein. Glycosylated gp120 expressed in mammalian cells retains the ability to bind CD4 and to react with various conformation-dependent, broadly neutralizing human monoclonal antibodies. The unglycosylated form of gp120 expressed in certain yeast cells or bacteria appears to fold differently from the glycosylated form. It also loses the ability to bind CD4 and to react with various conformation-dependent, broadly neutralizing human monoclonal antibodies. Primarily based on these observations, the glycosylated form of recombinant gp120 has been regarded as superior to the unglycosylated form for inclusion in candidate vaccines.

The HIV envelope protein is thought to be an oligomer on the surface of virions or virus-infected cells.[97-99] Oligomeric gp120 is anchored to the surface of the virion through interaction with oligomeric gp41. The exact number of gp120 and gp41 monomers involved in the oligomeric structure is unknown; the consensus appears to be that it is a trimer or a tetramer. An experiment was conducted in which mice were immunized with oligomeric or monomeric forms of recombinant HIV envelope proteins.[100] The oligomeric form of the recombinant envelope was found to elicit conformational antibodies targeting primarily the CD4 receptor binding site. In contrast, the monomeric form was found to elicit antibodies targeting V3. The oligomeric form of gp120 appears to direct the immune response more to the discontinuous, CD4 receptor binding site, instead of the "linear" V3 epitopes. Because the CD4 receptor binding site is a more universal target than V3, the preservation of the native conformation of HIV envelope proteins appears to be important in candidate vaccines.

It has been speculated that natural gp120 antibodies are elicited by monomeric gp120, although not by oligomeric gp120.[100] Presentation of fully assembled, oligomeric gp120 to the immune system must occur during natural infection, because HIV is known to replicate, albeit at different rates, throughout the course of infection.[101] It therefore appears that vaccines aimed at improving the antigenicity and immunogenicity will be more effective than those that are aimed solely at preserving the native conformation of the HIV envelope protein.

It has also been suggested that hypervariable regions of gp120 affect the antigenicity of this protein.[102] Deletion of V1, V2, and V3 from a recombinant gp120 protein was reported to have negligible effect on CD4 binding.[34] This observation raised the possibility of enhancing the accessibility of conserved regions of gp120 to the immune system by deleting hypervariable regions from gp120. Deletions introduced to several hypervariable regions were found to

increase the accessibility of some broadly neutralizing human monoclonal antibodies directed to the CD4 receptor binding site of gp120.[103] However, modifying gp120 antigenicity by this approach has some limitations. For instance, not all variable regions can be deleted without disturbing the overall conformation of gp120.[104] The accessibility of an epitope recognized by the antibody b12, which is known for its ability to neutralize a relatively large number of field isolates of HIV, was reduced by deletions introduced to three of the five hypervariable regions of gp120.[105,106]

A relatively large number of potential N-linked glycosylation sites have been demonstrated in gp120 (Fig. 32.1-1).[19] Carbohydrate moieties were reported to account for approximately 50% of the molecular mass of gp120.[39,107] Most, if not all, of the carbohydrate moieties found in the protein are believed to be N-linked sugars.[39,107–109] The N-linked sugars are thought to occur in many of the potential N-linked sites found in gp120. This would account for the difference between the predicted molecular weight of gp120 and that observed in SDS-polyacrylamide gels. One important role these N-linked sugars play is in the processing and folding of HIV envelope proteins as demonstrated by studies using inhibitors of N-linked glycosidases.[110–113]

The possibility that N-linked sugars mask the accessibility of certain gp120 antigenic epitopes to the immune system must be considered. It has been previously documented that carbohydrate moieties can affect the immune recognition of viral antigens. A neutralizing escape mutant of an influenza virus was found to have an N-linked sugar generated at the site targeted by a neutralizing monoclonal antibody.[114] In this case, a virus's ability to escape the immune

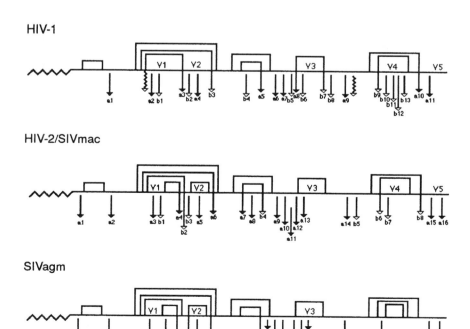

HIV-1

HIV-2/SIVmac

SIVagm

FIG. 32.1-1. Potential N-linked glycosolation sites of gp120 from HIV-1, HIV-2/SIV$_{mac}$, and SIV$_{agm}$. (Adapted from Human retroviruses and AIDS, 1991. Los Alamos, NM: Los Alamos National Laboratory, 1991.)

response is achieved through direct masking of the target site by the *N*-linked sugar. Other studies have demonstrated that the deglycosylated envelope proteins of murine leukemia virus and feline leukemia virus elicited neutralizing antibodies more effectively than their fully glycosylated counterparts.[115,116] This finding illustrates that the carbohydrate moieties of these viral glycoproteins can influence immune recognition. Evidence also indicates that modifications introduced to carbohydrate moieties of a virus glycoprotein, such as desialylation of HIV gp160, can redirect the immune response to an antigenic epitope that is mapped to a nonglycosylated protein segment.[117] This observation demonstrates that modification of the carbohydrate moieties of a virus glycoprotein can influence the accessibility of distal antigenic epitopes by the immune system.

If *N*-linked sugars of gp120 are evolutionarily conserved by HIV to evade host immune response, the removal of such sugars should not affect virus replication in vitro. This hypothesis was tested in a study in which substitutions removing potential *N*-linked glycosylation sites were introduced into gp120.[118] Mutations that removed individual *N*-linked glycosylation sites at most positions in the C-terminal half had negligible effects on HIV infectivity. The C-terminal half of gp120 is a functionally important region that contains the putative CD4 receptor binding domain and epitopes recognized by the broadly neutralizing human monoclonal antibodies previously mentioned. The finding that most *N*-linked sugars in the C-terminal region of gp120 are dispensable for HIV replication is further supported by the observation that the simultaneous removal of nine *N*-linked glycosylation sites, including the last six consecutive sites from the C-terminus of gp120, did not abolish the infectivity of the mutant viruses (unpublished observation).

It is conceivable that *N*-linked sugars in the N-terminal half of gp120 are necessary and sufficient for processing and transport of gp120 and that those in the C-terminal half are preserved to evade host immune response. This possibility is further supported by a correlation observed between the pathogenicity of primate lentiviruses in their natural hosts and the density of *N*-linked glycosylation sites in the C-terminal end of gp120 of these viruses. As shown in Figure 32.1-1, the density of *N*-linked glycosylation sites in the C-terminal end of gp120 is progressively reduced from the most pathogenic HIV-1 to the less pathogenic HIV-2[119] and to the least pathogenic SIV$_{agm}$ (see Fig. 32.1-1).[19,120]

The approach of selective deglycosylation may be useful for future vaccine design based on the modification of gp120. This approach can generate a conformationally relevant gp120 and may augment accessibility of antigenic sites otherwise unavailable to the the immune system.

New Technology

The approach of nucleic acid vaccination has attracted significant attention lately. Although the long-term safety of nucleic acid vaccination remains to be determined, this approach does have features, including presenting endogenously processed antigens to the immune system, stability, and low production cost, that are not always shared by the more conventional vaccines.

The feasibility of eliciting an immune response by introducing expression vectors to skin, muscle, or other tissues has been demonstrated in many studies.[121–127] For instance, antibodies were elicited in mice by introducing plasmids encoding human growth hormone gene or human α_1-antitrypsin gene to the skin.[121] Another example is the induction of CTLs in mice by intramuscular vaccination with a plasmid encoding the nucleoprotein of the influenza virus.[122]

The approach of nucleic acid vaccination may be particularly relevant to the design of subunit vaccines containing recombinant HIV envelope protein. Using available technologies, it is feasible to express the oligomeric form of recombinant HIV envelope protein, but the task of isolating and purifying the oligomeric HIV envelope protein is cumbersome, and it is not certain that a sufficiently high yield can be achieved to make such vaccine preparations affordable. An immune response directed to the oligomeric form of the HIV envelope protein can, in theory, be elicited by vaccination with a properly designed expression vector. Such an approach offers a less costly alternative to recombinant subunit protein or live attenuated vaccines.

In the absence of indicators of protection or an adequate animal model, the task of developing a DNA vaccine for HIV will be no less challenging than developing a conventional one. It was shown that nucleic acid vaccination elicited an immune response in animals that did not respond to conventional vaccines.[128] Although the exact mechanism by which the antigen was presented to the immune system of those animals is not well understood, this example illustrates that a nucleic acid vaccine should not be regarded merely as a convenient substitute for a conventional vaccine. It is possible that nucleic acid vaccination can be used to elicit an immune response to regions of HIV antigens that cannot be achieved by more conventional vaccines. In this regard, the usefulness of comparing the immunogenicity of a candidate DNA vaccine for HIV with that of recombinant subunit vaccines is dubious.

Another factor to be considered is that the level of expression for HIV structural proteins can vary according to cell types and animal species. Under most circumstances, the expression of HIV structural proteins depends on the Rev protein. The presence or absence of appropriate Rev-interacting cellular factors in the target tissues significantly influences the level of expression of the HIV structural proteins. For instance, cells of rodent origin do not efficiently support Rev-dependent expression of HIV structural proteins.[129] Preclinical studies in which rodent species are used to evaluate the immunogenicity of nucleic acid vaccines encoding HIV structural proteins may not predict the immunogenicity of such vaccine preparations in humans.

Vaccine Efficacy

Effective vaccines are available for several viral diseases. It is thought that these vaccines rarely prevent infection, but they are effective in preventing the pathologic consequence of the infection. One of the examples is the vaccination of cats against feline leukemia virus (FeLV), which, like HIV, is a retrovirus. Vaccination against FeLV does not prevent cats from being infected; it prevents cats from contracting FeLV-associated diseases by preventing viremia and limiting dissemination of FeLV to distant lymphoid tissues.[130] Based on this and other observations, it appears that preventing disease progression should be considered a valid measurement of the efficacy of an HIV vaccine. Such a vaccine may not generate sterilizing immunity, but it may delay disease progression by limiting the spread of HIV from the initial point of infection to distant lymphoid tissues.

Identification of immunologic factors linked to long-term nonprogression in HIV infection may prove helpful to the development of an HIV vaccine that is effective only in preventing disease. Although HIV infection has a high mortality rate, some infected individuals, who are often referred to as slow progressors or long-term nonprogressors, remain healthy for unusually long periods. It is not known if these persons will never progress to AIDS or if they will eventually develop symptoms of the disease. In either case, some studies have found that HIV isolated from slow progressors tend to show more intrasubject sequence divergence than those isolated from rapid progressors.[131] It was suggested that the larger degree of sequence divergence is the result of a more robust immune response that may also account for the slower rate of disease progression. Such observations suggest that vaccine preparations that elicit a stronger immune response are more likely to slow the rate of disease progression. Another study comparing gp120 sequence divergence between long-term nonprogressors and rapid progressors found that disproportionately more changes in constant region 3 and fewer in variable regions 1 through 4 of gp120 were associated with slower disease progression.[132] These findings suggest that one of the ways an HIV vaccine may help to slow the rate of disease progression is to focus selection pressure more on the constant region than on the variable regions of gp120. Some studies also suggest that HIV vaccine preparations that elicit broadly neutralizing antibodies or CTLs to HIV may also have the potential to delay progression to AIDS.[60,63,133]

Two HIV Epidemics

It has been suggested that the global spread of HIV falls into two types of epidemics.[134] The epidemic that occurs in North America and Western Europe involves approximately 1.5 to 2 million persons who are infected primarily by the subtype B of HIV. The major route of transmission in this epidemic is direct contact with blood, which occurs as the result of blood transfusion, intravenous drug use, or rectal microabrasions. The cells most likely to be exposed on contact are monocytes, lymphocytes, or both types. This epidemic appears to have reached a plateau.

The other epidemic, which occurs in Africa and Southeast Asia, involves approximately 15 to 20 million persons who are infected primarily by several HIV strains other than subtype B. The major route of transmission in this epidemic is heterosexual transmission. The cells most likely to be exposed on heterosexual contact are Langerhans' cells, which are abundant in the vagina and the foreskin. This epidemic appears to be expanding, and more persons among the at-risk population are likely to be infected. Although most HIV vaccine development efforts have focused on the epidemic occurring in North America and Western Europe, it is likely that substantial attention will be paid to the epidemic dominated by heterosexual transmission in the future.

It has been hypothesized that subtype B HIV might have been counterselected for heterosexual transmission, because such viruses have become adapted to transmission through direct blood contacts. In contrast, the non-B HIV subtypes, which have been involved in the epidemic dominated by heterosexual transmission, are thought to retain the ability to replicate efficiently in Langerhans' cells.[135] This hypothesis is supported by the observation that subtype C and subtype E viruses replicate more efficiently in Langerhans' cells in vitro.[135] Future HIV vaccine development efforts will likely benefit from studies that help to identify viral determinants linked to efficient replication in Langerhans' cells. The possibility that in vitro assays that use Langerhans' cells to demonstrate HIV neutralizing activity may provide a better estimation of the potency of a candidate HIV vaccine should be considered.

CONCLUSIONS

Conventional vaccine designs for viral diseases are largely based on attenuated virus, killed virus, or a molecular replica of the pathogen. Such approaches are unlikely to be directly applicable to HIV. Alternative vaccine design and development efforts that take unique properties of HIV pathogenesis and epidemiology into consideration will be necessary to optimize the risk-benefit ratio of a candidate HIV vaccine for the targeted population.

REFERENCES

1. Esparza J, Osmanov S, Kallings LO, Wigzell H. Planning for HIV vaccine trials: the World Health Organization perspective. AIDS 1991;5(Suppl 2):S159.
2. World Health Organization. Current and future dimensions of the HIV/AIDS pandemic: a capsule summary. Geneva: World Health Organization, 1991.
3. Hilleman MR. Vaccinology, immunology, and comparative pathogenesis of measles in the quest for a preventative against AIDS. AIDS Res Hum Retroviruses 1994;10:3.
4. Gallo RC, Salahuddin SZ, Popvic M, et al. Frequent detection and isolation of cytopathic retroviruses (HTLV-III) from patient with AIDS and at risk for AIDS. Science 1984;224:500.

5. Sarngadharan M, Popvic M, Bruch L, Schupbach J, Gallo RC. Antibodies reactive with human T-lymphotropic retroviruses (HTLV-III) in the serum of patients with AIDS. Science 1984;224:506.

6. Popvic M, Sarngadharan M, Read E, Gallo RC. Detection, isolation and continuous production of cytopathic retroviruses (HTLV-III) from patient with AIDS and pre-AIDS. Science 1984;224:497.

7. Schupbach J, Popovic M, Gilden RV, Gonda MA, Sarngadharan MG, Gallo RC. Serological analysis of a subgroup of human T-lymphotropic retroviruses (HTLV-III) associated with AIDS. Science 1984;224:503.

8. Ratner L, Haseltine W, Patarca R, et al. Complete nucleotide sequence of the AIDS virus, HTLV-III. Nature 1985;313:277.

9. Muesing MA, Smith DH, Cabradilla CD, Benton CV, Lasky LA, Capon DJ. Nucleic acid structure and expression of the human AIDS/lymphadenopathy retrovirus. Nature 1985;313:450.

10. Wain-Hobson S, Sonigo P, Danos O, Cole S, Alizon M. Nucleotide sequence of the AIDS virus, LAV. Cell 1985;40:9.

11. Sanchez-Pescador R, Power MD, Barr PJ, et al. Nucleotide sequence and expression of an AIDS-associated retrovirus (ARV-2). Science 1985;227:484.

12. Fast PE, Walker MC. Human trials of experimental AIDS vaccines. AIDS 1993;7(Suppl 1):S147.

13. Graham BS. Serological responses to candidate AIDS vaccines. AIDS Res Hum Retroviruses 1994;10(Suppl 2):S145.

14. Keefer MC, Belshe R, Graham B, McElrath J, Clements ML, Sposto R. Safety profile of HIV vaccination: first 1000 volunteers of AIDS vaccine evaluation group. NIAID AIDS Vaccine Clinical Trials Network. AIDS Res Hum Retroviruses 1994;10(Suppl 2):S139.

15. Allan J, Coligan JE, Barin F, et al. Major glycoprotein antigens that induce antibodies in AIDS patients are encoded by HTLV-III. Science 1985;228:1091.

16. Veronese FD, DeVico AL, Copeland TD, Oroszlan S, Gallo RC. Characterization of gp41 as the transmembrane protein coded by the HTLV-III/LAV envelope gene. Science 1985;229:1402.

17. Modrow S, Hahn BH, Shaw GM, Gallo RC, Wong-Staal F, Wolf H. Computer-assisted analysis of envelope protein sequences of seven human immunodeficiency virus isolates: prediction of antigenic epitopes in conserved and variable regions. J Virol 1987;61:570.

18. Starcich BR, Hahn BH, Shaw GM, et al. Identification and characterization of conserved and variable regions in the envelope gene of HTLV-III/LAV, the retrovirus of AIDS. Cell 1986;45:637.

19. Myers G, Korber B, Wain-Hobson S, Smith RF, Pavlakis GN. Human retroviruses and AIDS 1994: a compilation and analysis of nucleic acid and amino acid sequences. Los Alamos, New Mexico: Theoretical Biology and Biophysics, Los Alamos National Laboratory, 1994.

20. Putney SD, Matthews TJ, Robey WG, et al. HTLV-III/LAV-neutralizing antibodies to an E. coli-produced fragment of the virus envelope. Science 1986;234:1392.

21. Javaherian K, Langlois AJ, LaRosa GJ, et al. Broadly neutralizing antibodies elicited by the hypervariable neutralizing determinant of HIV-1. Science 1990;250:1590.

22. Emini EA, Schleif WA, Nunberg JH, et al. Prevention of HIV-1 infection in chimpanzees by gp120 V3 domain-specific monoclonal antibody. Nature 1992;355:728.

23. LaRosa GJ, Davide JP, Weinhold K, et al. Conserved sequence and structural elements in the HIV-1 principal neutralizing determinant. Science 1990;249:932.

24. Korber BT, Farber RM, Wolpert DH, Lapedes AS. Covariation of mutations in the V3 loop of human immunodeficiency virus type 1 envelope protein: an information theoretic analysis. Proc Natl Acad Sci USA 1993;90:7176.

25. Fouchier RAM, Groenink M, Kootstra NA, et al. Phenotype-associated sequence variation in the third variable domain of the human immunodeficiency virus type 1 gp120 molecule. J Virol 1992;66:3183.

26. De Jong J-J, De Ronde A, Keulen W, Tersmette M, Goudsmit J. Minimal requirements for the human immunodeficiency virus type 1 V3 domain to support the syncytium-inducing phenotype: analysis by single amino acid substitution. J Virol 1992;66:6777.

27. Wolinsky SM, Wike CM, Korber BTM, et al. Selective transmission of human immunodeficiency virus type-1 variants from mothers to infants. Science 1992;255:1134.

28. Zhu T, Mo H, Wang N, et al. Genotypic and phenotypic characterization of HIV-1 in patients with primary infection. Science 1993;261:1179.

29. Zhang LQ, MacKenzie P, Cleland A, Holmes EC, Leigh Brown AJ, Simmonds P. Selection for specific sequences in the external envelope protein of human immunodeficiency virus type 1 upon primary infection. J Virol 1993;67:3345.

30. Lasky LA, Nakamura G, Smith DH, et al. Delineation of a region of the human immunodeficiency virus type 1 gp120 glycoprotein critical for interaction with the CD4 receptor. Cell 1987;50:975.

31. Kowalski M, Potz J, Basiripour L, et al. Functional regions of the envelope glycoprotein of human immunodeficiency virus type 1. Science 1987;237:1351.

32. Olshevsky U, Helseth E, Furman C, Li J, Haseltine W, Sodroski J. Identification of individual human immunodeficiency virus type 1 gp120 amino acids important for CD4 receptor binding. J Virol 1990;64:5701.

33. Syu WJ, Huang JH, Essex M, Lee TH. The N-terminal region of the human immunodeficiency virus envelope glycoprotein gp120 contains potential binding sites for CD4. Proc Natl Acad Sci USA 1990;87:3695.

34. Pollard SR, Rosa MD, Rosa JJ, Wiley DC. Truncated variants of gp120 bind CD4 with high affinity and suggest a minimum CD4 binding region. EMBO J 1992;11:585.

35. Robinson JE, Holton D, Pacheco-Morell S, Liu J, McMurdo H. Identification of conserved and variant epitopes of human immunodeficiency virus type 1 (HIV-1) gp120 by human monoclonal antibodies produced by EBV-transformed cell lines. AIDS Res Hum Retroviruses 1990;6:567.

36. Posner M, Hideshima T, Cannon T, Mukherjee M, Mayer K, Byrn R. An IgG human monoclonal antibody that reacts with HIV-1 gp120 inhibits virus binding to cells, and neutralizes infection. J Immunol 1991;146:4325.

37. Thali M, Olshevsky U, Furman C, Gabuzda D, Posner M, Sodroski J. Characterization of a discontinuous human immunodeficiency virus type 1 gp120 epitope recognized by a broadly reactive neutralizing human monoclonal antibody. J Virol 1991;65:6188.

38. Thali M, Furman C, Ho DD, et al. Discontinuous, conserved neutralization epitopes overlapping the CD4-binding region of human immunodeficiency virus type 1 gp120 envelope glycoprotein. J Virol 1992;66:5635.

39. Leonard CK, Spellman MW, Riddle L, Harris R, Thomas JN, Gregory TJ. Assignment of intrachain disulfide bonds and characterization of potential glycosylation sites of the type 1 recombinant human immunodeficiency virus envelope glycoprotein (gp120) expressed in Chinese hamster ovary cells. J Biol Chem 1990;265:10373.

40. Trauger RJ, Ferre F, Daigle AE, et al. Effect of immunization with inactivated gp120-depleted human immunodeficiency virus type 1 (HIV-1) immunogen on HIV-1 immunity, viral DNA, and percentage of CD4 cells. J Infect Dis 1994;169:1256.

41. Sarin PS, Sun DK, Thornton AH, Naylor PH, Goldstein AL. Neutralization of HTLV-III/LAV replication by antiserum to thymosin alpha 1. Science 1986;232:1135.

42. Weber JN, Clapham PR, Weiss RA, et al. Human immunodeficiency virus infection in two cohorts of homosexual men: neutralising sera and association of anti-gag antibody with prognosis. Lancet 1987;1:119.

43. Okuda K, Inami S, Kanedo T. Strong synergistic effects of polyvalent vaccine for human immunodeficiency virus (HIV-1) infection. Abstract. Eighth International Conference on AIDS/III STD World Congress, Amsterdam, 1992.

44. Palker TJ, Clark ME, Langlois AJ, et al. Type-specific neutralization of the human immunodeficiency virus with antibodies to env-encoded synthetic peptides. Proc Natl Acad Sci USA 1988;85:1932.

45. Palker TJ, Matthews TJ, Langlois A, et al. Polyvalent human immunodeficiency virus synthetic immunogen comprised of envelope gp120 T helper cell sites and B cell neutralization epitopes. J Immunol 1989;142:3612.

46. Hart MK, Palker TJ, Matthews TJ, et al. Synthetic peptides containing T and B cell epitopes from human immunodeficiency virus envelope gp120 induce anti-HIV proliferative responses and high titers of neutralizing antibodies in rhesus monkeys. J Immunol 1990;145:2677.

47. Hart MK, Weinhold KJ, Scearce RM, Washburn EM, Clark CA, Palker TJ. Priming of anti-human immunodeficiency virus (HIV) CD8+ cytotoxic T cells in vivo by carrier-free HIV synthetic peptides. Proc Natl Acad Sci USA 1991;88:9448.

48. Wang CY, Looney DJ, Li ML, et al. Long-term high-titer neutralizing activity induced by octameric synthetic HIV-1 antigen. Science 1991;254:285.

49. Defoort JP, Nardelli B, Huang W, Ho DD, Tam JP. Macromolecular assemblage in the design of a synthetic AIDS vaccine. Proc Natl Acad Sci USA 1992;89:3879.

50. Coleman R, Stites D, Scillian J. The development of cytotoxic T-lymphocytes (CTL) in subjects immunized with HGP-30 A 30 amino acid subunit of HIV p17 core protein. (Abstract) J Cell Biochem 1992;(Suppl 16E):60.

51. Kahn J, Coleman R, Stites D. A phase I study of HGP-30, a 30 amino acid subunit of HIV p17 synthetic peptide analogue subunit vaccine in seronegative subjects. Abstract. Eighth International Conference on AIDS/III STD World Congress, Amsterdam, 1992.

52. Weber J, Kennedy A, Callow D, Zigmond A, Cheingsong-Popov R. A phase I study of the safety and immunogenicity of Ty-p24 VLP in healthy volunteers. Abstract. Eighth International Conference on AIDS/III STD World Congress, Amsterdam, 1992.

53. Hesselton RM, Mazzara GP, Panicali D, Sullivan JL. HIV-specific immune responses in rabbits. Abstract. Eighth International Conference on AIDS/III STD World Congress, Amsterdam, 1992.

54. Graham BS, Matthews TJ, Belshe RB, et al. Augmentation of human immunodeficiency virus type 1 neutralizing antibody by priming with gp160 recombinant vaccinia and boosting with rgp160 in vaccinia-naive adults. The NIAID AIDS Vaccine Clinical Trials Network. J Infect Dis 1993;167:533.

55. Montefiori DC, Graham BS, Zhou J, Bucco RA, Schwartz DH, Posner MR. V3-specific neutralizing antibodies in sera from HIV-1 gp160-immunized volunteers block virus fusion and act synergistically with human monoclonal antibody to the conformation-dependent CD4 binding site of gp120. NIH-NIAID AIDS Vaccine Clinical Trials Network [see comments]. J Clin Invest 1993;92:840.

56. Pincus SH, Messer KG, Schwartz DH, Lewis GK, Graham BS, Blattner WA. Differences in the antibody response to human immunodeficiency virus-1 envelope glycoprotein (gp160) in infected laboratory workers and vaccinees. J Clin Invest 1993;91:1987.

57. Goldenthal KL, Cavagnaro JA, Alving CR, Vogel FR. Safety evaluation of vaccine adjuvants: national cooperative vaccine development meeting working group. AIDS Res Hum Retroviruses 1993;9(Suppl 1):S47.

58. Alving CR, Detrick B, Richards RL, Lewis MG, Shafferman A, Eddy GA. Novel adjuvant strategies fro experimental malaria and AIDS vaccines. Ann N Y Acad Sci 1993;690:265.

59. Moore J, Anderson R. The WHO and why of HIV vaccine trials [see comment]. Nature 1994;372:313.

60. Cao Y, Qin L, Zhang L, Safrit J, Ho DD. Virologic and immunologic characterization of long-term survivors of human immunodeficiency virus type 1 infection. N Engl J Med 1995;332:201.

61. Moore JP, Cao Y, Qing L, et al. Primary isolates of human immunodeficiency virus type 1 are relatively resistant to neutralization by monoclonal antibodies to gp120, and their neutralization is not predicted by studies with monomeric gp120. J Virol 1995;69:101.

62. Koup RA, Safrit JT, Cao Y, et al. Temporal association of cellular immune responses with the initial control of viremia in primary human immunodeficiency virus type 1 syndrome. J Virol 1994;68:4650.

63. Rinaldo C, Huang X-L, Fan Z, et al. High levels of anti-human immunodeficiency virus type 1 (HIV-1) memory cytotoxic T-lymphocyte activity and low viral load are associated with lack of disease in HIV-1 infected long-term nonprogressors. J Virol 1995;69:5838.

64. Alcabes P, Munoz A, Vlahov D, Friedland GH. Incubation period of human immunodeficiency virus. Epidemiol Rev 1993;15:303.

65. Delwart EL, Shaper EG, Louwagie J, et al. Genetic relationships determined by a DNA heteroduplex mobility assay: analysis of HIV-1 env genes. Science 1993;262:1257.

66. Essex M. The AIDS vaccine challenge. Technol Rev 1994;97:23.

67. Steinhauer DA, Holland JJ. Rapid evolution of RNA viruses. Annu Rev Microbiol 1986;41:409.

68. Holland JJ, de la Torre JC, Steinhauer DA. RNA virus populations as quasispecies. Curr Top Microbiol Immunol 1992;176:1.

69. Wain-Hobson S. Human immunodeficiency virus type 1 quasispecies in vivo and ex vivo. Curr Top Microbiol Immunol 1992;176:181.

70. Goodenow M, Huet T, Saurin W, Kwok S, Sninsky J, Wain-Hobson S. HIV-1 isolates are rapidly evolving quasispecies: evidence for viral mixtures and preferred nucleotide substitutions. J Acquir Immune Defic Syndr 1989;2:344.

71. Meyerhans A, Cheynier R, Albert J, et al. Temoporal fluctuations in HIV quasispecies in vivo are not reflected by sequential HIV isolations. Cell 1989;58:901.

72. Coffin JM. HIV population dynamics in vivo: implications for genetic variation, pathogenesis, and therapy. Science 1995;267:483.

73. Wolfs TFW, De Jong J-J, Van Den Berg H, Tijnagel JMGH, Krone WJA, Goudsmit J. Evolution of sequences encoding the principal neutralization epitope of human immunodeficiency virus 1 is host dependent, rapid, and continuous. Proc Natl Acad Sci USA 1990;87:9938.

74. Simmonds P, Balfe P, Ludlam CA, Bishop JO, Leigh Brown AJ. Analysis of sequence diversity in hypervariable regions of the external glycoprotein of human immunodeficiency virus type 1. J Virol 1990;64:5840.

75. Balfe P, Simmonds P, Ludlam CA, Bishop JO, Leigh Brown AJ. Concurrent evolution of human immunodeficiency virus type 1 in patients infected from the same source: rate of sequence change and low frequency of inactivating mutations. J Virol 1990;64:6221.

76. Lamers SL, Sleasman JW, She JX, et al. Independent variation and positive selection in env V1 and V2 domains within maternal-infant strains of human immunodeficiency virus type 1 in vivo. J Virol 1993;67:3951.

77. Feinberg MB, Greene WC. Molecular insights into human immunodeficiency virus type 1 pathogenesis. Curr Opin Immunol 1992;4:466.

78. Wei X, Ghosh SK, Taylor ME, et al. Viral dynamics in human immunodeficiency virus type 1 infection. Nature 1995;373:117.

79. Ho DD, Neumann AU, Perelson AS, Chen W, Leonard JM, Markowitz M. Rapid turnover of plasma virions and CD4 lymphocytes in HIV-1 infection. Nature 1995;373:123.

80. Tersmette M, De Goede REY, Al BJM, et al. Differential syncytium-inducing capacity of human immunodeficiency virus isolates: frequent detection of syncytium-inducing isolates in patients with acquired immunodeficiency syndrome (AIDS) and AIDS-related complex. J Virol 1988;62:2026.

81. Tersmette M, Lange JMA, De Goede REY, et al. Association between biological properties of human immunodeficiency virus variants and risk for AIDS and AIDS mortality. Lancet 1989;i:983.

82. Tersmette M, Gruters RA, De Wolf F, et al. Evidence for a role of virulent human immunodeficiency virus (HIV) variants in the pathogenesis of acquired immunodeficiency syndrome: studies on sequential HIV isolates. J Virol 1989;63:2118.

83. Kuiken CL, De Jong J-J, Baan E, Keulen W, Tersmette M, Goudsmit J. Evolution of the V3 envelope domain in proviral sequences and isolates of human immunodeficiency virus type 1 during transition of the viral biological phenotype. J Virol 1992;66:4622.

84. Connor RI, Mohri H, Cao Y, Ho DD. Increased viral burden and cytopathicity correlate temporally with CD4+ T-lymphocyte decline and clinical progression in human immunodeficiency type 1–infected individuals. J Virol 1993;67:1772.

85. Schuitemaker H, Kootstra NA, De Goede RY, De Wolf F, Miedema F, Tersmette M. Monocytotropic human immunodeficiency virus type 1 (HIV-1) variants detectable in all stages of HIV-1 infection lack T-cell line tropism and syncytium-inducing ability in primary T-cell culture. J Virol 1991;65:356.

86. Schuitemaker H, Koot M, Kootstra NA, et al. Biological phenotype of human immunodeficiency virus type 1 clones at different stages of infection: progression of disease is associated with a shift from monocytotropic to T-cell-tropic virus populations. J Virol 1992;66:1354.

87. Hwang SS, Boyle TJ, Lyerly HK, Cullen BR. Identification of the envelope V3 loop as the primary determinant of cell tropism in HIV-1. Science 1991;253:71.

88. O'Brien WA, Koyanagi Y, Namazie A, et al. HIV-1 tropism for mononuclear phagocytes can be determined by regions of gp120 outside the CD4-binding domain. Nature 1990;348:69.

89. Shoida T, Levy JA, Cheng-Mayer C. Macrophage and T cell-line tropisms of HIV-1 are determined by specific regions of the envelope gp120 gene. Nature 1991;349:167.

90. Westervelt P, Trowbridge DB, Epstein LG, et al. Macrophage tropism determinants of human immunodeficiency virus type 1 in vivo. J Virol 1992;66:2577.

91. Reitz MS Jr, Wilson C, Naugle C, Gallo RC, Robert-Guroff M. Generation of a neutralization-resistant variant of HIV-1 is due to selection for a point mutation in the envelope gene. Cell 1988;54:57.

92. Agy MB, Frumkin LR, Corey L, et al. Infection of *Macaca nemestrina* by human immunodeficiency virus type-1. Science 1992;257:103.

93. Li J, Lord CI, Haseltine W, Letvin NL, Sodroski J. Infection of cynomolgus monkeys with a chimeric HIV-1/SIV$_{mac}$ virus that expresses the HIV-1 envelope glycoproteins. J Acquir Immune Defic Syndr 1992;5:639.

94. Chou MJ, Lee TH, Hatzakis A, Mandalaki T, McLane MF, Essex M. Antibody responses in early human immunodeficiency virus type 1 infection in hemophiliacs. J Infect Dis 1988;157:805.

95. Lee TH, Chou M-J, HUang J-H, et al. Association between antibody to envelope glycoprotein gp120 and the outcome of human immunodeficiency virus infection. Cold Spring Harbor: Cold Spring Harbor Laboratory, 1988:373.

96. Moore JP, Ho DD. Antibodies to discontinuous or conformationally sensitive epitopes on the gp120 glycoprotein of human immunodeficiency virus type 1 are highly prevalent in sera of infected humans. J Virol 1993;67:863.

97. Earl PL, Doms RW, Moss B. Oligomeric structure of the human immunodeficiency virus type 1 envelope glycoprotein. Proc Natl Acad Sci USA 1990;87:648.

98. Pinter A, Honnen WJ, Tilley SA, Bona C, Zaghouani H, Gorny MK. Oligomeric structure of gp41, the transmembrane protein of human immunodeficiency virus type 1. J Virol 1989;63:2674.

99. Schawaller M, Smith GE, Skehel JJ, Wiley DC. Studies with crosslinking reagents on the oligomeric structure of the env glycoprotein of HIV. Virology 1989;172:367.

100. Earl PL, Broder CC, Long D, et al. Native oligomeric human immunodeficiency virus type 1 envelope glycoprotein elicits diverse monoclonal antibody reactivities. J Virol 1994;68:3015.

101. Piatak M, Saag MS, Yang LC, et al. High levels of HIV-1 in plasma during all stages of infection determined by competitive PCR. Science 1993;259:1749.

102. Coffin JM. Genetic variation in AIDS viruses. Cell 1986;46:1.

103. Wyatt R, Sullivan N, Thali M, et al. Functional and immunologic characterization of human immunodeficiency virus type 1 envelope glycoproteins containing deletions of the major variable regions. J Virol 1993;67:4557.

104. Lee C-N, Robinson J, Mazzara G, Cheng Y-L, Essex M, Lee T-H. Contribution of hypervariable domains to the conformation of a broadly neutralizing epitope of human immunodeficiency virus type 1. AIDS Res Hum Retroviruses 1995;11:777.

105. Roben P, Moore JP, Thali M, Sodroski J, Barbas CF, Burton DR. Recognition properties of a panel of human recombinant Fab fragments to the CD4 binding site of gp120 that show differing abilities to neutralize human immunodeficiency virus type 1. J Virol 1994;68:4821.

106. Burton DR, Pyati J, Koduri R, et al. Efficient neutralization of primary isolates of HIV-1 by a recombinant human monoclonal antibody. Science 1994;266:1024.

107. Feizi T, Larkin M. AIDS and glycosylation. [Published erratum appears in Glycobiology 1991;1:315]. (Review) Glycobiology 1990;1:17.

108. Geyer H, Holschbach C, Hunsmann G, Schneider J. Carbohydrates of human immunodeficiency virus. J Biol Chem 1988;263:11760.

109. Mizuochi T, Spellman MW, Larkin M, Solomon J, Basa LJ, Feizi T. Carbohydrate structures of the human immunodeficiency virus (HIV) recombinant envelope glycoprotein gp120 produced in Chinese hamster ovary cells. Biochem J 1988;254:599.

110. Gruters RA, Neefjes JJ, Tersmette M, et al. Interference with HIV-induced syncytium formation and viral infectivity by inhibitors of trimming glucosidase. Nature 1987;330:74.

111. Walker BD, Kowalski M, Goh WC, et al. Inhibition of human immunodeficiency virus syncytium formation and virus replication by castanospermine. Proc Natl Acad Sci U S A 1987;84:8120.

112. Montefiori DC, Robinson WE, Mitchell WM. Role of protein N-glycosylation in pathogenesis of human immunodeficiency virus type 1. Proc Natl Acad Sci USA 1988;85:9248.

113. Li Y, Luo L, Pasool N, Kang CY. Glycosylation is necessary for the correct folding of human immunodeficiency virus gp120 in CD4 binding. J Virol 1993;67:584.

114. Skehel JJ, Stevens DJ, Daniels RS, Douglas AR, Knossow M, Wilson IA. A carbohydrate side chain on hemagglutinins of Hong Kong influenza viruses inhibits recognition by a monoclonal antibody. Proc Natl Acad Sci USA 1984;81:1779.

115. Elder JH, McGee JS, Alexander S. Carbohydrate side chains of Rauscher leukemia virus envelope glycoproteins are not required to elicit a neutralizing antibody response. J Virol 1986;57:340.

116. Alexander S, Elder JH. Carbohydrate dramatically influences immune reactivity of antisera to viral glycoprotein antigens. Science 1984;226:1328.

117. Benjouad A, Gluckman J-C, Rochat H, Montagnier L, Bahraoui E. Influence of carbohydrate moieties on the immunogenicity of human immunodeficiency virus type 1 recombinant gp160. J Virol 1992;66:2473.

118. Lee WR, Syu WJ, Bin D, et al. Non-random distribution of gp120 N-linked glycosylation sites critical for HIV-1 infectivity. Proc Natl Acad Sci USA 1992;89:2213.

119. Travers K, Mboup S, Marlink R, et al. Natural protection against HIV-1 infection provided by HIV-2 [see comments]. Science 1995;268:1612.

120. Hirsch VM, Myers G, Johnson PR. Genetic diversity and phylogeny of primate lentiviruses. In: Morrow WJW, Haigwood NL, eds. HIV molecular organization, pathogenicity and treatment. Amsterdam: Elsevier Science Publishers, 1993:221.

121. Tang DC, DeVit M, Johnston SA. Genetic immunization is a simple method for eliciting an immune response. Nature 1992;356:152.

122. Ulmer JB, Donnelly JJ, Parker SE, et al. Heterologous protection against influenza by injection of DNA encoding a viral protein Science 1993;259:1745.

123. Wang B, Ugen KE, Srikantan V, et al. Gene inoculation generates immune responses against human immunodeficiency virus type 1. Proc Natl Acad Sci USA 1993;90:4156.

124. Wolff JA, Ludtke JJ, Acsadi G, Williams P, Jani A. Long-term persistence of plasmid DNA and foreign gene expression in mouse muscle. Hum Mol Genet 1992;1:363.

125. Xiang ZQ, Spitalnik S, Tran M, Wunner WH, Cheng J, Ertl HC. Vaccination with a plasmid vector carrying the rabies virus glycoprotein gene induces protective immunity against rabies virus. Virology 1994;199:132.

126. Sedegah M, Hedstrom R, Hobart P, Hoffman SL. Protection against malaria by immunization with plasmid DNA encoding circumsporozoite protein. Proc Natl Acad Sci USA 1994;91:9866.

127. Raz E, Carson DA, Parker SE, et al. Intradermal gene immunization: the possible role of DNA uptake in the induction of cellular immunity to viruses. Proc Natl Acad Sci USA 1994;91:9519.

128. Schirmbeck R, Bohm W, Ando K, Chisari FV, Reimann J. Nucleic acid vaccination primes hepatitis B virus surface antigen–specific cytotoxic T lymphocytes in nonresponder mice. J Virol 1995;69:5929.

129. Trono D, Baltimore D. A human cell factor is essential for HIV-1 Rev action. EMBO J 1990;9:4155.

130. Essex M. The HIV-1 vaccine dilemma: lessons from the cat. J Natl Inst Health Res 1995;7:37.

131. Delwart EL, Sheppard HW, Walker BD, Goudsmit J, Mullins JI. Human immunodeficiency virus type 1 evolution in vivo tracked by DNA heteroduplex mobility assays. J Virol 1994;68:6672.

132. Wang WK, Essex M, McLane MF, et al. Pattern of gp120 sequence divergence linked to a lack of clinical progression in human immunodeficiency virus type 1 infection. Proc Nat Acad Sci USA 1996;93.

133. Pantaleo G, Menzo S, Vaccarezza M, et al. Studies in subjects with long-term nonprogressive human immunodeficiency virus infection. N Engl J Med 1995;332:209.

134. Cohen J. Differences in HIV strains may underlie disease patterns. Science 1995;270:30.

135. Soto-Ramirez LE, Renjifo B, McLane MF, et al. HIV-1 Langerhans' cell tropism associated with heterosexual transmission of HIV. Science 1996;271:1291.

AIDS: Biology, Diagnosis, Treatment and Prevention, fourth edition, edited by Vincent T. DeVita, Jr., Samuel Hellman, and Steven A. Rosenberg. Lippincott–Raven Publishers, © 1997

32.2

Clinical Trials of Human Immunodeficiency Virus Vaccines

Mary Lou Clements

IMMUNIZATION STRATEGIES

Immunizations are the most cost-effective public health intervention for control of infectious diseases. Instead of conferring sterilizing immunity (ie, complete protection against infection), highly effective vaccines confer immunity that eliminates the pathogen, resulting in protection against or amelioration of disease. Even more important than the benefit to the individual vaccine recipient is the effect of wide-scale immunization with effective live attenuated or nonreplicating vaccines, resulting in herd immunity and reduced transmission of infections such as those caused by *Haemophilus influenzae* type B, hepatitis B, measles, rubella, and poliovirus in communities.

Safe, effective human immunodeficiency virus (HIV) vaccines, combined with counseling, education, and behavioral modification, are needed to stem the rapid pandemic of HIV-1 infection resulting from sexual, vertical, and other routes of transmission. Because sterilizing immunity is unlikely to be achieved, a realistic goal for HIV vaccines is to provide sufficient immunity (or immunologic memory) that can be recalled rapidly and augmented in persons exposed to HIV and thereby restrict HIV replication and destroy virus-infected cells, resulting in a subclinical infection. Even a partially effective HIV vaccine may benefit populations at risk if vaccinated persons who become infected can maintain a level of viremia below the threshold needed for transmission to sexual partners and others.

Several immunization strategies to induce, augment, and broaden HIV-specific immune responses are under clinical investigation: prophylactic immunization of uninfected persons using preventive HIV vaccines; postexposure immunization (ie, immunotherapy) of HIV-infected persons; maternal immunization of infected women during pregnancy (ie, perinatal immunization) to diminish viremia and the likelihood of transmission of HIV to the infant; and postexposure immunization of neonates born to HIV-infected women.[1] Each investigational HIV vaccine requires extensive clinical evaluation to meet the requirements for licensure for each indication. This chapter focuses mainly on the clinical evaluation of preventive HIV vaccines.

REGULATORY REQUIREMENTS FOR CLINICAL DEVELOPMENT OF CANDIDATE VACCINES

To qualify for licensure in the United States, vaccines must meet the standards and requirements stated in the Code of Federal Regulations (Title 21, part 600) for safety, purity, potency, immunogenicity, and efficacy.[2] Preclinical tests must be conducted in vitro, in small animals, and sometimes in nonhuman primates to assess the safety, toxicity, and immunogenicity of a candidate vaccine. After the preclinical tests have been completed successfully, the sponsor (eg, investigator, university, commercial firm, government agency) can submit a Notice of Claimed Exemption for a New Drug to the U.S. Food and Drug Administration (FDA). The investigational vaccine is then referred to as an investigational new drug (IND).

The IND application must include descriptions of the composition, source, and manufacturing process of the vaccine; quality control and the methods used to test the vaccine's safety, purity, and potency; a summary of all laboratory and preclinical animal tests; a protocol detailing the clinical study and consent form approved by the local institutional review board; and names and qualifications of the clinical investigators. During a 30-day period, the IND application is reviewed by the FDA to determine whether human subjects will be exposed to unwarranted risks. Vaccine lots for

Mary Lou Clements, Johns Hopkins University, Center for Immunization Research, Hampton House 125, 624 North Broadway, Baltimore, MD 21205.

clinical trials must be produced according to standard good manufacturing practices. If the vaccine is safe and efficacious in clinical trials, an application for a product license application (PLA) can be submitted to the FDA. FDA approval for licensure is based on a satisfactory review of all data in the PLA, the results of confirmatory tests by the FDA on product samples from the manufacturer, and an inspection of the production facilities.

CLINICAL TESTING OF PREVENTIVE HIV VACCINE CANDIDATES

Clinical evaluation to determine the safety and immunogenicity of HIV vaccines in seronegative volunteers is usually conducted in a randomized, double blind, controlled fashion in phases. Phase I trials of HIV vaccines have been conducted in a dose-escalation manner, using a small number of volunteers who are at relatively low risk or intermediate risk for acquiring HIV infection to determine the optimal concentration of immunogen, number of doses, schedule of immunization, route of administration, and the duration of immune responses. Investigational adjuvants are also evaluated in phase I trials in which different concentrations of the adjuvant alone and in combination with different concentrations of the vaccine antigen are tested to determine the optimal concentration of each component in terms of tolerability and immunogenicity.

If the vaccine candidate is safe and immunogenic, a phase II study can be conducted with a larger number of volunteers, including persons from populations at high risk for acquiring HIV infection, to obtain additional information about the safety and immunogenicity of the vaccine. A study that is repeated to evaluate the safety and immunogenicity of a candidate vaccine in a small number of persons from a population with a high incidence of HIV infection is sometimes referred to as a phase I/II trial. Such trials can serve as pilot studies to assess the feasibility of conducting a phase III efficacy trial in a particular population.

Randomized, placebo-controlled phase III trials must be conducted to determine the safety and efficacy of a vaccine product when the correlates of protective immunity are unknown. Assessment of the protective efficacy of preventive HIV vaccines will require enrollment and long-term follow-up of several thousand volunteers at high risk for acquiring HIV infection.[3-6] The sample size will depend on the incidence of infection in the study population, the duration of the trial, the rate of attrition of trial participants, and other factors.[4-6] As with the development of non-HIV vaccines, criteria and milestones for proceeding from phase II to phase III trials to evaluate the safety and efficacy of a candidate vaccine should be determined in advance by the sponsor and the vaccine manufacturer. If the results of phase I and phase II trials indicate a candidate vaccine is safe and sufficiently immunogenic, and the sponsor and the manufacturer are willing, a phase III trial of HIV vaccines should be conducted to determine the level of efficacy of the vac-

cine based on one or more end points (eg, reduction in virus load or the severity of disease). Additional efficacy studies may be required to confirm a high level of efficacy of a candidate vaccine in other populations, particularly if the route of transmission is different, and to determine the duration of protective immunity conferred.

It is equally important to understand why a vaccine fails to confer full protection. Results of trials of partially effective or ineffective vaccines have provided valuable insight into the design of improved vaccines. For example, serotype-specific immunity may be required, the vaccine may need to be combined with a more potent adjuvant to augment or extend immunity for certain groups, and the vaccine may not protect against disease in certain populations or age groups because of greater exposure to the pathogen or a different route of transmission. Importantly, correlates of immunity may be identified when a vaccine confers partial immunity. For these reasons, experienced vaccine developers are usually willing to proceed with phase III trials with the realization that the vaccines tested may not be efficacious, additional efficacy studies may be required, and the vaccines tested may not be licensed.

HIV ANTIGENS USED AS IMMUNOGENS

Although the correlates of protective immunity are unknown, an effective HIV vaccine will probably need to induce neutralizing antibodies and cell-mediated immunity (especially CD8+ cytotoxic T lymphocyte [CTL] activity) to prevent the establishment of infection or to control a chronic HIV infection after transmission by virus-infected cells, free virus, or both.[1,5,7,8] Because the envelope of HIV contains epitopes for neutralizing antibodies and helper T cell and CTL responses,[9,10] gp160, gp120, or the V3 loop has been included as an immunogen in most candidate HIV vaccines. Induction of CD8+ CTLs requires presentation of target antigens associated with class I major histocompatibility complex (MHC) molecules.[11] This type of immunity can be induced safely by immunization with certain peptides, core proteins, and live recombinant poxvirus vectors expressing gene products, such as Env, Gag, Nef, and polymerase, that contain CTL epitopes.[9-12]

VACCINES UNDER CLINICAL INVESTIGATION

Phase I or I/II trials of preventive HIV vaccine candidates have been conducted in uninfected volunteers in the United States, United Kingdom, France, Switzerland, Australia, Japan, China, Thailand, and Brazil (Table 32.2-1). Since 1988, the U.S. National Institutes of Allergy and Infectious Diseases (NIAID) has supported a network of several academic institutions and corporations, referred to as the AIDS Vaccine Evaluation Group (AVEG), to evaluate the safety and immunogenicity of candidate HIV vaccines in phase I and II clinical trials.[1,12] By mid-1995, the NIAID-sponsored AVEG had initiated 23 multicentered safety and immunogenicity trials of 16 investigational vaccines involving more than 1700

TABLE 32-1. *HIV vaccine candidates in clinical trials*

HIV Strain and Immunogen Expression System	Adjuvant† or delivery system	Vaccine Manufacturer	Type and Phase of Trial	
			Preventive	Immunotherapy
HIV-IIIB*				
gp160 (baculovirus)	Alum	MicroGeneSys	I	I, II
gp160 (vaccinia)	Alum + DOC	ImmunoAG	I	I, II
gp160 (mammalian)	IFA	Universite Libre de Bruxelles	I	
gp120 (CHO)	Alum	Genentech	I	I
p24 (baculovirus)	Alum	MicroGeneSys		I
Vaccinia gp160‡	None	Bristol-Myers-Squibb/Oncogen	I	
Vaccinia gp160‡	None	Institut-Jacques Monod	I	
Vaccinia Env, Gag, Pol (TBC-3B)	None	Therion Biologics	I	
V3 peptide	ISA724	Universite Libre de Bruxelles	I	
Gag peptide	Lipopeptide	United Biomedical, Inc.	I	
p17 peptide (HGP30)	Alum	Viral Technologies	I	
p17 and p24 (yeast transposon)	Virus-like particles, alum	British Biotechnology Ltd.	I	
HIV-MN				
gp120 MN/gp41 LAI (mammalian)	Alum or IFA	Pasteur-Merieux/Transgene	I	
Canarypox gp160‡	None	Pasteur-Merieux-Connaught, Virogenetics	I	I
Canarypox Env, Gag, Protease‡	None	Pasteur-Merieux-Connaught, Virogenetics	I	
gp120 (CHO)	Alum	Genentech	I, II	I, II
gp120 (CHO)	QS21	Genentech	I	
V3	PPD conjugate	Swiss Serum & Vaccine Institute	I	
V3	Alum or IFA	Pasteur-Merieux/Transgene	I	
V3-MAPS	Alum	United Biomedical, Inc.	I	
V3-MAPS	Microparticulate	United Biomedical, Inc.	I	
HIV-SF2				
gp120 (yeast)	MF59 ± MTP-PE	Chiron/Biocine	I	I
gp120 (CHO)	MF59 ± MTP-PE	Chiron/Biocine	I	I
gp120 (CHO)	MF59	Chiron/Biocine	I, II	I
gp120 (CHO)	Multiple adjuvants†	Chiron/Biocine	I	
OTHERS				
V3-MAPS, clades A–E	Alum	United Biomedical, Inc.	I	
V3, MN, RE, and IIIB	Alum, KLH carrier	Yokohama City University	I	
Irradiated whole HIV, HZ321	IFA	Immune Response Corp.		I, II, III

DOC, deoxycholate; IFA, incomplete Freund's adjuvant; MF59 ± MTP-PE, microfluidized oil in water emulsion with or without muramyl tripeptide palmitodyl ethanolamine; KLH, keyhold limpet hemocyanin; MAPS, multiple antigen peptide system; CHO, Chinese hamster ovarian cells; PPD, purified protein derivative.

*The HIV IIIB strain includes isolates referred to elsewhere as LAI, LAV and BRU.

†Adjuvants included alum, monophoryl lipid A (MPL) in squalene (SAF2); alum, MF59 +/− MTP-PE, and lipid A-liposome encapsulated MPL with aluminum hydroxide.

‡After priming with live recombinant pox viruses expressing HIV gene products, volunteers were boosted with subunit gp160, with V3 loop peptide, or with both.

Data from Fast PE, Walker MC. Human trials of experimental AIDS vaccines. AIDS 1993;7:S147 and from Johnston MI. Candidate vaccines for the treatment of HIV infection. Pract Allergy Immunol 1994;9:6.

HIV-seronegative volunteers. The details of many of these AVEG studies have been reported elsewhere.[1,12–20]

The HIV immunogens tested in seronegative humans were derived initially from the HIV-1-IIIB strain (also referred to as HTLV-IIIB, LAI, LAV, or BRU strains) and later from HIV-MN or HIV-SF2 strains, which are more closely antigenically related to the clade B isolates recovered commonly from infected individuals in the United States and Europe. A combination of vaccine products rep-

resenting different clade B strains of HIV has also been tested. The only investigational vaccine tested that could be considered suitable antigenically for global trials contains V3 loop peptides representing five clades of HIV-1.

ADJUVANTS

Most HIV subunit or peptide HIV vaccine candidates have been formulated with alum, the only adjuvant licensed in the United States. Different adjuvants or antigen-presentation systems are needed to improve the capability of subunit and peptide vaccines to generate high titers of neutralizing antibodies and CD8+ CTLs.[7,21] To determine which adjuvants offer advantages in terms of tolerability and their ability to augment the vaccine's immunogenicity, the following adjuvants were combined with HIV-SF2 gp120 subunit vaccine and tested in seronegative volunteers[1,12]: alum, a microfluidized oil in water emulsion (MF59), MF59 with muramyl tripeptide palmitodyl ethanolamine (MTP-PE), incomplete Freund's adjuvant (IFA), monophosphoryl lipid A (MPL) in squalene (SAF2), and lipid A–liposome-encapsulated MPL with aluminum hydroxide. None of these adjuvants combined with this subunit vaccine appeared to offer a clear advantage over MF59 in terms of tolerability and the ability to induce significantly greater neutralizing antibody responses and CD8+ CTLs.[12] The MTP-PE and MPL-SAF2 adjuvants caused severe, self-limited, local and systemic reactions more often than other adjuvants, and they did not appreciably augment the neutralizing antibody responses.[12,22]

HIV-MN gp120 vaccine formulated with saponin (QS21), with or without alum, augmented the antibody responses to smaller (but not larger) concentrations of gp120 compared with alum alone.[12] HIV-IIIB and HIV-MN gp160 subunit vaccines formulated with deoxycholate and alum elicited strong, long-lasting gp160-specific lymphoproliferative responses.[13,23,24] Other novel antigen presentation systems under evaluation in AVEG trials include lipid moieties,[25] virus-like particles,[26] and microencapsulation of polymers of octameric HIV-MN V3 loop peptides that are administered orally in an effort to induce mucosal immune responses.

VACCINE REACTOGENICITY

Healthy HIV-seronegative volunteers 18 to 60 years of age who participate in AVEG trials of investigational vaccines are monitored for clinical and laboratory evidence of vaccine reactogenicity.[27] Local and systemic reactions are monitored during the week after each inoculation, and tests to evaluate hematologic, hepatic, and renal function and lymphoproliferative responses to recall antigens and mitogens are usually performed 2 weeks after each inoculation. All safety data are reviewed periodically by the AIDS Vaccine Data Safety and Monitoring Board.

The investigational HIV vaccines tested by the AVEG have been remarkably well tolerated by adults, children, and infants.[1,12,27] Self-limited, severe, local or systemic reactions to candidate vaccines in some volunteers have been associated mainly with certain investigational adjuvants, particularly MTP-PE, MPL-SAF2, deoxycholate, and acidic preparations of QS21.[12,22] Inoculation by scarification with live recombinant vaccinia gp160 resulted in a more prominent and longer-lasting lesion and regional lymphadenitis in vaccinia-naive volunteers than in vaccinia-immune volunteers, but these reactions were indistinguishable from those observed after

vaccination with the vaccinia virus parent.[17,28] An occlusive dressing was used to cover the inoculation site to prevent transmission of the vaccinia virus to unvaccinated contacts, especially those for whom vaccination with vaccinia virus is contraindicated, such as immunocompromised and HIV-infected persons and pregnant women. Live recombinant canarypox gp160, given by intramuscular injection, caused fewer local and systemic reactions than vaccinia gp160.[29] Moreover, canarypox virus recombinants are not transmissible, because the virus does not replicate in human cells.

The clinical and laboratory parameters monitored in the volunteers by the AVEG have remained normal[12,27] despite in vitro tests suggesting that HIV envelope glycoproteins might cause cytolytic activity against CD4 cells[30] and release cytokines that upregulate HIV gene expression[31] or cause antibody binding to CD4 cells that might enhance susceptibility to HIV infection and increase viral replication (ie, antibody-dependent enhancement [ADE]).[32] Antibodies reactive against an epitope of the HLA class I heavy chain[33] and ADE antibodies[34,35] were detected in recipients of 640 μg of baculovirus-expressed gp160/alum vaccine and in volunteers immunized with live vaccinia gp160 and with gp160/alum.[34] There is no in vivo evidence of disease caused by vaccine-induced ADE antibodies.[32] The numbers and percentages of CD4 and CD8 cells of uninfected vaccinees have remained stable, and lymphocyte blastogenic responses to mitogens and tetanus and *Candida* antigens have not been impaired.[1,12–20,22–24,27–29,36–41] The biologic relevance of ADE antibody and molecular mimicry elicited by HIV immunization is unknown.

Social discrimination is a concern for uninfected volunteers participating in HIV vaccine trials, because HIV vaccine recipients may develop a positive or indeterminate result in HIV antibody screening tests. Assays that use whole HIV lysates containing gp41 are more likely to detect antibodies to vaccine products containing gp160 than vaccines containing V3 loop peptides or gp120.[42] During the screening process, the risks of participating in HIV vaccine trials are discussed, including medical risks and social risks of acquiring antibody to HIV and possibly being identified falsely as HIV infected.[1,12] Only a few instances of social discrimination due to false-positive test results have been reported among the 1700 volunteers enrolled in the AVEG trials. Nevertheless, this risk has made it difficult to recruit uninfected volunteers for HIV vaccine trials.

IMMUNOGENICITY OF THE VACCINES EVALUATED IN VOLUNTEERS

Most of the vaccines tested in seronegative volunteers have elicited immunogen-specific binding antibodies in serum (and sometimes in saliva), as measured by ELISA, and HIV-specific lymphoproliferative responses, indicative of immunogen-specific B- and T-cell immune responses.[12–15,17–20,36–48] The level of vaccine-specific binding and neutralizing antibodies achieved has depended on the vaccine product and adjuvant formulation, dose of vaccine, the number of doses, and schedule of immunization. Maximal neutralizing antibody responses were usually achieved after three or four immunizations were given, and booster doses were administered at intervals of 3 to 6 months, rather than monthly.[12,18,24,47,49] Table 32.2-2 summarizes the functional immune responses after three to four immunizations with the highest dose of selected candidate HIV vaccines tested by the AVEG. The highest neutralizing antibody responses have been achieved by priming twice with live recombinant canarypox–HIV-MN gp160 and boosting twice with HIV-SF2 gp120/MF59.[50]

Selected serum samples from some vaccinees that neutralized tissue culture–grown HIV strains have failed to neutralize primary isolates of HIV, using a peripheral blood mononuclear cell (PBMC) assay.[12,14,29,42,51] However, this assay requires a set of conditions that do not mimic those in humans, such as stimulation of the patient's PBMCs in phytohemagglutinin and exposure of diluted sera to a high multiplicity of HIV strains. Whether the results of this in vitro neutralization assay or the results of in vivo neutralization studies, in which chimpanzees were immunized and subsequently challenged with primary isolates of HIV,[52] are predictors of protective immunity in humans remains to be determined in vaccine efficacy trials.

Recombinant HIV envelope vaccines have elicited CD4+ CTLs in a subset of volunteers,[53-57] but the role of CD4+ CTLs in vivo is unknown. In vitro, HIV vaccine-induced CD4+ CTLs (like CD8+ CTLs) can lyse virus-infected cells (but not innocent bystander CD4 cells) rapidly and efficiently[53] by a mechanism involving a preformed mediator that is functionally similar to the mechanism used by CD8+ CTLs.[58] Only a few vaccines have elicited HIV-specific CD8+ CTLs that could be detected transiently in human PBMCs on restimulation: live recombinant canarypox–HIV-MN gp160 in about 15% to 39% of volunteers[12,16,29,50]; vaccinia–HIV-IIIB gp160 in approximately 15% of vaccinia-naive volunteers[11,54,59]; and occasionally, V3 loop peptide conjugated to a purified protein derivative (PPD) carrier,[60] subunit HIV-SF2 gp120 formulated in MF59,[11] and synthetic p17.[41]

TABLE 32.2-2. *Neutralization antibody and cytotoxic T-cell responses of HIV-seronegative volunteers to selected HIV vaccine candidates*

HIV Strain and Dose of Vaccine	Manufacturer	Third Immunization		Fourth Immunization		Any Cytotoxic T-cell Response§	
		Proportion Responding	Reciprocal GMT (range)	Proportion Responding	Reciprocal GMT (range)	CD4+	CD8+
HIV-1 IIIB							
640 µg gp160	MicroGeneSys	5/19	8 (5–38)	9/19	11 (5–79)	+	–
200 µg gp160	ImmunoAG	3/20	7 (5–29)	14/18	21 (5–160)	+	–
300 µg gp120	Genentech	9/10	54 (5–168)	4/5	27 (5–90)	+	–
10^6–10^8 PFU/mL vaccinia gp160	Bristol Myers-Squibb						
and 640 µg gp160	MicroGeneSys			13/28†	12 (5–90)	++	++
HIV-1 MN							
500 µg V3	United Biomedical, Inc.	5/10	14 (5–102)			+/–	NA
600 µg gp120	Genentech	12/12	242 (90–978)	11/11	245 (78–486)	+	+/–
600 µg gp120‡	Genentech	26/27	319 (5–2048)		NA	+/–	+/–
10^6 TCID$_{50}$ canarypox gp160	Pasteur-Merieux/Virogenetics	4/11	12 (5–108)	4/10	13 (5–238)	++	++
HIV-1 SF2							
50 µg gp120	Biocine	7/7	233 (20–924)	6/6	102 (19–429)	+	+
50 µg gp120‡	Biocine	24/27	73 (5–1216)		NA	+/–	+/–
HIV-1 MN AND SF2							
10^6 TCID$_{50}$ canarypox gp160	Pasteur-Merieux/ Virogenetics	3/9 (MN)	12 (5–310)	9/9	354 (21–10,240)	++	++
and 50 µg SF gp120	Biocine	2/9 (SF2)	8 (5–93)	9/9	117 (23–438)		
10^7 TCID$_{50}$ canarypox gp160	Pasteur-Merieux Virogenetics	9/12 (MN)	43 (5–1223)			+++	+++
and 50 µg gp120	Biocine	10/19 (SF2)	15 (5–99)	28/28	165 (28–2560)		

GMT, geometric mean titer; NA, not available.

*The multiple-dose HIV-1 neutralization assay was performed using tissue culture–grown HIV strains as described in reference 18.

†Volunteers received three or four immunizations (one or two doses of vaccinia gp160 and one dose of gp160).

‡Data were obtained from a subset of participants in a phase II trial.

§ The score for cytotoxic T-cell response is an estimate, based on a score of ++++ for CTL responses in asymptomatic HIV-1 infected persons.

Subunit gp120 and gp160 Vaccines

As shown in Table 32.2-2, fully glycosylated HIV gp120 subunit products expressed in a Chinese hamster ovary cell system and formulated with alum[14,20] or with MF59[22] have generated serum neutralizing antibodies against tissue culture–grown homologous and heterologous HIV strains in higher titers and after fewer immunizations than yeast-expressed gp120/MF59 with or without MTP-PE,[12,39,61] baculovirus-expressed gp160/alum,[15,19] or vaccinia virus–expressed gp160/deoxycholate and alum.[13,24] Most recipients of three doses of 300 μg of HIV-IIIB gp120/alum, 300 μg or 600 μg of HIV-MN gp120/alum, and 25 μg or 50 μg of HIV-SF2 gp120/MF59 developed V3 loop and neutralizing antibody to the homologous HIV-1.[12,14,20,22,49] A fourth immunization with these vaccines broadened and increased the neutralizing antibody titers to different strains of HIV. Antibodies that block CD4 binding and antibodies that mediate antibody-dependent cellular cytotoxicity have also been observed in recipients of the fully glycosylated HIV-MN gp120/alum vaccine.[14]

The V3 loop and neutralizing antibody responses of adult volunteers immunized with HIV-IIIB gp120/alum, HIV-MN gp120/alum, and HIV-SF2/MF59 were remarkably similar to those observed in chimpanzees that had been immunized with the same products and subsequently resisted intravenous challenge with tissue culture–grown HIV or a primary isolate of HIV.[14,20,52,62] The postimmunization sera of all vaccinated chimpanzees failed to neutralize the PBMC-grown HIV-SF2 primary isolate, but all three immunized chimpanzees were protected against persistent HIV infection.[52] This finding suggests the PBMC assay for detection of neutralization of primary isolates is not sufficiently sensitive to predict in vivo protection against persistent HIV infection.

The gp160 vaccines tested by the AVEG have induced lower titers of homologous neutralizing antibody in a minority of the vaccinees and usually not until after administration of four or more immunizations with a high dose of vaccine.[12,13,19,24] The yeast-expressed, nonglycosylated HIV-SF2 gp120 (referred to as Env 2-3) formulated with MF59 with or without MTP-PE induced a low level of neutralizing antibodies in most subjects after three or four doses of this vaccine in an AVEG study,[61] but it had no effect in any of the subjects in another study.[39]

Live Vector Recombinant Vaccines

Immunization with a live recombinant poxvirus vector (eg, vaccinia virus, canarypox virus) expressing HIV gene products can prime the immune system for humoral and cell-mediated immune responses.[1,11,12] The priming effect of one or two doses of a live recombinant vaccinia or canarypox virus expressing HIV gp160 can be readily demonstrated by boosting once or twice with gp160, gp120, V3 loop peptide, or canarypox gp160.[11,12,18,29,47,50,59,63] As with other live virus vaccines, the dose of the live vector recombinant affects the infectivity and immunogenicity of these vaccines. All vaccinia-naive volunteers could be infected with one inoculation of 10^8 PFU/mL of vaccinia gp160 (HIVAC-1e), but two inoculations of 10^6 PFU/mL of HIVAC-1e were usually required to infect all vaccinees.[17] Even though canarypox virus is host-range restricted and therefore unable to replicate beyond a single cycle in human cells, priming with the higher dose (10^7 50% tissue culture infective dose [$TCID_{50}$]) of canarypox (ALVAC)–HIV-MN gp160 was more effective than priming with a 10-fold lower dose.[29,50] Volunteers primed with the higher dose of canarypox gp160 and boosted with gp120 developed HIV-specific CD4+ and CD8+ CTLs more frequently and higher titers of neutralizing antibodies to HIV-MN and HIV-SF2 (see Table 32.2-2).[50]

Prior immunity to vaccinia virus interferes with the immune responses induced by vaccinia-expressed gp160. The prime and boost combination of live recombinant HIVAC-1e and gp160 or gp120 has been much less immunogenic in persons previously vaccinated with smallpox vaccine than in vaccinia-naive individuals.[12,59] Even in vaccinia-naive volunteers, priming with vaccinia gp160 (HIVAC-1e) and boosting with subunit gp160 or gp120 subunit vaccines have induced only low levels of neutralization and CD4-blocking antibodies and CD8+ and CD4+ CTL activity in a subset.[12,18,54,57,59]

The first study to demonstrate that immune responses after immunization with live recombinant canarypox (ie, HIV-MN gp160) were not affected by preexisting immunity to vaccinia virus was conducted in France.[29] Twenty vaccinia-immune adults were immunized with 10^6 $TCID_{50}$ of canarypox–HIV-MN gp160 at 0 and 1 months and boosted with recombinant hybrid HIV-MN gp120/HIV-LAI gp41 subunit formulated with alum or IFA at 3 and 6 months. (The IFA adjuvant did not appear to alter the immune responses.) Neutralizing antibodies against HIV-MN were detected in 65% and 90% after the first and second booster with gp120/gp41, respectively, in titers up to 1 : 202; over one half still had neutralizing antibodies by 1 year. One half of the vaccinees also developed neutralizing antibodies against HIV-SF2. CD4+ or CD8+ CTLs were detected in as many as 39% of the 18 subjects tested. In contrast, very weak CD8+ CTLs were detected in 20% of 25 volunteers immunized with HIV-MN gp120/HIV-LAI gp41 in IFA or alum, some of whom were boosted with MN V3 peptide in alum or IFA.[64] The AVEG also found no difference in the ability of vaccinia-immune and vaccinia-naive volunteers to mount Env-specific CD8+ CTLs and neutralizing antibodies after priming with live recombinant canarypox gp160 and boosting with HIV-SF2 gp120/MF59.[12,16,50]

The combination of these two vaccines elicited CD8+ CTLs, CD4 blocking, and syncytia-inhibiting antibodies to HIV-MN more frequently and produced the highest levels of neutralizing antibodies to HIV-MN and HIV-SF2 observed in any AVEG trial (see Table 32.2-2). Considered together, these results indicated the HIV-SF2 gp120/MF59 subunit vaccine was a more effective booster immunization than the hybrid gp120/gp41 preparations in alum or IFA.[29]

In vaccinia-naive volunteers, the humoral immune responses appeared to be augmented by administering the HIVAC-1e twice and waiting for at least 6 months to boost with gp160.[18,47,59] Johnson and colleagues[10] found that the HLA class I–restricted CD8+ CTLs and the CD4+ CTLs induced by HIVAC-1e recognized at least five epitopes in relatively conserved regions of gp120 and gp41. The lymphoproliferative and binding antibody responses, but not neutralizing antibody, persisted for 1 year after the initial gp160 boost.[38] Reboosting with gp160 after 1 year elicited strong lymphoproliferative and binding antibody responses in all 12 vaccinees and low titers of neutralizing antibody in 4 vaccinees, but it produced no detectable CD8+ CTL activity.[38]

Peptide Vaccines

Two phase I trials of an octameric V3 loop peptide attached to a heptalysyl core (V3-MAPS) have been conducted by the AVEG. In the first trial, three immunizations with 500 µg of HIV-MN V3/alum induced low levels of neutralizing antibody titers against HIV-MN in 5 of 10 volunteers.[12,65] In the second trial, three doses of a multivalent V3/alum preparation containing the V3 from 15 strains, representing five major clades of HIV, elicited neutralizing antibodies to HIV-MN in only 5 of 15 vaccinees.[66] Both V3 peptide vaccines formulated in alum were minimally immunogenic.

In another trial in the United States, submicrogram doses of HIV-MN V3 peptide coupled to a PPD of *Mycobacterium tuberculosis*, administered intradermally at 0, 14, and 28 days to HIV-seronegative volunteers who were PPD skin-test positive or negative, induced homologous neutralizing antibodies and high affinity, long-lasting vaccine-specific IgG (mainly IgG3) in the sera of 8 of 9 volunteers.[60] IgA binding antibodies in serum and saliva were detected in most volunteers, and three vaccinees had HLA-B7–restricted MN-PPD–specific CTLs above background levels. The immunogenicity of this peptide was attributed to the PPD carrier.

A synthetic analog of p17, coupled to the carrier protein keyhole limpet hemocyanin (referred to as HGP30 vaccine) having an immunodominant T-cell epitope, elicited CD8+ CTLs in some seronegative volunteers in London.[41] In another trial in London, among 16 volunteers immunized with a yeast retrotransposon (Ty) p17/p24 virus-like particles/aluminum hydroxide, 11 developed anti-p24 antibodies, but only 5 mounted anti-p17 antibodies and none had Gag-specific responses.[37]

PHASE II TRIAL OF GP120 SUBUNIT VACCINES

The AVEG has conducted one phase II trial of the HIV-SF2 gp120/MF59 vaccine and the HIV-MN gp120/alum vaccine with 296 volunteers from low-risk and high-risk populations.[1,12] The high-risk participants included those using injection drugs, homosexual men engaging in unprotected

sexual intercourse, young adults 18 to 28 years with a recent sexually transmitted disease, and heterosexual partners of HIV-infected partners. The study participants underwent frequent, extensive counseling and education about HIV prevention, the experimental nature of the vaccine candidate, and the inclusion of a placebo in the trial. Behavioral changes among the participants were also monitored during the blinded trial and after the volunteers had been informed about whether they had received vaccine or placebo. The preliminary results of this trial indicated both gp120 vaccines were as safe and immunogenic in volunteers at high risk for acquiring HIV infection as in volunteers at a low risk for HIV infection.[12]

INTERCURRENT AND BREAKTHROUGH HIV INFECTIONS

It is not possible to acquire HIV infection from the investigational vaccines, nor can the results of a phase I or II trial determine whether a full immunization course with any of the investigational vaccines can confer protective immunity that alters the course of HIV infection. For this reason, volunteers participating in trials of investigational vaccines and adjuvants are counseled to avoid unprotected sexual or parenteral exposures. Despite the counseling, a small proportion of volunteers who have participated in phase I or II HIV vaccine trials, including some who claimed to have been at low risk for acquiring HIV infection initially, have become infected after engaging in high-risk behavior.[67,68] Based on a classification used in non-HIV vaccine trials, an infection is referred to as an intercurrent infection if it occurred in a placebo recipient or in a vaccinee before completion of the full course of immunizations or as a breakthrough infection if the vaccinee had received all scheduled immunizations before acquiring the infection.

By mid-1995, 20 of 1700 volunteers participating in several AVEG trials to evaluate a variety of doses of investigational HIV vaccines and adjuvant formulations had become infected with HIV.[12,67] These infected subjects had nine intercurrent infections (among four placebo recipients and five partially immunized subjects) and 11 breakthrough infections in volunteers who had received at least three immunizations of an investigational vaccine. The incidences of HIV infection were similar in the vaccinees and placebo controls (0.83 and 0.95 cases per 100 person-years, respectively). These infected volunteers are being followed closely to monitor their virologic and immunologic responses and their clinical courses.

A few breakthrough infections have been reported in other trials.[68,69] One of these volunteers who had received four injections with a low dose (25 µg) of HIV-SF2 gp120/MF59 vaccine over 1 year had had more than 230 different partners with whom he had oral sex (without condoms) or insertive or receptive anal intercourse (without condoms about 20% of the time) during the 17-month trial.[68] The IGPGRAF amino acid region of the V3 loop of the infecting virus was homologous to that in the gp120 vaccine. The immune responses induced by this dosage of vaccine were not sufficient to confer solid protection against infection resulting from the frequent intrarectal and oral challenges with HIV. Although the information obtained from this and other breakthrough infections occurring in phase I or II trials cannot be used to determine the efficacy of the vaccines, it may be possible to follow the infected vaccinated subjects and unvaccinated placebo recipients long term to obtain preliminary data on the antiviral effect of vaccine-induced immunity on virus load, disease progression, or both.

IMMUNOTHERAPY

Clinical trials of HIV vaccine products consisting of gp120, gp160, p24, p17, or inactivated HIV have been conducted using several hundred HIV-infected individuals, including some HIV-infected pregnant women and their infants (see Table 32.2-1). These vaccines appear to be quite safe, even when given repeatedly and at short intervals.[1,12,70–78] The baculovirus-expressed recombinant HIV-IIIB gp160 formulated in alum[70–74,77] and the whole inactivated HIV formulated in IFA have been tested most extensively.[76,79] In uncontrolled trials, the gp160 vaccine appeared to broaden binding antibody responses and boost cellular immune responses, as measured by lymphoproliferative responses, delayed-type hypersensitivity reactions, and CD4+ and CD8+ CTL activity.[71–74,80–82] The immune responses were more pronounced in those who received frequent booster immunizations and in those with higher CD4 levels.[71,74] Individuals who received six immunizations in the first year and a booster every 4 months thereafter maintained stable CD4 levels more noticeably during the first year than later.[71] In a controlled phase II trial conducted in Sweden, six doses of gp160 induced strong T-cell responses against a variety of HIV antigens and appeared to selectively increase the reactivity in the vaccinees to several non-HIV recall antigens.[72,73] Most of the 40 vaccinees had improved CD4 counts during the first year of the trial, and some had increases in neutralizing antibodies and antibody-dependent cellular cytotoxicity.

One controlled multicenter phase II trial of whole inactivated HIV formulated in alum has shown some evidence of an antiviral effect in asymptomatic HIV-infected persons.[76] Recipients of this inactivated HIV vaccine had a statistically significantly lower increase in viral DNA and stabilization in CD4 cells compared with placebo controls. Double blind, randomized, placebo-controlled, large-scale trials with long-term follow-up are needed to determine the clinical and antiviral effectiveness of immunotherapy. Such a phase III immunotherapy trial of an inactivated HIV vaccine will be conducted in the United States.

FUTURE TRIALS OF PREVENTIVE HIV VACCINES

Additional clinical trials will be required to identify more promising candidate HIV vaccines that are able to induce higher levels of antibodies that neutralize even primary isolates of HIV and strong CD8+ CTL activity in most uninfected volunteers. In the meantime, well-designed, placebo-controlled phase III efficacy trials of selected HIV vaccine candidates may provide answers to questions about the roles of different types of immunity induced by different HIV vaccines that cannot be addressed by in vitro assays, studies in imperfect animal models, and clinical trials with inadequate sample sizes.[5,83] Only two vaccine candidates have been tested in phase II trials sponsored by NIAID, and both have been found to be safe and immunogenic in several hundred low-risk and high-risk volunteers. However, the proposed criteria for proceeding from phase II trials to phase III trials sponsored by NIAID have changed as data have emerged and other priorities have competed for available funds. As a result, phase III efficacy trials of the gp120 vaccines in the United States have been delayed, despite the infrastructure that has been developed to conduct such trials and to search for correlates of immunity.[5]

The Global Programme on AIDS of the World Health Organization (WHO), in collaboration with two vaccine manufacturers and national scientists, is conducting phase I/II trials of the HIV-MN gp120/alum vaccine in Thailand and phase I/II trials of HIV-MN V3 peptide/alum vaccine in Thailand and Brazil. A consortium, consisting of the U.S. Department of Defense (DOD) scientists, a vaccine manufacturer, and Thai public health leaders and scientists, is developing a bivalent clade B HIV-SF2 gp120/MF59 and clade E gp120/MF59 vaccine to be tested in Thailand.[83] The WHO, NIAID, DOD, and several other organizations are also sponsoring research to prepare sites for vaccine efficacy trials in Thailand and other developing countries. This preparation includes virologic and epidemiologic surveillance, education and counseling, and phase I/II trials of candidate HIV vaccines and other interventions to reduce HIV transmission in populations with a high incidence of HIV infection.[3,5]

It is probably more feasible to conduct efficacy trials of HIV vaccine candidates in countries such as Thailand, where the incidence of HIV infection is high and the communities and the public health leaders consider the risk-benefit ratio favorable to HIV vaccine development. The Thai scientists and public health leaders, in collaboration with the WHO, the vaccine manufacturers, and DOD, are planning such trials to determine the role of immunity (ie, neutralizing antibodies and T-cell responses) induced by HIV clade B and E gp120 vaccines in reducing the rate of persistent infection, the virus load, and the disease burden in high-risk populations.

REFERENCES

1. Fast PE, Walker MC. Human trials of experimental AIDS vaccines. AIDS 1993;7:S147.
2. Parkman P, Hardegree MC. Regulation and testing of vaccines. In: Plotkin SA, Mortimer EA, eds. Vaccines. 2nd ed. Philadelphia: WB Saunders, 1994:889.
3. Esparaza J, Osmanov S, Kallings LO, et al. Planning for HIV vaccine trials: the World Health Organization perspective. AIDS 1991; 5:S159.

4. Dixon DO, Rida WN, Fast PE, Hoth DF. HIV vaccine trials; some design issues including sample size calculation. J Acquir Immune Defic Syndr 1993;6:485.
5. Hoth DF, Bolognesi DP, Corey L, Vermund SH. HIV vaccine development: a progress report. Ann Intern Med 1994;121:603.
6. Smith PG, Hayes RJ, Mulder DW. Epidemiological and public health considerations in the design of HIV vaccine trials. AIDS 1991;5:S105.
7. Karzon DT, Bolognesi DP, Koff WC. Development of a vaccine for the prevention of AIDS, a critical appraisal. Vaccine 1992;10:1039.
8. Sheppard H, Bridges SH, Mathieson BJ, Walker MC, Weinhold K. Conference on advances in AIDS vaccine development—1993. Summary: correlates of HIV immunity working group. AIDS Res Hum Retroviruses 1994;10:S171.
9. Berzofsky JA. Approaches and issues in the development of vaccines against HIV. J Acquir Immune Defic Syndr 1991;4:451.
10. Johnson RP, Hammond SA, Trocha A, Siliciano RF, Walker BD. Induction of a major histocompatibility complex class I–restricted cytotoxic T-lymphocyte response to a highly conserved region of human immunodeficiency virus type 1 (HIV-1) gp120 in seronegative humans immunized with a candidate HIV-1 vaccine. J Virol 1994;68:3145.
11. Walker MC, Walker BD, Mestecky J, Mathieson BJ. Conference on advances in AIDS vaccine development—1993. Summary: cytotoxic T cell immunity workshop. AIDS Res Hum Retroviruses 1994;10:S177.
12. Walker MC, Fast PE, Graham B, Belshe R, Dolin R. Phase I/II preventive vaccine trials. AIDS Res Hum Retroviruses 1995;11:1279.
13. Belshe RB, Clements ML, Dolin R, et al. Safety and immunogenicity of a fully glycosylated recombinant gp160 HIV-1 vaccine in human immunodeficiency virus type 1 vaccine in subjects at low risk of infection. J Infect Dis 1993;168:1387.
14. Belshe RB, Graham BS, Keefer MC, et al. Neutralizing antibodies to HIV-1 in seronegative volunteers immunized with recombinant gp120 from the MN strain of HIV-1. JAMA 1994;272:475.
15. Dolin R, Graham B, Greenberg S, et al. Safety and immunogenicity of an HIV-1 recombinant gp160 candidate vaccine in humans. Ann Intern Med 1991;114:119.
16. Egan MA, Pavlat WA, Tartaglia J, et al. Induction of human immunodeficiency virus type 1 (HIV-1)-specific cytolytic T lymphocyte responses in seronegative adults by a nonreplicating, host-range–restricted canarypox vector (ALVAC) carrying the HIV-1MN env gene. J Infect Dis 1995;171:1623.
17. Graham BS, Belshe RB, Clements ML, et al. Vaccination of vaccinia-naive adults with human immunodeficiency virus type 1 gp160 recombinant vaccinia virus in a blinded, controlled, randomized clinical trial. J Infect Dis 1992;166:244.
18. Graham BS, Matthews TJ, Belshe RB, et al. Augmentation of human immunodeficiency virus type 1 (HIV-1) neutralizing antibody by priming with gp160 recombinant vaccinia and boosting with rgp160 in vaccinia-naive adults. J Infect Dis 1993;167:533.
19. Keefer MC, Graham BS, Belshe RB, et al. Studies of high doses of a human immunodeficiency virus type 1 recombinant glycoprotein 160 candidate vaccine in HIV type 1-seronegative humans. AIDS Res Hum Retroviruses 1994;10:1713.
20. Schwartz DH, Gorse G, Clements ML, et al. Induction of HIV-1 neutralizing and syncytium-inhibiting antibodies in seronegative recipients of HIV-1 IIIB rgp120 subunit vaccine. Lancet 1993;342:69.
21. Alving CR, Glass M, Detrick B. Summary: adjuvants/clinical trials working groups. AIDS Res Hum Retroviruses 1992;8:1427.
22. Kahn JO, Sinangil F, Baenziger J, et al. Clinical and immunologic responses to human immunodeficiency virus (HIV) type 1SF2 gp120 subunit vaccine combined with MF59 adjuvant with or without muramyl tripeptide dipalmitoyl phosphatidylethanolamine in non–HIV-infected human volunteers. J Infect Dis 1994;170:1288.
23. Gorse GJ, Belshe RB, Newman FK, Frey SE. Lymphocyte proliferative responses following immunization with human immunodeficiency virus recombinant gp160. Vaccine 1992;10:383.
24. Gorse GJ, Schwartz DH, Graham BS, et al. HIV-1 recombinant gp160 vaccine given in accelerated dose schedules. Clin Exp Immunol 1994;98:178.
25. Deres K, Schild HJ, Wiesmuller KH, Jung G, Rammensee HG. In vivo priming of virus-specific cytotoxic T lymphocytes with synthetic lipopeptide vaccines. Nature 1989;342:561.
26. Rovinski B, Haynes JR, Cao SX, et al. Expression and characterization of genetically engineered human immunodeficiency virus-like particles containing modified envelope glycoproteins: implications for development of a cross-protective AIDS vaccine. J Virol 1992;66:4003.
27. Keefer MC, Belshe R, Graham B, et al. Phase I/II trials of preventive HIV vaccine candidates. Safety profile of HIV vaccination: first 1000 volunteers of AIDS Vaccine Evaluation Group. AIDS Res Hum Retroviruses 1994;10:S139.
28. Cooney EL, Collier AC, Greenberg PD, et al. Safety of and immunological response to a recombinant vaccinia virus vaccine expressing HIV envelope glycoprotein. Lancet 1991;337:567.
29. Pialoux G, Excler J-L, Riviere Y, et al. A prime-boost approach to HIV preventive vaccine using a recombinant canarypox virus expressing glycoprotein 160 (MN) followed by a recombinant glycoprotein 160 (MN/LAI). AIDS Res Hum Retroviruses 1995;11:373.
30. Siliciano RF, Lawton T, Knall C, et al. Analysis of host-virus interactions in AIDS with anti-gp120 T cell clones: effect of HIV sequence variation and a mechanism for CD4 cell depletion. Cell 1988;54:561.
31. Bollinger RC, Quinn TC, Liu AY, et al. Cytokines from vaccine-induced HIV-1 specific cytotoxic T lymphocytes: effects on viral replication. AIDS Res Hum Retroviruses 1993;9:1067.
32. Mascola JR, Mathieson BJ, Zack PH, et al. Summary report: workshop on the potential risks of antibody-dependent enhancement in human HIV vaccine trials. AIDS Res Hum Retroviruses 1993;9:1175.
33. De Santis C, Robbioni P, Longhi R, et al. Cross-reactive response to human immunodeficiency virus type 1 (HIV-1) gp120 and HLA class I heavy chains induced by receipt of HIV-1–derived envelope vaccines. J Infect Dis 1993;168:1396.
34. Montefiori DM, Graham BS, Kliks S, et al. Serum antibodies to HIV-1 in recombinant vaccinia virus recipients boosted with purified recombinant gp160. J Clin Immunol 1993;12:429.
35. Haubrich RH, Takeda A, Koff W, Smith G, Ennis FA. Studies of antibody-dependent enhancement of human immunodeficiency virus (HIV) type 1 infection mediated by Fc receptors using sera from recipients of a recombinant gp160 experimental HIV-1 vaccine. J Infect Dis 1992;165:545.
36. Clerici M, Tacket CO, Via CS, et al. Immunization with subunit human immunodeficiency virus vaccine generates stronger T helper cell immunity than natural infection. Eur J Immunol 1991;21:1345.
37. Martin SJ, Vyakarnam A, Cheingsong-Popov R, et al. Immunization of human HIV-seronegative volunteers with recombinant p17/p24: Ty virus-like particles elicits HIV-1 p24-specific cellular and humoral immune responses. AIDS 1993;7:1315.
38. McElrath MJ, Corey L, Berger D, et al. Immune responses elicited by recombinant vaccinia-human immunodeficiency virus (HIV) envelope and HIV envelope protein: analysis of the durability of responses and effect of repeated boosting. J Infect Dis 1994;169:41.
39. Wintsch J, Chaignat C, Braun DG, et al. Safety and immunogenicity of a genetically engineered human immunodeficiency virus vaccine. J Infect Dis 1991;163:219.
40. Tacket CO, Baqar S, Munoz C, et al. Lymphoproliferative responses to mitogens and HIV-1 envelope glycoprotein among volunteers vaccinated with recombinant gp160. AIDS Res Hum Retroviruses 1990;6:535.
41. Naylor PH, Sztein MB, Wada S, et al. Preclinical and clinical studies on immunogenicity and safety of the HIV-1 p17-based synthetic peptide AIDS vaccine—HGP-30-KLH. Int J Immunopharmacol 1991;13:117.
42. Graham BS. Serological responses to candidate AIDS vaccines. AIDS Res Hum Retroviruses 1994;10:S145.
43. Gorse GJ, Rogers JH, Perry JE, et al. HIV-1 recombinant gp160 vaccine induced antibodies in serum and saliva. Vaccine 1995;13:209.
44. Keefer MC, Bonnez W, Roberts NJ Jr, Dolin R, Reichman RC. Human immunodeficiency virus (HIV-1) gp160-specific lymphocyte proliferative responses of mononuclear leukocytes from HIV-1 recombinant gp160 vaccine recipients. J Infect Dis 1991;163:448.
45. Picard O, Achour A, Bernard J, et al. A 2-year follow-up of an anti-HIV immune reaction in HIV-1 gp160-immunized healthy seronegative humans: evidence for persistent cell-mediated immunity. J Acquir Immune Defic Syndr 1992;5:539.
46. Viscidi R, Ellerbeck E, Garrison L, et al. Characterization of serum antibody responses to recombinant HIV-1 gp160 vaccine by enzyme immunoassay. AIDS Res Hum Retroviruses 1990;6:1251.
47. Graham BS, Gorse GJ, Schwartz DH, et al. Determinants of antibody response after recombinant gp160 boosting in vaccinia-naive volunteers primed with gp160-recombinant vaccinia virus. J Infect Dis 1994;170:782.

48. Funkhouser A, Clements ML, Slome S, Clayman B, Viscidi R. Antibodies to recombinant gp160 in mucosal secretions and sera of persons infected with HIV-1 and seronegative vaccine recipients. AIDS Res Hum Retroviruses 1993;9:627.
49. Gorse GJ. Phase I/II trials of preventive HIV vaccine candidates. Dose and schedule: summary. AIDS Res Hum Retroviruses 1994;10:S141.
50. Clements ML, Schwartz D, Siliciano R, et al. HIV immunity induced by canarypox-MN gp160, SF2 gp120, or both. (Abstract) In: Scientific program and abstracts. Austin, TX: American Society for Virology, 1995:185.
51. Mascola JR, Snyder SW, Weislow OS, et al. Immunization with envelope subunit vaccine products elicits neutralizing antibodies against laboratory-adapted but not primary isolates of human immunodeficiency virus type 1. AIDS Res Hum Retroviruses (in press).
52. Berman PW, Eastman DJ, Nakamura GR, et al. Apparent protection of MN-rgp120 immunized chimpanzees from infection with a primary isolate of HIV-1. In: Vaccines 95. Molecular approaches to the control of infectious diseases. Plainview, NY: Cold Spring Harbor Laboratory Press, 1995:143.
53. Orentas RJ, Hildreth JEK, Obah E, et al. An HIV envelope protein vaccine induces CD4 human cytolytic T cells active against HIV-infected cells. Science 1990;248:1234.
54. Hammond SA, Bollinger RC, Stanhope PE, et al. Comparative clonal analysis of HIV-1 specific CD4 and CD8 cytolytic T lymphocytes isolated from seronegative humans immunized with candidate HIV-1 vaccines. J Exp Med 1992;176:1531.
55. Stanhope PE, Clements ML, Siliciano RF. Human cytolytic T-lymphocyte responses to an HIV-1 gp160 subunit vaccine. J Infect Dis 1993;168:92.
56. Stanhope PE,, Liu AY, Pavlat W, Pitha PM, Clements ML, Siliciano RF. An HIV-1 envelope protein vaccine elicits a functionally complex human CD4+ T cell response that includes cytolytic T lymphocytes. J Immunol 1993;150:4672.
57. Siliciano RF, Bollinger RC, Callahan KM, et al. Clonal analysis of T-cell responses to the HIV-1 envelope proteins in AIDS vaccine recipients. AIDS Res Hum Retroviruses 1992;8:1359.
58. Miskovsky EP, Liu AY, Pavlat W, et al. Studies of the mechanism of cytolysis by HIV-1–specific CD4+ human CTL clones induced by candidate AIDS vaccines. J Immunol 1994;153:2787.
59. Cooney EL, Corey L, Hu SL, et al. Enhanced immunity to human immunodeficiency virus (HIV) envelope elicited by a combined vaccine regimen consisting of priming with a vaccinia recombinant expressing HIV envelope and boosting with gp160-protein. Proc Natl Acad Sci USA 1993;90:1882.
60. Rubinstein A, Goldstein H, Pettoello-Mantovani M, Mizralhi Y, et al. Safety and immunology of a V3 loop synthetic peptide conjugated to purified protein derivative in HIV-seronegative volunteers. AIDS 1995;9:243.
61. Keefer MC, Graham BS, McElrath MJ, et al. Safety and immunogenicity of env 2-3, a human immunodeficiency virus type-1 candidate vaccine in combination with a novel adjuvant, MTP-PE/MF59. AIDS Res Hum Retroviruses (in press).
62. Berman PW, Eastman DJ, Wilkes DM, et al. Comparison of the immune response to recombinant gp120 in humans and chimpanzees. AIDS 1994;8:591.
63. Zagury D, Bernard J, Cheynier R, et al. A group specific anamnestic immune reaction against HIV-1. Nature 1988;332:728.
64. Salmon-Céron D, Excler JL, Sicard D, et al. Safety and immunogenicity of a recombinant HIV-1 gp160 followed by a V3 synthetic peptide in HIV negative volunteers. AIDS Res Hum Retroviruses 1995;11:1479.
65. Gorse GJ, Keefer M, Weinhold K, et al. Evaluation of HIV-1 MN V3 octameric peptide vaccine. Abstract. Presented at 7th Annual Meeting, National Cooperative Vaccine Development Groups for AIDS. Reston, VA, 1994.
66. Keefer MC, Lambert JS, Koff W, et al. A phase I study of multivalent HIV-1 peptide vaccine in HIV-1 seronegative subjects. Abstract. Presented at Infectious Diseases Society of America Annual Meeting. San Francisco, CA, 1995.
67. Belshe RB, Bolognesi DP, Clements ML, et al. HIV infection in vaccinated volunteers. (Letter) JAMA 1994;272:431.
68. Kahn JO, Steimer KS, Baenziger J, et al. Clinical, immunologic and virologic observations related to human immunodeficiency virus (HIV) type 1 infection in a volunteer in an HIV-1 vaccine clinical trial. J Infect Dis 1995;171:1343.
69. Corey L, McElrath J, Greenberg P, Mullins J. Acquisition of HIV and subsequent immunodeficiency despite vaccination. Abstract. Presented at Laboratory of Tumor Cell Biology Annual Meeting. Rockville, MD, 1994.
70. Birx DL, Redfield RR. HIV vaccine therapy. Int J Immunopharmacol 1991;13:129.
71. Johnston MI. Candidate vaccines for the treatment of HIV infection. Pract Allergy Immunol 1994;9:6.
72. Wahren B, Sandstrom E, Wigzell H. Properties of an HIV vaccine. Nature 1993;362:505.
73. Wahren B, Bratt G, Persson C, et al. Improved cell-mediated immune responses in HIV-1 infected asymptomatic individuals after immunization with envelope glycoprotein gp160. J Acquir Immune Defic Syndr 1994;7:220.
74. Redfield R, Birx DL, Ketter N, et al. A phase I evaluation of the safety and immunogenicity of vaccination with recombinant gp160 in patients with early human immunodeficiency virus infection. N Engl J Med 1991;324:1677.
75. Blick G, Crook SW, Buchanan S. Therapeutic vaccines in HIV infection. AIDS Reader 1993;3:114.
76. Trauger RJ, Ferre F, Daigle AE, et al. Effect of immunization with inactivated gp120-depleted human immunodeficiency virus type 1 (HIV-1) immunogen on HIV-1 immunity, viral DNA, and percentage of CD4 cells. J Infect Dis 1994;169:1256.
77. Zunich KM, Lane HC, Davey RT, et al. Phase I/II studies of the toxicity and immunogenicity of recombinant gp160 and p24 vaccines in HIV-infected individuals. AIDS Res Hum Retroviruses 1992;8:1335.
78. Gradon JD, Schooley RT, Schnittman SM. Report on the therapeutic vaccine workshop: National Cooperative Vaccine Development Group meeting. AIDS Res Hum Retroviruses 1993;9:S55.
79. Turner JL, Trauger RJ, Daigle AE, Carlo DJ. HIV-immunogen induction of HIV-1–specific delayed-type hypersensitivity: results of a double-blind adjuvant-controlled, dose-ranging trial. AIDS 1994;8:1429.
80. Kundu SK, Katzenstein D, Moses LE, Merigan TC. Enhancement of human immunodeficiency virus (HIV)-specific CD4 and CD8 cytotoxic T-lymphocyte activities in HIV-infected asymptomatic patients given recombinant gp160 vaccine. Proc Natl Acad Sci USA 1992;89:11204.
81. Nordlund S, Eriksson L, Volovitz F, et al. Improved cell-mediated immune responses in HIV-1–infected asymptomatic individuals after immunization with envelope glycoprotein gp160. J Acquir Immune Defic Syndr 1994;7:220.
82. Biselli R, Loomis LD, Del Bono V, Burke DS, Redfield RR, Birx DL. Immunization of HIV-infected patients with rgp160: modulation of anti-rgp120 antibody spectrotype. J Acquir Immune Defic Syndr 1994;7:1016.
83. Mascola JR, McNeil JG, Burke DS. AIDS vaccines: are we ready for human efficacy trials? JAMA 1994;272:488.

AIDS: Biology, Diagnosis, Treatment and Prevention, fourth edition, edited by Vincent T. DeVita, Jr., Samuel Hellman, and Steven A. Rosenberg. Lippincott–Raven Publishers, © 1997

CHAPTER **33**

Acquired Immunodeficiency Syndrome and Human Rights

Jonathan M. Mann

The relation between acquired immunodeficiency syndrome (AIDS) and human rights is essential for understanding the societal response to the pandemic. Two dimensions of this association have emerged in sequential fashion. First, violations of human rights have occurred against persons infected with the human immunodeficiency virus (HIV) and persons with AIDS; this is a *consequence* of the pandemic. Through an analysis of successes and failures in HIV prevention and the evolution of the pandemic, it has become evident that a lack of respect for human rights and dignity is also a *root cause* of the pandemic. These two aspects of human rights and AIDS—as effect and as cause—are essential for the design of more effective prevention and control efforts, and they will continue to have a profound impact on how public health authorities understand and conduct their mission of promoting and protecting population health.

To consider these complex and evolving associations, it is first necessary to summarize information about modern human rights. Human rights is not a subject usually taught in medical or public health schools, and health workers often have only a rudimentary knowledge of the subject.

BASIC HUMAN RIGHTS

The human rights movement has a long early history, including philosophic efforts to define the natural rights of all persons, international campaigns such as abolitionism against slavery, and issuance of key documents such as the Declaration of the Rights of Man and the Citizen in France (1789) and the U.S. Declaration of Independence.

The modern period of human rights started after the Second World War in response to the atrocities of the Holocaust

in Europe. The same determination to prevent recurrent human tragedy that led to the creation of the United Nations (1945) also resulted in a dramatic change in the definition and meaning of human rights. The promotion of human rights was identified as one of the four principal purposes of the United Nations. In 1948, and thanks in large part to Eleanor Roosevelt, the Universal Declaration of Human Rights was adopted by the U.N. General Assembly as "a common standard of achievement for all peoples and all nations."

All of the rights in the Universal Declaration are based on the central idea that "all human beings are born free and equal in dignity and rights." Accordingly, persons must not be discriminated against on the basis of race, sex, religion, social class, or other such categories. The Universal Declaration then lists the human rights. One reason for the power of human rights is their accessibility; according to Eleanor Roosevelt, the Universal Declaration was intended for ordinary persons, not just jurists or philosophers.

The rights described in the Universal Declaration are often divided into two categories. The civil and political rights deal with rights that protect the individual against the power of the state. These rights include the right not to be tortured or subjected to cruel, inhuman, or degrading treatment or punishment; the right not to be subjected to arbitrary interference with privacy, family, home, or correspondence; equality before the law; and the right to freedom of thought, conscience, and religion. Because much public health work involves governmental action, directly or indirectly, it is particularly important for public health workers to be cognizant of and literate about human rights. The second category involves economic, social, and cultural rights, including such areas as education, social security, work, and a standard of living "adequate for the health and well-being of himself and his family, including food, clothing, housing and medical care . . . ." The Universal Declaration does not call for economic equality; it instead mandates

Jonathan M. Mann, Francois-Xavier Bagnoud Professor of Health and Human Rights, Professor of Epidemiology and International Health, Harvard School of Public Health, Boston, MA .

a universal minimum, adequate to provide the necessities of life for all. These basic rights were further elaborated in two international covenants and then incorporated in a large number of treaties and declarations on specific issues (eg, discrimination against women, rights of children, refugees).

However, the modern view of human rights goes beyond a list. Several core principles apply to all internationally protected rights:

Rights are inherent in persons simply because they are human.

Rights are inalienable; they cannot be granted nor taken away by a government.

Rights are universal, applying equally to all persons in all places at all times. This also means that violations of rights in any country are of relevance to all.

Rights are individual and focus on the relationships between individuals and their governments.

Rights represent claims on society; governments must strive to realize these rights.

Rights are so important that they are generally considered to be inviolable; they "trump" other social goods, although public health may constitute an important exception.

Rights are inseparable and indivisible; there is no hierarchy of rights.

Human rights represent a set of beliefs about persons and what is required to promote and protect their well-being. Rights are a set of statements that cannot be proved or disproved empirically. Rights derive their legitimacy by having been agreed on and voted on by the nations of the world. Because the list of rights is human made and not derived from revelation or religious authority, it can change and evolve.

The human rights movement has changed dramatically since 1945. For the first time in history, a set of human rights has been defined at the international level, providing a universal, secular description of the preconditions for human well-being, and international and national institutions and organizations have been created to promote and protect these rights.

HUMAN RIGHTS VIOLATIONS AS A CONSEQUENCE OF THE PANDEMIC

In the early 1980s, discovery of AIDS prompted a public health response that was rather traditional, derived from the long history of efforts to prevent and control communicable diseases.[1,2]

Initially, many governments proposed instituting such classic public health measures as mandatory reporting, surveillance, contact tracing, isolation, and quarantine.[3] After an HIV antibody test became available, calls for mass and mandatory screening became widespread.[2] Compulsory or mass screening has been mandated for many groups in many countries, including commercial sex workers (eg, Indonesia, Belize); prisoners (eg, Hungary, Sri Lanka, Uruguay); injecting drug users (eg, Bulgaria, Thailand); homosexual men (eg, El Salvador, Philippines, former USSR); pregnant women (eg, Mexico, Papua New Guinea); persons with sexually transmitted diseases (eg, Dominican Republic; Vietnam); all hospitalized patients (eg, Burma, Nigeria); persons with hemophilia (eg, Kuwait, Panama); seafarers (eg, China, Tunisia); airline personnel (eg, former Czechoslovakia); and truck drivers (eg, Bhutan, Sudan).[2] The practice of requiring HIV testing for returning nationals, prospective immigrants, migrants, foreign students, tourists, and refugees has also been widespread.[2]

These measures, adopted and adapted in the context of traditional public health approaches to control communicable diseases in general and sexually transmitted diseases in particular, were often opposed on human rights grounds. In the past, such resistance to public health measures was somewhat unusual; in most countries, the primacy of public health protection over individual claims was recognized, in practice, in the law, or in both circumstances.[3]

In many industrialized countries, the AIDS epidemic emerged at a time of broader societal controversy and struggle for respect and realization of human rights. For example, in the United States, the civil rights movements of the 1960s, progress toward reducing gender discrimination, and the emerging gay rights movement helped emphasize the importance of human rights. The initial recognition of AIDS within the community of gay men in the United States and its rapid and unfortunate characterization as a "gay plague" brought a community with recent experience in fighting discrimination based on human rights principles into direct conflict with those public health authorities seeking to apply to the new problem of AIDS the prevention and control practices derived from traditional public health.

A new element was added that served to help reconcile the conflicting claims of public health and human rights. Public health officials became increasingly aware that persons suspected or confirmed to be HIV infected were subjected to coercive and discriminatory treatment, including dismissal from work or school; denial of health care; and imprisonment, beatings, or physical harassment. Fears of such treatment had become a major barrier to voluntary participation by persons at higher risk of HIV infection in HIV prevention programs. The justified fear of profound personal and social consequences led those most likely to be infected to avoid contact with governmental agencies, health clinics, or other settings in which knowledge of HIV status could become known to governmental authorities or to the public. Alternatively, when HIV testing services were offered in a manner that truly protected confidentiality (eg, by providing the person with a number so the linkage between a blood sample and a person could only be made by the tested person), the participation of higher-risk persons in testing programs increased.

This global experience prompted a reexamination of public health strategies, leading to a public health rationale for preventing discrimination toward HIV-infected persons and those with AIDS.[4] Recognition of the need to respect human rights and dignity in the design and conduct of HIV prevention programs emerged from practical field experience and concrete situations, rather than representing a "capitulation" to human rights advocates or an ideologic commitment to human rights. There was little or no tradition within the public health sector of special concern for or knowledge about human rights as a primary societal value.

The evolution of this concept can be delineated within the evolving policies of the World Health Organization (WHO), as part of the global AIDS strategy developed by that organization and approved by virtually all countries. In May 1987, in a consultation on HIV testing of international travelers, border controls and mandatory testing were rejected on purely pragmatic and operational grounds.[5] At the World Health Assembly in May 1987, the concept of the "third epidemic" of political, social, and cultural reaction to HIV and AIDS was identified as a vital part of the pandemic itself.[6] (The first epidemic was HIV infection; the second was the illness of AIDS, occurring years after the first).

In December 1987, a pamphlet issued by the WHO Global Program on AIDS stated that "AIDS prevention and control strategies can be implemented effectively and efficiently . . . in a manner that respects and protects human rights."[7] It continued, "there is no public health rationale to justify isolation, quarantine, or any discriminatory measures based solely on the fact that a person is suspected or known to be HIV-infected . . . [and] exclusion of persons suspected or known to be HIV-infected would be unjustified in public health terms and would seriously jeopardize . . . efforts to prevent the spread of HIV." The pamphlet concluded: "The avoidance of discrimination against persons known or suspected to be HIV-infected is important for AIDS prevention and control; failure to prevent such discrimination may endanger public health."[7]

After approval of this concept at the London AIDS Summit (January 1988), the World Health Assembly formally incorporated these ideas into WHO policy in May 1988. The Assembly Declaration reiterated the necessity for antidiscrimination and concluded that "respect for the human rights and dignity of HIV-infected people and people with AIDS . . . is vital to the success of national AIDS prevention and control programs."[8]

These policies were translated into programmatic terms through WHO's work to support and assist national AIDS programs throughout the world. By late 1988, more than 140 countries had received support from WHO in adapting a generic model of HIV prevention to specific national and community circumstances.[9] This model, described as the "prevention triad," included two elements adapted from traditional public health practice: information and education and the health and social services linked to the information (eg, condom supply, drug treatment services, confidential testing and counseling services). The third element was nondiscrimination toward HIV-infected persons and those with AIDS, identified as critical to the program's success as the other two elements.

Unfortunately, in many countries and communities, the objective of preventing such discrimination has frequently not been achieved. Discriminatory practices, officially sanctioned and unofficial, continue to occur, particularly in the domains of employment, access to health care, and housing. Discrimination continues within public health programs ostensibly created to help prevent HIV transmission and within society in general. This distinction is important, because many public health programs are created and implemented by state authorities, for whom the obligation to protect human rights and prevent discrimination is paramount.[1] Governmental responsibility for discrimination against HIV-infected persons and those with AIDS by nongovernmental bodies, such as private businesses, hospitals, schools, insurance schemes and other settings, depends in part on the extent to which these bodies are subject to governmental licensing and other regulation.

The governmental responsibility for "private" discrimination, occurring between individuals outside official settings is less clear. However, governments often play an important role in creating or sustaining the general conditions within which discrimination flourishes. This may occur through condoning or failing to protest discriminatory practices or by failing to provide victims with adequate channels for legal redress (this argument parallels recent thinking about the human rights dimensions of rape).[10]

The critical point is that for the first time, the principle of nondiscrimination became an integral part of an official strategy for preventing and controlling communicable disease or for any public health problem. Efforts to reduce HIV-related discrimination will continue to be important for effective HIV and AIDS prevention and control, as well as underscoring the pernicious and often unrecognized impact of other forms of health status–related discrimination, such as involves cancer, obesity, and various physical disabilities.[1]

HUMAN RIGHTS AS A ROOT CAUSE OF THE PANDEMIC

The second and more comprehensive understanding of the relation between AIDS and human rights emerged through two related analyses of the evolution of the pandemic and of successes and failures of HIV prevention programs.

The HIV or AIDS pandemic is an enormously complex mosaic, composed of many different epidemics at the national and community level.[2] However, as the pandemic has evolved within each society and globally, a new common denominator among the different epidemics gradually appeared. Because HIV's initial appearance within a society could occur through many different channels, the early history of each epidemic may be strikingly different, but just as the natural history of HIV-infected persons can only be clarified over time, so the societal natural history of the pandemic requires time (perhaps decades) to evolve.

The emerging commonality among epidemics worldwide can be described as a societal risk factor for HIV infection or as a critical source of vulnerability to HIV infection at a population level. Those populations at greatest risk within each society are those who before the arrival of the HIV pandemic were marginalized, stigmatized, and discriminated against.[11] For example, in the United States, the epidemic is moving steadily and increasingly into the "underclasses," including ethnic and racial minorities, residents of inner cities, the homeless, injection drug users, and women. In 1993, 55% of new AIDS cases were from minority populations.[12] That same year, the AIDS rate was about five times higher for African-American men and three times higher for Hispanic men than for white men; rates among African-American and Hispanic women were 15 and six times higher, respectively, than for white women.[12] Although 7% of new AIDS cases in the United States in 1985 were among women, this proportion had more than doubled (to 18%) by 1994.[13]

Similarly in France, the force of the AIDS epidemic focused on "les exclus"—those excluded from mainstream French society, including illegal immigrants, the poor, homeless, drug users, and others falling through the interstices of the social support net. In Brazil, although the epidemic first appeared among members of the elite society, HIV has become a raging epidemic among heterosexual men and women in the favelas (slums) surrounding Rio de Janeiro and Sao Paulo. Earlier observations of higher rates of HIV or AIDS among elites in Africa have proven to be temporary phenomena, replaced in most cases by a tremendous and expanding impact on poor and socially disadvantaged populations.

With time, the AIDS pandemic moves in a predictable direction within each society. Although the details vary, the common factor is epidemic intensification among those populations within each society who have traditionally been marginalized and discriminated against, among those whose human rights and dignity have been relatively less respected and protected.

These observations, identifying human rights and dignity as core issues for understanding the AIDS pandemic, have been complemented and reinforced by analysis of the successes and failures of HIV prevention programs worldwide. At one level, there have been important successes. When the prevention triad is sensitively and creatively implemented, HIV prevention can be as effective or even more effective than any public health programs seeking to influence behavior. Pilot projects and community-based programs have succeeded in changing sexual behaviors and reducing HIV incidence.[14,15] However, important failures have occurred at several levels. First, political commitment to AIDS prevention is plateauing or declining in many countries, even in the face of an expanding epidemic.[2] Second, a careful analysis of prevention strategies reveals major gaps, which are not directly related to resource availability, between theory and practice.

The Global AIDS Policy Coalition (GAPC) is an independent international research group based at the Harvard School of Public Health. The GAPC has highlighted the ways in which societal discrimination undermines and inter-

feres with each element of the prevention triad.[16] Marginalized groups are less likely to receive information and education adapted to their needs; they are less likely to have access to the range of health and social services needed to support HIV prevention; and they are less likely to organize effectively and otherwise participate in determining HIV or AIDS policy and resource allocations.

Another approach to the differences between programmatic intent and societal reality has focused on HIV infection and AIDS among women. Elias and Heise deconstructed the standard AIDS prevention strategy to demonstrate how the prevention objectives are out of touch with the realities of women's lives.[17] For example, they considered how the prevention recommendation to "reduce the number of sexual partners" fails for women on three levels. First, women's risk is highly dependent on their partner's sexual behavior. In Sao Paulo, Brazil, one half of new AIDS cases among women are among married, monogamous women; in Kigali, Rwanda, about one fifth of HIV-infected women had had only one lifetime sex partner. Second, having multiple sexual partners is often the key to survival in developing countries. Sexual partnerships provide women with access to resources, including education, credit, and jobs. Most commercial sex workers are involved with this activity for survival; reasons for entry into sex work often include having survived rape, being divorced or widowed, or having been rejected as infertile. Third, women are often unable to exercise control over their sexual activity, principally because of the threats of violence or divorce. Worldwide, between one third and one half of women report having been beaten by their partner and in such situations, women frequently do not have legal recourse or possibility for redress. Because divorce is often a unilateral decision by the man, leaving a women without property or social standing, the threat of divorce may be sufficient to lead a woman to have unwanted or unprotected sexual intercourse with her husband, even if both know he is HIV infected.[1]

These practical observations led to recognition that fundamental violations of human rights and dignity underlie the realities of women's lives, which create or heighten their vulnerability to becoming HIV-infected.[18] This form of analysis, quite similar to the discussions of reproductive health and rights that have transformed the global approach to population control, emphasize the critical linkage between human rights and health.[1] Taken together, these observations and analyses have prompted a substantial critique of the existing WHO global AIDS strategy.

AIDS, HUMAN RIGHTS, AND PUBLIC HEALTH

The first global AIDS strategy defined the problem of prevention and the reality of the pandemic in essentially individual terms. The goal was individual behavior change; the strategy involved providing the prevention triad of information and education, health and social services, and nondiscrimination toward HIV-infected persons and persons with AIDS to populations through national and community programs. Programs based on this approach have been highly successful at a community or pilot-project level.

However, such programs have encountered two fundamental problems. First, these programs, even when quite successful, have not been widely disseminated or generalized. For example, a successful project for reducing HIV incidence among commercial sex workers in Nairobi had been copied in only one other city in Kenya as of mid-1993, and effective needle-exchange programs in the United States still face formidable barriers to widespread application. This striking failure to apply lessons learned about HIV prevention suggests that something about these projects is resisted by governments or societies.

The second problem is that, despite these efforts, the pandemic continues to expand. According to estimates of the GAPC, the cumulative number of HIV-infected persons worldwide increased from about 100,000 in 1980 to 10 million in 1990 and 26 million (including 23 million adults and 3 million children) by January 1, 1995. Although few HIV infections had occurred in southeast Asia as of the mid-1980s, by 1995, an estimated 4.5 million persons had become HIV-infected, which is more than twice the number infected in all the industrialized countries combined. GAPC projections for the year 2000, although difficult and highly uncertain, estimate about 60 to 80 million cumulative infections.

In the face of an expanding and dynamic pandemic, the limited success of the existing, program-based, individual-focused strategy is challenged by new awareness of the societal dimensions of vulnerability to HIV. The tragic dilemma of the married, monogamous woman in East Africa who cannot refuse unwanted or unprotected intercourse from her husband, even when she knows he is HIV-infected, symbolizes the limits of what public health programs based on information and education and health and social services can provide. Her vulnerability stems directly from the status of her rights and dignity. Throughout the world and for many persons, real choices regarding HIV prevention are tightly constrained by societal respect or lack of respect for human rights.

In 1993, the GAPC published a booklet entitled, *Towards a New Health Strategy for AIDS,* which integrated human rights and HIV prevention.[16] By viewing vulnerability to HIV as a consequence of programmatic inadequacy and underlying human rights status, a new, two-part AIDS strategy was proposed. First, existing approaches, based on the prevention triad, needed to be strengthened, including careful attention to eliminating discrimination within the design and implementation of such programs. For example, societally marginalized and discriminated-against groups need to be sought out and included in information or education efforts and the organization of relevant health and social services. The second part of the new strategy was based on the concept that "to the extent that societies can reduce discrimination and promote respect for rights and dignity, they will be successful in preventing HIV transmission [and] caring for those who are infected and ill . . . ."[16]

Societal "risk reduction" was proposed, based on recognition of the central importance of promoting human rights to reduce vulnerability to HIV. First, the basic forms of discrimination and human rights violations within a community need to be identified. Using the example cited previously, discrimination against women is a universal societal problem, although assuming different forms and expressions in different societies. Second, the pathways through which such violations put persons at increased risk of HIV infection must be identified. Violations of women's rights to nondiscrimination, to equal standing before the law, and to equality in marriage and divorce place women in a highly vulnerable position, depriving them of the ability to make and effect free and informed choices about their sexual practices. Third, specific steps can then be taken to reduce HIV vulnerability by directly addressing the human rights issues. In several countries, women's groups have sought to change laws governing property distribution after divorce, as well as laws on marriage and inheritance, as part of anti-AIDS efforts.[2,19] These efforts must be closely linked with other community-development and rights promotion activities, often coming from outside the health sector.

This approach proposes a transformation of public health or, perhaps more accurately, a return to first principles. The U.S. Institute of Medicine has defined public health as "assuring the conditions in which people can be healthy."[20] Awareness that societal factors are the principal determinants of health status is not new.[21] However, public health has often chosen to work entirely within the societal status quo. AIDS has helped rearticulate the need to consider disease as linked with societal structures and thereby to address the underlying societal factors—the status of realization of human rights and respect for dignity—in addition to strengthening traditional public health programs. It is neither necessary nor desirable to choose between traditional public health programs and promoting human rights and dignity; both are necessary, and both require short- and long-term commitments.

This approach goes beyond preventing AIDS. As summarized by the GAPC, "The central insight from a decade of hard work against AIDS is that societal discrimination is at the root of individual and community vulnerability to AIDS—and to other major health problems of the modern world. This joins HIV/AIDS work to the larger global movement for health . . . . A careful analysis of the major causes of preventable illness, disability and premature death—including cancer, heart disease, injuries and violence, and infectious diseases—shows that, like HIV/AIDS, they are linked to societal discrimination and lack of respect for fundamental human rights and dignity."[16]

CONCLUSION

The AIDS epidemic is the first major pandemic to occur in the modern era of human rights.[1] Global experience with HIV prevention has uncovered two critical associations between human rights and AIDS prevention. First, discrimination occurring as an effect of the pandemic, directed principally toward HIV-infected persons and those with AIDS, was found to be counterproductive in public health terms. Accordingly, antidiscrimination was explicitly included in the WHO global AIDS strategy. Second, the lack of respect for human rights and dignity within each society was identified as a root cause of vulnerability to HIV. Efforts to protect and promote human rights are an integral part of a new strategy for preventing and controlling the pandemic. For the first time in history, public health officials have a dual responsibility: to protect public health and to respect and promote human rights and dignity. These insights have great importance for the future of public health, because they mandate attention to the reality of the preeminent importance of society for health.

REFERENCES

1. Mann JM, Gostin L, Gruskin S, et al. Health and human rights. Health Hum Rights 1994;1:6.
2. Mann JM, Tarantola D, Netter T, eds. AIDS in the world. Cambridge: Harvard University Press, 1992.
3. Gostin L, Curran WJ. Legal control measures for AIDS: reporting requirements, surveillance, quarantine, and regulation of public meeting places. Am J Public Health 1987;77:214.
4. Mann, JM. AIDS: discrimination and public health. (Doc. WHO/GPA/DIR/88.3) Geneva, Switzerland: World Health Organization, 1988.
5. World Health Organization. Report of the consultation on international travel and HIV infection, Geneva, 2–3 March 1987. (Doc. WHO/SPA/GLO/87.1) Geneva, Switzerland: World Health Organization, 1987.
6. The Panos Institute. AIDS and the third world. London: Panos Institute, 1986:57.
7. World Health Organization. Social aspects of AIDS prevention and control programmes. Geneva 1987 (Doc. WHO/SPA/GLO/87.2) Geneva, Switzerland: World Health Organization, 1987.
8. World Health Assembly. Avoidance of discrimination against HIV-infected persons and people with AIDS. Resolution WHA Geneva, Switzerland: World Health Assembly, 41.24, 13 May 1988.
9. Mann JM, Kay K. Confronting the pandemic: the World Health Organization's Global Programme on AIDS, 1986–89. AIDS 1991;5(Suppl2):S221.
10. Romany C. State responsibility goes private: a feminist critique of the public/private distinction in international human rights law. In: Cook RJ, ed. Human rights of women: national and international perspectives. Philadelphia: University of Pennsylvania Press, 1994:85.
11. Mann JM. AIDS: the personal and global challenges of renewal. Working paper series no. 3. Cambridge: Francois-Xavier Bagnoud Center for Health and Human Rights, March 1995.
12. Centers for Disease Control. AIDS among racial/ethnic minorities—United States, 1993. MMWR 1994;43:644.
13. Centers for Disease Control. Update: AIDS among women—United States, 1994. MMWR 1995;44:81.
14. World Health Organization. Effective approaches to AIDS prevention: report of a meeting, Geneva 26–29 May 1992. (Doc. WHO/GPA/IDS/93.1). Geneva, Switzerland: World Health Organization, 1993.
15. Choi KH, Coates TJ. Prevention of HIV infection. AIDS 1994;8:1371.
16. Global AIDS Policy Coalition. Towards a new health strategy for AIDS. Cambridge, 1993.
17. Elias C, Heise L. The development of microbicides: a new method of HIV prevention for women. Working papers 1993, no. 6. New York: The Population council, 1993.
18. duGuerny J, Sjoberg E. Inter-relationship between gender relations and the HIV/AIDS epidemic: some possible considerations for policies and programmes. AIDS 1993;7:1027.
19. Patten W, Ward AJ. Empowering women to stop AIDS in Cote d'Ivoire and Uganda. Harvard Hum Rights J 1993;6:210.
20. Institute of Medicine. The future of public health: summary and recommendations. Washington, DC: National Academy Press, 1988.
21. Evans RG, Barer ML, Marmor TR, eds. Why are some people healthy and others not? New York: Aldine de Gruyter, 1994.

AIDS: Biology, Diagnosis, Treatment and Prevention, fourth edition, edited by Vincent T. DeVita, Jr., Samuel Hellman, and Steven A. Rosenberg. Lippincott–Raven Publishers, © 1997

CHAPTER 34

Human Immunodeficiency Disease: Ethical Considerations for Clinicians

Christine Grady

Ethical questions present some of the most vexing problems associated with human immunodeficiency virus (HIV) infection and the numerous and varied efforts to understand, prevent, control, and treat it. Ethics is a branch of philosophy concerned with values related to human conduct, the rightness or wrongness of certain actions, and the goodness or badness of the motives or ends of such actions.[1] Ethics invites us to use reasoned analytic and critical approaches and precedents to answer questions about how we ought to behave in given situations and why. Because most human behavior and human endeavor is value laden and has ethical, legal, social, economic, and political implications, there is often conflict or uncertainty about the ethical or right thing to do.

Conflict may exist within an individual or between two or more individuals, groups, or institutions. Facing and resolving these conflicts is complicated and often involves significant turmoil and discomfort. "Ethical issues involve uncertainty and conflicting responses about what we should or should not do, about the values we must maintain and those we must sacrifice. Of course, that is all so abstract. Phrasing ethical issues in statements and questions is a linguistic transformation of conflicts that rage in the bodies, minds, and hearts of people. Value conflicts are most visible in the faces of people who suffer."[2].

Ethical analysis helps in the development of morally and socially appropriate solutions to problems or conflicts of value. Theories and principles of ethics guide us in searching for and appraising solutions to ethical problems, as do legal and ethical precedents. Ethical theories organize our

analyses in different ways, depending on the focus of the theory. Theories define what it means to act morally and attempt to articulate and justify principles that can guide moral decisions and be used as standards for the evaluation of actions and policies.[3]

Four moral principles—respect for autonomy, nonmaleficence, beneficence, and justice—are accepted as central to biomedical ethics and are often used as general action guides within which there is room for interpretation and judgment in specific cases (Table 34-1).[1,4] However, faced with the life circumstances and dilemmas of individual patients and families, clinicians may find the principles difficult to apply, interpret, or rank. Some have argued that a principle-based approach to ethics is inadequate to the complex, human dimensions of many bioethical dilemmas. A "care ethic," built on the understanding that individuals are unique, that relationships and their value are crucial in moral deliberations, and that emotions and character traits have a role in moral judgment,[5] may add an important dimension to ethical guidance for clinicians. Several questions that incorporate and build on the principles may be helpful in considering the ethical dimensions of individual and aggregate choices, regardless of the theory espoused (Table 34-2).

The outcome of ethical reflection and analysis does not preclude the possibility that reasonable people can disagree. However, "the process of debate and scrutiny . . . is likely to produce the kind of thoughtful judgment that is always more valuable than simplistic conclusions reached without the benefit of careful, sustained reflection and discourse."[6]

Ethical analysis can help to determine and to judge our individual and collective responses to the HIV epidemic. Determining ethically appropriate responses to the HIV epidemic and putting those responses into motion have posed formidable challenges for our society. The National Commission on AIDS repeatedly lamented that "America is (still) doing poorly . . . after a decade of unreasoning fear

Christine Grady, Assistant Director for Clinical Science, National Institute of Nursing Research, National Institutes of Health, Building 31, Room 5B10, Bethesda, MD 20892-2178.

TABLE 34-1. *Principles of biomedical ethics*

Nonmaleficence—a duty to avoid harming or injuring other people. "We ought to act in ways that do not cause needless harm or injury to others."
Beneficence—duty to promote the good of another or contribute to their welfare, this duty is inherent in the role of all health care professionals. "We ought to act in ways that promote the welfare of other people."
Respect for autonomy—Respect for the liberty, privacy and self-determination of individuals. "We ought to act in ways that respect, and do not interfere with, the decisions and actions of autonomous individuals."
Justice (distributive)—fairness, equity in the distribution of benefits/burdens "We ought to act in ways that promote fairness in the distribution of benefits and burdens."

From Beauchamp T, Childress J. Principles of Biomedical ethics. 4th ed. New York: Oxford University Press, 1994; Gillon R. Principles of health care ethics. New York: John Wiley & Sons, 1994.

and cruel indifference to the AIDS epidemic . . . ."[7] We may ask ourselves: have we confronted acquired immunodeficiency syndrome (AIDS) with compassion, concern, and responsible action or with anger, blame, and disengagement? Have our policies been guided by rational, informed thought and reflection or by fear and anxiety? Are we treating those who are infected with respect and dignity or as outcasts stripped of their rights and unable to get the care they need? Are we appropriately balancing the rights and welfare of individuals within our society with the rights and welfare of society as a whole?

WHAT IS THE NATURE OF ETHICAL PROBLEMS FACED IN HIV INFECTION?

Many of the ethical issues that confront us in the context of HIV infection are not new. Some authorities have argued that the majority of issues that have occupied bioethicists over the last several decades are issues we are struggling with in HIV. "In some ways it may be said that to know the acquired immunodeficiency syndrome in all of its moral manifestations and relations is to learn biomedical ethics, or at least a great deal of its scope and ambitions."[8]

Issues such as confidentiality, discrimination, prenatal testing, abortion, individual freedom versus public compulsion, access to health care, justice in health care, informed consent and patient decision making, advance directives, decisions about life-sustaining care, euthanasia, suicide, the conduct of clinical trials, access to experimental therapies, and scientific integrity have emerged as pertinent to HIV infection. Aspects of the HIV epidemic have defined unique dimensions to some of these ethical questions and demanded attention. Some of the uniqueness stems from the fact that HIV is an infectious, chronic, and lethal disease in an era when infectious diseases are generally treatable. HIV primarily affects young persons in the prime of their lives, most of whom have been infected through socially unac-

ceptable behaviors that are not well understood or approved of by some health care providers. In the United States, HIV infection is increasingly concentrated in "socially disadvantaged" groups,[9] encouraging an attitude that has already had a powerful influence on ethical discourse in HIV disease, a misguided perception that HIV is "their" problem, not particularly dangerous to or relevant to "us." Ethical questions also are confounded by the fact that HIV is a global epidemic that is expanding dramatically; that access to health care is unequal in the United States and around the world; that preventing HIV requires changing behaviors that are notoriously resistant to change; and that caring for those affected is complicated, demanding, and expensive.

In considering some of the particular ethical issues of HIV treatment and prevention, three distinct but related spheres[10] can be identified: issues related to prevention and the public health, issues related to the delivery of health care and provision of care to individuals, and issues related to biomedical and behavioral research. From the myriad issues that could be addressed, I have selected issues that remain problematic for health care professionals in the United States

PUBLIC HEALTH, CONTROL, AND PREVENTION OF HIV INFECTION

An often cited struggle in the HIV epidemic is conflict between the rights and civil liberties of individuals and the public health or the common good. Given the traditional and predominant values in our liberal society, the basic conflict could be restated: to what extent can individual autonomy and privacy be compromised to protect or benefit the health of others? When does protection of the public health justify overriding individual rights and liberties? Individuals living in society normally relinquish some liberty for the benefit of the public health (eg, compulsory vaccinations, speed limits, restrictions on smoking). Faced with a crisis, such as war, natural disaster, or epidemic, increased curtailment of civil liberties may be justified. Rational and ethical decisions

TABLE 34-2. *Consideration of the ethical dimensions of choices or chosen solutions*

What are the potential benefits and who will benefit (beneficence)?
What art the potential risks and who will be harmed (nonmaleficence)?
Who makes or ought to make the decisions (respect for autonomy)?
What is the fairest thing to do (that which distributes benefits and burdens most equitably, justice)?
What other moral principles should be applied (confidentiality, fidelity, solidarity)?
What rights and responsibilities should be protected or adhered to?
What are the unique needs of the individual (care)?
What relationships should be taken into account (care)?
What virtues should be considered or encouraged?

about policies that curtail civil liberties require consideration of the consequences of such policies on the health, welfare, and rights of individuals and the public, as well as an accurate evaluation of the effectiveness of such policies in promoting or protecting the public health.[11]

In the early years of the HIV epidemic, traditional public health measures used in the past and thought to be beneficial to the public health, such as screening, testing, reporting, contact tracing, isolation, and quarantine were vigorously challenged on the grounds that they violated individual liberty and privacy rights without demonstrable benefit to the public health. Despite universal agreement that stopping AIDS was a worthy goal, HIV disease was recognized as different from many other infectious diseases, especially with respect to the mode of transmission, usual course, and fatal outcome. Because of these factors and the prominent values in U.S. society, HIV was given an "exceptionalist" status.[12] Efforts to control HIV concentrated on education and voluntary behavior change.[13,14] Some argued that implementation of public health policies perceived as coercive and an infringement of privacy could actually be harmful to the public health by driving underground those who were most at risk of HIV infection.[9,15,16] If so, then defense of the public health and protection of civil liberties are not at odds; they are compatible and interdependent. It has been argued that the most effective means of protecting the public health from HIV is by respecting the rights and autonomy of individuals and empowering them to make responsible choices.[17]

HIV Testing

Tension between individual rights and the public health has been apparent in persistent debates surrounding testing for HIV antibody. Early advocates of testing believed that knowledge of HIV status would be an important motivator of behavioral change necessary to reduce transmission and therefore of benefit to the public health. Although there was some evidence of behavior changes by those who knew their serostatus,[18,19] there was no evidence that mandatory testing would lead to voluntary changes in risk-taking behaviors, and there was some evidence that it might not (eg, mandatory premarital testing in Illinois resulted in a 22.5% decrease in applications for marriage licenses).[11] Other advocates of mandatory universal testing saw it as prerequisite to isolation or mass quarantine, options ethically and practically reprehensible.[20] Opponents of mandatory testing argued that the deleterious consequences for an individual of being identified as HIV infected—which included possible discrimination in jobs, insurance, and housing; psychologic distress; and violence and hate crimes—outweighed any possible public health or individual benefit.[21]

A broad consensus emerged and remains that testing should be conducted only with the specific voluntary consent of individuals who have received adequate information and counseling.[22] Compulsory programs to identify the presence of HIV infection were, in general, deemed unacceptable. Respect for autonomy is central to this consensus, because informed consent, protection of confidentiality, and protection against discrimination are all prominent considerations. Despite this standard of voluntary testing, many clinicians and hospitals did and do test patients without their informed consent,[23] believing that protection of health care workers and sound diagnostic work justifies such screening.[9] There are a number of groups in the United States for whom testing is compulsory, including members of the military, State Department, Peace and Job Corps, immigrants and foreign visitors, and some prisoners. The informed consent of these individuals for testing is not sought, not necessarily because they are more dangerous to the public health, but because they are more subject to social control.[24] In other contexts, the rationale for testing is not protection of the health of others but cost savings (eg, HIV testing required by health and life insurance companies). Mandatory testing of donors of blood, organs, and semen is not controversial because recipients cannot otherwise protect themselves, and it is believed to be in everyone's interest to have an HIV-free blood and organ supply.[11]

As benefits to the individual of being tested increased (ie, early intervention and opportunistic infection prophylaxis[25,26]) and protection against some of the negative consequences of testing had been put in place (eg, the American with Disabilities Act[27]), the risk-benefit calculus changed in the direction of increased individual benefit. Politically active gay organizations, previously opposed to testing, now encourage individuals to be tested.[9,12] Physicians and public health officials encourage routine HIV testing of patients deemed to be at risk.[28,29]

"Testing for HIV antibody should be strongly recommended when it will benefit the patient or the patient's contacts or when it will minimize the risk for transmission of the virus or protect the public health."[29] This recommendation is accompanied by the caveats that the patient must give consent after being appropriately informed and counseled by trained personnel; that the provision of care must not be in any way contingent on consent to be tested or the results of the test; and that appropriate safeguards for the confidentiality of the test results must be in place.[30] Clinicians should recommend HIV testing as a diagnostic modality to individuals who may be at risk of HIV infection, for whom the risk-benefit assessment is favorable, and from whom voluntary informed consent can be obtained.

Prenatal Testing

If the only consideration in decisions about prenatal HIV testing were possible benefits and risks to the woman herself, respect for autonomy would trump, and pregnant women would simply be included in the voluntarist consensus described earlier. However, the prospect of benefit to the offspring of an HIV infected woman or prevention of harm to society by preventing transmission to offspring through the identification of infected pregnant women makes this a distinct situation. The principle of nonmaleficence assumes greater power "when the recipient of the potential harm is an unconsenting future child whose health and welfare may be unalterably affected."[31] It is accepted public health practice to test pregnant women for syphilis and hepatitis B and to screen newborns for phenylketonuria and other metabolic diseases. Many argue that consistent with this practice all pregnant women and newborns should be HIV tested because of potential benefit to the baby. Others argued that testing without consent is treating the mother solely as a vector and not as a person with autonomy and privacy rights of her own. As suggested by Bayer in 1991, potential benefit to the fetus and newborn was a forceful argument even before the evidence that antiretroviral interventions can reduce the rate of perinatal transmission: "The promise—with little evidentiary basis—that early intervention might protect the fetus or at least enhance the life prospects of babies at risk for HIV had begun to override concerns about the coercive identification of infected women, most of whom were black or Hispanic, as well as about the potential burdens of exclusion from housing, social services, and health care itself that might be imposed on those so identified."[13]

The societal values of reproductive freedom and respect for the autonomy of the woman, coupled with the possibility that compulsory testing could actually result in a decrease in the number of disadvantaged women who seek prenatal care and therefore potentially harm to the mother and the baby, argue strongly for routine but voluntary prenatal testing for HIV.[32] The Institute of Medicine,[33] the Working Group on HIV testing for pregnant women and newborns at Johns Hopkins and Georgetown Universities,[34] the Centers for Disease Control and Prevention,[35] and others have urged routine testing of pregnant women; however, they oppose imposing testing on women or their newborns without the woman's informed consent. Despite this consensus, pregnant women are often tested without their knowledge, while at the same time in places where HIV seroprevalence is relatively high, HIV testing is not even routinely offered to poor pregnant women because of its cost.[9]

The success of zidovudine during pregnancy in reducing the rate of perinatal HIV transmission[36] has been seen by some as sufficiently altering the balance between benefits to offspring and rights of the mother to favor mandatory prenatal screening. Bayer contends, however, that mandatory HIV screening of pregnant women remains objectionable, ethically and practically, because mandatory treatment of competent adults is not acceptable.[37] If the ultimate purpose of prenatal testing is to empower women to make informed choices on behalf of themselves or their babies rather than to serve a public health goal of preventing the birth of infected newborns, routine voluntary prenatal testing with informed consent is appropriate and adequate. Mandatory testing of pregnant women would not be ethical unless access to the therapy and support indicated were guaranteed

if the test were positive. Preferable to mandatory screening would be a policy that mandated that every pregnant woman be offered voluntary HIV testing with the assurance that, if positive, she would have access to at least zidovudine therapy during pregnancy and for the newborn or to some more comprehensive package of medical, nutritional, and social services before, during, and after delivery of the child.

HIV Testing of Newborns and Blinded Testing

Because approximately 75% of newborns who are seropositive at birth due to the transfer of maternal antibody are not infected, the claim has been made that testing newborns is really a devious way of identifying infected women.[38] Debates about HIV testing of newborns have also been entangled in the controversy surrounding blinded seroprevalence testing. Blinded or unlinked seroprevalence testing of blood specimens collected for other purposes and stripped of identifiers has been seen as vital for estimating the scope of the HIV epidemic, thereby enabling the planning and provision of targeted prevention programs and needed medical and social services.

Since the mid-1980s, the Centers for Disease Control and Prevention (CDC) has conducted blinded seroprevalence surveillance in selected populations, including newborns in 44 states, and among clients of public health clinics, sexually transmitted disease clinics, drug treatment centers, family planning clinics, tuberculosis clinics, runaway and homeless shelters, sentinel hospitals, and some colleges.[39] Blinded testing is extremely valuable in epidemiologic research but has no role in the care of individuals; it is of benefit to society but not directly to the tested individuals. Opponents of blinded testing have argued that the practice is deceitful, "affronts respect for the individual . . . exploits vulnerable populations, affronts equity concerns, and fails to provide test subjects with any benefits."[40] Blinded testing as a research tool has been reviewed by several groups and been found to be ethically acceptable for several reasons. The information is important to the welfare of society, may not be obtainable in any other way, and is obtained without harm to the individual because no extra blood is drawn, infected individuals cannot be identified, and anonymous or confidential testing is widely available for those who want to know their serostatus.[41]

Controversy persists, however, particularly related to blinded testing of newborns.[42] The controversy has been fueled by the rejection on ethical grounds of blinded seroprevalence testing in Europe[41,43] and by the Newborn Infant HIV Notification Act, a bill (H.R. 1289) introduced in 1995 in the U.S. Congress by Rep. Gary Ackerman (D-NY) that would require disclosure of any newborn HIV test results to the mother or legal guardian. Amid public debate, the CDC suspended its program of newborn seroprevalence testing.[44]

Although blinded testing does not offer benefit to the individual, participation in blinded seroprevalence testing does not preclude testing any individual infant after obtaining the informed consent of the mother. HIV testing should be routinely offered and encouraged for infants born to infected or high-risk mothers but should be done with the mother's informed consent. Routine voluntary testing of pregnant women should remain a crucial and early step in reducing neonatal HIV infection, so antiretroviral therapy can begin prenatally.

Disclosure of HIV Status

Closely related to decisions about testing are decisions about disclosing information about HIV infection. It is widely accepted that the individual being tested should be informed of HIV test results and the implications thereof out of respect for his or her autonomy and welfare. The infected person has an ethical obligation to inform others at risk. More controversial is when it may be justifiable to disclose confidential information about the HIV status of an individual without their consent or against their wishes.

Maintenance of the confidentiality of patient information is the responsibility of all health care providers and is a classic requirement of health professional ethics. Maintaining patient confidentiality respects patients' privacy and control over personal information and encourages persons to seek care and candidly discuss problems with health care providers, fostering trust in the health care provider–patient relationship. Disclosure of confidential information about HIV infection may violate privacy, jeopardize trust, and put the individual at risk of serious discrimination. Nonetheless, the obligation of health care workers to maintain patient confidentiality is not absolute. In the United States, health care workers have a legal and ethical duty to report child abuse, gunshot wounds, and certain infectious diseases, even if in doing so they breach the confidentiality of some patients. This duty is founded on the principle of nonmaleficence because of tangible risk to third parties and overrides the duty to protect confidentiality.

Those most clearly at risk of HIV infection are sexual and needle-sharing partners of an infected individual. The primary strategy for protecting third parties from risk of HIV infection should be to empower the infected individual to inform relevant parties of their risk. This strategy accords with the principle of respect for autonomy and stresses the responsibility of the infected individual to be nonmaleficent and to respect the autonomy of others by notifying those they place at risk. With proper counseling, encouragement, and follow-up, most HIV-infected persons do inform their at-risk partners (ie, voluntary partner notification).[45] Debate has centered primarily on the smaller number of infected individuals who are not capable or not willing to inform partners at risk. In a study by Cameron and colleagues,[46] although most subjects knew that informing at-risk partners was the right thing to do, not all had done so. Physicians should have and in most states do have by law the discretion to inform or to request that the appropriate public health authorities inform sexual or needle-sharing partners, espe-

cially when the third party does not know he or she is at risk of infection. This is referred to as "permission or privilege to warn." Lo and colleagues argue that, although by law it is a "privilege," ethically, it is required to notify partners who are unknowingly at grave risk.[45] The decision to inform others at risk over the wishes of the infected individual, although justified by protecting innocent third parties, is a serious one, because of the many potentially grave negative consequences of disclosure of HIV status. In addition to discrimination and stigma, a decision to override the individual's confidentiality could further harm the individual by affecting the trust that may exist in the health care professional–patient relationship and by putting the infected person in jeopardy of violence.[47]

The Limits of Autonomy

Respect for individual autonomy has been apparent in many policy decisions and laws regarding testing and partner notification and in driving efforts to enact antidiscrimination laws, mandate informed consent before testing, and protect the confidentiality of medical information. Some have expressed concern about whether this same respect will extend to the "newer groups" of HIV infected patients, who are concentrated in socially and economically deprived communities and traditionally subject to harsher social controls.[9] Fear of contagion and the possibility of draconian measures to control HIV may also be exacerbated by the reemergence of tuberculosis associated with HIV infection, especially multidrug-resistant tuberculosis. Creative and innovative approaches to respect the rights of individuals and maximize benefit to individuals and the public health (not one at the expense of the other) while preventing HIV and containing the epidemic must continually be sought.

PROVISION OF HEALTH CARE TO HIV-INFECTED INDIVIDUALS

Health Care Services

Persons with HIV infection need a broad range of health care services from diagnosis to death. Despite variability in the HIV disease experience, the usual trajectory includes a lengthy period of few or no physical symptoms, often after a brief, acute episode, and ultimately, a period of multisystem clinical disease and death. Primary care, careful immunologic monitoring, antiretroviral therapy, prophylaxis and treatment of opportunistic diseases, psychologic and social support, home care, and terminal care are some of the services that may be needed throughout the course of HIV disease. Needed therapy, care, and services depend on the stage of disease, presenting clinical problems, the premorbid health status, and the social situation of the infected person.

Prevalent weaknesses, deficiencies, and inequities in the U.S. health care delivery system have been demonstrated by our inability to provide comprehensive and appropriate services to all HIV-infected persons.[9] HIV-infected individuals have been denied treatment by individual practitioners and by health care institutions. The complex and often expensive treatment and care needs of persons with HIV disease have been unevenly addressed and attended to. Lack of health insurance, forfeiture of insurance because of job loss, and the well-documented inadequacies and inconsistencies in Medicaid coverage, availability, and reimbursement have all contributed to these inadequacies.[48] An increasing number of HIV-infected persons are poor, inner-city dwellers, including many homeless persons, who have limited access to quality health care services or the means to pay for them. Major legislative proposals for health care reform that include a provision for universal access could improve access to needed health services for many HIV-infected persons. However, the trend toward managed care and capitation may make it more difficult for persons with HIV disease to get the often complex and expensive care and treatment they need. In the words of the 1993 National Research Council report: "The calls for adequate ongoing medical care for HIV infected persons reflect and reinforce other current demands for an overall reordering of staffing and reimbursement priorities in American health care."[9]

Decisions About Treatment

Within the scope of what is available and affordable, it is generally agreed that decisions about treatment and care are made by autonomous individuals after receiving adequate and realistic information from the health care professional or team. As is true for any autonomous adult, an HIV-infected adult has the right to choose among alternative therapies, choose to withdraw from therapy, or choose not to be treated. Ensuring that patients have the information they need to make informed decisions about treatment, research, diagnostic tests, and care is a demonstration of respect for the individual and fulfills a health care provider's legal and ethical obligation. Health care providers further demonstrate care and respect for their patients by empowering and supporting them in making treatment and care decisions, including advanced directives, decisions about life-sustaining therapies, research participation, or choice of providers.

Advance Directives

An advance directive is a means of expressing wishes and making decisions about health care that will come into effect if and when the patient becomes unable to make decisions. Two forms of advance directive are in common usage and sanctioned by statute in most states: the durable power of attorney for health care (DPA) and the living will. The U.S. Patient Self-Determination Act (PSDA), which became effective in December 1991, requires health care institutions to inform clients of their rights to make decisions regarding treatment and medical care, including the right to refuse medical or surgical treatment and the right to formulate advance directives.[49] In particular, the PSDA requires health care institutions to establish policies regarding advance directives, provide information and education to patients and staff, and to document advance directives and discussions about them. "Advance directives are precautionary tools to prevent intractable problems regarding end of life decisions when AIDS patients are incapacitated."[50]

The DPA, which allows a surrogate appointed by the individual to make decisions about treatment and care when the individual is not able, may be very important for the HIV-infected person who has a lover, friend, or family member who without a DPA would have no legal standing and could be excluded from decision making. Generally, persons can best discuss and decide what they want when given time for reflection. Providing early opportunities for discussion and planning for difficult decisions about treatment and the end of life demonstrates caring and respect for HIV-infected individuals. Early discussion is extremely important in HIV disease, because almost 70% of AIDS patients develop neuropsychiatric disorders, including AIDS dementia.[51]

Euthanasia and Physician-Assisted Suicide

The idea that individuals with serious and terminal illnesses, including but not limited to AIDS, should have the option of choosing to end their lives with or without the assistance of health care providers has gained considerable attention and some level of public acceptance. Public opinion surveys demonstrate strong support for the idea that a physician should help a patient die by means of euthanasia or assisted suicide when that individual has a terminal illness, a short expected survival, and a consistently expressed desire for assistance.[52] Ballot initiatives formalizing this type of terminal care have appeared in several states, and one such initiative, the Death with Dignity Act, was passed by voters in Oregon in 1994 (the initiative is on hold because of a constitutional challenge).[53]

Proponents argue that assistance in dying respects the autonomy of patients and provides benefit with little risk by access to a way to relieve a patient's suffering accompanied by procedural safeguards, including assessment of decision-making capacity and certification of the nature of the terminal illness and brief expected survival, often by two physicians.[54] Opponents argue that there is a significant moral line between killing and allowing to die, that abuses of involuntary euthanasia could occur, and that hastening death as a primary objective of an intervention is inconsistent with the fundamental ethic of medical practice and could result in distrust or confusion about the role of health care providers.[53,55] Dr. Jack Kevorkian has continued to receive widespread publicity, and as of late 1995, impunity in Michigan, for assisting in the deaths of as many as 47 variously diagnosed persons, including some without terminal illnesses.

A related issue is that of rational suicide, whereby a patient who is not depressed and understands the consequences is clear about his or her intent and plan to commit suicide but does not necessarily request assistance from a health care provider. The ethics of suicide has been debated for thousands of years.[56] If suicide is not morally acceptable, assisted suicide also is not, but what about the well-considered plans of a rational person who does not want to suffer? The probability of suicide is higher in persons with AIDS than in those with most other chronic diseases,[57] and many persons with AIDS have suicide plans without ever implementing them. Battin points out that, although we do not know the extent to which it is practiced, access to the means to commit suicide is widely available to AIDS patients, especially in the gay community.[58] When faced with an HIV patient's suicide plans, the health care provider may struggle with how to balance respect for autonomous decision making and protection from harm.

Some critics of suicide or euthanasia for persons with AIDS argue that attending adequately to an individual's need for pain reduction, comfort, support, and control usually would obviate the desire to end his or her life through assisted or unassisted methods. Consideration of alternatives and the provision of quality palliative care should be part of health care providers' response to terminally ill AIDS patients. The hospice model has contributed significantly to achieving this end.

BIOMEDICAL AND BEHAVIORAL RESEARCH

Current U.S. regulations and codes of ethics that guide research with human subjects emphasize protection of the rights and welfare of individual participants of research. These regulations emerged from an extensive and colorful history of human subjects research that often violated the rights of individuals, was sometimes done without their knowledge or consent, was risky, and often intentionally used captive, accessible, and vulnerable groups of persons.[59] The Nuremberg Code, which was established at the Nuremberg trials of Nazi war crimes, proclaimed individual informed consent central to ethical research.[60] Subsequent exposures of experiments in the United States, such as the Willowbrook hepatitis studies, the Tuskegee syphilis study, and others thought to violate the rights of participants, sparked public outrage and Congressional action and led to the creation in 1974 of the National Commission for the Protection of Human Subjects of Biomedical and Behavioral Research, whose work has been singularly influential in shaping U.S. regulations and the many codes of research ethics that have ensued.

The most important elements of the U.S. regulations (found in the Code of Federal Regulations Title 45, part 46) include protection of subjects from unreasonable risk, the informed consent of subjects to ensure their voluntary participation, exclusion or increased safeguards for subjects perceived to be vulnerable, and prior review and approval of all human subjects research by a review committee (ie, Institutional Review Board). The regulations are based on principles identified in the *Belmont Report* by the National Commission as most relevant to the conduct of human subjects research: respect for persons, beneficence, and justice.[61] The Commission also explicated a distinction between research designed to produce socially necessary, generalized knowledge and therapy designed to benefit an individual.

The HIV epidemic has been the catalyst for a major reexamination of research ethics and drug development.[9,62-67] "Controversy has never been absent from the drug development process nor is the ethics of human subjects research a closed topic. Nonetheless, whatever carefully crafted consensus once existed has broken down."[68]

AIDS activists, sometimes in collaboration with ethicists and clinicians, challenged tradition and the status quo and brought some of the difficult issues in clinical research to the forefront. Rather than being protective, they argued that research regulations and traditions were discriminatory and paternalistic. They also advocated for a shift in emphasis away from protection from risk (ie, nonmaleficence) toward autonomy and beneficence, perceiving participation in research to be an opportunity, benefit, or even a right. Rather than paternalistic protection from risks that others have decided are too great, activists argued for increased autonomy and personal control in choosing for themselves what risks were acceptable, through participation in research and through earlier access to experimental drugs and interventions. Excluding certain vulnerable groups from research for their own protection was described as discrimination, denial of a potentially beneficial opportunity, and therefore unjust.

Through challenging government and academic practices and rules and raising issues for public scrutiny and discussion, AIDS activists have achieved some success in changing the regulatory process for drug development and the conduct of clinical trials.[69] Studies have been written with more flexible entry criteria so as not to categorically exclude women, children, or individuals with multiple complications of disease. Surrogate end points (eg, CD4 counts, viral measures) rather than clinical end points (eg, opportunistic diseases, death) have been accepted for some clinical trials, such as those that led to the approval of dideoxyinosine (ddI). The Public Health Service has allowed some investigational drugs to be made available through a "parallel track" program. The use of placebos in clinical trials was opposed by some commentators, based on the argument that reasonable persons faced with a fatal disease like HIV would accept a drug that might help them, even if it was not proven.[70] Activists and community members demanded a role in decision making about when a clinical trial should begin and end and how it should be designed.[67] For example, all committees of the AIDS Clinical Trials Group, a large network of institutions conducting HIV clinical treatment trials, have community representation, and most institutions involved in HIV research have community advisory boards. Consortia of community providers willing to conduct research in primary care settings have been established (eg, Community consortium for clinical research, Community Programs for Clinical Research in AIDS).

Although the landscape of clinical research in HIV has changed, how far the changes will go and the extent to which they will influence the conduct of or regulations guiding clinical research remains to be seen. Some formidable and unique ethical problems in conducting HIV research remain.

Trial Design

Because of the natural history of HIV, clinical end points are difficult to achieve in clinical trials, for logistic and ethical reasons. At the speed with which scientific developments occur, keeping someone on a trial for many years may deprive them of the opportunity for newer, more effective therapies, but evaluating surrogate markers that do not correlate well with morbidity or mortality or stopping the trial before end points are reached could render data about treatment efficacy invalid and the trial useless. This is also an important problem for vaccine trials.

Subject Recruitment

Researchers are seeking participants for clinical trials, but doctors are usually not seeking more HIV patients. For some persons, entering a research trial may be the only way to obtain needed health care or treatment. Persons with few options may even perceive participation in phase I research as potentially therapeutic. Legislation[71] and guidelines from the National Institutes of Health mandate a systematic effort to recruit adequate numbers of women and ethnic minorities into clinical trials. How do all of these factors influence the ability of an individual to autonomously "volunteer" for participation in research? And who takes care of the research participants who have few or no other health care options when they withdraw from participation in research?

Resource Allocation in Research

There has been considerable debate about whether HIV is unique or just another disease. Should it get a proportionate share of resources or more because it is new and infectious? The response of the research community to HIV was initially characterized as slow, but this was followed by a rapid increase in dollars allocated to HIV research. In an era of shrinking budgets and belt-tightening, there is some backlash against the amount of money designated for HIV-related research. There has also been disagreement about the appropriate distribution of research dollars among different research interests within the HIV research community. How should resources be divided between prevention (eg, vaccines, behavioral research) and treatment; between basic

and applied research; between research on antiretrovirals and that on immunomodulating therapies; between anti-HIV therapy and treatment of opportunistic diseases?

Scientific Integrity and Conflict of Interest

In addition to competition for resources, all scientists, including HIV scientists, are under enormous pressure to be productive and to publish. Individual scientists in cooperation with their research institution accept responsibility for ensuring the integrity of their research program. Public attention to instances of scientific misconduct has raised the level of public distrust of scientists and the government and has affected morale among scientists.[72]

TABLE 34-3. *National Commission on AIDS: Principles to guide the future response to the epidemic*

1. Leadership is essential. Leadership in any context entails developing a vision of the response needed, establishing a plan to realize it, and accepting responsibility for its fulfillment. Leadership in response to AIDS also provides the visible affirmation of the inclusion of people affected by HIV disease in the community.
2. Access to basic health care, including preventive, medical, and social services, should be a right for all. Our nation must find ways to finance that care for all.
3. The U.S. must have a vital and responsive public health system. This means rebuilding an adequately supported public health "infrastructure" with a sufficient number of trained personnel to carry out the primary public health functions of surveillance, assessment and analysis, and prevention. All levels—federal, state, and local—must have the necessary capacity to fill their designated roles.
4. The best science will yield the best strategies, but science cannot flourish where it is blocked or constrained for ideologic reasons or political convenience, nor can it contribute properly where it is underfunded or its lessons ignored in program design.
5. To the greatest extent possible, health care solutions must avoid disease specificity. Solutions should offer a broad continuum of comprehensive services to those with problems of chronic, relapsing disease. Strategies should recognize that the health of entire communities often depends on the health of the least advantaged.
6. Partnerships are necessary. Collaboration between all levels of government, with the business community, the religious community, the voluntary not-for-profit sector, and community-based organizations is essential to providing a coordinated response. A broad array of persons, including people with HIV disease, AIDS advocates, health professionals, and community representatives, must be included in formulating prevention, care, and research strategies.
7. The human face of AIDS should be ever before us. Respecting personal dignity and autonomy, respecting the need for confidentiality, reducing discrimination, and minimizing intrusiveness should all be touchstones in the development of HIV and AIDS policies and programs.

National Commission on AIDS. AIDS: An expanding tragedy. Washington, DC, 1993:12.

CONCLUSION

The National Commission on AIDS included in its 1993 report a list of "Principles to Guide the Future Response to the Epidemic."[9] These are listed in Table 34-3.

This chapter has explored several ethical issues relevant to HIV disease and of importance to health care providers. Ethical reflection and discourse on these issues is necessary to find morally and socially acceptable solutions. Employing the bioethical principles of respect for persons, beneficence, nonmaleficence, justice, and care, which are visible in the National Commission's set of principles, and adding a dose of courage, strength, wisdom, and solidarity may serve to direct our discourse and responses in the right direction.

REFERENCES

1. Beauchamp T, Childress J. Principles of biomedical ethics. 4th ed. New York: Oxford University Press, 1994.
2. Tsoukas C, Roy D. Ethics and AIDS. Proceedings from a North American conference on care of terminally ill people with AIDS. : National Hospice Organization, U.S. and Palliative Care Foundation, Ottawa, Canada, 1987:91.
3. Munson R. Intervention and reflection: basic issues in medical ethics. 4th ed. Belmont, CA: Wadsworth Publishing, 1992.
4. Gillon R. Principles of health care ethics. New York: John Wiley & Sons, 1994.
5. Noddings N. Caring: a feminine approach to ethics and moral education. Berkeley: University of California Press, 1984.
6. Reamer F. AIDS: the relevance of ethics. In: Reamer F, ed. AIDS and ethics. New York: Columbia University Press, 1991:13.
7. National Commission on AIDS, AIDS: an expanding tragedy. Washington, DC: National Consensus on AIDS, 1993:1.
8. Murphy T, Walters L. The moral significance of AIDS. J Med Phil 1994;19:519.
9. National Research Council. The social impact of AIDS in the United States. Washington, DC: National Academy of Sciences Press, 1993.
10. Walters L. Ethical issues in the prevention and treatment of HIV infection and AIDS. Science 1988;239:597.
11. Childress J. Mandatory HIV screening and testing. In: Reamer F, ed. AIDS and ethics. New York: Columbia University Press, 1991:50.
12. Bayer R. Public health policy and the AIDS epidemic: an end to HIV exceptionalism. N Engl J Med 1991;324:1500.
13. Bayer R. AIDS, public health and civil liberties: consensus and conflict in policy. In: Reamer F, ed. AIDS and ethics. New York: Columbia University Press, 1991:26.
14. Harris J, Holm S. If only AIDS were different! Hastings Cent Rep 1993;23:6.
15. Lo B. Clinical Ethics and HIV-related illnesses: issues in therapeutic and health services research. Med Care Rev 1990;47:15.
16. Lo B. Ethical dilemmas in HIV infection. J Am Podiatr Med Assoc 1990;80:26.
17. Pinching A. AIDS: health care ethics and society. In: Gillon R, ed. Principles of health care ethics. New York: John Wiley & Sons, 1994:903.
18. Cates W, Handsfield H. HIV counseling and testing: does it work? Am J Public Health 1988;78:1533.
19. McKusker J, Stoddard A, Mayer K, Zapka J, Morrison C, Saltzman S. Effects of antibody test knowledge on subsequent sexual behaviors in a cohort of homosexually active men. Am J Public Health 1988;78:462.
20. Macklin R. Predicting dangerousness and the public health response to AIDS. Hastings Cent Rep 1986:16.
21. Lo B, Steinbrook R, Cooke M, Coates T, Walters E, Hulley S. Voluntary screening for HIV infection: weighing the benefits and harms. Ann Intern Med 1989;110:727.
22. Public Health Service Guidelines for counseling and antibody testing to prevent HIV infection and AIDS. MMWR 1987;36:509.
23. Lewis C, Montgomery K. The HIV testing policies of U.S. hospitals. JAMA 1990;264:2764.
24. Bayer R, Levine C, Wolf S. HIV antibody screening: an ethical framework for evaluating proposed programs. JAMA 1986;256:1768.
25. Volberding P, Lagakos S, Koch M. Zidovudine in asymptomatic HIV infection: a controlled trial in persons with less than 500 CD4+ cells/mm³. N Engl J Med 1990;322:941.
26. Fischl M, Dickinson G, LaVoie L. Safety and efficacy of sulfamethoxazole and trimethoprim chemoprophylaxis for *Pneumocystis carinii* pneumonia in AIDS. JAMA 1988;259:1185.
27. Gostin L. The AIDS litigation project JAMA. 1990;263:2086.
28. Rhame F, Maki D. The case for wider use of testing for HIV infection. N Engl J Med 1989;320:1248.
29. American College of Physicians. Position paper: human immunodeficiency virus (HIV) infection. Ann Intern Med 1994;120:310.
30. American College of Physicians. Position paper: human immunodeficiency virus (HIV) infection. Ann Intern Med 1994;120:314.
31. Levine C. AIDS and the ethics of human subjects research. In: Reamer F, ed. AIDS and ethics. New York: Columbia University Press, 1991:77.
32. Nolan K. Ethical issues in caring for pregnant women and newborns at risk for human immunodeficiency virus infection. Semin Perinatol 1989;13:55.
33. Hardy L, ed. HIV screening of pregnant women and newborns. Committee on prenatal and newborn screening for HIV infection, Institute of Medicine. Washington, DC: National Academy Press, 1991.
34. Faden R, Geller G, Acuff K, et al for the Working Group on HIV testing of pregnant women and newborns. HIV infection, pregnant women, and newborns: a policy proposal for information and testing. JAMA 1990;264:2416.
35. Centers for Disease Control. Guidelines for prophylaxis against Pneumocystis carinii pneumonia for children infected with HIV. MMWR 1991;40(RR-2):1.
36. Connor E, Sperling R, Gelber R, et al. Reduction of maternal-infant transmission of human immunodeficiency virus type 1 with zidovudine treatment. N Engl J Med 1994;331:1173.
37. Bayer R. Ethical challenges posed by zidovudine treatment to reduce vertical transmission of HIV. N Engl J Med 1994;331:1223.
38. Fleischman A, Post L, Dubler N. Commentary: mandatory newborn screening for human immunodeficiency virus. Bull N Y Acad Med 1994;71:4.
39. Pappaioanou M, Dondero T, Peterson L, Onorato I, Sanchez C, Curran J. The family of seroprevalence surveys: objectives, methods and uses of sentinel surveillance for HIV in the U.S. Public Health Rep 1990;105:113.
40. Isaacman S. HIV surveillance testing: taking advantage of the disadvantaged. Am J Public Health 1993;83:597.
41. Bayer R. The ethics of blinded HIV surveillance testing. Am J Public Health 1993;83:496.
42. Leo J. Mother's privacy vs. baby's health. Washington Times April 25, 1995:A21.
43. Gillon R. Testing for HIV without permission. Br Med J 1987;294:821.
44. Editorial. Washington Post June 17, 1995:A16.
45. Lo B. Ethical dilemmas in HIV infection: what have we learned? Law Med Health Care 1992;20:92.
46. Cameron M, Crisham P, Lewis D. The nature of ethical problems experienced by persons with acquired immunodeficiency syndrome: implications for nursing ethics education and practice. J Prof Nurs 1993;9:327.
47. North R, Rothenberg, K. Partner notification and the threat of domestic violence against women with HIV infection. N Engl J Med 1993;329:1194.
48. Shacknai D. Wealth = health: the public financing of AIDS care. In: Hunter N, Rubinstein W, eds. AIDS agenda: emerging issues in civil rights. New York: New Press, 1992:147.
49. Yellen S, Elpern E, Burton L. Patient concerns about advance directives. In: Monagle J, Thomasma D, eds. Health care ethics: critical issues. Rockville, MD: Aspen, 1994:109.
50. Fletcher J, Wispelwey B. AIDS and ethics: clinical, social, and global. In: Broder S. Merrigan T, Bolognesi D, eds. Textbook of AIDS medicine. Baltimore: Williams & Wilkins, 1994:853.
51. Price R, Brew B. AIDS dementia complex. J Infect Dis 1988;158:1079.

52. Cooke M. Patient rights and physician responsibility: four problems in AIDS care. In: Volberding P, Jacobson M, eds. AIDS clinical reviews 1993/4. New York: Marcel Dekker, 1994:253.

53. Pellegrino E. Ethics. JAMA 1995;273:1674.

54. Miller F, Brody H. Professional integrity and physician-assisted death. Hastings Cent Rep 1995;25:8.

55. American Medical Association. Report of the Council on Ethical and Judicial Affairs, "Decisions near the end of life," 1991, report B. Chicago: American Medical Association, 1991.

56. Cooke M. Patient rights and physician responsibility: four problems in AIDS care. In: Volberding P, Jacobson M, eds. AIDS clinical reviews 1993/4. New York: Marcel Dekker, 1994:261.

57. Marzuk P, Tierney H, Tardiff K. Increased risk of suicide in persons with AIDS JAMA 1988;259:1333.

58. Battin M. Going early, going late: the rationality of decisions about suicide in AIDS. J Med Philos 1994;19:571.

59. Rothman D. Ethics and human experimentation—Henry Beecher revisited. N Engl J Med 1987;317:1195.

60. Nuremberg Code (1949). In: Annas G, Grodin M, eds. The Nazi doctors and the Nuremberg Code: human rights and human experimentation. New York: Oxford University Press, 1992.

61. National Commission for the Protection of Human Subjects of Biomedical and Behavioral Research. The Belmont Report: ethical principles and guidelines for the protection of human subjects of research. Washington DC: U.S. Government Printing Office, 1979.

62. Annas G. Faith (healing), hope, and charity at the FDA: the politics of AIDS drug trials. In: Gostin L, ed. AIDS and the health care system. New Haven: Yale University Press, 1990:183.

63. Arno P, Feiden K. Against the odds: the story of AIDS drug development. New York: Harper-Collins, 1992.

64. Freedman B. Suspended judgment: AIDS and the ethics of clinical trials: learning the right lessons. Control Clin Trials 1992;13:1.

65. Levine C. Has AIDS changed the ethics of human subjects research? Law Med Health Care 1988;16:3.

66. Levine C. AIDS and the ethics of human subjects research. In: Reamer F, ed. AIDS and ethics. New York: Columbia University Press, 1991:77.

67. Bayer R. AIDS, ethics, and activism. In: Bluger R, Bobby E, Fineberg H, eds. Society's choices: social and ethical decision making in biomedicine. Washington, DC: National Academy Press, 1995:458.

68. Levine C, Dubler N, Levine R. Building a new consensus: ethical principles and policies for clinical research on HIV/AIDS. IRB: a review of human subjects research 1991;13:1.

69. Merrigan T. You can teach an old dog new tricks—how AIDS trials are pioneering new strategies. N Engl J Med 1990;323:1341.

70. Rothman D, Edgar H. Scientific rigor and medical realities: placebo trials in cancer and AIDS research. In: Fee E, Fox D, eds. AIDS: the making of a chronic disease. Berkeley: University of California Press, 1992:194.

71. NIH Revitalization Act of 1993 (Public Law 103-43) and the NIH Guidelines on the Inclusion of Women and Minorities as Subjects in Clinical Research. Bethesda, MD: National Institutes of Health, August 1994.

72. Benditt J. Conduct in Science. Science 1995; 268:1705.

PART VIII

HIV Infection and the Health Care Worker

AIDS: Biology, Diagnosis, Treatment and Prevention, fourth edition, edited by Vincent T. DeVita, Jr., Samuel Hellman, and Steven A. Rosenberg. Lippincott–Raven Publishers, © 1997

CHAPTER 35

Occupational Risk of Human Immunodeficiency Virus Infection in Health Care Workers

Ruthanne Marcus and David M. Bell

Considerable progress has been made in understanding the occupational risk of human immunodeficiency virus (HIV) infection among health care workers (HCWs) and in developing and evaluating measures to prevent exposures to blood, which is the most important source of HIV transmission in health care settings. Assessment of risk requires information derived from multiple sources, including surveillance data, seroprevalence studies of HCWs and patients, prospective studies that assess the risk of seroconversion after an exposure to HIV-infected blood, and studies of the frequency and preventability of blood contacts.

Factors influencing the risk to an individual HCW over a lifetime career include the risk of HIV transmission after a single blood contact, the prevalence of HIV infection among patients treated by the worker, and the number and types of blood contacts experienced by the worker. In this chapter, we review the data on occupationally acquired HIV infection in HCWs, including information on these three determinants of risk. We also outline the progress and future directions for development of preventive measures. We summarize information regarding HIV transmission to patients in health care settings, transmissions that should be preventable if recommended infection control measures are followed.

SURVEILLANCE OF AIDS AND OCCUPATIONALLY ACQUIRED HIV INFECTION AMONG HEALTH CARE WORKERS

In the United States, two databases in the National HIV and AIDS Surveillance System of the Centers for Disease Control and Prevention (CDC) have been useful for monitoring reports of HCWs with HIV infection or acquired immunodeficiency syndrome (AIDS).[1,2] Both rely on information provided by state and local health departments to the CDC. AIDS case surveillance data, which have been collected since the early 1980s, indicate whether the person reported with AIDS had been employed in a health care setting. In 1991, the CDC formally initiated surveillance of HCWs reported with occupationally acquired HIV infection, regardless of whether they met the AIDS case definition.

As of December 31, 1994, the CDC had received reports of 304,651 adults with AIDS for whom information on previous employment in health care was available; of these persons, 14,591 (4.8%) had been employed in health care settings. In comparison, approximately 5.7% of the U.S. labor force is employed in health services.[3] HCWs are not overrepresented among reported cases of AIDS. Of the HCWs with AIDS, 93% reported one or more nonoccupational risks for acquiring HIV. The remaining 7% did not report a nonoccupational risk factor; most of these cases are still under investigation to determine the mode of transmission. The proportion of these workers with undetermined risks who may have acquired HIV infection from an occupational exposure cannot be determined; those with possible occupational transmission are included in the data described in the following sections.

Ruthanne Marcus, Yale University School of Medicine, Division of Epidemiology and Public Health, 60 College Street, New Haven, CT 06520.

David M. Bell, HIV Infections Branch, Hospital Infections Program, Mailstop E-68, Centers for Disease Control and Prevention, Atlanta, Georgia 30333.

TABLE 35-1. *U.S. health care workers with documented and possible occupationally acquired HIV infection, reported through December 1994*

Occupation	Number of Documented Occupational Transmissions	Number of Possible Occupational Transmissions
Dental worker, including dentist		6
Embalmer or morgue technician		2
Emergency medical technician or paramedic		9
Health aide or attendant	1	9
Housekeeper or maintenance worker	1	7
Laboratory technician, clinical	15	14
Laboratory technician, nonclinical	2	1
Nurse	13	20
Physician, nonsurgical	6	9
Physician, surgical		3
Respiratory therapist	1	2
Technician, dialysis	1	2
Technician, surgical	2	1
Technician or therapist other than those listed above		4
Other health care occupations		2
Total	42	91

Centers for Disease Control and Prevention. HIV/AIDS surveillance report. Atlanta, GA: Centers for Disease Control and Prevention 1994;6:21.

Cases in the surveillance database for occupationally acquired HIV infection are classified as "documented" or "possible" cases. With one exception, persons classified as having documented cases have evidence of HIV seroconversion (ie, conversion from documented HIV seronegative to seropositive status) temporally associated with an occupational percutaneous, mucous membrane, or cutaneous exposure. In the one exception, a person who worked with concentrated HIV was determined by HIV DNA sequence analysis to be infected with this HIV strain, although the time and route of exposure were not determined (Ciesielski C, CDC: personal communication).

Persons classified as having possible cases of occupational infection have been investigated by state and local health departments and are without identifiable behavioral or transfusion risks. Each reported percutaneous or mucocutaneous occupational exposure to blood or body fluids or laboratory solutions containing HIV. However, HIV seroconversion temporally associated with an occupational exposure was not documented.

As of December 31, 1994, 42 documented and 91 possible cases of occupationally acquired infection among HCWs in the United States were reported to the CDC (Table 35-1).[1] Of the 42 persons with documented cases, 38 were exposed to HIV-infected blood, one was exposed to visibly bloody fluid from a patient with HIV infection, one to an unspecified fluid, and two to concentrated HIV in a laboratory. Thirty-six (86%) workers sustained percutaneous injuries, four (10%) had mucocutaneous exposures, one (2%) had both percutaneous and mucocutaneous exposures, and one had an unknown route of exposure to concentrated virus. Thirty-six documented cases resulted from percutaneous injuries with needles or other sharp objects; all of the nee-

dles had hollow bores (Ciesielski C, CDC: personal communication).

The CDC is also aware of at least 20 cases of occupationally acquired infection reported from outside the United States.[4-6] Documented transmission of HIV from a patient to a HCW in a clinical setting has always been by mean of occupational exposure to blood, with three possible exceptions: in one case, a nurse was exposed to visibly bloody pleural fluid[7]; another case involved visibly bloody abscess fluid; and in the third case, a hospital housekeeping worker was injured with a discarded needle attached to a syringe that had contained an unknown fluid.

Although friends and relatives providing nursing and custodial care to HIV-infected patients at home are not classified as HCWs, it is important to recognize that these caregivers have occasionally acquired HIV infection during these activities. In one case, a mother acquired HIV infection while providing extensive nursing care without gloves to her infant son (eg, drawing blood, removing intravenous catheters, emptying and changing ostomy bags). In two additional cases, caregivers became infected while providing nursing care at home to terminally ill adults with AIDS. In both cases, skin contact with body secretions and excretions occurred; blood exposure may also have occurred but was not documented.[8]

SURVEYS OF SEROPREVALENCE AMONG HEALTH CARE WORKERS

It is likely that data from passive surveillance systems do not reflect the full extent of occupationally acquired HIV infection. Some cases may not be recognized or documented, particularly if exposures are not reported at the time of occurrence.[9] Concerns about worker confidentiality may inhibit reporting to public health authorities. For this reason, cross-sectional studies of HIV seroprevalence in groups of HCWs provide important additional information on the risk of occupationally acquiring HIV infection (Table 35-2). Such studies must be interpreted carefully, taking into account whether the enrolled HCWs are representative of the population being studied and whether information is available to assess the possibility of occupational and nonoccupational exposure to HIV. Voluntary seroprevalence surveys, even if anonymous, are subject to a variety of selection biases; for example, persons who already know their HIV test results may decline to participate. Nevertheless, these surveys may be extremely useful in identifying previously unsuspected HIV infection.

In one of the largest studies, Chamberland and colleagues evaluated 8519 HCWs who donated blood in six urban regions in the United States between March 1990 and August 1991; three (0.04%) workers were HIV seropositive.

Two workers reported nonoccupational risks for HIV infection and the third was lost to follow-up.[10]

Two large, voluntary, anonymous seroprevalence surveys of surgeons have been conducted. The first was conducted by the CDC in collaboration with the American Academy of Orthopaedic Surgeons (AAOS) at the AAOS annual meeting in 1991.[11] Of the 3420 orthopedic surgeons who participated (48% of those eligible), two (0.06%; upper limit of 95% confidence interval [CI] = 0.18%) were HIV seropositive. These two seropositive surgeons reported nonoccupational risks for HIV infection on the anonymous questionnaires that were linked to their blood specimens. Among the 108 surgeons who reported nonoccupational risks, the HIV seroprevalence was 1.8% (upper limit of 95% CI = 5.7%). Of the 3267 surgeons who did not report nonoccupational risks for HIV infection, none was HIV seropositive (upper limit of 95% CI = 0.092%). Of the 45 participants who did not respond to the question on risk factors, none was HIV seropositive.

TABLE 35-2. *HIV seroprevalence in selected groups of health care workers*

Worker Group	Number Tested	Number (%) Positive	Number Positive With Community Risk	Prevalence, Excluding Seropositives With Community Risk*	Reference
Orthopedic surgeons	3,420	2 (0.06)	2	0.00	11
Surgeons in high AIDS incidence areas—USA	770	1 (0.13)	0	0.14	12
Medical personnel in U.S. Army Reserve	58,394	138 (2.37)	NA	NA	13
Dentists					
San Francisco	304†	0 (0)	†	0	15
Sacramento	89	0 (0)	0	0	107
USA 1986 annual meeting and New York City	1,132†	1 (0.09)	†	0.09	14
USA—1987 annual meeting	1,195	0 (0)	0	0	16
USA—1988 annual meeting	1,165	1 (0.09)	0	0.09	16
USA—1989 annual meeting	1,480	1 (0.07)	0	0	16
USA—1990 annual meeting	1,466	1 (0.07)	0	0	16
USA—1991 annual meeting	1,642	0 (0)	0	0	‡
USA—1992 annual meeting	1,812	0 (0)	0	0	‡
USA—1993 annual meeting	2,035	0 (0)	0	0	‡
USA—1994 annual meeting	1,687	0 (0)	0	0	‡
Denmark	961	0 (0)	0	0	108
Dental assistants (New York City and Sacramento)	176	0 (0)	0	0	14,107
Dental hygienists (New York City and Sacramento)	167	0 (0)	0	0	14,107
Hemodialysis staff (New York, Paris, Chicago, Brussels, Florence)	356	0 (0)	0	0	18, 19, 20, 21, 22
Blood donors, USA—six urban regions	8,519	3 (0.04)	0–1	0–0.01	10
Morticians					
Massachusetts	133	1 (0.75)	1	0	23
Maryland	130	1 (0.77)	1	0	24

NA, not available.
*Values are percentages
†Persons with community risk not included.
‡C. Siew, American Dental Association, personal communication.

Based on questionnaire data, opportunities for occupational exposure were assessed for the 3267 HIV seronegative surgeons who did not report nonoccupational risks. These surgeons spent approximately 11,837 years of training and practice in areas of high AIDS incidence during 1979–1991 (20% of the group's total years of training and practice); 1201 participants performed or assisted at an estimated 6822 surgical procedures on patients with known HIV infection or AIDS. During their careers, the participants reported a total of 162 percutaneous injuries with sharp objects contaminated with blood from patients with known HIV infection or AIDS.

A second seroprevalence survey of surgeons was conducted by Panlilio and colleagues in 1991 and 1992 among surgeons on the general surgery, obstetrics and gynecology, or orthopedic services in 21 hospitals in two areas of high HIV prevalence in the United States.[12] Of the 770 surgeons who participated (27% of those eligible), one was HIV seropositive (0.13%, upper 95% CI = 0.62%). This surgeon did not report a nonoccupational risk factor on the accompanying questionnaire. The surgeon reported having practiced general surgery for at least 25 years and having received three percutaneous injuries involving patients with HIV or AIDS and at least five injuries involving patients with risk factors for HIV infection.

Cowan and colleagues at Walter Reed Army Institute of Research analyzed data from the mandatory HIV testing program for members of the U.S. Army Reserve; these personnel spend about 90% of their time working in civilian settings.[13] Among physicians, surgeons, and dentists, the HIV seroprevalence was 0 of 263 women and 3 of 3084 men. Among all of the 58,349 reservists employed in a medical field, 138 (2.37 per 1000 tested; 95% CI = 2.02 to 2.83) were HIV seropositive. In contrast, 925 of 619,112 nonmedical reservists (1.49 per 1000 tested; 95% CI = 1.41 to 1.60) were HIV seropositive. The higher rate of HIV infection in medical workers resulted primarily from infections among never-married men. Because no information on possible risk factors was reported, it is unknown whether these men acquired infection occupationally.

Several seroprevalence surveys of dentists have been conducted, mostly during annual meetings of the American Dental Association. These surveys, as well as surveys of dental hygienists and dental chairside assistants, have also found low rates of infection among persons not reporting behavioral or transfusion risks.[14–17] In the most detailed published report, Klein and colleagues tested 1309 dental workers, including 1132 dentists and 177 dental hygienists and assistants, over half of whom practiced in areas of the United States reporting a large number of AIDS cases. Fifteen percent of the participants had treated patients with AIDS; 72% had treated patients at risk for HIV infection. One (0.08%) dentist without behavioral risks for HIV infection tested seropositive from the group of 1309 dental workers. This dentist worked in an area of the United States with a high prevalence of HIV infection and reported treating patients at increased risk for HIV infection.[14]

Workers in hemodialysis units have also been evaluated because of the recognized high risk of hepatitis B virus infection in such workers in the past. Combining results from several small studies, none of 356 dialysis workers tested was HIV seropositive.[18–22]

In two studies of morticians in the northeast United States, the combined HIV seroprevalence was 2 (0.8%) of 263; both seropositive morticians reported nonoccupational risks for HIV infection.[23,24]

Relatively few seroprevalence surveys have been conducted among HCWs in developing countries, where the HIV seroprevalence among patients is high and resources for infection control are limited. In the few studies that have been conducted, rates of HIV infection in medical workers were similar to those in the community.[25–27]

RISK OF HIV SEROCONVERSION AFTER EXPOSURE

Several prospective cohort studies have assessed the risk of HIV infection in HCWs after a documented exposure to HIV-infected blood.[28–35] These studies have consistently indicated that the risk of acquiring HIV infection after a percutaneous exposure to HIV-infected blood is approximately 0.3%. In the largest study, the CDC's ongoing Surveillance of Health Care Workers Exposed to HIV-Infected Blood, HCWs in more than 200 hospitals in the United States are enrolled and tested at the time of exposure and at least 6 months later. As of March 31, 1995, of 1373 workers enrolled after a percutaneous exposure (ie, needle stick or cut with a sharp object) to HIV-infected blood, four (0.29%; upper limit of 95% CI = 0.66%) seroconverted to HIV positive. In a published report of a similar study conducted in Italy, the results of 14 prospective studies, including the CDC study, were aggregated; of 3628 HCWs with a percutaneous exposure to HIV-infected blood, nine (0.25%; 95% CI = 0.12% to 0.47%) became infected.[35]

The risk estimate of 0.3% represents an average of many types of percutaneous exposures to blood from source patients in various stages of HIV infection. It is likely that there are subsets of exposures for which the risk is higher or lower than 0.3%. Determination of the risks associated with those subsets would be of tremendous value in counseling exposed workers and in targeting and evaluating preventive measures. Unfortunately, the prospective studies have insufficient statistical power to stratify the risk of infection based on various factors hypothesized to be important, including the size (large versus small gauge) or type (hollow versus solid bore) of needle, the depth or severity of exposure, the volume of blood involved, the titer (or a surrogate for titer) of HIV in the blood, and other factors, including the use of postexposure antiretroviral chemoprophylaxis.

Several investigators have performed in vitro studies to compare the volumes of blood transferred in needle-stick injuries. They have found that the volume is greater for more deeply penetrating injuries; for hollow-bore needles than for solid-bore needles; and when the needle does not pass through glove material.[36,37] Because these differences in volume are generally within one order of magnitude, Gerberding suggested that the most important determinant of transmission risk is likely to be the titer of HIV in the source patient's blood, which may vary by several orders of magnitude over the course of HIV infection.[38,39] It is also possible that the HCW's immune response may be important.[40]

Retrospective case-control methods have been used to identify risk factors for seroconversion among HCWs with percutaneous exposures to HIV-infected blood. Cardo and coworkers[41] compared 31 HCWs with occupationally acquired HIV infection reported to national surveillance systems with 679 control HCWs who did not seroconvert but who had been followed prospectively in a different CDC project after exposure to HIV-infected blood (previously discussed). Analysis using logistic regression identified several potential risk factors that were statistically significant, including a "deep" injury (adjusted odds ratio [OR] = 16.1), visible blood on the device causing the injury (OR = 5.2), injury by a needle placed directly in a vein or artery (OR = 5.1), the source patient being in the terminal stage of AIDS (OR = 6.4), and the lack of zidovudine postexposure use by the HCW (OR = 0.2). (See Chap 37).

Assessment of the risk of HIV transmission after a mucous membrane or skin exposure has been more difficult because of the low number of seroconversions among workers with such exposures enrolled in prospective studies. In a report from Italy, one HCW seroconverted after extensive contact of the eyes, mouth, and hands with a large amount of blood from an asymptomatic source patient; aggregating this study with five others, Ippolito and colleagues estimated the risk after a mucous membrane exposure at 0.09% (1 of 1107; 95% CI = 0.006% to 0.50%).[35]

The risk after a skin exposure to HIV-infected blood is believed to be less than after other types of exposure, but it has not been precisely quantified because no HCWs enrolled in these prospective studies have seroconverted after an isolated skin exposure. In the largest study of HCWs with skin contact with HIV-infected blood, none of 2712 workers at the National Institutes of Health Clinical Center who recalled such contact seroconverted (0%; upper limit of 95% CI = 0.11%).[30] At the same institution, Fahey and colleagues reported no HIV seroconversions among HCWs who estimated having had 20,028 skin contacts with blood from all patients, including an estimated 6528 contacts with HIV-infected blood.[42]

To evaluate the possibility of delayed seroconversion, several investigators have used the polymerase chain reaction (PCR) to examine specimens from HIV antibody-negative HCWs more than 6 months after exposure to HIV-infected blood.[29,30,43,44] In one study, 3 of 133 HCWs with a history of parenteral exposure to HIV-infected blood had one or more positive PCR test results; after 3 or 4 years, all three were PCR negative, and all remain seronegative, p24 antigen negative, culture negative, and clinically

healthy.[29] These data, combined with data on several hundred HCWs who have remained seronegative when tested 2 years or longer after exposure,[28–30] suggest that seroconversion (if it occurs) more than 6 months after occupational exposure is likely to be uncommon.

HIV SEROPREVALENCE AMONG PATIENTS

The second factor influencing the occupational risk of HIV infection is the prevalence of HIV infection among the patients receiving care. The risk of infection influenced by the level of infected patients, and the use of infection control precautions may be altered depending on the HCWs' perceptions of the HIV prevalence in their patients. In several studies of patient seroprevalence, the HIV seropositive status of most positive patients was unknown to HCWs at the time of treatment.[45,47,53]

In the United States, seroprevalence surveys among groups of patients have found that the rates vary widely by geographic area, the patient's age, sex, race or ethnicity, presenting clinical condition, and other factors.[46] Despite these variations, these studies demonstrate that infection with HIV (and other bloodborne pathogens) is found among patients in all areas of the United States and in patients with a wide variety of clinical conditions.

For example, in the CDC Sentinel Hospital Surveillance System, blood samples of patients treated in 20 acute-care hospitals were tested anonymously for HIV antibody. Of 195,829 blood samples tested, the overall HIV seroprevalence in the participating hospitals was 4.7%.[47] Rates varied from 0.2% to 14.2%, depending on the geographic location of the hospital.

Serosurveys of surgical patients have also revealed variations in HIV seroprevalence, depending on the patient population. Surgical and obstetric patients at Westchester County Medical Center, a tertiary care hospital near New York City, were tested blindly for HIV, hepatitis B virus, and hepatitis C virus. Among patients undergoing 1062 surgical procedures, the HIV seroprevalence was 1.6%.[48] Operations involving women between the ages of 25 and 44 years had the highest seroprevalence rates for any of the three viruses (17.2%), for HIV-1 (6.7%), and for HCV (15.3%). At the Johns Hopkins Hospital in Baltimore, the HIV seroprevalence was 0.4% among 4087 elective surgery patients, who were predominantly white (approximately 80%) and resided outside of the City of Baltimore (60%).[49] Of 2004 trauma surgery patients in Wichita, Kansas, 0.15% were HIV seropositive.[50] Women delivering at hospitals in Boston and New York City have had an HIV seroprevalence of approximately 2%.[51,52]

Several studies of HIV seroprevalence have been conducted in emergency department patients.[45,53–59] In a CDC study, blinded HIV antibody testing was conducted of left-over blood specimens from 20,382 emergency department patients in six hospitals, one inner-city and one suburban hospital in each of three cities in the United States with a high AIDS incidence. Seroprevalence rates per 100 patient visits were 4.1 to 8.9 in the inner-city emergency departments, 6.1 in one suburban emergency department, and 0.2 and 0.7 in the other two suburban hospitals. Rates were highest among patients between 15 and 44 years of age, males, blacks, and patients presenting with pneumonia. The percentage of patients whose HIV infection was unknown was 66% to 70% among inner-city emergency departments, 40% in the suburban emergency department with a higher seroprevalence, and 76% to 91% in the other two suburban emergency departments.[45]

Kelen and colleagues found that of 2522 patients presenting to the Johns Hopkins Hospital Emergency Department in 1988, 6% were HIV seropositive.[54,55] High rates of HIV infection were found among victims of penetrating trauma; however, this has not been the case in every emergency department studied,[45,59] illustrating the variability of HIV seroprevalence among different patient populations. Kelen also found that 18% of the patients studied were seropositive for hepatitis C virus and that 5% were positive for hepatitis B surface antigen; 24% were infected with at least one of these three agents.

The prevalence of HIV among hemodialysis patients[22,60–62] has ranged from 0% to 39%, depending on the city where the dialysis unit was located and the patient population treated. For example, centers that treated a large proportion of intravenous drug users had higher rates of HIV infection among the patients.

Collectively these findings underscore the need for universal precautions (see Chap. 36.1).

EPIDEMIOLOGY OF BLOOD CONTACT

Researchers have prospectively studied the nature and frequency of blood contact among workers in a variety of health care settings, including in surgical and obstetric suites, emergency departments, on hospital wards, in dental clinics, and in pre-hospital emergency medical services. These studies, plus information obtained in questionnaire surveys,[11,63–66] are useful for assessing risk factors for blood contact and for targeting preventive measures. Based on prospective studies of the frequency of blood exposure per procedure performed or per shift worked by each HCW, annual rates of blood contact have been estimated for workers in various occupational groups in the United States (Table 35-3). All of these figures are estimates that are clearly not applicable to every worker in each occupational group. Moreover, not all exposures may be comparable; for example, most of the surgeons' exposures result from solid-bore suture needles. Solid-bore needles inject a smaller quantity of blood[67,68] and are probably less likely to transmit infection than are hollow-bore needle exposures, which are more likely to be sustained by other HCWs, such as physicians and nurses on medical wards.

Several observational studies have found at least one sharp injury in 1.3% to 15.4% of surgical procedures

observed.[69–76] The frequency of injury varies with the procedure performed, duration of the procedure, and workers' technique (eg, using fingers instead of instruments to hold tissue). For example, Tokars and coworkers observed 99 percutaneous injuries during 95 (6.9%) of 1382 general, orthopedic, gynecologic, cardiac, and trauma surgical procedures.[71] Of the 99 injuries, 76 (80%) were caused by suture needles; 46 (46%) were associated with use of fingers rather than an instrument to hold tissue being sutured; and 62 (63%) affected the nondominant hand, primarily the distal forefinger. Injuries occurring on this portion of the hand may be prevented by the use of a barrier such as a thimble. Other potentially preventive measures such as blunted suture needles and puncture-resistant gloves may also be indicated to reduce the frequency of percutaneous injuries during surgery.

Injury rates varied by occupation and subspecialty, with residents and attending surgeons experiencing the highest rates (2.5 and 2.1 per 100 person-procedures, respectively); circulating nurses sustained no percutaneous injuries. At least one percutaneous injury was observed during 10% of gynecologic procedures.[71]

In these same surgical and obstetric studies, the rates of mucocutaneous blood contact ranged from 6.4% to 50.4%, depending on the study methodology, the definition of a blood contact, procedures observed, and the use of infection control precautions.[69–77] Gerberding found that the factors affecting the risk of blood contact were the length of the procedure, the volume of blood loss, and whether the operation involved major vascular or intraabdominal gynecologic surgery.[75] The risk of exposure was not influenced by the surgeon's prior knowledge of the patient's serostatus or risk of HIV infection.[71,75]

Hands were the most frequent area of contact identified by Tokars.[77] However, surgeons wearing two pairs of gloves had 72% fewer hand contacts than those wearing one pair. Other studies have also found the frequency of blood contact on hands to be reduced by double gloving.[78–81] Body contacts have been associated with increased amount of estimated blood loss; face contacts were most frequently observed during orthopedic procedures.[77] Panlilio found that more than one half of obstetricians' contacts might have been prevented by the use of barriers such as face shields, impervious gowns, and impervious shoe covers; one half of the midwives' contacts might have been prevented by the use of gowns.[72] Other protective measures, such as face shields, could be useful for preventing mucous membrane and eye contact.[77]

The frequency of blood contact among hospital emergency department workers has also been studied prospectively.[45] In a CDC study of six hospitals, blood contact varied by procedure observed; for example, blood contacts were highest during thoracotomy (63%) and lowest during phlebotomy (2%). Gloves significantly reduced the rate of blood contact; for example, the relative risk of blood contact for ungloved compared with gloved emergency department

TABLE 35-3. *Annual estimates of the frequency of blood contact by health care workers*

Investigator	Occupation Studied	Total Number of Blood Contacts* per Year	Number of Percutaneous Blood Contacts per Year	Reference Used to Derive Annual Estimate
Tokars	Surgeon	81–135	8–13	71
Panlilio	Obstetrician	77	4	72
Cleveland	Dentist	NA	4	82
Wong	Physician on medical ward	31.2	1.8	66
Smith	Nurse on medical ward	NA	0.98	†
Tokars	Surgical scrub assistant	7–12	0.6–1.0	71
Marcus	Hospital emergency department worker	24.2	0.4	45
Marcus	Pre-hospital emergency medical worker	12.3	0.2	109

NA, not available.
*Percutaneous, mucous membrane, or skin contact, based on prospective studies.
†H. Smith, University of Pennsylvania, personal communication.

workers was 19.8 for obtaining an arterial blood gas, 13.0 for inserting an intravenous line, and 5.4 for phlebotomy.

In a study of dental personnel, 0.33 injuries per dentist-month were observed. In this same study, no injuries were reported in over 4000 outpatient oral surgery procedures.[82]

Most documented cases of HIV seroconversion have involved hollow-bore needle devices used for drawing blood or intravascular access. In recent years, attention has been focused on the frequency and preventability of injuries associated with these devices. Among 326 needle-stick injuries reported to the employee health service at a university hospital, Jagger and associates found that 17.8% occurred before or during use of the needle-bearing device, 69.6% occurred after use but before disposal, and 13.2% occurred during or after disposal.[83] One third of injuries involved recapping, which was often reportedly done to avoid a competing hazard, such as disassembling a device with an exposed needle or carrying uncapped items to a disposal box. When injury rates were estimated based on the number of devices purchased, the highest rates of injury were for items that required disassembly after use. Among 2248 percutaneous injuries reported in the CDC's multicenter surveillance project of HCWs exposed to HIV-infected blood, the greatest percentage (44%) also occurred after use of a device but before disposal; 38% occurred during use of the device, 10% during disposal, and 7% at other or unknown times (Cardo DM: unpublished CDC data). These data suggest that a large proportion of needle-stick injuries related to phlebotomy and intravenous lines could be prevented with new or modified medical devices. Training, changes in work practices and improved access to needle disposal containers are also important,[66,84,85] but they have not been uniformly successful in reducing injury rates.[86]

Several researchers have estimated the cumulative risk to HCWs of HIV infection.[45,75,87–89] For example, Gerberding estimated that a worker at San Francisco General Hospital will become infected with HIV every 8 years.[75] Howard pre-

dicted that 47 of the approximately 18,000 Fellows of the American College of Surgeons would become infected with HIV during their surgical careers.[88] Such calculations are most likely to be accurate when the prevalence of HIV infection in the patient population is well defined, the frequency of blood contact (especially sharps exposures) is established, and the use of infection control practices is ascertained.

Aerosols

True aerosols, unlike larger droplets, are particles less than 100 μm in diameter that may remain suspended in air for extended periods. Although inhalation of particles of aerosolized blood may pose a theoretical risk of bloodborne pathogen transmission, no case of such transmission has been documented. Transmission of bloodborne pathogens by aerosols would require generation of aerosolized particles of blood, the presence of infective bloodborne pathogens in these aerosolized particles, and the deposition of a sufficient number of infective blood particles in the respiratory tract or on the mucous membranes of a susceptible host to cause infection. In studies conducted in dental operatories and in hemodialysis units, hepatitis B surface antigen was not detected in the air during treatment of patients infected with hepatitis B virus.[90] Aerosolized HIV has been detected in laboratory studies,[91] although these studies should not be interpreted to mean that HIV is aerosolized in a clinical setting or that HIV is transmitted by this route. Large HIV seroprevalence surveys of surgeons have provided no evidence of a significant risk for HIV transmission by the aerosol route.[11,12] Until further research is conducted, the possibility of occupational transmission of HIV through aerosolized blood should be considered theoretical.

HIV Transmission to Patients

HIV transmission to six patients of a dentist with AIDS has been reported.[92,93] Investigations of 22,171 patients of 51 other HIV-infected HCWs (representing 17% of the patients treated by these HCWs during the periods under investigation) have not identified other episodes of HCW-to-patient transmission of HIV.[94] These data confirm the assessments of the CDC and others that the risk of such transmission is very small.[95,96]

A potentially greater risk to patients is HIV transmission from other patients because of the failure of health care facilities or HCWs to adhere to recommended infection control precautions. In developing countries with limited resources for infection control, HIV transmission has occurred because of the reuse of intravenous infusion tubing,[97] inadequately sterilized needles, and syringes[98,99] and because of, in dialysis units, inadequate disinfection practices and suspected reuse of dialyzers, needles, and syringes.[100,101] In more developed countries, patient-to-patient transmission has resulted from inadvertent reinjection of HIV-infected material into the wrong patients during nuclear medicine procedures.[102,103] Transmission among patients was reported in a surgeon's office in Australia[104] and probably also occurred on a pediatric ward in New York City.[105] Although the mechanisms of transmission in Australia and New York City could not be identified retrospectively, failure to adhere to recommended precautions was presumed.

FUTURE RESEARCH

Additional research is needed to define more precisely the risk for seroconversion after exposure to HIV-infected blood, the frequency and preventability of occupational blood contacts, and the efficacy and toxicity of postexposure prophylaxis. Studies are also needed to assess the effect of preventive measures, including new or improved medical devices, work practices, and personal protective equipment in preventing blood contact without adversely affecting patient care.[83,106]

REFERENCES

1. Centers for Disease Control and Prevention. HIV/AIDS surveillance report. Atlanta, GA: Centers for Disease Control and Prevention 1994;6:21.
2. Chamberland ME, Conley LJ, Bush TJ, Ciesielski CA, Hammett TA, Jaffe HW. Health care workers with AIDS: national surveillance update. JAMA 1991;266:3459.
3. Bureau of Labor Statistics. Employment and earnings, volume 35. Washington, DC: U.S. Department of Labor, 1988:13.
4. Marcus R, Kay K, Mann JM. Transmission of human immunodeficiency virus (HIV) in health-care settings worldwide. Bull World Health Organ 1989;67:577.
5. Perez L, de Andres R, Fitch K, Najera R. HIV seroconversions following occupational exposure in European health care workers. Abstract PO-C18-3040. Presented at the IX International Conference on AIDS, Berlin, June 1993.
6. Tait DR, Pudifin DJ, Gathiram V, Windsor IM. HIV seroconversions in health care workers, Natal, South Africa. Abstract PoC 4141. Presented at the VIII International Conference on AIDS, Amsterdam, July 1992.
7. Oksenhendler E, Harzic M, Le Roux J-M, et al. HIV infection with seroconversion after a superficial needlestick injury to the finger. (Letter) N Engl J Med 1986;315:582.
8. Centers for Disease Control and Prevention. Human immunodeficiency virus transmission in household settings—United States. MMWR 1994;43:347.
9. Mangione CM, Gerberding JL, Cummings SR. Occupational exposure to HIV: frequency and rates of underreporting of percutaneous and mucocutaneous exposures by medical housestaff. Am J Med 1991;90:85.
10. Chamberland M, Petersen LR, Munn VP, et al. Human immunodeficiency virus infection among health care workers who donate blood. Ann Intern Med 1994;121:269.
11. Tokars JI, Chamberland ME, Schable CA, et al, for the American Academy of Orthopaedic Surgeons Serosurvey Study Committee. A survey of occupational blood contact and HIV infection among orthopedic surgeons. JAMA 1992;268:489.
12. Panlilio AL, Shapiro CN, Schable CA, et al. Serosurvey of human immunodeficiency virus, hepatitis B virus, and hepatitis C virus infection among hospital-based surgeons. J Am Coll Surg 1995;180:16.
13. Cowan DN, Brundage JF, Pomerantz RS, Miller RN, Burke DS. Human immunodeficiency virus infection among members of the U.S. Army Reserve Components with medical and health occupations. JAMA 1991;265:2826.
14. Klein RS, Phelan JA, Freeman K, et al. Low occupational risk of human immunodeficiency virus infection among dental professionals. N Engl J Med 1988;318:86.
15. Gerberding JL, Nelson K, Greenspan D, et al. Risk to dental professionals from occupational exposure to human immunodeficiency virus: follow-up. Abstract 698. In: Program and Abstracts of the Interscience Conference on Antimicrobial Agents and Chemotherapy, New York, October 4–7, 1987.
16. Gruninger SE, Siew C, Chang S-B, et al. Human immunodeficiency virus type 1 infection among dentists. J Am Dental Assoc 1992;123:57.
17. Siew C, Gruninger SE, Chang S-B, Clayton R. Seroprevalence of hepatitis B and HIV infection among oral surgeons. (Abstract 1431) J Dent Res 1994;73:281.
18. Goldman M, Leisnard C, Vanherweghem J-L, et al. Markers of HTLV-III in patients with end stage renal failure treated by haemodialysis. Br Med J 1986;293:161.
19. Peterman TA, Lang GR, Mikos NJ, et al. HTLV-III/LAV infection in hemodialysis patients. JAMA 1986;255:2324.
20. Comodo N, Martinelli F, De Majo E, et al. Risk of HIV infection on patients and staff of two dialysis centers: seroepidemiological findings and prevention trends. Eur J Epidemiol 1988;4:171.
21. Assogba U, Ancelle Park RA, Rey MA, Barthelemy A, Rottembourg J, Gluckman JC. Prospective study of HIV 1 seropositive patients in hemodialysis centers. Clin Nephrol 1988;29:312.
22. Chirgwin K, Rao TKS, Landesman SH. HIV infection in a high prevalence hemodialysis unit. AIDS 1989;3:731.
23. Turner SB, Kunches LM, Gordon, et al. Occupational exposure to human immunodeficiency virus (HIV) and hepatitis B virus (HBV) among embalmers: a pilot seroprevalence study. Am J Public Health 1989;79:1425.
24. Gershon RR, Vlahov D, Farzedegan H, Alter MJ. Occupational risk of human immunodeficiency virus, hepatitis B virus, and hepatitis C virus infections among funeral service practitioners in Maryland. Infect Control Hosp Epidemiol 1995;16:194.
25. Mann JM, Francis H, Quinn TC, et al. HIV seroprevalence among hospital workers in Kinshasa, Zaire: lack of association with occupational exposure. JAMA 1986;256:3099.
26. N'Galy B, Ryder RW, Bila K, et al. Human immunodeficiency virus infection among employees in an African hospital. N Engl J Med 1988;319:1123.
27. Lu S-L, Sow I, Coll E, et al. HIV-1, HIV-2, and HBV serologic status among Dakar hospital workers. Abstract 9009. Presented at the IV International Conference on AIDS, Stockholm, Sweden, June 12–16, 1988.
28. Tokars JI, Marcus R, Culver DH, et al, for the CDC Cooperative Needlestick Surveillance Group. Surveillance of HIV infection and zidovudine use among health-care workers after occupational exposure to HIV-infected blood. Ann Intern Med 1993;118:913.
29. Gerberding JL. Incidence and prevalence of human immunodeficiency virus, hepatitis B virus, hepatitis C virus, and cytomegalovirus among health care personnel at risk for blood exposure: final report from a longitudinal study. J Infect Dis 1994;170:1410.
30. Henderson DK, Fahey BJ, Willy M, et al. Risk for occupational transmission of human immunodeficiency virus type 1 (HIV-1) associated with clinical exposures: a prospective evaluation. Ann Intern Med 1990;113:740.

31. McEvoy M, Porter K, Mortimer P, Simmons N, Shanson D. Prospective study of clinical, laboratory, and ancillary staff with accidental exposures to blood or body fluids from patients infected with HIV. Br Med J 1987;294:1595.

32. Heptonstall J, Gill ON, Porter K, Black MB, Gilbart VL. Health care workers and HIV: surveillance of occupationally acquired infection in the United Kingdom. Communicable Disease Report 1993;3:R147.

33. Lot F, Abiteboul D, Bouvet E, et al. Surveillance of occupationally acquired HIV infection in France. Abstract PO-C18-3039. IX International Conference on AIDS, Berlin, Germany, 1993.

34. Francioli P, Saghafi L, Raselli P. Exposures of health care workers (HCW) to blood during various procedures: results of two surveys before and after the implementation of universal precautions (UP). Abstract TC 602. Sixth International Conference on AIDS, San Francisco, CA, 1990.

35. Ippolito G, Puro V, De Carli G, Italian Study Group on Occupational Risk of HIV Infection. The risk of occupational human immunodeficiency virus infection in health care workers. Arch Intern Med 1993;153:1451.

36. Mast ST, Woolwine JD, Gerberding JL. Efficacy of gloves in reducing blood volumes transferred during simulated needlestick injury. J Infect Dis 1993;168:1589.

37. Bennett NT, Howard RJ. Quantity of blood inoculated in a needlestick injury from suture needles. J Am Coll Surg 1994;178:107.

38. Gerberding JL. Management of occupational exposures to blood-borne viruses. N Engl J Med 1995;332:444.

39. Ho DD, Moudgil T, Alam M. Quantitation of human immunodeficiency virus type 1 in the blood of infected persons. N Engl J Med 1989;321:1621.

40. Clerici M, Levin JM, Kessler HA, et al. HIV-specific T-helper activity in seronegative health care workers exposed to contaminated blood. JAMA 1994;271:42.

41. Centers for Disease Control and Prevention. Case-control study of HIV seroconversion in health care workers after percutaneous exposure to HIV-infected blood. MMWR 1995;44:929.

42. Fahey BJ, Koziol DE, Banks SM, Henderson DK. Frequency of non-parenteral occupational exposures to blood and body fluids before and after universal precaution training. Am J Med 1991;90:145.

43. Wormser GP, Joline C, Bittker S, Forsetter G, Kwok S, Sninsky JJ. Polymerase chain reaction for seronegative health care workers with parenteral exposure to HIV-infected patients. N Engl J Med 1989;321:1681.

44. Henry K, Campbell S, Jackson B, et al. Long-term follow-up of health care workers with work site exposure to human immunodeficiency virus. JAMA 1990;263:1765.

45. Marcus R, Culver DH, Bell DM, et al. Risk of human immunodeficiency virus infection among emergency department workers. Am J Med 1993;94:363.

46. Centers for Disease Control and Prevention. National HIV serosurveillance summary—results through 1992. Publication No. HIV/NCID/11–93/036. Atlanta: U.S. Department of Health and Human Services, Public Health Service, 1993.

47. Janssen RS, St. Louis ME, Satten GA, et al. HIV infection among patients in U.S. acute-care hospitals: strategies for the counseling and testing of hospital patients. N Engl J Med 1992;327:445.

48. Montecalvo MA, Lee MS, DePalma H, et al. Seroprevalence of human immunodeficiency virus-1, hepatitis B virus and hepatitis C virus in patients having major surgery. Infect Control Hosp Epidemiol 1995;16:627.

49. Charache P, Cameron JL, Maters AW, et al. Prevalence of infection with human immunodeficiency virus in elective surgery patients. Ann Surg 1991;214:562.

50. Mullins JR, Harrison PB. The questionable utility of mandatory screening for the human immunodeficiency virus. Am J Surg 1993;166:676.

51. Donegan SP, Steger KA, Recla L, et al. Seroprevalence of human immunodeficiency virus in parturients at Boston City Hospital: implications for public health and obstetric practice. Am J Obstet Gynecol 1992;167:622.

52. Krasinski K, Borkowsky W, Bebenroth D, et al. Failure of voluntary testing for human immunodeficiency virus to identify infected parturient women in a high-risk population. (Letter) N Engl J Med 1988;318:185.

53. Kelen GD, Fritz S, Qaqish B, et al. Unrecognized human immunodeficiency virus infection in emergency department patients. N Engl J Med 1988;318:1645.

54. Kelen GD, DiGiovanna T, Bisson L, Kalainov D, Sivertson KT, Quinn TC. Human immunodeficiency virus infection in emergency patients: epidemiology, clinical presentations, and risk to health-care workers: the Johns Hopkins experience. JAMA 1989;262:516.

55. Kelen GD, Green GB, Purcell RH, et al. Hepatitis B and hepatitis C in emergency department patients. N Engl J Med 1992;326:1399.

56. Jui J, Modesitt S, Fleming D, et al. Multicenter HIV and hepatitis B seroprevalence study. J Emerg Med 1990;8:243.

57. Schweich PJ, Fosarelli PD, Duggan AK, Quinn TC, Baker JL. Prevalence of human immunodeficiency virus seropositivity in pediatric emergency room patients undergoing phlebotomy. Pediatrics 1990;89:660.

58. Rhee KJ, Albertson TE, Kizer KW, Hughes MJ, Ascher MS. The HIV-1 seroprevalence rate of injured patients admitted through California emergency departments. Ann Emerg Med 1991;20:969.

59. Baraff LJ, Talan DA, Torres M. Prevalence of HIV antibody in a non-inner-city university hospital emergency department. Ann Emerg Med 1991;20:782.

60. Marcus R, Favero MS, Banerjee S, et al. Prevalence and incidence of human immunodeficiency virus among patients undergoing long-term hemodialysis. Am J Med 1991;90:614.

61. Baltimore-Boston Collaborative Study Group. Human immunodeficiency virus infection in hemodialysis patients. Arch Intern Med 1988;148:617.

62. Johnston BL, Poole CL, Zito DR, Normansell DE, Westervelt FB, Farr BM. Cohort study of human immunodeficiency virus (HIV) antibody testing among patients receiving long-term dialysis at a university hospital. Am J Infect Control 1988;16:235.

63. Hussain SA, Latif ABA, Choudhary AAAA. Risk to surgeons: a survey of accidental injuries during operations. Br J Surg 1988;75:314.

64. Lowenfels AB, Mehta V, Levi DA, Montecalvo MA, Savino JA, Wormser GP. Reduced frequency of percutaneous injuries in surgeons: 1993 versus 1988. AIDS 1995;9:199.

65. Willy ME, Dhillon GL, Loewen NL, Wesley RA, Henderson DK. Adverse exposures and universal precautions practices among a group of highly exposed health professionals. Infect Control Hosp Epidemiol 1990;11:351.

66. Wong ES, Stotka JL, Chinchilli VM, Williams DS, Stuart CG, Markowitz SM. Are universal precautions effective in reducing the number of occupational exposures among health care workers? A prospective study of physicians on a medical service. JAMA 1991;265:1123.

67. Mast ST, Woolwine JD, Gerberding JL. Efficacy of gloves in reducing blood volumes transferred during simulated needlestick injury. J Infect Dis 1993;168:1589.

68. Bennett NT, Howard RJ. Quantity of blood inoculated in a needlestick injury from suture needles. J Am Coll Surg 1994;178:107.

69. Rudnick J, Chamberland M, Panlilio A, et al. Blood contacts during obstetrical procedures. Infect Control Hosp Epidemiol 1994;15:349.

70. Panlilio AL, Foy DR, Edwards JR, et al. Blood contacts during surgical procedures. JAMA 1991;265:1533.

71. Tokars JI, Bell DM, Marcus R, et al. Percutaneous injuries during surgical procedures. JAMA 1992;267:2899.

72. Panlilio AL, Welch BA, Bell DM, et al. Blood and amniotic fluid contact sustained by obstetric personnel during deliveries. Am J Obstet Gynecol 1992;167:703.

73. Popejoy SL, Fry DE. Blood contact and exposure in the operating room. Surg Gynecol Obstet 1991;172:480.

74. Quebbeman EJ, Telford GL, Hubbard S, et al. Risk of blood contamination and injury to operating room personnel. Ann Surg 1991;214:614.

75. Gerberding JL, Littell C, Tarkington A, Brown A, Schecter WP. Risk of exposure of surgical personnel to patients' blood during surgery at San Francisco General Hospital. N Engl J Med 1990;322:1788.

76. Robert L, Short L, Chamberland M, et al. Percutaneous injuries (PIs) sustained during gynecologic surgery (GS). (Abstract) Infect Control Hosp Epidemiol 1994;15:349.

77. Tokars JI, Culver DH, Mendelson MH, et al. Skin and mucous membrane contacts with blood during surgical procedures: risks and prevention. Infect Control Hosp Epidemiol (in press).

78. Rose DA, Ramiro NZ, Perlman JL, Schecter WP, Gerberding JL. Two gloves or not two gloves? Intraoperative glove utilization at San Francisco General Hospital. Infect Control Hosp Epidemiol 1994;15:P37.
79. Cohn GM, Seifer DB. Blood exposure in single versus double gloving during pelvic surgery. Am J Obstet Gynecol 1990;162:715.
80. Telford GL, Quebbeman EJ. Assessing the risk of blood exposure in the operating room. Am J Infect Control 1993;21:351.
81. Quebbeman EJ, Telford GJ, Wadsworth K, Hubbard S, Goodman H, Gottlieb MS. Double gloving: protecting surgeons from blood contamination in the operating room. Arch Surg 1992;127:213.
82. Cleveland JL, Lockwood SA, Gooch BF, et al. Percutaneous injuries in dentistry: an observational study. J Am Dent Assoc 1995;126:745.
83. Jagger J, Hunt EH, Brand-Elnagger J, Pearson RD. Rates of needlestick injury caused by various devices in a university hospital. N Engl J Med 1988;319:284.
84. Beekmann SE, Vlahov D, Koziol DE, McShalley ED, Schmitt JM, Henderson DK. Temporal association between implementation of universal precautions and a sustained, progressive decrease in percutaneous exposures to blood. Clin Infect Dis 1994;18:562.
85. Haiduven DJ, DeMaio TM, Stevens DA. A five-year study of needlestick injuries: significant reduction associated with communication, education, and convenient placement of sharps containers. Infect Control Hosp Epidemiol 1992;13:265.
86. Linnemann C, Cannon C, De Ronde M, et al. Effect of educational programs, rigid sharps containers, and universal precautions on reported needlestick injuries in health-care workers. Infect Control Hosp Epidemiol 1991;12:214.
87. Hagen MD, Meyer KB, Kopelman RI, Pauker SG. Human immunodeficiency virus infection in health care workers: a method for estimating individual occupational risk. Arch Intern Med 1989;149:1541.
88. Howard RJ. Human immunodeficiency virus testing and the risk to the surgeon of acquiring HIV. Surg Gynecol Obstet 1990;171:22.
89. Orient JM. Assessing the risk of occupational acquisition of the human immunodeficiency virus: implications for hospital policy. South Med J 1990;83:1121.
90. Petersen NJ. An assessment of the airborne route in hepatitis B transmission. Ann N Y Acad Sci 1980;353:157.
91. Johnson GK, Robinson WS. Human immunodeficiency virus-1 (HIV-1) in the vapors of surgical power instruments. J Med Virol 1991;33:47.
92. Ciesielski C, Marianos D, Ou CY, et al. Transmission of human immunodeficiency virus in a dental practice. Ann Intern Med 1992;116:798.
93. Ciesielski CA, Marianos DW, Schochetman G, Witte JJ, Jaffe HW. The 1990 Florida dental investigation. The press and the science. Ann Intern Med 1994;121:886.
94. Robert LM, Chamberland ME, Cleveland JL, et al. Investigations of patients of health care workers infected with HIV: the Centers for Disease Control and Prevention database. Ann Intern Med 1995;122:653.
95. Centers for Disease Control. Recommendations for preventing transmission of human immunodeficiency virus and hepatitis B virus to patients during exposure prone procedures. MMWR 1991;40(RR-8):1.
96. Bell DM, Shapiro CN, Culver DH, Martone WJ, Curran JW, Hughes JM. Risk of hepatitis B and human immunodeficiency virus transmission to a patient from an infected surgeon due to percutaneous injury during an invasive procedure: estimates based on a model. Infect Agents Dis 1992;1:263.
97. Avila C, Stetler HC, Sepulveda J, et al. The epidemiology of HIV transmission among paid plasma donors, Mexico City, Mexico. AIDS 1989;3:631.
98. Pokrovsky W. Localization of nosocomial outbreak of HIV infection in Southern Russia in 1988–1989. Abstract PoC 4138. Presented at VIII International Conference on AIDS, Amsterdam, July 1992.
99. Patrascu IV, Constantinescu StN, Dublanchet A. HIV-1 infection in Romanian children. Lancet 1990;335:672.
100. Dyer E. Argentinian doctors accused of spreading AIDS. Br Med J 1993;307:584.
101. Velandia M, Fridkin SK, Cardenas V, et al. Transmission of human immunodeficiency virus in a dialysis center, Colombia. (Abstract 25) Infect Control Hosp Epidemiol 1995;16:P20.
102. Lange JMA, Boucher CAB, Hollak CE, et al. Failure of zidovudine prophylaxis after accidental exposure to HIV-1. N Engl J Med 1990;322:1375.
103. Centers for Disease Control. Patient exposures to HIV during nuclear medicine procedures. MMWR 1992;41:575.
104. Chant K, Lowe D, Rubin G, et al. Patient-to-patient transmission of HIV in private surgical consulting rooms (letter). Lancet 1993;342:1548.
105. Blank S, Simonds RJ, Weisfuse I, et al. Possible nosocomial transmission of HIV. Lancet 1994;344:512.
106. Rhodes RS, Bell DM, eds. Prevention of transmission of bloodborne pathogens. Surg Clin North Am 1995;75:1047.
107. Flynn NM, Pollet SM, Van Horne JR, et al. Absence of HIV antibody among dental professionals exposed to infected patients. West J Med 1987;146:439.
108. Ebbesen P, Melbye M, Scheutz F, et al. Lack of antibodies to HTLV III/LAV in Danish dentists. (Letter) JAMA 1986;256:2199.
109. Marcus R, Srivastava PU, Bell DM, et al. Occupational blood contact among prehospital providers. Ann Emerg Med 1995;25:776.

AIDS: Biology, Diagnosis, Treatment and Prevention, fourth edition, edited by Vincent T. DeVita, Jr., Samuel Hellman, and Steven A. Rosenberg. Lippincott–Raven Publishers, © 1997

CHAPTER 36 Safety Precautions

36.1 Universal Precautions in the Health Care Setting

Elizabeth A. Bolyard and David M. Bell

With the emergence of acquired immune deficiency syndrome (AIDS) as a clinical entity and reports of occupational transmission as a result of exposure to blood from patients infected with human immunodeficiency virus (HIV), health care workers (HCWs) in clinical settings have become more cognizant of the risks of infection with HIV and other bloodborne pathogens, such as hepatitis B (HBV) and C viruses and human T-cell lymphotropic virus type I.[1-3] This chapter discusses the various methods and techniques recommended to prevent the transmission of bloodborne pathogens.

HISTORY OF ISOLATION PRECAUTIONS

Isolation was practiced for hospitalized patients with infectious diseases in the United States as early as 1877, when recommendations were made to place patients with infectious diseases in separate facilities, referred to as infectious disease hospitals. As time progressed, separate units within these facilities were designated for the care of patients with specific infectious diseases. Aseptic practices, including handwashing, were introduced to prevent transmission of infections among the patients in the infectious disease hospitals. Gradually adopted by general hospitals, the practices while caring for patients with transmissible infections included separate isolation cubicles and the use of barrier precautions such as wearing gowns, washing hands, and disinfecting contaminated objects. Widespread adoption of isolation and barrier precautions in general hospitals, as well as the advent of effective antibiotic therapy for many serious infections, led to the closing of infectious disease hospitals in the 1950s and 1960s.

In the 1970s, the Centers for Disease Control and Prevention (CDC) published detailed recommendations to assist hospitals with isolation practices. These recommendations used a system of seven isolation categories that were determined by the epidemiologic features of the diseases grouped in each category: strict isolation, respiratory isolation, protective isolation, enteric precautions, wound or skin precautions, discharge precautions and blood precautions.

The isolation recommendations were updated and modified in 1983 to allow hospitals to choose a category system or a disease-specific system; in both systems, the use of the components of isolation (eg, private room, gowns, masks, gloves) were based on the epidemiologic features of transmission of a specific disease or infection. In the category system, because of the recognition that AIDS was probably caused by a bloodborne agent, the CDC recommended that patients with AIDS be treated using the (now obsolete) isolation category of "blood and body fluid precautions," requiring that precautions be taken to prevent contact with blood and other body fluids thought capable of transmitting bloodborne viruses.[4]

Implementation of blood and body fluid precautions required the HCWs to know or suspect that the patient had a particular infection. Recognition that the infection status of many patients with HIV and other bloodborne pathogens would be unknown to HCWs and others potentially exposed to blood in the workplace led CDC to recommend the use of blood and body fluid precautions routinely, regardless of whether the patient was known to be infected with HIV or HBV.[5] Recommendations were also published for hemodialysis,[6] ophthalmologic procedures,[7] clinical laboratory procedures,[8] and dentistry.[9]

Elizabeth A. Bolyard, Prevention Activity, HIV Infections Branch, Hospital Infections Program, National Center for Infectious Diseases, Centers for Disease Control and Prevention, CDC-Mailstop E-68, 1600 Clifton Road, Atlanta, GA 30333.

David M. Bell, HIV Infections Branch, Hospital Infections Program, National Center for Infectious Diseases, Centers for Disease Control and Prevention, CDC-Mailstop E-68, 1600 Clifton Road, Atlanta, GA 30333.

In 1987, after three HCWs were reported to have acquired HIV after mucocutaneous exposures to blood,[10] CDC published the "Recommendations for Prevention of HIV Transmission in Health Care Settings."[11] These recommendations, updated in 1988,[12] are based on the principle of *universal precautions* (UP), which assumes that blood, certain other body fluids, and tissues of all patients should be considered potentially infectious. These documents emphasized that blood was the single most important source of HIV, HBV, and other bloodborne pathogens in the occupational setting and that infection control efforts for preventing transmission of bloodborne pathogens in health care settings must focus on preventing exposures to blood. The importance of HBV immunization was also emphasized. UP is intended to protect HCWs and patients from infection with bloodborne pathogens in health care settings. UP is not intended to prevent transmission of all pathogens; additional precautions are necessary to prevent transmission of other infectious agents.

In 1987, an alternative system of isolation called *body substance isolation* (BSI) was proposed by infection control experts in two university hospitals.[13] BSI incorporates the principle of universality (ie, for all patients) contained in the CDC UP recommendations, but it extends those recommendations to cover all moist and potentially infectious body substances, such as blood, feces, urine, sputum, saliva, wound drainage, and other body fluids. This system is intended to prevent transmission of a variety of infectious agents in addition to bloodborne pathogens. Under BSI, gloving is recommended before contact with mucous membranes and nonintact skin and for anticipated contact with moist body substances. Hands are to be washed after glove removal only when the hands are visibly soiled. As is the case for UP, additional precautions are needed to prevent the transmission of airborne infections (eg, tuberculosis). The advantages and disadvantages of these systems and comparisons of the various isolation practices have been discussed elsewhere.[14–16]

In 1991, the Occupational Safety and Health Administration (OSHA) published a standard regarding occupational exposure to bloodborne pathogens.[17] Unlike CDC recommendations, OSHA standards have the force of law and must be adhered to by most employers in the United States. The standard, based on the concept of UP, mandates precautions to protect HCWs from the transmission of bloodborne pathogens. It does not address protection for patients.

In 1995, the CDC's Hospital Infection Control Practices Advisory Committee (HICPAC) published a revised and updated system of infection control that synthesized the major features of UP and BSI, called *standard precautions,* and applied the system to all patients receiving care in hospitals, regardless of their diagnosis or presumed infection status. Standard precautions apply to blood, all body fluids, secretions, excretions, nonintact skin, and mucous membranes, regardless of whether they contain or are contaminated with visible blood. Transmission-based precautions are recommended for patients documented or suspected to be infected with highly transmissible or epidemiologically important pathogens for which the standard precautions may not be adequate to interrupt transmission in hospitals (eg, airborne precautions for patients with infectious pulmonary tuberculosis).[18] Hospitals may wish to follow the more comprehensive precautions in this guideline to prevent transmission of non-bloodborne pathogens.

ELEMENTS OF UNIVERSAL PRECAUTIONS

UP should be followed if there is potential for contact with blood and other body fluids containing visible blood. Table 36.1-1 lists the fluids to which UP does and does not apply. UP applies to semen and vaginal secretions, because these fluids have been implicated in the sexual transmission of HIV and HBV, although not in occupational transmission from patient to HCW. UP also applies to tissues and to amniotic, cerebrospinal, pericardial, peritoneal, pleural, and synovial fluids, from which HIV or HBV has been isolated but from which transmission to HCWs has not been documented. Epidemiologic studies in the health care setting are inadequate to assess the potential risk to HCWs from occupational exposures to these fluids. UP does not apply to feces, nasal secre-

TABLE 36.1-1. *Universal precautions: associated body fluids*

Fluids to Which Universal Precautions Apply	Fluids to Which Universal Precautions Do Not Apply Unless They Contain Visible Blood
Blood	Feces
Semen	Nasal secretions
Vaginal fluid	Sputum
Amniotic fluid	Sweat
Cerebrospinal fluid	Tears
Pericardial fluid	Urine
Peritoneal fluid	Vomitus
Pleural fluid	
Synovial fluid	
Breast milk*	
Saliva†	

*Precautions are needed only in special circumstances, such as breast milk banking.
†Precautions are recommended only for dentistry, because saliva is often contaminated with blood.

tions, sputum, sweat, tears, urine, or vomitus unless they contain visible blood, because epidemiologic studies have demonstrated that the risk of HIV and HBV transmission from exposures to these fluids is extremely low or nonexistent. Some of these fluids and excretions represent a potential source for nosocomial and community-acquired infections with other pathogens.

Human breast milk has been implicated in perinatal transmission of HIV, and hepatitis B surface antigen (HBsAg) has been isolated from breast milk, but occupational exposure to human breast milk has not been implicated in the transmission of HIV or HBV infection to HCWs. Although UP does not apply to human breast milk, gloves may be worn by HCWs when exposures to breast milk may be frequent, such as breast milk banking.[12]

UP does not apply to saliva. Although HBV DNA has been found in the saliva of some persons infected with HBV and HBsAg-positive saliva has been shown to be infectious when injected into experimental animals and in human bite exposures, HBsAg-positive saliva has not been shown to be infectious when applied to oral mucous membranes in experimental primate studies. Epidemiologic studies suggest that the potential for salivary transmission of HIV is remote. Routine infection control practices, including the use of gloves when performing a digital examination of mucous membranes and during endotracheal suctioning and handwashing after exposure to saliva, should further minimize the risk, if any, for salivary transmission of HIV and HBV. Special precautions are recommended for dentistry, because occupationally acquired HBV infection has occurred in dental workers and contamination of saliva with blood is predictable during dental procedures (see Chap. 36.3).

UP emphasizes the use of appropriate barrier precautions (eg, gloves, gowns, and facial protection) routinely to prevent mucocutaneous blood contact. The precautions also emphasize the need for prevention of percutaneous injuries through care in the use of needles and other sharp instruments and during disposal of these devices, including the use of conveniently placed sharps disposal units. Proper handwashing, linen and waste handling, and disinfection and sterilization of instruments and other reusable equipment are recommended. A discussion of each of these practices follows.

Handwashing and Gloves

Handwashing is frequently called the single most important measure for preventing the spread of infection. Hands should be washed between patient contacts; after contact with blood, bloody fluids, secretions, excretions, and contaminated equipment or articles; and after removal of gloves. Handwashing with plain soap cleans the hands and removes transient microbial flora. No epidemiologic evidence has indicated that antiseptic handwashing products offer additional benefit in the prevention of transmission of bloodborne viruses.[12,19,20]

When UP is applied, gloves are worn to provide a protective barrier and prevent gross contamination of the hands when touching blood, body fluids that contain blood, mucous membranes, and nonintact skin and when performing procedures in which blood or body fluid contact is likely to occur, such as during venipuncture for delivery of intravenous fluids, endoscopy, suturing lacerations, handling specimens, insertion of catheters and diagnostic devices, and cleaning soiled equipment. It is unnecessary to wear gloves when performing procedures in which blood or body fluid contact is unlikely to occur, such as giving intramuscular injections to cooperative patients, changing lightly soiled diapers, bathing patients with intact skin, or delivering oral medications. Gloves can provide a protective barrier from other pathogens when contacting body secretions and excretions. However, gloves do not normally prevent penetrating injuries due to needles or other sharp objects.

Gloves should be changed when contaminated and as soon as possible if they are torn or punctured. Gloves should also be changed between patient contacts, because they can be colonized by pathogenic microorganisms.[21] When gloves have not been changed between patient contacts, outbreaks of bacterial infections and HBV occurred.[22-25] Wearing gloves does not replace the need for handwashing, because gloves may have small inapparent defects or be torn during use, and hands can become contaminated during removal and use of gloves.[18,21,26,27]

Standards for medical gloves have been established by the U.S. Food and Drug Administration. Gloves cannot offer absolute protection against hand-blood contact but, when combined with other measures, including handwashing after removing the gloves, they greatly reduce the frequency of blood contact with hands.

The selection of gloves should be based on the task being performed. Studies of the penetrability of various glove materials under conditions of use and when using various test materials, including viral particles, bacteria, blood, and water, have been difficult to interpret owing to variations in test methods and the effect of latex and chemicals on the recovery of virus.[28] Several studies, using water-fill stress or dye tests to evaluate examination gloves, have demonstrated that vinyl gloves had more leaks than latex gloves. The clinical implication remains uncertain, however. Three studies using simulated or actual clinical situations have shown that vinyl and latex examination gloves offer similar protection against penetration against bacteria.[26,27,29] There remains no evidence that demonstrates differences in barrier effectiveness between intact latex or vinyl gloves.

Vinyl and latex gloves should not be washed or disinfected, because increased penetration of liquids through undetected holes in the glove may occur and because some disinfectants may cause deterioration of the glove material. Utility gloves can be decontaminated and reused, but they should be discarded if there is evidence of deterioration.

Allergic reactions to latex and rubber utility gloves, as well as to condoms and other medical devices containing latex, have been reported by HCWs and patients. In one report, the incidence of latex allergy among 512 HCWs was found to be 2.9% or 4.5%, depending on the testing method used.[30] In another study of 40 HCWs reporting allergic reactions, 85% had positive skin test reactions to latex allergens, and 47.5% showed increased IgE antibodies to latex.[31] Reactions appear to occur more commonly in persons with histories of other atopic disease and can include rhinitis, contact urticaria, asthma, eczema, and anaphylaxis. It has also been reported that latex allergens absorb to cornstarch particles inside latex gloves, although not in vinyl gloves. Wearing vinyl or synthetic gloves or using glove liners has been recommended to prevent allergic reactions.[32]

Protective Gowns

Gowns of woven and nonwoven fabrics, plastic aprons, and laboratory coats are worn to prevent contamination of clothing and protect the skin of personnel from blood and body fluid exposure. Gowns or plastic aprons should be worn during procedures that are likely to generate splashes of blood or other body fluids, such as vaginal deliveries, angioplasty, cutting or drilling of bone, colonoscopy, cleaning soiled instruments, and emptying containers of body fluids. Whenever possible, gowns should be changed when heavily soiled.

The OSHA bloodborne pathogens standard requires that personal protective equipment not permit blood or other potentially infectious materials to pass through the barrier under normal conditions of use and for the duration of time the protective equipment is used. There have been a number of controversies regarding gowns, including the relative merits of disposable or reusable gowns and different gown materials. CDC recommendations state that gowns should provide an "effective barrier," but the CDC has no recommendations regarding gown design, type of materials used, or how these materials should be tested.

Selection of gowns should be based the type of procedure being performed while wearing the gown, taking into account the extent and sites of possible blood contact. Differences in the site and extent of blood skin contact depend on the type of surgical procedure being performed.[33-35]

Some gowns are lined or specially treated to make them impermeable to liquids, although the efficacy of these treatments may not be absolute.[35] Cloth laboratory coats may not be adequate to prevent penetration of liquids when performing laboratory procedures.[36] Factors to consider when selecting gowns[35,37] and the methods for determining the barrier efficacy of gowns[38] have been published. Leg coverings, boots, or shoe covers may provide additional protection to the skin when splashes or large quantities of potentially infective material are present or anticipated.

Masks and Protective Eyewear

A mask that covers the nose and mouth and protection for the eyes, such as goggles, glasses with solid side shields, or a face shield, are worn to protect the mucous membranes of the nose, mouth, and eyes during procedures and care activities that are likely to generate splashes or sprays of blood or body fluids, such as operative procedures, obstetric deliveries, manipulation of arterial devices, centrifugation of blood, and emergency treatment of trauma cases. A variety of devices are available and can be worn in combination, and their selection should be based on the likelihood of or amount of splashing or spattering that may occur during a specific procedure, the length of time they are to be worn, their ability to prevent blood exposure, worker comfort, and worker acceptability.

Protection From Needles and Sharp Instruments

Percutaneous injuries represent the greatest risk of transmission of HIV and other bloodborne pathogens to HCWs (see Chap. 35). Careful work practices, including the safe handling and disposal of needles and sharp instruments, are recommended to reduce the likelihood of sharp injuries; in recent years, a variety of devices with safety features intended to reduce injuries have been marketed.

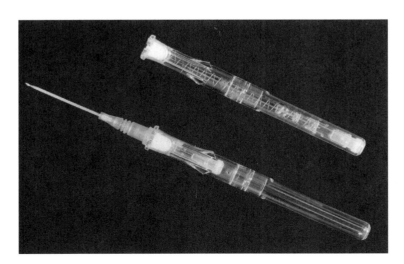

FIG. 36.1-1. An intravenous catheter with a spring-loaded retractable needle. Before the needle is fully withdrawn from the catheter, the plastic button of the safety barrel is pushed, which causes the needle to retract into the barrel and be locked into place. (Display of a particular brand of device is for illustration purposes only and does not imply endorsement by the Public Health Service or the U.S. Department of Health and Human Services.) (Photograph courtesy of Becton Dickinson Vascular Access, Sandy, UT.)

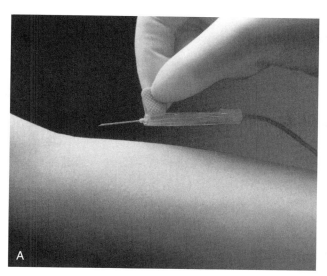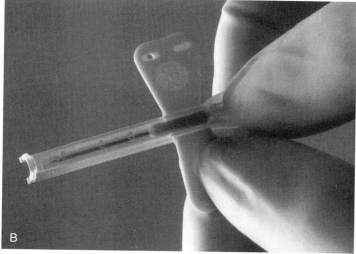

FIG. 36.1-2. (A) Example of winged intravenous needle with a resheathing safety device. (B) After the needle is withdrawn, the protective shield is pushed forward over the device. The shield is designed to lock into place, covering the tip of the needle. (Display of a particular brand of device is for illustration purposes only and does not imply endorsement by the Public Health Service or the U.S. Department of Health and Human Services.) (Photograph courtesy of Becton Dickinson Vascular Access, Sandy, UT.)

Care should be taken to prevent injuries when using needles, scalpels, and other sharp instruments or devices; when handling sharp instruments after procedures; when cleaning used instruments; and when disposing of used needles. Used needles should never be recapped or otherwise manipulated using both hands or any other technique that involves directing the point of a needle toward any part of the body. A one-handed "scoop" technique or a mechanical device designed for holding the needle sheath should be employed. Used needles from disposable syringes should not be removed by hand, nor should they be bent, broken, or otherwise manipulated by hand. Reusable sharps should be placed in puncture-resistant containers for transport to reprocessing areas.

Changes in the design of needle-bearing medical devices are likely to reduce injuries in common procedures such as venipuncture and the delivery of intravenous solutions and medications. Technologic innovations include methods for resheathing syringes and needle-catheter stylets, self-blunting or recessed needles, retractable lancets, and needle-less intravenous systems. Figures 36.1-1 and 36.1-2 show examples of two needle-bearing devices with safety features that must be activated by the worker. Some of these new devices have been shown to reduce needle-stick injuries.[39-44] The development and implementation of devices with safety features offer the most promising avenue for further reduction of needle-stick injuries. It is important, however, that these sometimes costly devices be evaluated for their efficacy in preventing injuries, user acceptability, and impact on patient care. Some devices have been redesigned because of problems identified during use. Needle-less intravenous systems [Fig. 36.1-3] have been associated with bloodstream infection in some patients receiving prolonged intravenous therapy.[45,46] As discussed in Chapter 36.2, changes in surgical instruments and techniques have been effective in reducing sharps injuries during surgical and obstetric procedures. Factors to consider when evaluating these devices have been described elsewhere.[39,47-49]

Disposal of Sharp Objects and Contaminated Waste

Between 7% and 31% of percutaneous injuries reported in various studies have been related to disposal of sharp objects, excluding recapping.[47,50] Many of the injuries result from overfilled, poorly designed, or poorly placed sharps disposal units. These injuries occur to workers using the sharps for medical procedures and to workers who handle linens and waste. Used disposable syringes and needles, scalpel blades, and other sharp items should be placed in puncture-resistant containers located as close as is practical to the area in which the items were used.

Consideration should be given to several factors when selecting sharps disposal containers, including the type, size, and volume of sharps requiring disposal in a particular area; ease of use; size of disposal opening; the patient population being cared for; areas that may require special considerations for placement of disposal units (eg, pediatrics, psychiatry); and how the unit will be discarded or incinerated, including consideration of local waste regulations. Evaluation of a variety of technical qualities of the disposal units is also important.[51]

The method of disposal of contaminated waste should be based on the likelihood of contamination with infective material, whether injury could result from waste handling (eg, needles, sharp instruments), and the amount of contamination that has occurred. Handling and disposal of waste that may be contaminated with bloodborne pathogens

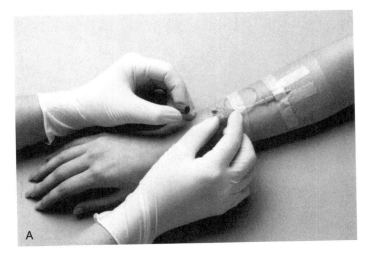

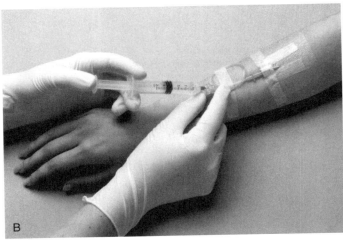

FIG. 36.1-3. Example of a needle-less intravenous access valve. (**A**) The sterile cap covering the valve is removed. (**B**) Then a syringe is attached that depresses the valve, allowing fluid to be injected into the vein. After the syringe is removed, the valve closes, preventing leakage from the vein. A sterile cap is then reapplied on the valve. (Display of a particular brand of device is for illustration purposes only and does not imply endorsement by the Public Health Service or the U.S. Department of Health and Human Services.) (Photograph courtesy of B. Braun Medical, Inc., Bethlehem, PA.)

should be in accordance with OSHA regulations and state and local laws.

Handling of Linens

Although soiled linen may be contaminated with pathogenic microorganisms, the risk of disease transmission is negligible if linen is handled, transported, and laundered in a manner that limits the transfer of microorganisms. Soiled linens should be handled as little as possible and placed in bags that prevent leakage at the location where the linens were used and during transport to the laundry. Patient care workers should be taught to separate sharps from linens before placing the soiled linen into soiled linen containers. Workers who transport, sort, or place soiled linens from health care settings in washing machines should wear barriers such as gloves to prevent contact with body fluids. The methods for handling, transporting, and laundering of soiled linens are determined by hospital policy and any applicable regulations. Normal laundry cycles are adequate to prevent transmission of bloodborne viruses.

Disinfection, Sterilization, and Waste Management

Standard sterilization and disinfection procedures for patient care equipment and environmental surfaces are adequate to inactivate bloodborne pathogens and have been described in other publications.[11,12,52,53] Specific recommendations for the inactivation of HIV are discussed in Chapter 36.5.

CDC recommendations for disinfecting environmental surfaces contaminated with blood include the use of an Environmental Protection Agency (EPA)–approved germicide or a 1 : 100 dilution of household bleach (or ¼ cup bleach to 1 gallon of tap water).

EFFICACY OF UNIVERSAL PRECAUTIONS IN PREVENTING BLOOD CONTACTS

The efficacy of UP in preventing blood contacts has been assessed in several settings. A study that evaluated reports of percutaneous exposure to blood over a 7-year period at the National Institutes for Health Clinical Center found a sustained decrease in parenteral exposure rates after the implementation of UP. The decrease occurred in many categories of HCWs and was consistent using several different denominators.[54] In a prospective questionnaire study of physicians on medical wards, the needle-stick injury rates declined from 0.39 to 0.15 per physician per patient-care–month after implementation of UP, a decline the researchers speculated may have been caused, in part, by a sharps disposal unit in every room.[55] Several studies have reported decreased needle-stick injury rates ranging from 60% to 75% over 3- to 4-year periods after implementation of sharps disposal units in patient rooms when done in conjunction with education regarding UP.[54,56,57] One study showed a 60% decrease among housekeeping personnel during the year after the placement of sharps disposal units in patient rooms, with a further reduction in those injuries in subsequent years.[54] Significant reduction of needle-stick injuries among nursing personnel after the introduction of sharps disposal units was attributed to the prevention of injuries due to recapping.

A survey that used paired questionnaires before and after the institution of UP found a reduction of approximately 50% in estimated annual rates of nonparenteral exposures to blood and body substances.[58] In one observational study of 9793 procedures performed by emergency department workers in six hospitals, skin-blood contact rates were 11.2 per 100 procedures for ungloved workers and 1.3 for gloved workers.[59] In a prospective questionnaire study of physicians on medical wards, the implementation of UP resulted in a decrease in the rate of blood contacts from 5.07 to 2.66 per physician per patient-care–month, primarily resulting from the reduction in skin contacts because of glove use.[55]

In general, UP appears to have been more effective in reducing mucocutaneous exposures than percutaneous injuries; continued reports of injuries with needles and other sharp objects have led to calls for technologic innovations to enhance the safety of these devices.[40]

PRECAUTIONS OUTSIDE THE HOSPITAL SETTING

Caring for HIV-Infected Persons in the Home

Care for HIV-infected persons in the home is often provided by family members and friends who do not have professional training in health care. Although several studies have found no evidence for HIV transmission in households due to casual contact,[60] there have been eight published reports of HIV transmission in household settings that were not associated with sexual contact, injection drug use, or breast feeding. Of these eight reports, five were associated with documented or probable blood contact. In the sixth report, HIV infection was diagnosed in a boy after his younger brother died of AIDS, although the mechanism of transmission was not determined. Two reports involved nursing care of terminally ill persons with AIDS in which a blood exposure may have occurred but was not documented; in both reports, skin contact with body secretions and excretions occurred.[61]

Professional health care providers should be aware of the potential for HIV transmission in the home and should provide training and education in infection control for HIV-infected persons and those who live with or provide care to them in the home. Such training should be an integral and ongoing part of the health care plan for every person with HIV infection.

The CDC has published a brochure, *Caring for Someone with AIDS: Information for Friends, Relatives, Household Members, and Others Who Care for a Person with AIDS at Home*. This brochure is available free from the CDC National AIDS Clearinghouse, P.O. Box 6003, Rockville, MD 20849-6003; telephone (800) 458-5231 or (301) 217-0023. The brochure includes recommendations that needles and sharp objects be handled with care and disposed of in puncture-proof containers and kept out of the reach of children and visitors. Bandages should be used to cover cuts, sores, or breaks on exposed skin of persons with HIV infection and of persons providing care. Persons who provide such care should wear gloves when there is a possibility of direct contact with HIV-infected blood or other body fluids, secretions, or excretions. Because urine and feces may contain a variety of pathogens, including HIV, persons providing nursing care to HIV-infected persons should wear gloves during contact with these substances. Even when gloves are worn, hands should be washed after contact with blood and other body fluids, secretions, or excretions.

Specialized Settings

Additional recommendations have been published for some specialized settings such as laboratories,[62,63] dental settings,[64] hemodialysis units,[65] and emergency services (ie, first responders).[66] Special considerations for surgery, dentistry, and emergency departments are discussed in Chapters 36.2, 36.3, and 36.4, respectively.

PREVENTION OF TRANSMISSION OF OTHER INFECTIONS, INCLUDING PULMONARY TUBERCULOSIS

Persons with HIV infection may present to health care facilities with a variety of infections, some of which may be severe because of the immunocompromised status of the patient. Depending on the pathogen, isolation precautions may or may not be necessary to prevent transmission of these infections from patients to HCWs and other patients. The appropriate precautions, based on the system of precautions in use in the health care facility, should be followed by HCWs caring for patients with transmissible infections.[4,13,18]

The incidence of pulmonary infection caused by *Mycobacterium tuberculosis* has increased worldwide since 1985. One of the reported reasons for this increase is the concomitant epidemic of HIV infections.[67,68] Persons with HIV infection are at high risk of developing active pulmonary tuberculosis through reactivation of latent tuberculosis infection or through primary infection. Once infected, HIV-infected persons are much more likely to develop disease than persons with competent immune systems. Mortality rates from tuberculosis among HIV-infected persons have been high.

M tuberculosis is carried in airborne particles (ie, droplet nuclei) that can be generated when persons with active pulmonary or laryngeal disease sneeze, cough, speak, or sing. These particles can remain airborne for long periods and can be transmitted by the airborne route. Outbreaks of tuberculosis among patients and HCWs have been reported in health care facilities.

In 1994, the CDC revised the guidelines for control of tuberculosis in health care facilities.[69] The fundamental measures for controlling *M tuberculosis* transmission are reiterated in this document and include administrative measures, engineering controls, and personal protective equipment. The administrative measures are intended primarily to reduce the risk for exposing uninfected persons to persons who have infectious tuberculosis. These measures include developing and implementing effective written policies and protocols to ensure the rapid identification, isolation, diagnostic evaluation, and treatment of persons likely to have tuberculosis; implementing effective work practices among HCWs in the health care facility, such as correctly wearing respiratory protection and keeping doors to isolation rooms closed; educating, training, and counseling HCWs about tuberculosis; and screening HCWs for tuberculosis infection and disease.

Engineering controls are expected to prevent the spread and reduce the concentration of infectious droplet nuclei. These controls include direct source control using local exhaust ventilation, controlling the direction of airflow to prevent contamination of air in areas adjacent to the infectious source, diluting and removing contaminated air through general ventilation, and air cleaning by air filtration or ultraviolet germicidal irradiation.

Administrative measures and engineering controls minimize the number of areas in the health care facility where exposure to infectious tuberculosis may occur, and they reduce, but do not eliminate, the risk in those few areas where exposure to *M tuberculosis* can still occur, such as rooms in which patients with known or suspected infectious tuberculosis are being isolated and treatment rooms in which cough-inducing or aerosol-generating procedures are performed on such patients. Because persons entering such rooms may be exposed to *M tuberculosis*, they should wear personal respiratory protection while in the rooms.

The recommendations concerning the type of personal respiratory protection necessary for HCW protection have been controversial in the United States, in part because of separate mandates for federal agencies and different methods used for certifying respirators.[70] In the 1994 guideline, the CDC specified standard criteria for respiratory protection devices for protection against transmission of tuberculosis. In 1995, the National Institute for Occupational Safety and Health (NIOSH) published a new respiratory protection certification rule[71] that provides for certification of nine classes of respirators that will meet or exceed the CDC standard criteria for respiratory protection against tuberculosis. The NIOSH certified that N95 through P100 series respirators are acceptable for use.

EDUCATION OF HEALTH CARE WORKERS

All HCWs should be provided information regarding the risk of occupational transmission of bloodborne pathogens, a thorough explanation of the practices of UP and the barriers and devices available for their protection, and protocols to follow if an exposure occurs. This education should be tailored to the various needs for protection in different settings and should be provided using the language of fluency, culture, and educational level of the target audience.

COMPLIANCE WITH UNIVERSAL PRECAUTIONS

HCWs continue to have various rates of compliance with UP. Questionnaire surveys and some observational studies have reported incomplete HCW compliance with UP practices.[72-74] A few studies have described the reasons for the noncompliance, including perceived barriers or impediments to compliance (eg, time, inaccessible equipment, decreased dexterity, comfort); attitudes regarding HIV-infected patients (eg, perception of risk of acquiring disease, perception of severity of disease, knowledge of persons with AIDS); and organization-level variables (eg, availability of equipment, performance feedback, safety climate).[72,75,76] These data underscore the need for the development of protective measures that do not depend on worker compliance (eg, engineering controls such as safer needle-bearing devices). Establishment of an organizational climate emphasizing safety and elimination of barriers to compliance is essential, and practical methods of altering behavior to promote compliance with UP and other infection control recommendations are needed.

REFERENCES

1. Short LJ, Bell DM. Risk of occupational infection with bloodborne pathogens in operating and delivery room settings. Am J Infect Control 1993;21:343.
2. Alter MJ. Occupational exposure to hepatitis C virus: a dilemma. Infect Control Hosp Epidemiol 1994;15:742.
3. Centers for Disease Control and Prevention. Recommendations for counseling persons infected with human T-lymphotropic virus, types I and II. MMWR 1993;42(RR-9):1.
4. Garner JS, Simmons BP. CDC guideline for isolation precautions in hospitals. Am J Infect Control 1984;12:103.
5. Centers for Disease Control. Recommendations for preventing transmission of infection with human T-lymphotropic virus III/lymphadenopathy-associated virus in the workplace. MMWR 1985;34:681.
6. Centers for Disease Control. Recommendations for providing dialysis treatment to patients infected with human T-lymphotropic virus III/lymphadenopathy-associated virus. MMWR 1986;35:376.
7. Centers for Disease Control. Recommendations for preventing possible transmission of human T-lymphotropic virus type III/lymphadenopathy-associated virus from tears. MMWR 1985; 34:533.
8. Centers for Disease Control. Acquired immune deficiency syndrome (AIDS): precautions for clinical and laboratory staffs. MMWR 1982;31:577.

9. Centers for Disease Control. Recommended infection control practices for dentistry. MMWR 1986;35:237.

10. Centers for Disease Control. Update: human immunodeficiency virus infections in health-care workers. MMWR 1987;36:285.

11. Centers for Disease Control. Recommendations for prevention of HIV transmission in health-care settings. MMWR 1987;36(Suppl 2):1S.

12. Centers for Disease Control. Update: universal precautions for prevention of transmission of human immunodeficiency virus, hepatitis B virus, and other bloodborne pathogens in health-care settings. MMWR 1988;37:377.

13. Lynch P, Jackson MM, Cummings J, Stamm WE. Rethinking the role of isolation practices in the prevention of nosocomial infections. Ann Intern Med 1987;107:243.

14. Jackson MM, Lynch P. An attempt to make an issue less murky: a comparison of four systems for infection precautions. Infect Control Hosp Epidemiol 1991;12:448.

15. Garner JS, Hughes JM. Options for isolation precautions. Ann Intern Med 1987;107:248.

16. Weinstein RA, Kabins SA. Isolation practices in hospitals. Ann Intern Med 1987;197:781.

17. Department of Labor, Occupational Safety and Health Administration. 29 CFR Part 1910.1030: occupational exposure to bloodborne pathogens; final rule. Fed Regist 1991;56:64175.

18. Garner JS. Hospital infection control practices advisory committee. Guideline for isolation precautions in hospitals. Am J Infect Cont 1996;24:24.

19. Garner JS, Favero MS. Guideline for handwashing and hospital environmental control. Atlanta: U.S. Department of Health and Human Services, Public Health Service, Centers for Disease Control, 1985.

20. Larson E. APIC guideline for use of topical antimicrobial products. Am J Infect Control 1988;16:253.

21. Doebbeling BN, Pfaller MA, Houston AK, Wenzel RP. Removal of nosocomial pathogens from the contaminated glove: implications for glove reuse and handwashing. Ann Intern Med 1988;109:394.

22. Maki DG, McCormick RD, Zilz MA, Stoltz SM, Alvarado CJ. An MRSA outbreak in a SICU during universal precautions: new epidemiology for nosocomial MRSA: downside for universal precautions (UPs). Abstract no. 473. Presented at the 30th Interscience Conference on Antimicrobial Agents and Chemotherapy, Atlanta, GA, 1990:165.

23. Patterson JE, Vecchio J, Pantelick EL, et al. Association of contaminated gloves with transmission of *Acinetobacter calcoaceticus* var. *anitratus* in an intensive care unit. Am J Med 1991;91:479.

24. Vickers J, Painter MJ, Heponstall J, Yusof JHM, Craske J. Hepatitis B outbreak in a drug trials unit: investigation and recommendations. Community Dis Rep CDR Rev 1994;4:R1.

25. Burkeholder B, Zaza S, Shapiro C, Salkind K. Hepatitis B virus transmission among nursing home patients in Ohio. Abstract no. 1405. Presented at the 32nd Interscience Conference on Antimicrobial Agents and Chemotherapy, Anaheim, CA, 1992:345.

26. Korniewicz DM, Laughton BE, Cyr WH, Lytle CD, Larson E. Leakage of virus through used vinyl and latex examination gloves. J Clin Microbiol 1990;28:787.

27. Olsen RJ, Lynch P, Coyle MB, Cummings J, Bokete T, Stamm WE. Examination gloves as barriers to hand contamination in clinical practice. JAMA 1993;270:350.

28. Lytle CD, Truscott W, Budacz AP, Venegas L, Routson LB, Cyr WH. Important factors for testing barrier materials with surrogate viruses. Appl Environ Microbiol 1991;57:2549.

29. Kornewicz DM, Laughon BE, Butz A, Larson E. Integrity of vinyl and latex procedure gloves. Nurs Res 1989;38:144.

30. Turjanmaa K. Incidence of immediate allergy to latex gloves in hospital personnel. Contact Derm 1987;17:270.

31. Bubak ME, Reed CE, Fronsway AF, et al. Subspecialty clinics, allergenic diseases, allergic reactions among health care workers. Mayo Clin Pract 1992;67:1075.

32. Jaeger D, Kleinhaus D, Czuppon AB, Baur X. Latex-specific proteins causing immediate-type cutaneous, nasal, bronchial and systemic reactions. J Allergy Clin Immunol 1992;89:759.

33. Quebbeman EJ, Telford GL, Hubbard S, et al. Risk of blood contamination and injury to operating room personnel. Ann Surg 1991;214:614.

34. Tokars JI, Culver DH, Mendelson MH, et al. Skin and mucous membrane contacts during surgical procedures: risk and prevention. Infect Control Hosp Epidemiol 1995;16:703.

35. Telford GL, Quebbeman EJ. Assessing the risk of blood exposure in the operating room. Am J Infect Control 1993;21:351.

36. Jagger J, Detmer DE, Cohen ML, Scar PR, Pearson RD. Reducing blood and body fluid exposures among clinical laboratory workers. Clin Lab Manage Rev 1992;September-October:415.

37. Belkin NL. Surgical gowns and drapes as aseptic barriers. Am J Infect Control 1988;16:14.

38. McCullough EA. Methods for determining the barrier efficacy of surgical gowns. Am J Infect Control 1993;21:368.

39. Chiarello L. New York State Department of Health report to the legislature: pilot study of needlestick prevention devices. Albany: New York State Health Department, March, 1992.

40. Jagger K. Hunt EH, Pearson RD. Sharp injuries in the hospital: causes and strategies for prevention. Am J Infect Control 1990;18:227.

41. Gartner K. Impact of a needleless intravenous system in a university hospital. Am J Infect Control 1992;20:75.

42. Younger B, Hunt EH, Robinson C, McLemore C. Impact of a shielded safety syringe on needlestick injuries among healthcare workers. Infect Control Hosp Epidemiol 1993;13:349.

43. Robert L, Short L, Chamberland M, et al. Reduction of blood contacts (BCs) and percutaneous injuries (PIs) during gynecological surgical procedures (GSPs). Presented at the Annual Meeting of The Society for Healthcare Epidemiology of America. (Abstract 45) Infect Control Hosp Epidemiol 1995;16(4, part 2):23.

44. Robert L, Short L, Chamberland M, et al. Impact of safety devices (SDs) to reduce percutaneous injuries during phlebotomy (PIPs). Presented at the Annual Meeting of The Society for Healthcare Epidemiology of America. (Abstract 50) Infect Control Hosp Epidemiol 1995;16:24.

45. Danzig LE, Short L, Collins K, et al. Bloodstream infections associated with a needleless intravenous infusion system in patients receiving home infusion therapy. JAMA 1995;273:1862.

46. Maki DG, Stolz R, McCormick R, Spiegel C. Possible association of a commercial needleless system with central venous catheter-related bacteremia. Abstract J201. The 34th Interscience Conference on Antimicrobial Agents and Chemotherapy, Orlando, FL, 1994:195.

47. Jagger J, Hunt EH, Brand-Elnaggar J, Pearson R. Rates of needlestick injury caused by various devices in a university hospital. N Engl J Med 1988;318:284.

48. ECRI. Needlestick prevention devices. Health Devices 1991;20:154.

49. American Hospital Association. Implementing safer needle devices. American Hospital Association. Item no. 196310. Chicago: American Hospital Association, 1992.

50. Wellman AC, Short LJ, Mendelson MH, Lillenfeld DE, Engin MS, Rodriguez M. Disposal-related sharps injuries at a New York City teaching hospital. Infect Control Hosp Epidemiol 1995;16:268.

51. ECRI. Sharps disposal containers. Health Devices 1993;22:359.

52. Favero MS, Bond WW. Sterilization, disinfection, and antisepsis in the hospital. In: Manual of clinical microbiology. Washington, DC: American Society for Microbiology, 1991:183.

53. Rutala WA. APIC guideline for selection and use of disinfectants. Am J Infect Control 1990;18:99.

54. Beekmann SE, Vlahov D, Koziol DE, McShalley ED, Schmitt JM, Henderson DK. Temporal association between implementation of universal precautions and a sustained, progressive decrease in percutaneous exposures to blood. Clin Infect Dis 1994;18:562.

55. Wong ES, Stotka JL, Chinchilli VM, Williams DS, Stuart CG, Markowitz SM. Are universal precautions effective in reducing the number of occupational exposures among health care workers? A prospective study of physicians on a medical service. JAMA 1991;265:1123.

56. Linnemann CC, Cannon C, DeRonde M, Lanphear B. Effect of educational programs, rigid sharps containers, and universal precautions on reported needlestick injuries in health care workers. Infect Control Hosp Epidemiol 1991;12:214.

57. Haiduven DJ, DeMaio TM, Stevens DA. A five year study of needlestick injuries: significant reduction associated with communication, education, and convenient placement of sharps containers. Infect Control Hosp Epidemiol 1992;13:265.

58. Fahey BI, Koziol DE, Bands SM, Henderson DK. Frequency of nonparenteral occupational exposures to blood and body fluids before and after universal precautions. Am J Med 1991;90:145.

59. Marcus R, Culver DH, Bell DM, et al. Risk of human immunodeficiency virus infection among emergency department workers. Am J Med 1993;94:393.

60. Simonds RJ, Rogers MF. HIV transmission—bringing home the message. (Editorial) N Engl J Med 1993;329:1883.
61. Centers for Disease Control and Prevention. Human immunodeficiency virus transmission in household settings—United States. MMWR 1994;43:347.
62. The National Committee for Clinical Laboratory Standards. Protection of laboratory workers from infectious disease transmitted by blood, body fluids, and tissue. 2nd ed. NCCLS document M29-T2. Villanova, Pennsylvania: NCCLS, 1992.
63. Centers for Disease Control. 1988 Agent summary statement for human immunodeficiency virus and report on laboratory-acquired infection with human immunodeficiency virus. MMWR 1988;37(Suppl 4):1.
64. Centers for Disease Control and Prevention. Recommended infection-control practices for dentistry. MMWR 1993;41(RR-8):1.
65. Favero MS, Alter MJ, Bland LA. Dialysis-associated infections and their control. In: Bennett JB, Brachman P, eds. Hospital infections. 3rd ed. Boston: Little, Brown, 1992:375.
66. Centers for Disease Control. Guidelines for prevention of transmission of human immunodeficiency virus and hepatitis B virus to health-care and public-safety workers. MMWR 1989;38(Suppl 6):1.
67. Centers for Disease Control. Tuberculosis and human immunodeficiency virus infection: recommendations of the advisory committee for the elimination of tuberculosis (ACET). MMWR 1989;38:236.
68. Ravigilone MC, Snider DE, Kochi A. Global epidemiology of tuberculosis: morbidity and mortality of a worldwide epidemic. JAMA 1995; 273:220.
69. Centers for Disease Control and Prevention. Guidelines for preventing the transmission of *Mycobacterium tuberculosis* in health-care facilities, 1994. MMWR 1994;43(RR-13):1.
70. Jarvis WR, Bolyard EA, Bozzi CJ, et al. Respirators, recommendations, and regulations: the controversy surrounding protection of health care workers from tuberculosis. Ann Intern Med 1995;122:142.
71. Department of Health and Human Services. Respiratory Protection Devices, Final Rule and Notice, 42 CFR Part 84. Fed Regist 1995; 60(110):30335.
72. Kelen GD, DiGiovanna TA, Celentano DD, et al. Adherence to universal (barrier) precautions during interventions on critically ill and injured emergency department patients. J Acquir Immune Defic Syndr 1990;3:987.
73. Willy ME, Dhillon GL, Loewen NL, Wesley RA, Henderson DA. Adverse exposures and universal precautions practices among a group of highly exposed health professionals. Infect Control Hosp Epidemiol 1990;11:351.
74. Henry K, Campbell S, Collier P, O'Boyle-Williams C. Compliance with universal precautions and needle handling and disposal practices among emergency department staff at two community hospitals. Am J Infect Control 1994;22:129.
75. O'Boyle-Williams C, Campbell S, Henry S, Collier P. Variables influencing worker compliance with universal precautions in the emergency department. Am J Infect Control 1994;22:138.
76. Gershon RM, Curbow B, Kelen G, Celantano K, Lears K, Vlahov D. Correlates of attitudes concerning human immunodeficiency virus and acquired immunodeficiency syndrome among hospital workers. Am J Infect Control 1994;22:293.

AIDS: Biology, Diagnosis, Treatment and Prevention, fourth edition, edited by Vincent T. DeVita, Jr., Samuel Hellman, and Steven A. Rosenberg. Lippincott–Raven Publishers, © 1997

36.2

Safety Precautions: Special Considerations for Surgeons

Louise J. Short and Daniel R. Benson

Occupational transmission of viral hepatitis has been recognized in the United States since 1948, when the New York State Workmen's Compensation Board granted its first compensation award for serum-transmitted hepatitis to a blood bank employee.[1] Since then clarification of markers for hepatitis B virus (HBV), the emergence of the human immunodeficiency virus (HIV) epidemic, and the discovery of hepatitis C virus have heightened concern about exposure of health care workers to blood and body fluids. These exposures vary in risk of potential transmission of bloodborne pathogens and include, from highest to lowest risk, percutaneous injuries (eg, needle-stick injury, cut with another sharp object); mucous membrane contacts (eg, primarily by splash); and skin contacts (eg, direct contact, soakage through personal protective equipment). The epidemiology of these exposures and their associated risks have been extensively described in chapter 35.

According to the principles of universal precautions recommended by the Centers for Disease Control and Prevention (CDC), blood, certain other body fluids, all visibly bloody body fluids, and tissue from all patients should be considered potentially infected with bloodborne pathogens (see Chap. 36.1).[2] This chapter focuses on strategies for preventing blood and body fluid exposures in surgical settings. These strategies are approached from an occupational safety and health perspective, using an industrial hygiene (IH) hazard abatement model. Within the IH model, there is a hier-

archy of controls commonly applied to reduce and eliminate occupational hazards and exposures in nonmedical settings. This hierarchy consists of engineering controls, work practice controls, personal protective equipment, and administrative controls.

STRATEGIES FOR PREVENTING BLOOD AND BODY FLUID EXPOSURES IN SURGICAL SETTINGS

Engineering Controls

The IH approach emphasizes elimination of exposures by removal or substitution with less hazardous materials. This principle can be applied to prevention of percutaneous injuries in surgical settings, most of which result from suture needles and scalpels. Reduction of exposure to these instruments can be achieved by use of existing technology, new safety devices, or a combination of these. For example, in terms of existing technology laparoscopic techniques can be substituted for open procedures, probably minimizing risk of blood and body fluid exposure for surgical staff and morbidity for patients. Lasers and ultrasonic dissectors may be used in selected cases to minimize dissection with sharp instruments, and staplers can be used for skin closure and in gastrointestinal and other types of surgery to eliminate the need for suturing at certain stages of a procedure. The judicious use of electrocautery rather than a scalpel for cutting may also help to decrease percutaneous injuries.[3]

Many new engineering controls (ie, safety devices) to prevent percutaneous injuries by hollow- and solid-bore needles and scalpels have become available. Examples of such devices for use in the operating room include blunt-tipped suture needles, finger protective strips, magnetic passing trays, shielded scalpels, and cushions that hold nee-

Louise J. Short, HIV Infections Branch, Hospital Infections Program, National Center for Infectious Diseases, Centers for Disease Control and Prevention, 1600 Clifton Road, Mailstop E-68, Atlanta, GA 30333.

Daniel R. Benson, University of California at Davis, Sacramento, California.

dles while the surgeon repositions the holder or ties knots.[4] For most of these devices, there are few data on efficacy in preventing exposures, adverse patient effects, or user acceptability. It is important that any evaluation of safety devices to reduce percutaneous injuries take into account all three of these outcomes.[5]

A safety device that has generated a high degree of interest within the surgical community and for which some evaluation data have been collected is the blunt-tipped suture needle (Fig. 36.2-1). Blunt-tipped needles have been used successfully for many years in certain types of procedures, such as liver surgery. Blunt-tipped needles are available in several different sizes and suture materials, and their application to other areas of surgery is being assessed.[6–9]

A CDC study performed in cooperation with three New York City hospitals measured the effect of blunt-tipped needles in reducing percutaneous injuries to gynecologic personnel. Preliminary analyses revealed that blunt-tipped suture needle use increased from 1% to 55% of all suture needle use between first and fifth (last) quarters of the study. There was a concomitant significant decrease in suture needle-related percutaneous injuries per 1000 procedures: from 5.8 in the first study quarter to 1.0 in the last study quarter. No percutaneous injuries occurred with the blunt-tipped suture needle; in contrast, injury rates per 1000 needles used were 2.1 and 14.2, respectively, for standard suture needles and straight needles (used in some institutions to close skin).[10]

Preliminary data have revealed no difference between standard and blunt-tipped suture needles for patient outcomes, including blood loss, operative time, and returns to the operating room. Although user acceptability was not formally assessed by questionnaire, anecdotal reports indicate that many surgeons could not discern the difference between standard and blunt-tipped suture needles except while suturing more delicate tissues such as peritoneum, for which they occasionally reported tissue tears and increased blood loss (CDC: unpublished data).

Work Practice Controls

The second line of defense against workplace hazards in the IH model is work-practice controls. In the surgical setting, this largely involves technique modification. For example, some surgeons have attempted to create protocols for specific procedures, such as abdominal hysterectomies and cesarean sections, which incorporate step-by-step modifications for minimizing use of sharps.[3] In addition, certain surgical techniques have been shown in epidemiologic studies to correlate with increased risk of percutaneous injury. For example, epidemiologic data reveal that a technique strongly associated with percutaneous injury is the use of fingers to hold tissue while the surgeon or a coworker is suturing or cutting.[11] Injuries occurring in such circumstances may be minimized by substituting forceps or other instruments for the use of fingers. Measures to reduce exposures that intuitively make sense, but for which few data have been collected on efficacy, include the following items, which have been suggested by the American Academy of Orthopaedic Surgeons (AAOS) Task Force on AIDS and Orthopaedic Surgery.[12]

1. Awareness and caution are necessary at all times. Before a long or difficult case, it may be wise for the entire surgical team to discuss the procedure and the potential for blood contact.
2. Oral announcements before sharps are passed alert the entire team, and the use of a passing tray or basin, particularly a magnetic one, may help to reduce risk of exposure (Fig 36.2-2).
3. Sharp instruments ideally should be protected on the Mayo stand to prevent accidental wounds; suture needles loaded and left upright before the surgeon is ready to use them may create an unnecessary hazard. Loading and unloading needles using an instrument instead of fingers may help to reduce percutaneous injuries (Fig. 36.2-3).[4]

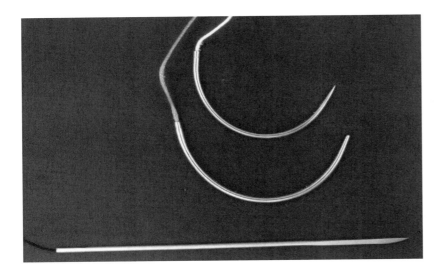

FIG. 36.2-1. Three types of suture needles (*top to bottom*): standard curved needle with a sharp point, blunt-tipped needle, and straight needle.

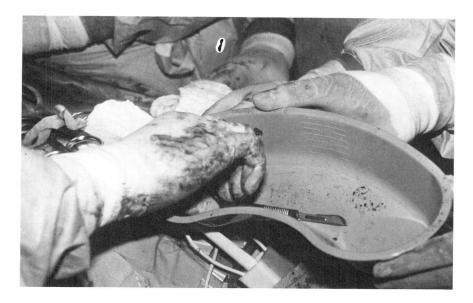

FIG. 36.2-2. When asking for sharp instruments, such as a scalpel, the surgeon should request them orally. An announcement should be made by the scrub personnel that the sharp instrument is being passed. The use of an intermediate tray, such as this basin, protects the surgeon or his team members from being cut as the instrument is being passed across the field.

4. Stapling or other nonsuture techniques may prevent percutaneous injuries during wound closure. In particular, it would be wise to avoid the use of straight needles, which are associated with very high injury rates.[10]
5. Two surgeons should avoid simultaneously suturing the same wound.
6. For tying sutures, instrument ties and pop-off needles offer alternatives to hand ties. If hand ties are needed, the needle can be removed from the suture before tying (Fig. 36.2-4).
7. Digital palpation of needle tips and suturing in confined spaces should be avoided when possible. If the surgeon needs to digitally examine sharp fracture fragments or wires, extra caution should be used. Exposures to internal wires and pins can be minimized by covering these items with pieces of tubing or cork stoppers (Figs. 36.2-5 and 36.2-6).

Personal Protective Equipment

Personal protective equipment is the third element in the IH hierarchy of controls to protect the worker. Gloves and other protective equipment have been worn in the operating room for decades to protect patients from infection; however, increasingly the efficacy of these barriers in reducing blood contacts has become an occupational health concern for health care workers.

Gloves

The effectiveness of gloves in decreasing blood-hand contact may depend on several factors, including the type of gloves used, the number of gloves used, and glove integrity over time.

Many different types of gloves are available for use in surgery, including latex, orthopedic (ie, slightly thicker

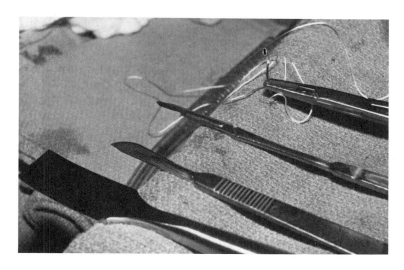

FIG. 36.2-3. Sharp instruments, such as osteotomes and scalpels, should be protected on the Mayo stand. If they are left hanging over the edge, as illustrated in this example, accidental skin penetration is likely to occur. Additionally, suture needles should not be loaded and placed on the Mayo stand in an upright position before they are needed. If a member of the operating team should accidentally place a hand or an arm on the Mayo stand, skin penetration is possible.

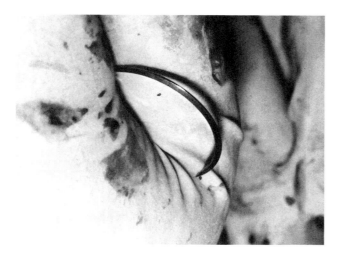

FIG. 36.2-4. When tying suture, instrument-tie or other no-touch techniques should be used if possible. If hand ties are necessary, the needle should be removed from the suture before tying. Tying with the needle in hand, such as demonstrated here, is dangerous and unnecessary.

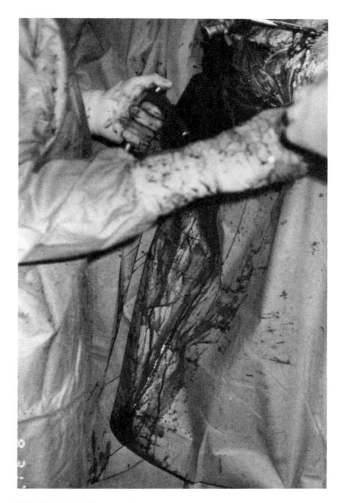

FIG. 36.2-5. When probing deep wounds where sharp bony fragments are present, the surgeon should be careful not to puncture his glove and skin. The use of a cloth or Kevlar glove between the two layers of latex gloves may help to prevent skin puncture in cases such as this.

latex), Kevlar, cloth, and chain-link. Several gloves and glove liners have been marketed as "cut resistant" (although not necessarily puncture-proof); however, these claims must be balanced against these products' acceptability by surgical staff. Although several reports in the literature examine different types of glove and glove-liner combinations within individual specialties, no large controlled studies have compared the efficacy of different types of products in preventing blood contacts or addressed their relative ease of use.

Several studies have shown that double and triple gloving significantly decreases the risk of perforation of the glove worn closest to the skin. Many studies have assessed rates of blood contact in single- and double-gloved surgical personnel and found significantly lower rates in double-gloved personnel.[13–15] Some of these studies have also assessed the acceptability of double gloving by surgeons and found that most surgeons did not perceive tactile sensation to be significantly altered with double gloves.[13,14]

Although blood-skin contamination of the hands may be preventable by double gloving and more frequent glove changes, the risk of disease transmission associated with these contacts is lower than that associated with a percutaneous injury. At least one study has shown that rates of percutaneous injury and blood contact were reduced for surgical personnel using double gloves. Preliminary analyses of 1472 gynecologic procedures showed that the number of blood-hand contacts per 100 surgeon-procedures was significantly higher (24.2) for single-gloved surgeons than double-gloved surgeons (2.1).[16] The number of percutaneous injuries per 100 surgeon-procedures was 2.6 for those who were single gloved versus 1.3 for those who were double gloved (CDC, unpublished data). Wearing double gloves

may reduce inner glove perforation rates and prevent percutaneous injuries; however, these data may be confounded by the fact that more safety-conscious personnel may be more likely to wear double gloves.

Double gloving may also reduce the risk of disease transmission by decreasing the volume of blood associated with a percutaneous injury. Several in vitro studies have shown that the amount of blood transferred by hollow-bore or solid (eg, suture) needles may be significantly decreased when needles are passed through two, rather than one, pair of gloves.[17,18]

The third factor in assessing the efficacy of gloves as a protective barrier is integrity over time. One large observational study of 1382 surgical procedures to assess the frequency of blood contacts in five surgical specialties showed that the incidence of blood-hand contacts was strongly related to procedure duration (ie, the longer the procedure, the more contacts were likely to occur).[15] Another study at San Francisco General Hos-

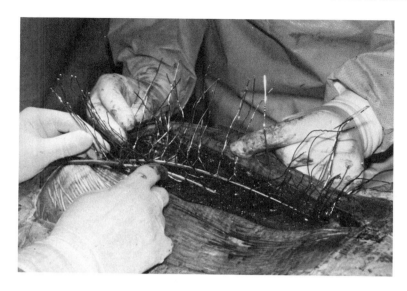

FIG. 36.2-6. In cases that involve the use of a large number of wires or other sharp instrumentation, great care must be taken to prevent skin puncture. The use of cloth or Kevlar gloves is also helpful in these cases, to prevent accidental sticks. In this case—a patient with spinal curvature—a Luque rod with multiple wires is being used to secure the spine to a rod. With this number of wires present, members of the surgical team can accidentally puncture their gloves and skin.

pital showed that the likelihood of gloves perforating during a procedure increases with time worn and that changing gloves hourly may decrease the risk of a blood contact.[13,19]

Given these data, many investigators have been exploring methods to detect intraoperative breaks in latex glove integrity. At least three such methods have been proposed. The first is direct inspection of gloves; however, small perforations can easily be missed. The second method relies on electrical current or resistance; loss of latex glove integrity interrupts resistance across the glove and allows current to flow.[20-23] However, there are some difficulties with this method in clinical settings. The size of the smallest detectable hole is unknown, and very small breaks in latex may go undetected. Moreover, current through the hole must be of a great enough magnitude to be distinguishable from current through the remainder of the glove. Some investigators have suggested that this type of monitoring may be of more practical value in quality assurance and glove manufacturing.[24] The third method for monitoring glove integrity uses color pigments; when fluid is present on the inner glove a colored indicator shows that the outer glove has been perforated.[25,26]

All three methods are still being tested, and there is no definite evidence that intraoperative monitoring of glove integrity is more effective in preventing blood contacts than is wearing double gloves or changing gloves on an hourly basis. At present CDC has no recommendations on methods for intraoperative monitoring of glove integrity or on double gloving.

Body and Facial Protection

Selection of appropriate personnel protective equipment for a particular procedure depends on a number of factors, including urgency of the procedure (ie, elective versus emergency), type of procedure, expected operative time, anticipated blood loss, skill of the operator, comfort, cost of the garments or equipment selected, potential adverse effects on patients (eg, a gown that limits movement, goggles that fog very easily), whether the equipment generates increased medical waste, and the roles of those participating in the procedure (eg, some studies have found that surgeons and first assistants have higher blood contact rates than do scrub and circulating nurses and anesthesiologists).[15,27,28]

A study of five surgical specialties (cardiac, general, gynecology, orthopedics, and trauma) to assess the frequency and preventability of blood-skin contacts in surgical personnel revealed that higher rates of blood-body (eg, torso, arm, leg) contacts were most closely correlated with greater amounts of blood loss during a procedure. Procedures associated with a significantly higher rate of blood-body contacts included cardiac surgery (excluding coronary artery bypass surgery), intestinal procedures, open reduction or internal fixations, and abdominal and other trauma surgery.[15]

Many different types of reusable and disposable surgical gowns are available. These gowns vary by fabric type and extent and type of reinforcement. There are several different laboratory tests available to evaluate the potential for "strike-through" or blood-body contacts with various gown materials, as well as the potential for virus penetration.[29-31] However, many surgical personnel advocate evaluation of gown performance in the operating room, because it is impossible to simulate the exact stresses that are placed on the fabric when worn. They suggest in-use evaluations that include collection of data by trained personnel using a standardized data collection form to assess gown comfort and to record incidences of blood strike-through on scrubs or skin.[27,32] One such study found significant differences in gowns based on the material, degree of reinforcement, and design of the gowns.[33]

Data from at least one study show that blood-facial contacts may be more common in orthopedics than in other surgical specialties.[15] The study concluded that facial and eye contacts vary by worker, specialty, and procedure and that they can largely be prevented by the use of barrier precautions. Another study, assessing blood-facial contacts among obstetricians, found that 50% of face shields were contaminated with blood during cesarean section, as were 32% during vaginal deliveries. A large percentage of these contacts were undetected by surgeons at the time of the procedure.[34] Options for facial protection other than standard surgical masks include face shields, hoods, and helmets.

In addition to adhering to the CDC's principles of universal precautions, the surgeon and operating team should wear the best available garments that offer protection against blood contact. This protective gear should be considered on a case by case basis. The AAOS[12] suggests that the following protective material be considered:

1. Knee-high, waterproof surgical shoes or boots and leg covers should be worn if considerable blood or fluid is expected to be present. Routine shoe covers can be worn over knee-high covers to prevent slipping on wet operating room floors (Fig. 36.2-7).
2. A water-impervious gown should be considered, and if none is available, a waterproof apron can be worn under the gown.
3. A head cover that maximizes head and skin coverage and extends down to protect the lower portion of the face is ideal.
4. Protective eyewear should include at least safety eyeglasses with side shields, if not goggles or a face shield (Fig. 36.2-8).
5. Standard surgical masks can be worn. If the mask is splattered or moist, it should be changed. If splatter is expected, a face shield may prevent the mask from becoming contaminated.
6. Given the known data about glove and gown integrity, the surgical team should consider checking periodically (hourly) to see if gloves and other barrier precautions are intact or contaminated with blood and other body fluids.

At the completion of the surgical procedure, the AAOS[12] recommends that the following precautions should be considered:

1. Bloody outer gloves should be removed before the patient's wound is washed and a dressing is applied. If necessary, the surgeon can don a clean pair of gloves to apply the dressing.
2. The boots, if bloody, should be removed before the gloves are taken off. To avoid contamination of other areas of the operating suite, the surgeon should not leave the operating room with blood-soaked shoe covers (Figs. 36.2-9 and 36.2-10).
3. The surgical team members should remove all blood-contaminated clothing in a manner that avoids contact with blood. Gowns and gloves can be removed as a unit, keeping the bloody side rolled within. They should then be placed in proper containers for infectious waste (Fig. 36.2-11).

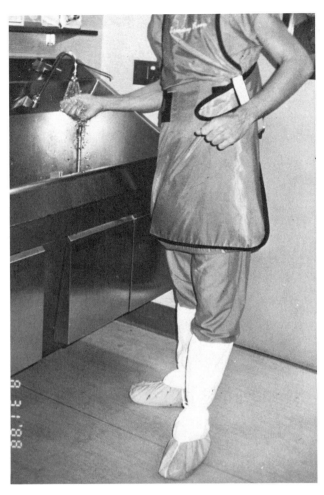

FIG. 36.2-7. While performing a surgical procedure where a great deal of blood or fluid is expected to contaminate the floor or sheets, the health-care worker should wear knee-high, fluid-impervious boots. The surgeon in this photograph has knee-high boots, which are supplemented by usual shoe covers to prevent slipping on the fluid-covered floor.

4. The surgical team members should not touch anything (eg, telephone, cabinets) with bloody gloves.
5. After surgery, the surgical team members should wash hands, forearms, and face with antiseptic soap at the surgical scrub sink.

Training surgeons to use engineering controls, work-practice controls, and personal protective equipment to the fullest benefit for surgeon and patient can be a significant challenge. A variety of strategies have been employed, ranging from didactic presentations to one-on-one training in the operating room.[35] One study provided a community-based program for surgeons and obstetrician-gynecologists that included a lecture and slide show on the risk of occupational transmission of bloodborne pathogens and an accompanying videotape on the use of blunt-tipped suture needles and double gloving. A survey of attitudes before and after the pre-

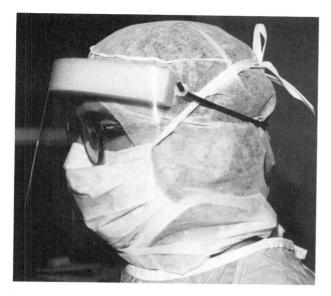

FIG. 36.2-8. Eye protection is important to prevent splatter of the eyes. Full glasses or goggles are good, but a face shield is better. The welder's-type mask used by this surgeon will prevent splatter to the face, particularly if a high-speed drill or saw is being used. Additionally, the head cover should enclose the lower portion of the face and the neck. The standard nurse's cap is not adequate to cover exposed skin.

sentation showed that 64% were double gloving before and that 96% were willing to try it after; it also showed that 3% were using blunt-tipped needles before but that 85% were willing to try these needles after.[36] Similarly, a CDC study showed that after a didactic training program on risk and prevention of blood-skin contacts with double gloving, this practice increased from 27% to 48% among house staff and attending surgeons in obstetrics and gynecology.[10]

Preliminary results from a CDC study assessing surgical technique changes after one-on-one training in the operating room or didactic training have shown that certain "risky" techniques occur less frequently in procedures if the primary surgeon or first assistant has received such training. These techniques include holding tissue with fingers while suturing or cutting, allowing sharps to remain on the field when not in use, and retrieving or returning instruments directly to the scrub nurses' table without announcement to the scrub nurse.

Administrative Controls

Administrative controls are adjunct controls in the IH model; they are to be used with other controls. They include policies such as rotation of workers to minimize exposure; in the operating room this may translate to not allowing surgical staff to work more than a certain number of hours without sufficient time off (this is likely of benefit to patients as well). Another type of administrative control is an operating room committee composed of representatives from several departments (eg, nursing, attending staff, resi-

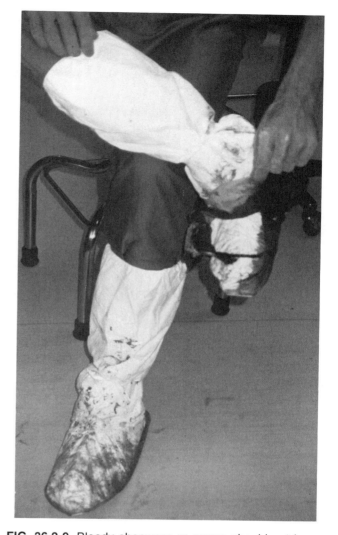

FIG. 36.2-9. Bloody shoewear or gowns should not be removed with bare hands, as the surgeon demonstrates in this case. The gloves should be left on until all contaminated materials have been removed. Additionally, bloody boots and gowns should be removed before leaving the operating room. Surgical team members should not walk through surgical corridors with bloody boots, because of the risk of contamination.

dents) who set and enforce policies and procedures, including certain laws or standards. For example, the Occupational Safety and Health Administration's Bloodborne Pathogen Standard promulgated in December 1991[37] mandates several precautions for diminishing transmission of bloodborne pathogens in occupational settings, including use of universal precautions and administration of HBV vaccine at the employers' expense, to all persons with potential occupational exposure to blood and body fluids.

The risk of occupational transmission of HBV is much higher than that of HIV[38] and has been correlated with several factors, including level of exposure to blood and body fluids, the degree of contact with contaminated sharp instru-

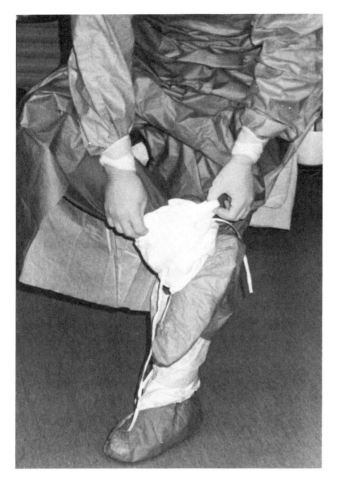

FIG. 36.2-10. This example demonstrates the surgeon properly removing his shoe covers while still wearing gloves. The shoe covers in this case have not been contaminated with visible blood, but the technique is correct.

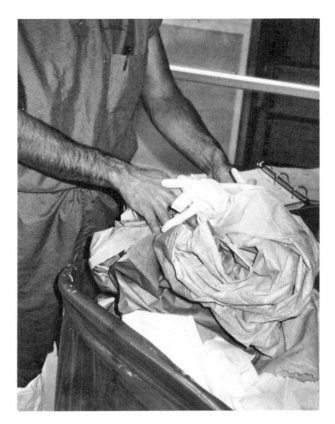

FIG. 36.2-11. The surgical gown and gloves should be removed as a unit, keeping the contaminated, bloody side rolled within, and should then be placed in proper containers for infectious waste. These are usually colored red or yellow, depending on your hospital.

ments, and length of employment in an occupation with frequent blood and needle exposure.[39] Vaccination, the most efficacious method for preventing occupational acquisition of HBV, is especially important for surgical staff, who frequently come into contact with blood. Before licensure of hepatitis B vaccine in 1981, seroepidemiologic studies revealed a higher prevalence of HBV markers among surgical personnel compared with other groups of health care workers.[40-43]

Despite the wide availability of the vaccine and the mandate of the bloodborne pathogen standard, additional efforts are needed to ensure that practicing surgeons are vaccinated. Two seroprevalence studies performed among surgeons since licensure of HBV vaccine revealed that 26% to 33% reported having received no doses of HBV vaccine. In both of these studies, age was inversely related to the proportion of surgeons vaccinated (ie, more house staff and younger surgeons were vaccinated than older surgeons), and infected.[44,45]

Vaccination of surgeons is also important in preventing surgeon-to-patient transmission of HBV. Clusters of trans-

missions of HBV from surgeons to patients continue to be reported.[46-49] Some cases have led health officials in the United Kingdom to recommend that HBV-infected surgeons who are hepatitis B e-antigen positive, correlating with an increased degree of infectiousness, should be prohibited from performing exposure-prone procedures. These are defined as procedures in which "the workers' gloved hands may be in contact with sharp instruments, needle tips, and sharp tissues (spicules of bone or teeth) inside a body cavity, wound, or confined anatomical space where the hands or fingertips may not be visible at all times."[50] Acquisition of HBV may have deleterious effects on a surgeon's career as well as his or her health.

CONCLUSIONS

Appropriate application of the IH model to the surgical setting, including engineering controls, work practices, personal protective equipment, and administrative controls, should help surgical staff to greatly decrease percutaneous, mucous membrane, and skin contacts with blood. These strategies may be applied in the traditional operating room and during labor and delivery, in the emergency room, and in outpatient surgical settings. Reducing the incidence of blood contact may have a positive psychologic effect on all members of the operating team and reduce the risk of blood-borne pathogen transmission to surgical personnel. All surgical personnel should be vaccinated against HBV, because this is the one bloodborne pathogen for which disease acquisition can be almost entirely prevented.

REFERENCES

1. Leibowitz S, Greenwald L, Cohen I, Litwins J. Serum hepatitis in a blood bank worker. JAMA 1949;140:1331.
2. Centers for Disease Control. Recommendations for prevention of HIV transmission in health-care settings. MMWR 1987;36(Suppl 2S).
3. Lewis F, Short L, Howard J, Jacobs A, Roche N. Epidemiology of injuries by needles and other sharp instruments: minimizing sharps injuries in gynecologic and obstetric operations. Surg Clin North Am 1995;75:1105.
4. Gerberding JL. Procedure-specific infection control for preventing intraoperative blood exposure. Am J Infect Control 1993;21:364.
5. Quebbeman EJ, Short LJ. How to select and evaluate new products on the market. Surg Clin North Am 1995;75:1159.
6. Montz FJ, Fowler JM, Farias-Eisner R, Nash TJ. Blunt needles in fascial closure. Surg Gynecol Obstet 1991;173:147.
7. Miller SS, Sabharwal A. Subcuticular skin closure using a blunt needle. Ann R Coll Surg Engl 1994;76:281.
8. DeWeese JD. Avoiding puncture wounds in the operating room. (Letter to the editor) N Engl J Med 1992;327:1461.
9. Davis M. Blunt-tipped suture needles. (Letter to the editor) Infect Control Hosp Epidemiol 1994;15:224.
10. Robert LM, Short LJ, Chamberland ME, et al. Reduction of blood contacts and percutaneous injuries during gynecologic surgical procedures. (Abstract) Infect Control Hosp Epidemiol 1995;16(Suppl):23.
11. Tokars JI, Bell DM, Culver DH, et al. Percutaneous injuries during surgical procedures. JAMA 1992;267:2899.
12. American Academy of Orthopaedic Surgeons. Recommendations for the prevention of human immunodeficiency virus (HIV) transmission in the practice of orthopedic surgery. Park Ridge, IL: American Academy of Orthopaedic Surgeons, 1989.
13. Gerberding JL, Quebbeman EJ, Rhodes R. Hand protection. Surg Clin North Am 1995;75:1133.
14. Quebbeman EJ, Telford GL, Wadsworth K, Hubbard S, Goodman H, Gottlieb M. Double gloving—protecting surgeons from blood contamination in the operating room. Arch Surg 1992;127:213.
15. Tokars JI, Culver DH, Mendelson MH, et al. Skin and mucous membrane contacts during surgical procedures: risk and prevention. Infect Control Hosp Epidemiol 1995;16:703.
16. Robert LM, Short LJ, Chamberland ME, et al. Interventions to reduce blood contact and percutaneous injuries during gynecologic procedures (abstract). Infect Control Hosp Epidemiol 1995;16:23.
17. Mast ST, Woolwine JD, Gerberding JL. Efficacy of gloves in reducing blood volumes transferred during simulated needlestick injury. J Infect Dis 1993;168:1589.
18. Bennett NT, Howard RJ. Quantity of blood inoculated in a needlestick injury from suture needles. J Am Coll Surg 1994;178:107.
19. Rose DA, Ramiro N, Perlman J, et al. Usage patterns and perforation rates for 6396 gloves from intra-operative procedures at San Francisco General Hospital. (Abstract) Infect Control Hosp Epidemiol 1994;15:349.
20. Burbridge E. Clinical experience with the NOVATEC "surgic alert" monitor. (Abstract) Infect Control Hosp Epidemiol 1994;15:341.
21. Rifkin CH, Tedesco SA, Lansing NC. Surgical glove failure during general surgical operations. (Abstract) Infect Control Hosp Epidemiol 1994;15:348.
22. Bennett JK. The feasibility of using electrical means for monitoring barrier integrity in natural rubber latex gloves. (Abstract) Infect Control Hosp Epidemiol 1994;15:341.
23. Cox MJ, Edlich RF. New advances in electronic devices for hole detection. (Abstract) Infect Control Hosp Epidemiol 1994;15:342.
24. Stampfer JF, Kissane RJ, Martin LS. Electrical conductivity as a test for the integrity of latex gloves. J Clin Engineer 1994;Nov/Dec:476.
25. Fay MF, Denton WG. Reducing the risk of cross contamination using a new patented glove puncture glove indicator system to detect barrier breach. (Abstract) Infect Control Hosp Epidemiol 1994;15:343.
26. Manson TM, Edlich RF. A colored inner glove for enhanced protection and hole detection. (Abstract) Infect Control Hosp Epidemiol 1994;15:347.
27. Fry DE, Telford GL, Fectau DL, Sperling RS, Meyer AA. Prevention of blood exposure: body and facial protection. Surg Clin North Am 1995;75:1141.
28. Quebbeman EJ, Telford GL, Hubbard S, et al. Risk of blood contamination and injury to operating room personnel. Ann Surg 1991;214:614.
29. McCullough EA. Methods for determining the barrier efficacy of surgical gowns. Am J Infect Control 1993;21:368.
30. Flaherty AL, Wick TM. Prolonged contact with blood alters surgical gown permeability. Am J Infect Control 1993;21:249.
31. Smith JW, Nichols RL. Barrier efficiency of surgical gowns: are we really protected from our patients' pathogens? Arch Surg 1991;126:756.
32. Telford GL, Quebbeman, EJ. Assessing the risk of blood exposure in the operating room. Am J Infect Control 1993;21:351.
33. Quebbeman EJ, Telford GL, Hubbard S, et al. In-use evaluation of surgical gowns. Surg Gynecol Obstet 1992;174:369.
34. Kouri DL, Ernest JM. Incidence of perceived and actual face shield contamination during vaginal and cesarean delivery. Am J Obstet Gynecol 1993;169:312
35. Raucher B, Stein J, Roche N, et al. OB/GYN personnel exposure to body fluids: educational strategies for prevention. Abstract. Presented at the First National Conference on Human Retroviruses and Related Infections, American Society for Microbiology, Washington D.C., 1993.
36. Davis M. Safe surgery for the nineties. (Abstract) Infect Control Hosp Epidemiol 1994;15:342.
37. Department of Labor, Occupational Safety and Health Administration. 29 CFR Part 1910.1030: occupational exposure to bloodborne pathogens; final rule. Fed Regist 1991;56:64175.
38. Short LJ, Bell DM. Risk of occupational infection with blood-borne pathogens in operating and delivery room settings. Am J Infect Control 1993;21:343.
39. Shapiro CN. Occupational risk of infection with hepatitis B and hepatitis C virus. Surg Clin North Am 1995;75:1047.
40. Denes AE, Smith JL, Maynard JE, Doto IL, Berquist KR, Finkel AJ. Hepatitis B infection in physicians: results of a nationwide seroepidemiologic survey. JAMA 1978;239:210.
41. Hadler SC, Doto IL, Maynard JE, et al. Occupational risk of hepatitis B infection in hospital workers. Infect Control 1985;6:24.
42. Janzen J, Tripatzis I, Wagner U, Schllieter M, Muller-Dethard E, Wolters E. Epidemiology of hepatitis B surface antigen (HBsAg) and antibody to HBsAg in hospital personnel. J Infect Dis 1978;137:261.
43. Smith JD, Maynard JE, Berquist KR, et al. Occupational risk of hepatitis B among physicians and dentists. J Infect Dis 1976;133:705.
44. Shapiro CN, Tokars JI, Chamberland ME, et al. Hepatitis B vaccine use and hepatitis B virus and hepatitis C virus infections among orthopaedic surgeons. J Bone Joint Surg (in press).
45. Panlilio AL, Shapiro CN, Schable CA, et al. Serosurvey of human immunodeficiency virus, hepatitis B virus, and hepatitis C virus infection among hospital-based surgeons. J Am Coll Surg 1995;180:16.
46. Harpaz R, Van Seidlin L, Averhoff F, et al. Transmission of hepatitis B virus to multiple patients from a surgeon without evidence of inadequate infection control. N Engl J Med 1996;334:549.
47. Heptonstall J, Collins M, Smith I, et al. Restricting practice of HBeAG positive surgeons: lessons from hepatitis B outbreaks in England, Wales, and Northern Ireland 1984-93. (Abstract) Infect Control Hosp Epidemiol 1994;15:344.
48. Johnston BL, Langille DB, LeBlanc JC, et al. Transmission of hepatitis B related to orthopedic surgery. (Abstract) Infect Control Hosp Epidemiol 1994;15:352.
49. Bell DM, Shapiro CN, Ciesielski CA, Chamberland ME. Preventing bloodborne pathogen transmission from health care workers to patients: the CDC perspective. Surg Clin North Am 1995;75:1189.
50. United Kingdom Department of Health, The Advisory Group on Hepatitis. Protecting healthcare workers and patients from hepatitis B. London, August 1993.

*AIDS: Biology, Diagnosis, Treatment and
Prevention, fourth edition,* edited by Vincent T.
DeVita, Jr., Samuel Hellman, and Steven A.
Rosenberg. Lippincott–Raven Publishers, © 1997

36.3

Special Considerations for Dentistry

Jennifer L. Cleveland and Donald W. Marianos

Although the underlying principles to prevent occupational disease transmission are common to all medical settings, including dentistry, the unique nature of most dental procedures, instrumentation, and patient care settings may require specific strategies directed to the prevention of transmission of bloodborne pathogens among dental workers and their patients. Available data suggest that the risk for bloodborne disease transmission among workers and patients in the dental setting is low. Nevertheless, during dental procedures, dental workers and patients may be exposed to a variety of microorganisms in blood or in oral or respiratory secretions. Because the potential exists for disease transmission in dental settings, specific strategies for reducing these risks have been developed and are presented in this chapter. First, we consider some of the factors unique to dental settings that influence the risk of occupational human immunodeficiency virus (HIV) transmission during dental procedures.

RISK OF HIV TRANSMISSION AMONG DENTAL WORKERS AND PATIENTS

Evaluating the risk of HIV transmission in health care settings, including dental settings, requires data from surveillance activities of health care workers (HCWs), HIV seroprevalence studies among HCWs and patients, and prospective studies that evaluate the risk of seroconverting after an exposure to HIV-infected blood and that attempt to define the frequency and circumstances of blood contacts in health care settings. These determinants of risk have been

discussed previously in Chapter 35, and this chapter focuses on available data specific to dental settings. Although the exact risk of transmission of bloodborne pathogens has not been quantified in dental settings by precise epidemiologic studies, several published reports provide information suggesting that the risk of infection of dental workers and patients during dental procedures is low.

Transmission of HIV From Patient to Dental Worker

As of June 1995, 143 HCWs had been reported to the Center for Disease and Prevention's (CDC) national surveillance system for occupational transmission of HIV.[1] No dental workers (ie, dentists, dental hygienists, or dental assistants) were among the 46 documented seroconversions associated with a documented exposure to HIV infected blood. Among the remaining 97 possible cases of occupational acquisition of HIV, six were classified as dental workers. For these six, no other risk for infection, such as a behavioral or transfusion risk, could be identified during follow-up investigations. Each of the six reported past percutaneous or mucous membrane exposure to blood or body fluids in the dental setting, but seroconversion resulting from a specific occupational exposure was not documented.

HIV Seroprevalence Among Dental Workers

HIV seroprevalence data of dentists has been collected at annual meetings of the American Dental Association (ADA) and in high acquired immunodeficiency syndrome (AIDS) incidence areas (Table 36.3-1).[2-5] These studies indicate very low HIV seroprevalence, ranging from 0 to less than 1% for these workers. A major limitation of these data is that the extent of exposure to HIV of the dentists tested is unknown. Nevertheless, these surveys are helpful in that they do not suggest a high rate of previously undetected HIV infection among the dentists studied.

Jennifer L. Cleveland, Oral Health Program, Centers for Disease Control and Prevention, 4770 Buford Hwy MS F-10, Chamblee, GA, 30341.

Donald W. Marianos, Oral Health Program, Centers for Disease Control and Prevention, 4770 Buford Hwy MS F-10, Chamblee, GA, 30341.

TABLE 36.3-1. *HIV seroprevalence among U.S. dentists*

Investigator	Location	Number Tested	Number Positive (%)
Flynn	Sacramento	89	0 (0)
Klein	1986 ADA meeting and New York City	1132*	1 (0.09)
Gruninger	1987 ADA meeting	1195	0 (0)
Gruninger	1988 ADA meeting	1165	1 (0.09)
Gruninger	1989 ADA meeting	1480	0 (0)
Gruninger	1990 ADA meeting	1466	0 (0)
Siew	1992 AAOMS meeting	321	0 (0)

*Dentists with community risk were excluded.
AAOMS, American Association of Oral and Maxillofacial Surgeons; ADA, American Dental Association.

Transmission of HIV From Dental Worker to Patients

Transmission of HIV to a patient during an invasive procedure performed by a dentist with AIDS was reported in 1990.[6] Follow-up epidemiologic and laboratory investigations strongly suggest that HIV subsequently was transmitted during dental care to an additional five patients before the dentist's death in 1991. Although the precise mechanism of HIV transmission in the Florida dental practice may never be identified, available evidence continues to suggest that transmission occurred from the dentist to his patients. This cluster remains the only documented instance of HCW-to-patient transmission of HIV. Further evidence supporting a very small risk of HIV transmission to patients comes from retrospective investigations of patients of other HIV-infected dental workers.

Blood Contacts During Dental Procedures

Occupational blood exposures, including percutaneous, skin, and mucous membrane exposures, may present to dental workers and patients some risk of infection with a bloodborne pathogen. Understanding the nature, frequency, and circumstances of occupational blood exposures specific to dental procedures is important in evaluating the risk of disease transmission to dental workers and patients. We know from experience that percutaneous exposures pose the greatest risk for infection.[8] Most available data on occupational blood exposures in dentistry have focused on percutaneous injuries.

Frequency of Injuries to Dental Workers

Retrospective, observational, and prospective studies of injuries among general dentists, oral surgeons, and dental hygienists and assistants have been conducted by the ADA, CDC, and academic teaching institutions (Table 36.3-2).[9–15] Since the first studies conducted at the Health Screening Program of the ADA's annual meetings, the number of sharps injuries reported by dentists has been decreasing. For example, in 1987, dentists reported having about one injury in the past month.[9] This estimate showed a gradual decrease until 1991, when dentists reported having about one injury

every 3 months. This decrease occurred at about the same time as dentists began routinely wearing gloves. Changes in work practices, including careful handling and disposal of sharps, using one-handed needle recapping, and using instruments instead of fingers to retract tissues during anesthetic injections and suturing, may have resulted in fewer injuries. Most studies among U.S. dental workers, including general dentists, oral surgeons, and dental hygienists and assistants, are finding frequencies of approximately 0.3 injuries per month, or about three to four injuries per year.

These studies also have found that injury rates among dental workers are probably less than among general surgical personnel. For example, data from a recent CDC prospective observational study among general dentistry and oral surgery residents in New York City found that dental residents experienced about two injuries per 1000 hours of observation,[11] a much lower rate of percutaneous injuries than general surgery personnel who, in another CDC study, experienced 34 injuries per 1000 hours of observation.[16]

Factors Associated With Injuries Among Dental Workers

The types of instruments or devices most commonly associated with injuries among dentists participating in the ADA's self-reported surveys or prospective study were dental burs, followed by syringe needles and sharp instruments (including laboratory knives).[9–10] Similar to the observational study of dental residents conducted by the CDC,[11] most of these injuries occurred to the dentists fingers or hand and were extraoral (ie, occurred while the worker's hands were outside the patient's mouth). The latter factor is important when considering the risk of the contaminated instrument again coming in contact with the patient. Although extraoral injuries may place the worker at risk for infection, injuries that occur outside the patient's mouth should allow the worker time to replace a contaminated instrument with a sterile one and time to tend to the wound and to replace damaged gloves when necessary.

With the exception of syringe needles, devices associated with injuries among oral surgeons differ from those among general dentists. More than half of the oral surgeons in a 1992 self-reported study disclosed that wire was associated

TABLE 36.3-2. *Studies of percutaneous injuries among U.S. dental workers*

Investigation	Study	Number of Injuries/month	Dental Worker
Siew, 1991	Self-report	0.29	General dentists
Gooch, 1992	Self-report	0.31	Oral surgeons
Siew, 1992	Prospective/self-report	0.28	General dentists and specialists
Cleveland, 1993	Prospective/observational	0.33	General dentistry and oral surgery residents
Malvitz, 1993	Self-report	0.30	Dental hygienists*
	Self-report	0.44	Dental assistants*

*Sample sizes were less than 150.

with most injuries, followed by syringe needles and suture needles.[12] Injuries were reported to have occurred more frequently during fracture reductions. One prospective study examined injuries to oral surgeons during outpatient and inpatient procedures.[13] No injuries were recorded during 521 outpatient procedures; however, four injuries occurred during operating room procedures. Consistent with previous self-reports, two of the four injuries involved wires used during fracture reductions. No other procedure-specific associations have been observed among the different categories of dental personnel, but procedure-specific injury data are limited. No association with the experience of the dentist, as measured by years in practice, has been reported.

Prevention of Occupational Blood Exposures

Strategies to prevent occupational blood exposures in dentistry and oral surgery require the development of improved engineering controls, safer work practices, and improved personal protective equipment. Briefly, some of the strategies include the use of safer devices, such as self-sheathing hollow-bore needles and dental units with designs that shield burs in handpieces placed in the unit. Modified work practices should discourage potentially uncontrolled movements of instruments, such as scalers or laboratory knives, under force or the use of fingers to retract or suture tissue in the operative field. Placement of cork or other covers on exposed wires should be explored as a preventive measure during oral surgery procedures. Because most injuries involve the fingers and hands, the continued development of personal protective equipment such as puncture-resistant gloves and thimbles may be important. Once developed, these preventive interventions must be evaluated to determine if sharps injuries among dental workers are reduced without adversely affecting patient care.

Hepatitis B Virus Transmission as a Model for HIV Transmission

Examining transmission patterns for hepatitis B virus (HBV) can be useful in understanding the risks for occupational transmission of HIV in health care settings. HBV seroprevalence among dentists and oral surgeons has decreased since the 1970s and early 1980s (Tables 36.3-3 and 36.3-4)[17–22] Among general dentists, infection rates decreased from prevaccine levels of 14% in 1972 to 9% in 1989 and remained level until 1992. Although levels of infection are generally higher among oral surgeons than general dentists, the percentage of oral surgeons showing serologic evidence of past or current HBV infection decreased from 26% in 1981 to 20% in 1992. These declines may reflect the increased use of hepatitis B vaccine as well as the increased use of universal precautions by dentists over the same period. For example, in 1972, only 6% of dentists attending the Health Screening Program at the ADA meeting reported using gloves.[15] In 1986, 20% of dentist's participating in the ADA's quarterly survey of dental practice reported routine glove use; by 1991 this percentage had increased dramatically to 91%.[23] Since the availability of the vaccine in 1982, reported hepatitis B vaccination rates among dentists increased dramatically from 17% in 1983 to 85% in 1992.

Since the early 1970s, nine clusters involving over 300 cases of HBV transmission from infected dental workers to patients have been identified.[24] Since 1987, no cases of dental worker to-patient transmission of HBV has been reported. This may reflect increasing levels of immunity among dental workers due to increased use of hepatitis B vaccine and increased compliance with universal precautions.

Patient-to-Patient Transmission

Reusable medical or dental instruments contaminated with blood or tissue during use have the potential to transmit infection to a subsequent patient if these instruments are not appropriately cleaned and disinfected or sterilized after each

TABLE 36.3-3. *Hepatitis B seroprevalence among U.S. dentists* *

Investigation	American Dental Association Meeting	Infection Past or Current (%)	Vaccinated (%)
Moseley	1972	14	0
Siew	1983	15	17
Siew	1985	12	37
Gruninger	1989	9	72
Cleveland	1992	9	85

*General dentists and some specialists.

TABLE 36.3-4. *Hepatitis B seroprevalence among U.S. oral surgeons*

Investigation	AAOMS Meeting	Infection, Past or Current (%)	Vaccinated (%)
Reingold	1981	26	0
Siew	1992	20	81

AAOMS, American Association of Oral and Maxillofacial Surgeons.

use. However, no incidents that confirm the transmission of a bloodborne disease through contaminated dental equipment, such as a handpiece or anesthetic syringe, have been reported. Patient-to-patient transmission of HBV has been identified and reported in other health care settings.[25] These reports involved transmission by acupuncture needles and spring-loaded fingerstick devices.

HIV in Saliva

Trace amounts of HIV are infrequently isolated from saliva of HIV-infected persons. No epidemiologic evidence exists, however, to indicate that saliva is an effective medium for HIV transmission.[26] HIV titers in saliva are much lower than in blood, and several studies have demonstrated HIV inhibitory activity in human saliva. At least two mechanisms have been identified as contributors of this inhibitory process; saliva can inhibit the infectivity of free virus and, to a lesser extent, virus within cells. Despite the absence of clinical evidence of HIV transmission by the oral route, most dental procedures produce various amounts of blood in the oral cavity. For this reason, continued adherence to recommended infection control practices is essential during delivery of dental services.

INFECTION CONTROL PRACTICES FOR DENTISTRY

Historical Background

The first infection control guidelines for dentistry were issued by the ADA in 1978.[27] Their development was a response to increased awareness and understanding of HBV transmissions occurring in dentistry. These guidelines stressed the use of sterilization for instruments, rather than chemical disinfection, and emphasized the need for wearing gloves while treating patients. In 1986, the CDC issued the first federal recommendations for infection control in dentistry.[28] Since then, the guidelines have been updated several times to reflect new data, materials, technology, and equipment.[29-31] As the importance of written infection control policies has been recognized, other organizations and institutions have developed their own or have adapted existing ADA or CDC guidelines. The Occupational Safety and Health Administration published a final ruling on occupational exposure to bloodborne pathogens in 1991; this set of regulations establishes certain infection control practices intended to increase worker safety and minimize occupational acquisition of bloodborne pathogens by all HCWs.[32]

Principles of Infection Control

The goal of all dental infection control procedures is to eliminate or minimize the possibility of infectious disease transmission. Dental patients and dental workers may be exposed to a variety of microorganisms through blood or through oral or respiratory secretions. Infections may be transmitted in dental settings through several routes, including direct contact with blood or other potentially infectious body fluids or indirect contact by means of contaminated instruments, equipment, or environmental surfaces. Contact with airborne contaminants in droplets, spatter, or aerosols of infectious fluids also may transmit infection.

Infection through any of these routes requires all three of the following conditions: a susceptible host, a pathogen with sufficient infectivity and numbers to cause infection, and an appropriate portal through which the pathogen may enter the host. Infection control procedures are intended to eliminate one or more of these conditions, thereby breaking the "chain of infection." Because all infected persons cannot be identified by medical history, physical examination, or laboratory tests, the CDC recommends that all patients be treated as if they were infectious, and proper infection control procedures should be used on all patients at all times while they are receiving dental care.[33] Specific actions also have been recommended to reduce the risk of tuberculosis transmission in dental and other ambulatory health care facilities.[34,35]

As part of a comprehensive infection control program, dental workers should adhere to four basic principles of dental infection control:

- Take action to stay healthy.
- Avoid contact with blood.
- Limit the spread of blood.
- Make objects safe for use.

Principle 1: Take Action to Stay Healthy

This principle is listed first to emphasize the importance of dental workers maintaining their own health. Because a susceptible host is required for an infection to occur, dental workers can protect themselves from several infections such as hepatitis B by becoming immunized.[36,37] Another component of this principle is prompt and appropriate postexposure management, as discussed in Chapter 37.

Proper handwashing removes microorganisms and helps diminish the likelihood of infection. For most routine dental procedures, handwashing with plain soap and water is adequate.[38] For surgical procedures, an antimicrobial product should be used. To ensure that handwashing is effective, fingernails should be kept short and rings or false fingernails should not be worn when providing dental care. Hands should be washed before and after treating each patient, before glove placement, after glove removal, after bare-handed touching of contaminated objects, and before leaving the dental operatory.

Principle 2: Avoid Contact with Blood

Avoiding contact with blood and other potentially infectious body fluids is an effective way to prevent the occurrence of infection. This principle is best accomplished by wearing appropriate protective coverings and by avoiding injuries.

Medical gloves always must be worn whenever the potential exists for contacting blood, blood-contaminated saliva, or mucous membranes. Sterile gloves should be used when performing surgical procedures; nonsterile gloves are appropriate for examinations and other nonsurgical procedures. Medical gloves should be changed between patients and should never be washed, disinfected, or sterilized for reuse.[34,39]

Chin-length plastic face shields or surgical masks and protective eyewear should be worn when splashing or spattering of blood or other body fluids is likely, as is common in dentistry. When used, masks should be changed between patients or during patient treatment if it becomes wet or moist. Face shields or protective eyewear should be cleaned and, when visibly soiled, disinfected between patients. Protective attire should be worn when clothing is likely to be soiled with blood or other body fluids.

Contaminated sharp items, such as needles, scalpels, and wires, should be considered potentially infective and handled with care to prevent injuries. Needles should never be recapped or otherwise manipulated using both hands or using any other technique that involves directing the point of a needle toward any part of the body. When recapping is indicated, a one-handed "scoop" technique (Fig. 36.3-1) or a mechanical device designed for holding the needle sheath should be employed. Bending or breaking needles before disposal is not recommended.

Accidental injuries do occur in dentistry, and for that reason, each dental office should have a written policy for their management. That policy should include a written log for recording appropriate information about the injury, follow-up action, and an explanation of how the injury occurred. Postexposure management of occupational exposures to blood are discussed in Chapter 37.

Principle 3: Limit the Spread of Blood

The spread of blood and saliva contaminated with blood can be minimized by planning ahead and anticipating the treatment needs of each patient. Impervious-backed paper, aluminum foil, or plastic covers should be used to protect items and surfaces such as light handles or x-ray equipment that may become contaminated during use and that are difficult or impossible to clean and disinfect. Between patients, the coverings should be removed and discarded and then replaced by new covering. The use of rubber dams, high-velocity air evacuation, and proper patient positioning can minimize the formation of droplets, spatter, and aerosols during patient treatment.

Principle 4: Make Objects Safe for Use

Cleaning, disinfection, and sterilization are all decontamination processes. These processes differ in the number and types of microorganisms killed. Selection of the proper decontamination process depends on the use of the instrument or equipment to be decontamination (see Chap. 36.5).[40-43]

Cleaning is the first step in all decontamination procedures; it removes debris and reduces the number of microorganisms present. Sterilization kills all microbial life and is the most effective decontamination process available. Disinfection is a process that kills disease-causing microorganisms, although not necessarily all microorganisms. Some nonpathogenic microorganisms may remain on an object after disinfection; the number and type depend on the level of disinfection used. There are three levels of disinfection:

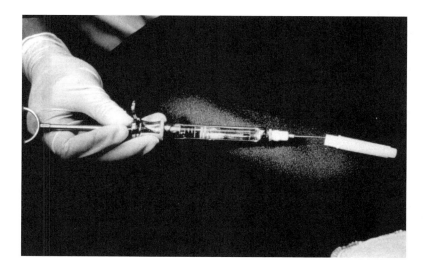

FIG. 36.3-1. Recapping an anesthetic syringe needle using the one-handed "scoop" technique.

Low-level disinfection does not kill bacterial spores or *Mycobacterium tuberculosis* var. *bovis,* a test microorganism used to classify the strength of disinfectant chemicals.

Intermediate-level disinfection does kill *M tuberculosis* var.*bovis,* which indicates that the process also kills more easily kill organisms such as HBV and HIV.

High-level disinfection kills some bacterial spores; it does kill *M tuberculosis* var. *bovis,* as well as other bacteria, fungi, and viruses.

As with other medical and surgical instruments, dental instruments are classified into three categories—critical, semicritical, and noncritical—depending on their use and their risk of transmitting infection (Fig. 36.3-2 through 36.3-4). It is important for each dental practice to classify all instruments as follows:

Critical instruments, used to penetrate soft tissue or touch bone, include forceps, scalpels, bone chisels, scalers, and burs. They should be sterilized after each use.

Semicritical instruments do not penetrate soft tissue or touch bone, but they do contact oral tissues. Examples include mirrors and amalgam condensers; they should be sterilized after each use. If sterilization is not feasible because the instrument will be damaged by heat, the instrument should receive, at minimum, high-level disinfection.

Noncritical instruments or medical devices come into contact only with intact skin and include x-ray tube heads and protective eyewear. Because noncritical surfaces have a relatively low risk of transmitting infection, they may be reprocessed between patients with intermediate-level or low-level disinfection or with detergent and water washing, depending on the degree and nature of contamination.

Methods of Sterilization or Disinfection of Dental Instruments

Cleaning is the first step in all instrument reprocessing. Persons decontaminating dental instruments should wear heavy-duty (ie, reusable utility) gloves, rather than examination or surgical gloves. All critical and semicritical dental instruments that are heat stable should be sterilized between patients by steam under pressure (ie, autoclaving), dry heat, or chemical vapor, following the instructions of the manufacturers of the instruments and the sterilizers. Periodic (at least weekly) use of biologic indicators (ie, spore tests) to verify proper functioning of sterilization cycles is recommended.

In all dental settings, indications for the use of liquid chemical germicides to sterilize instruments are limited. Use of these products may require up to 10 hours of exposure to a liquid chemical agent registered with the U.S. Environmental Protection Agency (EPA) and cleared for marketing as a medical instrument germicide by the Food and Drug Administration (FDA) as a sterilant-disinfectant. When using any of these chemicals to achieve high-level disinfection of heat-sensitive semicritical medical and dental instruments, the manufacturer's directions regarding appropriate concentration and exposure time should be followed.

Cleaning and Disinfection of Environmental Surfaces

After each patient and at the completion of the work day, counter tops and the dental unit surfaces that may have become contaminated with patient material should be cleaned using an appropriate cleaning agent and water.

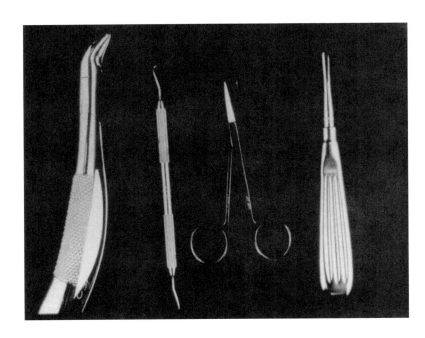

FIG. 36.3-2. Examples of critical items for needle manipulation. From left to right: extraction forceps, curette, scissors, and elevator.

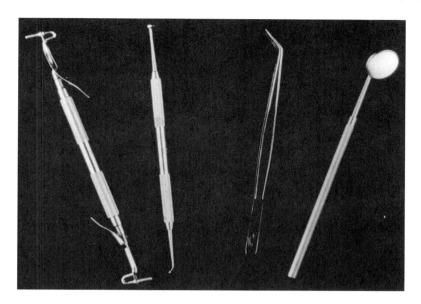

FIG. 36.3-3. Examples of semicritical items. From left to right: amalgam dispenser, amalgam burnisher, cotton forceps, and mirror.

Those surfaces should then be disinfected using an appropriate chemical germicide. Germicides registered with the EPA as a hospital disinfectant and labeled for tuberculocidal activity are recommended for disinfecting surfaces contaminated with patient material. Fresh solutions of sodium hypochlorite (ie, household bleach) in concentrations ranging from 500 to 800 ppm of chlorine ($\frac{1}{4}$ cup of bleach to 1 gallon of water) also are effective on environmental surfaces that have been cleaned of visible contamination and that will not become corroded from chlorine solutions.

Low-level disinfectants (ie, EPA-registered as hospital disinfectants) that are not labeled for tuberculocidal activity are appropriate for general housekeeping purposes such as cleaning of floors and walls.

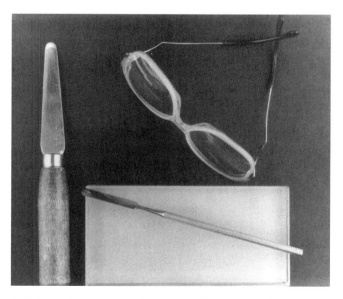

FIG. 36.3-4. Examples of noncritical items. From left to right: spatula, glass slab, and protective eyewear.

Use and Care of Handpieces

Internal surfaces of high-speed handpieces, low-speed handpiece components, and prophylaxis angles have the potential to become contaminated with patient material during use. This retained material may then be expelled during subsequent use.[44-46] It is therefore recommended that all high-speed dental handpieces, low-speed handpiece components used intraorally, and reusable prophylaxis angles be reprocessed between patients using a heating process (eg, autoclaving, dry heat, heat and chemical vapor) capable of sterilization. Manufacturers' instructions for cleaning, lubrication, and sterilization should be followed closely to ensure the effectiveness of the sterilization process and the longevity of the handpiece.

Antiretraction valves (ie, one-way flow check valves) should be installed in dental unit water lines to prevent fluid aspiration and to reduce the risk of transfer of potentially infective material.[47] Routine maintenance of these valves is necessary. It is also recommended that high-speed handpieces should be run to discharge water and air for a minimum of 20 to 30 seconds after use on each patient. This process is intended to aid in the physical flushing out of patient material that may have entered the turbine and air or water lines.[37] There is evidence that overnight or weekend microbial accumulation in dental unit water lines can be reduced by removing the handpiece and allowing the water lines to run and discharge water for several minutes at the beginning of each clinic day.[48]

Single-Use Disposable Instruments

All single-use disposable instruments such as prophylaxis angles, tips for high-speed evacuators, and saliva ejectors, should be used for one patient only and discarded appropriately. These items are neither designed nor intended to be cleaned, disinfected, or sterilized for reuse.

Disposal of Waste Materials

Blood, suctioned fluids, or other liquid waste may be poured carefully into a drain connected to a sanitary sewer system. Disposable needles, scalpels, or other sharp items should be placed intact into puncture-resistant containers before disposal. Solid waste contaminated with blood or other body fluids should be placed in sealed, sturdy, impervious bags to prevent leakage of the contained items. All contained solid waste should then be disposed of according to requirements established by local, state, or federal regulatory agencies.

APPLICATION OF RECOMMENDED INFECTION-CONTROL PRACTICES FOR DENTISTRY

In all settings where dental treatment is provided, emphasis should be placed on consistent adherence to recommended infection-control practices. The following five strategies may provide guidance for the dental practitioner to achieve this goal.

First, for each dental office, a dentist or other staff member should be assigned the responsibility for the office's infection control program. This person should have a thorough understanding of the principles of infection control and should be familiar with standard operating procedures in the office.

Second, there should be initial training and retraining of the dental staff in the principles of infection control and in standard operating procedures in the office.

Third, a written infection control policy for the office should be developed. This policy should include the use of hepatitis B vaccinations; safe work practices, such as handwashing and careful handling of sharp instruments; personal protective equipment; engineering controls, such as rigid containers for disposal of sharps; adequate decontamination procedures; and reporting and follow-up of occupational exposure incidents. The latter policy ensures that exposed workers receive appropriate counseling and testing and postexposure prophylaxis when indicated. Prompt reporting of occupational exposures can help to identify and alter specific work practices that may increase the risk for future exposures

Fourth, a checklist for standard office procedures may assist the dental staff in establishing and ensuring that patterns of performance for each infection control process are followed consistently. For example, one check list may be followed for operatory cleanup between patients, another for cleaning and sterilizing instruments, and another for the use of protective covers and handwashing.

Fifth, it is important for each dental office to maintain adequate records. Such records may include sterilizer spore test results and injury reports, including occupational exposures to blood.

Periodically, in-office procedures can be compared with written infection control policies and instructions to ensure that the practices are applied consistently by all dental staff. These strategies, together with a thorough understanding of infection control principles, can create an environment that protects dental workers and patients from the risk of infection.

The primary goal of all infection control precautions is to reduce blood contact, thereby minimizing bloodborne pathogen transmission to dental workers or patients. Although numerous studies examining dental-specific risks for occupational exposures have been reported, little research has been conducted to examine specific prevention strategies. Additional studies are needed for the development and evaluation of improved designs for dental instruments, equipment, and personnel protective equipment. More efficient reprocessing techniques should be considered in the design of future dental instruments and equipment. Systematic evaluations must be ongoing to ensure that new technologies can improve the safety of dental treatment without compromising the quality of patient care.

ACKNOWLEDGEMENTS

The authors gratefully acknowledge the contributions of Drs. Dolores Malvitz and Barbara Gooch, Oral Health Program, and Walter Bond and Elizabeth Bolyard, Hospital Infections Program, Centers for Disease Control and Prevention.

BIBLIOGRAPHY

Centers for Disease Control and Prevention. Guidelines for preventing the transmission of *Mycobacterium tuberculosis* in health-care facilities, 1994. MMWR 1994;43(RR-13):1.
Centers for Disease Control and Prevention. Guidelines for prevention of transmission of human immunodeficiency virus and hepatitis B virus to health-care and public-safety workers. MMWR 1989;38(Suppl S-6):1.
Centers for Disease Control and Prevention. Hepatitis B virus: a comprehensive strategy for eliminating transmission in the United States through universal childhood vaccination. MMWR 1991;40(RR-13):1.
Centers for Disease Control and Prevention. Recommended infection-control practices for dentistry, 1993. MMWR 1993;41(RR-8):1.
Centers for Disease Control and Prevention. Recommendations for preventing transmission of human immunodeficiency virus and hepatitis B virus to patients during exposure-prone invasive procedures. MMWR 1991;40(RR-8):1.
Ciesielski C, Marianos D, Chin-Yih Ou, et. al. Transmission of human immunodeficiency virus in a dental practice. Ann Intern Med 1992;116:798.
Cleveland JL, Gooch BF, Bolyard EA, Simone PM, Mullan RJ, Marianos DW. TB infection control recommendations from the CDC, 1994: considerations for dentistry. J Am Dent Assoc 1995;126:593.
Cottone JA, Molinari JA. State-of-the-art infection control in dentistry. J Am Dent Assoc 1991;122:33.
Department of Labor, Occupational Safety and Health Administration. 29 CFR Part 1910.1030: occupational exposure to bloodborne pathogens; final rule. Fed Regist 1991;56:64004.
Favero MS, Bond WW. Chemical disinfection of medical and surgical materials. In: Block SS, ed. Disinfection, sterilization, and preservation. 4th ed. Philadelphia: Lea & Febiger, 1991:617.
Fox PC. Anti-HIV-1 activity in human saliva. In: Greenspan DG, Greenspan JS, eds. Oral manifestations of HIV infection. Chicago: Quintessence, 1995:130.
Larsen EL. APIC guideline for handwashing and hand antisepsis in health care settings. Am J Infect Control 1995;23:251.

Miller CH, Palenik CJ. Sterilization, disinfection and asepsis in dentistry. In: Block SS, ed. Disinfection, sterilization, and preservation. 4th ed. Philadelphia: Lea & Febiger, 1991:676.

Robert LM, Bell DM. HIV transmission in the health-care setting. Infect Dis Clin North Am 1994;8:319.

U.S. Department of Health and Human Services. Infection control file: practical infection control in the dental office. Atlanta: Centers for Disease Control and Prevention/Food and Drug Administration, 1993. (Available through the U.S. Government Printing Office, Washington, DC or the National Technical Information Services, Springfield, VA.)

REFERENCES

1. Centers for Disease Control and Prevention. HIV/AIDS surveillance report. 1995;7:15.
2. Flynn NM, Pollet SM, Van Horne JR, Elvebakk R, Harper SD, Carlson JR. Absence of HIV antibody among dental professionals exposed to infected patients. West J Med 1987;146:439.
3. Klein RS, Phelan JA, Freeman K, et al. Low occupational risk of human immunodeficiency virus infection among dental professionals. N Engl J Med 1988;318:86.
4. Gruninger SE, Siew C, Chang S-B, et al. Human immunodeficiency virus type 1 infection among dentists. J Am Dent Assoc 1992;123:57.
5. Siew C, Gruninger S, Chang S-B, Clayton R. Seroprevalence of hepatitis B and HIV infection among oral surgeons. (Abstract 1431) J Dent Res 1994;73:281.
6. Ciesielski C, Marianos D, Chin-Yih Ou, et.al. Transmission of human immunodeficiency virus in a dental practice. Ann Intern Med 1992;116:798.
7. Robert LM, Chamberland ME, Cleveland JL, et.al. Investigation of patients of health-care workers infected with HIV: the CDC database. Ann Intern Med 1995;122:653.
8. Bell DM. Human immunodeficiency virus transmission in health care settings: risk and risk reduction. Am J Med 1991;91(Suppl 3B):294.
9. Siew C, Chang S-B, Gruninger SE, Verrusio AC, Neidle EA. Self-reported percutaneous injuries in dentists: implications for HBV, HIV transmission risk. J Am Dent Assoc 1992;123:37.
10. Siew C, Gruninger SE, Miaw C, Neidle EA. Percutaneous injuries in practicing dentists. J Am Dental Assoc 1995;126:1227.
11. Cleveland JL, Lockwood SA, Gooch BF, Chamberland ME, and the Dental Cooperative Study Group. Percutaneous injuries during dental procedures: an observational study. J Am Dent Assoc 1995;126:745.
12. Gooch BF, Siew C, Cleveland JL, Gruninger S, Lockwood SA. Occupational exposures reported by oral surgeons—United States, 1992. (Abstract 85) J Dent Res 1995;74:22.
13. Carlton JE, Dodson TB, Cleveland JL, Lockwood SA. The risk of percutaneous injury in oral and maxillofacial surgery. J Oral Maxillofac Surg 1995;53(Suppl 4):110.
14. Gooch BF, Cardo DM, Marcus R, et. Al. Percutaneous exposures to HIV-infected blood among dental workers enrolled in the CD needlestick study. J Am Dent Assoc 1995;126:1237.
15. Malvitz DM, Siew C, Cleveland JL, Gruninger SE. Hepatitis B exposure and vaccination among dental hygienists and dental assistants. J Am Dent Hyg Assoc (in press).
16. Tokars J, Bell DM, Culver DH, et al. Percutaneous injuries during surgical procedures. JAMA 1992;267:2899.
17. Moseley JW, Edwards VM, Casey G, Redeker AG, White E. Hepatitis B virus infection in dentists. N Engl J Med 1975;293:729.
18. Siew C, Gruninger SE, Mitchell EW, Burrell KH. Survey of hepatitis B exposure and vaccination in volunteer dentists. J Am Dent Assoc 1987;114:457.
19. Gruninger S, Siew C, Chang S, et.al. Hepatitis B, C, and HIV infection among dentists. (Abstract 2131) J Dent Res 1991;70:532.
20. Cleveland J, Siew C, Lockwood S, et.al. Trends in hepatitis B vaccination among US dentists, 1983–1992. (Abstract 891) J Dent Res 1995;74:123.
21. Reingold AL, Kane MA, Wightower AW. Failure of gloves and other protective devices to prevent transmission of hepatitis B virus to oral surgeons. JAMA 1988;259:2558.
22. Siew C, Gruninger S, Chang S, Clayton R. Seroprevalence of hepatitis B and HIV infection among oral surgeons. (Abstract 1431) J Dent Res 1994;73:281.
23. Nash KD. How infection control procedures are affecting dental practice today. J Am Dent Assoc 1992;123:67.
24. Bell DM, Shapiro CN, Gooch BF. Preventing HIV transmission to patients during invasive procedures. J Public Health Dent 1993;53:170.
25. Robert LM, Bell DM. HIV transmission in the health-care setting. Infect Dis Clin North Am 1994;8:319.
26. Fox PC. Anti-HIV-1 activity in human saliva. In: Greenspan DG, Greenspan JS, eds. Oral manifestations of HIV infection. Chicago: Quintessence, 1995:130.
27. Council on Dental Materials and Devices and Council on Dental Therapeutics. Infection control in the dental office. J Am Dent Assoc 1978;97:673.
28. Centers for Disease Control. Recommended infection-control practices for dentistry. MMWR 1986;35:237.
29. Centers for Disease Control. Recommendations for prevention of HIV in health-care settings. MMWR 1987;36:2S.
30. Centers for Disease Control and Prevention. Recommended infection-control practices for dentistry, 1993. MMWR 1993;41(RR-8):1.
31. U.S. Department of Health and Human Services. Infection control file: practical infection control in the dental office. Atlanta: Centers for Disease Control and Prevention/Food and Drug Administration, 1993. (Available through the U.S. Government Printing Office, Washington, DC or the National Technical Information Services, Springfield, VA.)
32. Department of Labor, Occupational Safety and Health Administration. 29 CFR Part 1910.1030, occupational exposure to bloodborne pathogens; final rule. Fed Regist 1991;56:64004.
33. Centers for Disease Control. Update: universal precautions for prevention of transmission of human immunodeficiency virus, hepatitis B virus, and other bloodborne pathogens in health-care settings. MMWR 1988;37:377.
34. Centers for Disease Control and Prevention. Guidelines for preventing the transmission of *Mycobacterium tuberculosis* in health-care facilities, 1994. MMWR 1994;43(RR-13):1.
35. Cleveland JL, Gooch BF, Bolyard EA, Simone PM, Mullan RJ, Marianos DW. TB infection control recommendations from the CDC, 1994: considerations for dentistry. J Am Dent Assoc 1995;126:593.
36. Centers for Disease Control and Prevention. Hepatitis B virus: a comprehensive strategy for eliminating transmission in the United States through universal childhood vaccination. MMWR 1991;40(RR-13):1.
37. Centers for Disease Control. Immunization recommendations for health-care workers. Atlanta: Centers for Disease Control, Division of Immunization, Center for Prevention Services, 1989.
38. Larsen EL. APIC guideline for handwashing and hand antisepsis in health care settings. Am J Infect Control 1995;23:251.
39. Adams D, Bagg J, Limaye M, Parsons K, Absi EG. A clinical evaluation of glove washing and re-use in dental practice. J Hosp Infect 1992;20:153.
40. Favero MS, Bond WW. Chemical disinfection of medical and surgical materials. In: Block SS, ed. Disinfection, sterilization, and preservation. 4th ed. Philadelphia: Lea & Febiger, 1991:617.
41. Miller CH, Palenik CJ. Sterilization, disinfection, and asepsis in dentistry. In: Block SS, ed. Disinfection, sterilization, and preservation. 4th ed. Philadelphia: Lea & Fegiber, 1991:676.
42. Rutala WA. APIC guideline for selection and use of disinfectants. Am J Infect Control 1990;18:99.
43. Favero MS, Bond WW. Transmission and control of laboratory-acquired hepatitis infection. In: Fleming DO, ed. Laboratory safety, principles and practices. 2nd ed. Washington, DC: ASM Press, 1995:19.
44. Lewis DK, Boe RK. Cross infection risks associated with current procedures for using high-speed dental handpieces. J Clin Microbiol 1992;30:401.
45. Crawford JJ, Broderius RK. Control of cross infection risks in the dental operatory: prevention of water retraction by bur cooling spray systems. J Am Dent Assoc 1988;116:685.
46. Lewis DL, Arens M, Appleton SS, et al. Cross-contamination potential with dental equipment. Lancet 1992;340:1252.
47. Bagga BSR, Murphy RA, Anderson AW, Punwani I. Contamination of dental unit cooling water with oral microorganisms and its prevention. J Am Dent Assoc 1984;109:712.
48. Scheid RC, Kim CK, Bright JS, Whitely MS, Rosen S. Reduction of microbes in handpieces by flushing before use. J Am Dent Assoc 1982;105:658.

AIDS: Biology, Diagnosis, Treatment and Prevention, fourth edition, edited by Vincent T. DeVita, Jr., Samuel Hellman, and Steven A. Rosenberg. Lippincott–Raven Publishers, © 1997

36.4

Special Considerations for Emergency Personnel

Gabor D. Kelen

EPIDEMIOLOGY OF HIV-1 AS IT RELATES TO EMERGENCY MEDICINE

In the United States, there are more than 500,000 allied emergency personnel: physicians, nurses, and prehospital care providers; this figure does not include ancillary staff, fire-fighters, or police. Emergency medicine is a procedure- and intervention-oriented specialty. Its very nature implies frequent patient contact and potential exposure to blood and body fluids in uncontrolled or poorly controlled circumstances. By most estimates, approximately 1 million residents of the United States are infected with human immunodeficiency virus type 1 (HIV-1),[1] and a large proportion are unaware of their infection. Considering that there are 100 million emergency department patient visits each year in the United States,[2] with approximately 10% of these involving prehospital care providers, the potential for exposure to HIV-1 for emergency personnel is considerable.

The implications of the acquired immunodeficiency syndrome (AIDS) epidemic were not well appreciated among emergency personnel until the spring of 1987, when much publicity was given to two reports. The first was a report by the Centers for Disease Control and Prevention (CDC) describing the first known cases of occupational transmission of HIV-1 after nonparenteral exposures.[3] One of those transmissions occurred from a resuscitation attempt in an emergency department setting. Two weeks later, a publication from the Johns Hopkins emergency department revealed that 6 (3.0%) of 203 critically ill and injured patients had unsuspected HIV-1 infection.[4] All six of these patients were transported by ambulance and required procedures in the prehospital setting. All six were bleeding on arrival to the emergency department and required invasive procedures. With these two reports, the potential impact of the AIDS epidemic for emergency personnel began to be widely appreciated.

Despite the heightened awareness of HIV-1 among emergency personnel after those two reports, many practitioners interpreted the emergency department–based study as implying that the potential for occupational exposure to HIV-1 was restricted to a narrowly defined cohort of patients. All six HIV-1 seropositive patients in that study were young black males between the ages of 25 and 34 years of age and presented with trauma; 5 of these 6 patients presented with penetrating trauma.[4] We observed that many emergency personnel took precautions only when dealing with such patients.

Although it was realized that occult HIV-1 among patients was not likely to be so confined, subsequent emergency department–based studies were aimed at determining whether it was possible to identify patients with unrecognized HIV-1 infection based on ascertainable features in the clinical setting. It was thought that such identification would aid practitioners in determining under what selective circumstances precautions were necessary.

A large follow-up serosurvey conducted at Johns Hopkins in 1987 revealed that 119 (5.2%) of 2302 of the general emergency department patient population were HIV-1 seropositive. Seventy-seven percent of those seropositive or 4% percent of the general emergency department population were unaware of their HIV infections.[5] The restricted associations with HIV-1 infection seen in the first study did not hold. Although occult HIV-1 infection also predominated among young black men in the follow-up study, HIV-1 infection was widely distributed among all races, both sexes, and across a wide age range. Unlike the initial study, HIV-1 infection was not limited to patients with certain clinical conditions but was present in significant proportions (2.8% to 16.7%) among all categories of presenting medical

Gabor D. Kelen, Department of Emergency Medicine, Marburg 190, The Johns Hopkins Hospital, 600 N. Wolfe Street, Baltimore, MD 21205.

problems. A third general emergency department serosurvey conducted in 1988 at Johns Hopkins demonstrated that even rigorous risk factor assessment failed to identify 27% of those with unrecognized HIV-1 infection.[6] The data from these latter two studies imply that patients harboring HIV-1 infection cannot be readily identified in an emergency department setting based on ascertainable variables such as demographics, clinical condition, and even risk factor assessment. That patients with unrecognized HIV-1 infection are not readily identified has been a finding common to all emergency department–based HIV-1 serosurveys.[7–12]

Although the Johns Hopkins emergency department population is the best defined, there have been other emergency department or trauma center serosurveys from other parts of the country (Table 36.4-1). These serosurveys have reported HIV seroprevalence rates of less than 1% to more than 11%.[7–22]

HIV seroprevalence has been rising among emergency department patient populations since serosurveys were first undertaken. In the Johns Hopkins Hospital emergency department, HIV seroprevalence was first found to be 3.0% among those critically ill and injured in 1986[4] and 5.2% among the general emergency department population in 1987.[5] In subsequent serosurveys of the general emergency department population, HIV seroprevalence rose to 6.0% in 1988,[6] 8.9% in 1989,[10] and 11.3% in 1992.[22]

Emergency practitioners in suburban and nonendemic areas may be the most complacent regarding the risk of occupational transmission of bloodborne infections. However, some case reports show that occupational transmissions have occurred in settings with HIV-1 infection rates as low as 2.5 per 1000 persons.[23] The continued increase in emergency department visits by HIV-infected patients has not been restricted to inner-city facilities in AIDS endemic areas. Studies from non–inner-city emergency departments have shown that the seroprevalence of HIV and other bloodborne infections is not trivial[8–10,15,16,18,19] and can be substantial. It was observed as early as 1989 that new AIDS cases have been decreasing concentrated in regions of the country previously recognized for their high prevalence of AIDS.[24]

Although much of the attention has focused on HIV, hepatitis B virus (HBV), hepatitis C virus (HCV), and other bloodborne viruses constitute a considerable nosocomial risk. Johns Hopkins' investigators found seroprevalences of 5% of hepatitis B surface antigen (HBsAg),[25] 18% for HCV,[25] and more than 1% for human T-cell lymphotropic virus type I/II[26] among the same emergency department patient population that was surveyed for HIV.

POTENTIAL MODES OF OCCUPATIONAL TRANSMISSION

HIV has been isolated from blood,[27] serum,[28] semen,[29] vaginal secretions,[30] saliva,[31] breast milk,[32] tears,[33] urine,[34] cerebrospinal fluid,[35] synovial fluid,[36] amniotic fluid,[37] alveolar fluid,[38] bone marrow,[39] and brain.[39] HIV nucleic acids, but not HIV itself, has been detected in feces.[40] However, transmission has been documented only from blood and blood products,[41] semen,[42] vaginal secretions,[41] in utero exposure, possibly from breast milk or breast-feeding,[43] and from transplanted tissue and organs.[44–46] Although one early report

TABLE 36.4-1. *Hospital emergency department–based HIV-1 serosurveys*

Location	Facility	Patient Population	Year	HIV Seroprevalence (%)	Reference
Baltimore	Inner-city	ED, critically ill and injured	1986	3.0	Baker[4]
Balitmore	Inner-city	General ED	1987	5.2	Kelen[5]
Preoria	Urban	ED, trauma	1987	0.4	Zeman[8]
Baltimore	Inner-city	Pediatric ED	1987	2.8	Schweich[13]
Baltimore	Trauma center	Trauma patients	1987–88	1.1–6.0	Soderstrom[12]
New Orleans	Inner-city	Trauma	1987–88	6.0	Risi[14]
		General ED		2.9	
Baltimore	Inner-city	General ED	1988	6.0	Kelen[6]
Detriot	Inner-city	ED, critically ill and injured	1988	6.0	Lewandowski[7]
Chicago	Inner-city	General ED	1988	7.2	Zalut[9]
	Suburban	General ED	1988	0.4	
California	3 High AIDS areas	General ED	1988	2.5	Rhee[15]
	3 Intermediate AIDS areas	General ED		0.9	
	4 Low AIDS areas	General ED		0.5	
Portland	7 Hospitals	General ED	1988	0.5	Jui[16]
New York City	Inner-city	General ED	1988	10.8	Schoembaum[17]
3 U.S. Cities	Inner-city	General ED	1989	4.2–8.9	Marcus[10]
	Suburban	General ED	1989	0.4–6.4	
Minneapolis	City	General ED	1989	1.3	Strum[11]
Los Angeles	Suburban	General ED	1989	4.5	Baraff[18]
Seattle	Prehospital setting	Cardiac arrest victims	1989–1990	0.8	CDC[19]
Italy	6 Urban hospitals; 4 cities	General ED	1991	0.7	Carli[20]
New Orleans	Inner-city	General ED	1991–1992	5.6	Ernst[21]
Baltimore	Inner-city	General ED	1992	11.3	Kelen[22]

CDC, Centers for Disease Control and Prevention; ED, emergency department.

suggested possible transmission from saliva,[47] accumulated evidence indicates that this is a highly unlikely mode of transmission, and no documented cases have been forthcoming. Although, casual contact has been raised as a mode of transmission, blood contact is likely in reported cases,[48–50] and it should be a concern for medical practitioners only from this perspective.

Most occupational transmissions of HIV-1 are from needle-stick injuries or other mishaps with sharp instruments. Initially, it was thought that infiltration or injection of patients' infected blood was necessary to transmit the virus.[51,52] However, cases of superficial needle-stick injuries[53,54] and nonparenteral exposures[1,55] have resulted in nosocomial transmission. A case of occupational transmission occurred in a laboratory worker who worked with concentrated virus but had no known percutaneous, direct skin, or mucous membrane exposures.[56] Although there were minor breaks in compliance with Biosafety Level 3 precautions, the laboratory worker routinely wore gloves and a gown. Whether or not appropriate precautions were taken, the latter case illustrates that it is possible to become infected with HIV-1 without realizing that an exposure has taken place—a situation of concern for emergency practitioners.

Exposure to blood has been the predominant infectious medium in occupational transmission. At least one reported case involved another body fluid; the needle-stick injury occurred after pleurocentesis, but even this transmission medium was described as having been bloody.[54]

RISKS TO EMERGENCY HEALTH CARE WORKERS

Risk Assessment

Risk of occupational transmission of HIV-1 can be assessed from data that fall into three categories: health care workers with AIDS,[57] estimates from surveillance studies,[58–64] and case reports.[3,23,51–56,59,60,64–68] These subjects are covered in detail in elsewhere in the text. Modes of transmission of HIV-1 are similar to that for HBV, and emergency department personnel have been shown to have among the highest rates of occupationally acquired HBV.[69,70]

As of 1995, the CDC had reported 40 health care providers as having occupationally acquired HIV-1 in the United States[71] Of these, 24 are documented by seroconversion. The remaining 16 occurred under significantly compelling circumstances for which, even though documentation of seroconversion was not possible, alternate explanations are not readily apparent. Most of these 40 cases are from percutaneous exposure with contaminated sharp instruments. Some of these occupational transmissions occurred during emergencies or procedures commonly performed in emergency departments.[3,52,58]

The risk of occupational transmission of HIV-1 after percutaneous exposure from a blood-contaminated sharp instrument is generally accepted to be approximately 0.25% (95%

confidence interval [CI] of 0.12% to 0.47%).[72] Mucous membrane risk of transmission is estimated at 0.09% (95% CI of 0.006% to 0.5%). However, only one case of HIV transmission after mucous membrane exposure has been documented in surveillance studies in the world, and that one occurred in Italy.[72] Of 949 documented cases of mucous membrane exposure to HIV-1 in the United States, none has resulted in seroconversion.[72] These figures were derived from metanalysis of several surveillance studies. Only 10 of the reported cases of occupationally related seroconversions in the United States come from surveillance studies.[58–60,64,72]

The numbers of health care providers with occupational transmission of HIV-1 are underestimated. A study by Tandberg and associates revealed significant underreporting of needle-stick injuries in a cohort of emergency department providers in the greater Albuquerque area.[73] Emergency department physicians among this group reported less than one eighth of their needle-stick injuries, but nurses and prehospital providers failed to report a third of such exposures. Skin contacts are probably underreported to an even greater extent. If this behavior is prevalent, it could be a major problem for emergency providers, because a large proportion of HIV-infected patients are those whose infections are not diagnosed at presentation.[4–7,10,22,24,74]

Two studies employing different methods assessed the risk of HIV infection among emergency department providers. The CDC emergency department collaborative study (based on observed data) calculated that 1 of every 40 full-time emergency department physicians or nurses can expect an HIV-positive percutaneous blood contact annually in high HIV seroprevalence emergency department, and 1 in every 575 in low HIV seroprevalence emergency departments. The annual occupational risk of HIV infection was estimated to be 0.0008% to 0.026% in an area of high HIV seroprevalence and 0.0005% to 0.0002% in a low-seroprevalence area.[10] Wears and colleagues used a Monte Carlo technique to estimate cumulative risk that included factors such as use of universal precautions and changing rates of HIV infection over time. Their mode calculated a median 30-year commutative emergency department physician career risk of 1.4% for high-prevalence areas not using universal precautions and 0.1% for low-prevalence areas. Assuming a presumed effectiveness of 40% for universal precautions, the model estimates a 30% effective decrease in risk if precautions are routinely followed.[75]

Exposures

Eighty percent or more of the documented nosocomial transmissions are from needle-stick or sharp-instrument injuries.[41] Forty percent of injuries with sharp instruments are considered preventable, and many are considered related to inferior device design.[76] Many of these exposures occur during recapping of needles. A large proportion of needle-stick injuries and exposures are related to disposal of sharp objects and instruments, but only a few occur during patient management.[76–78] There are data to indicate that new workers are at the greatest risk of sustaining sharp instrument injuries.[78]

There are limited but increasing data available regarding exposures during emergency procedures or patient care. An early Johns Hopkins emergency department study reported circumstances under which potential exposure to undiagnosed HIV-1 infection might occur and associated patient seroprevalence rates (Table 36.4-2).[5] In a later study, Johns Hopkins researchers reported 32 instances of unprotected emergency department health care provider exposure to blood and 16 instances of unprotected exposures to other body fluids during a 6-week, 24-hour per day direct observational study.[6] Precautions taken were not generally assessed. However, an investigation in the same emergency department conducted at the same time assessed emergency department providers' compliance with universal precautions during the care of critically ill or injured patients. The overall glove use rate was 64% to 85% in situations in which skin exposure to blood was a possibility.[79] In the CDC multicenter emergency department study, observers found a 4% aggregate rate of blood exposures, of which 98% were skin contacts.[10] Exposures during arterial blood sampling were 20 times higher during ungloved procedures than during gloved procedures, demonstrating the efficacy of using gloves for such procedures. Using a self-report questionnaire, Jagger and colleagues at the University of Virginia Health Sciences Center determined a rate of 54% for intact skin exposures, 1.5% nonintact skin, and 0.87% mucous membrane–blood or body fluids contacts per full-time employee per year, with 93% of the contacts from blood.[80]

One study examined the epidemiology of needle-stick injuries among prehospital emergency personnel, drawing the sample population from the St. Louis, Missouri, EMS

TABLE 36.4-2. *Exposure of health care workers to unrecognized HIV in 2275 emergency department patients with unknown HIV status*

Exposure	Number Seropositive (%)
Patients bleeding on arrival	268 (6.0)
Exposure to patients' body fluids	1892 (4.3)
Performance of major emergency invasive procedure*	99 (5.0)
Placement of intravenous lines before arrival at hospital	239 (3.8)
Patients with altered level of consciousness at presentation	291 (5.8)
Patients admitted to hospital	854 (4.1)
Patients admitted to operating suite directly from emergency room	65 (4.6)

*Central line placement, venous cutdown, thoracotomy, thoracostomy tube placement, intubation, transvenous or transthoracic pacing, or pericardiocentesis.

Reproduced with permission from Kelen GD, Fritz Sr, Qaquh Br, et al. Unrecognized human immunodeficiency virus infection in emergency department patients. N Engl J Med 1988;318:1645.

system.[78] An incidence of 145 injuries per 1000 employee-years, with 43% of injuries reported by personnel employed less than 1 year. The Portland Fire Rescue and Emergency Services, during a 2-year period in 1988 and 1989, reported 4.4 exposures for every 1000 EMS calls. Of the exposures, only 14% were needle sticks, 15% were considered exposures to nonintact skin, and 24% were "respiratory only" exposures.[81] The CDC cooperative study of prehospital providers calculated 1.25 blood or body fluid contacts (0.02 percutaneous) per 100 patients attended. Based on the data, the annual rate of exposures is estimated to be 12.3 per year, of which only 0.2 would be percutaneous.[82]

In teaching hospitals, the emergency department is frequently considered an excellent site for medical student, nursing, paramedic, and resident training. However, there is evidence that needle-stick injuries are highest among students and that they decrease during training.[83,84]

UNIVERSAL PRECAUTIONS APPLIED TO EMERGENCY MEDICINE

In 1983, the CDC recommended that precautions be taken in treating patients with known or suspected infection with bloodborne pathogens.[85] Two years later, the CDC advanced the concept of [86] This concept states that "all patients should be assumed to be infectious for HIV-1 and other bloodborne pathogens." In 1987, a few months after the CDC report of the three seroconversions among HCWs with nonparenteral exposures to HIV-1 and the Johns Hopkins emergency department seroprevalence data, the CDC consolidated its universal precautions recommendations.[67] Recommendations that included situations specific to prehospital care workers and public-safety workers (eg, fire-fighters, law enforcement, correctional facility staff) have been made.[57]

Although the CDC initially recommended that all patients' bodily fluids be considered infectious,[86] a revision recommended that only potential contact with blood and certain fluids need be of concern.[87] Precautions are recommended for those body media from which HIV-1 or HBV transmission could occur: blood, amniotic fluid, pericardial fluid, peritoneal fluid, synovial fluid, cerebrospinal fluid, semen, vaginal secretions, and any body fluid visibly contaminated with blood. Occupational transmission of HIV-1 has been documented from blood,[3,23,51–53,55,59,60,64–68] bloody pleural fluid,[54] and concentrated virus,[56] and semen and vaginal secretions have been implicated in the sexual transmission of HIV-1 but not in nosocomial transmission. Hepatitis B surface antigen has been detected in synovial fluid,[88] amniotic fluid,[89] and peritoneal fluid.[90] Exposure to other body fluids (eg, feces, nasal secretions, sputum, sweat, tears, urine, vomitus, breast milk, saliva) are not considered infectious because of a lack of epidemiologic evidence of transmission, although HIV-1 has been isolated from some of these substances.[31,33,34] Saliva is considered a potential infectious medium for dentists because of frequent contamination with blood.[57] Although not specifically stated, this caveat should hold for emergency practitioners also, because oral conditions and procedures frequently involve blood.

There are two potential limitations for following infection control recommendations in a discriminatory manner in the emergency setting. One is of general concern, and the other is specific to emergency practice. First, documentation of transmission from body fluid exposures is difficult at best, and in our experience, they are unlikely to be reported[73] and may even go unrecalled. Second, emergency practitioners cannot always know in advance if body fluids will be tainted with visible blood. In recognition of this, the CDC issued a specific caveat advocating following universal precautions "under uncontrolled emergency circumstances," during which all body fluids should be treated as potentially infectious.[57] In the prehospital or emergency department settings, few circumstances involving major procedures can be considered controlled. In patients with serious illness or injury, a relatively benign situation can instantaneously change to an uncontrolled situation in which the patient begins to bleed profusely or requires immediate intervention in the form of major procedures. Emergency providers frequently cannot anticipate body fluids or blood exposure. The Occupational Safety and Health Administration has issued regulations for emergency responders, including fire fighters and law enforcement personnel.[91]

Based on the CDC guidelines, we had previously made recommendations regarding barrier precautions in emergency settings according to a simple classification (Table 36.4-3).[79] The recommendations were based on the reasonable possibility of the procedure or intervention resulting in exposure to blood or blood-tinged body fluids or the degree of active bleeding by the patient from injuries or bleeding iatrogenically induced from previous procedures. Procedures have been classified as examination, minor, or major on the basis of the potential extent of exposure as a result of the procedure itself (see Table 36.4-3).[79] Major procedures are based on the reasonable possibility of generating profuse bleeding, spray or aerosolization of blood, or bloody body fluids as a result of performing the procedure. For example, placing a nasogastric tube is not considered a major procedure. However, practitioners of emergency medicine can easily recall many instances in which the procedure induces nasal bleeding along with severe coughing and sneezing, resulting in the wide spray of blood. All major trauma cases, critically ill patients, and all resuscitations by definition are opportunities for significant exposure to blood, and maxi-

mum barrier precautions should be followed regardless of what intervention or procedure is contemplated.

The concepts of appropriate barrier precautions for routine emergency department procedures have been based on data from Johns Hopkins (Table 36.4-4).[92] Kelen and colleagues directly observed over 2500 procedures performed on over 1000 patients and documented blood contacts of health care providers body areas. Some basic procedures such as lumbar puncture, local infiltration, wound irrigation, and placement of urinary catheters resulted in blood or body fluid contacts to a provider's face. Similarly, procedures not normally expected to have contact with the body area, such as arterial blood gas procurement, local infiltration of anesthetic, and basic suturing, were found to result in such contacts. Accordingly, recommendations have been proposed (Table 36.4-5).

Data regarding the protective quality of gloves have been published. Johnson and colleagues calculated that the puncture of single gloves would result in successful culture of HIV in 90% of cases. Double or triple gloves reduced the ability to successfully culture HIV to 23% to 63% of cases, depending on other factors. An interposed Kevlar glove impregnated with nonoxynol-9 reduced the ability to culture HIV to 0%.[93]

The mechanisms of glove failure have been investigated in emergency departments. Investigators in the Johns Hopkins emergency department observed that at least pinhole defects could be expected at a rate of 1% for unworn surgical gloves, and the rate was increased to 8% by simply taking them on and off. Higher rates of defects correlated with use for longer than 20 minutes (13.7%), use for major procedures such as central line (12.7%) and thoracotomy tube insertion (28.%), and use for handing surgical instruments (11.7%).[94] Gloves used in caring for critically ill patients, who often require multiple procedures, resulted in failure rates of 24%. The use of two pairs of gloves resulted in defects in both pairs (inner and outer) in only 2% of cases.

The choice of surgical gloves may also have an effect on preventing exposures. Unused surgical gloves are likely to have some antiviral properties, and general examination gloves may fare as well.[95]

Technology advancements such as sheathed catheters should assist in preventing HIV exposures. One high-risk situation deserves special mention. Many emergency thoracotomies are performed in emergency departments. The risk of percutaneous exposure for HCWs is very high given the emergency situation, working in the confinements of a body

TABLE 36.4-3. *Precautions expected under given circumstances*

	Clinical Situation				
Intervention	No Bleeding	Active Bleeding	Profuse Bleeding	Major Trauma	Resuscitation
Examination		Gloves	All*	All	All
Minor procedure	Gloves	Gloves	All	All	All
Major procedure	All	All	All	All	All

*All barrier methods, including gloves, gown, mask, and eye protection.

TABLE 36.4-4. *Classification of interventions for appropriate barrier attire*

Examination	Minor Procedure	Major Procedure
Patient physical examination	Phlebotomy	Arterial canalization
Pelvic examination*	Venous cannulation	Central venous catheter
Splinting	Arterial sampling	placement
Casting	Intramuscular injection	Swan-Ganz placement
Fracture or dislocation reduction	Foley catheter placement	Cricothyroidotomy
Ocular tonometry	Local anesthesia	Culdocentesis
Electrocardiogram lead placement	Nerve blocks	Nasogastric tube placement
Spinal immobilization	Arthrocentesis	Endotracheal suctioning
Cardiopulmonary resuscitation[†]	Lumbar puncture	Tracheal Intubation (oral or nasal)
Cardioversion[‡]	Thoracentesis	Foreign body removal
Defibrillation[§]	Pericardiocentesis	Gastric lavage
External cardiac pacing	Paracentesis	Incision and drainage[#]
Patient extrication	Intraosseous catheter	Nasal packing
	placement	Peritoneal lavage
		Internal temporary cardiac pacing (transthoracic or transvenous)
		Wound repair[¶]
		Wound irrigation
		Cut-down
		Sigmoidoscopy
		Precipitous vaginal delivery
		Thoracostomy
		Thoracotomy

*If patient complains of bleeding or bleeding can possibly be encountered, all precautions should be taken.

[†]This is technically an examination, but because it always implies a resuscitation effort, risk of blood exposure from other providers activities or a bleeding patient is considerable; therefore, all precautions are required.

[‡]Cardioversion in an of itself is a benign procedure. However, a reasonable expectation under emergency conditions is that it may fail requiring a resuscitation effort. Therefore all precautions would be prudent.

[§]Implies a resuscitation effort.

[#]Requires irrigation.

cavity, and the resultant sharp edges of the dissected bony anatomy. Rather than using suture needles, which may require blind digital guidance, cardiac stapling may allow control of bleeding in a difficult situation.[96]

Precautions to Prevent Reverse Transmission

Since the early 1990s, the concerns of possible transmission of HIV and other bloodborne infections to patients from practitioners has come to the forefront. The CDC and the American Medical Association had sponsored a number of open forums on this issue, and virtually all medical societies debated the issue and arrived at a position. The CDC issued recommendations in 1991.[97]

This issue has been explored in great depth by the American College of Emergency Physicians and the Society for Academic Emergency Medicine. The College undertook a detailed evaluation of the literature on bloodborne transmission of infectious agents to patients from providers, including CDC assessments, and a careful assessment of procedures considered within the practice of emergency medicine. The College concluded that emergency physicians perform only two procedures that could construe a conceivable risk of reverse transmission of bloodborne

infectious disease. The first of these, blind, digitally guided intraoral nerve block, was deleted from the procedure armamentarium of emergency practice, because alternate modes of facial and intraoral nerve block techniques were available. The second procedure was emergency thoracotomy. This procedure is undertaken only as a last heroic effort in emergency situations for patients who are otherwise dead or would surely die. It is reasoned that the risk of reverse transmission is immaterial if the patient, who would otherwise die, is saved by the procedure.

Look-back studies of up to 20,000 patients treated by HIV-infected practitioners, including many surgeons and other practitioners engaging in practices involving potential reverse exposure, have not revealed any documented transmissions.[98] The practice of the Florida dentist remains the only known situation in which such transmissions have occurred.

Compliance With Precautions

Unfortunately, even as the risks in emergency settings become better defined and recognized, initial assessments of compliance with universal precautions (particularly barrier precautions) has not been encouraging. In one northeastern

TABLE 36.4-5. *Recommendations of appropriate precautions for emergency department procedures*

Procedures	Gloves	Gown	Eye and Face Protection	Feet Protection
SHARP INSTRUMENTS				
Arterial blood gas	y*	y		
Central line	y	y	a†	y
Incision and drainage	y	y	a	y
Wound irrigation	y	y	y	y
Intravenous placement	y	y		
Local Infiltration	y	y	y	
Lumbar puncture	y	a	y	
Chest tube	y	y	y	y
Phlebotomy without intravenous placement	y	a		
Intramuscular Injection				
Suturing	y	y	a	a
NONSHARP INSTRUMENTS				
Urinary catheter	y	y	y	
Cardiopulmonary resuscitation	y	a	a	a
Intubation	y	y	a	
Examination of the bleeding patient		y	y	n‡
Nasogastric tube		y	a	y
Pelvic examination		n	n	
Specimen handling				

*Yes. Blank spaces indicate usually unnecessary.
†Suggested; actual frequency of potential contacts is small.
‡Generally no, unless other factors need to be considered, such as profuse bleeding or multiple simultaneous procedures.
Adapted from Kelen GD, Hansen KN, Green GB, Tang N, Chandana G. Determinants of emergency department procedure- and condition-specific universal (barrier) precaution requirements for optimal provider protection. Ann Emerg Med 1995;25:743.

inner-city emergency department–based study in which universal precautions criteria were strictly applied, appropriate barrier precautions were followed only 44% of the time during management of patients with critical illnesses or injuries.[79] The rate of compliance was only 19% for interactions with profusely bleeding patients and only 16% during the performance of major procedures. Other studies applying less stringent criteria have reported even lower rates of compliance. Hammond and colleagues found that surgical residents at the University of Miami–Jackson Memorial Medical Center were in compliance with strict universal precautions during only 16% of the trauma resuscitations.[99] Baraff and Talan at the University of California–Los Angeles Medical Center emergency department[100,101] and Campbell and associates[102] at St. Paul-Ramsey Medical Center emergency department in Minneapolis found a similar lack of compliance. A survey of emergency medicine residencies revealed that barrier attire was available in 82% of responding programs but was consistently used at only 16%.[103]

Reasons for failure to comply have been sought. Providers in emergency department settings have indicated that barrier protection is time consuming to put on and interferes with the skillful performance of procedures.[79,99] Others have indicated lack of familiarity with protocols.[99]

Two studies have evaluated methods to improve compliance with barrier universal precautions in an emergency department setting. One study from a university teaching hospital that has an HIV-1 seroprevalence rate of approximately 1% found that intensive educational efforts were associated with only moderate or insignificant increases in observed compliance.[101] Researchers at Johns Hopkins reported a substantial increase in compliance with universal precautions among emergency department staff after implementation of policy with a monitoring component.[104] Overall compliance improved from 44% to 73%, with rates of compliance reaching 80% for personnel under the emergency department's control. Improved compliance has been shown to decrease but not eliminate nonparenteral exposures.[105] A self-reported decrease of approximately 50% in blood contact and other exposures after universal precautions training is also encouraging.[105]

Adherence to barrier universal precautions is expensive,[106] and it is legitimate to question its effectiveness given the costs.[107] This is especially true, because much of the costs go for disposable items that protect only against nonparenteral exposures. The greater problem is from needle-stick exposures. The value of barrier protection beyond wearing gloves may prove minimal. However, most costs required for adequate barrier protection are consumed by gloves.[106]

HIV-1 is just one of the important transmissible infections that providers confront in the workplace, and other infections such HBV, HCV, HTLV-I/II, other retroviruses,

Epstein-Barr virus, and cytomegalovirus are perhaps just as important and, in some cases (eg, HBV), easier to transmit.[57] Hepatitis B vaccine is considered an important adjunct to universal precautions.[87,108] John Hopkins researchers reported that, in 1988, almost 25% of their general emergency department patient population were infectious with HIV-1, HBV (ie, surface antigen testing), or HCV.[25] A general dictum followed in emergency practice is to assume the worst until proven otherwise. Similarly, it is prudent to strictly observe all aspects of universal precautions, including barrier protection, until they are demonstrated to be of low utility.

Emergency providers with possible exposure to HIV-1 should follow the guidelines set forth by the CDC[57] and local institutional policy. Management of persons exposed to HBV should be undertaken independently.[109] These issues are discussed in detail elsewhere in the text.

As the AIDS epidemic continues to grow and is no longer restricted to large urban centers, the potential risk for occupational acquisition of HIV-1 for emergency personnel will grow. Even though the risk of seroconversion after parenteral exposure to HIV-1 is probably less than 1%, as the seroprevalence of HIV-1 in patient populations increases, the number of exposures will probably increase. The best protection against HIV-1 and other bloodborne pathogens at this time is to follow the universal precautions. However, the industry needs to address the problems inherent in current barrier technology and device design.

REFERENCES

1. Centers for Disease Control. HIV prevalence estimates and AIDS case projections for the United States: report based on a workshop. MMWR 1990;39(RR-16);5.
2. United States General Accounting Office. Emergency departments: unevenly affected by growth and change in patient use. Report to the Chairman, Subcommittee on Health for Families and the Uninsured, Committee on Finance, U.S. Senate. HRD-93-4. Washington, DC: Government Accounting Office, 1993;2.
3. Centers for Disease Control. Update: human immunodeficiency virus infections in health-care workers exposed to blood of infected patients. MMWR 1987;36:285.
4. Baker JL, Kelen GD, Sivertson KT, Quinn TC. Unsuspected human immunodeficiency virus in critically ill emergency patients. JAMA 1987;257:2609.
5. Kelen GD, Fritz S, Qaqish B, et al. Unrecognized human immunodeficiency virus infection in emergency department patients. N Engl J Med 1988;318:1645.
6. Kelen GD, DiGiovanna T, Bisson L, Kalainov D, Sivertson KT, Quinn TC. Human immunodeficiency virus infection in emergency patients: epidemiology, clinical presentations, and risk to health care workers: The Johns Hopkins experience. JAMA 1989;262:516.
7. Lewandowski D, Ognjan A, Rivers E, Pohlod D, Belian B, Saravolatz D. HIV-1 and HTLV-I seroprevalence in critically ill resuscitated emergency department patients. Abstract Th AP9:142. Presented at the Fifth International Conference on AIDS, Montreal, Canada,1989.
8. Zeman MG, Mayhue FE. Occupational risk of HIV infection. (Letter) Ann Emerg Med 1989;18:798.
9. Zalut T, Cooper MA, Wainstein J, et al. (Abstract) Prevalence of HIV-positive patients in multiple emergency department settings. Ann Emerg Med 1990;19:611
10. Marcus R, Culver DH, Bell DM, et al. Risk of human immunodeficiency virus infection among emergency department workers. Am J Med 1993;94:363.
11. Strum JT. HIV prevalence in a Midwestern emergency department. Ann Emerg Med 1991;20:272.
12. Soderstrom CA, Furth PA, Glasser D, Dunning RW, et al. HIV infection rates in trauma center treating predominantly rural blunt trauma victims. J Trauma 1989;29:1526-30
13. Schweich PJ, Fosarelli PD, Duggan AK, Quinn TC, et al. Prevalence of human immunodeficiency virus seropositivity in pediatric emergency room patients undergoing phlebotomy. Pediatrics 1990;86:660.
14. Risi GF, Gaumer RH, Weeks S, et al. Human immunodeficiency virus: risk of exposure among health care workers at a southern urban hospital. South Med J 1989;82:1079.
15. Rhee KJ, Albertson TE, Kizer KW, Huges MJ, Ascher MS and the California HIV-1 emergency department seroprevalence study group. The HIV-1 seroprevalence rate of injured patients admitted through California emergency departments. Ann Emerg Med 1991;20:969.
16. Jui J, Modesitt S, Fleming D, Stevens P, Wayson B, et al. Multicenter HIV And hepatitis B seroprevalence study. J Emerg Med 1989;8:243.
17. Schoenbaum EE, Webber MP. The underrecognititon of HIV Infection in women in an inner-city emergency room. Am J Public Health 1993;83:363.
18. Baraff LJ, Talan DA, Torres M. Prevalence of HIV antibody in a non-inner-city university hospital emergency department. Ann Emerg Med 1991;20:782.
19. Centers for Disease Control. HIV seroprevalence among adults treated for cardiac arrest before reaching a medical facility—Seattle, Washington, 1989–1990. MMWR 1992;41:381.
20. De Carli G, Puro V, Binkin NJ, Ippolito M. Risk of human immunodeficiency virus infection for emergency department workers. J Emerg Med 1993;12:737.
21. Ernst AA, Farley TA, Martin DH. Screening and empiric treatment for syphilis in an inner-city emergency department. Acad Emerg Med 1995;2:765.
22. Kelen GD, Hexter DA, Hansen KN, Tang N, Pretorius S, Quinn TC. Trends in infection among an inner-city department patient population; Implications for emergency department based HIV-screening programs. Clin Infect Dis 1995;21:867.
23. Wallace MR, Harrison WO. HIV seroconversion with progressive disease in health care worker after needlestick injury. Lancet 1988; 1:1454
24. Centers for Disease Control. AIDS and human immunodeficiency virus infection in the United States: 1988 Update. MMWR 1989;38:S4.
25. Kelen GD, Green GB, Purcell RH, Chan DW, Qaqish BF, Sivertson KT, Quinn TC. Infectious hepatitis (HBsAg and HCV) in an emergency department patient population: epidemiology and implications for health care personnel. N Engl J Med 1992;326:1399.
26. Kelen GD, DiGiovanna TA, Lofy L, et al. HTLV I-II infection among patients in an inner-city emergency department. Ann Intern Med 1990;113:368.
27. Gallo RC, Salahuddin SZ, Popovic M, et al. Frequent detection and isolation of cytopathic retroviruses (HTLV-III) for patients with AIDS and at risk for AIDS. Science 1984;224:500.
28. Michaelis B. Levy JA. Recovery of human immunodeficiency virus from serum. JAMA 1987;257:1327.
29. Levy JA, Hoffman AD, Kramer SM, Landis JA, Shimabukuro JM, Oshiro LS. Isolation of lymphocytopathic retroviruses from San Francisco patients with AIDS. Science 1984;226:449.
30. Vogt MW, Witt DJ, Craven DE, et al. Isolation of HTLV-III/LAV from cervical secretions of women at risk for AIDS. Lancet 1986;1:525.
31. Groopman JE, Salahuddin SZ, Sarngadharan MG, et al. HTLV-III in saliva of people with AIDS-related complex and healthy homosexual men at risk for AIDS. Science 1984;226:447.
32. Thiry L, Sprecher-Goldberger S, Jonckheer T, et al. Isolation of AIDS virus from cell-free breast milk of three healthy virus carriers (Letter) Lancet 1985;2:981.
33. Fujikawa LS, Salahuddin SZ, Palestine AG, Masur H, Nussenblatt RB, Gallo RC. Isolation of human T-lymphotropic virus type III from the tears of a patient with the acquired immunodeficiency syndrome. Lancet 1985;2:529.
34. Levy JA, Kaminski LS, Morrow WJW, et al. Infection by the retrovirus associated with the acquired immunodeficiency syndrome. Ann Intern Med 1985;103:694.
35. Levy JA, Shimabukuro J, Hollander H, Mills J, Kaminsky L. Isolation of AIDS-associated retroviruses from cerebrospinal fluid and brain of patients with neurological symptoms. Lancet 1986;5;2:586.

36. Withrington RH, Cornes P, Harris JRW, et al. Isolation of human immunodeficiency virus from synovial fluid of a patient with reactive arthritis. Br Med J 1987;294:484.

37. Mundy DC, Schinazi RF, Gerber AR, Nahmias AJ, Randall HW. Human immunodeficiency virus isolated from amniotic fluid. Lancet 1987;2:459.

38. Ziza J-M, Brun-Vezinet F, Venet A, et al. Lymphadenopathy-associated virus isolated from bronchoalveolar lavage fluid in AIDS-related complex with lymphoid interstitial pneumonitis. N Engl J Med 1985;313:183.

39. Salahuddin SZ, Markham PD, Popovic M, et al. Isolation of infectious human T-cell leukemia/lymphotropic virus type III (HTLV-III) from patients with acquired immunodeficiency syndrome (AIDS) or AIDS-related complex (ARC) and from health carriers: a study of risk groups and tissue sources. Proc Natl Acad Sci USA 1985;82:5530.

40. Yoken RH, Li S, Perman J, Visicidi, R. Persistent diarrhea and fecal shedding of retroviral nucleic acids in children infected with human immunodeficiency virus. J Infect Dis 1991;164:61.

41. Centers for Disease Control. Update: acquired immunodeficiency syndrome and human immunodeficiency virus infection among health care workers. MMWR 1988;37:229.

42. Stewart GJ, Tyler JPP, Cunningham AL, Barr JA, Driscoll GL, Gold J. Transmission of human T-cell lymphotropic virus type III (HTLV-III) by artificial insemination by donor. Lancet 1985;2:581.

43. Ziegler JB, Cooper DA, Johnson RD, Gold J. Postnatal transmission of AIDS-associated retrovirus from mother to infant. Lancet 1985;1:896.

44. Centers for Disease Control. Transmission of HIV through bone transplantation: Case report and public health recommendations. MMWR 1988;37:597.

45. Centers for Disease Control. Human immunodeficiency virus infection transmitted from an organ donor screened for HIV antibody—North Carolina. MMWR 1987;36:306.

46. Quarto M, Germinario C, Fontana A, Barbuti S. HIV transmission through kidney transplantation from a living related donor. N Engl J Med 1989;320:1754.

47. Salahuddin SZ, Groopman JE, Markham PD, et al. HTLV-III in symptom-free seronegative persons. Lancet 1984;2:1418.

48. Centers for Disease Control. Human immunodeficiency virus transmission in household settings—United States. MMWR 1994;43:347.

49. Centers for Disease Control. HIV transmission between two adolescent brothers with hemophilia. MMWR 1993;42:948.

50. Fitzgibbon JE, Gaur S, Frenkel LD, et al. Transmission from one child to another of human immunodeficiency virus type 1 with a zidovudine-resistance mutation. N Engl J Med 1993;329:1835.

51. Anonymous. Needlestick transmission of HTLV-III from a patient infected in Africa. Lancet 1984;2:1376.

52. Stricof RL, Morse DL. HTLV-III/LAV seroconversion following a deep intramuscular needlestick injury. (Letter) N Engl J Med 1986;314;1115.

53. Neisson-Vernant C, Arfi S, Mathez D, Leibowitch J, Monplaisir N. Needlestick HIV seroconversion in a nurse. (Letter) Lancet 1986;2:814.

54. Oksenhendler E, Harzic M, Le Roux JM, Rabian C, Clauvel JP. HIV infection with seroconversion after a superficial needlestick injury to the finger. (Letter) N Engl J Med 1986;315:582.

55. Gioannini P, Sinicco A, Cariti G, Lucchini A, Paggi G, Giachino O. HIV infection acquired by a nurse. Eur J Epidemiol 1988;4:119.

56. Weiss SH, Goedert JJ, Gartner S, et al. Risk of human immunodeficiency virus infection among laboratory workers. Science 1988;239:68.

57. Centers for Disease Control. Guidelines for prevention of transmission of human immunodeficiency virus and hepatitis B virus to health-care and public-safety workers. MMWR 1989;38:S6.

58. Marcus R and the CDC Cooperative Needlestick Surveillance Group. Surveillance of health care workers exposed to blood from patients infected with the human immunodeficiency virus. N Engl J Med 1988;319:1118.

59. Gerberding JL, Bryant-Leblanc CE, Nelson K, et al. Risk of transmitting the human immunodeficiency virus, cytomegalovirus, and hepatitis B virus to health care workers exposed to patients with AIDS and AIDS-related conditions. J Infect Dis 1987:156:1.

60. Henderson DK, Fahey BJ, Saah AJ, Schmitt JM, Lane HC. Longitudinal assessment of risk for occupational/nosocomial transmission of human immunodeficiency virus, type 1 in health care workers. Abstract 634. Presented at the International Conference on AIDS and Associated Cancers, Los Angeles, 1988.

61. Kuhls TL, Viker S, Parris NB, Barakian A, Sullivan-Bolyai J, Cherry JD. Occupational risk of HIV, HBV and HSV-2 infections in health care personnel caring for AIDS patients. Am J Public Health 1987;77:1306.

62. McEvoy M, Porter K, Mortimer P, Simmons N, Shanson D. Prospective study of clinical, laboratory, and ancillary staff with accidental exposures to blood or body fluids from patients infected with HIV. Br Med J 1987;294;1595.

63. Health and Welfare Canada. National surveillance program on occupational exposures to HIV among health-care workers in Canada. Can Med Assoc J 1988;138:31.

64. Ramsey KM, Smith EN, Reinarz JA. Prospective evaluation of 44 health care workers exposed to human immunodeficiency virus-1, with one seroconversion. (Abstract) Clin Res 1988;36:22A.

65. Michelet C, Cartier F, Ruffault A, Amus C, Genetet N, Thomas R. Needlestick HIV infection in a nurse. Abstract. Presented at the Fourth International Conference on AIDS, Stockholm, June 12–16, 1988.

66. Centers for Disease Control. Update: acquired immunodeficiency syndrome and human immunodeficiency virus infection among health care workers. MMWR 1988;37:229.

67. Centers for Disease Control. Recommendations for prevention of HIV transmission in health care settings. MMWR 1987;36(Suppl 2S):1S.

68. Centers for Disease Control. Apparent transmission of human T-lymphotropic virus type III/lymphadenopathy-associated virus from a child to a mother providing health care. MMWR 1986;35:76.

69. Dienstag JL, Ryan DM. Occupational exposure to hepatitis B virus in hospital personnel: infection or immunization? Am J Epidemiol 1982;115;26.

70. Kunches LM, Craven DE, Werner BG, Jacobs LM. Hepatitis B exposure in emergency medicine personnel: prevalence of serologic markers and need for immunization. Am J Med 1982;75:269.

71. State of Maryland. Occupational exposure to human immunodeficiency virus. A review of current management. Community Dis Bull 1990.

72. Ippolito G, Puro V, De Carli G. The risk of occupational human immunodeficiency virus infection in health care workers. Italian Multicenter Study. Arch Intern Med 1993;153:1451.

73. Tandberg D, Stewart KK, Doezema D. Under-reporting of contaminated needlestick injuries in emergency health care workers. Ann Emerg Med 1990;20:66.

74. Apprahamian C, Walker SB, Quebbeman JE, Bergstein JM, Sasse EA, Wittmann DH. Use of medical center facilities by human immunodeficiency virus (HIV)-positive patients. J Trauma 1990;30:745.

75. Wears RL, Vukich DJ, Winton CN, Fluskey LL, MacMath TR, Li S. An analysis of emergency physicians' cumulative career risk of HIV infection. Ann Emerg Med 1991;20:749.

76. Jagger J, Hunt EH, Brand-Elnaggar J, Pearson RD. Rates of needlestick injury caused by various devices in a university hospital. N Engl J Med 1988;319:284.

77. Wormser GP, Joline C, Duncanson F. Needle-stick injuries during the care of patients with AIDS. N Engl J Med 1984;310:1461.

78. Hochreiter MC, Barton LL. Epidemiology of needlestick injury in emergency medical service personnel. J Emerg Med 1988;6:9.

79. Kelen GD, DiGiovanna TA, Celentano DD, et al. Adherence to universal (barrier) precautions during interventions on critically ill and injured emergency department patients. J Acquir Immune Defic Syndr 1990;3:987.

80. Jagger J, Powers RD, Day JS, Detmer DE. Epidemiology and prevention of blood and body fluid exposures among emergency department staff. J Emerg Med 1994;12:753.

81. Reed E, Daya MR, Jui J, Grellman K, et al. Occupational infectious disease exposures in EMS personnel. J Emerg Med 1993;11:9.

82. Marcus R, Srivastava PU, Bell DM, et al. Occupational blood contact among prehospital providers. Ann Emerg Med 1995;25:776.

83. McGeer A, Simor AE, Low DE. Epidemiology of needlestick injuries in house officers. J Infect Dis 1990;162:961.

84. Yassi A, McGill M. Determinants of blood and body fluid exposure in a large teaching hospital: hazards of the intermittent intravenous procedure. Am J Infect Control 1991;19:129.

85. Garner JS, Simmons BP. Guideline for isolation precautions in hospitals. Infect Control 1983;4:245.

86. Centers for Disease Control. Recommendations for preventing transmission of infection with human T-lymphotropic virus type III/lymphadenopathy-associated virus in the workplace. MMWR 1985;34;681.

87. Centers for Disease Control. Universal precautions for prevention of transmission of human immunodeficiency virus, hepatitis B and other blood borne pathogens in health-care settings. MMWR 1988;37:377.

88. Onion DK, Crumpacker CS, Gilliland BC. Arthritis of hepatitis associated with Australia antigen. Ann Intern Med 1971;75:29.

89. Lee AKY, Ip HMH, Wong VCW. Mechanisms of maternal-fetal transmission of hepatitis B virus. J Infect Dis 1978;138:668.
90. Bond WW, Petersen NJ, Gravelle CR, Favero MS. Hepatitis B virus in peritoneal dialysis fluid: a potential hazard. Dial Transplant 1982;11:592.
91. Occupational Safety and Health Administration. 3130: Occupational exposure to bloodborne pathogens: precautions for emergency responders. Report 1-27. Washington, DC: U.S. Department of Labor, 1992.
92. Kelen GD, Hansen KN, Green GB, Tang N, Chandana G. Determinants of emergency department procedure- and condition-specific universal (barrier) precaution requirements for optimal provider protection. Ann Emerg Med 1995;25:743.
93. Johnson GK, Nolan T, Wuh HC, Robinson WS. Efficacy of glove combinations in reducing cell culture infection after glove puncture with human immunodeficiency virus type 1. Infect Control Hosp Epidemol 1991;12:435.
94. Hansen K, Korniewicz D, Larson E, Green GB, Kelen G. Loss of glove integrity during common ED procedures. Poster abstract PoC 4547. Presented at the Eighth International Conference on AIDS, Amsterdam, Netherlands, 1992:C336.
95. Dalgleish AG, Malkovsky M: Surgical gloves as a mechanical barrier against human immunodeficiency viruses. Br J Surg 1988;75:171.
96. Macho JR, Markison RE, Schecter WP. Cardiac stapling in the management of penetrating injuries of the heart: rapid control of hemorrhage and decreased risk of personal contamination. J Trauma 1993;34:711.
97. Centers for Disease Control. Recommendations for preventing transmission of human immunodeficiency virus and hepatitis B virus to patients during exposure-prone invasive procedures. MMWR 1991;40(RR-8):1.
98. Centers for Disease Control. Update: investigations of persons treated by HIV-infected health-care workers—United States. MMWR 1993;42:329.
99. Hammond JS, Eckes JM, Gomez GA, Cunningham DN. HIV, trauma and infection control: universal precautions are universally ignored. J Trauma 1990;30:555.
100. Baraff LJ, Talan DA. Compliance with universal precautions in a university hospital emergency department. Ann Emerg Med 1989;18:654.
101. Talan DA, Baraff LJ. Effect of education on the use of universal precautions in a university hospital emergency department. Ann Emerg Med 1990;19:1322.
102. Campbell S, Maki M, Henry K. Compliance with universal precautions among emergency department personnel. Abstract, book 2:99. Presented at the Sixth International Conference on AIDS, San Francisco, 1989.
103. Huff JS, Basala M. Universal precautions in emergency medicine residencies. (Letter) Ann Emerg Med 1989;18:654.
104. Kelen GD, Green G, Fortenberry C, et al. Substantial improvement in adherence to universal precautions in an emergency department following administrative changes. (Abstract) Ann Emerg Med 1990;19:481.
105. Fahey BJ, Koziol DE, Banks SM, Henderson DK. Frequency of nonparenteral occupational exposures to blood and body fluids before and after universal precautions training. Am J Med 1991;90:145.
106. Doebbeling BD, Wenzel RP. The direct costs of universal precautions in a teaching hospital. JAMA 1990;264:2083.
107. Bartlett JG. Panel: AIDS and hepatitis B: can we make the workplace safe? Response. Proceedings from the Third National Forum on AIDS and Hepatitis B. Bethesda, MD: National Foundation for Infectious Diseases, 1989:3.
108. Immunization Practices Advisory Committee. Recommendations for protection against viral hepatitis. MMWR 1985;34:313.
109. Centers for Disease Control. Protection against viral hepatitis. Recommendations of the Immunization Practices Advisory Committee (ACIP). MMWR 1990;39(RR-2):1.

AIDS: Biology, Diagnosis, Treatment and Prevention, fourth edition, edited by Vincent T. DeVita, Jr., Samuel Hellman, and Steven A. Rosenberg. Lippincott–Raven Publishers, © 1997

36.5

Sterilization and Disinfection Strategies for Medical Instruments and Equipment

Martin S. Favero

This article describes the general procedures used in health care facilities to sterilize or disinfect instruments or to decontaminate items, devices, and environmental surfaces. These standard procedures have been devised using relatively stringent criteria and are more than adequate for sterilizing or disinfecting instruments, devices, and other items contaminated with blood or other body fluids from persons infected with bloodborne pathogens, including human immunodeficiency virus (HIV) and hepatitis B virus (HBV).

The effective use of antiseptics, disinfectants, and sterilization procedures in health care settings is important in the prevention of hospital-acquired infections. Historically, physical agents, such as moist heat in the form of steam autoclaves or dry heat sterilizers, have played the predominant role for sterilizing devices, equipment, and supplies in hospitals. Gaseous sterilization by ethylene oxide is also popular for sterilizing heat-sensitive items. Several newly developed, low-temperature sterilization procedures can be used instead of ethylene oxide sterilization. These include vapor-phase hydrogen peroxide, plasma, peracetic acid, and low-temperature steam plus formaldehyde. Liquid chemical germicides formulated as sterilants have also been available for many years but are used primarily to disinfect rather than sterilize medical devices.[1]

The choice of which sterilization or disinfection procedure or which specific chemical germicide should be used for sterilization, disinfection, or antisepsis or for environmental sanitization depends on several factors. No single chemical germicide or procedure is adequate for all pur-

poses. Factors that should be considered in the selection of a specific sterilization or disinfection procedure include the degree of microbiologic inactivation required for the particular device, the nature and physical composition of the device being treated, and the cost and ease of using a particular procedure.[1–5]

REGULATION OF CHEMICAL GERMICIDES

In the United States, chemical germicides are regulated by two governmental agencies: the Environmental Protection Agency (EPA) and the Food and Drug Administration (FDA). Chemical germicides formulated as sterilants or disinfectants had been regulated by the EPA, but the EPA and FDA have agreed that products intended for use on specific medical devices (eg, hemodialysis machines, endoscopes, high-speed dental handpieces) will be regulated by the FDA. The EPA requires manufacturers of chemical germicides formulated as sanitizers, disinfectants, hospital disinfectants, or sterilant-disinfectants (ie, sporocides) to test these products by using specific, standardized assay methods for microbicidal potency, stability, and toxicity to humans. For chemical germicides intended for use on medical devices, rather than environmental or housekeeping surfaces, the FDA requires that manufacturers submit a premarket application that may include additional data on microbicidal activity and device or chemical compatibility and detailed instructions to the user regarding the "safe and effective use" of the product. The FDA regulates all sterilization devices such as steam or ethylene oxide autoclaves and dry heat ovens. The FDA also regulates chemical germicides formulated as antiseptics, preservatives, or drugs to be used on or in the human body to inhibit or kill microorganisms on the skin.

The Centers for Disease Control and Prevention (CDC) does not approve, regulate, or test chemical germicides for-

Martin S. Favero, Associate Director for Laboratory Science, Hospital Infections Program, National Center for Infectious Diseases, Centers for Disease Control and Prevention, 1600 Clifton Road Northeast, MSA-07, Atlanta, GA 30333.

mulated as disinfectants or antiseptics. The CDC recommends broad strategies for the use of sterilants, disinfectants, and antiseptics to prevent transmission of infections in the health care environment.[2]

The definitions of sterilization, disinfection, antisepsis, and other related terms, such as decontamination and sanitization, are generally accepted in the scientific community, but some of these terms are misused. It is important to understand the definition and inferred capabilities of each term and the related procedure.

STERILIZATION

The definition of sterilization depends on the vantage point from which the term is viewed. I choose to view this term somewhat like a hologram and define it in the context of the state of sterilization, the procedure of sterilization and the application of sterilization.

An item, device, or solution is considered to be sterile when it is completely free of all living microorganisms. This state of sterility is the objective of the sterilization procedure, and when viewed in this context, the definition is a categorical and absolute one; an item is sterile, or it is not.

A sterilization procedure is one that kills all microorganisms, including high numbers of bacterial endospores. Sterilization can be accomplished by heat, ethylene oxide gas, other low-temperature systems referred to previously, irradiation (in industry), and several liquid chemical sterilants. A sterilization procedure from an operational standpoint is defined as a process, after which the probability of a microorganism surviving on an item is less than one chance in a million (10^{-6}). This approach is used by the medical device industry to sterilize large quantities of medical devices.

Sterilization procedures used in industry are much more sophisticated and controlled than the procedures used in health care facilities. However, steam autoclaves, ethylene oxide sterilizers, and dry heat sterilization ovens used in health care facilities have operational protocols that are verified by the manufacturer to accomplish sterilization, and all the variables that control for the inactivation of microorganisms are automated or built into simple controls in the devices.

The application of the sterilization process involves the strategy associated with a particular medical device or solution and the context of its exposure to humans. In 1972, Spalding[6] proposed that the nature of device and equipment sterilization and disinfection could be understood more readily if medical devices, equipment, and surgical materials were divided into three categories based on the risk of infection involved in their use. Briefly, devices that are exposed to sterile areas of the body, such as blood, require sterilization; devices that touch mucous membranes may be sterilized or disinfected; and devices or items that touch skin or environmental surfaces can be sanitized with a low-level disinfectant or cleaned with soap and water.

In the context of these categories, Spalding also classified chemical germicides by activity level. The activity levels are listed in Table 36.5-1 and delineated in the following paragraphs.

High-level disinfection kills vegetative microorganisms but not necessarily high numbers of bacterial spores. Chemical germicides used in this procedure are, by Spalding's definition, capable of accomplishing sterilization; they kill all microorganisms, including a high number of bacterial spores when the contact time is relatively long (6 to 10 hours). As high-level disinfectants, however, they are used for a relatively short period (10 to 30 minutes). These chemical germicides are registered with the EPA as sterilant-disinfectants.

Intermediate-level disinfection kills vegetative microorganisms, including *Mycobacterium tuberculosis*, all fungi, and most viruses. These chemical germicides often correspond to EPA approved hospital disinfectants that are also tuberculocidal.

Low-level disinfection kills most vegetative bacteria except *M tuberculosis*, some fungi, and some viruses. These chemical germicides usually are approved by EPA as hospital disinfectants or sanitizers.

The relation between the EPA's system of classification and the CDC's recommendation for strategies of sterilization and disinfection is shown in Table 36.5-2. Table 36.5-3 lists the comparative resistance of various classes of microorganisms to chemical germicides.

Decontamination renders a device, item, or material safe to handle; safe means reasonably free of the probability of transmission of infection. The decontamination process sometimes is a sterilization procedure such as steam autoclaving. Often this may be the most cost-effective procedure for decontaminating a device or an item. However, cleaning with soap and water may be equally effective. When chemical germicides are used for decontamination, they can range in activity from sterilant-disinfectants, which may be used to decontaminate spills of highly infectious agents in research or clinical laboratories, to low-level

TABLE 36.5-1. *Levels of germicidal action*

	Bacteria				Viruses	
Level	Vegetative Bacteria	Tubercle Bacillus	Spores	Fungi	Lipid and Medium-sized	Nonlipid and Small
High	+	+	+	+	+	+
Intermediate	+	+	±	+	+	±
Low	+	−	−	±	+	−

+ kills all; - does not kill; ± kills some.

TABLE 36.5-2. *Centers for Disease Control and Prevention and Environmental Protection Agency classification schemes for sterilants, disinfectants, and sanitizers*

EPA Product Classification	Type of Device or Surface	CDC Process Classifications
Sterilant or disinfectant	Critical (surgical instruments, catheters, implants)	Sterilization (sporicidal chemical, prolonged contact time)
	Semicritical (some endoscopes, endotracheal tubes, laryngoscopes)	High-level disinfection (sporicidal chemical, short contact time)
Hospital disinfectant (with label claim for tuberculocidal activity)	Noncritical (large blood spills, contaminated control knobs of dialysis machines, blood pressure cuffs)	Intermediate-level disinfection
Hospital disinfectant; sanitizer	Noncritical (exterior of machines, bed pans, floors)	Low-level disinfection or soap and water

disinfectants or sanitizers, which are used to decontaminate environmental surfaces.

An *antiseptic* has antimicrobial activity and is formulated to be used on or in living tissue to inhibit or destroy microorganisms. Often, the distinction between an antiseptic and a disinfectant is not made; however, the differences are great, and their applications are substantially different. A *disinfectant* is a chemical germicide that is formulated for use solely on medical devices, instruments, or environmental surfaces. An antiseptic is a chemical germicide that is formulated for use solely on or in living tissues. Some chemical germicidal agents, such as iodophors, can be used as active ingredients in disinfectants and in antiseptics. However, the precise formulations are significantly different, they are used differently, and the germicidal efficacy of each formulation differs substantially. Consequently, disinfectants should never be used as antiseptics and vice versa.

VIRAL INACTIVATION

Viruses can be inactivated by a variety of chemical germicides. Studies on inactivation of HBV and HIV have shown that neither virus is unusually resistant.[7,8] In 1977, it was proposed that the resistance level of HBV be considered to be between that of the tubercle bacillus and bacterial spores, although nearer that of the former.[8] In 1977, this type of rationale appeared reasonable, and it was believed that the most conservative approach would be to recommend at least high-level disinfection for all types of medical devices known or suspected of being contaminated with HBV. Subsequently, two studies employing direct chimpanzee inoculation with disinfectant-treated human serum with high titers of HBV showed that a variety of intermediate- to high-level disinfectant chemicals were effective inactivators of the virus in relatively short exposure times and at low temperatures.[9,10] The high-level disinfectants included two glutaraldehyde-based products, 500 mg/L of free chlorine from sodium hypochlorite, an iodophor product, 70% isopropanol, 80% ethanol, and dilutions of glutaraldehyde as low as 0.1%.

Several studies on the effect of various chemical and physical agents on HIV have shown that HIV is relatively sensitive to chemical germicides. In the human body, cell-free HIV

usually enters the CD4+ T lymphocyte and can become latent in the cell or replicate, resulting in a new virus being released into the surrounding milieu, where virus may infect other CD4+ cells. The number of HIV-infected cells per milliliter of blood in an infected individual is estimated to be between 10 and 10,000 during the course of the disease. The titer per milliliter of cell-free virus is estimated to be about 1000 or less. Cell-free HIV and HIV-infected cells may be present in the circulating blood. In the laboratory, cell-free HIV can be cultured in CD4+ T cells and T-cell lines. Generally, the virus-containing supernatant fluid is harvested. The titer of cell-free virus in supernatant culture fluid ranges from 10^4 to 10^6/mL, and after centrifugation, it is 10^6 to 10^8/mL, concentrations that are much higher than those naturally occurring in blood of infected patients. The amounts of protein and other organic materials in laboratory tissue culture fluid are usually less than that found in blood.[10-14]

TABLE 36.5-3. *Descending order of resistance to germicidal chemicals*

Bacterial Spores
Bacillus subtilis
↓
Mycobacteria
Mycobacterium tuberculosis var. *bovis*
↓
Nonlipid or Small Viruses
poliovirus
↓
Fungi
Trichophyton spp.
↓
Vegetative Bacteria
Pseudomonas aeruginosa
↓
Lipid or Medium-Sized Viruses
herpes simplex virus
hepatitis B virus
human immunodeficiency virus

Adapted from Favero MS, Bond WW. Sterilization, disinfection and antisepsis in the hospital. In: Manual of clinical microbiology. Washington, DC: American Society for Microbiology, 1991:183.

Laboratory-based inactivation studies have been performed by mixing high-titer virus-containing fluid and disinfectant for various periods. Sattar and Springthorpe[14] summarized the results of many of these, which show that HIV is susceptible to a wide variety of chemical disinfectants.

Conventional disinfection and sterilization strategies and protocols can be used for items or environments that are potentially or actually contaminated with blood and body fluid from patients infected with bloodborne viruses. These conventional procedures are conservative. Extraordinary protocols or use of more potent chemical germicides are unnecessary. For general housekeeping purposes, such as cleaning floors, walls, and other similar environmental surfaces in surgical suites, wards, and other areas in health care facilities, any EPA-approved hospital-grade disinfectant-detergent can be used.

HOUSEKEEPING CONSIDERATIONS

Methods

Surfaces such as walls, floors, table tops, and telephones have not been associated with transmission of infections to patients or health care workers.[1-3] Extraordinary attempts to disinfect or sterilize these environmental surfaces are unnecessary, but cleaning should be done routinely.

Disinfectant-detergent formulations registered by the EPA can be used for cleaning environmental surfaces, but the actual physical removal of microorganisms by scrubbing is probably at least as important as any antimicrobial effect of the germicidal agent used. No hospital protocol dealing with sterilization, disinfection, and housekeeping procedures needs to be changed because of concerns about contamination with HIV or HBV.[1]

Decontamination is a process that renders contaminated material, devices, and surfaces safe to handle, eliminating or significantly reducing the risk of infection transmission. For decontaminating spills of blood and other body fluids, the CDC recommends the use of chemical germicides that are approved for use as hospital disinfectants. Sites within health care facilities or laboratories that have become significantly contaminated with blood or body fluids may warrant the use of chemical germicides that are tuberculocidal. This strategy is relatively conservative and requires common sense judgment in assessing risk levels according to the size and location of the blood or body fluid spill. Because the CDC does not recommend specific commercial products, the EPA system of classification for label claim registration has been used for guidance on product selection, such as a hospital disinfectant with a claim of tuberculocidal activity (see Table 36.5-2). Users typically choose chemical germicides that have intermediate to high levels of germicidal activity (eg, sodium hypochlorite bleach, iodophors, phenolics) rather than low levels of activity (eg, quaternary ammonium compounds). A product with tuberculocidal activity is indicated, because mycobacteria are comparatively resistant to chem-

ical germicides and the descriptor "tuberculocidal" can be used as a surrogate indicator of potency. It is not used because of a concern for the transmission of M tuberculosis from environmental surfaces.

Protocols for housekeeping, laundry, sanitization, disinfection, and sterilization used in health care facilities are relatively conservative and do not need to be changed because of concerns about HIV or HBV contamination.

Handling of Infectious Waste

The CDC has published recommendations for the identification, handling, transport, storage, and disposal of infectious waste.[2,7] However, there is no evidence to suggest that most hospital waste is any more infective than residential waste, and there is no epidemiologic evidence that hospital waste has caused disease in the community as a result of improper disposal.

Identifying wastes for which special precautions are indicated is largely a matter of judgment about the relative risk of disease transmission. The most practical approach to the management of infectious waste is to identify those wastes with the potential for causing infection during handling and disposal and for which some special precautions appear prudent. Hospital wastes for which special precautions appear prudent include microbiology laboratory waste, pathology department waste, needles and sharps, and blood specimens or blood products.

Although any item that has had contact with blood, exudates, or secretions may be potentially infective, it is not usually considered practical or necessary to treat all such waste as infective. In general, infectious waste should be incinerated or should be decontaminated before disposal in a sanitary landfill. Bulk blood, suctioned fluids, excretions, and secretions may be carefully poured down a drain connected to a sanitary sewer. Other infectious wastes may be ground and flushed into a sanitary sewer. Universal precautions[15,16] are not intended to alter these basic recommendations for waste management. Health care professionals should refer to the local governmental body that regulates waste for exact requirements that pertain to the disposal of infectious wastes.

REFERENCES

1. Favero MS, Bond WW. Sterilization, disinfection and antisepsis in the hospital. In: Manual of clinical microbiology. Washington, DC: American Society for Microbiology, 1991:183.
2. Garner JL, Favero MS. Guidelines for handwashing and hospital environment control. Health and Human Services publication 00-1117. Atlanta: Centers for Disease Control, 1985.
3. Rutala WA. Guideline for selection and use of disinfectants. Am J Infect Control 1990;18:99.
4. Bruch MK, Larson E. Regulation of topical antimicrobials: history, status and future perspective. Infect Control Hosp Epidemiol 1989;10:505.
5. Zanowiak P, Jacobs MR. Topical anti-infective products. In: Handbook of nonprescription drugs. 7th ed. Washington, DC: American Pharmaceutical Association, 1982:92.
6. Spaulding EH. Chemical disinfection and antisepsis in the hospital. J Hosp Res 1972;9:5.

7. Bond WW, Petersen NJ, Favero MS. Viral hepatitis B: aspects of environmental control. Health Lab Sci 1977;14:235.
8. Bond WW, Favero MS, Petersen NJ, Ebert JW. Inactivation of hepatitis B virus by intermediate- to high-level disinfectant chemicals. J Clin Microbiol 1983;18:535.
9. Kobayashi H, Tsuzuki M, Koshimizu K, et al. Susceptibility of hepatitis B virus to disinfectants and heat. J Clin Microbiol 1984; 20:214.
10. Resnik L, Veren K, Salahuddin SF, Tondreau S, Markham PD. Stability and inactivation of HTLV-III/LAV under clinical and laboratory environments. JAMA 1986;255:1887.
11. McDougal JS, Cort SP, Kennedy MS, et al. Immunoassay for the detection and quantitation of infectious human retrovirus, lymphadenopathy-associated virus (LAV). J Immunol Methods 1985;76:171.
12. Martin LS, McDougal JS, Loskoski SL. Disinfection and inactivation of the human T lymphotrophic virus type III lymphadenopathy-associated virus. J Infect Dis 1985;152:400.
13. Spire B, Barre-Sinoussi F, Montagnier L, Chermann JC. Inactivation of lymphadenopathy associated virus by chemical disinfectants. Lancet 1984;2:899.
14. Ho DD, Moudgil T, Alam M. Quantitation of human immunodeficiency virus type 1 in the blood of infected persons. N Engl J Med 1989;3211621.
15. Sattar SA, Springthorpe VS. Survival and disinfectant inactivation of the human immunodeficiency virus: a critical review. Rev Infect Dis 1991;13:430.
16. Centers for Disease Control. Recommendations for prevention HIV transmission in health-care settings. MMWR 1987;36:1.

AIDS: Biology, Diagnosis, Treatment and Prevention, fourth edition, edited by Vincent T. DeVita, Jr., Samuel Hellman, and Steven A. Rosenberg. Lippincott–Raven Publishers, © 1997

CHAPTER 37

Postexposure Management

Denise M. Cardo and David M. Bell

Health care workers (HCWs) are potentially at risk for occupational exposures to blood and certain other body fluids containing bloodborne pathogens, including human immunodeficiency virus (HIV).[1-4] Although exposure prevention is the optimal strategy for protecting HCWs,[5-7] exposures are likely to continue to occur. Appropriate postexposure management must be included in programs to prevent transmission of bloodborne infections. Exposures to blood and body fluids may require evaluation and management of possible exposure to bloodborne pathogens, such as HIV, hepatitis B and C viruses,[8,9] tetanus prophylaxis,[10] but this chapter focuses only on the issues regarding HIV.

An occupational exposure that may place a worker at risk of HIV infection has been defined by the U.S. Public Health Service (PHS) as "a percutaneous injury (eg, a needle stick or a cut with a sharp object), contact of mucous membranes, or contact of skin (especially when the exposed skin is chapped, abraded, or afflicted with dermatitis or the contact is prolonged or involving an extensive area) with blood, tissues, or other body fluids to which universal precautions apply, including semen, vaginal secretions, or other body fluids contaminated with visible blood, because these substances have been implicated in the transmission of HIV infection; cerebrospinal fluid, synovial fluid, and amniotic fluid, because the risk of transmission of HIV from these fluids has not yet been determined; and laboratory specimens that contain HIV (eg, suspensions of concentrated virus) during the performance of job duties."[11]

RISK OF TRANSMISSION OF HIV AFTER AN OCCUPATIONAL EXPOSURE

Available information on the risk of transmission of HIV after an occupational exposure is reviewed in detail in Chap-

ter 35. Briefly, prospective studies of HCWs who have had occupational exposure have estimated that the risk of HIV infection after percutaneous exposure to HIV-infected blood is approximately 0.3% (upper limit of 95% confidence interval [CI] = 0.6%),[1-4] and after a mucous membrane exposure, it is 0.09% (upper limit of 95% CI = 0.5%).[12] Cases of transmission of HIV infection after skin exposures have also been documented; the risk of transmission after exposures to skin, whether intact or nonintact, has not been precisely quantified.[13] In one study, the upper limit of 95% CI for HIV transmission after skin exposure to HIV-infected blood was 0.04%.[7] The risk of transmission after occupational exposure to potentially infectious tissues or fluids other than blood (ie, fluids for which universal precautions are recommended) has not been quantified.

Laboratory and epidemiologic studies have suggested that a variety of factors may increase or decrease the probability of HIV transmission after an individual occupational exposure, such as the volume of blood transferred and the titer of the virus in the specimen. In vitro studies have demonstrated that less blood is transferred across membranes by a needle that passes through gloves or is of smaller gauge or solid rather than hollow bore.[14-17] The titer of virus in the specimen is likely to be an important determinant for transmission; it may vary by several orders of magnitude, depending on the stage of illness of the source patient and whether the source patient was taking antiviral drugs to which the virus was sensitive.[18] A retrospective case-control study to identify risk factors for HIV seroconversion among HCWs after a percutaneous exposure to HIV-infected blood has shown that HCWs were more likely to become infected if they were exposed to a larger quantity of blood, represented in the study as presence of visible blood on the device before injury, deep injury, and a procedure that involved a needle placed directly in the source patient's vein or artery. In this study, transmission of HIV was also associated with injuries in which the source patient was terminally ill with acquired immunodeficiency syn-

Denise M. Cardo, National Center for Infectious Diseases, Centers for Disease Control and Prevention, CDC Mailstop E-68, 1600 Clifton Road, Atlanta, GA 30333.

David M. Bell, Centers for Disease Control and Prevention, CDC Mailstop E-68, 1600 Clifton Road, Atlanta, GA 30333.

drome (AIDS); this may be attributable to the increased titer of HIV in blood that is known to accompany late stages of illness.[19]

Host defenses may also influence the risk of transmission. A study demonstrated an HIV-specific helper T cell immune response when peripheral blood mononuclear cells from a small number of HCWs exposed to HIV who did not seroconvert were stimulated in vitro by HIV. Although there may be several explanations for this observation, one possibility is that host immune responses may sometimes be able to prevent establishment of HIV infection after a percutaneous exposure.[20]

Available data for risk of occupational transmission of HIV come from studies with HIV-1. No cases of occupational transmission of HIV-2 have been reported. Until further information regarding occupational exposures to HIV-2 become available, postexposure management for exposures to HIV-2 should follow the same recommendations as those for HIV-1. Simian immunodeficiency virus (SIV) is similar to HIV-2. One case of occupationally acquired infection has been reported after a percutaneous exposure to blood from a macaque infected with SIV.[21]

POSTEXPOSURE MANAGEMENT PROGRAM

Each institution should adopt an appropriate postexposure management plan for exposure to blood and bloodborne pathogens. This plan should include an explanation of what constitutes an occupational exposure that may place a worker at risk of HIV infection, procedures for promptly reporting and evaluating such exposures, and recommended follow-up management of the exposed worker, including the possible use of antiviral agents.[11,22,23]

Reporting Exposures

In several studies, 40% to 90% of percutaneous injuries were not reported; underreporting rates varied among different institutions and occupations.[24–26] The prompt reporting of exposures is essential for management of the exposed workers and for identification of continuing hazards and evaluation of preventive measures.

Reporting systems should include access to expert consultants and measures to safeguard the confidentiality of exposed workers. Some institutions have found it useful to implement hotlines staffed by expert clinicians 24 hours each day to coordinate reporting and initial management of exposed workers.[9,22,27] For institutions where exposures to bloodborne pathogens are relatively uncommon, hotlines may not be cost effective; other solutions, such as having protocols in emergency departments or programs in association with larger hospitals, may be considered.

HCWs must understand the importance of reporting all exposures as soon as possible after they occur, because certain interventions that may be indicated must be initiated promptly to be effective. Prompt and complete reporting

depends on appropriate education of workers and a supportive and nonpunitive response by employers. Educational programs for workers, including orientation and inservice activities, should be provided to discuss the importance of properly reporting exposures and to familiarize HCWs with their personal risk of occupational exposure to HIV, measures to prevent these exposures, and the principles of postexposure management.[9,11,23]

Evaluation and Initial Management of the Exposed Worker

On reporting an exposure, the worker should be evaluated and counseled regarding the risk of HIV infection; the procedures for postexposure management, including the availability of potentially useful antiviral agents such as zidovudine (ZDV); the need for follow-up evaluation; and precautions to prevent HIV transmission to others during the follow-up period. Optimally, workers should be familiarized with these procedures before the exposure occurs.[11]

Each incident of occupational exposure to blood or body fluids that may contain HIV should be treated as rapidly as possible. Local treatment of the exposed site should be administered as necessary. Puncture wounds and other cutaneous injuries should be washed with soap and water. Exposed oral and nasal mucosa should be decontaminated by vigorous flushing with water. Eyes should be irrigated with clean water, saline, or sterile irrigants designed for this purpose.[11] No scientific evidence indicates that the use of antiseptics for wound care offers additional benefit in reducing the risk of transmission of HIV; however, their use is not contraindicated. The use of caustic agents such as bleach or the injection of disinfectants or antiseptics into the wound that cause tissue trauma is not recommended. Although speculative prophylactic treatments, including local applications of glucocorticoids, have been proposed, no evidence of benefit has been demonstrated.[9] Some of these treatments may interfere with host defenses.[28–29]

Efforts should be made to identify and evaluate clinically and epidemiologically the source individual for evidence of HIV infection. The source patient should be informed of the incident and tested for serologic evidence of HIV infection after consent is obtained in accordance with state and local laws. If consent cannot be obtained from the source individual (eg, because the individual is unconscious), policies should be developed for testing source individuals in compliance with applicable laws. Confidentiality of the source patient should be maintained at all times.[11]

Data to be collected should include relevant factors to evaluate the exposure and to provide information on the patterns of exposures in the institution for future preventive strategies. Data should be recorded in a confidential medical record and include demographic information about the exposed worker, the date and time of exposure, a detailed account of the exposure (eg, type of exposure, amount and type of fluid or material, type and purpose of device, gauge of needle, presence of visible blood on device, severity of exposure, circumstances of exposure), a description of infection-control precautions (eg, gloves, eye protection, masks), conditions of the source person (eg, stage of disease, use of antiretroviral drugs), and details about counseling, postexposure management, and follow-up plans.[9,11,27]

The psychologic impact of an occupational HIV exposure on the HCW should be considered during counseling and follow-up; experts have found that supportive counseling is an important part of management.[9,22,23,27] Because of the possibility of incubating HIV infection, to prevent further transmission to his or her contacts, the HCW should be advised to refrain during the follow-up period from donating blood, semen, or organs and to refrain from breast-feeding if safe and effective alternatives to breast-feeding are available. To prevent HIV transmission to sexual partners, all exposed HCWs, including pregnant women, should abstain from or use latex condoms during sexual intercourse throughout the follow-up period.[11]

Follow-up Management

If the source individual has AIDS, is known to be HIV-seropositive, or refuses testing, the HCW should be evaluated clinically and serologically for evidence of HIV infection as soon as possible after the exposure (ie, baseline evaluation) and, if seronegative, should be retested periodically for at least 6 months (eg, at 6 weeks, 3 months, and 6 months) to determine whether HIV infection has occurred.[11] The routine use of polymerase chain reaction (PCR), viral culture, or p24 antigen test to detect infection in the HCW is not generally recommended.[9,30] False-positive PCR test results have been observed in HCWs, even when the test was performed under stringent conditions.[30] In one case of occupational transmission of HIV after a percutaneous exposure, antibody test results were positive before the HIV genome was detectable by PCR.[4]

The PHS recommends serologic follow-up for at least 6 months after exposure, although some hospitals elect to perform HIV testing until 1 year after exposure. Because of reports of delayed seroconversion in some studies of homosexual men, several investigators have used PCR to examine specimens from HCWs after exposure to HIV-infected blood to assess the possibility of delayed seroconversion.[31-33] Data from these examinations, combined with data on several hundred HCWs who have remained seronegative when tested 2 or more years after exposure, suggest that seroconversion beyond 6 months after an occupational exposure, if it occurs, is uncommon.[1,4,30,31]

The HCW should be advised to report and seek medical evaluation for any acute illness that occurs during the follow-up period. Such illness, particularly if characterized by fever, rash, myalgia, fatigue, malaise, or lymphadenopathy, may be indicative of acute HIV infection, drug reaction, or another medical condition. In 50% to 70% of patients with primary HIV infection, an acute retroviral syndrome develops approximately 3 to 6 weeks after the exposure.[34]

If the source individual is HIV seronegative and has no clinical manifestations of AIDS or HIV infection, no further HIV follow-up of the exposed HCW is necessary, unless there is epidemiologic evidence to suggest that the source individual may have recently been exposed to HIV.[11] Transmission of HIV from occupational exposures to patients with early infection who had not yet seroconverted has been reported.[12] If the source patient is HIV negative and the probability of infection is low, the HCW can be reassured that HIV transmission is extremely unlikely.[27] If the source patient cannot be identified, decisions regarding appropriate follow-up should be individualized, based on factors such as whether the potential sources are likely to include an individual at increased risk of HIV infection.[11] If the HCW is subsequently found to be HIV seropositive, medicolegal and financial compensation issues may be greatly simplified if seroconversion can be shown to be temporally associated with an occupational exposure. Consequently, obtaining a serum specimen from the HCW promptly after exposure for testing or storage should be considered, regardless of the follow-up that is decided on.

During all phases of follow-up, the confidentiality of the HCW and the source patient must be protected.

POSTEXPOSURE CHEMOPROPHYLAXIS

Zidovudine

Reverse transcriptase inhibitors such as ZDV have been shown to have clinical benefit in HIV-infected patients.[35-37] Although their mechanism of antiviral action does not suggest that they would be ideal chemoprophylactic agents,[38,39] they have been considered for prophylaxis after an occupational exposure. The ideal prophylactic agent should exert its effect before the virus is incorporated into the genome of the target cell. Although ZDV and other reverse transcriptase inhibitors exert their antiviral activity only afterward, they may prevent early viral dissemination and could potentially be important for postexposure prophylaxis.

Animal Studies

The attempts to assess the efficacy of postexposure chemoprophylaxis in animal models have yielded inconclusive results. Data involving studies of laboratory animals must be interpreted with caution, because they have often been derived by using nonhuman retroviruses having pathogenic mechanisms different from those of HIV infection in humans. The lack of a good animal model for HIV infection in humans is a major problem. To ensure an adequate viral challenge, as documented by a high infection rate in the untreated animals, most of the studies have relied on intravenous injection of a large viral inoculum—an exposure which bears little resemblance to most needle-stick exposures in health care settings.[40–48]

Ruprecht and colleagues demonstrated that ZDV administered 4 hours after inoculation with Rauscher murine leukemia virus suppressed viremia.[40] Tavares and associates showed that ZDV apparently prevented feline leukemia virus infection when administered to cats immediately after the virus exposure; however, no sensitive techniques for detecting proviral DNA (eg, PCR) were used to definitely exclude infections.[41] Although these studies using murine and feline retroviruses suggest that ZDV may alter the course of these retroviral infections when given immediately after the exposure to the virus, they are of limited value, because these viruses have pathogenic mechanisms different from those of HIV in humans.

Some studies with SIV showed that ZDV did not prevent SIV infection in monkeys injected with moderate or high inocula or with a rapidly lethal variant of SIV, even when ZDV was combined with interferon and administered before virus inoculation.[42–44] When lower challenge doses of SIV were used and ZDV was begun before exposure, one of six monkeys in the highest-dose treatment group in one study did not become infected.[45] In a study with infant monkeys inoculated with a low dose of SIV, Van Rampey and colleagues demonstrated that infant monkeys pretreated with ZDV 2 hours before virus inoculation remained uninfected during the study.[46]

In studies using immunodeficient mice that had received transplants of human hematolymphoid organs (SCID-hu mice), McCune and associates observed that HIV infection was suppressed during the use of ZDV, but infection was detected in all animals after discontinuation of ZDV. Because the mice were exposed to HIV by intrathymic injection of a sizable virus inoculum, the relevance of this experiment to percutaneous exposures in HCWs is unclear.[47] In a subsequent study, the SCID-hu mice were treated with ZDV at different times after intravenous infection with a standard dose of HIV and the effects of ZDV in suppressing the HIV infection were shown to be time dependent. When ZDV was given within 2 hours of injection, viral replication was suppressed in all animals 2 weeks later, but the investigators did not determine whether infection was present after ZDV was discontinued.[48]

Human Studies

Little information exists with which to assess the efficacy of postexposure ZDV for humans. Because of the relatively low rate of seroconversion after an occupational exposure to HIV-infected blood, a prospective trial involving many thousands of exposed workers would be necessary to have the statistical power to assess the efficacy of postexposure prophylaxis.[1] The Burroughs-Wellcome Company sponsored a prospective, double-blind, randomized, placebo-controlled study to evaluate 6 weeks of ZDV prophylaxis involving HCWs who had experienced occupational exposures to HIV-infected blood; however, this trial was terminated prematurely because of low enrollment.[49]

Results from a randomized, double-blind, placebo-controlled trial of the efficacy and safety of ZDV in reducing the risk of maternal-infant HIV transmission (Protocol 076) have shown that a regimen consisting of ZDV given antepartum and intrapartum to the mother and to the newborn for 6 weeks reduced the risk of transmission by approximately two thirds.[50,51] In this trial, the protective effect of ZDV was only partly explained by reduction of the HIV titer in maternal blood, suggesting that ZDV may also have had a direct protective effect on the fetus or infant postexposure.[52]

A retrospective case-control study of HIV seroconversion to identify risk factors for HIV-seroconversion among HCWs after a documented percutaneous exposure to HIV-infected blood has found that the use of postexposure ZDV by the exposed HCW was associated with a lower likelihood of seroconversion (odds ratio = 0.21, 95% CI = 0.06–0.57).[19]

Failures of Zidovudine to Prevent Infection

Failure of ZDV to prevent HIV infection in humans when administered postexposure has been reported in at least 13 instances.[1,11,53–61] In five instances, the exposures involved injection of a larger quantity of HIV-infected blood than would be expected from a needle stick. They include two instances of accidental intravenous inoculation of HIV-infected blood or other body fluid during nuclear medicine procedures,[53,54] one blood transfusion,[11] one suicidal self-inoculation,[55] and one assault on a prison guard with a needle syringe.[56]

Tokars and collaborators summarized data for eight HCWs who became infected with HIV despite ZDV treatment after percutaneous exposure to HIV-infected blood (Table 37-1).[1] In these cases, ZDV was begun 30 minutes to 12 hours (median, 1.75 hours) after exposure and was used in doses of 800 to 1200 mg/day (median, 1000 mg/day) for 8 to 54 days (median, 21 days). Among these eight documented failures of ZDV postexposure, three involved source patients who had no known history of ZDV use and were therefore less likely to be infected with ZDV-resistant HIV. For two of the eight cases, laboratory studies were conducted to assess possible ZDV resistance of the infecting strain. In one case (case 5), the source patient was not known to have taken ZDV before the exposure. Because the infecting strain could not be isolated from the HCW's blood, the Centers for Disease Control and Prevention (CDC) performed direct sequencing of the HIV reverse transcriptase gene (amplified by PCR) from the HCW's peripheral blood mononuclear cells. No mutations were found at positions known to be associated with ZDV resistance, suggesting that the strain was probably sensitive to ZDV.[1] In the other case (case 3), the source patient had been receiving ZDV for 18 months at the time of the exposure. The HIV isolated from the HCW showed substantially decreased sensitivity to ZDV.[60]

TABLE 37-1. *Reported instances of failure of postexposure zidovudine to prevent HIV infection in health care workers following percutaneous exposure to HIV-infected blood*

Country	Year	Sharp Object	Hours to First Dose	Regimen* Mq.	Regimen* Days	Onset of Retroviral Illness	Time Seroconversion Documented[†]	Source Patient on ZVD
South Africa	1992	IV cannula	0.5	1200	42	No	6 Weeks	No
United States	1991	22-gauge phlebotomy needle	0.75	800	10	Week 2	3 Months	Yes
Western European country	1992	18–20-gauge IV cannula	1	1000	42	Week 2	56 Days	Yes
France	1990	Phlebotomy needle	1.5	1000	21	Day 16	52 Days	Yes
United States	1992	21-gauge syringe needle	2	1000	17	Week 6	6 Months	No
United States	1990	16-gauge IV cannula	3–7	1000	8	Day 36	94 Days	Yes
Australia	1990	Hollow needle	6	1000	54	Week 5	6 Weeks	Yes
South Africa	1990	Lancet	12	1200	21	Day 17	24 Days[‡]	No

*Regimens are expressed as milligrams of zidovudine per day and number of days taken. Report 5: 500 mg per day for 1 day, then 1000 mg per day for 16 additional days.

[†]By enzyme immunoassay and western blot.

[‡]At 24 days, enzyme immunoassay reactive and Western blot weakly positive. At 3 months, enzyme immunoassay had higher optical density reading and Western blot had strongly positive bands.

Tokars JI, Marcus R, Culver DH, et al. Surveillance of human immunodeficiency virus (HIV) infection and zidovudine use among healthcare workers with occupational exposure to HIV-infected blood. Ann Int Med 1993,118:915.

The emergence of ZDV-resistant strains of HIV from AIDS patients previously treated with ZDV has been reported by several researchers.[62–66] ZDV-resistant HIV can be transmitted and can cause primary infections.[67–69] An exposure to a strain of HIV already resistant to ZDV could potentially explain some failures of attempted prophylaxis with ZDV. These case reports indicate that, if ZDV is protective, any protection afforded is not absolute.

Toxicity

Information about the toxicity of orally administered ZDV comes primarily from animal studies and from studies of HIV-infected patients who were treated with ZDV.[70] Prolonged treatment is associated with hematologic toxicity (eg, anemia, granulocytopenia, thrombocytopenia), myopathy, nausea, fatigue, insomnia, and headaches.[70]

Serious toxicity associated with short-course ZDV therapy in healthy persons appears to be rare. In several prospective studies, the most commonly reported symptoms and signs of acute toxicity included nausea, vomiting, headache, malaise, fatigue, anemia, and granulocytopenia.[1,49,71–74] These adverse effects have subsided with dose reduction or discontinuation of ZDV.

In a placebo-controlled trial (Burroughs-Wellcome), nausea, vomiting, and arthralgia were reported more commonly among HCWs taking ZDV than among those taking placebo.[49] In a CDC surveillance project of prospective evaluation of HCWs exposed to HIV-infected blood, information was available for 310 (89%) of 348 HCWs who took ZDV and for 475 of workers who did not. Side-effect information was collected at the 6-week follow-up visit. Overall,

230 (74%) HCWs who took ZDV postexposure reported one or more symptoms during the 6 weeks after beginning prophylaxis, compared with 127 (25%) workers who did not. The most frequent symptoms reported among the HCWs who took ZDV were nausea (50%), malaise or fatigue (33%), headache (25%), vomiting (11%), or myalgia or arthralgia (10%). Ninety-nine (32%) HCWs did not complete their planned regimen of ZDV because of adverse symptoms.[1]

Investigators at the University of California at San Francisco and the National Institutes of Health are conducting a prospective open-label trial to evaluate postexposure ZDV toxicity at 19 U.S. centers. In preliminary results, among 148 HCWs exposed to HIV-infected blood or body fluids who completed an average of 30 weeks of follow-up, 52 (35%) discontinued the drug before 28 days because of moderate to severe subjective toxicities, including fatigue (74%), nausea (58%), headaches (41%), insomnia (26%), and anorexia (25%). Mild decreases of hemoglobin and absolute neutrophil counts were observed; these mild objective toxicities did not correlate with the reported subjective symptoms.[71]

In the Italian Multicentre Study on occupational risk of HIV infection, all HCWs enrolled at the 30 centers participating in the study who decide to take ZDV are followed periodically for at least 2 weeks after interruption of the drug to monitor ZDV toxicity. Fifty-six percent of the 211 HCWs who took prophylactic ZDV developed side effects. The most frequent reactions reported were nausea (40%), asthenia (17%), vomiting (15%), headache (9%), or gastric pain (8%); most adverse effects began within the first 10 days of prophylaxis. In 29 (14%) cases, toxicity led to prophylaxis interruption; in 9 cases, side effects resolved after reduction from the initial dose. Major hematologic side effects were rare: anemia in 5 cases (2.5%) and neutropenia in 1 case (0.5%). All hematologic side effects were observed within 10 days of beginning prophylaxis, which was continued at 1000 mg per day for 3 to 4 weeks without further decrease in hematologic values.[72]

Forseter and coworkers evaluated the safety, tolerability, and acceptability of a ZDV postexposure regimen offered in a daily dose of 1200 mg for 42 days. Adverse events occurred in 44 (73%) of 60 HCWs taking ZDV; the most frequent events were nausea (47%), headache (35%), and fatigue (30%). Among 60 (53%) of 113 HCWs who took ZDV, 21 (35%) completed the recommended dose; 18 (30%) HCWs stopped treatment because of clinical adverse reactions. Minor changes in laboratory parameters (eg, decrease of hematocrit, hemoglobin level, white cell count) were observed, but none were clinically significant.[73]

Minimal short-term toxicity was observed among the infants who received ZDV during Protocol 076; the level of hemoglobin at birth in the infants in the ZDV group was significantly lower than that in the infants in the placebo group. However, by 12 weeks of age, hemoglobin values in the two groups were similar. The long-term effects on mother and infant are unknown.[51]

For healthy persons not infected with HIV, the risk of long-term toxicity, including teratogenic and carcinogenic effects, is unknown. Vaginal tumors, including carcinomas, have been observed in mice receiving doses of ZDV that the Food and Drug Administration has determined resulted in plasma levels in mice approximately equal to plasma levels in human receiving a dose of 200 mg of ZDV every 4 hours.[11]

ZDV has a direct effect on the developing mouse embryo.[75] However, it is not known whether ZDV can cause fetal harm when administered to a pregnant woman or whether it can affect reproductive capacity. In limited studies of the outcomes of newborns of HIV-infected mothers treated with ZDV during pregnancy, adverse outcomes specifically attributable to this drug were not observed.[76] Data from Protocol 076 provide no evidence of an increased risk of birth defects from exposure to ZDV in utero after 14 weeks of gestation; however, larger numbers of exposed infants need to be evaluated.[51,52] The PHS recommends that pregnancy should be avoided throughout the time ZDV is taken.[11]

Current Practice

The proportion of enrolled HCWs using ZDV in a CDC surveillance prospective project, which includes over 200 health care facilities in the United States, increased from 5% in the fourth quarter of 1988 to 50% in the third quarter of 1990 and remained stable subsequently, averaging 35% to 40% during 1993. Physicians, dentists, and medical students were more likely to use ZDV than were other health care professionals, as were HCWs with percutaneous injury compared with those exposed through contact of mucous membranes or skin. In this project, ZDV was prescribed by collaborating investigators in doses ranging from 200 to 1800 mg/day (median, 1000 mg/day) and for periods of 1 to 180 days (median, 42 days). The interval from exposure to first dose of ZDV ranged from less than 5 minutes to 17 days (median, 4 hours).[1]

Theoretical models designed to evaluate the cost effectiveness of the use of ZDV postexposure demonstrated that ZDV, if moderately effective and when confined to workers who sustain percutaneous exposures to blood from known HIV sources, can be cost effective.[77,78] Protocols for prophylaxis have been established by many hospitals and institutions.

US Public Health Service Recommendations

In March 1996, a workshop was co-sponsored by CDC and the National Foundation for Infectious Diseases to discuss chemoprophylaxis after occupational exposures to HIV. Based in part on the input received at this workshop, the PHS is currently developing updated recommendations for chemoprophylaxis after occupational exposures to HIV. These recommendations are expected to be published in Morbidity and Mortality Weekly Report in 1996. In a previous statement, published in 1990, the PHS recommended that HCWs who may be at risk for occupational exposure be aware of the considerations that pertain to the use of ZDV postexposure. Ideally, HCWs should be familiarized with these considerations before exposure to facilitate prompt and rational decision making after exposure. These include the postexposure risk of HIV infection and the factors that have been postulated to influence this risk; the limitations of current knowledge of the efficacy of ZDV as postexposure prophylaxis; the apparent need to begin prophylaxis promptly if prophylaxis is given the relatively frequent short-term toxicity; the lack of knowledge of potential long-term toxicity; and the need for postexposure follow-up, regardless of whether ZDV is taken.[11]

GOALS AND TRENDS

The prevention of occupationally acquired HIV infection requires measures to reduce exposures and appropriate postexposure management. Experimental models have shown a possible window between the exposure and infection that represents an opportunity to interfere with the development of infection.

As new antiretroviral agents are developed and are shown to be effective in the treatment of established HIV infection, these agents should be evaluated for efficacy and toxicity when used for postexposure prophylaxis. Such evaluation and improved understanding of the initial events in the pathogenesis of infection will require development of appropriate animal models and collaboration among many groups of investigators to pool information on exposed workers.

REFERENCES

1. Tokars JI, Marcus RA, Culver DH, et al. Surveillance of human immunodeficiency virus (HIV) infection and zidovudine use among health care workers with occupational exposure to HIV-infected blood. Ann Intern Med 1993;118:913.
2. Marcus R, CDC Cooperative Needlestick Study Group. Surveillance of health-care workers exposed to blood from patients infected with the human immunodeficiency virus. N Engl J Med 1988;319:1118.
3. Gerberding JL, Bryant-LeBlanc CE, Nelson K, et al. Risk of transmitting the human immunodeficiency virus, cytomegalovirus, and hepatitis B virus to health care workers exposed to patients with AIDS and AIDS-related conditions. J Infect Dis 1987;156:1.
4. Henderson DK, Fahey BJ, Willy M, et al. Risk for occupational transmission of human immunodeficiency virus type 1 (HIV-1) associated with clinical exposures: a prospective evaluation. Ann Intern Med 1990;113:740.
5. Centers for Disease Control and Prevention (CDC). Recommendations for prevention of HIV transmission in health-care settings. MMWR 1097;36:2S.
6. Occupational Safety and Health Administration (OSHA). Occupational exposure to bloodborne pathogens; final rule. Fed Regist 1991;56:64175.
7. Fahey BJ, Koziol DE, Banks SM, Henderson DK. Frequency of non-parenteral occupational exposures to blood and body fluids before and after universal precautions training. Am J Med 1991;90:145.
8. Centers for Disease Control and Prevention (CDC). Protection against viral hepatitis: recommendations of the immunization practices advisory committee (ACIP). MMWR 1990;39(RR-2):1.
9. Gerberding JL. Management of occupational exposures to blood-borne viruses. N Engl J Med 1995;332:444.
10. Centers for Disease Control and Prevention (CDC). Immunization practices advisory committee. Diphtheria, tetanus, and pertussis: recommendations for vaccine and other preventive measures. MMWR 1991;40(RR-10):1.
11. Centers for Disease Control and Prevention (CDC). Public health service statement on management of occupational exposure to human immunodeficiency virus, including considerations regarding zidovudine postexposure use. MMWR 1991;39(RR-1):1.
12. Ippolito G, Puro V, DeCarli G, Italian Study Group on Occupational Risk of HIV. The risk of occupational human immunodeficiency virus in health care workers. Arch Intern Med 1993;153:1451.
13. Centers for Disease Control and Prevention (CDC). Update: human immunodeficiency virus infections in health care workers exposed to blood of infected patients. MMWR 1987;36:285.
14. Shirazian D, Herzlich BC, Mokhtarian F, Grob D. Needlestick injury: blood, mononuclear cells, and acquired immunodeficiency syndrome. Am J Infect Control 1992;20:133.
15. Gaughwin MD, Gowans E, Ali R, Burrell C. Blood needles: the volumes of blood transferred in simulations of needlestick injuries and shared use of syringes for injection of intravenous drugs. AIDS 1991;5:1025.
16. Napoli VM, McGowan E. How much blood is in a needlestick? J Infect Dis 1987;155:828.
17. Mast S, Woolwine J, Gerberding J. Efficacy of gloves on reducing blood volumes transferred during simulated needlestick injury. J Infect Dis 1993;168:1589.
18. Ho DD, Mougil T, Alam M. Quantitation of HIV type 1 in the blood of infected persons. N Engl J Med 1989;321:1622.
19. Centers for Disease Control and Prevention. Case-control study of HIV seroconversion in health care workers after percutaneous exposure to HIV-infected blood—France, United Kingdom, and United States, January 1988–August 1994. MMWR 1996;44:929.
20. Clerici M, Levin JM, Kessler HA, et al. HIV-specific T-helper activity in seronegative health care workers exposed to contaminated blood. JAMA 1994;271:42.
21. Khabbaz RF, Heneine W, George JR, et al. Brief report: infection of a laboratory worker with simian immunodeficiency virus. N Engl J Med 1994;330:172.
22. Henderson DK. Postexposure chemoprophylaxis for occupational exposure to human immunodeficiency virus type 1: current status and prospects for the future. Am J Med 1991;91:3125.
23. World Health Organization (WHO). Global program on AIDS: report of the consultation on action to be taken after occupational exposure of health care workers to HIV. Geneva: World Health Organization, 1989.
24. Short L, Chamberland M, Srivastava P, et al. Impact of safety devices to reduce percutaneous injuries during phlebotomy. Abstract 50. The Fifth Annual Meeting of Society for Healthcare Epidemiology of America. Infect Control Hosp Epidemiol 1995;16:24.
25. Mangione CM, Gerberding JL, Cummings SR. Occupational exposure to HIV: frequency and rates of underreporting of percutaneous and mucocutaneous exposures by medical housestaff. Am J Med 1991;90:85.
26. Hamory BH. Underreporting of needlestick injuries in a university hospital. Am J Infect Control 1983;11:174.
27. Gerberding JL, Henderson DK. Management of occupational exposures to bloodborne pathogens: hepatitis B virus, hepatitis C virus, and human immunodeficiency virus. Clin Infect Dis 1992;14:1179.
28. Sprecher E, Becker Y. Herpes simplex virus type 1 pathogenicity in footpad and ear skin of mice depends on Langerhans cell density, mouse genetics, and virus strain. J Virol 1987;61:2515.
29. Kalter DC, Gendelman HE, Meltzer MS. Monocytes, dendritic cells, and Langerhans cells in human immunodeficiency virus infection. Dermatol Clin 1991;9:415.
30. Gerberding JL. Incidence and prevalence of HIV, hepatitis B virus, hepatitis C virus, and cytomegalovirus among health care personnel at risk for blood exposure: final report from a longitudinal study. J Infect Dis 1994;170:1410.
31. Horsburgh CR, Ou CY, Jason J, et al. Duration of human immunodeficiency virus infection before detection of antibody. Lancet 1989;2:637.
32. Wormser GP, Joline C, Bittker S, Forseter G, Kwok S, Sninsky JJ. Polymerase chain reaction for seronegative health care workers with parenteral exposure to HIV-infected patients. N Engl J Med 1989;321:1681.
33. Henry K, Campbell S, Jackson B, et al. Long-term follow-up of health care workers with work-site exposure to human immunodeficiency virus. (Letter) JAMA 1990;263:1765.
34. Pontaleo G, Graziosi C, Fauci A. The immunopathogenesis of human immunodeficiency virus infection. N Engl J Med 1993;5:327.
35. Fischl MA, Richman DD, Grieco MH, et al. The efficacy of azidothymidine (AZT) in the treatment of patients with AIDS and AIDS-related complex: a double-blind, placebo-controlled trial. N Engl J Med 1987;317:185.
36. Volberding PA, Lagakos SW, Koch MA, et al. Zidovudine in asymptomatic human immunodeficiency virus infection. N Engl J Med 1991;322:941.
37. Fischl MA, Richman DD, Hansen M, et al. The safety and efficiency of zidovudine (AZT) in the treatment of subjects with mildly symptomatic human immunodeficiency virus type-1 (HIV) infection. Ann Intern Med 1990;112:727.
38. Yarchoan R, Mitsuya H, Myers C, Broder S. Clinical pharmacology of 3'-azido-2',3'-dideoxythimidine (zidovudine) and related dideoxynucleosides. N Engl J Med 1989;321:726.
39. Kamali F. Clinical pharmacology of zidovudine and other 2',3'-dideoxynucleoside analogues. Clin Invest 1993;71:392.
40. Ruprecht RM, O'Brien LG, Rossoni LD, Nusinoff-Lehrman S. Suppression of mouse viraemia and retroviral disease by 3'-azido-3'-deoxythymidine. Nature 1986;323:467.
41. Tavares L, Roneker C, Johnston D, Lehrman SN, de Noronha F. 3'-Azido-3'-deoxythymidine in feline leukemia virus-infected cats: a model for therapy and prophylaxis of AIDS. Cancer Res 1987;47:3190.
42. McClure HM, Anderson DC, Fultz P, Klumpp SA, Schinazi RF. Prophylactic effects of AZT following exposure of macaques to an acutely lethal variant of SIV (SIV/SMM/PBj-14). Abstract TCO42. Fifth International Conference on AIDS, Montreal, 1989:522.
43. Fazely F, Haseltine WA, Rodger RF, Ruprecht RM. Postexposure chemoprophylaxis with ZDV or ZDV combined with interferon: failure after inoculating rhesus monkeys with a high dose of SIV. J Acquir Immune Defic Syndr 1991;4:1093.
44. Lundgren B, Bottiger D, Ljungdahl-Stahle E, et al. Antiviral effects of 3'-fluorothymidine and 3'-azidothymidine in cynomolgus monkeys infected with simian immunodeficiency virus. J Acquir Immune Defic Syndr 1991;4:489.
45. Tsai CC, Follis KE, Grant R, et al. Effect of dosing frequency on zidovudine prophylaxis against simian immunodeficiency virus in *Macaca facicularis*. Abstract 58. Program and Abstracts, 32nd Interscience Conference on Antimicrobial Agents and Chemotherapy (Anaheim). Washington, DC: American Society for Microbiology, 1992:120.

46. Van Rompay KK, Marthas ML, Ramos RA, et al. Simian immunodeficiency virus (SIV) infection of infant rhesus macaques as a model to test antiretroviral drug prophylaxis and therapy: oral 3'-azido-3'-deoxythymidine prevents SIV infection. Antimicrob Agents Chemother 1992;36:2381.

47. McCune JM, Namikawa R, Shih CC, Rabin L, Kaneshima H. Suppression of HIV infections in AZT-treated SCID-hu mice. Science 1990;247:564.

48. Shih C-C, Kaneshima H, Rabin L, et al. Postexposure prophylaxis with zidovudine suppresses human immunodeficiency virus type 1 infection in SCID-hu mice in a time-dependent manner. J Infect Dis 1991;163:625.

49. LaFon SW, Mooney BD, McMullen JP, et al. A double-bind, placebo-controlled study of the safety and efficacy of retrovir (zidovudine, ZDV) as a chemoprophylactic agent in health care workers exposed to HIV. Abstract 489. Program and Abstracts, 30th Interscience Conference on Antimicrobial Agents and Chemotherapy in Atlanta. Washington, DC: American Society for Microbiology, 1990:167.

50. Centers for Disease Control and Prevention. Recommendations of the U.S. Public Health Service task force on the use of zidovudine to reduce perinatal transmission of HIV. MMWR 1994;43(RR-11):1.

51. Connor EM, Sperling RS, Gelber R, et al. Reduction of maternal-infant transmission of HIV type 1 with zidovudine treatment. N Engl J Med 1994;331:1173.

52. Sperling RS, Shapiro DE, Coombs R, et al. Maternal plasma HIV-1 RNA and the success of zidovudine (ZDV) in the prevention of mother-child transmission. Abstract LB1. The Third Conference on Retroviruses and Opportunistic Infections in Washington, DC. Washington, DC: American Society for Microbiology, 1996:161.

53. Centers for Disease Control and Prevention (CDC). Patient exposures to HIV during nuclear medicine procedures. MMWR 1992;41:575.

54. Lange JMA, Boucher CAB, Hollak CEM, et al. Failure of prophylactic zidovudine after accidental exposure to HIV-1. N Engl J Med 1990;322:1375.

55. Durand E, LeJenne C, Hugues FC. Failure of prophylactic zidovudine after suicidal self-inoculation of HIV-infected blood. (Letter) N Engl J Med 1991;324:1062.

56. Jones PD. HIV transmission by stabbing despite zidovudine prophylaxis. (Letter) Lancet 1992;338:884.

57. Tait DR, Pudifin DJ, Gathiram V, Windsor IM. HIV seroconversions in health-care workers, Natal, South Africa. Abstract PoC 4141. Seventh International Conference on AIDS, Amsterdam, 1992:268.

58. Lot F, Abiteboul D. Infections professionnelles par le V.I.H. en France: le point au 31 mars 1992. Bull Epidemiol Hebdomadaire 1992;26:117.

59. Looke DF, Grove DI. Failed prophylactic zidovudine after needlestick injury. (Letter) Lancet 1990;335:1280.

60. Anonymous. HIV seroconversion after occupational exposure despite early prophylactic zidovudine therapy. (Letter) Lancet 1993;341:1077.

61. Coutellier A, Desmoulius C, Veron M, Herson S. Failure of zidovudine prophylaxis after occupational needlestick injury. Abstract PO-B26-2074. Ninth International Conference on AIDS, Berlin, 1993:481.

62. Smith MS, Koerber KL, Pagano JS. Zidovudine-resistant human immunodeficiency virus type 1 genomes detected in plasma distinct from viral genomes in peripheral blood mononuclear cells. J Infect Dis 1993;167:445.

63. Land S, McGavin C, Lucas R, Birch C. Incidence of zidovudine-resistant human immunodeficiency virus isolated from patients before, during, and after therapy. J Infect Dis 1992;166:1139.

64. Larder BA, Kemp SD. Multiple mutations in HIV-1 reverse transcriptase confer high-level resistance to zidovudine (AZT). Science 1989;246:1155.

65. Larder BA, Kellam P, Kemp SD. Zidovudine resistance predicted by direct detection of mutations in DNA from HIV-infected lymphocytes. AIDS 1991;5:137.

66. Kellan P, Boucher CA, Larder BA. Fifth mutation in human immunodeficiency virus type 1 reverse transcriptase contributes to the development of high-level resistance to zidovudine. Proc Natl Acad Sci USA 1992;89:1934.

67. Erice A, Mayers DL, Strike DG, et al. Primary infection with zidovudine-resistant human immunodeficiency virus type 1. N Engl J Med 1993;328:1163.

68. Hermans P, Sprecher S, Clumeck N. Primary infection with zidovudine resistant HIV. (Letter to the editor) N Engl J Med 1993;329:1123.

69. Fitzgibbon JE, Gaur S, Frenkel LD, Laraque F, Edlin BR, Dubin DT. Transmission from one child to another of human immunodeficiency virus type 1 with a zidovudine-resistance mutation. N Engl J Med 1993;329:1835.

70. Richman DD, Fischl MA, Grieco MH, et al. The toxicity of AZT in the treatment of patients with AIDS and AIDS-related complex: a double-blind, placebo-controlled trial. N Engl J Med 1987;317:192.

71. Fahrner R, Beekman S, Koziol DE, Gerberding JL, Henderson DK. Safety of zidovudine administered as post-exposure chemoprophylaxis to health care workers sustaining occupational exposures to HIV. Abstract I154. Thirty-Fourth Interscience Conference on Antimicrobial Agents and Chemotherapy in Orlando. Washington, DC: American Society for Microbiology, 1994:132.

72. Puro P, Ippolito G, Guzzanti E, et al. Zidovudine prophylaxis after accidental exposure to HIV: the Italian experience. AIDS 1992;6:963.

73. Forseter G, Joline C, Wormser GP. Tolerability, safety, and acceptability of zidovudine prophylaxis in health care workers. Arch Intern Med 1994;154:2745.

74. Schmitz SH, Scheding S, Voliotis D, Rasokat H, Diehl V, Schrappe M. Side effects of AZT prophylaxis after occupational exposure to HIV-infected blood. Ann Hematol 1994;69:135.

75. Toltzis P, Marx CM, Kleinman N, Levine E, Schmidt EV. Zidovudine-associated embryonic toxicity in mice. J Infect Dis 1991;163:1212.

76. Sperling RS, Shatton P, O'Sullivan M, et al. A survey of zidovudine use in pregnant women with human immunodeficiency virus infection. N Engl J Med 1992;326:857.

77. Ramsey SD, Nettleman MD. Cost-effectiveness of prophylactic AZT following needlestick injury in health care workers. Med Decis Making 1992;12:142.

78. Allen UD, Read S, Gafni A. Zidovudine for chemoprophylaxis after occupational exposure to HIV-infected blood: an economic evaluation. Clin Infect Dis 1992;14:822.

AIDS: Biology, Diagnosis, Treatment and Prevention, fourth edition, edited by Vincent T. DeVita, Jr., Samuel Hellman, and Steven A. Rosenberg. Lippincott–Raven Publishers, © 1997

CHAPTER 38

Societal Impact of the Acquired Immunodeficiency Syndrome Epidemic

Harvey V. Fineberg

The societal dimensions of acquired immunodeficiency syndrome (AIDS) can be understood in at least three ways. First, any entity we recognize as a disease has a biologic impact and a socially constructed meaning. This social construction is reflected in part by the progression of names assigned to the affliction (eg, from gay-related immunodeficiency to AIDS) and, more significantly, by the metaphoric meanings attached to the disease. As Susan Sontag explains,

> Although the way in which disease mystifies is set against a backdrop of new expectations, the disease itself . . . arouses thoroughly old-fashioned kinds of dread. Any disease that is treated as a mystery and acutely enough feared will be felt morally, if not literally, contagious . . . . Contact with someone afflicted with a disease regarded as a mysterious malevolency inevitably feels like a trespass; worse, like the violation of a taboo.[1]

Although she was referring to cancer, Sontag's words apply even more appropriately to AIDS, a disease that is literally as well as morally contagious.[2]

Societal dimensions may refer to social causes of the epidemic—those conditions of poverty, unemployment, hopelessness, and family breakdown that promote behavior such as injecting drug use and indifference to personal risk. René Dubos reminded us that, just as the fire can be doused by water but not caused by the absence of water, the existence of a biologic preventive or cure does not necessarily deny the social origins of disease.[3] Many circumstances of modern life facilitated the transformation of AIDS from isolated infection to widespread epidemic: urbanization in

sub-Saharan Africa, patterns of prostitution in Thailand, gay liberation in the United States, and the importation and use of blood clotting factors in France, among many other examples. The same capacity for technology that promises scientific solutions to the epidemic also made possible the blood processing and jet travel that contributed to the spread of disease.

The societal dimensions of AIDS may be seen as the consequences of the epidemic. In an important sense, we are all living with AIDS. Regardless of which of us is actually infected with the virus, AIDS affects all of us in ways obvious and subtle. Although every disease has personal and social consequences, the association of AIDS with contagion, intimacy, sexuality, morality, and youthful mortality lend it special poignancy and prominence as a social concern. The epidemic has touched our daily lives; our families, schools, and communities; our cultural and health care institutions; our churches, businesses, and community agencies; our courts of law and prisons; and our military services and government at all levels. Social scientists have explored AIDS from a host of analytic perspectives, including historical,[4,5] political,[6] and anthropologic.[7] Just as AIDS influences the conduct of our social institutions, so the responses of these institutions define the social reality of AIDS.[8]

In this chapter, I review public attitudes and the social response to AIDS, examine the effects of the epidemic on health care, and summarize some of the economic, legal, and policy consequences of the disease. Although the social consequences of AIDS have been profound for many developing countries,[9–11] the focus in this chapter is on conditions and responses in the United States. What unfolds illustrates the interplay of biologic and social reality, samples enlightened and mean-spirited reactions, and highlights the social construction and expression of disease. What follows depicts the social context of illness.

Harvey V. Fineberg, Harvard School of Public Health, 677 Huntingdon Avenue, Boston, MA 02115-6023.

PUBLIC ATTITUDES, UNDERSTANDING, AND BEHAVIOR

Americans recognize AIDS as an extremely serious threat to health. By 1993, 26% of Americans reported that they personally knew someone who had died from AIDS.[12] When asked what they regarded as the most serious health risk in the United States, almost twice as many (36%) choose AIDS as choose cancer (19%).[13] However, the proportion that rank AIDS first declined from 68% in 1987.[14] Nearly 6 (59%) in 10 say they are somewhat concerned or very concerned that they or another family member could get AIDS.[15] Nearly one half (49%) believe the country is losing ground against AIDS.[15] The proportion who favor more funding for AIDS declined from 70% in 1990 to 45% in 1994, but only 15% think too much is being spent on AIDS research.[14,16]

More than a decade after the recognition of AIDS, almost 5 of 6 Americans report that they know a lot (45%) or at least something (39%) about the disease.[12] Nearly everyone knows you can get AIDS by having sex with someone of the opposite sex (96%) or from a blood transfusion (98%).[12] However, misunderstanding persists about the modes of transmission. For example, 28% believe it is possible for someone to get AIDS when they donate their own blood, and about 18% believe AIDS can be transmitted by a mosquito or another insect.[12] Unsurprisingly, persons with higher educational levels and socioeconomic status are more likely to answer questions about human immunodeficiency virus (HIV) transmission correctly.[17] The principal source of information (ie, print or electronic media) appears to be less predictive of knowledge about HIV transmission.[17]

Americans are strong supporters of education to prevent AIDS.[14] Ninety-three percent of Americans favor school-based education about AIDS,[18] and by 1993, 57% favored providing high school students with access to condoms,[19] up from about 40% in 1988.[14] Although those who attend church regularly are less likely to favor AIDS education, even among fundamentalists, most support AIDS education programs.[20]

Approximately one half (49%) of all Americans say they have taken steps to avoid getting AIDS, most often limiting sexual partners, using condoms, or abstaining from sex.[12] Awareness of popular figures who are infected with HIV appears to influence the willingness of many individuals to take action to protect themselves. After the basketball star, Magic Johnson, revealed that he was infected with HIV, 60% to 70% of adults polled said his statement would make them more likely to practice safer sex, talk with a son or daughter about AIDS, or limit the number of sex partners.[21]

More than 90% of Americans believe patients with AIDS should be treated with compassion. However, the number drops to 73% if the individual contracted AIDS through homosexual relations and to 70% if the disease was contracted by intravenous drug use.[14] AIDS appears to have sharpened the attitudes of most Americans toward gays, with 30% feeling more sympathetic and 33% feeling less sympathetic toward homosexuals as a result of the epi-demic.[22] Perhaps related, 16% of Americans believe AIDS is punishment from God for immoral sexual behavior.[23] Even several years after the Americans With Disabilities Act made the practice illegal, 28% of Americans believe an employer should be allowed to refuse to hire someone who is HIV positive.[24] Fifty-two percent believe an employer has a right to know whether an employee is HIV positive or has AIDS.[25] About three fourths of Americans would prohibit foreigners and tourists who carry the AIDS virus from entering the United States.[26]

Overall, Americans regard AIDS as a very significant health problem, although less dire than was perceived in the late 1980s. There is strong endorsement of education to prevent AIDS and substantial support for continued government funding to combat AIDS. Some misperceptions about ways of contracting AIDS persist. A growing number know someone personally who has died of AIDS, and about one half the adult population are acting to protect themselves from exposure to the virus. Although most feel compassion for persons with AIDS, a minority view the disease as the deserved result of immoral behavior.

During the past decade, AIDS has come to be construed more as a familiar, endemic disease problem than as a novel, epidemic crisis. In the first decade of the epidemic, social commentators and public health officials frequently talked about the dual epidemics of disease and fear. Today, the more prevalent combination is disease and complacency, which is perhaps even more treacherous. Although there has been a gradual abatement in the overall rate of increase in AIDS cases in the United States since 1989, the epidemic continues to intensify among injecting drug users (IDUs) and among women.[27] In most of the world, heterosexual spread of HIV predominates, and there is no reason to expect this mode of spread to fail to gain in the United States. The dual challenge today is to attain public understanding and support for special attention to populations currently at risk and to strengthen and sustain the vigilance and behavioral patterns that will protect everyone from exposure to HIV.

MEDIA COVERAGE

In contrast to the regular increase in AIDS cases and reasonably smooth increase in professional publications about the disease, coverage of AIDS on television and in newspapers has been episodic.[28,29] A steadily expanding epidemic does not make news. The first flurry of attention in the popular media occurred in connection with the 1983 editorial by Dr. Anthony Fauci that raised the possibility that AIDS might be transmissible by "routine close contact." Interest in the media subsequently subsided until the July 1985 revelation that actor Rock Hudson was undergoing treatment for the disease. The media reported on the search for scientific breakthroughs and on government action and inaction in the face of the epidemic, stories that evoked a combination of hope and despair. Television coverage grew again from early-1986 through mid-1987, reflecting Surgeon General Koop's report, the first public statement on AIDS by President Reagan, and the third international conference on AIDS in Washington, D.C. Then coverage diminished again, reflecting the cycle of newsworthiness of any topic.

The writers, editors, and producers in the media are also members of the public, and the choices of these opinion leaders reflect as well as shape public attitudes. The consequences of words and images in the media reverberate through personal choices and public policy. As Dorothy Nelkin explains,

> The metaphors and images used to describe a situation can point the finger of blame and imply responsibility. Is AIDS a crisis or a problem? A plague or a disease? Is it a gay disease or a disease related to certain behaviors? Is it an STD or a viral disease? Are those with AIDS victims or people with an illness? Is testing an intrusion on civil liberties or a protection of public health? Is fear of AIDS a phobia or simply a concern? Selective use of language can trivialize an event or render it important; marginalize some groups, empower others; define an issue as an urgent problem or reduce it to a routine.[29]

VOLUNTEERISM AND SOCIAL ACTIVISM

In accord with the long tradition of volunteerism in America, AIDS prompted the establishment of numerous local and national organizations in the private sector. Many individuals responded with compassion, dedication, time, and money to a new, deadly disease and especially to illness and death of friends and loved ones. They created organizations to meet the needs for education, prevention, advocacy, services to patients and families, and funding for research. Such grass-roots organizations as the Shanti Project in San Francisco, the Gay Men's Health Crisis, Inc., in New York City, and the AIDS Action Committee in Boston provided crucial support and structure for assisting persons with AIDS. Consortia of private sector funders and such dedicated foundations as the American Foundation for AIDS Research and the Pediatric AIDS Foundation initiated innovative research and service programs before or beyond what government was prepared to do.

One of the most lasting legacies of the AIDS epidemic may be the shaping of a new role for social activism in patient advocacy, physician practices, the conduct of clinical research, pharmaceutical regulation and pricing, government funding, and public policies toward disease. Patients and volunteer activists influenced many aspects of the social response to AIDS, and their influence has extended indirectly to the regulatory and medical response to other diseases as well.

Several factors together created the conditions for a new and dramatic form of social activism in the case of AIDS.[30] AIDS first became evident in the early 1980s among male homosexuals, a group with a strong sense of identity and a decade's experience with sexual liberation. In the early years, homosexual groups strongly resisted intrusions on their sex-

ual freedoms and concentrated on care of individuals stricken with the disease. By 1987, more than 20,000 Americans had died of AIDS, three fourths of whom had probably contracted the virus through sex with other men. Thousands more homosexuals had been tested and knew they were HIV positive, but efforts to find new drugs appeared to be languishing in the federal research-regulatory pipeline. A precipitating event came in 1987, when, speaking in Greenwich Village, Larry Kramer exhorted gay men to demand research for AIDS treatments, saying they were doomed unless they took action. Soon after, chapters of Act Up (AIDS Coalition To Unleash Power) formed in a number of cities around the United States and, eventually, in other countries as well. Although many other organizations have advocated ardently and successfully in behalf of AIDS patients and to promote AIDS research, Act Up established a new level of confrontation and civil disobedience in a matter of health.

Act Up members employed tactics ranging from disruption of the New York Stock Exchange, to mass demonstrations at the Food and Drug Administration (FDA) headquarters, to heckling and shouting down the Secretary of Health and Human Services at an AIDS conference.[30] Such behavior earned the organization much enmity, including criticism from others in the gay community. At the same time, the activists stimulated the expedited drug approval process adopted by FDA for life-threatening diseases, led Burroughs-Wellcome to lower the price of zidovudine, and helped shape the conduct of clinical trials of AIDS drugs.[30] Along with others, members of Act Up helped promote the strong federal investment in AIDS research. Most of the time, members of the organization sought the limelight, seeing publicity as key to their strategy. However, they also worked behind the scenes, as in negotiations about the drug ddI involving FDA and Bristol-Myers.[31] Kramer, a writer, articulated the way extremists can open the door for more moderate elements:

> There has to be room for civil disobedience or even more extreme forms of activism. When you have an extreme group of activists it makes it easier for the center to negotiate. With us out there asking for the moon, the moderates can get a few stars . . . .[31]

As years passed and some successes were realized, many AIDS activists have grown less strident and more mainstream, more often partners of clinical scientists and public health officials than opponents. Many of the early demonstrators have been lost to the disease, and the nature of the AIDS epidemic has also evolved. Only about one half of the current cases of AIDS in the United States are men who contracted the virus from sex with other men, and although large cities (>500,000 persons) still contain more than 80% of cases, the caseload is increasing even more rapidly in smaller cities.[27]

AIDS was a dominant, life or death agenda for the homosexual community, which brought a capacity for organization and intensity of focus not shared by others, such as IDUs, affected by the epidemic. The AIDS activists also benefited from the growing awareness of patient rights and emphasis on patient self-determination. For the most part, other organized health interests lack the previous political agenda and group consciousness that characterized AIDS activists.[30] However, patient lobbyists for such diseases as breast cancer and Alzheimer's disease have learned from the methods and successes of the AIDS groups.[30] As they sought to influence decisions about AIDS, the AIDS activists have indelibly marked the processes of health policy and research in the United States.

ECONOMIC PERSPECTIVE

The costs of a disease bear on individuals and families, on institutions (eg, hospitals, businesses), and on communities and society as a whole. When assessing the economic burden of a disease such as AIDS on society, it is customary to account for the direct costs of illness (ie, medical bills) and for the indirect costs (ie, lost future earnings) attributable to each case of the disease. A more complete accounting would also include induced costs (ie, non–disease-realated expenses induced by the illness). Within a country such as the United States, AIDS has an uneven geographic distribution and a concomitantly uneven distribution of portions of its economic burden.[32]

The ability of persons with AIDS to continue working and earning income depends on the mental and physical demands of their jobs.[33] A systematic study of AIDS patients in Boston found 76% employed at the time of their diagnosis and 53% still employed 16 months later, although one third of these were on disability or sick leave.[33] The loss of earnings had reduced monthly income by an average of 75%.

The costs of AIDS borne by business and government are substantial. To businesses in the United States, the expected 5-year costs of an HIV-infected employee range up to $32,000.[34] These include expenditures for health insurance; short-term and long-term disability benefits; recruiting, hiring, and training costs; life insurance; and retirement benefits. Between 1986 and 1993, the life and health insurance industries paid out approximately $7.7 billion in AIDS-related claims.[35] In 1993, AIDS accounted for approximately 3% of all private life insurance payments and 1.5% of private health insurance claims. In fiscal year 1995, the federal government spent $633 million through the Ryan White Act for care of AIDS patients in metropolitan areas with heavy patient caseloads. The number of eligible areas grew from 16 in 1991 to 42 in 1995.[36] These funds are in addition to expenditures through Medicare and Medicaid. The National Institutes of Health research budget for HIV amounted to $1.338 billion in fiscal year 1995. An additional $590 million was spent on surveillance and prevention through the Centers for Disease Control and Prevention (CDC) and $186 million for housing of persons with AIDS.[37]

The annual, direct cost of medical care for AIDS patients in the United States is estimated to be about $10 billion.[38] Although a substantial sum, this is just 1% to 2% of all national health care expenditures. Over the years of the epidemic, the proportion of AIDS patients covered by public insurance (ie, Medicaid or Medicare) has been growing.[39] AIDS, like other severe, chronic diseases, tends to impoverish as it debilitates, and a growing proportion of AIDS patients are poor before they become infected or fall ill. By fiscal year 1993, Medicaid (a combined federal and state program) accounted for more than $2.5 billion of costs of care for AIDS patients, or about one fourth of all health care expenditures for AIDS. Medicare added approximately an additional $385 million. These funds covered about 60,000 beneficiaries. The figures are projected to rise to more than $4.5 billion and 80,000 beneficiaries by 1997.[38]

With advances in treatment, the lifetime cost of care for an individual infected with HIV has tended to increase over the past decade, although estimates of lifetime treatment costs have ranged widely, from $40,000 to $140,000.[39-45] In some circumstances, the cost effectiveness of care has not shown continuous improvement over time. In one San Francisco study, for example, the cost effectiveness of intensive care for patients with *Pneumocystis carinii* pneumonia and severe respiratory failure improved during the first 8 years of the epidemic, but it then worsened because of diminished survival and increased hospital costs. For the years between 1989 and 1991, this study found that the cost per year of life saved had exceeded $215,000.[46]

The largest, longitudinal study of the use of health services by HIV-infected patients is the AIDS Cost and Services Utilization Survey (ACSUS) conducted by the Agency for Health Care Policy and Research in 1991 through 1992. This study of almost 2000 patients classified each as asymptomatic, HIV symptomatic, or having AIDS. From the accumulated data, Hellinger estimated the lifetime cost of treating a person with HIV from the time of infection until death to be approximately $119,000.[45] The cost of care before the development of AIDS was $50,000, and the cost after the development of AIDS was $69,000. The rise in costs overall were ameliorated by decreasing reliance on inpatient care. In a survey of hospital use and costs, Andrulis and coworkers found that 35% of HIV-related admissions and 29% of HIV-related inpatient costs were accumulated by patients before the development of AIDS.[47] After the onset of clinical disease, a high proportion of costs appears to be concentrated in the period immediately preceding death.[48]

The indirect costs of the AIDS epidemic—those attributable to loss of productivity due to morbidity and premature mortality—rose with the size of the epidemic through the 1980s. By 1991, the indirect costs in the United States were estimated to have exceeded $55 billion.[49] This amounted to almost 12% of the estimated indirect costs of all illnesses.[49] By comparison, AIDS accounted for 5.3% of the total loss of productivity due to illness in Canada in 1991.[50] The indirect costs are disproportionately large compared with the fraction of all deaths caused by AIDS, because such a large proportion of those who succumb to HIV die as young adults who would otherwise have had many productive years ahead of them.

In the case of AIDS, the induced costs range over a wide spectrum. They include, for example, the cost of blood screening, of research, of promoting AIDS awareness in many settings, and of universal precautions in health care facilities. Universal precautions have triggered additional expenses, such as those associated with increased allergic reactions to latex used in protective gloves.[51] In fairness, there may also be induced benefits and savings, such as a reduction in hepatitis transmission because of universal precautions or a reduction in unwanted pregnancy because of increased use of condoms. AIDS has the special property of increasing the occurrence and severity of other diseases, such as tuberculosis, which also have costs. The expenses connected with volunteer support are substantial; the value of volunteer care at home for a person with AIDS exceeds $25,000 per year.[52] Especially telling in personal terms are induced costs related to the care of children whose parents are lost to the epidemic. By the year 2000, 80,000 children and adolescents in the United States will have lost their mothers to AIDS.[53]

Economic costs are no measure of the burden of an epidemic such as AIDS, but they do represent one important index of social consequence. In parts of the world where national income is much lower and the prevalence of AIDS much higher than in the United States, the economic and demographic impact of the epidemic is considerable.[54] Within the United States, the economic impact of AIDS in high-prevalence geographic areas has been ameliorated by funds provided through the Ryan White Act. Although the economic costs of AIDS are notable, they remain relatively small compared with overall health expenditures and national income in the United States.

HEALTH CARE AND HEALTH CARE WORKERS

As a disease process in individuals, HIV infection is a chronic condition, with complications often deferrable and then manageable when they occur, although ultimately fatal. In the population, AIDS is now endemic, the sum of a set of overlapping epidemics according to the mode of spread: homosexual sex, heterosexual sex, injecting drug use, or blood exposure. As the front-line social institution coping with illness, the health care system has responded to AIDS in individuals and to the epidemic overall. With advances in knowledge and therapy (eg, prophylaxis, treatment of opportunistic infection) and shifts in the dominant modes of disease spread (eg, increasing numbers of women, IDUs, the poor) the patterns of treatment, financing, and expected costs have likewise evolved.

As is frequently true in medical care, the pattern of services received by patients with HIV infection varies with the socioeconomic, racial, and insurance status of the patient. Reporting on patterns of care found in the ACSUS study, Mohr observed that, regardless of stage of disease, a higher proportion of black, low-income, and unemployed persons were admitted to hospital than persons in other race, income, or employment categories.[55] Overall, 46% of the participants in ACSUS used

informal home services, and IDUs were as likely to use informal home services as other patients. (The cost of such services donated by family members or from volunteer support agencies is not reflected in the cost estimates reported.) White, higher-income, insured AIDS patients were more likely than their counterparts to use psychologic counseling and to have taken advantage of dental services.

A smaller, national sample of patients recruited from outpatient settings and through community-based service organizations found 29% with no insurance, 39% with private insurance, and 41% covered by some form of public insurance.[56] Clinics were the source of services for 95% of the uninsured or publicly insured but only 47% of those with private insurance. In a Massachusetts comparison, AIDS patients who are IDUs had 42% longer lengths of stay and 38% higher costs compared with non-IDU male AIDS patients.[57] In a San Francisco study, men without health insurance used outpatient services less often than men with fee-for-service insurance or managed care plans.[58] The men without insurance also used prophylaxis for P carinii less often (63%) than those with fee-for-service (93%) or managed care (83%) insurance. In this study, as in ACSUS, there was not much difference in the use of zidovudine between the insured and uninsured. Lower incomes also tend to translate into worse outcomes of illness. In a Canadian study, AIDS patients whose annual incomes were below Canadian $10,000 had a 63% higher age-adjusted mortality rate than patients who were financially better off.[59]

The impact of AIDS on health care extends beyond the care of patients who are infected with HIV. Universal precautions to prevent the spread of HIV have permanently altered the interface between all patients and their health care providers. They have also added costs for supplies, disposal, and training, which do not appear on the AIDS account because they are spread over all hospital or clinic operations. In a decade of many substantial changes in medicine, AIDS has added to the stresses of practice for many physicians, nurses, and other health care workers, especially because of the fear of infection, sense of futility from the inability to cure patients, and the youth of so many terminally ill patients.[60,61] If a health care worker is stuck by a needle pulled from an HIV-infected patient, the estimated risk of transmission is about 0.3%.[62] The ultimate lethality of AIDS, as well as the more immediate personal and professional consequences of HIV infection, make that small likelihood loom large.

The legal and moral obligations of physicians and hospitals to care for HIV-infected patients are clear. Federal regulations prohibit hospital discrimination against HIV-infected patients if the hospital accepts Medicare or Medicaid payments, and the Americans With Disabilities Act of 1990 provides many added protections.[63] The rights and opportunities of the HIV-infected doctor or nurse are more problematic, in part because of the attitudes of many patients. Americans believe it is very likely (23%) or somewhat likely (40%) that they can get infected by being cared for by a doctor or other health professional who has the AIDS virus.[23] The actual risk of HIV transmission from an infected health care worker to a patient is exceedingly small unless invasive procedures are performed without following universal precautions.[62,64] Although the American Medical Association (AMA) recommends that HIV-infected physicians continue to practice as long as there is no risk to their patients, more than one half of persons who had seen a physician in the previous 5 years would switch doctors if they knew their physician carried the AIDS virus.[65]

The questions of HIV testing of health care workers, possible restrictions on infected practitioners, and disclosure of HIV status to patients illustrate the web of legal, ethical, civil rights, privacy, professional responsibility and patient rights issues that are evoked by AIDS.[66,67] At least 16 states have enacted statutes related to HIV-infected health care workers; some statutes give patients the right to know if they have been exposed to body fluids of an infected health care worker and even to insist on HIV testing of the health care worker in cases of such exposure.[68] After the CDC issued guidelines for infected health workers in 1991, the federal government required all states to comply with the guidelines or their equivalent to retain eligibility to receive assistance under the Public Health Service Act.[68] Although the CDC guidelines give special attention to "exposure-prone procedures," it proved difficult in practice to identify such procedures apart from the specifics of precautions being taken in each case. The guidelines were subsequently interpreted as being consistent with New York Department of Health rules that instead declared any limitations on practice to be "determined on a case-by-case basis after consideration of the factors that influence transmission risk."[68,69]

The CDC guidelines expressly oppose mandatory HIV testing of health care workers, a position endorsed by virtually every professional association. The AMA recommends that physicians who perform procedures that could place patients at risk voluntarily determine their HIV status at periodic intervals, and if they know they are infected, they are urged to disclose their status to a confidential review committee.[70] The most celebrated case of possible HIV transmission from a health professional to patients involved a Florida dentist,[71–74] and the American Dental Association advises HIV-infected dentists who elect to continue performing invasive procedures to make a public disclosure of their HIV status.[68] Thoughtful medical and legal commentators disagree about whether a patient's right to know or a physician's right to privacy should take precedence in the case of an HIV-infected doctor.[75,76]

The obligations of doctors and patients to one another are not symmetric. Granted that the actual risks of transmission from doctor to patient are remote, cannot a patient still legitimately choose a personal physician on grounds, such as gender or race, for which it would be unethical for a doctor to accept or reject a patient? Even if a physician is not obliged to make a public declaration of seropositive status, should a doctor disclose the truth about her or his HIV status if asked directly by a patient? Such questions highlight the special dilemma of physician-patient relationships in the era of AIDS.

SOCIAL POLICY

After early years of ambivalence and official silence, a succession of national policy assessments and reports have marked the nation's experience with the AIDS epidemic. Surgeon General C. Everett Koop released his Report on AIDS in October, 1986, and nearly 2 years later, a shortened, simplified version introduced plain talk about sex education into virtually every American household.[77,78] The Presidential Commission on the HIV Epidemic, chaired by Admiral James Watkins, issued its comprehensive report in June of 1988. This document advanced nearly 600 recommendations dealing with a full range of research, prevention, care, financing, and legal and civil rights issues.[79] An act of Congress in November 1988 established the National Commission on AIDS "for the purpose of promoting the development of a national consensus on policy concerning acquired immune deficiency syndrome . . . and of studying and making recommendations for a consistent national policy concerning AIDS."[80] For the next 5 years, the National Commission, co-chaired by David Rogers and June Osborn, conducted hearings in cities around the country and issued a series of reports. Some dealt broadly with issues such as leadership and governmental responsibility, prevention strategies, civil rights, medical care, and financing,[81–84] and others focused on particular aspects of the epidemic, such as the growing disease burden in rural America,[85] HIV in correctional facilities,[86] and the special challenge of drug abuse plus HIV infection.[87] Along the way, the Institute of Medicine, National Research Council, and National Academy of Sciences issued several influential reports on coping with AIDS,[88–90] numerous guidelines emerged from the Public Health Service, and myriad analyses and recommendations emanated from the academic community, professional organizations, foundations and citizen groups.

Enactment of several pieces of federal legislation and regulatory decisions have strengthened the capacity of the nation to contend with AIDS and reaffirmed the rights and improved the lives of persons who are infected with HIV. Among these significant federal actions are sustained funding of research and prevention activities, expansion of clinical trials to community-based settings, and fast-tracking of regulatory review for potentially valuable new drugs. The Fair Housing Amendments Act of 1988 extended to the private sector protection for persons with handicaps, which was interpreted by the Department of Housing and Urban Development to include persons with HIV infection.[83] The Ryan White Act of 1990 has provided supplemental funds for areas with disproportionate numbers of patients with AIDS, and the Americans With Disabilities Act of 1990 extended many civil rights protections to persons with HIV infection.

Despite repeated calls for greater coherence in the design and conduct of a national strategy against AIDS, at no time has an entity emerged with comprehensive authority to execute all aspects of a national AIDS program. Within and across a number of federal agencies, however, there have been substantial moves toward coordination of planning and activities. For example, following the advice of citizen interest groups and the Institute of Medicine, the National Institutes of Health appointed a single director with authority over all funding for AIDS throughout the institutes.[91] Similarly, the CDC consolidated under a single center responsibility for AIDS, sexually transmitted diseases, and tuberculosis programs.[92]

State legislatures, which control or influence so many aspects of public health, have enacted much AIDS-related legislation.[93] The topics covered by state laws and regulations include treatment, research, and education requirements; blood screening; case finding; restrictions on movement or activity of infected persons; and antidiscrimination. Many states explicitly endorsed the confidentiality of records and requirement of informed consent for AIDS testing.[93] Much discussion about mandatory HIV antibody testing resulted in few laws mandating tests, and in at least one case where mandatory premarital testing was instituted, it was subsequently repealed.

Debates over national policy toward AIDS reflect and amplify differences in social values and priorities. Perhaps no area is more revealing in this respect than policies about HIV antibody testing. Decisions about testing arise in the military; in prisons; in connection with employment, insurance, and medical care; before marriage and during pregnancy; and in association with travel and immigration. The issues involve the right to know and the right not to know, freedom from discrimination and preservation of privacy, and protecting the health of the individual and of others. Advocates of mandatory testing see it as a way of protecting the uninfected by identifying the sources of risk and believe public health officials reluctant to apply widespread testing are abrogating their responsibility to protect the public. Most health officials and AIDS interest groups have strenuously resisted mandatory testing on the grounds that it serves no health objective, needlessly adds cost, violates individual rights, and would do more harm than good.

The shifting course of immigration law and policy illustrates the nation's ambivalence toward mandatory testing.[83] Before 1987, the Public Health Service had authority to designate diseases on the list of "dangerous contagious diseases" that warranted exclusion from entry into the country. By amendment to the Supplemental Appropriations Act of 1987 (P.L. 100-71), the Congress directed the President to add HIV infection to this list. This gave the United States the world's broadest legal exclusion of persons with HIV infection, and the law could be applied to resident aliens as well as to applicants for immigration.[94,95] This action prompted several countries and a number of national and international organizations to boycott the Sixth International AIDS Conference in San Francisco in June 1990 and prompted demonstrations at the meeting. After strenuous criticism by many individuals and organizations and recommendations from the National AIDS Commission, the Congress enacted a new immigration law in October 1990 (P.L. 101-649). This legislation directed the Secretary of Health and Human Ser-

vices to replace the previous list of "dangerous contagious diseases" with a new list of "communicable diseases of public health significance." The Secretary determined that sexually transmitted diseases, including HIV, should not be grounds for excluding aliens from entry into the United States, and the new list proposed in January 1991 contained only tuberculosis. However, on May 31, the day before the proposed regulation would have taken effect, it was withdrawn in favor of an interim rule that reinstated the earlier list for the indefinite future. In 1990, the United States became the first country expressly to repeal a law excluding persons with HIV infection, only to revert in 1991, by regulation, to mandatory testing and exclusion.

Sensible decisions about testing for HIV antibody depend in the first instance on clear thinking about the purposes of testing. These purposes determine some of the options and requirements for testing. The goal of surveillance, for example, is consistent with anonymous testing, which would be incompatible with testing for the purpose of individual patient care. Expanding knowledge of the epidemiology and pathogenesis of HIV provides a basis for defining attainable health objectives and for periodically reconsidering policies such as testing for HIV antibody. This is well illustrated by the evolving rationale over the years for testing pregnant women and newborns.

HIV transmission occurs in 15% to 30% of children born to women infected with HIV in the United States.[96] This translated into a cumulative number of 14,920 infants infected between 1978 and 1993.[96] As early as 1985, case reports suggested the possibility of transmission through breast-feeding, later confirmed by large prospective studies in Europe.[97-101] The earliest arguments in favor of HIV testing of pregnant women were to enable appropriate counseling and avoidance of breast-feeding. The CDC recommended in 1985 that HIV antibody testing and counseling be directed to women known to be at increased risk for HIV infection (eg, IDUs).[102] In the infected newborn, the most frequent early threat to survival is *P carinii* pneumonia, which can be prevented by early prophylaxis.[103] This realization provided a sound medical basis for the identification of infants at risk through testing of newborns or of their mothers during pregnancy. An even more compelling reason for identifying HIV infection in pregnant women arose from the findings of a clinical trial (ie, AIDS Clinical Trials Group Protocol 076) released in late 1994. This study found that a regimen of zidovudine in a pregnant woman and early infancy reduced vertical transmission of HIV by two thirds, from 25.5% to 8.3%.[104] Although many questions remained unanswered by this trial,[105] these results represented the first biologic intervention that prevented transmission of HIV. The CDC subsequently released new guidelines that called for universal counseling and voluntary testing for HIV among all pregnant women in the United States.[106]

Lest there be any mistake about its emphasis on the nonmandatory nature of accepting an HIV antibody test in the proposed policy, the CDC included the word *voluntary* in the title of its report and explained just before the recommendations that they "stress the need for a universal counseling and voluntary testing program for pregnant women."[106] This accommodates the right of a woman whose fears of discrimination, abandonment, or violence may lead her to decline to be tested despite the medical advantages to herself or her offspring.[107] It also recognizes that a decision to accept zidovudine treatment may not be without long-term risk to the mother or infant. Moreover, the CDC points to several studies that have demonstrated that routine, voluntary testing can achieve high rates of acceptance.[108–110] However, mandatory screening of pregnant women would be consistent with the responsibility of public health (and the interests of the state) to protect newborns against medical harm from decisions by their parents. There is also a compelling humanitarian argument to prevent the suffering of AIDS in as many newborns as possible, which also would save net costs to society.[111] Universal and automatic screening could help reduce any stigma from testing.[111]

Mandatory testing may find favor in those motivated by humanitarian and health concerns, as in those whose intention is to identify, label, and ostracize. In the case of pregnant women, the medical advantages of knowledge of HIV status are clear and compelling, but preserving the rights of individual choice and avoiding the risk of discrimination are also powerful concerns. The public's health will be served by making the availability of HIV tests to pregnant women a routine part of medical practice (even legally required of health providers) in association with counseling, while retaining the rights of the patient to accept or decline the routinely offered test. This area of evolving policy demonstrates the interplay of advancing medical knowledge, technical capabilities, social interests, and individual rights.

In many issues of AIDS policy, contending values and convictions (eg, the value of privacy and civil rights versus the belief that acts which introduce the AIDS virus demonstrate moral depravity) mix with facts and health consequences. As the AIDS epidemic reveals new epidemiologic trends and as knowledge of the efficacy and cost of interventions unfolds against the backdrop of evolving social values and judgments, the societal dimensions of AIDS will continue to be reshaped. This is the inevitable, continuing brew of social policy in a democratic society.

The arrival of AIDS mocked medical hubris and firmly upended the false expectation that the advent of vaccines and antimicrobials would relegate infectious diseases to historical interest only. The continuing reality of HIV has been absorbed into everyday life—in our closest personal relations; in our homes, schools, and businesses; in our legislatures, courts, and prisons; in our health care institutions; and as represented in art, theater, film, and television. In its darker side, AIDS resonates to the fear and anxiety of past epidemics: stigmatized minorities, prejudice against homosexuals and other marginalized populations, indifference to the suffering of others, blaming victims for harboring a dread disease, attacks on individual rights, unwarranted violations of privacy, and exclusions from work and from school. AIDS also prompts ennobling personal sacrifice, devotion, and generosity; awareness and education about sex and sexuality; remarkable scientific discovery; and innovative social responses at the grass-roots and government levels. AIDS is a social and cultural phenomenon as much as a biologic and medical condition.

The era of modern microbiology was heralded by the demonstration of specific bacterial causes for specific diseases. In the century since the pioneering bacteriology of Pasteur, Koch, and others, this effort has ramified to the study of helminthic, protozoal, fungal, bacterial, and viral origins of disease. Any infectious organism that takes hold in a population represents for that species an ecologic and evolutionary success; the very presence of an infection is prima facie evidence of the suitability of the organism to its environment and of the suitability of the environment to the organism. The emergence of infection may be seen in terms of the dynamic equilibrium of a relevant ecologic system.[112] From an ecologic perspective, the cause of a disease is much more than the necessary presence of a particular organism. The biologic, behavioral, environmental, and social dimensions of a disease are all legitimate aspects of its cause, expression, and consequence. The socially constructed meaning of AIDS, the social factors that contribute to its spread, and the societal and institutional responses to the disease are all part of a wider nexus of cause and effect present with any disease but revealed with special force and clarity in AIDS, the epidemic of our age.

ACKNOWLEDGMENTS

The author thanks Karen Donelan and Deborah Wexler for their assistance in gathering materials for this chapter. Dr. Mary E. Wilson provided valuable comments and suggestions.

REFERENCES

1. Sontag S. Illness as metaphor. New York: Farrar, Straus & Giroux, 1977:6.
2. Fineberg HV. The social dimensions of AIDS. Scientific American 1988;259:128.
3. Dubos R. Mirage of health: utopias, progress, and biological change. 3rd ed. New Brunswick, NJ: Rutgers University Press, 1993.
4. Fee E, Fox DM. The contemporary historiography of AIDS. J Soc History 1989;23:303.
5. Brandt AM. The syphilis epidemic and its relation to AIDS. Science 1988;239:375.
6. Bayer R. Private acts, social consequences. New York: The Free Press, 1989.
7. Singer M. AIDS and the health crisis of the U.S. urban poor; the perspective of critical medical anthropology. Soc Sci Med 1994;39:931.
8. Berk RA, ed. The social impact of AIDS in the U.S. Cambridge, MA: Abt Books, 1988.
9. Mann JM, Tarantola DJM, Netter TW, eds. AIDS in the world. Cambridge, MA: Harvard University Press, 1992.
10. Danziger R. The social impact of HIV/AIDS in developing countries. Soc Sci Med 1994;39:905.
11. Hamilton KA. The HIV and AIDS pandemic as a foreign policy concern. Washington Q 1993;17:201.
12. CBS News/New York Times 1993, June 1–3, 1993. Storrs, CT: Roper Center for Public Opinion Research, 1993.

13. Marttila & Kiley Inc., April 14–19, 1993. Storrs, CT: Roper Center for Public Opinion Research, 1993.

14. Blendon RJ, Donelan K, Knox RA. Public opinion and AIDS: lessons for the second decade. JAMA 1992;267:981.

15. Princeton Survey Research Associates, March 16–21, 1994. Storrs, CT: Roper Center for Public Opinion Research, 1994.

16. Hart and Teeter Research companies, January 15–18, 1994. Storrs, CT: Roper Center for Public Opinion Research, 1994.

17. LeBlanc AJ. Examining HIV-related knowledge among adults in the U.S. J Health Soc Behav 1993;34:23.

18. Yankelovich Partners Inc., January 22–25, 1993. Storrs, CT: Roper Center for Public Opinion Research, 1993.

19. Hart and Teeter Research Companies, April 17–20, 1993. Storrs, CT: Roper Center for Public Opinion Research, 1993.

20. Greeley AM. Religion and attitudes towards AIDS policy. Sociology and Social Research 1991;75:129.

21. Rogers RF, Singer E, Imperio J. Poll trends: AIDS—an update. Public Opin Q 1993;57:92.

22. Princeton Survey Research Associates/Newsweek, February 3–4, 1994. Storrs, CT: Roper Center for Public Opinion Research, 1993.

23. Princeton Survey Research Associates, November 6–December 4, 1992, Storrs, CT: Roper Center for Public Opinion Research, 1992.

24. Louis Harris and Associates, March 3–April 28, 1993. Storrs, CT: Roper Center for Public Opinion Research, 1993.

25. Response Analysis Corporation, November 13–December 13, 1992. Storrs, CT: Roper Center for Public Opinion Research, 1992.

26. Los Angeles Times, February 18–19, 1993. Storrs, CT: Roper Center for Public Opinion Research, 1993.

27. Centers for Disease Control and Prevention. HIV/AIDS surveillance report. 1995;7.

28. Colby DC, Cook TE. Epidemics and agendas: the politics of nightly news coverage of AIDS. J Health Politics Policy Law 1991;16:215.

29. Nelkin D. AIDS and the news media. Milbank Q 1991;69:293.

30. Wachter RM. AIDS, activism, and the politics of health. N Engl J Med 1992;326:128.

31. Pally M. AIDS activism: a conversation with Larry Kramer. Tikkun 1990;5:22.

32. Bloom DE, Glied S. The evolution of AIDS economic research. Health Policy 1989;11:187.

33. Massagli MP, Weissman JS, Seage GR III, Epstein AM. Correlates of employment after AIDS diagnosis in the Boston health study. Am J Public Health 1994;84:1976.

34. Farnham PG, Gorsky RD. Costs to business for an HIV-infected worker. Inquiry 1994;31:76.

35. American Council of Life Insurance (ACLI) and the Health Insurance Association of America (HIAA). AIDS-related claims survey. Washington, DC: ACLI/HIAA, 1994.

36. U.S. General Accounting Office. Improving funding equity under the Ryan White CARE Act of 1990 (GAO/T-HEHS-95-91). Washington, DC: U.S. General Accounting Office, 1995.

37. AIDS Action Council. AIDS action network information. September 30, 1994.

38. Department of Health and Human Services. Financing health care for people with AIDS and HIV: the role of the Health Care Financing Administration. Washington, DC: Department of Health and Human Services, 1993.

39. Green J, Arno P. The medicaidization of AIDS. JAMA 1990;264:1261.

40. Bloom DE, Carliner G. The economic impact of AIDS in the United States. Science 1988;239:604.

41. Hay JW, Osmond DH, Jacobson MA. Projecting the medical costs of AIDS and ARC in the United States. J Acquir Immune Defic Syndr 1988;1:466.

42. Scitovsky AA. Studying the cost of HIV-related illnesses: reflections on a moving target. Milbank Q 1989;67:318.

43. Hellinger F. Forecasting the medical care costs of the HIV epidemic: 1991–1994. Inquiry 1991;28:213.

44. Hellinger F. Forecasts of the costs of medical care for persons with HIV: 1992–1995. Inquiry 1992;29:356.

45. Hellinger F. The lifetime cost of treating a person with HIV. JAMA 1993;270:474.

46. Wachter RM, Luce JM, Safrin S, Berrios DC, Charlebois E, Scitovsky AA. Cost and outcome of intensive care for patients with AIDS, *Pneumocystis carinii* pneumonia, and severe respiratory failure. JAMA 1995;273:230.

47. Andrulis DP, Weslowski VB, Hintz E, Spolarich AW. Comparisons of hospital care for patients with AIDS and other HIV-related conditions. JAMA 1992;267:2482.

48. Fleishmann JA, Mor V, Laliberte LL. Longitudinal patterns of medical service use and costs among people with AIDS. Health Serv Res 1995;30:403.

49. Scitovsky AA, Rice DP. Estimates of the direct and indirect costs of acquired immunodeficiency syndrome in the United States, 1985, 1986, and 1991. Public Health Rep 1987;102:5.

50. Hanvelt RA, Ruedy NS, Hogg RS, et al. Indirect costs of HIV/AIDS mortality in Canada. AIDS 1994;8:F7.

51. Bubak ME, Reed CE, Fransway AF, et al. Allergic reactions to latex among health-care workers. Mayo Clin Proc 1992;67:1075.

52. Ward D, Brown MA. Labor and cost in AIDS family caregiving. West J Nurs Res 1994;16:10.

53. Michaels D, Levine C. Estimates of the number of motherless youth orphaned by AIDS in the United States. JAMA 1992;268:3456.

54. Garnett GP, Anderson RM. No reason for complacency about the potential demographic impact of AIDS in Africa. Trans R Soc Trop Med Hyg 1993;87(Suppl 1):19.

55. Mohr PE. Patterns of health care use among HIV-infected adults: preliminary results. Washington, DC: Agency for Health Care Policy and Research, United States Department of Health and Human Services, 1994.

56. Fleishman JA, Mor V. Insurance status among people with AIDS: relationships with sociodemographic characteristics and service use. Inquiry 1993;30:180.

57. Seage GR III, Hertz, T, Stone VE, Epstein AM. The effects of intravenous drug use and gender on the cost of hospitalization for patients with AIDS. J Acquir Immune Defic Syndr 1993;6:831.

58. Katz MH, Chang SW, Buchbinder SP, Hessol NA, O'Malley P, Doll LS. Health insurance and use of medical services by men infected with HIV. J Acquir Immune Defic Syndr Hum Retroviruses 1995;8:58.

59. Hogg RS, Strathdee SA, Craib KJP, O'Shaughnessy MV, Montaner JSG, Schechter MT. Lower socioeconomic status and shorter survival following HIV infection. Lancet 1994;344:1120.

60. Cotton DJ. The impact of AIDS on the medical care system. JAMA 1988;260:519.

61. Center for Washington Area Studies. AIDS care in six Washington, D.C. area hospices: satisfactions and stresses among professional caregivers. Washington, DC: The George Washington University, 1993.

62. Centers for Disease Control and Prevention (CDC). Recommendations for preventing transmission of human immunodeficiency virus and hepatitis B virus to patients during exposure-prone invasive procedures. Atlantic Information Services, 1992.

63. Rubenstein WS. The Americans With Disabilities Act: what it means for people living with AIDS. ACLU, New York: American Civil Liberties Union, January 1995.

64. Robert LM, Chamberland ME, Cleveland JL, et al. Investigations of patients of health care workers infected with HIV: the Centers for Disease Control and Prevention database. Ann Intern Med 1995;122:653.

65. Gerbert B, Maguire BT, Hulley SB, Coates TJ. Physicians and acquired immunodeficiency syndrome: what patients think about human immunodeficiency virus in medical practice. JAMA 1989;262:1969.

66. Gostin L. The HIV-infected health care professional: public policy, discrimination and patient safety. Arch Intern Med 1991;151:663.

67. Miike L, Ostrowsky J, Behney C, Hewitt M. HIV in the health care workplace. Washington, DC: Office of Technology Assessment of the United States Congress, 1991.

68. Craig RT, Bryant LL. HIV-infected health workers: debating the issues. Colorado: State Legislative Report, 1992;17:1.

69. New York State Department of Health. Policy statement and guidelines to prevent transmission of HIV and hepatitis B through medical/dental procedures. Albany, NY: New York State Department of Health, 1992.

70. American Medical Association. Digest of AMA HIV/AIDS policy. Chicago: American Medical Association, 1994.

71. Centers for Disease Control and Prevention. Possible transmission of human immunodeficiency virus to a patient during an invasive dental procedure. MMWR 1990;39:489.

72. Centers for Disease Control and Prevention. Update: transmission of HIV infection during an invasive dental procedure—Florida. MMWR 1991;21.

73. Centers for Disease Control and Prevention. Update: transmission of HIV infection during invasive dental procedures—Florida. MMWR 1991;40:377.

74. Weiss SH. HIV infection and the healthcare worker. Med Clin North Am 1992;76:269.

75. Angell M. A dual approach to the AIDS epidemic. N Engl J Med 1991;324:1498.

76. Brennan T. Transmission of the human immunodeficiency virus in the health care setting-time for action. N Engl J Med 1991;324:1504.

77. U.S. Surgeon General. The Surgeon General's report on acquired immune deficiency syndrome. Washington, DC: US Department of Health and Human Services, 1986.

78. Understanding AIDS: a message from the Surgeon General. Washington, DC: US Department of Health and Human Services, 1988.

79. Report of the Presidential Commission on the human immunodeficiency virus epidemic, Washington, DC: The Commission, June 24, 1988.

80. Public Law 100-607, Subtitle D—national commission on acquired immune deficiency syndrome. In: AIDS: an expanding tragedy; the final report of the National Commission on AIDS. Washington, DC, November 4, 1988.

81. Failure of U.S. health care system to deal with the HIV epidemic. Washington, DC: National Commission on AIDS, 1989.

82. Leadership, legislation and regulation. Washington, DC: National Commission on AIDS, 1990.

83. America living with AIDS: transforming anger, fear, and indifference into action. Washington, DC: National Commission on AIDS, 1991.

84. AIDS: an expanding tragedy. Washington, DC: National Commission on AIDS, 1993.

85. Research, the workforce and the HIV epidemic in rural America. Washington, DC: National Commission on AIDS, 1990.

86. HIV disease in correctional facilities. Washington, DC: National Commission on AIDS, 1991.

87. The twin epidemics of substance use and HIV. Washington, DC: National Commission on AIDS, 1991.

88. Institute of Medicine, National Academy of Sciences. Confronting AIDS: directions for public health, health care and research. Washington, DC: National Academy Press, 1986.

89. Miller HG, Turner CF, Moses LE, eds, for the Committee on AIDS Research and the Behavioral, Social, and Statistical Sciences, Commission on the Behavioral and Social Sciences and Education, National Research Council. AIDS: the second decade. Washington, DC: National Academy Press, 1990.

90. The social impact of AIDS in the United States. Washington, DC: National Academy Press, 1993.

91. Cohen J. New AIDS chief takes charge. Science 1994;263:1364.

92. National Center for HIV, STD, and TB Prevention, Centers for Disease Control and Prevention. Washington, DC: US Department of Health and Human Services 1995 Fact book.

93. Gostin LO. Public health strategies for confronting AIDS: legislative and regulatory policy in the United States. JAMA 1989;261:1621.

94. Gilmore N. Medical and political aspects of travel for HIV-positive persons. In: Lobel HO, Steffen R, Kozarsky PE, eds. Travel medicine 2: proceeding of the second Conference on International Travel Medicine, Atlanta, CA, May 9–12, 1991:207.

95. Gostin LO, Cleary PD, Mayer KH, Brandt AM, Chittenden EH. Screening immigrants and international travellers for the human immunodeficiency virus. N Engl J Med 1990;322:1743.

96. Davis SF, Byers RH Jr, Lindegren MS, Caldwell MB, Karon JM, Gwinn M. Prevalence and incidence of vertically acquired HIV infection in the United States. JAMA 1995;274:952.

97. Ziegler JM, Johnson RO, Cooper DA, et al. Postnatal transmission of AIDS-associated retrovirus from mother to infant. Lancet 1985;1:896.

98. Lepage P, Van de Perre P, Caraël M, et al. Postnatal transmission of HIV from mother to child. Lancet 1987;2:400.

99. Weinbreck P, Loustaud, Denis FV, et al. Postnatal transmission of HIV infection. Lancet 1988;1:482.

100. European Collaborative Study. Risk factors for mother-to-child transmission of HIV-1. Lancet 1992;339:1007.

101. The HIV Infection in Newborns French Collaborative Study Group. Comparison of vertical human immunodeficiency virus type 2 and human immunodeficiency virus type 1 transmission in the French prospective cohort. Pediatr Infect Dis J 1994;271:1925.

102. Centers for Disease Control. Recommendations for assisting in the prevention of the perinatal transmission of human T-lymphotropic virus type III/lymphadenopathy-associated virus and acquired immunodeficiency syndrome. MMWR 1985;34:721.

103. Simonds RJ, Lindegren ML, Thomas P, et al. Prophylaxis against *Pneumocystis carinii* pneumonia among children with perinatally acquired human immunodeficiency virus infection in the United States. N Engl J Med 1995;332:786.

104. Connor EM, Sperling RS, Gelber R, et al. Reduction of maternal-infant transmission of human immunodeficiency virus type 1 with zidovudine treatment. N Engl J Med 1994;331:1173.

105. Peckham C, Gibb D. Mother-to-child transmission of the human immunodeficiency virus. N Engl J Med 1995;333:298.

106. Centers for Disease Control and Prevention. U.S. Public Health Service recommendations for human immunodeficiency virus counseling and voluntary testing for pregnant women. MMWR 1995;44(RR-7):1.

107. Voelker R. Foes of mandatory maternal HIV testing fear guidelines will lead to reprisals. JAMA 1995;273:977.

108. Barbacci M, Repke JT, Chaisson RE. Routine prenatal screening for HIV infection. Lancet 1991;337:709.

109. Lindsay MK, Peterson HB, Feng TI, Slade BA, Willis S, Klein L. Routine antepartum human immunodeficiency virus infection screening in an inner-city population. Obstet Gynecol 1989;74:289.

110. Cozen W, Mascola L, Enguidanos R, et al. Screening for HIV and hepatitis B virus in Las Angeles County prenatal clinics: a demonstration project. J Acquir Immune Defic Syndr 1993;6:95.

111. Wilfert CM. Mandatory screening of pregnant women for the human immunodeficiency virus. Clin Infect Dis 1994;19:664.

112. Wilson ME. Infectious diseases: an ecological perspective. Br Med J 1995;311:1681.

Subject Index

Page numbers followed by f *indicate figures;*
page numbers followed by t *indicate tabular material.*

A

Abscess
  cerebral, toxoplasmic, 339
  Monro's, 394
ABT-538. *See* Ritonavir
Acid-base disorders, 424
Acquired immunodeficiency syndrome
    (AIDS). *See also* HIV infection
  case definition, 203-204
  community-based response to. *See*
      Community resources
  diagnosis, 177-193
  historical perspective, 3-4
  human rights and, 627-632. *See also*
      Human rights
  infectious etiology, 4
  Kaposi's sarcoma. *See* Kaposi's
      sarcoma
  malignancies, 319-327. *See also*
      Lymphoma; *specific*
      malignancies
  origin, 3-12
    denial of HIV etiology, 11
    distribution and transmission of HIV-
        1 subtypes, 6-8, 7f, 8f, 8t
    diversion among human lentiviruses,
        5
    emergence of disease phenotypes, 8-9
    HIV-1, 5-6, 7f
    HIV-2, 10-11
    human retroviruses, 4-5
    infectious etiology, 4
    simian AIDS, 9-10
  risk groups, 3-4
  serologic tests, 177-189
  simian AIDS, 9-10
  societal dimensions, 709-716
  surveillance case definition, 138-139
  transfusion-associated, epidemiologic
      analyses, 154, 154t
  virologic tests, 189-193
Act Up (AIDS Coalition to Unleash
    Power), 553, 559-560, 711

Acute abdomen, 383-384
Acyclovir
  combination therapy, AZT plus, 505
  for herpes simplex virus, 269t, 271
  renal complications, 424t
  for varicella-zoster virus, in pediatric
      AIDS, 450
  for zoster, 276
ADCC (antibody-dependent cytotoxicity),
    92, 94, 95t
Adenovirus
  gastrointestinal infection, 369
  in pediatric AIDS, 450
Adjuvants, HIV vaccines, 619-620
Adolescence
  condom use in United States, 141
  HIV-1 transmission, 147-157
    injecting drug users, 152-154
    rare/putative modes, 156-157
    sexual transmission, 147-152
    transfusion therapy, 154-155
Adrenal insufficiency, 423
Advocacy
  financial advocates, 563
  for injecting drug users, 558
  legal services and advocacy, 563-564
AEGIS World HQ, 563t
Aerosolized blood, 651-652
Africa
  HIV-2 in, 6t, 128
  Kaposi's sarcoma, 295
  North, HIV-1 infection, 112
  seroprevalence of HIV-1 and HIV-2, 6t
  sub-Saharan, HIV infection,
      109-110, 111f
  West
    HIV-1 infection, 130t
    HIV-2 infection, 128, 130, 130t
    map, 129f
African-American population. *See*
    Race/ethnicity
Age/aging
  HIV-1 transmission, 106, 107f, 150

HIV-2 infection, 10
AIDS Action Council, 556
AIDS bulletin boards, 563t
AIDS Clinical Trial Group (ACTG), 454
AIDS Clinical Trials Information Service,
    560t
AIDS Coalition to Unleash Power. *See* Act
    Up
AIDS Community Demonstration
    Projects, 579
AIDS dementia complex, 333-338, 340t
  cerebrospinal fluid examination,
      336-337
  in children, 335-336
  classification and terminology, 334
  clinical features, 334-336, 336t, 547t
  epidemiology, 337
  etiology, 338
  histopathology, 337-338
  motor abnormalities, 335
  natural history, 337
  neuroimaging studies, 336
  neuropathology, 337-338
  neuropsychologic testing, 336
  pathogenesis, 338
  risk factors, 337
  staging scheme, 335t
  treatment, 338
  WHO/AAN classification, 334
AIDS Directory, 562t
AIDS Info BBS, 563t
AIDS Network, 555
AIDS-related complex (ARC), 203. *See*
    also HIV infection, intermediate
AIDS Research, 554
AIDS Resource Center, 556
AIDS Treatment News, 558-559, 559t
AL-721, 561
Alcohol abuse, HIV transmission and, 570
Allograft transplantation, HIV
    transmission, 155
Alovudine. *See* FLT
Alveolitis, lymphocytic, 417

for *Pneumocystis carinii* pneumonia, 217t, 219, 219t
Pregnancy
  HIV testing
    ethical issues, 635-636
    social policy, 715-716
  vertical transmission of HIV-1, 104, 142. *See also* Human immunodeficiency virus, HIV-1, vertical (mother-child) transmission
Pr55^gag, 52
Principle neutralizing domain (determinant) (PND), HIV vaccine development, 606, 606t
Probenecid, AZT interations, 489
Procarbazine, for AIDS-related lymphoma, 325t
Proctitis, herpes simplex virus, 368
Progressive multifocal leukoencephalopathy (PML), 208, 340t, 341
Project Inform, 558
  PI Perspectives Newsletter, 559t
  Treatment Hotline, 560t
Prostate gland, in cryptococcosis, 233, 235
Protease, HIV-1, 57
Protease inhibitors, 469-470
  clinical pharmacokinetics, 484-485
  clinical trials, 501
  combination therapy, RT inhibitors plus, 504-505
  mechanism of action, 500-501
  resistance to, 501
  structure, 469f
Protein binding, drug activity and, 484
Protein S, 437
Pruritus, 398
Pseudomonas aeruginosa, infection, 261
Psoriasis, in HIV infection, 206, 394-395
  clinical features, 394-395
  etiology, 395
  treatment, 395
Psychiatric issues, 541-548. *See also* Counseling; Psychosocial issues
  at-risk person, 543-545
    HIV-1 antibody testing, 543-544
    seroconversion and disclosure, 544
    social support and interventions for recently seropositive persons, 544-545
  seropositive persons, 545-547
    anxiety, 546-547
    cognitive deficits, 547
    depression, 545-546
    neuropsychologic functioning, 547
  symptomatic infection, AIDS, and terminal illness, 547-548
Psychosocial issues
  continued high-risk behavior in at-risk populations, 199-200

depression, 545-546
HIV antibody testing, 543-544
mental health outcomes, resources and vulnerabilities, 542, 543t
seroconversion and disclosure of serostatus, 544
seropositive persons, 545-547
stage of infection and, 542t
suicide potential assessment, recently seropositive persons, 545
in symptomatic infection, AIDS, and terminal illness, 547-548
"worried well," 543
Psychotic disorders, 547t
Public health, human rights of HIV-infected persons and, 628, 630-631
Pulmonary hypertension, 417
Pulmonary lymphoid hyperplasia (PLH)/lymphocytic interstitial pneumonitis (LIP) complex, 413. *See also* Lymphocytic interstitial pneumonitis
Punctuated equilibrium theory, HIV infection, 124
PWA Coalition Newsline & SIDAAhora, 559t
Pyrazinamide, for tuberculosis, 253t
Pyrimethamine
  prophylactic, for toxoplasmic encephalitis, 223
  for toxoplasmic encephalitis, 223t
Pyrimethamine-dapsone, prophylactic, for *Pneumocystis carinii* pneumonia, 220t, 221
Pyrimethamine-sulfadoxine
  adverse cutaneous reactions, 399
  prophylactic, for Pneumocystis carinii pneumonia, 220t, 221

Q

Quinolinic acid, cerebrospinal fluid
  in AIDS dementia complex, 337
  in pediatric AIDS, 449

R

R0 31-8959. *See* Saquinavir
Rabbit, HIV studies, 19
Race/ethnicity
  bisexual behavior and, 140
  depression and suicide and, 545-546
  disparity in HIV rates, 138
    homosexual/bisexual men, 139
    injecting drug users, 140
  drug disposition and, 488
  pediatric AIDS and, 444
  sexual risk of HIV infection, 150-151
Radiation therapy
  Kaposi's sarcoma, 309
  primary CNS lymphoma, 326

splenic irradiation, for thrombocytopenia, 431
Radiculomyelitis
  cytomegalovirus, 272
  sacral, herpes simplex virus type 2 and, 268
Radioimmunoprecipitation assay, 185-187
Radionuclide studies
  in Kaposi's sarcoma, pulmonary, 407-408
  in lymphocytic interstitial pneumonitis, 414
Rapid latex agglutination assay, 187
Rash, in pediatric AIDS, 455t
Recombination, naturally recombinant HIV-1 strains, 120
Rectum. *See* Anorectum
Reiter's syndrome, HIV-associated, 395-396
Rejection, fear of, disclosure and, 535
Research
  American Medical Foundation (1982), 554-555
  Community Research Initiative, 557
  ethical issues, 639-640
  HIV prevention, limitations of literature, 580-581
  San Francisco County Community Consortium (1985), 557
Respiratory infection
  bacterial, 260-262
    pneumonia, 260-261
    sinusitis, 261-262
  Pneumocystis carinii pneumonia, 215-221
Respiratory isolation, for suspect tuberculosis, 255
Respiratory syncytial virus, in pediatric AIDS, 450
Respiratory tract
  bronchogenic carcinoma, 411-413
  Hodgkin's disease, 411
  inflammatory airway disorders, 417
  interstitial pneumonitis, 413-417
  Kaposi's sarcoma, 405-410
  lymphoma, 410-411
Reticulum cells, bone marrow, in HIV infection, 436
Retina, depigmentation, DDI and, 453
Retinal necrosis, acute, varicella zoster virus infection and, 276
Retinitis, cytomegalovirus, 272
  in pediatric AIDS, 450, 453
  treatment, 273-274
Retinoids, in Kaposi's sarcoma, 311
Retrovir. *See* AZT
Retrovirus(es). *See also specific viruses*
  complex, 46
  genome and virion structure, 46
  genotype relatedness, 7f
  groups, 29